COMPREHENSIVE REVIEW
OF PSYCHIATRY

COMPREHENSIVE REVIEW
OF PSYCHIATRY

Editor-In-Chief
RAJESH R. TAMPI, M.D., M.S.

Director, Geriatric Psychiatry Fellowship Program
Department of Psychiatry, Yale University School of Medicine
Co-Service Manager, Geriatric Services, Yale New Haven Psychiatric Hospital
New Haven, Connecticut

Associate Editors
SUNANDA MURALEE, M.D.

Fellow, Child and Adolescent Psychiatry
Yale Child Study Center, Yale University School of Medicine
New Haven, Connecticut

NATALIE D. WEDER, M.D.

PGY 4 Resident
Department of Psychiatry, Yale University School of Medicine
New Haven, Connecticut

Assistant Editor
Heath Penland, M.D.

Private Practice
Greenville, Texas

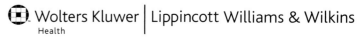
Wolters Kluwer | Lippincott Williams & Wilkins
Health

Philadelphia · Baltimore · New York · London
Buenos Aires · Hong Kong · Sydney · Tokyo

Acquisitions Editor: Charles W. Mitchell
Managing Editor: Sirkka E. Howes
Marketing Manager: Kimberly Schonberger
Production Editor: Bridgett Dougherty
Manufacturing Manager: Kathleen Brown
Design Coordinator: Steve Druding
Compositor: Aptara, Inc.

The publisher is not responsible (as a matter of product liability, negligence, or otherwise) for any injury resulting from any material contained herein. This publication contains information relating to general principles of medical care that should not be construed as specific instructions for individual patients. Manufacturers' product information and package inserts should be reviewed for current information, including contraindications, dosages, and precautions.

Printed in the United States of America

Library of Congress Cataloging-in-Publication Data
Comprehensive review of psychiatry / editor-in-chief, Rajesh R. Tampi ; associate editors, Sunanda Muralee, Natalie D. Weder ; assistant editor, Heath Penland.
    p. ; cm.
  Includes bibliographical references and index.
  ISBN-13: 978-0-7817-7176-4
  ISBN-10: 0-7817-7176-5
  1. Psychiatry—Examinations, questions, etc.   I. Tampi, Rajesh R.
  [DNLM: 1. Mental Disorders—Examination Questions.   2. Nervous System Diseases—Examination Questions.   WM 18.2 C7375 2008]
  RC457.C66 2008
  616.890076–dc22   2008002509

The publishers have made every effort to trace the copyright holders for borrowed material. If they have inadvertently overlooked any, they will be pleased to make the necessary arrangements at the first opportunity.

To purchase additional copies of this book, call our customer service department at (800) 638-3030 or fax orders to (301) 824-7390. International customers should call (301) 714-2324.

Visit Lippincott Williams & Wilkins on the Internet: http://www.LWW.com. Lippincott Williams & Wilkins customer service representatives are available from 8:30 am to 6:00 pm, EST.

10 9 8 7 6 5 4 3 2 1

To our son, Vaishnav Sai Tampi, and our parents, Dr. Rajagopalan and Mrs. Sreedevi Tampi and Mr. Parakkat and Mrs. Vimala Muralee, whose love and support make anything possible.
—Drs. Rajesh Tampi and Sunanda Muralee

To Juan, for showing me what love and commitment can mean.
—Dr. Natalie Weder

To my wife, Tu, and daughter, Ava, for your strength, love, and all you have given me.
To Mom and Dad, for teaching me to become the man I am.
—Dr. Heath Penland

PREFACE

The scientific developments in the field of psychiatry and neurology are so astounding that it is impossible for many individuals to keep pace with the latest developments. This situation gets further complicated for students of psychiatry and neurology, who have to balance a very busy clinical workload with the pressures of academic and personal life. Added to this mix is the pressure of passing peer accepted examinations in these specialties. These examinations are complex and need extensive preparation. The subject matter is broad and there are no clear guidelines or texts to help in their preparation. Examinees usually have to use numerous sources to master the essential data needed to do well on them. This preparation also comes at a very high financial cost to the individual. To ease this burden, my colleagues and I have compiled a list of 2,000 questions and answers in psychiatry (1,250) and neurology (750). They have been developed from the most current information available in the field. These questions and answers cover topic areas tested on most professional examinations in psychiatry and neurology. This book has been specifically written for the busy professional who does not have the time to access numerous resources necessary to pass their peer accepted examinations. It is intended to be a one-stop shop to obtain that information. Those readers who want to explore a particular topic area can obtain further knowledge from the references that we have provided after each answer.

This project has been a labor of love for all of us. We have spent many hours developing and refining these questions and answers. They have been written in a format that will aid in the preparation for most professional examinations in psychiatry and neurology. Each question and answer is a review on one topic area in either psychiatry or neurology. Although this book is primarily targeted for postgraduate students in psychiatry or neurology, it will also be helpful to other professionals in psychiatry and neurology who want to gain knowledge, but don't have the luxury of time or money to review multiple sources of information.

We sincerely hope that this book will be helpful to our readers. Given the rapid growth in these fields, we intend to revise the information available in subsequent editions of the book. We wish those readers who are taking examinations in psychiatry and neurology, the very best of luck. For those of you reading this book for knowledge, we commend you for your interest.

Rajesh R. Tampi, M.D., M.S.
Editor-In-Chief

CONTRIBUTORS

Rehan Aziz, MD
Fellow
Geriatric Psychiatry
Department of Psychiatry
Yale University School of Medicine
New Haven, Connecticut

Matthew E. Barnas, MD
Clinical Assistant Professor
New Jersey Medical School—U.M.D.N.J.
Attending Psychiatrist
Geriatric Psychiatry Outpatient Service
Veteran's Administration New Jersey Health Care System
East Orange Campus
East Orange, New Jersey

Michael B. Greenspan, MD
PGY 4 Resident
Department of Psychiatry
Yale University School of Medicine
New Haven, Connecticut

Constance Guille, MD
PGY 3 Resident
Department of Psychiatry
Yale University School of Medicine
New Haven, Connecticut

Miyun Kang, MD
Instructor
Department of Psychiatry
Yale University School of Medicine
New Haven, Connecticut
Staff Psychiatrist
Department of Mental Hygiene
Veterans Administration Medical Center
West Haven, Connecticut

Joshua Kantrowitz, MD
Fellow
Schizophrenia Research
Department of Psychiatry
Albert Einstein College of Medicine
Bronx, New York
Nathan S. Kline Institute for Psychiatric Research
Orangeburg, New York
Department of Psychiatry
New York University
New York, New York

Karin E. Dymond Kerfoot, MD, FRCPC
Attending Psychiatrist
Department of Psychiatry
Yale University School of Medicine
New Haven, Connecticut

Prem Kumar Kunjukrishnan, MBBS, MRCPsych
Consultant
Department of Old Age Psychiatry
Fieldhead Hospital
Yorkshire, United Kingdom

Christina J. Lee, MD
PGY 3 Resident
Department of Psychiatry
Yale University School of Medicine
New Haven, Connecticut

Shruti Mutalik, MD
PGY 1 Resident
Department of Psychiatry
Beth Israel Medical Center
New York, New York

Yann Poncin, MD
Associate Research Scientist
Yale Child Study Center
Yale University School of Medicine
New Haven, Connecticut

Alicia A. Romeo, MD
PGY 4 Resident
Department of Psychiatry
Yale University School of Medicine
New Haven, Connecticut

Abhay K. Singh, MD
Clinical Assistant Professor of Psychiatry
University of Vermont
Burlington, Vermont
Chairman, Attending Psychiatrist
St. Mary's Regional Medical Center
Lewiston, Maine

Caren B. Teitelbaum, MD
PGY 4 Resident
Department of Psychiatry
Yale University School of Medicine
New Haven, Connecticut

Kirsten Matthews Wilkins, MD
Assistant Professor
Department of Psychiatry
Yale University School of Medicine
New Haven, Connecticut
Attending Psychiatrist
Veterans Administration Medical Center
West Haven, Connecticut

Solomon S. Williams, MD
Assistant Professor of Psychiatry
Texas A&M University
Psychiatrist
Central Texas Veterans Health Care System
Temple, Texas

The editors also wish to thank the following colleagues for their contribution to this project:

Gauri Khatkhate, MD
Attending Psychiatrist
Hines Veterans Administration Medical Center
Maywood, Illinois

Barbra Lesh, MD
Attending Psychiatrist
Buffalo, New York

Boris Lorberg, MD
Fellow
Child and Adolescent Psychiatry
Massachusetts General Hospital
Department of Psychiatry
Harvard Medical School
Boston, Massachusetts

Lori A. Lowthert, MD
PGY 4 Resident
Department of Psychiatry
Yale University School of Medicine
New Haven, Connecticut

Prakash K. Thomas, MD
Lecturer
Yale Child Study Center
Yale University School of Medicine
New Haven, Connecticut

We have divided this book into ten booklets of 200 questions and answers each. Each booklet has 125 questions in psychiatry and 75 questions in neurology. Each booklet is an independent workbook that covers all the representative topic areas in these fields. It contains questions pertaining to each of the following areas:

A. Psychiatry:

  I. Development through the life cycle: 8 questions
  II. Neuroscience: 8 questions
  III. Behavioral and social sciences: 5 questions
  IV. Epidemiology and public policy: 6 questions
  V. Diagnostic procedures: 8 questions
  VI. Psychiatric disorders: 40 questions
  VII. Treatment of psychiatric disorders: 45 questions
  VIII. Special topics: 5 questions

B. Neurology:

  I. Basic science aspects of neurologic disorders: 20 questions
  II. Incidence and risks of neurologic disorders: 5 questions
  III. Diagnostic procedures related to neurologic disorders: 12 questions
  IV. Clinical evaluation of neurologic disorders: 25 questions
  V. Management and treatment of neurologic disorders: 13 questions

Readers taking professional examinations in psychiatry or neurology, must time their testing efforts per booklet to 180 minutes or less. This exercise should be done to get the feel of a real examination, where, the information has to be processed under time pressure.

Based on the level of complexity of these questions, we feel that a score of 80% or more correct answers per booklet is outstanding. On the other hand, a score of <65% indicates the need for further improvement in the level of knowledge. We have provided a grading system that should help readers gauge their level of knowledge.

Correct answers per booklet	Grade
> 80%	Outstanding
75%–80%	Excellent
70%–74.9%	Very Good
65%–69.9%	Good
60%–64.9%	Fair
<60%	Poor

Readers who score <65% and are taking professional examinations in the near future should thoroughly read the answers provided and also use the references to further strengthen their knowledge base. The average length of time needed to completely review the information provided in this book is about 10 weeks.

CONTENTS

Questions

1. A mother brings her child to your office for an initial visit. The child is wandering around the office by himself, is able to go up and down the stairs without help, and can build a tower of six cubes. If this child did not show any developmental problems, approximately how old would he be?
   - **A.** 15 months
   - **B.** 18 months
   - **C.** 24 months
   - **D.** 36 months
   - **E.** 48 months

2. Which one of the following choices correctly describes electrical signal transmission in the neuronal synapses?
   - **A.** They are mediated by the direct flow of current between two neurons.
   - **B.** They are mediated by the release of the neurotransmitter at a gap junction and there is a delay in transmission.
   - **C.** Transmission is typically both unidirectional and bidirectional.
   - **D.** They are mediated by the release of the neurotransmitter at a terminal bouton into the synaptic cleft and there is a delay in transmission.
   - **E.** They are mediated by the release of neurotransmitters at a gap junction and there is a minimal delay in transmission.

3. J. B. Skinner's operant conditioning is based on which of the following principles?
   - **A.** The stimulus becomes paired with a response.
   - **B.** The response becomes paired with a consequence.
   - **C.** There is no pairing of a response or consequence.
   - **D.** The subject is passive.
   - **E.** None of the above.

4. Who coined the term *catatonia*?
   - **A.** Jung
   - **B.** Adler
   - **C.** Erikson
   - **D.** Freud
   - **E.** Kahlbaum

5. A 50-year-old white man with a 30-year history of schizophrenia is admitted to the hospital for sudden onset of confusion, fever, tachycardia, hypertension tremors, and rigidity. He had recently been switched from olanzapine 10 mg qhs to haloperidol 25 mg/day PO. You diagnose the patient with neuroleptic malignant syndrome (NMS) and recommend treatment in the intensive care unit (ICU). When you write your multiaxial classification according to DSM-IV-TR, NMS should be coded on which axis of this classification system?
   - **A.** Axis I
   - **B.** Axis II
   - **C.** Axis III
   - **D.** Axis IV
   - **E.** Axis V

6. Which one of the following patients diagnosed with bipolar disorder has the highest risk of developing a rapid cycling subtype of this disorder?
   - **A.** A 35-year-old woman with lithium-resistant bipolar disorder I recently started on amitriptyline
   - **B.** A 46-year-old woman with bipolar disorder II on maintenance treatment with lithium
   - **C.** A 23-year-old treatment-naïve man presenting with his first episode of mania
   - **D.** A 42-year-old woman with a long-standing history of bipolar disorder II presenting with a depressive episode
   - **E.** A 70-year-old man with a recent diagnosis of bipolar disorder I who was started on lithium

7. A patient with a history of cocaine dependence is involved in an outpatient treatment program. After refraining from any cocaine use for 9 months, she runs into an old buddy and goes on a 4-day cocaine binge, resulting in absence from work and fights between herself and her partner. After the binge, she returns to continue with her treatment. What is her most accurate current diagnosis?
   - **A.** Cocaine Abuse
   - **B.** Cocaine Dependence, Sustained Partial Remission
   - **C.** Cocaine Dependence, Sustained Full Remission
   - **D.** Cocaine Dependence, Early Partial Remission
   - **E.** Cocaine Dependence, Early Full Remission

8. A 32-year-old woman presents to her primary care physician, complaining of debilitating exhaustion for the past 8 months. She is on leave from her job as a bank teller and has been doing only a minimal amount of cooking, cleaning, and laundry. The

patient denies any history consistent with a mood, anxiety, psychotic, or substance use disorder. Her screening physical examination and subsequent medical investigations fail to show any abnormalities. What is her most likely diagnosis?

A. Somatization Disorder
B. Conversion Disorder
C. Hypochondriasis
D. Undifferentiated Somatoform Disorder
E. Somatoform Disorder Not Otherwise Specified (NOS)

9. Which of the following statements is true regarding dissociative screening scales?

A. The Dissociative Experiences Scale (DES), developed by Eve Bernstein Carlson and Frank Putnam in the mid-1980s, has 28 items and the overall score can range from 0 to 100.
B. The Child Dissociative Checklist (CDC) is a parent-caretaker-teacher 100-item report measure used for children in the age group of 3 to 10 with scores ranging from 0 to 100.
C. The Adolescent Dissociative Experiences Scale (A-DES) has 10 items with a 0 to 5 answer format and does not include depersonalization and derealization.
D. The Peritraumatic Dissociative Experiences Questionnaire (PDEQ), developed by Marmar et al., has 30 items and the overall score can range from 0 to 100.
E. The Dissocative Experiences Scale (DES), developed by Marmar in the mid-1980s, has 28 items and the overall score can range from 0 to 100.

10. Which is the selective serotonin reuptake inhibitor (SSRI) with the longest half-life (t 1/2)?

A. Sertraline
B. Citalopram
C. Escitalopram
D. Fluoxetine
E. Paroxetine

11. What percentage of patients diagnosed with depression do not have an adequate response to a first trial of an antidepressant?

A. 0% to 15%
B. 15% to 30%
C. 30% to 45%
D. 45% to 60%
E. 60% to 75%

12. In which of the following conditions is benzodiazepines contraindicated?

A. Agitation in cocaine withdrawal
B. Agitation in amphetamine overdose
C. Alcohol-induced delirium
D. Agitation in inhalant intoxication
E. Acute episode of posthallucinogen perception disorder

13. A 25-year-old man was hospitalized for his first episode of psychosis and was started on haloperidol (Haldol). After 3 days, the nursing staff calls you because his upper body is contorting and he is in obvious pain and is frightened. Of the following, which would be the best medication to help relieve his suffering?

A. Propanolol
B. Olanzapine
C. Quetiapine
D. Benztropine
E. Risperidone

14. A 35-year-old concert pianist with bipolar disorder who is doing well on lithium monotherapy comes to see you today for a follow-up appointment. He states that he is doing well and usually does not have any side effects from his medication aside from a mild tremor. However, he has noticed that the tremor becomes more pronounced just prior to any large performance. At a recent concert, his tremor was so bad that he was unable to perform certain pieces of music and had to modify his performance to a technically less difficult piece. During the physical examination, you note a mild intension tremor, but otherwise he has an unremarkable neurological examination. His lithium level is within normal range. You modify his lithium medication regimen to the minimally effective dose and ask him to avoid caffeine prior to his performances. In addition to these modifications, which of the following medications taken 30 minutes before his performance may lessen his tremor?

A. Citalopram
B. Hydrochlorothiazide
C. Propranolol
D. Alprazolam
E. Benztropine

15. The highest rates of completed suicides are seen among which one of the following groups?

A. White men, 55 to 75 years
B. White men, >75 years
C. White men, 25 to 55 years
D. Black men, 55 to 75 years
E. Black men, >75 years

16. Which one of the following statements is NOT TRUE regarding adult neurogenesis?

A. It occurs in the subventricular and subgranular zones.

B. Stress suppresses neurogenesis.
C. Antidepressant treatment increases neurogenesis in the adult hippocampus.
D. Brain derived neurotropic factor (BDNF) causes increased neurogenesis following intrahippocampal infusion in adult rats.
E. Antidepressant treatment has no effect on BDNF expression.

17. Which of the following pairs of a clinical feature and its underlying cause is matched correctly for Sturge-Weber syndrome?
A. Cluster headaches: calcification in the brain
B. Hemiparesis: cerebral lesions surrounded by sclerosis
C. Epilepsy: bilateral vascular calcification
D. Port-wine stain: extremely thin cutaneous layer
E. Learning disabilities: vascular malformations of the face

18. Regarding the heredity of diseases with excessive trinucleotide repeats, all of the following are true EXCEPT:
A. Fragile X syndrome is inherited via sex-linked transmission.
B. Huntington's disease is inherited via autosomal dominant transmission.
C. Myotonic dystrophy is inherited via autosomal dominant transmission.
D. Friedreich's ataxia is inherited via autosomal dominant transmission.
E. The spinocerebellar atrophies are inherited via autosomal dominant transmission.

19. A 50-year-old healthy white man is brought to the emergency room (ER) of a major teaching hospital following a motor vehicle accident. He was riding a motorcycle when he fell and hit his head on the road. He was not wearing a helmet at the time of the accident and he is presently comatose and unable to give any further history. During the examination in the ER, his eyes are found to be looking to the left and he has a right hemiplegia. A computed tomography (CT) scan of the brain confirms injury to which of the following structures?
A. Right cerebral hemisphere
B. Left cerebral hemisphere
C. Left pons
D. Left medulla
E. Right medulla

20. A 67-year-old man presents to a neurologist for evaluation. As he walks from the waiting room to the examining room, the neurologist observes that his gait is unsteady and has a wide base. As he introduces himself, his speech is noted to be irregular with

prolonged pauses and difficulty separating adjacent sounds. While reaching for a pen to complete some forms, the patient is seen to have a tremor that is absent at rest. Based on these observations alone, the neurologist suspects a lesion in which area?
A. Posterior columns of the spinal cord
B. Cerebellum
C. Pons
D. Left frontal lobe
E. Right parietal lobe

21. A 45-year-old woman with a history of chronic paranoid schizophrenia has been admitted to the inpatient psychiatric unit for an acute psychotic episode. Prior to her hospitalization, she had been stable on olanzapine 5 mg qhs. On stabilization, she reports, "I often just don't see things and then I bump into them." She is concerned that this may be a side effect of her medication. Members of the staff have also noticed this problem and have reported that they frequently see her bumping into the corner of walls. She denies dizziness, palpitations, shortness of breath, or fatigue. Her blood pressure and pulse are 139/85 and 72 beats/minute sitting and 136/85 and 76 beats/minute standing. Your next step in management is to:
A. Stop her olanzapine
B. Decrease the olanzapine and supplement it with risperidone
C. Obtain a magnetic resonance imaging (MRI)
D. Perform a thorough neurological examination
E. Check liver function tests (LFTs) and a complete blood count (CBC) with differential

22. Which one of the following is the classic clinical triad of tuberous sclerosis?
A. Skin lesions, chest pain, and headache
B. Seizures, mental retardation, and skin lesions
C. Seizures, chest pain, and headache
D. Mental retardation, chest pain, and headache
E. Skin lesion, chest pain, and headache

23. A 19-year-old woman who is playing baseball with her friends accidentally gets hit on the head with the bat. Within a few hours she develops progressively severe headache, vomiting, and a change in her mental status. This patient is taken to the nearby hospital and, by the time she gets to the emergency department, she is found to be unresponsive with a heart rate of 50 beats/minute, a blood pressure of 190/110 mm Hg, and irregular breathing. What is the most likely cause of this patient's presentation?
A. Chronic subdural hematoma
B. Acute subarachnoid hemorrhage

C. Acute epidural bleed
D. Concussion
E. Acute carotid-cavernous fistula

24. Which of the following patients with gait problems is suffering from cerebellar ataxia?
    A. A 29-year-old man who stands with his feet wide apart, walks with titubation, and falls down when asked to place his feet together
    B. A 41-year-old man with his spine bent forward while walking, who takes small steps, and does not swing his arms while walking
    C. A 35-year-old man who takes wide steps, lifting his legs higher than normal, and when asked to stand with his feet together and eyes open, he is able to remain stable, but looses balance when asked to close his eyes
    D. A 32-year-old man who shows sudden rapid movements of his arms and trunk while walking, which are accentuated by walking
    E. A 10-year-old boy who stands with marked lumbar lordosis and shows a waddling motion of his pelvis when walking

25. Which one of the following statements is TRUE about myasthenia gravis?
    A. Acetylcholine receptor antibodies are detected in approximately 70% of the ocular form of the illness.
    B. Acetylcholine receptor antibodies are detected in 80% to 90% of patients with generalized myasthenia gravis.
    C. Antibodies against muscle-specific receptor tyrosine kinase (MuSK) are seen in approximately one third of the patients without acetylcholinesterase antibodies.
    D. Antititin (antistriatal muscle antibodies) are present in approximately 30% of adult patients with myasthenia gravis and 80% of patients who have thymomas.
    E. All of the above.

26. Which one of the following drugs is not helpful in the treatment of trigeminal neuralgia?
    A. Carbamazepine
    B. Gabapentin
    C. Baclofen
    D. Clonazepam
    E. Acetaminophen

27. Which of the following is NOT a characteristic of adults in Erickson's epigenetic stage of generavity versus stagnation?
    A. They have a greater incidence of depression than younger adults.

B. There is an overall increase in the use of alcohol in this stage.
C. The age range is generally 40 to 60 years.
D. The ability to live independently is a key task.
E. They may think about failures and disappointments in their life.

28. Which of the following correctly describes conduction speed down and action potential?
    A. Conduction is slower in myelinated axons than it is in unmyelinated axons of the same diameter.
    B. Conduction is slower in unmyelinated axons with smaller diameters than it is in unmyelinated axons with larger diameters.
    C. Myelin sheathing is typically continuous down the length of the axon.
    D. Smaller axon diameters lead to smaller resistance to current flow.
    E. Myelin sheaths are formed by astrocytes.

29. Who is regarded as the founder of rational emotive behavioral therapy (REBT)?
    A. Paul Meehl
    B. Albert Ellis
    C. Starke Hathaway
    D. J. Charnley McKinley
    E. Sigmund Freud

30. Which one of the following is the MOST COMMON cause of malpractice claims in psychiatry?
    A. Incorrect treatment
    B. Attempted or completed suicide
    C. Incorrect diagnosis
    D. Improper supervision
    E. Medication error or drug reaction

31. While working in the ER, you are asked to evaluate a 34-year-old man complaining of nonspecific visual and auditory hallucinations. He is seeking voluntary admission to an inpatient psychiatry unit. You evaluate the patient and note the following on his mental status examination: he has multiple gang tattoos on his body, is casually dressed, and relates appropriately with no psychomotor abnormalities. He reports anxious mood and displays congruent affect. His thought process is linear and goal directed; he denies homicidal or suicidal ideation. Although he endorses auditory and visual hallucinations, he does not appear to be responding to internal stimuli. Cognition is intact; he scores 30/30 on the Folstein Mini Mental State Examination (MMSE). His social history is significant for someone with a history of multiple incarcerations, and he is engaged in ongoing illegal activities. ER staff members report overhearing the patient mention he is being sought by rival gang members who wish to harm the patient because of a

transgression. His vital signs are within normal limits. His urine toxicology is negative, and he has been medically cleared. Which of the following choices is the most likely diagnosis to account for his current presentation?

A. Factitious Disorder
B. Somatization Disorder
C. Malingering
D. Lewy Body Dementia
E. Conversion Disorder

32. What is the most common type of obsession in patients with obsessive-compulsive disorder (OCD)?
A. Worries about contamination
B. Intrusive sexual thoughts
C. Religious obsessions
D. Hoarding
E. Preoccupation with body image

33. A parent insists that her young child must donate one of his Christmas presents to a local charity. The following week, the mother gets angry at the child for giving away his new pencil crayons to a classmate. This example most closely illustrates which etiological theory of schizophrenia?
A. Schizophrenogenic mother
B. High expressed emotion
C. Double bind hypothesis
D. Decathexis theory
E. None of the above

34. Who introduced the term *conversion* to psychiatric theory?
A. Paul Briquet
B. Jean-Martin Charcot
C. Sigmund Freud
D. Thomas Sydenham
E. Emil Kraeplin

35. A 53-year-old woman from Puerto Rico starts exhibiting convulsivelike movements at her husband's funeral. She cries out loudly and curses. Following this, she falls down and lies still for a while. After this episode, she has no memory of the event. This has never happened to her before and she has no family history of epilepsy. What is the most likely diagnosis?
A. Ataque de nervios
B. Depersonalization disorder
C. Dissociative convulsions
D. Dissociative amnesia
E. Adjustment disorder

36. A 62-year-old woman was admitted to the hospital after developing sudden onset of vomiting, abdominal pain, bilateral hand tremor, dysarthria, and ataxia.

An electrocardiogram (EKG) done in the ER showed QTc prolongation and diffuse T-wave inversions. The patient's family member reports that she has a history of bipolar disorder and has been on lithium and lamotrigine for several years. The patient was recently started on aspirin and an ACE-inhibitor for coronary artery disease. What is the most likely cause of her symptoms?
A. Lamotrigine toxicity due to the addition of aspirin
B. Lithium toxicity due to the ACE-inhibitor
C. Lithium toxicity due to aspirin
D. Lithium toxicity due to a lamotrigine-lithium interaction
E. Renal failure due to aspirin

37. What percentage of clinical response to SSRIs occurs at the starting dosage?
A. At least 50%
B. At least 60%
C. At least 70%
D. At least 80%
E. At least 90%

38. Which one of the following choices is recommended as maintenance therapy for the prevention of recurrent depression in patients 70 years or older with major depression that had an initial response to treatment with paroxetine and interpersonal psychotherapy?
A. Paroxetine and monthly interpersonal psychotherapy
B. Paroxetine and clinical management
C. Monthly interpersonal psychotherapy
D. Clinical management only
E. Donepezil and memantine

39. You are doing cognitive therapy with a 33-year-old patient with depression who forgot to bring her homework to the session. Her automatic thought in response to her forgetting is "I am an idiot." Which of the following describes this type of thought?
A. Labeling
B. Projection
C. Emotional reasoning
D. Reaction formation
E. Intellectualization

40. A 28-year-old woman has recently been diagnosed with bipolar disorder and will need long-term treatment with a mood stabilizer. Before starting lithium monotherapy you counsel your patient regarding the signs and symptoms of lithium toxicity as well as other common side effects and potential long-term adverse effects from lithium therapy. She asks how likely it is that she will develop hypothyroidism in the future. You explain that although we are

unable to predict who will develop hypothyroidism and that we will need to continue to monitor her thyroid hormones throughout her treatment, the likelihood of developing hypothyroidism is greater than the general population while receiving lithium therapy. What percentage of patients will develop hypothyroidism while on long-term lithium therapy?

A. 0.3%
B. 1.3%
C. 5%
D. 8%
E. 10%

41. You are on the consultation-liaison service and are called by the oncology service to evaluate a 37-year-old woman for confusion. After an evaluation and looking through her chart, you suspect that the patient's symptoms may be due to metastases from her primary cancer. Which of the following is the type of cancer that is most likely to metastasize to the brain?

A. Melanoma
B. Lung
C. Breast
D. Colon
E. Rectum

42. A patient presents with the loss of sensation and weakness of his right hand and arm. He has non-fluent speech, but retained comprehension. He has difficulty seeing, is clumsy, and appears ataxic. His symptoms are most likely due to an abnormal blood supply to the brain from which of the following blood vessels?

A. Left posterior cerebral artery
B. Right middle cerebral artery
C. Right internal carotid artery
D. Left middle cerebral artery
E. Right posterior inferior cerebellar artery

43. Which one of the following is most commonly seen in the brain lesions of patients with multiple sclerosis (MS)?

A. Axonal plaques
B. Neurofibrillary tangles
C. Hirano bodies
D. Granulovacuolar degeneration
E. All of the above

44. Which one of the following statements about Friedreich's Ataxia (FA) is NOT true?

A. Friedreich's ataxia accounts for approximately 50% of inherited ataxias.
B. Incidence among North Americans is approximately 1.5 per 100,000 cases per year.

C. Gait ataxia is a frequent initial finding, with both legs affected simultaneously.
D. Pes cavus foot deformity and kyphoscoliosis develop variably in the course.
E. Cardiomyopathy is demonstrable in less than 10% of Friedreich's ataxia patients.

45. Which one of the following electroencephalogram (EEG) patterns is seen in hepatic encephalopathy?

A. Triphasic waves
B. Periodic lateralized epileptiform discharges (PLEDs)
C. Periodic complexes
D. Predominant delta waves
E. Predominant B waves

46. A woman with history of a recent stroke presents to a neurologist for follow-up. As she is sitting in the office, she looks down at her lap, where her left hand is resting. She becomes quite confused and upset, claiming that she has found a hand and she does not know whose it is or how it got there. Based on this incident, what is the most likely location of this patient's injury?

A. Right occipital lobe
B. Right parietal lobe
C. Left parietal lobe
D. Left frontal lobe
E. Right temporal lobe

47. A 50-year-old man with AIDS presents with right-sided hemiparesis. He has no other focal deficits. An MRI indicates that he has a brain tumor and consultation with the neurology service suggests that this is an aggressive tumor. Which of the following tumors is it likely to be?

A. Oligodendroglioma
B. Primary cerebral lymphoma
C. Cerebellar astrocytoma
D. Medulloblastoma
E. Pituitary adenoma

48. What is the most common sports-related traumatic brain injury?

A. Subarachnoid hemorrhage
B. Contusion
C. Concussion
D. Subdural hematoma
E. Epidural hematoma

49. What is the main function of the Glasgow Coma Scale?

A. Predict morbidity
B. Predict mortality
C. Predict recovery

D. Predict development of early complications
E. Predict development of late complications

50. An 18-year-old man comes to your office with a 6-month history of unsteady gait. During your physical examination, you ask the patient to stand straight with his feet together. He is able to remain stable, but when asked to close his eyes, he immediately becomes unstable and needs to hold on to a nearby chair to prevent him from falling. Which part of the brain is most likely involved in the patient's symptoms?
    A. Cerebellum
    B. Frontal cortex
    C. Dorsal columns
    D. Temporal cortex
    E. Optic nerve

51. A 28-year-old black woman treated with steroids for neurosarcoidosis complains of a 4-month history of headaches, polyuria, and increasing memory impairment. You would consider all the following possibilities more readily for her symptoms EXCEPT:
    A. Hydrocephalus
    B. Hypercalcemia
    C. Diabetes insipidus
    D. Granulomatous meningitis
    E. Hepatic encephalopathy

52. You have been treating a 75-year-old man with idiopathic Parkinson's disease and depression. Since his last visit, he has been started on Sinemet (levodopa/carbidopa) by his neurologist to reasonably good effect. Parkinson's disease and depression are his only health problems. Which of the following antidepressants would you want to ensure that the patient is not taking?
    A. Sertraline
    B. Phenelzine
    C. Venlafaxine
    D. Amitriptyline
    E. Paroxetine

53. All of the following are normal, nonpathologic changes in an aging brain EXCEPT:
    A. Decrease in the weight of the brain
    B. Enlargement of the ventricles
    C. Lewy bodies
    D. Widening of sulci
    E. Decrease in the blood flow to the brain

54. The presenilin-1 (PS-1) gene, a major locus for Alzheimer's disease in early onset familial Alzheimer's disease, is found on which one of the following chromosomes?
    A. Chromosome 1

B. Chromosome 21
C. Chromosome 19
D. Chromosome 14
E. None of the above

55. Which one of the following is NOT a projective personality test?
    A. Rorschach
    B. Thematic Apperception Test (TAT)
    C. Draw-A-Person Test
    D. Apperceptive Personality Test (APT)
    E. Minnesota Multiphasic Personality Inventory (MMPI)

56. Which one of the following choices is generally NOT part of the accepted standard for information disclosure for any given psychiatric treatment?
    A. Description of the fee schedule for the visits
    B. Description of the illness
    C. Nature and purpose of proposed treatments
    D. Risks and benefits of the proposed treatment
    E. Other therapeutic options and their risks and benefits

57. While working in the ER, you are asked to evaluate a 34-year-old man complaining of nonspecific visual and auditory hallucinations. He is seeking voluntary admission to an inpatient psychiatry unit. You evaluate the patient and note the following on his mental status examination: he has multiple gang tattoos on his body, is casually dressed, and relates appropriately with no psychomotor abnormalities. He reports anxious mood and displays congruent affect. His thought process is linear and goal directed; he denies homicidal or suicidal ideation. Although he endorses auditory and visual hallucinations, he does not appear to be responding to internal stimuli. His cognition is intact; he scores 30/30 on the Folstein MMSE. His social history is significant for someone with a history of multiple incarcerations, and he is engaged in ongoing illegal activities. ER staff members report overhearing the patient mention he is being sought by rival gang members who wish to harm the patient because of a transgression. His vital signs are within normal limits. His urine toxicology is negative, and he has been medically cleared. If you decide that this individual is malingering, how would you code your diagnosis in the DSM-IV-TR multiaxial system?
    A. Factitious Disorder NOS on axis I
    B. Malingering as a "V code" on axis I
    C. Malingering as a "V code" on axis II
    D. "Antisocial traits" on axis I
    E. Malingering is not coded in the DSM-IV-TR diagnostic system.

58. A 17-year-old single man of African origin presents to your clinic for a consultation. He has been sent for evaluation by his primary care physician. He had presented to his primary clinician's office with a 2-month history of memory problems, burning feeling in his head, visual symptoms, and fatigue. A complete workup for any infectious, inflammatory, and metabolic causes of his symptoms has been negative. A neurological consultation and further investigations with MRI of the brain, lumbar puncture (LP), and EEG have not shown any abnormalities. A trial of analgesics, vitamins, and nutritional supplements has not ameliorated his symptoms. The patient is not able to attend school because of his symptoms. The history obtained from the patient's mother indicates that they recently moved to the United States from Nigeria. The patient has been having a difficult time adjusting to his new cultural environment, especially at school. Given the patient's history and presentation, what is the most likely culture bound syndrome (CBS)?
A. Koro
B. Latah
C. Amok
D. Pibloktog
E. Brain fag

59. An 18-year-old single man recently diagnosed with schizophrenia is referred to you for consultation. He was recently fired from his job at a fast food restaurant and his clinical picture has been dominated by positive symptomatology. His cousin has also been diagnosed with schizophrenia. The patient is asking about his prognosis. Which of the following would be considered a good prognostic factor in his case?
A. Predominant positive symptoms
B. Young age at onset
C. Family history of schizophrenia
D. Bizarre delusions
E. Poor premorbid psychosocial functioning

60. The DSM-IV-TR criteria for somatization disorder include the occurrence of which of the following sets of symptoms?
A. Two pain, four gastrointestinal, one sexual, and one pseudoneurological
B. Four pain, two gastrointestinal, one sexual, and one pseudoneurological
C. Four pain, two gastrointestinal, one respiratory, and one pseudoneurological
D. Two pain, four gastrointestinal, one respiratory, and one pseudoneurological
E. Four pain, two gastrointestinal, one respiratory, and one sexual

61. Which of the following drugs have been shown to improve cataplexy?
A. Phenobarbitone
B. Modafinil
C. Amphetamines
D. Benzodiazepines
E. Amitriptyline and fluoxetine

62. Major depressive disorder frequently requires more than one step of treatment to elicit a remission of symptoms. In level 2 of the Sequenced Treatment Alternatives to Relieve Depression (STAR*D) trial, the authors found which one of the following statements true with regard to augmenting citalopram?
A. Buspirone produced a greater reduction in the number of and severity of symptoms and had fewer side effects and adverse reactions than sustained-release bupropion.
B. Sustained-release bupropion produced a greater reduction in the number of and severity of symptoms and had fewer side effects and adverse reactions than buspirone.
C. Sustained-release bupropion and buspirone produced an equal reduction in the number of and severity of symptoms and had an equivalent dropout rate.
D. Neither buspirone nor sustained-release bupropion appeared to be useful in clinical settings.
E. Sustained-release bupropion produced a greater reduction in the number of and severity of symptoms, but had a greater dropout rate due to side effects and adverse reactions than buspirone.

63. Which SSRI is most commonly associated with extrapyramidal symptoms?
A. Citalopram
B. Escitalopram
C. Fluoxetine
D. Paroxetine
E. Sertraline

64. You are asked to evaluate a patient on the neurology service who is severely agitated and paranoid. The patient was originally admitted for uncontrolled seizures and has a long history of a poorly controlled seizure disorder. You determine that the patient is suffering from persecutory delusions secondary to an untreated bipolar disorder with psychotic features. You recommend starting a mood stabilizer and antipsychotic medication and advise the neurology service to avoid which antipsychotic medication?
A. Fluphenazine
B. Haloperidol

C. Chlorpromazine
D. Risperidone
E. Perphenazine

65. You are working in the psychiatric ER and are called to see a patient who has come to the ER because he has been having suicidal thoughts. All of the following approaches to your interaction with the patient should be included in the initial assessment EXCEPT:
    A. Asking the patient whether or not he hears voices
    B. Asking about recent stressors
    C. After completing your interview, calling collaterals to assess his risk
    D. After completing the interview, starting the patient on an antidepressant
    E. Asking about the patient's pain level

66. Which one of the following is TRUE of tardive dyskinesia (TD)?
    A. The rate of developing spontaneous TD in an otherwise healthy young adult with schizophrenia is about 0.05% per year.
    B. The risk of TD is highest only in the first year of treatment with typical antipsychotics.
    C. Approximately 5% of the patients develop TD in the first 3 years of treatment with typical antipsychotics.
    D. The risk of an elderly patient developing TD in the first year of treatment with typical antipsychotics is about five times higher than in a younger patient.
    E. All of the above.

67. Which of the following choices reflect an ethical dilemma?
    A. Autonomy versus justice
    B. Autonomy versus shame and doubt
    C. Basic trust versus basic mistrust
    D. Initiative versus guilt
    E. None of the above

68. A patient arrives at your office with incomprehensible speech. He can follow commands and can repeat phrases. Which one of the following types of speech impairment does he have?
    A. Wernicke's aphasia
    B. Broca's aphasia
    C. Conduction aphasia
    D. Transcortical motor aphasia
    E. Transcortical sensory aphasia

69. Which one of the following areas, when disturbed, is thought to cause an inability to learn new information (anterograde amnesia) or recall recently acquired memories (retrograde amnesia) in patients with Korsakoff's syndrome?
    A. Mammillary bodies
    B. Cingulate gyrus
    C. Presubiculum
    D. Hippocampus
    E. Fornix

70. All of the following are examples of mitochondrial-transmitted disorders EXCEPT:
    A. Cytochrome-C oxidase deficiency
    B. Leigh's syndrome (subacute necrotizing encephalomyelopathy)
    C. Movements of the eye, lactic acidosis, strokelike episodes (MELAS)
    D. Myoclonic epilepsy with ragged red fibers (MERRF)
    E. Progressive supranuclear palsy

71. When rapid eye movement (REM) rhythm is seen on an EEG recording during the daytime, it indicates which one of the following conditions?
    A. Sleep deprivation
    B. Normal pattern
    C. Dementia
    D. Delirium
    E. None of the above

72. A 34-year-old woman presents with new onset blindness. An examination reveals weakness in the left leg and paresthesias in both hands. The diagnosis of MS is suspected. Which one of the following is a true statement of the radiological evaluation of MS?
    A. Early in the disease, a CT scan is rarely normal.
    B. MS plaques typically have a round, bull's eye appearance.
    C. The presence of lesions on MRI is highly correlated with the clinical picture.
    D. The sensitivity of MRI in detecting MS is approximately 50%.
    E. Focal white matter hyperintensities on MRI are highly suggestive of MS.

73. A 70-year-old white man with a history of hypertension and insulin dependant diabetes mellitus is brought to the ER of a major teaching hospital following an episode of sudden loss of consciousness. He was in his usual state of health until about 2 hours ago when he suddenly complained of a headache, vomited, and lost consciousness as he was talking to his wife. During the examination in the ER, his eyes are found to be looking to the right and he has a right hemiplegia. His blood pressure is recorded at 220/120 mm Hg and his blood sugar is 120 mg%. All

metabolic and infectious workups are normal at the present time. The CT scan of the brain confirms a hemorrhage in which of the following structures?

A. Right cerebral hemisphere
B. Left cerebral hemisphere
C. Left pons
D. Left medulla
E. Right medulla

74. A 26-year-old white man was hit from behind while driving on the highway. After the accident, the patient complains of severe neck pain that radiates to his shoulders and head, as well as weakness and loss of deep tendon reflexes (DTRs) in both arms. What is this patient's most likely diagnosis?

A. A herniated cervical intervertebral disc due to whiplash injury
B. Posttraumatic delirium due to a contusion
C. Damage to the brachial plexus
D. A soft tissue neck injury
E. A spinal epidural hematoma

75. A 74-year-old woman with a history of Parkinson's disease is referred for a psychiatric consultation due to worsening psychotic symptoms. A complete medical workup failed to find any organic etiology for her auditory hallucinations and paranoid delusions. Which of the following antipsychotic medications would be most appropriate in treating this patient's symptoms?

A. Haloperidol
B. Risperidone
C. Quetiapine
D. Ziprasidone
E. Perphenazine

76. The police brought a 54-year-old man to the ER who they found asleep in the street near the ER. He was very confused and was able to give them only limited personal information and was unable to state how he got there. Although he had two empty bottles of Vodka in his coat pocket and he smelled liked alcohol, he scored zero on a breath analyzer test, which indicated that he was not intoxicated. On examination, he appears disheveled and malnourished. Laboratory testing indicated that he is dehydrated and has low total protein and albumin levels. His blood sugar is 90 mg%. He scores 5/30 on an MMSE. You also notice that he has nystagmus on extreme lateral gaze and gait instability. Which one of the following drugs should be given prior to the treatment of his dehydration with dextrose saline IV?

A. Potassium chloride
B. Vitamin C

C. Vitamin B_{12} injections
D. Oral thiamine
E. Parenteral thiamine IV

77. A recently unemployed 45-year-old man arrives at your clinic with a 2-year history of hypersomnolence, mildly depressed mood, and fatigue. He used to go hiking until 3 years ago, when had to stop because of significant arthritis. You suspect borreliosis, which is confirmed by laboratory investigations and a further neurological consultation. Your psychosocial assessment also reveals significant domestic tension. You would do all the following EXCEPT:

A. Treat with antibiotics
B. Treat with antidepressants
C. Psychological therapy
D. Advise vocational rehabilitation
E. Antipsychotic treatment

78. A 28-year-old woman with a history of generalized seizure disorder has been stable on carbamazepine and seizurefree for 2 years. She asks about the possibility of discontinuing her antiepileptic medication. Which of the following would be the most accurate statement about the potential for seizure recurrence?

A. There are no tests that can help guide this decision.
B. After withdrawal of anticonvulsants, the patient has a 10% to 20% chance of seizure recurrence at 30 months.
C. After withdrawal of anticonvulsants, the patient has a 30% to 40% chance of seizure recurrence at 30 months.
D. After withdrawal of anticonvulsants, the patient has a 70% to 80% chance of seizure recurrence at 30 months.
E. The chance for seizure recurrence is idiosyncratic, and the epidemiological studies have been contradictory.

79. Which one of the following choices is a normal change seen in the elderly?

A. Decrease in psychomotor speed
B. Inability to learn new tasks
C. A significant decrease in intelligence quotient (IQ) starting at 70 years of age
D. Changes in vocabulary
E. Impairments in social functioning due to cognitive decline

80. Which one of the following statements is NOT TRUE regarding neuronal signaling?

A. The usual method for communication among neurons is either molecular or electrical.

B. The four classes of molecular signals are the monoamines, amino acids, peptides, and neurotrophic factors.
C. There is heterogeneity among the multiple subtypes of receptors for a particular neurotransmitter.
D. A single neuron usually releases only a single type of molecular signal.
E. None of the above.

81. Which one of the following is a test of general intellectual functioning?
    A. Shipley Scale
    B. California Verbal Learning Test II
    C. Benton Visual Retention Test
    D. Boston Naming Test (Revised)
    E. Wisconsin Card Sorting Test

82. Based on the American Psychiatric Association (APA) Task Force's recommendations on the pretreatment evaluation for Electroconvulsive therapy (ECT), which of the following is NOT CORRECT?
    A. A psychiatric history and examination documenting the need for ECT
    B. An evaluation by a judge for determining the capacity to consent for ECT
    C. A medical review determining the risks and contraindications for ECT
    D. An anesthesia evaluation and clearance for ECT
    E. A written informed consent for the ECT

83. While working in the emergency department, a 66-year-old Spanish-speaking woman arrives seeking psychiatric services. Accompanying the patient are her 70-year-old husband and her 40-year-old son. The patient speaks no English. Her husband speaks fluent Spanish and a fair amount of English; her son is completely fluent in both Spanish and English. Ideally, what is the most advisable approach to assessing this patient?
    A. Conduct the interview without assistance from anyone. Any interpreter used will interfere with your therapeutic alliance.
    B. Conduct the interview with assistance from the patient's husband. He has the most consistent interaction with the patient, thus he is the most familiar with her condition.
    C. Conduct the interview with assistance from the patient's son. He spends less time with the patient overall, but he is more fluent in both languages and will translate better.
    D. Conduct the interview with assistance from an interpreter (employed by the hospital). The husband and son should not be used as interpreters because they may distort the patient's complaints.

E. Do not evaluate the patient; instead advise the family to seek a Spanish-speaking psychiatrist in the community.

84. A 21-year-old man who returned home from fighting in Iraq a year ago comes to your office because of the following problems. Since being home, he has continued to suffer from his combat experience. He no longer enjoys being with his family and feels empty. He does not want to talk about what he experienced and feels estranged from his family and friends. He does not think that he will be able to get married and will probably die young. Once a cheerful teenager with little anxiety, he is frequently irritable with those around him and easily startled. He also has difficulty falling asleep and, when he does sleep, he frequently has horrible nightmares. Based on the patient's history alone, which of the following diagnoses are you least concerned that he might have?
    A. Agoraphobia
    B. Schizophrenia
    C. Alcohol Dependence
    D. Major Depression
    E. Panic Disorder

85. Which of the following is NOT considered one of Kurt Schneider's first-ranked criteria for schizophrenia?
    A. Audible thoughts
    B. Thought broadcasting
    C. Delusional perceptions
    D. Loose associations
    E. Made impulses

86. What are the most common locations of imagined defects in body dysmorphic disorder?
    A. Stomach and waist
    B. Breasts and genitals
    C. Arms and legs
    D. Face and hair
    E. Neck and shoulders

87. Which one of the following choices is a supporting feature for the diagnosis of dementia with Lewy bodies?
    A. Visual hallucinations
    B. Changing levels of alertness
    C. Cogwheeling
    D. Repeated falls
    E. Resting tremor

88. Which of these antidepressants has the highest relative potency for blocking the reuptake of dopamine?
    A. Nefazodone
    B. Bupropion

C. Sertraline

D. Paroxetine

E. Nortriptyline

89. A 45-year-old woman with a history of dysthymic disorder recently started taking sertraline 75 mg/day PO. She now complains of sudden onset of myoclonus, diaphoresis, diarrhea, shivering, and worsened anxiety. On physical examination, she has a low-grade fever and exhibits hyperreflexia. Further history reveals that she has been taking St. John's wort, valerian, and multivitamins over the counter for the past 9 months. What is the most likely diagnosis?

A. NMS

B. Malignant hyperthermia

C. Lethal catatonia

D. Serotonin syndrome

E. Anticholinergic toxicity

90. Which of the following are the most appropriate steps in the initial management of a patient with NMS?

A. Hydration, cooling blanket, cardiac and renal function monitoring

B. Cooling blanket, dialysis, hydration, cardiac monitoring

C. Hydration, administer baclofen IV, restraints, cardiac monitoring

D. Administer lorazepam IV, hydration, measure urine output

E. Administer diphenhydramine IV, cooling blankets, cardiac monitoring

91. A psychiatrist has made arrangements to begin dialectical behavioral therapy for a patient diagnosed with borderline personality disorder. Which of the following represents the correct order of the therapy's first-stage targets?

A. Decreasing therapy-interfering behaviors, decreasing suicidal behaviors, decreasing quality-of-life interfering behaviors, increasing behavior skills

B. Decreasing suicidal behaviors, decreasing therapy-interfering behaviors, decreasing quality-of-life interfering behaviors, increasing behavior skills

C. Decreasing suicidal behaviors, decreasing therapy-interfering behaviors, increasing behavior skills, decreasing quality-of-life interfering behaviors

D. Decreasing suicidal behaviors, increasing behavior skills, decreasing therapy-interfering behaviors, decreasing quality-of-life interfering behaviors

E. Decreasing suicidal behaviors, increasing behavior skills, decreasing quality-of-life interfering behaviors, decreasing therapy-interfering behaviors

92. Which one of the following is most likely to have a good response to treatment with opioids?

A. Patients with tonic pain

B. Patients with neuropathic pain

C. Patients with phasic pain

D. Patients with cognitive impairment

E. Patients with high levels of psychological distress

93. A 75-year-old widowed woman with major depression is discharged home after a 2-week hospitalization for worsening symptoms of depression. You want to follow her in your out-patient clinic to ensure appropriate continuity of care. On discussion with her, you become aware that she will not be able to make the copayment for the clinic visits. What is the next appropriate step to ensure appropriate follow-up for this patient?

A. You should not follow her in your clinic as she cannot make the copayment.

B. It is your duty to provide follow-up, so follow her even if she cannot make the copayment.

C. Do not arrange any psychiatric follow-up as she cannot make the copayment.

D. Check with her insurance company about the copayment policy before making the follow-up appointment.

E. Refer her back to her primary clinician only as she cannot make the copayment for the psychiatric follow-up.

94. All of the following are signs of an upper motor neuron (UMN) lesion EXCEPT:

A. Extensor plantar response

B. Weakness

C. Rigidity

D. Atrophy

E. Spasticity

95. The basal ganglia constitutes a group of nuclei associated with motor and learning functions. Which of the following is not part of the nuclei that comprise the basal ganglia?

A. Caudate

B. Globus pallidus

C. Putamen

D. Ventral striatum

E. Hypothalamus

96. All of the following statements regarding mitochondrial disorders are true EXCEPT:
    A. The majority of mitochondrial DNA disorders affect the nervous system.
    B. Clumping of the mitochondria in muscle fibers is a frequent occurrence.
    C. Lactic acidosis is a commonly observed feature with these disorders.
    D. Cytochrome-C oxidase is the least commonly affected respiratory complex.
    E. Most protein components of the respiratory chain come from the nucleus.

97. Which one of the following choices is NOT TRUE about MRI of the brain?
    A. Better definition of anatomic structures and greater sensitivity to pathologic lesions
    B. Multiplanar capability displaying dimensional information and relationships between structures
    C. Better demonstration of physiologic processes, such as blood flow and cerebrospinal fluid (CSF) motion
    D. Better demonstration of special properties of tissue, such as water diffusion or biochemical makeup
    E. Poorer visualization of the posterior fossa and intraspinal lesions

98. A 36-year-old man with a 10-year history of epilepsy is undergoing evaluation for surgical removal of his seizure focus. Which of the following statements is correct about the use of positron emission tomography (PET) for the evaluation of seizures?
    A. PET imaging is especially useful in the evaluation of frontal lobe epilepsy in the absence of EEG abnormalities.
    B. Temporal lobe hypometabolism is seen in approximately 25% of patients with temporal lobe seizures.
    C. Extratemporal lobe hypometabolism is not relevant to the evaluation of temporal lobe seizures.
    D. Severe interictal hypometabolism of the affected temporal lobe is associated with better postoperative seizure control.
    E. PET imaging is not useful in the evaluation of infantile spasms.

99. A 75-year-old man is brought to the ER by ambulance after he was found on the floor of his house by his wife. He has a history of hypertension and noninsulin dependant diabetes mellitus. History obtained from the family indicates that he has not been very compliant with his medications for hypertension and diabetes. The blood pressure recorded in the ER is 200/100 mm Hg and a nonfasting blood sugar level is 300 mg%. The rest of the history is unremarkable. When you go to see the patient, you see an obese white man who is lying in the hospital bed. He is mute and quadriplegic, but appears to be able to move his eyes. On further examination, it becomes clear that he is able to understand what you are saying to him and he is trying to communicate by using eye movements. An MRI of the brain reveals an infarction in which of the following structures?
    A. Cerebral cortex
    B. Thalamus
    C. Cerebellum
    D. Internal capsule
    E. Basis pontis

100. What is the most important factor in predicting the late development of posttraumatic epilepsy?
    A. The severity of the initial injury
    B. The patient's age
    C. The appearance of a seizure within hours after the injury
    D. The patient's gender
    E. Family history of epilepsy

101. A 16-year-old boy arrives at the office complaining of gait and balance problems that seem to be worsening as time goes by. His past medical history is significant for scoliosis. On physical examination, the patient has ataxia, weakness with loss of DTRs of both legs, impaired position sense, and mild diminished bilateral visual acuity. What is this patient's most likely diagnosis?
    A. Multiple sclerosis
    B. Guillain-Barré syndrome
    C. Refsum's disease
    D. Friedrich's ataxia
    E. Amyotrophic lateral sclerosis

102. What is the cause of spinocerebellar ataxias?
    A. Chromosomal trisomy
    B. Chromosomal monosomy
    C. Parental imprinting
    D. Trinucleotide repeat expansion
    E. Spontaneous mutation

103. A 50-year-old homeless man is brought to the ER by the police after he was found wandering in a confused manner. Information from the homeless shelter reveals that he has been drinking alcohol excessively for the past 12 months. The physical examination reveals glossitis and a weeping eczematous rash of the face and neck with hyperpigmentation. The diagnostic workup included the following: mean

corpuscular volume, 106 fL; normal leukocyte and platelet counts; normal renal function test results; elevated gamma GT, serum alanine aminotransferase, and serum aspartate aminotransferase. Chest radiograph, EKG, and serial creative kinase determinations were normal. An additional workup included the following tests, the results of which were normal: serum thyrotropin, cortisol, vitamin B, folate, iron studies, and rapid plasma reagin test; stool cultures and examinations for ova and parasites; sequential blood cultures for bacteria, mycobacteria, and fungi. The mental state examination reveals visual hallucinations and illusions with disorientation. Your immediate management will include the following EXCEPT:

A. Treat for delirium tremens
B. Parenteral thiamine
C. Social work assessment
D. Niacin supplementation
E. Dietary assessment

104. A 27-year-old HIV-positive man presents with fever and acute onset of psychotic symptoms. His meningeal signs are positive. An LP reveals 200 cells/cubic mm and CSF sugars as 20 mg/dL. The diagnosis is established by finding certain organisms in the counting chamber centrifuge sediment of the CSF. What is the treatment of choice?

A. Fluconazole, stopped after CSF is sterilized, or amphotericin B/flucytosine
B. Fluconazole, stopped 3 months after CSF is sterilized, or amphotericin B/flucytosine
C. Fluconazole, stopped 6 months after CSF is sterilized, or amphotericin B/flucytosine
D. Flucytosine, stopped after CSF is sterilized
E. Flucytosine, stopped 3 months after CSF is sterilized

105. Which one of the following statements best describe REM sleep in the elderly?

A. Shorter REM periods
B. More frequent REM periods
C. Overall decrease in REM sleep
D. All of the above
E. None of the above

106. Which one of the following statements is TRUE regarding neurotransmitters?

A. There are seven classic monoamine neurotransmitters.
B. The monoamine neurotransmitters are present in a large percentage of neurons.
C. The amino acid neurotransmitters are present in a small percentage of neurons.

D. There are approximately 10 identified putative neuropeptide neurotransmitters.
E. None of the above.

107. Which one of the following is NOT a test for executive function?

A. Wisconsin Card Sorting Test
B. Category Test
C. Trail-Making Test
D. Delis-Kaplan Test
E. Judgment of line orientation

108. Which one of the following statements regarding a suicide risk assessment is NOT TRUE?

A. It is a process and not an event.
B. It should be part of all standard psychiatric assessments.
C. Obtaining a no-harm contract is essential.
D. It requires frequent updating.
E. It should always evaluate risk and protective factors.

109. You recently began treating an individual with a diagnosis of major depression. There is no previous history of hypomania, mania, or psychosis. Shortly after starting the patient on antidepressant therapy, a manic episode ensues (the patient "switches" to mania). Based only on the information given, what is this patient's diagnosis now according to DSM-IV-TR?

A. Major depressive disorder with atypical features
B. Bipolar I Disorder
C. Bipolar II Disorder
D. Bipolar Disorder NOS
E. Schizoaffective disorder

110. Which one of the following is not part of the five stages describing the reactions of a person to their impending death as proposed by Dr. Kubler-Ross?

A. Acceptance
B. Depression
C. Anger
D. Bargaining
E. Reaction formation

111. A 30-year-old woman is brought to the emergency department (ED) by her husband. She recently returned early from a trip overseas during which she began to hear voices and developed a belief that locals had implanted a microchip in her brain for surveillance purposes. She has no mood symptoms and does not abuse substances. She was well when she left for her trip 2 weeks ago. She has no psychiatric history and had previously been functioning

well as a high school teacher. What is her most accurate current diagnosis?

A. Schizophrenia
B. Delusional Disorder
C. Schizophreniform Disorder
D. Psychotic Disorder NOS
E. Brief Psychotic Disorder

112. A 25-year-old woman presents for obstetrical evaluation. She states that she is pregnant and shows many objective signs of pregnancy, including increased abdominal girth, cessation of monthly periods, nausea, and breast enlargement. She indicates that she can feel intermittent movement of the fetus. To the physician's later surprise, the patient's pregnancy test is negative and an ultrasound shows an empty uterus. According to the DSM-IV-TR, what is this patient's diagnosis?

A. Somatization disorder
B. Conversion disorder
C. Hypochondriasis
D. Undifferentiated somatoform disorder
E. Somatoform disorder NOS

113. A primary care physician asks for your professional opinion regarding one of his patients. The patient is a 16-year-old girl with a height of 5'4" and a current weight of 98 lb. The patient has been refusing to eat everything except rice cakes and diet soda, insisting that she is fat and extremely fearful that any increased intake will cause her to gain excessive weight. The physician's records indicate that the patient was an average weight for her height at the age of 12, when she experienced menarche. Over the past few years, she has continued to have regular menstrual periods approximately every month. She is not currently taking any medications or herbal supplements. Based on this information, what is her most accurate diagnosis?

A. Anorexia Nervosa, Restricting Type
B. Anorexia Nervosa, Binge-eating/Purging Type
C. Bulimia Nervosa, Purging Type
D. Bulimia Nervosa, Nonpurging Type
E. Eating Disorder NOS

114. A 65-year-old man with a history of recurrent major depressive disorder has been psychiatrically stable on nortriptyline for the last 12 years. He arrives at the clinic complaining of poor mood, decreased energy, interrupted sleep, and loss of appetite for the last several weeks. He has tolerated the medication well, although with occasional dry mouth and episodic bouts of dizziness. He takes 125 mg of nortriptyline daily. The serum level, drawn the same day as his visit to the clinic, is 164 ng/mL. What should be the next step in treating this patient's depression?

A. Decrease nortriptyline to 100 mg daily
B. Augment nortriptyline with escitalopram at 20 mg daily
C. Augment nortriptyline with fluoxetine at 20 mg daily
D. Discontinue nortriptyline and start sertraline at 75 mg daily
E. Increase nortriptyline to 150 mg daily

115. A 36-year-old man with a history of seizures and schizoaffective disorder (bipolar type) was recently admitted to the hospital for worsening auditory hallucinations. He was restarted on his usual dose of haloperidol 10 mg daily. He was tolerating this medication well before he discontinued it on his own accord 2 weeks prior to admission to the hospital. The severity and frequency of the patient's auditory hallucinations decreased, but he developed extrapyramidal symptoms within in a few days. Which of the following events is most likely to have occurred to cause this problem?

A. Phenytoin was added to his treatment regimen during this admission.
B. He stopped smoking during this admission.
C. Sertraline was discontinued from his treatment regimen during this admission.
D. Buspirone was discontinued from his treatment regimen during this admission.
E. He had used a hallucinogen a day prior to this admission and it was still in his body and interacting with the haloperidol.

116. You have been seeing a 34-year-old woman with schizophrenia in your outpatient clinic for several months. Her symptoms associated with schizophrenia have been fairly well controlled on haloperidol 10 mg daily, but the patient has expressed concern regarding the long-term side effects of haloperidol. Recognizing the chronic nature of her disease and the need for long-term treatment, you decide to change her antipsychotic to an atypical antipsychotic medication. She returns to your office and states that she is doing well, but has recently noticed discharge from her breasts. Which of the following antipsychotic medication is this patient likely taking?

A. Olanzapine
B. Quetiapine
C. Ziprasidone
D. Risperidone
E. Perphenazine

117. Which medication used in the treatment of alcohol dependence is most closely based on the behavioral concept of "aversion?"
    A. Acamprosate
    B. Naltrexone
    C. Disulfiram
    D. Lorazepam
    E. Buspirone

118. A 75-year-old white man is admitted to the hospital for a fall and hip fracture. He has a history of chronic pain and has been prescribed propoxyphene hydrochloride at 65 mg PO twice daily for the last 5 years with excellent pain control. He is otherwise healthy and is cognitively intact. His only other medication is enteric coated aspirin at 81 mg PO daily. He has no history of pain medication abuse. His laboratory workup is negative. His blood alcohol level is zero and the urine drug screen is positive for opiates only. He has an open reduction and internal fixation of his left hip fracture. The aspirin he is taking is held back during the first 2 postoperative days to reduce the risk of bleeding. For good pain control during the postoperative period, the surgeon switches him to codeine at 60 mg PO twice daily with 15 mg PO every 4 hours as needed. He is also started on subcutaneous heparin for deep vein thrombosis prophylaxis. He appears to do well for the first 24 hours and denies being in any pain. However, he then starts getting confused, agitated, and is hallucinating. A psychiatric consultation is called for the evaluation of this man's confusion. He is very confused and scores a 15 on the MMSE. The medical workup, including a chest x-ray and CT scan of his head, is normal. Careful review of the chart indicates that he has had a total of three doses of codeine at 60 mg and two 15-mg tablets in a 36-hour period. Which of the following choices is the most possible cause of his confusion?
    A. Too little pain medication postoperatively resulting in uncontrolled pain and delirium.
    B. Too much pain medication postoperatively and resultant delirium.
    C. Aspirin withdrawal.
    D. Cerebrovascular accident and resultant delirium.
    E. Codeine potentiates the metabolism of propoxyphene and resulting delirium.

119. Among the leading cause of death in the United States, suicide is ranked at which position?
    A. 5th
    B. 6th
    C. 7th
    D. 8th
    E. 9th

120. Which of the following tests would be most sensitive in detecting an ischemic infarct within the first few hours?
    A. Noncontrast head CT
    B. Contrast enhanced head CT
    C. Diffusion weighted MRI
    D. Cerebral angiogram
    E. Carotid ultrasound

121. A young man was brought in by the police after being found in the park. He was confused and became combative when the police approached him. He was apprehended and brought to the ER for evaluation. While examining him, he appears intoxicated and tells you that it looks like your face is melting. You presume he has ingested lysergic acid diethylamide (LSD) and ask for a toxicology screen. Which one of the following receptors does LSD affect to produce these symptoms?
    A. Mu-opioid receptor
    B. Dopamine type 2 (D2) receptor
    C. Serotonin type 2A (5-HT2A) receptor
    D. N-methyl-D-aspartate acid (NMDA) receptor
    E. Gamma-aminobutyric acid (GABA) type A

122. Which of the following is the most common genetic abnormality seen in velocardiofacial syndrome?
    A. Microdeletion of band 13 on the short arm of chromosome 22
    B. Microdeletion of band 11 on the short arm of chromosome 22
    C. Microdeletion of band 11 on the long arm of chromosome 22
    D. Microdeletion of band 13 on the long arm of chromosome 22
    E. Microdeletion of variable band on the long arm of chromosome 22

123. An MRI of the brain would be the diagnostic imaging modality of choice for which one of the following conditions?
    A. Clinical suspicion of Alzheimer's disease
    B. Fear of enclosed spaces
    C. Clinical suspicion of an intracranial hemorrhage
    D. Clinical suspicion of progressive multifocal leukoencephalopathy
    E. Clinical suspicion of a meningioma

124. Which one of the following is a common clinical characteristic of peripheral vertigo?
    A. Patients often present with intermittent vertigo.
    B. Tinnitus is usually absent.
    C. Patients often present with ataxia.
    D. Patients often present with vertical nystagmus.
    E. The vertigo is usually mild in severity.

125. Which one of the following is the correct mode of inheritance for neurofibromatosis 1?

- **A.** X-linked recessive
- **B.** X-linked dominant
- **C.** Y linked
- **D.** Autosomal recessive
- **E.** Autosomal dominant

126. A 64-year-old man on several medications for asthma, diabetes, and recurrent deep vein thrombosis who is treated with warfarin now presents to the ED complaining of a first episode of generalized tonic–clonic seizures. During your evaluation, the patient reports a 2-week history of progressively worsening headaches, drowsiness, and lightheadedness. He has a vague recollection of having hit his head after getting out of his car a few weeks ago. Physical examination is essentially normal. What would be the most likely finding on a CT scan of the head that explains his symptoms?

- **A.** An epidural hematoma
- **B.** A subarachnoid hemorrhage
- **C.** A subdural hematoma
- **D.** A frontal lobe tumor
- **E.** A temporal lobe tumor

127. A 14-year-old wheelchair-bound boy is brought to the office by his mother. His mother reports that he had difficulties walking as a small child, and his condition has slowly progressed to the point where he needs to be in a wheelchair. During the interview, the patient seems inattentive and sad. He has slurred speech with a slow rate, and he presents with significant myoclonic jerks. On physical examination, the DTRs are diminished, but the Romberg's sign is absent. What is this illness mode of inheritance for this illness?

- **A.** Autosomal dominant
- **B.** Multifactorial
- **C.** Spontaneous
- **D.** Autosomal recessive
- **E.** X-linked recessive

128. A 24-year-old white woman with no previous history of psychiatric or neurological illness arrives at a neurology clinic with a 3-month history of fluctuating facial muscle weakness, which gets progressively worse with exertion. She reports that by evening her eyelids are drooping and she has blurred vision. Her family has also noticed the eyelid droop. She has no other complaints and her physical examination is normal. Her mother corroborates her recollection of accounts and states that her daughter has always been a healthy person. All the necessary investigations confirm the diagnosis of myasthenia gravis. When meeting with the patient and her mother to discuss the treatment plan, the neurologist can make which one of the following statements?

- **A.** Approximately 90% of patients initially presenting with purely ocular symptoms eventually develop a more generalized form of the disease.
- **B.** Most patients evolve to their weakest within the first year of the onset of symptoms.
- **C.** Patients usually do not develop severe generalized weakness with respiratory failure or inability to swallow.
- **D.** Severe respiratory and bulbar weakness only develops after the development of ocular or extremity weakness.
- **E.** Patients with mild weakness do not require therapy with immunosuppressive or immunomodulating agents.

129. Which one of the following is NOT a classic feature of pellagra?

- **A.** Death
- **B.** Dermatitis
- **C.** Dactylitis
- **D.** Dementia
- **E.** Diarrhea

130. A 24-year-old man is newly diagnosed with primary generalized epilepsy and started on lamotrigine. Ten days after beginning treatment, he calls your office complaining of a maculopapular rash on his trunk. You advise him to stop taking the lamotrigine and make an appointment to see him immediately. After assuring yourself that the rash does not require emergent treatment, you and the patient agree that the medication should be switched and prescribe which of the following treatments as an antiepileptic?

- **A.** Gabapentin
- **B.** Valproic acid
- **C.** Phenytoin
- **D.** Carbamazepine
- **E.** Phenobarbital

131. Which one of the following statements is NOT TRUE about elder abuse?

- **A.** It occurs in about 25% of elderly Americans.
- **B.** The victims are usually very old and frail.
- **C.** The abusers are often financially dependant on the victim.
- **D.** The abuser often lives with the victim.
- **E.** The abusers and the victims often deny or minimize the abuse.

132. Which of the following responses is NOT TRUE about the interaction between structural brain lesions and immune response?

- **A.** Lesions of the anterior hypothalamus result in a decrease in thymic and splenic cell number, splenic mitogen responsiveness, antigen responsiveness, and the number of natural killer cell activation (NKCA).
- **B.** Bilateral lesions of the hippocampus and the amygdala are associated with an increase in the thymic and splenic mitogen responsiveness, but with no change in thymic or splenic cell number.
- **C.** Left-sided neocortical lesions have been associated with a decrease in the number of splenic T-cells, T-cell mitogen proliferation, T-cell cytotoxicity, and NKCA.
- **D.** Right-sided neocortical lesions have been associated with either no change or an increase in the number of splenic T-cells, T-cell mitogen proliferation, T-cell cytotoxicity, and NKCA.
- **E.** Right-sided and left-sided neocortical lesions decrease the B-cell and macrophage-mediated immune response.

133. Which one of the following statements regarding no-harm suicide contracts is NOT TRUE?

- **A.** They have legal validity.
- **B.** They should never replace a risk assessment.
- **C.** They are designed to encourage patients to ask for help.
- **D.** They have no clinical utility.
- **E.** Some patients refuse to sign them to stay longer in the hospital.

134. Which one of the following is not a rating scale for a mood disorder?

- **A.** Hamilton Depression Scale (HAM-D)
- **B.** Young's Mania Rating Scale (YMRS)
- **C.** Beck Depression Inventory (BDI)
- **D.** Simpson-Angus Rating Scale (SARS)
- **E.** Montgomery-Asberg Depression Rating Scale (MADRS)

135. Which of the following conditions is not classified as a dyssomnia in the DSM-IV-TR?

- **A.** Nightmare Disorder
- **B.** Narcolepsy
- **C.** Circadian Rhythm Sleep Disorder
- **D.** Primary Insomnia
- **E.** Primary Hypersomnia

136. Which one of the following is NOT a risk factor for the development of a delusional disorder?

- **A.** Young age
- **B.** Sensory impairment
- **C.** Family history
- **D.** Recent immigration
- **E.** Social isolation

137. Which one of the following choices is NOT TRUE of paraphilias?

- **A.** It was initially labeled as "perversions" by Sigmund Freud.
- **B.** It is characterized by an impairment of sexual response.
- **C.** It is characterized by a significant deviation in the erotic stimulus or activity.
- **D.** It is more common in men.
- **E.** It is characterized by intensely arousing fantasies, sexual urges, or behaviors that involve nonhuman objects.

138. According to the DSM-IV-TR, the research criteria for binge-eating disorder includes all of the following EXCEPT:

- **A.** Recurrent episodes of binge eating
- **B.** Marked distress regarding binge eating
- **C.** Binge eating occurring, on average, at least 2 days per week for 6 months
- **D.** Binge eating associated with compensatory behaviors (e.g., purging, fasting)
- **E.** Binge eating not occurring exclusively during the course of anorexia nervosa

139. A 76-year-old woman on the oncology service who has a history of metastatic breast cancer is evaluated for an acute change in mental status by the psychiatry consultation service. She is found to be delirious. Her vital signs are within normal limits. She has no history of recent fevers. She has been maintained on a fentanyl patch for the last 6 months for pain. Her most recent labs show white blood cells (WBC) 8.0, Hct 37, Plts 250, Na 136, K 4.0, Bun 15, Cre 1.0, Ca 10.1, and albumin 4.0. Her urinalysis is unremarkable. Her head CT and chest radiograph are within normal limits. Last night she had difficulty sleeping and received 50 mg of amitriptyline. What is the most likely cause of her delirium?

- **A.** Alcohol withdrawal
- **B.** Brain metastases
- **C.** Amitriptyline
- **D.** Fentanyl patch
- **E.** Occult infection

140. A 30-year-old man with a history of schizophrenia and medication noncompliance was readmitted to the hospital after threatening to kill his neighbors because he believed they were poisoning his water. Due to his history of medication noncompliance, a trial of fluphenazine decanoate was considered. He tolerated several doses of oral fluphenazine, but then began to complain of tongue "thickness" and difficulty swallowing. Several hours later he was found to have severe muscular rigidity and cramping in the musculature of his neck and back with opisthotonos. Benztropine 2 mg IM was administered. Twenty minutes later there was no improvement and he continued to have severe dystonic reaction. Which of the following medications should be given next to treat his symptoms?

A. Propranolol
B. Dantrolene
C. Baclofen
D. Lorazepam
E. Repeat dose of benztropine

141. According to data from the National Institute of Mental Health (NIMH) Clinical Antipsychotic Trials of Intervention Effectiveness Study (CATIE), which one of the following antipsychotic medications were patients least likely to discontinue due to lack of efficacy?

A. Olanzapine
B. Quetiapine
C. Ziprasidone
D. Risperidone
E. Perphenazine

142. A 44-year-old man finds that he is preoccupied with playing video lottery terminals (VLT). He has tried to cut back on his daily trips to the casino, but finds that he is unable to do so. He recently became very angry with his wife when she confronted him about this behavior and threatened that he would leave her if she mentioned it again. He has called in "sick" to his place of employment on several occasions and recently borrowed money from his brother in order to pay several debts. Which of the following behavioral principle offers the best explanation for the maintenance of his gambling behavior?

A. Classical conditioning
B. Negative reinforcement
C. Continuous reinforcement
D. Partial reinforcement
E. Punishment

143. A 45-year-old man is started on monotherapy of a drug, a few days following which he develops copious salivation, causing pooling of saliva in the oral cavity, and drooling. He has noticed that he often wakes up with a wet pillow, causing him tremendous social embarrassment. Which of the following drugs is he most likely to be taking?

A. Quetiapine

B. Risperidone
C. Olanzapine
D. Clozapine
E. Venlafaxine

144. Anosognosia may result from a lesion affecting which one of the following areas of the brain?

A. Dominant parietal lobe
B. Nondominant parietal lobe
C. Occipital lobe
D. Dominant temporal lobe
E. Nondominant temporal lobe

145. Neurotransmitter systems consist of densely packed neurons that provide diffuse projections to areas of the brain in order to modulate function. Which of the following groups of neurons is not correctly paired with the appropriate anatomical location?

A. Dopaminergic neurons/substantia nigra
B. Cholinergic neurons/basal forebrain
C. Serotonergic neurons/raphe nuclei
D. Noradrenergic neurons/locus coeruleus
E. Cholinergic neurons/ventral tegmental area

146. Which one of the following is NOT TRUE of PET scans?

A. PET scans recognize the site of positron annihilation.
B. PET scans require exposing the patient to radiation.
C. PET scans always require an intravenous access to introduce the radionucleotide.
D. PET scans are technically complex to perform and have a high financial cost.
E. PET scans are useful noninvasive measurements of the living human brain.

147. Which of the following is a common characteristic of sensory ataxia?

A. Patients frequently present with dysarthria.
B. Patients are unable to stand with feet together and eyes closed.
C. Patients usually present with nystagmus.
D. Patients have normal proprioception.
E. Ankle reflexes are usually normal.

148. A 61-year-old man presents with a transient ischemic attack (TIA). His symptoms resolve completely in 15 minutes. He sees you the next day, and you tell him that he is at risk of having another cerebrovascular event in the future. Which of the following statements about the pharmacological treatment of his condition is NOT TRUE?

A. A statin medication should be prescribed, even if lipid levels are normal.

B. The addition of dipyridamole, clopidogrel, or ticlopidine to aspirin will greatly reduce the risk of stroke when compared to either alone.

C. Aspirin monotherapy reduces by 13%, at most, the progression or recurrence of stroke.

D. Warfarin treatment is preventative if there is a clear embolic source.

E. Antihypertensive agent should be prescribed only if blood pressure is elevated.

149. Which of the following might be seen in the brain of a healthy 80-year-old person without dementia?

A. No neuropathological changes
B. Neuritic plaques
C. Neurofibrillary tangles
D. Cortical atrophy
E. All of the above

150. Which one of the following statements is TRUE regarding chronic stress, major depression, and immunity?

A. There is an increase in the number of monocytes in chronic stress and major depression.
B. There is a reduction in the CD4 to CD8 ratio in chronic stress and major depression.
C. There is no change in the percentage of natural killer cells in chronic stress and major depression.
D. There is no change in the B lymphocyte count in chronic stress and major depression.
E. There is no change in the T lymphocyte count in chronic stress and major depression.

151. Which one of the following neuropsychological tests is considered the gold standard for intellectual assessment?

A. Wechsler Adult Intelligence Scale
B. Shipley Scale
C. California Verbal Learning Test
D. Delis-Kaplan Executive Function System
E. Fuld's Object Memory Test

152. Which of the following substances does not have an associated withdrawal syndrome defined in the DSM-IV-TR?

A. Heroin
B. Nicotine
C. Caffeine
D. Cocaine
E. Alcohol

153. Which one of the following stages is not described as a part of the normal adult sexual response cycle?

A. Latency
B. Desire
C. Excitation

D. Plateau
E. Resolution

154. Which one of the following statements regarding the diagnosis of factitious disorders using DSM-IV-TR criteria is TRUE?

A. There is intentional production or feigning of physical or psychological signs or symptoms.
B. The motivation for the behavior is to assume the sick role.
C. External incentives for the behavior are absent.
D. There are three predominant types based on the type of symptom presentation.
E. All of the above.

155. Potential medical complications of eating disorders include all EXCEPT which of the following?

A. Arrhythmias
B. Fertility problems
C. Heat intolerance
D. Peripheral neuropathies
E. Dental caries

156. Fluoxetine is Food and Drug Administration (FDA) approved for the treatment of all of the following conditions EXCEPT:

A. Major depressive disorder
B. Bulimia nervosa
C. Panic disorder
D. Premenstrual dysphoric disorder
E. Generalized anxiety disorder

157. You are asked by a colleague to consult on one of his patients who he sees in his outpatient clinic. The patient has a long history of schizoaffective disorder (bipolar type with a tumultuous course of illness mainly due to mood instability). The outpatient psychiatrist has trialed several mood stabilizer medications with adequate dosages and duration with poor results. However, throughout his illness, his psychotic symptoms have been well controlled with haloperidol 10 mg daily. Recently the patient's mood has stabilized, but he is now complaining of worsening auditory hallucinations. The addition of which one of the following medications to his medication regimen is the most likely cause of his symptoms?

A. Warfarin
B. Carbamazepine
C. Atorvastatin
D. Hydrochlorothiazide
E. Valproate

158. According to data from the NIMH Clinical Antipsychotic Trials of Intervention Effectiveness Study (CATIE), which one of the following antipsychotic medications were patients most likely to discontinue due to weight gain and metabolic derangements?

A. Olanzapine
B. Quetiapine
C. Ziprasidone
D. Risperidone
E. Perphenazine

159. A 42-year-old man returns to your clinic today for a follow-up appointment and medication management. He has a long history of bipolar disorder and his mood his been euthymic on lithium 1,500 mg daily. At today's visit his blood pressure is 155/95. On review of his last three visits, his blood pressures have ranged between 150 and 160/90 and 95. Knowing your patient is unlikely to follow-up with his primary care physician for antihypertensive treatment, you decide to start him on an antihypertensive medication. Which of the following medications would likely result in lithium toxicity and thus should be avoided in treating your patient's blood pressure?

A. Verapamil
B. Hydrochlorothiazide
C. Amlodipine
D. Metoprolol
E. Losartan

160. Which of the following is NOT associated with an increased intensity of benzodiazepine withdrawal symptoms?

A. Abrupt discontinuation of benzodiazepines
B. Use of short half-life benzodiazepines
C. Prolonged treatment with benzodiazepines
D. Higher doses of benzodiazepines
E. Gradual taper of benzodiazepines

161. A 60-year-old man presents with incoordination, an intention tremor, and a wide-based gait. In addition, which one of the following symptoms would you expect to see along with the previously described symptoms?

A. Paresis
B. Hyperreflexia
C. Dysdiadochokinesia
D. Homonymous hemianopsia
E. Aphasia

162. A 24-year-old female medical student is experiencing debilitating migraines, which often occur several times per month. She is concerned that she will be unable to cope with the upcoming demands of her training as a senior medical student and as a resident. Other than pharmacological treatment, which of the following techniques have been shown to be useful in the treatment of migraine headaches?

A. Biofeedback
B. Eye movement desensitization and reprocessing
C. Systematic desensitization
D. Implosion
E. Aversion therapy

163. You evaluate a 35-year-old patient in your neurology clinic for "odd movements." After a careful history, physical examination, and blood tests, you make a diagnosis of early Huntington's disorder. From the family history, you learn that the patient's parent died when she was a baby, and she has two younger sisters. The patient asks you not to discuss the patient's diagnosis with her siblings, but offers no reason for this decision. What is the ethically correct way to proceed?

A. You comply with the patient's request without any further discussion.
B. You ask the patient's husband for permission to contact the relatives.
C. You decide that the risk outweighs confidentiality and decide to contact the siblings.
D. You educate the patient about Huntington's disease, including genetic testing.
E. You call for an ethics conference at your hospital to discuss the case.

164. All of the following changes in the cardiovascular system occur with age EXCEPT:

A. Blood vessels thicken and become less distensible.
B. Sympathetic nervous activity decreases.
C. Maximum heart rate decreases.
D. Systolic blood pressure increases.
E. Cardiac output declines.

165. Dysfunction of which one of the protein receptors has been implicated in the development of attention deficit and hyperactivity syndrome?

A. Dopamine
B. Serotonin
C. Thyroid hormone
D. Gamma-aminobutyric acid
E. Norepinephrine

166. The Wisconsin Card Sorting Test is a useful assessment tool primarily for which one of the following functions?

A. Language
B. Retrieval and storage of information
C. Attention and immediate recall of information
D. Visuospatial skills
E. Volition, motivation, planning, and execution

167. An 18-year-old man is brought to the ED by the police after assaulting a passerby. The patient is slurring his speech and appears unsteady. On physical examination, he is found to have nystagmus, generalized muscle weakness, and depressed reflexes. He sluggishly complains that he is seeing double. Which class of substances is most likely to have caused his intoxication syndrome?

A. Inhalants
B. Benzodiazepines
C. Opioids
D. Hallucinogens
E. Amphetamines

168. Which one of the following statements is NOT TRUE about gender identity?

A. Biological factors play an important role in the development of gender identity.
B. Gender identity is an individual's perception and awareness of being male or female.
C. It is usually established by 3 years of age.
D. It depends on the sex in which an individual is reared.
E. Once established, it is very resistant to change.

169. Which one of the following facts regarding Munchausen syndrome is INCORRECT?

A. The term was coined by Richard Asher.
B. It is also called chronic factitious disorder with predominantly physical signs and symptoms.
C. The terms *hospital hoboes, hospital addicts,* and *professional patients* have been used to describe it.
D. Its presentation is characterized by pseudologic fantastica and peregrination.
E. It constitutes approximately 25% of all factitious disorder cases.

170. A 20-year-old woman is brought to the ED by police. In the process of being arrested for shoplifting junk food at a local grocery store, the woman had become agitated and told police that she was going to kill herself. On a full psychiatric evaluation, you learn that the patient has been binge eating almost daily for the past 6 months. She tells you that by abusing laxatives and diuretics, her weight has remained stable. In the ED, her weight is found to be 135 lb. and her height is measured at 5'5''. What is her approximate body mass index (BMI) and weight status?

A. BMI = 18, underweight
B. BMI = 22.5, healthy weight
C. BMI = 27, overweight
D. BMI = 29.5, overweight
E. BMI = 32, obese

171. Which one of the following drugs has the shortest half-life (t 1/2)?

A. Olanzapine
B. Risperidone
C. Quetiapine
D. Ziprasidone
E. Aripiprazole

172. A 54-year-old homeless man with a history of schizophrenia was admitted to the hospital with shortness of breath, fever, and productive cough. He was found to have a right lower lobe consolidation on a chest x-ray and sputum positive for acid fast bacilli. A culture confirmed a diagnosis of tuberculosis and drug sensitivities indicated a drug-resistant form of tuberculosis requiring ciprofloxacin as part of his antibiotic regimen. Antipsychotic medications that should be avoided while he is on this antibiotic regimen include which one of the following?

A. Thioridazine
B. Mesoridazine
C. Pimozide
D. All the above
E. None of the above

173. A 22-year-old man is brought to the ER by his friends from a local club in a comatose state. On examination, he is found to be bradycardic (pulse rate of 45 beats/minute) and is unresponsive to painful stimuli. His friends claim that he lost consciousness about 45 minutes after the oral ingestion of a club drug. He is also hypoventilating (respiratory rate of 6 breathes/minute) and having jerky movements of his arms and legs. Within a few minutes of arrival at the ER, he stops breathing. Which one of the following choices indicates the correct treatment plan for this patient's condition?

A. Establishing an airway, intravenous access, atropine, oxygen supplementation
B. Establishing an airway, intravenous access, atropine, oxygen supplementation, flumazenil
C. Establishing an airway, intravenous access, atropine, oxygen supplementation, naloxone
D. Establishing an airway, intravenous access, atropine, oxygen supplementation, activated charcoal
E. Establishing an airway, intravenous access, atropine, oxygen supplementation, physostigmine

174. A 25-year-old woman was admitted to the hospital after 1 week of decreased need for sleep, flight of ideas, increased irritability, and starting fights at work resulting in the loss of her job. She is diagnosed with bipolar disorder and started on lithium. During the course of 2 weeks, her mood stabilized; however, she is now complaining of increased frequency in urination, which is disruptive to her daily activities and interfering with her new job as a taxi cab driver. Urinalysis, electrolytes, blood urea nitrogen, and creatinine are all within normal limits. You determine that she is likely experiencing polyuria, a common side effect associated with lithium. You adjust her lithium to the minimally effective dose and change her dosing to once a day at bedtime, but she continues to complain of increased frequency of urination. Which of the following can be helpful in the treatment of this burdensome side effect?

A. Amiloride
B. Oxybutynin
C. Benztropine
D. Bladder training
E. Kegel exercises

175. Which of the following benzodiazepines is preferred for use in the elderly?

A. Lorazepam
B. Clonazepam
C. Diazepam
D. Alprazolam
E. Flurazepam

176. Which one of the following findings may be demonstrated in the CSF of a patient with MS?

A. Increased glucose
B. Decreased glucose
C. Decreased protein
D. Oligoclonal bands
E. Decrease WBCs

177. A 43-year-old married woman has been on leave from her job as a nursing assistant for the past 7 months after sustaining a lower back injury at work. She has been treated with several different medications, the majority of which she did not tolerate and which were largely ineffective in managing her pain. The patient is very concerned about issues of medication dependence and would like to pursue nonpharmacological management options. Recommended behavioral and cognitive therapies for the management of chronic pain include all of the following EXCEPT:

A. Relaxation
B. Imagery
C. Hypnosis
D. Meditation
E. Aversion

178. A couple brings their 5-year-old child into your pediatric neurology clinic for an assessment of developmental delay. On examination, you note that the pa-

tient has macrocephaly, a prominent forehead, large prominent ears, and a long, narrow face, and learn that the child has tested in the moderately mentally retarded range. You make a probable diagnosis of Fragile X syndrome, and educate the parents about the genetic inheritance pattern of the disease. Which of the following statements about the Fragile X inheritance pattern is true?

A. The patient's unaffected brother's children are at risk of being carriers of Fragile X premutation.
B. The patient's sons will be at risk of having Fragile X disorder.
C. All of the couple's sons will have Fragile X syndrome.
D. For unaffected parents, the risk of passing on a full mutation is greater for a father to a daughter than for a mother to a son.
E. The patient's daughters are not at risk of being a carrier of Fragile X disorder.

179. According to the Epidemiological Catchment Area (ECA) Study, what is the estimated lifetime prevalence of alcohol use disorders in the United States?

A. 7%
B. 13.5%
C. 22.5%
D. 33%
E. 46%

180. Which one of the following is the most common type of sexual dysfunction in women?

A. Sexual arousal disorders
B. Hypoactive sexual desire disorder
C. Orgasmic disorders
D. Sexual pain disorders
E. None of the above

181. A 27-year-old man, with an unstable self-image, is impulsive and reckless. He has never had a close relationship lasting more than a few weeks at any time. He often makes suicidal threats. He gets very angry easily and has earned the reputation of being manipulative. Which of the following defense mechanisms are most likely to be observed in this person?

A. Projective identification, primitive idealization, splitting, turning against the self
B. Projection, isolation, splitting, turning against the self, acting out
C. Dissociation, projective identification, fantasy, acting out
D. Splitting, acting out, rationalization, turning against the self
E. Projective identification, primitive idealization, rationalization, acting out

182. Which of the following is the most common comorbid disorder found in patients with anorexia nervosa?
    A. Major depressive disorder
    B. Social phobia
    C. Bipolar disorder
    D. OCD
    E. Alcohol abuse

183. Selegiline Transdermal System (STS) was recently approved for the treatment of a major depressive disorder by the FDA. It comes in three strengths: a 6 mg/24-hour patch, a 9 mg/24-hour patch, and a 12 mg/24-hour patch. Which of the following statements regarding dietary modifications with monoamine oxidase inhibitors (MAOIs) is true for STS?
    A. Dietary modifications are not necessary with the 6 mg/24-hour patch, but are required for the 9 mg/24-hour and the 12 mg/24-hour patches.
    B. Dietary modifications are not necessary with the 6 mg/24-hour and the 9 mg/24-hour patches, but are required for the 12 mg/24-hour patch.
    C. Dietary modifications are not necessary with the 6 mg/24-hour, the 9 mg/24-hour, or the 12 mg/24-hour patches.
    D. Dietary modifications are necessary for all of the patches.
    E. This is a trick question! Selegiline is not an MAOI.

184. What is the mechanism of action of the illicit drug that can be synthesized using potassium cyanide?
    A. Release of monoamines from storage sites in axon terminals
    B. Inhibition of reuptake of monoamines
    C. NMDA blockade
    D. Increasing the flow of chloride ions by binding to the GABA receptor complex
    E. Phosphodiesterase inhibition

185. Which of the following drugs DOES NOT exacerbate acute intermittent porphyria?
    A. Meprobamate
    B. Chloral hydrate
    C. Ethchlorvynol
    D. Phenobarbital
    E. Chlorpromazine

186. An elderly gentleman is evaluated in the ED after being found at his home confused, slurring his speech, and having difficulty walking. He has a history of bipolar disorder and is taking lithium among other medications. On physical examination, he is found to be hypotensive, bradycardic, and ataxic. A course tremor is also noted. His serum lithium level is 3.5. He is admitted to the hospital and dialysis is started immediately. His family is concerned regarding his prognosis and specifically want to know what effects may be permanent as a result of lithium toxicity. Potential long-term adverse effects from lithium toxicity include which of the following?
    A. Cerebellar ataxia
    B. Tremor
    C. Peripheral neuropathy
    D. Downbeat nystagmus
    E. Benign intracranial hypertension (pseudotumor cerebri)

187. Which of the following statements regarding the use of SSRIs for the treatment of OCD is TRUE?
    A. The starting dose for OCD is less than the starting dose for depression.
    B. Target symptoms worsen before they improve once treatment with an SSRI is started.
    C. The maintenance dose for OCD may be higher than the maintenance dose for depression.
    D. The onset of response is quicker in OCD than in depression.
    E. If a patient fails to respond to one SSRI, they will likely fail to respond to all of the SSRIs.

188. Which of the following vitamins in excess can lead to a peripheral neuropathy?
    A. Cyanocobalamin (vitamin B_{12})
    B. Thiamine (vitamin B_1)
    C. Niacin (vitamin B_3)
    D. Pyridoxine (vitamin B_6)
    E. Tocopherol (vitamin E)

189. Which one of the following statements about the brain of patients with Alzheimer's disease (AD) is NOT TRUE?
    A. Compared to age matched controls, the brain of a patient with Alzheimer's disease is more atrophic.
    B. The areas of the cortex governing motor, sensory, and visual functioning are preferentially affected.
    C. Consequent to the atrophy, the lateral and third ventricles are dilated.
    D. Plaques and tangles are the most conspicuous histological feature in the brain of these patients.
    E. Of all histological features, loss of neuronal synapses correlates most closely with dementia.

190. A 33-year-old woman presents with double vision and profound weakness. On physical examination, you see ptosis in her right eye and that she has

difficulty smiling. You administer edrophonium and her strength, ptosis, and difficulty smiling briefly resolve. What is the mechanism of action of edrophonium?

A. It inhibits the metabolism of dopamine.
B. It inhibits the reuptake of norepinephrine.
C. It inhibits the metabolism of acetylcholine.
D. It enhances the release of acetylcholine.
E. It enhances the release of norepinephrine.

191. As a practicing psychiatrist, you diagnose a patient with polysubstance dependence and decide to proceed with motivational interviewing. Motivational interviewing incorporates ALL of the following principles EXCEPT?

A. Expressing empathy
B. Giving advice
C. Developing discrepancy
D. Rolling with resistance
E. Supporting self-efficacy

192. Which is the most common type of male sexual dysfunction?

A. Hypoactive sexual desire disorder
B. Erectile disorders
C. Premature ejaculation
D. Sexual pain disorders
E. None of the above

193. Belief in clairvoyance and telepathy fall in the list of diagnostic features for which of the following personality disorders?

A. Histrionic Personality Disorder
B. Schizoid Personality Disorder
C. Schizotypal Personality Disorder
D. Narcissistic Personality Disorder
E. Paranoid Personality Disorder

194. What is the gold standard for confirmation of Munchausen's syndrome by proxy?

A. Covert video surveillance after consultation with a legal counsel
B. Reviewing collateral information
C. Structured Clinical Interview for DSM Disorders (SCID)
D. Munchausen's syndrome rating scale
E. Separation from primary caregiver

195. All of the following statements are true regarding neurofibromatosis type I (NF-1) EXCEPT:

A. Neurofibromas are subcutaneous growths along peripheral nerves.
B. Lisch nodules are yellow to brown nodules on the iris.

C. NF-1 is inherited in an autosomal dominant pattern.
D. A café au lait spot is pathognomonic of neurofibromatosis.
E. Neurofibromas can compress the spinal cord.

196. Which one of the following statements regarding the cyclic adenosine monophosphate (cAMP) system is NOT TRUE?

A. Generation of cAMP is controlled by the balance between the activity of adenylyl cyclase and phosphodiesterase.
B. The activity of adenylyl cyclase is regulated by G proteins.
C. There are two classes of G proteins called G_s and G_i, depending on whether they stimulate or inhibit cAMP formation.
D. cAMP-dependent protein kinase is also referred to as *protein kinase A* (PKA).
E. Suppression of the cAMP system enables the regulation of gene expression.

197. A 19-year-old woman with a history of epilepsy presents to her primary medical doctor because several of her family members have been diagnosed with tuberculosis. The patient has a positive purified protein derivative (PPD) test result, but no active signs of infection. Her doctor plans to start her on isoniazid (INH) and calls her neurologist who has been prescribing phenytoin to control her seizures to tell her that he is starting this new medication. Which one of the following is the most appropriate approach given the addition of isoniazid to this patient's medication regimen?

A. Decrease the dose of phenytoin
B. Increase the dose of phenytoin
C. Increase the dose of phenytoin and augment with cimetidine
D. Maintain the current dose of phenytoin
E. Increase the dose and augment with carbamazepine

198. A 50-year-old man with a history of panic disorder and seizure disorder has been well-managed on phenytoin for many years. During a period of increased stress at work and trouble in his marriage, he develops symptoms including feelings of worthlessness, fatigue, anhedonia, decreased appetite, and insomnia. He consults with a physician who places him on fluoxetine. Three weeks later, the man is brought to an ER by concerned coworkers. He appears sedated and confused, has an ataxic gait and slurred speech, and complains of diplopia. On his history, he denies any alcohol or illicit drug use. On examination, he is noted to have tremor and nystagmus. Which of the following is the most likely explanation?

A. The patient has most likely been drinking, and his symptoms represent acute alcohol intoxication.

B. The patient is experiencing symptoms of fluoxetine toxicity precipitated by drug-drug interaction with phenytoin.

C. The patient is experiencing symptoms of phenytoin toxicity precipitated by drug-drug interaction with fluoxetine.

D. The patient is experiencing seizure activity related to decreased phenytoin levels precipitated by drug-drug interaction with fluoxetine.

E. The patient is experiencing a panic attack precipitated by his recent increased stressors.

199. Use of valproate during pregnancy is associated with significantly increased risk of which one of the following fetal malformations?

A. Neural tube defects
B. Limb phocomelia and amelia
C. Ebstein's anomaly
D. Staining of the teeth
E. Uterine abnormalities

200. LP is a useful procedure for diagnosis of which one of the following conditions?

A. Huntington's disease
B. Meningitis
C. MS
D. Alzheimer's disease
E. Intracranial mass

Answers

1. Answer: C. This child is approximately 24 months old. At his age, he should be able to run without falling and go up and down the stairs. His separation anxiety is starting to diminish, and he should be able to build a tower with six or seven cubes. An 18-month-old child can walk without falling frequently, but is unable to run freely and can only build a tower of three or four cubes. A 36 month old can ride a tricycle, build a tower of nine or ten cubes, and is able to copy a circle or cross. A 15 month old can usually walk without support.

Kaplan HI, Sadock BJ. *Kaplan & Sadock's Synopsis of Psychiatry*. 8th ed. Philadelphia: Lippincott Williams & Wilkins; 1998:29.

2. Answer: D. Cells transmit electrical signals either via an electrical synapse or chemical synapse. With cells that communicate via electrical synapses, there is minimal delay at the synapse because they communicate via the direct flow of current. These cells are typically joined by less than 3 nm gap junctions and are bidirectional. On the other hand, with cells that communicate via chemical synapses, the presynaptic cell releases a transmitter at the terminal bouton, which alters the postsynaptic membrane potential, the release of the transmitter contributing significantly to a synaptic delay.

Berne RM, Levy MN. *Physiology*. 4th ed. St. Louis: Mosby; 1998:43, 47–48.

3. Answer: B. J. B. Skinner's theory of learning is called operant or instrumental conditioning. In this form of learning, a behavior is followed by a response. Thus, the learning occurs as a consequence of action. In this form of learning, the participant is active and behaves in a way to get a positive response. Pavlov's classical conditioning depends on the repeated pairing of a neutral conditioned stimulus with a stimulus that evokes a response (unconditioned stimulus). This pairing of a conditioned and unconditioned stimulus results in the neutral stimulus evoking a response called the conditioned response. In classical conditioning, the participant is passive and the behavioral reinforcement is not under its control.

Kaplan HI, Sadock BJ. *Kaplan & Sadock's Synopsis of Psychiatry*. 8th ed. Philadelphia: Lippincott Williams & Wilkins; 1998:148–151.

4. Answer: E. Karl Ludwig Kahlbaum's monograph, "Die Katatonie oder das Spannungsirresein," characterized catatonia as a specific disturbance in motor functioning that represents a phase in a progressive illness that includes stages of mania, depression, and psychosis and that typically ends in dementia. Carl Jung described, *collective unconscious*, *archetypes*, *complexes*, *introverts*, *extroverts*, *persona*, *animus*, *anima*, and *individuation*. Alfred Adler, the founder of individual psychology, coined the term *inferiority complex*. Erik Erickson described the *epigenetic principles*, which describe the development of an individual in sequential and clearly defined stages. Sigmund Freud is the originator of psychoanalysis and has described various theories and models of the mind including topographical and structural models.

1. Kaplan HI, Sadock BJ. *Kaplan & Sadock's Synopsis of Psychiatry*. 8th ed. Philadelphia: Lippincott Williams & Wilkins; 1998:206–239.
2. Taylor MA, Fink M. Catatonia in psychiatric classification: a home of its own. *Am J Psychiatry*. 2003; 160:1233–1241.

5. Answer: A. According to the DSM-IV-TR, NMS (333.92) should be coded on axis I of the multiaxial classification system. In the multiaxial classification system, axis I should include clinical conditions or other conditions that may be a focus of clinical attention. Conditions that fall under the category of other "conditions that may be a focus of clinical attention" include: NMS, psychological factors affecting medical conditions, medication-induced movement disorders, other medication induced movement disorders, and additional conditions that may be a focus of clinical attention, such as noncompliance with treatment. Axis II includes personality disorders/mental retardation. Axis III includes general medical conditions. Axis IV includes psychosocial and environmental problems, and axis V includes global assessment of functioning.

American Psychiatric Association. *Quick Reference to the Diagnostic Criteria from DSM-IV-TR*. Washington, DC: American Psychiatric Association; 2000:132.

6. Answer: A. Rapid cycling (four or more affective episodes a year) occurs more commonly in women with bipolar disorder. The use of an antidepressant, especially tricyclics, has been associated with the development of rapid cycling. Other consistent risk factors are hypothyroidism and the number of affective episodes during the course of illness. Patients with rapid cycling tend to have a weaker response to lithium in comparison to other patients with bipolar disorder.

1. Kupka RW, Luckenbaugh DA, Post RM, et al. Comparison of rapid-cycling and non-rapid-cycling bipolar disorder based on prospective mood ratings in 539 outpatients. *Am J Psychiatry*. 2005;162:1273–1280.
2. Sadock BJ, Sadock VA. *Kaplan and Sadock's Comprehensive Textbook of Psychiatry*. 8th ed. Philadelphia: Lippincott Williams & Wilkins; 2005:1690.

7. Answer: D. Substance abuse cannot be diagnosed if the patient has ever met the criteria for substance dependence in that class of substance. The first 1 to 12 months of remission is designated "early." Following 12 months of remission, the designation of "sustained" is given. "Full" remission indicates that no criteria for substance abuse or dependence have been met in that time period. The "partial" specifier is used if one or more of the criteria for abuse or dependence have been met, but the full criteria for dependence have not been met.

American Psychiatric Association. *Quick Reference to the Diagnostic Criteria from DSM-IV-TR*. Washington, DC: Author; 2000:105–151.

8. Answer: D. According to the DSM-IV-TR, patients with undifferentiated somatoform disorder present with one or more physical complaints lasting at least 6 months that are below the threshold for the diagnosis of somatization disorder. Two symptom patterns in undifferentiated somatoform disorder have been proposed: those involving the autonomic nervous system and those involving the experience of fatigue/weakness. The latter has also been described as "neurasthenia" and may overlap with chronic fatigue syndrome.

1. American Psychiatric Association. *Quick Reference to the Diagnostic Criteria from DSM-IV-TR*. Washington, DC: American Psychiatric Association; 2000:229–236.
2. Sadock BJ, Sadock VA. *Kaplan and Sadock's Synopsis of Psychiatry*. 9th ed. Philadelphia: Lippincott Williams and Wilkins; 2003:658–659.

9. Answer: A. The DES, which was developed by Eve Bernstein Carlson and Frank Putnam in the mid-1980s, has 28 items and the overall score can range from 0 to 100. The PDEQ, which was developed by Charles R. Marmar et al., assesses dissociative experiences at the time of the traumatic event, and the most widely used version is the PDEQ ten-item self-report version (PDEQ-10-SRV). The CDC is a parent–caretaker–teacher 20-item report measure using a

three-point scale, used for children from 5 to 12 years of age, with scores ranging from 0 to 40. The A-DES is an adolescent-oriented version of the DES with 30 items on a 0 to 10 answer format, which also includes questions regarding depersonalization and derealization in its questionnaire.

Sadock BJ, Sadock VA. *Kaplan and Sadock's Comprehensive Textbook of Psychiatry*. 8th ed. Philadelphia: Lippincott Williams & Wilkins; 2005:1850–1851.

10. Answer: D. The SSRI with the longest half-life (t 1/2) is fluoxetine; it has a t 1/2 of approximately 2 to 5 days. Its metabolite norfluoxetine has a t 1/2 of 7 to 10 days. Citalopram has a t 1/2 of 35 hours, and escitalopram has a t /12 of 30 hours. Sertraline has a t 1/2 of 24 hours and its metabolite, desmethylsertraline, has a t 1/2 of 2 to 4 days. Paroxetine and fluvoxamine have the shortest t 1/2 among the SSRIs; their t 1/2 is approximately 15 to 20 hours (THINK WITHDRAWAL!).

Albers LJ, Hahn RK, Reist C. *Handbook of Psychiatric Drugs*. Laguna Hills: Current Clinical Strategies Publishing; 2005:6–15.

11. Answer: C. Approximately 30% to 45% of patients diagnosed with depression do not have an adequate response to a first trial of an antidepressant. Patient-related and treatment-related risk factors that have been identified and increase the chances of nonresponse to antidepressant treatment include: disease severity, coexisting medical or psychiatric disorders, such as alcohol abuse or anxiety, and a possible familial predisposition to a poor response to antidepressants in which serotonin transporter gene polymorphisms may play a role.

Keller MB. Issues in treatment-resistant depression. *J Clin Psychiatry*. 2005;66(suppl 8):5–12.

12. Answer: D. Benzodiazepines are contraindicated in inhalant intoxication because they potentiate the effects of inhalants. They can be used in all the other conditions.

Sadock BJ, Sadock VA. *Kaplan and Sadock's Comprehensive Textbook of Psychiatry*. 8th ed. Philadelphia: Lippincott Williams & Wilkins; 2005:1254.

13. Answer: D. The patient is experiencing an opisthotonic reaction to haloperidol (Haldol), which is an acute dystonic reaction. Of these, benztropine (Cogentin) is the most appropriate treatment for acute dystonia. (Another good choice is diphenhydramine.) Although a treatment for akathisia, propanolol would not be a good choice for an acute dystonic reaction. Although a change in medications after an acute dystonic medication is not necessarily warranted as long as the dystonic reaction is treated and the patient remains on the antiparkinsonian medication, the experience is often disturbing enough for patients to request a medication change. Depending on the clinical circumstances, quetiapine, olanzapine, or risperidone may ultimately be an appropriate alternative medication for this patient; however, the first thing to do would be to relieve the acute dystonic reaction by giving, for example, benztropine.

Schatzberg A. *Manual of Clinical Psychopharmacology*. 4th ed. Arlington: American Psychiatric Publishing; 2003:213–215.

14. Answer: C. A β-adrenergic blocker, such as propranolol, can help reduce tremors in patients taking lithium. It can be taken a half hour prior to an activity where tremors can interfere with functioning or taken daily to constantly suppress tremors. Before treating tremors, it is important to complete a neurological exam to rule out other possible etiologies for tremors as well as to check the lithium level, because tremors can be a sign of lithium toxicity. Antidepressants and diuretics can increase lithium levels, which would likely worsen the tremors. Alprazolam and benztropine would not help decrease tremors and alprazolam is likely to impair coordination.

Rosenbaum JF, Arana GW, Hyman SE, et al. *Handbook of Psychiatric Drug Therapy*. 5th ed. Philadelphia: Lippincott Williams and Wilkins; 2005:142.

15. Answer: B. Highest rates of completed suicides are seen in white men over the age of 75 years. Although they only constitute 10% of the total population, they account for 25% of suicides. The rates in those older than 75 years is >3 times the rate among younger people. Presence of multiple medical problems, loneliness, hopelessness, psychiatric disorders, substance abuse, and a prior history of suicide attempts are all major risk factors for suicide.

1. Kaplan HI, Sadock BJ. *Kaplan & Sadock's Synopsis of Psychiatry*. 8th ed. Philadelphia: Lippincott Williams & Wilkins; 1998:864–872.
2. O' Connell H, Chin AV, Cunningham C, et al. Recent developments: suicide in older people. *BMJ*. 2004;329:895–899.

16. Answer: E. Adult neurogenesis is an ongoing process in the subventricular zone, resulting in granule cells in the olfactory bulb, and in the subgranular zone, resulting in granule cells in the adult hippocampus. Stress results in suppression of neurogenesis, possibly through sustained elevations of cortisol in brains with dysfunctional regulation of the Hypothalamo-pituitary-adrenal axis (HPA) axis. Antidepressant treatments increase neurogenesis. An-

tidepressants increase expression of BDNF, which itself, increases neurogenesis.

1. Duman RS. Depression: a case of neuronal life and death? *Biol Psychiatry*. 2004;56:140–145.
2. Scharfman H, Goodman J, Macleod A, et al. Increased neurogenesis and the ectopic granule cells after intrahippocampal BDNF infusion in adult rats. *Exp Neurol*. 2005 Apr;192(2):348–356.
3. Russo-Neustadt AA, Beard RC, Huang YM, et al. Physical activity and antidepressant potentiate the expression of specific brain-derived neurotropic factor transcripts in the rat hippocampus. *Neuroscience*. 2000;101(2):305–312.

17. Answer: B. Sturge-Weber syndrome is typically characterized by calcification of vessels in one cerebral hemisphere. Vascular malformations of the face, not thin skin, cause a port-wine stain. Cluster headaches are not a usual feature of Sturge-Weber syndrome. Although patients with this disease can have learning disabilities and mental retardation, these are not caused by facial vascular malformations. Sclerotic lesions in the brain can lead to neurologic problems, such as hemiparesis.

Kaufman DM. *Clinical Neurology for Psychiatrists*. 5th ed. Philadelphia: WB Saunders; 2001:332.

18. Answer: D. All of the previously described diseases are excessive trinucleotide repeat (ETR) disorders. Unlike the others types of diseases in this group, Friedreich' s ataxia is inherited via autosomal recessive transmission. The early onset form (teen years) is caused by a mutation on chromosome 9q13–2. The later onset type (20 to 30 years) is also caused by a mutation on chromosome 9. In the vast majority of cases, mutation is an example of a GAA trinucleotide repeat within an intron. The mutation affects the protein frataxin by decreasing its level and function.

1. Kaufman DM. *Clinical Neurology for Psychiatrists*. 5th ed. Philadelphia: WB Saunders; 2001:24–25, 610.
2. Ropper A, Brown R. *Adams and Victor' s Principles of Neurology*. 8th ed. New York: McGraw-Hill; 2005:932–933.

19. Answer: B. The patient has had an injury to the left cerebral hemisphere. When there is damage to one frontal gaze center or its descending fiber tract, the eyes drift toward the involved cerebral hemisphere due to unopposed action of the remaining frontal gaze center (i.e., the eyes appear to look at a destructive hemispheric lesion and look away from the resulting hemiplegia). In pontine lesions where there is damage to the paramedian pontine reticular formation (PPRF) and to the descending pyramidal tract fibers that cross the midline in the medulla, eyes look away from the side of the destructive pontine lesion, but look toward the hemiplegia. Damage to the medulla involves the nuclei and the initial portion of the cranial nerves IX through XII, the descending corticospinal, and the ascending sensory and sympathetic nervous system. Lesions to the medulla result in bulbar palsy, lateral medullary infarction of Wallenberg, and locked-in syndrome.

1. Goetz C. *Textbook of Clinical Neurology*. 2nd ed. Philadelphia: WB Saunders; 2003:7–8.
2. Kaufman DM. *Clinical Neurology for Psychiatrists*. 5th ed. Philadelphia: WB Saunders; 2001:49, 304–306.

20. **Answer: B.** This patient has an ataxic gait, scanning speech, and an intention tremor, which are characteristic of cerebellar lesions. Scanning speech is also seen in bulbar and pseudobulbar palsy. Formal testing for an intention tremor includes finger-to-nose and heel-to-shin tests. Another cerebellar sign is dysdiadochokinesia, which is difficulty in performing rapid alternating movements.

Kaufman DM. *Clinical Neurology for Psychiatrists*. 5th ed. Philadelphia: WB Saunders; 2001:16–21.

21. **Answer: D.** The patient is presenting with symptoms consistent with bilateral hemianopsia, which is likely a chromophobe pituitary adenoma compressing the optic chiasm. (Prolactinomas are usually microscopic in size when diagnosed.) This is not a side effect of olanzapine. Although olanzapine can cause sedation and orthostatic hypotension, the patient denies fatigue and does not have orthostatic hypotension. At this point, there is no indication to check liver function or obtain a complete blood count. One may confirm the cause of the findings by requesting an MRI of the brain for ruling out a pituitary tumor. However, the first stage in management of this patient's complaints is to confirm the findings by a thorough neurological examination.

1. Kaufman DM. *Clinical Neurology for Psychiatrists*. 5th ed. Philadelphia: WB Saunders; 2001:518–520.
2. Schatzberg A. *Manual of Clinical Psychopharmacology*. 4th ed. Arlington: American Psychiatric Publishing; 2003:196.

22. **Answer: B.** The classical triad of tuberous sclerosis is skin lesions, seizures, and mental retardation. Depigmented macules are usually present at birth and persist through life. Three or more macules measuring 1 cm or more in length are diagnostic. Facial adenoma sebaceum are usually never present at birth, but are clinically evident by the age of 4. Yellowish-brown elevated plaques called *Shagreen patches* are usually found in the lumbosacral region after the age of 10 years. *Café au lait* spots and small fibromas may be seen after puberty. Seizures and mental retardation indicate a diffuse encephalopathy. The younger the

patient is when the seizures begin, the greater the risk of mental retardation. However, focal neurological examination is usually normal. Hamartomas of the retina or optic nerve are also observed in approximately half the number of patients.

1. Kaufman DM. *Clinical Neurology for Psychiatrists*. 5th ed. Philadelphia: WB Saunders; 2001:49, 329.
2. Rowland LP. *Merritt's Neurology*. 11th ed. Philadelphia: Lippincott Williams & Wilkins; 2005:724–731.

23. **Answer: C.** This patient is presenting with the classic Cushing's triad, which consists of rising blood pressure, bradycardia, and respiratory irregularity. It is usually seen in patients who sustain an epidural hemorrhage and are experiencing a dangerously high intracranial pressure. Epidural hemorrhages are most commonly encountered after a temporal or parietal fracture and present with headaches, vomiting, aphasia, and seizures that can progress to coma. Death is imminent unless there is a rapid surgical intervention. A chronic subdural hematoma does not have such a drastic progression and is frequently seen in elderly patients. A concussion is a mild impairment in mental status with or without loss of consciousness that does not involve intracranial bleeding. An acute subarachnoid hemorrhage presents with sudden onset of extremely severe headache, neck stiffness and fever, and is usually caused by a ruptured aneurysm. The most common sports-related head trauma is a concussion, which causes a short change in mental status with or without loss of consciousness. An acute carotid-cavernous fistula involves the laceration of the internal carotid artery and causes a pulsating exophthalmos and a painful orbit; the eye may become immobile.

1. Kaufman DM. *Clinical Neurology for Psychiatrists*. 5th ed. Philadelphia: WB Saunders; 2001:276–277, 581–595.
2. Rowland LP. *Merritt's Neurology*. 11th ed. Philadelphia: Lippincott Williams & Wilkins; 2005: 483–500.

24. **Answer: A.** Patients with cerebellar ataxia need to keep their legs far apart from each other to keep their balance. They tend to fall when their feet are together whether their eyes are open or closed. They usually feel more comfortable walking with support and tend to fall when walking in tandem. Patients with Parkinson's disease usually have a shuffling gait with small steps and loss of the normal arm swing. Patients with sensory ataxia, which results from a loss of sensory perception, are unable to know where their limbs are positioned. They are able to remain stable with their feet together and their eyes open, but they tend to lose balance when their eyes are closed (positive Romberg sign). Patients with chorea

have sudden and abrupt movements of the trunk and extremities that are unpredictable and tend to worsen while walking. The gait in muscular dystrophy is characterized by weakness of the trunk and the proximal part of the legs. Patients have lumbar lordosis, a positive Gower's sign, and a need to walk with their legs wide apart.

Rowland LP. *Merritt's Neurology*. 11th ed. Philadelphia: Lippincott Williams & Wilkins; 2005: 783–852.

25. Answer: E. Acetylcholine receptor antibodies are detected in 70% of the ocular form of the illness and in 80% to 90% of patients with generalized myasthenia gravis. Antibodies directed against the MuSK are seen in approximately one third of patients without acetylcholine receptor antibodies. Antititin (antistriatal muscle antibodies) are present in approximately 30% of the adult patients with myasthenia gravis and in 80% of patients who have thymomas. Approximately, 70% of patients with myasthenia gravis have thymic hyperplasia and 10% of those patients have thymoma. Thymomas are more common in patients older than 50 years of age and are usually malignant.

Samuels MA. *Manual of Neurologic Therapeutics*. 7th ed. Philadelphia: Lippincott Williams & Wilkins; 2004:260–265.

26. Answer: E. Analgesics like acetaminophen are useful in the treatment of other types of headaches, but not trigeminal neuralgia. Anticonvulsant medications like phenytoin, carbamazepine, lamotrigine, sodium valproate, and gabapentin are the mainstay of the treatment for this condition. Other drugs useful in the treatment include muscle relaxants like baclofen and benzodiazepines like clonazepam. Most patients can be treated effectively with medications and there may be spontaneous remission of symptoms especially early in the illness.

1. Kaufman DM. *Clinical Neurology for Psychiatrists*. 5th ed. Philadelphia: WB Saunders; 2001:214–215.
2. Samuels MA. *Manual of Neurologic Therapeutics*. 7th ed. Philadelphia: Lippincott Williams & Wilkins; 2004:351.

27. Answer: D. The ability to live independently is a major task of Erickson's stage of identity versus role diffusion, which usually occurs earlier than the stage of generativity versus stagnation. The age range for generativity is generally between 40 to 60 years. There is an increase in the risk of depression and alcohol use at this stage than in younger adults.

Sadock BJ, Kaplan H. *Synopsis of Psychiatry*. 9th ed. Philadelphia: Lippincott Williams & Wilkins; 2003:214–216.

28. Answer: B. Myelin, which is formed by Schwann cells and oligodendrocytes, increases conduction velocity down an axon. Myelination is not continuous down the axon. An action potential jumps between breaks in the myelination (nodes of Ranvier), which have a significant amount of voltage-gated sodium channels and enable the action potential to regenerate and spread to the next node. (This kind of "jumping" conduction is called salutatory conduction.) Thus, the myelin sheathing is not continuous. Assuming no difference in myelination, conduction is faster in axons of greater diameter than axons of smaller diameters, because there is less resistance to current flow than in axons with a smaller diameter.

Kandel ER, Schwartz JH, Jessel TM. *Principles of Neural Science*. 4th ed. New York: McGraw-Hill; 2000:20, 146–149.

29. Answer: B. Albert Ellis is the founder of REBT, which is a form of cognitive behavioral therapy. Paul Meehl, Starke Hathaway, and J. Charnley McKinley invented the Minnesota and Multiphasic Personality Inventory (MMPI). Sigmund Freud is the founder of psychoanalysis.

1. Ellis A. Why I (really) became a therapist. *J Clin Psychol*. 2005;61:945–948.
2. Ellis A. Remembering and honoring Paul Meehl. *J Clin Psychol*. 2005;61:1231–1232.

30. Answer: A. The most common reason for a malpractice claim is incorrect treatment (33%), followed by attempted or completed suicide (20%), and incorrect diagnosis (11%). Claims for improper supervision and medication errors are less common at 7% of the cases. Other less common causes are improper commitment (5%), breach of confidentiality (4%), unnecessary hospitalization (4%), and abandonment, electroconvulsive therapy, or third-party injury (4%).

Sadock BJ, Sadock VA. *Kaplan and Sadock's Comprehensive Textbook of Psychiatry*. 8th ed. Philadelphia: Lippincott Williams & Wilkins; 2005:3970.

31. Answer: C. According to DSM-IV-TR, malingering "is the intentional production of false or exaggerated physical or psychological symptoms, motivated by external incentives." This patient's mental status examination does not correlate with his presenting complaints and history. The incentive associated with hospital admission is avoidance of the rival gang members who wish to harm him. DSM advises to consider a diagnosis of malingering when there are medicolegal issues involved in the patient's case (a lawsuit), when there is a discrepancy between subjective disability and the objective findings, when there is a lack of cooperation with assessment and treatment, or in the presence of antisocial personality disorder. This individual has a history suggestive of antisocial personality disorder: previous incarcerations, ongoing illegal behavior, secondary personal gain associated with his symptoms, and admission to the hospital. With factitious disorder, external incentives are absent. Somatization disorder would require multiple systemic complaints. A person with conversion disorder might be indifferent to their symptoms (la belle indifference), their symptoms would not be intentionally produced, and their symptoms would be more responsive to suggestion or hypnosis. An individual with Lewy body dementia would be expected to be older and would have a history of motor and cognitive disturbance in addition to possible visual hallucinations.

American Psychiatric Association. *DSM-IV-TR, Diagnostic and Statistical Manual of Mental Disorders*. 4th ed. Washington, DC: American Psychiatric Association; 2000: 739.

32. Answer: A. Patients with OCD are most commonly worried about being contaminated and need to compulsively wash themselves or clean their environment. The second most common pattern of obsessions is doubt (forgetting to lock the car, leaving the door open) with checking patterns, followed by intrusive thoughts that are not followed by compulsions, and a need for a specific symmetry.

1. Juang YY, Liu CY. Phenomenology of obsessive-compulsive disorder in Taiwan. *Psychiatry Clin Neurosci*. 2001;55:623–627.
2. Kaplan HI, Sadock BJ. *Kaplan & Sadock's Synopsis of Psychiatry*. 8th ed. Philadelphia: Lippincott Williams & Wilkins; 1998:613.

33. Answer: C. The double bind hypothesis of schizophrenia was proposed by Gregory Bateson and Donald Jackson. It suggested that children who receive conflicting parenting messages withdraw into a psychotic state to escape the confusion of the double bind, ultimately resulting in schizophrenia. The clinical example given in this question illustrates the concept of the double bind, which is not currently accepted as a causal explanation for schizophrenia. The schizophrenogenic mother (derived from early psychoanalytic formulations of schizophrenia), expressed emotion within families (high levels of which have been shown to increase relapse rates in schizophrenic patients), and the decathexis theory (originally proposed by Freud) have all been offered as causal explanations for the development of schizophrenia.

1. Gabbard GO. *Psychodynamic Psychiatry in Clinical Practice*. 4th ed. Arlington: American Psychiatric Publishing; 2005:183–187.
2. Sadock BJ, Sadock VA. *Kaplan and Sadock's Synopsis of Psychiatry*. 9th ed. Philadelphia: Lippincott Williams & Wilkins; 2003:483–484.

34. Answer: C. Sigmund Freud introduced the term *conversion*, which was based on his work with Anna O. Freud hypothesized that the symptoms of conversion disorder reflect unconscious conflicts. Paul Briquet and Jean-Martin Charcot noted the influence of heredity on conversion symptoms and highlighted their common association with a traumatic event. The syndrome, now called somatization disorder, was previously referred to as Briquet's syndrome. Thomas Sydenham observed that psychological factors were involved in the pathogenesis of somatization disorder. Emil Kraeplin (of "dementia precox" fame) coined the term *dysmorphophobia*, which is a term that is now replaced in the DSM-IV-TR by body dysmorphic disorder.

1. Gabbard GO. *Psychodynamic Psychiatry in Clinical Practice*. 4th ed. Arlington: American Psychiatric Publishing; 2005:542.
2. Sadock BJ, Sadock VA. *Kaplan and Sadock's Synopsis of Psychiatry*. 9th ed. Philadelphia: Lippincott Williams & Wilkins; 2003:643–653.

35. Answer: A. Ataque de nervios is an example of a trance state disorder form of dissociative disorder NOS. Somatic symptoms, including seizurelike convulsive movements, may be seen. Crying, cursing, self-harm, or harm to others, may be seen. These episodes are usually followed by partial or complete amnesia. Interpersonal conflicts or loss are common stressors seen in this condition. From a demographic standpoint, females who are 45 years of age or older; who are widowed, divorced, or separated; who are of low-income socioeconomic status; and who have less than a high school education are more likely to have attacks of ataque de nervios. The estimated lifetime prevalence rate in Puerto Rico is approximately 14%. In depersonalization disorder, there are recurrent feelings of being detached from one's body, which causes significant distress or impairment. In dissociative convulsions, features of convulsions, such as tongue biting and urinary/fecal incontinence may be seen. In dissociative amnesia, the unavailable memories are usually related to routine information that is a part of day-to-day conscious awareness. Adjustment disorder does not involve amnesia or dissociative symptoms.

Sadock BJ, Sadock VA. *Kaplan and Sadock's Comprehensive Textbook of Psychiatry*. 8th ed. Philadelphia: Lippincott Williams & Wilkins; 2005: 1845, 1894, 1870–1871, 1860–1861, 2055, 2056.

36. Answer: B. This patient is presenting with lithium toxicity. It is most possibly due to the recent addition of an ACE-inhibitor, which has been reported to decrease lithium clearance and cause toxicity. Although most non-steroidal anti-inflammatory drugs (NSAIDs) have been reported to have dangerous interactions with lithium, aspirin has not been reported to produce toxicity. The major risk of using lamotrigine is the development of severe dermatological reactions, especially when used in combination with valproic acid, started at higher doses, or titrated rapidly. Valproic acid inhibits the metabolism of lamotrigine and increases its level in the blood.

1. Hsu CH, Liu PY, Chen JH, et al. Electrocardiographic abnormalities as predictors for over-range lithium levels. *Cardiology*. 2005;103:101–106.
2. Juurlink DN, Mamdani MM, Kopp A, et al. Drug-induced lithium toxicity in the elderly: a population-based study. *J Am Geriatr Soc*. 2004;52:794–798.

37. **Answer: E.** Unlike many tricyclic antidepressants, SSRIs do not have a linear-response curve and thus higher dosages do not necessarily result in increased effectiveness. At least 90% of the clinical response to SSRIs occurs at the starting dose. Higher doses tend to mainly increase adverse effects. Sertraline is the most likely to be raised above its starting dose, 50 mg/day to 150 to 200 mg/day, whereas paroxetine is the most likely to be continued at its starting dose of 20 mg/day.

Sadock BJ, Sadock VA. *Kaplan and Sadock's Synopsis of Psychiatry*. 9th ed. Philadelphia: Lippincott Williams & Wilkins; 2002:1094–1095.

38. **Answer: B.** In patients 70 years or older with major depression, monthly interpersonal psychotherapy does not help prevent recurrence of major depression. Paroxetine and clinical management is the best treatment option.

Renolds CF, Dew MA, Pollock BG, et al. Maintenance treatment of major depression in old age. *N Engl J Med*. 2006;354:1130–1138.

39. **Answer: A.** Of these choices, labeling and emotional reasoning are the only two that are cognitive distortions. In this scenario, the patient is using a fixed, global label ("idiot") to describe herself, which is a generalization that is highly unlikely to be true. Emotional reasoning involves incorrectly inferring that something is true based on the way that one feels (e.g., believing that feeling that one cannot perform a task implies that one actually cannot perform the task). Projection, reaction formation, and intellectualization are all defense mechanisms.

1. Beck J. *Cognitive Therapy: Basics and Beyond*. New York: Guilford Press; 1995:119.
2. McWilliams N. *Psychoanalytic Diagnosis: Understanding Personality Structure in the Clinical Process*. New York: Guilford Press; 1994:108, 123–124, 131–133.

40. **Answer: C.** Approximately 5% of patients receiving long-term lithium therapy will develop hypothyroidism compared to 0.3% to 1.3% of the general population who will develop noniatrogenic hypothyroidism. A patient with antithyroid antibodies prior to starting lithium therapy will have a greater chance of developing hypothyroidism.

Rosenbaum JF, Arana GW, Hyman SE, et al. *Handbook of Psychiatric Drug Therapy*. 5th ed. Philadelphia: Lippincott Williams and Wilkins; 2005:144.

41. **Answer: B.** Lung cancers are the primary cancers most likely to metastasize to the brain, with breast cancers being the second most common, with melanoma third, colon cancers fourth, rectal cancers fifth, and renal cancers sixth in order of occurrence.

Wyszynski AA, Wyszynski B, eds. *Manual of Psychiatric Care for the Medically Ill*. Arlington: American Psychiatric Publishing; 2005:8.

42. **Answer: D.** A lesion in the middle cerebral artery territory will result in contralateral hemiparesis and contralateral hemisensory loss of the face, arm, and hand. If a lesion develops in the dominant hemisphere, which is typically the left side, aphasia also can be seen. A contralateral homonymous hemianopsia also can occur as well as limb ataxia, astereognosis, and agraphesthesia. A lesion in the posterior cerebral artery territory would not result in arm and hand weakness. A lesion involving the internal carotid artery territory could resemble a middle cerebral artery lesion; however, the lesion here is on the left. A posterior inferior cerebellar artery lesion would not present with the previously mentioned symptoms and would include ipsilateral facial sensory loss, contralateral pain and temperature loss, and ipsilateral Horner's syndrome (ptosis, miosis, and anhidrosis).

Kandel ER, Schwartz JH, Jessell TM. *Principles of Neural Science*. 3rd ed. Connecticut: Appleton and Lange; 1991:1045–1046.

43. **Answer: A.** Axonal plaques are areas of the nervous system where the axons have become demyelinated in MS. Neurofibrillary tangles, Hirano bodies and granulovacuolar degeneration are all seen in Alzheimer's disease and not in MS.

1. Kaufman DM. *Clinical Neurology for Psychiatrists*. 5th ed. Philadelphia: WB Saunders; 2001:369.
2. Rowland LP. *Merritt's Neurology*. 11th ed. Philadelphia: Lippincott Williams & Wilkins; 2005:772–774.

44. **Answer: E.** Cardiomyopathy is seen in more than 50% of Friedreich's ataxia cases. Many of these patients die of a cardiac arrhythmia or congestive heart failure. A minority of patients may abruptly become

ataxic after febrile illness, and infrequently one leg may become clumsy before the other. Hand incoordination is a later finding with dysarthria occurring even further in the course of the illness.

Ropper A, Brown R. *Adams and Victor's Principles of Neurology.* 8th ed. New York: McGraw-Hill; 2005:932–933.

45. Answer: A. Triphasic waves are generalized bisynchronous waves that occur in brief runs. Half the patients with triphasic waves have hepatic encephalopathy with the other half having other toxic-metabolic encephalopathies like uremic encephalopathy. PLEDs are seen in acute destructive cerebral lesions. They are characterized by recurrent focal epileptiform discharges (1 to 2 cycles per second [cps]) in the setting of focally slow/attenuated background activity. PLEDs are seen in acute cerebral infarction, cerebral abscess, and anoxia. Periodic complexes are seen in subacute sclerosis panencephalitis and Creutzfeld-Jakob disease where patients present with myoclonic jerks. Beta waves (13 to 25 cps) are usually seen in frontal and central regions. They become prominent when the people become anxious, concentrate, or use sedative-hypnotic medications. Delta waves (1 to 3 cps) are seen in children or when people enter deep sleep and are usually absent in awake, alert, and healthy adults. The presence of diffuse delta waves on an EEG recording suggests a metabolic abnormality or degenerative illness.

1. Kaufman DM. *Clinical Neurology for Psychiatrists.* 5th ed. Philadelphia: WB Saunders; 2001:226–231.
2. Rowland LP. *Merritt's Neurology.* 11th ed. Philadelphia: Lippincott Williams & Wilkins; 2005: 79–84.

46. Answer: B. This patient is demonstrating "alien hand syndrome," an extreme form of hemi-inattention in which the patient believes that he or she does not possess his or her hand (usually the left) and that it is moving either independently or under someone else's power. The limb maintains some basic sensory and motor functions and may perform simple tasks, but the patient does not feel aware or in control of these. Hemi-inattention refers to the neglect of sensory stimuli, including visual and tactile, which originate from the patient's left side. It is generally the result of injury to the nondominant parietal lobe cortex and the underlying thalamus and reticular activating system.

Kaufman DM. *Clinical Neurology for Psychiatrists.* 5th ed. Philadelphia: WB Saunders; 2001:185–186.

47. Answer: B. Primary cerebral lymphomas occur in patients who are immuonsuppressed, including patients with AIDS. They are typically aggressive and patients often present with focal findings, evidence of intracranial pressure, or confusion. All of the tumors listed are primary brain tumors. Oligodendrogliomas are rare tumors, which typically grow slowly; cerebellar astrocytomas tend to occur in children. Astrocytoma and medulloblastomas typically occur in the cerebellum. One would not typically expect a pituitary adenoma to cause a right-sided hemiparesis; these patients usually present with bilateral hemianopsia.

1. Goetz C. *Textbook of Clinical Neurology.* 2nd ed. Philadelphia: WB Saunders; 2003:1028–1029.
2. Kaufman DM. *Clinical Neurology for Psychiatrists.* 5th ed. Philadelphia: WB Saunders; 2001:153, 512.

48. Answer: C. The most common sports-related head trauma is a concussion, which causes a short change in mental status with or without loss of consciousness. A contusion is less common and involves minor intracranial bleeding. An epidural hematoma is most commonly seen after a temporal bone fracture, subdural hematomas are frequently seen in elderly people, and subarachnoid hemorrhages are usually the result of a ruptured aneurysm.

1. Delaney JS, Abuzeyad F, Correa JA, et al. Recognition and characteristics of concussions in the emergency department population. *J Emerg Med.* 2005;29:189–197.
2. Kaufman DM. *Clinical Neurology for Psychiatrists.* 5th ed. Philadelphia: WB Saunders; 2001:581–595.

49. Answer: B. The Glasgow Coma Scale is used in the ER and other acute care settings to predict the patient's risk of mortality. It consists of three different sections, which include motor, eye, and verbal components. In patients with Glasgow Coma Scale scores of less than 8, the mortality rates can be as high as 71%. Although this scale is useful in grading the severity of a case, and thereby predicts the risk of complications, its most useful function is to assess the outcome or risk of mortality.

1. Lieh-Lai MW, Theodoru AA, Sarnaik AP, et al. Limitations of the Glasgow Coma Scale in predicting outcome in children with traumatic brain injury. *J Pediatr.* 1992;120:195–199.
2. Moore L, Lavoie A, Camden S, et al. Statistical validation of the Glasgow Coma Score. *J Trauma.* 2006:60:1238–1243.

50. Answer: C. Lesions in the afferent fibers of peripheral nerves, dorsal roots, or dorsal columns of the spinal cord present with sensory ataxia. Patients are unaware of their leg positioning and, therefore, loose balance when they close their eyes (positive Romberg sign). Patients with cerebellar ataxia have balance problems when their feet are held together, regardless of whether their eyes are open or closed. The frontal and temporal cortices are not involved in gait.

1. Pearce JMS. Romberg and his sign. *Eur Neurol.* 2005;53:210–213.

2. Rowland LP. *Merritt's Neurology*. 11th ed. Philadelphia: Lippincott Williams & Wilkins; 2005: 783– 852.

51. Answer: E. Involvement of the central nervous system (CNS) occurs in 5% of the patients with sarcoidosis. The parts most frequently involved are the cranial nerves, meninges, hypothalamus, and pituitary. Granulomatous meningitis affects mainly the basal brain regions. Involvement of the hypothalamus and third ventricular region leads to somnolence, obesity, hyperthermia, memory difficulties, or a change of personality. Pituitary involvement may present as menstrual disturbances, diabetes insipidus, and other endocrine disturbances. Neurosarcoidosis is often accompanied by mental disturbance. Hydrocephalus may arise as a consequence of basal meningitis or CSF obstruction due to granulomatous masses. Metabolic disturbances, such as hypercalcemia and renal failure, may contribute to psychiatric symptoms as does steroid therapy. Although liver involvement occurs in 90% of the cases, liver dysfunction is not usually clinically important. Only 20% to 30% of the patients have hepatomegaly or biochemical evidence of liver dysfunction.

1. Lishman WA. *Organic Psychiatry*. 3rd ed. Boston: Blackwell Science; 1996:763–765.
2. Stern, Barney J. Neurological complications of Sarcoidosis. *Curr Opinion Psychiatry*. 2004;17:311–316.

52. Answer: B. Monoamine oxidase A inhibitors should not be taken with levodopa because doing so could precipitate a hypertensive crisis. For this reason, phenelzine is contraindicated when a patient is taking levodopa.

Katzung BG. *Basic and Clinical Pharmacology*. 8th ed. New York: McGraw-Hill; 2001:467–468.

53. Answer: C. As the brain ages, there is a decrease in the weight of the brain with widening of sulci and an enlargement of the ventricles. There is also slight reduction in the blood flow to the brain. Lewy bodies are inclusion bodies that are found in neurons of the cerebral cortex and are associated with Lewy body dementia. They are also found in the basal ganglia of patients with Parkinson's disease.

1. Kaufman DM. *Clinical Neurology for Psychiatrists*. 5th ed. Philadelphia: WB Saunders; 2001:141.
2. Sadock BJ, Kaplan H. *Synopsis of Psychiatry*. 9th ed. Philadelphia: Lippincott Williams & Wilkins; 2003:52.

54. Answer: D. The PS-1 on chromosome 14 has been recognized as a major locus for Alzheimer' s disease in early onset familial Alzheimer's disease, contributing to as many as 70% of the cases. A coding DNA sequence showing high homology to the PS-1 gene on chromosome 14 was found to map within the chromosome 1 region of interest for Alzheimer' s disease, which was subsequently named presenilin-2 (PS-2). Missense mutations have been found in PS-2 in several families with early onset Alzheimer's disease. Individuals with Down syndrome (trisomy 21) develop an early onset dementia that is clinically and histopathologically indistinguishable from Alzheimer's disease. For this reason, chromosome 21 was considered to be an excellent candidate region for initial genetic studies of Alzheimer's disease. A number of missense mutations identified near or within the β-amyloid sequence of the Amyloid precursor protein (APP) on chromosome 21 are present in families with early onset Alzheimer's disease. A linkage study using markers in late-onset Alzheimer's disease families found a susceptibility gene on the long arm of chromosome 19. A candidate gene known to map to this is the apolipoprotein E (apoE) lipoprotein gene.

1. Kaufman DM. *Clinical Neurology for Psychiatrists*. 5th ed. Philadelphia: WB Saunders; 2001:139.
2. Sadock BJ, Sadock VA. *Kaplan and Sadock's Comprehensive Textbook of Psychiatry*. 8th ed. Philadelphia: Lippincott Williams & Wilkins; 2005:257–258.

55. Answer: E. MMPI is an example of objective personality testing, whereas Rorschach, TAT, Draw-A-Person, and APT are all examples of projective personality tests.

Jacobson JL, Jacobson AM. *Psychiatric Secrets*. 2nd ed. Philadelphia: Hanley and Belfus; 2001:21–25.

56. Answer: A. Although it is important for patients to be aware of the fee schedule for their visits, it is not part of the accepted standard of information disclosure for any given psychiatric treatment. The five main elements in the accepted standard for information disclosure are diagnosis, available treatments, consequences of these treatments, alternative treatments, and their risks and prognosis.

1. Gutheil TH, Applebaum PS. *Clinical Handbook of Psychiatry and the Law*. 3rd ed. Philadelphia: Lippincott Williams & Wilkins; 2000:210–211.
2. Sadock BJ, Sadock VA. *Kaplan and Sadock's Comprehensive Textbook of Psychiatry*. 8th ed. Philadelphia: Lippincott Williams & Wilkins; 2005:3972.

57. Answer: B. In DSM-IV-TR, malingering is described as an "additional condition that may be the focus of clinical attention," and is recorded as a "V code" on axis 1. Most "V codes" are documented on axis I with the exception of borderline intellectual functioning, which is recorded on axis II. Malingering and other "V codes" are not considered mental disorders. Other examples include: noncompliance with treatment, bereavement, religious, or spiritual problem. Personality traits, personality disorders, defense mechanisms, mental retardation, and borderline intellectual function are all coded on axis II.

American Psychiatric Association. *DSM-IV-TR, Diagnostic and Statistical Manual of Mental Disorders.* 4th ed. Washington, DC: American Psychiatric Association; 2000: 739–742.

58. Answer: E. This patient is presenting with a culture bound syndrome called "Brain fag." It is usually seen in male students from Nigeria and Saharan Africa and it is thought to be caused by stress at school. These patients usually complain of unpleasant feelings in the head, visual problems, poor memory, fatigue, and sleepiness. It is thought to be a form of anxiety, depression, or somatoform disorder, which responds well to relaxation therapy, antidepressants, and anxiolytics. Koro is a CBS seen in Malaysia and South East Asia, which is characterized by symptoms of anxiety with the fear that the genitalia will be retracted completely into the abdomen and then the person would die. Latah is a CBS seen in Malaysia and is characterized by hypersensitivity to sudden fright, echopraxia, echolalia, command obedience, and a trancelike state and is commonly seen in women of lower socioeconomic status. Amok is another CBS seen in Malaysia and is characterized by brooding, homicidal frenzy, exhaustion, and amnesia. Pibloktoq, also called "Arctic Hysteria," is seen in Eskimos in the Arctic and sub-Arctic regions and is more common in women. It is characterized by severe agitation/excitement and is followed by seizures and a transient coma after which the victim sleeps for many hours and then resumes normal function.

1. Gaw AC. *Concise Guide to Cross-Cultural Psychiatry.* Washington, DC: American Psychiatric Publishing; 2004: 73–97.
2. Kaplan HI, Sadock BJ. *Kaplan & Sadock's Synopsis of Psychiatry.* 8th ed. Philadelphia: Lippincott Williams & Wilkins; 1998:499.

59. Answer: A. Late onset, obvious precipitating factors, acute onset, good premorbid functioning, mood symptoms, being married, family history of mood disorders, good support systems, and predominant positive symptoms are all considered good prognostic factors in schizophrenia. Poor prognostic factors include young age at onset, lack of precipitating factors, insidious onset, poor premorbid functioning, family history of schizophrenia, poor support systems, and predominant negative symptoms.

Sadock BJ, Sadock VA. *Kaplan and Sadock's Synopsis of Psychiatry.* 9th ed. Philadelphia: Lippincott Williams & Wilkins; 2003:485.

60. Answer: B. The DSM-IV-TR criteria for somatization disorder include a history of many physical complaints beginning before the age of 30 years, impairment in functioning, and the occurrence of four pain symptoms, two gastrointestinal symptoms, one sexual (or reproductive) symptom, and one pseudoneurological symptom. The symptoms cannot be intentionally produced or feigned.

American Psychiatric Association. *Quick Reference to the Diagnostic Criteria from DSM-IV-TR.* Washington, DC: American Psychiatric Association; 2000:229–236.

61. Answer: E. Tricyclic antidepressants and SSRIs have been shown to be beneficial in cataplexy. Amphetamines and modafinil improve wakefulness, and hence target symptoms of narcolepsy, not cataplexy. Benzodiazepines and phenobarbitone are obviously contraindicated in narcolepsy-cataplexy.

Sadock BJ, Sadock VA. *Kaplan and Sadock's Comprehensive Textbook of Psychiatry.* 8th ed. Philadelphia: Lippincott Williams & Wilkins; 2005:2033.

62. Answer: B. Buspirone is a partial agonist at the postsynaptic 5-hydroxytryptamine1A (5-HT$_{1A}$) receptor. As an augmentation agent, it works to enhance the activity of SSRIs through the 5-HT$_{1A}$ receptors. Bupropion produces its antidepressant effects by blocking the reuptake of dopamine and norepinephrine. Unlike buspirone, it is an antidepressant monotherapy agent. The evidence for efficacy of either medication for augmentation of SSRIs, up till this point, has been derived from case reports, case series, and small, inconclusive placebo-controlled trials. In the STAR*D trial, sustained-release bupropion produced a greater reduction in the number of and severity of symptoms and had fewer side effects and adverse reactions than buspirone. Although, rates of remission on the Hamilton Rating Scaled for Depression (HSRD-17) were 29.7% for sustained release bupropion and 30.1% for buspirone.

Trivedi MH, Fava M, Wisniewski SR, et al. Medication augmentation after the failure of SSRIs for depression Multicenter Study. Randomized controlled trial. *N Engl J Med.* 2006;354:1243–1252.

63. Answer: C. Tremor is seen in 5% to 10% percent of patients taking SSRIs, a frequency two to four times that of placebo. SSRIs may cause akathisia, dystonia, tremor, cogwheel rigidity, torticollis, opisthotonos, gait disorders, and bradykinesia. Also cases of tardive dyskinesia have been reported. Patients with Parkinson's disease or spasticity may experience some worsening of their motor symptoms when taking an SSRI. Extrapyramidal effects are most closely associated with fluoxetine, particularly at doses

>40 mg/day. The pathogenesis of such adverse reactions is unknown, but it has been hypothesized that they may be caused by serotonergically mediated inhibition of dopaminergic transmission.

1. Coulter DM, Pillans PI. Fluoxetine and extrapyramidal side effects. *Am J Psychiatry*. 1995;152:122–125.
2. Sadock BJ, Sadock VA. *Kaplan and Sadock's Synopsis of Psychiatry*. 9th ed. Philadelphia: Lippincott Williams & Wilkins; 2002:1099.

64. Answer: C. Dopamine receptor antagonists have been shown to lower seizure threshold and this effect is greater with low-potency antipsychotic medications. Clinically, those with a history of seizure disorders are at greater risk of this adverse effect thus it is preferable to use a high-potency antipsychotic medication in patients with seizure disorders.

Sadock BJ, Sadock VA. *Kaplan & Sadock's Comprehensive Textbook of Psychiatry*. 8th ed. Philadelphia: Lippincott Williams & Wilkins; 2005:16, 31.

65. Answer: D. Generally, it makes sense to wait on starting an antidepressant for a patient who presents to the ER in this manner until clinicians have managed to do a more thorough evaluation. It does make sense, however, to order a CBC with differential, chemistry panel (including LFTs), thyroid functions tests, rapid plasma reagin (RPR), EKG, and urine toxicology so that this information will be available before the patient is started on an antidepressant. All of the other choices are essential parts of the interview process. Of note, one wants to particularly ascertain whether the patient is experiencing command auditory hallucinations, the content of the hallucinations, and how long the patient has been hearing them. Also of note, untreated pain, once treated, can result in an alleviation of suicidal ideation.

Bernstein C, Ishak WW, Weiner E, et al. *On Call Psychiatry*. 2nd ed. Philadelphia: WB Saunders; 2001:73–80.

66. Answer: D. Schizophrenia is associated with spontaneous TD rate in otherwise healthy young adults of about 0.5% per year when compared to the normal population. After the age of 60 years, spontaneous TD occurs at about 0.5% per year in the general population. The risk of TD is highest in the first 5 years of treatment with typical antipsychotics, and the incidence of decreases after this period. Approximately 20% of patients develop TD in the first 3 years of treatment with typical antipsychotics. In the elderly, the risk of TD in patients with schizophrenia who are treated with typical antipsychotics is as high as 29%, and rises to approximately 63% after 3 years. The risk of an elderly patient developing TD in the first year is approximately five times higher than a younger patient who is treated with a typical antipsychotic.

Shirzadi AA, Ghaemi SN. Side effects of atypical antipsychotics: extrapyramidal symptoms and the metabolic syndrome. *Harv Rev Psychiatry*. 2006;14:152–164.

67. Answer: A. The best known principles in medical ethics are those described by philosophers Tom Beauchamp, James Childress and Raanon Gillon. The four ethical principles described by them include: autonomy, beneficence, nonmaleficence, and justice. They described these four principles as being pertinent in any medical ethical problem (i.e., prima facie). In each case, the relevant ethical principles should be considered, weighed appropriately, and a conclusion should be reached only after appropriately balancing these principles. Autonomy versus shame and doubt and basic trust versus basic mistrust are Erikson's epigenetic stages and not ethical dilemmas.

1. Gelder MG, Lopez-Ibor JJ, Andreasen N. *New Oxford Textbook of Psychiatry*. Oxford: Oxford University Press; 2000:30.
2. Stern TA, Herman JB. *Massachusetts General Hospital Psychiatry Update and Board Preparation*. 2nd ed. New York: McGraw-Hill; 2004:29.

68. Answer: D. In transcortical motor aphasia, repetition and comprehension are intact but speech is nonfluent. In Wernicke's aphasia, repetition and comprehension are impaired and speech is fluent. In Broca's aphasia, speech is nonfluent and repetition is impaired, whereas comprehension is intact. In conduction aphasia, repetition is impaired, comprehension is spared, and speech is fluent. In transcortical sensory aphasia, speech is fluent, comprehension is impaired, and repetition is intact.

Stern TA, Herman JB. *Massachusetts General Hospital Psychiatry Update and Board Preparation*. 2nd ed. New York: McGraw-Hill; 2004:278.

69. Answer: A. In Korsakoff's syndrome, demyelination of nerve fibers in multiple brain structures disrupts the Papez circuit and leads to disturbances in episodic memories in chronic alcoholics with poor nutrition. In Korsakoff's syndrome, demyelination occurs primarily in the mammillary bodies and the dorsomedial and laterodorsal thalamic nuclei and thus interrupting the Papez circuit. This interruption leads to anterograde amnesia and retrograde amnesia. The Papez circuit includes the hippocampus, fornix, mammillary bodies, anterior nucleus of the thalamus, cingulate gyrus, and presubiculum.

Budson AE, Price BH. *Memory: Clinical Disorders. Encyclopedia of Life Sciences*. London: Macmillian Publishers; 2001:1–3.

70. **Answer: E.** Progressive external ophthalmoplegia is another mitochondrial-transmitted disorder, in addition to cytochrome-C oxidase deficiency, Leigh's syndrome (subacute necrotizing encephalomyelopathy), MELAS, and MERRF. Progressive supranuclear palsy is considered a "Parkinson's plus" neurodegenerative disorder; in familial cases it is transmitted in autosomal dominant fashion. Mitochondrial DNA is inherited almost exclusively through maternal lineage from the female ovum. Mitochondrial DNA does not recombine, permitting accumulation of mutations through maternal lines. Replication and distribution of mitochondrial DNA is not mitotic; contributions from various mitochondria pass to progeny.

Ropper A, Brown R. *Adams and Victor's Principles of Neurology*. 8th ed. New York: McGraw-Hill; 2005:798, 841–845.

71. **Answer: A.** REM activity seen on EEG recording during the daytime indicates either one of the following; sleep deprivation, withdrawal from REM suppressing drugs like alcohol, cocaine, hypnotics, tricyclic antidepressants, and amphetamines or narcolepsy. During stage 1 of sleep when the subject is going from being awake to falling asleep, alpha rhythm disappears and is replaced by waves of low voltage and slower activity. During stage 2 of sleep, sleep spindles (symmetric, sinusoidal waves of 12 to 14 cps) appear. During stages 3 and 4 of sleep, high-voltage slow waves called delta waves appear. REM sleep is characterized by low-voltage waves similar to those seen in stage 1 of sleep and is associated with REM and atonia. REM rhythm is not usually seen during EEG recordings. Dementia is usually characterized by the slowing of background alpha waves from 10 to 12 cps to 8 cps followed by a disorganized pattern in advanced cases. In delirium, there is loss of alpha activity with the development of theta and delta activity.

1. Kaufman DM. *Clinical Neurology for Psychiatrists*. 5th ed. Philadelphia: WB Saunders; 2001:226–231.
2. Rowland LP. *Merritt's Neurology*. 11th ed. Philadelphia: Lippincott Williams & Wilkins; 2005: 79–84.

72. **Answer: B.** MRI is the imaging modality of choice in the evaluation of MS, with approximately 85% sensitivity, although the clinical correlation of disability with specific lesions is generally considered poor. MS plaques are typically round in appearance and look like a bull's eye. Focal white matter intensities are a common nonspecific finding often found on an MRI. Contrast enhanced CT scans can be used to evaluate MS, but early in the disease, they are often normal.

Orrison WW. *Neuroimaging*. Philadelphia: WB Saunders; 2000:800–805.

73. **Answer: C.** This patient has had a hemorrhage in the left pons. Hypertensive hemorrhages are commonly seen in basal ganglia, thalamus, pons, and cerebellum. They occur suddenly and produce headache, nausea, and vomiting. Patients with pontine lesions usually lose consciousness suddenly, because there is damage to the PPRF and to the descending pyramidal tract fibers that cross the midline in the medulla. In these lesions, the eyes look away from the side of the destructive pontine lesion, but look toward the hemiplegia. Because of the overlaps with the midbrain reticular formation, conjugate gaze examination is of vital importance in comatose patients. In damage to one frontal gaze center or its descending fiber tract, the eyes drift toward the involved cerebral hemisphere due to unopposed action of the remaining frontal gaze center (i.e., the eyes appear to look at a destructive hemispheric lesion and look away from the resulting hemiplegia). Damage to the medulla involves the nuclei and the initial portion of the cranial nerves IX through XII, the descending corticospinal, ascending sensory system, and sympathetic nervous system. Lesions to the medulla results in bulbar palsy, lateral medullary infarction of Wallenberg, and locked-in syndrome.

1. Goetz C. *Textbook of Clinical Neurology*. 2nd ed. Philadelphia: WB Saunders; 2003:7–8.
2. Kaufman DM. *Clinical Neurology for Psychiatrists*. 5th ed. Philadelphia: WB Saunders, 2001:49, 304–306.

74. **Answer: A.** This patient is presenting with a herniated cervical intervertebral disk caused by a whiplash injury. Patients with whiplash injury usually present with neck pain, headaches of the muscular contraction type, dizziness, and sometimes with paresthesias. Brachial plexus injuries are commonly seen in newborns that experienced trauma during childbirth and present with loss of sensation and weakness of an arm. A soft tissue neck injury would not cause loss of DTRs. Spontaneous epidural hematomas are rare and usually present with the sudden onset of spinal pain followed by myelopathy.

1. Ewans RW. Some observations on whiplash injuries. *Neurol Clin*. 1992;10:975–997.
2. Hsieh CF, Lin HJ, Chen KT, et al. Acute spontaneous cervical spinal epidural hematoma with hemiparesis as the initial presentation. *Eur J Emerg Med*. 2006;13:36–38.
3. Kaufman DM. *Clinical Neurology for Psychiatrists*. 5th ed. Philadelphia: WB Saunders, 2001:581–595.

75. **Answer: C.** The use of dopamine antagonists in patients with Parkinson's disease, with the exception of quetiapine and clozapine, will worsen the patient's

motor symptoms associated with the underlying illness of Parkinson's disease.

Rosenbaum JF, Arana GW, Hyman SE, et al. *Handbook of Psychiatric Drug Therapy.* 5th ed. Philadelphia: Lippincott Williams & Wilkins; 2005:24.

76. Answer: E. This patient has acute Wernicke's encephalopathy (WE). WE is a neuropsychiatric syndrome usually seen in alcoholic patients that can lead to permanent neuropsychiatric deficits, if left untreated. The classic triad (ataxia, confusion, and ophthalmoplegia) only occurs in approximately 10% of the cases. Parenteral thiamine is the treatment of choice for the acute treatment of WE. Parenteral administration is better because there is a risk of poor absorption of thiamine from the gut, especially in chronic alcoholics due to erosive gastritis. There is also the need for a rapid increase in the level of thiamine in the brain to prevent permanent neuropsychiatric damage. Although alcoholics tend to have a poor diet and may benefit from the administration of vitamins, the corner stone in treatment of WE is the replacement of thiamine.

1. Rowland LP. *Merritt's Neurology.* 11th ed. Philadelphia: Lippincott Williams & Wilkins; 2005: 39, 156.
2. Thomson AD, Christopher CH, Cook RT, et al. The Royal College of Physicians report on alcohol: guidelines for managing Wernicke's encephalopathy in the accident and emergency department. *Alcohol.* 2002;37:513–521.

77. Answer: E. Borreliosis is often described as the "great new imitator" owing to its widespread multisystemic effects. This patient classically describes stage 3 of persistent infection with borreliosis, which includes arthritis, acrodermatitis, and neurological manifestations (neuroborreliosis). The most common form of chronic CNS involvement is a subtle encephalopathy affecting sleep, mood, or memory. Psychiatric disturbances include anxiety, affective symptoms especially depression, somatization disorder, dementia, and rarely psychosis. Occasionally patients are left with chronic fatigue or fibromyalgia. The various manifestations of borreliosis are usually successfully treated with oral antibiotic therapy, except for objective neurological abnormalities which require intravenous therapy. Psychotropic medications may be helpful as an adjunct to medical treatments for Lyme disease. Most commonly used are anxiolytics, low-dose antidepressants for pain and sleep, and higher-dose antidepressants for major depression. Given that Lyme disease can cause conduction abnormalities, it is of particular importance to obtain an EKG before starting treatment with tricyclic antidepressants. Family therapy may be indicated especially where a sick child is concerned. Couple ther-

apy may be indicated in some cases as most patients report a significant loss of libido. In this case, antipsychotic treatment is not indicated in the absence of psychosis.

Lishman WA. *Organic Psychiatry.* 3rd ed. Boston: Blackwell Science; 1996:369.

78. Answer: C. There are only a few firm rules to guide physicians in the withdrawal of anticonvulsants. An abnormal EEG would be relative contraindication to stopping treatment. Several large epidemiological studies have had similar results, such as after 2 years of seizurefree monotherapy, there is a 33% to 40% chance of recurrence with discontinuation. With continuation, the rate is approximately 20%.

1. Callaghan N, Garrett A, Goggin T. Withdrawal of anticonvulsant drugs in patients free of seizures for two years. *N Engl J Med.* 1988;318:942–946.
2. Ropper AH, Brown RH. *Adams and Victor's Principles of Neurology.* 8th ed. New York: McGraw-Hill; 2005:294.
3. Specchio LM, Tramacere L, LaNeve A, et al. Discontinuing antiepileptic drugs in patients who are seizure-free on monotherapy. *J Neurol Neurosurg Psychiatry.* 2002;72:22–25.

79. Answer: A. As people age, their psychomotor speed declines. Although the elderly take longer to learn new tasks, their ability to learn is usually intact. IQ remains stable till the 80s, and there can be benign forgetfulness or memory problems with simple data, but this should not significantly impact social functioning.

Sadock BJ, Kaplan H. *Synopsis of Psychiatry.* 9th ed. Philadelphia: Lippincott Williams & Wilkins; 2003:52,339.

80. Answer: D. A single neuron can release multiple different types of molecular signals and can have receptors for multiple different molecular signals. The usual method for communication among neurons is either molecular or electrical. The four common classes of molecular signals are the monoamines, amino acids, peptides, and neurotrophic factors. Usually, there is heterogeneity among receptors so that there are multiple subtypes of receptors for a particular neurotransmitter.

Sadock BJ, Sadock VA. *Kaplan and Sadock's Comprehensive Textbook of Psychiatry.* 8th ed. Philadelphia: Lippincott Williams & Wilkins; 2005:1–2.

81. Answer: A. Shipley Scale and Wechsler Intelligence Scales are tests of general intellectual functioning. Shipley Scale is a 20-minute pencil and paper test that measures vocabulary and open-ended verbal abstraction. Wechsler Adult Intelligence Scale-Third Edition (WAIS-III) is useful in evaluating the general intellectual functioning in age ranges 16 to

89 years. The WAIS-III uses complex verbal and visuospatial tasks that are then normatively summarized as verbal IQ (VIQ), performance IQ (PIQ), and full-scale IQ. It indicates the person's long-standing abilities and current functioning. It is more helpful to characterize an individual's intellectual function in terms of the range of functioning—borderline, low average, average, high average, and superior—than just denoting the specific value itself. Analyzing the discrepancy between VIQ and PIQ and examination of the patterns of performance across various aspects of the test help us understand the underlying brain pathology. California Verbal Learning Test II and Benton Visual Retention Test are tests of memory and not general intellectual functioning. Boston Naming Test-Revised is a test of language and the Wisconsin Card Sorting Test is a test of executive functioning.

Sadock BJ, Sadock VA. *Kaplan and Sadock's Comprehensive Textbook of Psychiatry*. 8th ed. Philadelphia: Lippincott Williams & Wilkins; 2005:869–870.

82. Answer: B. The APA Task Force on ECT recommended the following procedures to be carried out prior to the administration of ECT: a psychiatric history and examination that documents the need for ECT, a medical review determining the risks factors and contraindications for ECT, an anesthesia evaluation and clearance for ECT, a written informed consent for the ECT, and an evaluation by the physician administering the ECT. Although not the absolute standard of care for ECT treatments, they may be used as evidence of the standard of care in malpractice suits involving ECT. An evaluation by a judge is necessary only when the treating physicians determine that the patient does not have the capacity to consent for such a procedure.

Sadock BJ, Sadock VA. *Kaplan and Sadock's Comprehensive Textbook of Psychiatry*. 8th ed. Philadelphia: Lippincott Williams & Wilkins; 2005:3973.

83. Answer: D. The patient should be evaluated promptly. Ideally, family members should not be used as interpreters, because they may distort the patient's complaints. Generally, when an interpreter is needed, the person should be a disinterested third party and unknown to the patient. The translator should translate verbatim.

Sadock BJ, Sadock VA. *Kaplan and Sadock's Comprehensive Textbook of Psychiatry*. 8th ed. Philadelphia: Lippincott Williams & Wilkins; 2005:834.

84. Answer: B. Posttraumatic stress disorder is associated with major depression, anxiety disorders (including agoraphobia and panic disorder as well as others), substance use disorder, and other mood disorders.

Of the choices listed, schizophrenia is the one that does not fall into one of those categories of disorders.

1. American Psychiatric Association. *DSM-IV-TR, Diagnostic and Statistical Manual of Mental Disorders*. 4th ed. Washington, DC: American Psychiatric Association; 2000:218–220.
2. Sadock BJ, Sadock VA. *Kaplan and Sadock's Comprehensive Textbook of Psychiatry*. 8th ed. Philadelphia: Lippincott Williams & Wilkins; 2005:1776.

85. Answer: D. "Loose associations" is not considered one of the Schneiderian first-rank symptoms. Schneider's eight first-rank symptoms include: audible thoughts, voices arguing and/or discussing, voices commenting, somatic passivity experiences, thought withdrawal (or other experiences of influenced thought), thought broadcasting, delusional perceptions, and all other experiences involving volition, made affects, and made impulses.

Sadock BJ, Sadock VA. *Kaplan and Sadock's Synopsis of Psychiatry*. 9th ed. Philadelphia: Lippincott Williams & Wilkins; 2003:472–473.

86. Answer: D. The most common locations of imagined defects in Body Dysmorphic Disorder involve the face and hair. Facial flaws, including those involving the nose, eyes, lips, chin, and facial skin are common, in addition to concern about one's hair.

Sadock BJ, Sadock VA. *Kaplan and Sadock's Synopsis of Psychiatry*. 9th ed. Philadelphia: Lippincott Williams & Wilkins; 2003:654.

87. Answer: D. To make the diagnosis of probable Lewy Body Dementia, *two* of the following core features must be present: fluctuating levels of attention and alertness, recurrent visual hallucinations and parkinsonian features (cogwheeling, bradykinesia, and resting tremor). Supporting features include: repeated falls, syncope, sensitivity to neuroleptics, systematized delusions, and hallucinations in other modalities (auditory, tactile, gustatory, etc.).

Sadock BJ, Sadock VA. *Kaplan and Sadock's Comprehensive Textbook of Psychiatry*. 8th ed. Philadelphia: Lippincott Williams & Wilkins; 2005:1084.

88. Answer: C. Increases in dopamine from reuptake blockade can have an antiparkinsonian effect. However, they can also cause psychomotor agitation and aggravation of psychosis. Sertraline appears to have the highest relative potency among antidepressants for blocking the reuptake of dopamine; although it has significant dopamine uptake blocking effects, these are considerably weaker than its serotonin uptake blocking properties. Sertraline has one active metabolite, demethylsertraline, which may continue to exert pharmacological effects once sertraline has been metabolized. Amoxapine has the greatest relative affinity among antidepressants for blocking dopamine receptors.

1. Carrasco JL, Sandner C. Clinical effects of pharmacological variations in selective serotonin reuptake inhibitors: an overview. *Int J Clin Pract*. 2005;59:1428–1434.
2. Tasman A, Kay J, Lieberman JA. *Psychiatry Therapeutics*. 2nd ed. England: John Wiley and Sons; 2003:310–311.

89. Answer: D. St. John's wort is a popular first-line agent for the treatment of mild depression and anxiety in Germany. In the United States, it is considered a food supplement and does not have any FDA approved indications. In several trials, it has not been significantly more effective than placebo in the treatment of major depression. It has mild serotonin reuptake-blocking properties, may inhibit COMT (catechol-O-methyltransferase), and may enhance GABA receptors. The most common side effects are gastrointestinal upset, photodermatitis, and fatigue. There have been rare reports of serotonin syndrome when used alone or with an SSRI and, hence, clinicians are advised against using it with an SSRI. St. John's wort is also an inducer of cytochrome P450 3A3/4 and can enhance the metabolism of protease inhibitors in AIDS patients. Serotonin syndrome is characterized by diaphoresis, hyperthermia, hypertension, tachycardia, nausea, diarrhea, hyperreflexia, myoclonus, restlessness, tremor, incoordination, muscular rigidity (in more severe cases), clonus, seizures, confusion, agitation, anxiety, hypomania, insomnia, hallucinations, and headaches. Patients with anticholinergic toxicity have normal reflexes with mydriasis, agitated delirium, dry oral mucosa, hot-dry-red skin, urinary retention, and absent bowel sounds. Hyperactive bowel sounds, neuromuscular abnormalities, diaphoresis, and normal skin color help distinguish serotonin syndrome from anticholinergic toxicity. Malignant hyperthermia is a pharmacogenetic disorder characterized by increased concentrations of carbon dioxide, hypertonicity, hyperthermia, and metabolic acidosis, which occurs in susceptible individuals within minutes after exposure to inhalational anesthetic agents. Severe skeletal muscle rigidity and hyporeflexia distinguish this condition from serotonin syndrome. NMS is an idiopathic reaction to dopamine antagonists which has a slow onset, bradykinesia/akinesia, "lead pipe" muscular rigidity, hyperthermia, fluctuating consciousness, and autonomic instability. Symptoms of neuroleptic malignant syndrome typically evolve during several days, in contrast to the rapid onset and hyperkinesia of serotonin syndrome. Knowledge of the precipitating drug helps to distinguish between the syndromes (i.e., dopamine antagonists produce bradykinesia, whereas serotonin agonists produce hyperkinesia).

1. Boyer EW, Shannon M. The serotonin syndrome. *N Engl J Med* 2005;352:1112–1120.
2. Schatzberg A, Cole J, DeBattista C. *Manual of Clinical Psychopharmacology*. 5th ed. 2005: 576–579, 582–583.
3. Sternbach H. Serotonin syndrome: how to avoid, identify, and treat dangerous drug interactions. *Curr Psychiatry*. 2003;2:14–24.

90. Answer: A. Initial management includes hydration, cooling blankets, and cardiac and renal function monitoring. Dialysis would not be indicated since antipsychotic medications are highly protein bound and deposit in peripheral tissue. Baclofen, lorazepam, and diphenhydramine are not indicated in the treatment of neuroleptic malignant syndrome. Dantrolene acts as a direct muscle relaxant thus decreasing muscle rigidity, secondary hyperthermia, and tachycardia. Bromocriptine acts centrally and is thought to decrease symptoms associated with neuroleptic malignant syndrome.

Rosenbaum JF, Arana GW, Hyman SE, et al. *Handbook of Psychiatric Drug Therapy*. 5th ed. Philadelphia: Lippincott Williams & Wilkins; 2005:44.

91. Answer: B. Dialectical behavior therapy (DBT) was developed by Marsha Linehan for the treatment of patients with borderline personality disorder. The first-stage hierarchy of primary behavior targets in DBT involves decreasing suicidal behaviors, decreasing therapy-interfering behaviors (such as therapy nonattendance, remaining mute, and extreme hostility), decreasing quality-of-life interfering behaviors (such as substance abuse, high-risk sexual behaviors, and criminal behaviors), then increasing behavioral skills (including core mindfulness, interpersonal effectiveness, emotional regulation, distress tolerance, and self-management).

1. Linehan MM. *Cognitive-Behavioral Treatment of Borderline Personality Disorder*. New York: Guilford Press; 1993:124–179.
2. Sadock BJ, Sadock VA. *Kaplan and Sadock's Synopsis of Psychiatry*. 9th ed. Philadelphia: Lippincott Williams & Wilkins; 2003:954–955.

92. Answer: A. Although it is difficult to predict the response of pain to opioids, some predictors of poor response include the presence of neuropathic pain, phasic pain (e.g., incident pain), cognitive impairment, and high levels of psychological distress in a patient. Another important indicator of poor response is a history of substance abuse. Patients with chronic or tonic pain usually respond better to treatment with opioids.

Barash PG, Cullen BF, Stoelting RK. *Clinical Anesthesia*. 5th ed. Philadelphia: Lippincott Williams & Wilkins; 2006:1459.

93. Answer: D. The next best step would be to check with the patient's insurance company about copayment policy before making the follow-up appointment with your clinic. The AMA policy, E-6.12: Forgiveness or Waiver of Insurance Copayments, states that physicians should be aware that forgiveness or waiver of copayments may violate the policies of some insurers, both public and private; other insurers may permit forgiveness or waiver if they are aware of the reasons for the forgiveness or waiver. Routine forgiveness or waiver of copayments may constitute fraud under state and federal law. Physicians should ensure that their policies on copayments are consistent with applicable law and with the requirements of their agreements with insurers. This patient requires adequate psychiatric follow-up and it needs to be arranged after appropriate consultation with her insurance company.

American Medical Association. Available at http://www. ama-assn.org/apps/pf_new/pf_online? Accessed August 26, 2006.

94. Answer: D. Signs of an UMN lesion include an extensor plantar response (Babinski sign present), weakness, spasticity, rigidity, and hyperactive deep tendon reflexes. Atrophy would be a characteristic of a lower motor neuron lesion as well as hypoactive deep tendon reflexes, the absence of a Babinski sign, weakness, and flaccidity.

Kaufman DM. *Clinical Neurology for Psychiatrists*. 5th ed. Philadelphia: WB Saunders; 2001:5.

95. Answer: E. The basal ganglia is made up of the following nuclei: caudate, globus pallidus, putamen, and ventral striatum. The hypothalamus is considered part of the limbic system and not the basal ganglia.

Stern, TA, Herman, JB. *Massachusetts General Hospital Psychiatry Update and Board Review Preparation*. 2nd ed. New York: McGraw-Hill; 2004:266.

96. Answer: D. Of the five complexes that make up the respiratory chain, cytochrome-C oxidase (complex IV) is the one most often disordered. Its deficient function gives rise to lactic acidosis, seen in many mitochondrial diseases. Also common is mitochondrial clumping in muscle, resulting in the observed "ragged red fibers." Most of the mitochondrial DNA disorders affect the nervous system prominently, at times exclusively. The majority of protein components of the respiratory chain come from nuclear DNA, which allows for Mendelian inheritance of some mitochondrial diseases.

1. DiMauro S, Schon EA. Mitochondrial respiratory-chain diseases. *N Engl J Med*. 2003;348:2656–2668.

2. Ropper A, Brown R. *Adams and Victor's Principles of Neurology*. 8th ed. New York: McGraw-Hill; 2005:798–799, 841–845.

97. Answer E. MRI is now the neuroimaging method of choice for most intracranial and intraspinal lesions. The advantages of MRI are that it provides better soft tissue contrast providing finer definition of anatomic structures and sensitivity to pathologic lesions. It also provides dimensional information and relationship between structures and has the ability to demonstrate physiologic processes such as blood flow and CSF motion. It is also helpful in demonstrating special properties of tissue, such as water diffusion or biochemical makeup using the magnetic resonance spectroscopy (MRS). It is also the neuroimaging method of choice for the visualization of the posterior fossa and intraspinal lesions. The lack of ionizing radiation is also a distinct advantage over the CT scan. Disadvantages of the MRI include the need for patient cooperation; duration (20 minutes to 60 minutes) of imaging process. Contraindications for MRI are the presence of metallic implants like cardiac pacemakers, cochlear implants, older-generation aneurysm clips, metallic foreign bodies in the eye, and implanted neurostimulators.

Rowland LP. *Merritt's Neurology*. 11th ed. Philadelphia: Lippincott Williams & Wilkins; 2005: 73.

98. Answer: D. Functional imaging techniques, such as PET, are useful for localizing the surgical focus in the presurgical evaluation of epileptic patients. PET is especially useful in the evaluation of temporal lobe epilepsy, showing temporal lobe hypometabolism in 60% to 90% of patients with temporal lobe seizures. The sensitivity is 95% when an EEG is used. The yield is considerably lower for extratemporal seizures with a sensitivity of 56% when compared to EEG. Moreover, severe interictal hypometabolism of the affected temporal lobe is associated with better postoperative seizure control, and evidence of extratemporal hypometabolism is associated with postoperative seizures. Last, PET imaging is useful in the evaluation of infantile spasms, showing focal metabolic changes due to cortical dysplasias.

Orrison WW. *Neuroimaging*. Philadelphia: WB Saunders; 2000:934–935.

99. Answer: E. This patient is suffering from a condition known as locked-in syndrome. Locked-in syndrome is caused by the infarction of the corticobulbar and corticospinal tracts in the basis pontis (sparing the tegmentum). There is paralysis of limbs and lower cranial nerves, but patients have intact eye movements. This syndrome is caused by an occlusion of a branch of the basilar artery. Patients are usually awake, alert, and have normal cognition. They are mute because of the bulbar palsy and the quadriplegia is caused by the infarction of the corticospinal tract. They often try to communicate via eye movements. EEG recordings in these patients are usually normal.

1. Kaufman DM. *Clinical Neurology for Psychiatrists*. 5th ed. Philadelphia: WB Saunders; 2001:49, 279.
2. Rowland LP. *Merritt's Neurology*. 11th ed. Philadelphia: Lippincott Williams & Wilkins; 2005:302.

100. **Answer: A**. Traumatic brain injury is responsible of 20% of the cases of symptomatic epilepsy. The most important factor in the development of posttraumatic seizures is the severity of the traumatic brain injury. Other risk factors include focal intracranial lesions and prolonged alteration in consciousness.

1. Garga N, Lowenstein DH. Posttraumatic epilepsy: a major problem in desperate need of major advances. *Epilepsy Curr*. 2006;6:1–5.
2. Salazar AM, Jabbari B, Vance SC, et al. Epilepsy after penetrating head injury. I. Clinical correlates: a report of the Vietnam head injury study. *Neurology*. 1985;35:1406–1414.

101. **Answer: D**. This patient is presenting with the classical clinical picture of Friedrich's ataxia. This illness has an autosomal recessive mode of inheritance and is thought to be due to a mitochondrial overload of iron that impairs mitochondrial respiratory activity. Patients usually develop symptoms during adolescence, which include ataxia, cardiomyopathy, leg weakness, and visual abnormalities. Multiple sclerosis is a white matter disease that is more common in women and frequently presents with painful unilateral impairment in visual acuity or ataxia and is not usually associated with scoliosis. Guillain-Barré syndrome is an acute inflammatory demyelinating polyradiculoneuropathy and consists of ascending weakness and loss of sensation that can end in respiratory depression. It is sometimes preceded by a gastrointestinal or respiratory infection. In amyotrophic lateral sclerosis, there is damage of both upper and lower motor neurons and it tends to occur in older patients. Refsum's disease is a rare entity characterized by retinitis pigmentosa, ataxia, deafness, and bony changes.

1. Gibberd FB, Feher MD, Sidey MC, et al. Smell testing: an additional tool for identification of adult Refsum's disease. *J Neurol Neurosurg Psychiatry*. 2004,75:1334–1363.
2. Goetz C. *Textbook of Clinical Neurology*. 2nd ed. Philadelphia: WB Saunders; 2003:741–756.
3. Kaufman DM. *Clinical Neurology for Psychiatrists*. 5th ed. Philadelphia: WB Saunders; 2001:1–100.

102. **Answer: D**. Spinocerebellar ataxias are a group of autosomal dominant disorders that usually present with progressive ataxia. The cause is an unstable trinucleotide expansion that can present in a diverse range of repeat units. Expansions of DNA repeats are the cause of several disorders including Fragile X syndrome, myotonic dystrophy, Huntington's disease, and the spinocerebellar ataxias.

1. Goetz C. *Textbook of Clinical Neurology*. 2nd ed. Philadelphia: WB Saunders; 2003:741–754.
2. Mirkin SM. DNA structures, repeat expansions and human hereditary disorders. *Curr Opin Struct Biol*. 2006;16:351–358.

103. **Answer: C**. The patient's presentation suggests delirium tremens which requires sedation with benzodiazepines and thiamine supplementation, the latter to prevent the development of WE. Because he is likely to have been subsisting primarily on alcohol rather than a balanced diet, a dietary assessment is essential. The presence of the rash suggests possible pellagra, which can be determined by 24-hour urine 5 HIAA, urinary N-methyl-nicotinamide, urinary pyridone, serum niacin, serum tryptophan, and serum NAD and NADP, all of which may be reduced. Ishii and Nishihara 1 suggest that when an alcoholic patient develops extrapyramidal signs in addition to mental and gastrointestinal symptoms, nicotinic acid deficiency must be suspected even in the absence of skin lesions. Neither a history of alcohol use nor homelessness alone has a strong positive predictive value for a diagnosis of pellagra. Homelessness coupled with alcoholism in patients who do not obtain meals from shelter-based meal programs, however, appears to identify a group at special risk. Psychosocial assessment may be undertaken at a later stage when his symptoms have resolved.

1. Ishii N, Nishihara Y. Pellagra among chronic alcoholics: clinical and pathological study of 20 necropsy cases. *J Neurol Neurosurg Psychiatry*. 1981;44:209–215.
2. Lishman WA. *Organic Psychiatry*. 3rd ed. Boston: Blackwell Science; 1996:573–574.
3. Stefan G Kertesz. Pellagra in 2 Homeless Men. *Mayo Clinic Proc*. 2001;76:315–318.

104. **Answer: B**. The patient has cryptococcal meningitis. Diagnosis is made by culture on Sabouraud's medium, by the detection of a cryptococcal antigen in the CSF, or by negative staining of the fungal capsule by India ink. The treatment is either amphotericin B/flucytosine (to prevent development of flucytosine resistance) or fluconazole, which is considered by several authorities as the drug of choice. Fluconazole should be continued for 3 months after CSF is sterilized, which is considered the best

monitoring endpoint of successful treatment. In relapsing cases, suppressive therapy of 200 mg/day PO of fluconazole is given.

Lewis RP. *Merritt's Neurology*. 11th ed. Philadelphia: Lippincott Williams & Wilkins; 2005:229–230.

105. Answer: D. Advancing age is associated with an increase in the prevalence of sleep disorders. This is also true for REM sleep, which is more frequent but much shorter, resulting in an overall reduction in the total time spent in REM sleep.

Sadock BJ, Kaplan H. *Synopsis of Psychiatry*. 9th ed. Philadelphia: Lippincott Williams & Wilkins; 2003: 1326.

106. Answer: E. The six classic monoamine neurotransmitters are serotonin, epinephrine, norepinephrine, dopamine, acetylcholine, and histamine. The monoamine neurotransmitters are present in only a small percentage of neurons localized in the small nuclei in the brain. The amino acid neurotransmitters on the other hand are widely distributed in the brain. There are more than 100 different putative neuropeptide neurotransmitters that have been identified to date.

Sadock BJ, Sadock VA. *Kaplan and Sadock's Comprehensive Textbook of Psychiatry*. 8th ed. Philadelphia: Lippincott Williams & Wilkins; 2005:1–2.

107. Answer: E. Judgment of line orientation, Rey-Osterreith Complex Figure Test, and Clock drawing are all tests of visuospatial functioning. Judgment of line orientation tests the subject's ability to judge angles of lines on a page presented in a match-to-sample format. Wisconsin Card Sorting Test, Category Test, Trail-Making Test, and Delis-Kaplan Test are all tests of executive functioning. *Executive function* is the term used to explain behaviors and refers to higher-level cognitive abilities that enable an individual to successfully engage in independent goal-directed behavior. These capacities are most commonly linked to the frontal cortex and they guide complex behavior over time through planning, decision making, and self-monitoring of judgments and impulses. Executive functions include planning, initiation of independent activities, sequencing, organizing, abstraction, and response inhibition. Defective executive functioning involves a cluster of deficits and not just one deficit. Deficits are usually associated with damage to the prefrontal cortex, as well as interconnected cortical and subcortical brain structures. Other tests of executive functioning include the Word Fluency Task, Stroop Tests, and the Porteus mazes.

1. Alzheimer's Disease Research Center. Executive func-

tions. Available at http://memory.ucsf.edu/Education/Topics/execfunction.html. Accessed August 30, 2006.
2. Sadock BJ, Sadock VA. *Kaplan and Sadock's Comprehensive Textbook of Psychiatry*. 8th ed. Philadelphia: Lippincott Williams & Wilkins; 2005:869–870.

108. Answer: C. Obtaining a no-harm contract is not an essential part of the suicide risk assessment. Suicide risk assessment is a process and not an event and should be part of all standard psychiatric assessments. It requires frequent updating and should evaluate for risks and protective factors for suicide. These risk assessments have three basic parts including identifying the patient at risk, assessing the overall risk for suicide and providing safety and treatments for these patients at risk.

1. Gutheil TH, Applebaum PS. *Clinical Handbook of Psychiatry and the Law*. 3rd ed. Philadelphia: Lippincott Williams & Wilkins; 2000:63–67, 78–79.
2. Sadock BJ, Sadock VA. *Kaplan and Sadock's Comprehensive Textbook of Psychiatry*. 8th ed. Philadelphia: Lippincott Williams & Wilkins; 2005:3973–3794.

109. Answer: D. Some consider antidepressant-induced mania or hypomania to be a "Bipolar III disorder" (which is not recognized by DSM-IV-TR). Using DSM-IV-TR criteria, this patient is diagnosed with "Bipolar disorder NOS" at this time.

Sadock BJ, Sadock VA. *Kaplan and Sadock's Comprehensive Textbook of Psychiatry*. 8th ed. Philadelphia: Lippincott Williams & Wilkins; 2005:1640.

110. Answer: E. Reaction formation is a defense mechanism usually associated with the anal phase of libidinal development characterized by shame and disgust in relation to anal impulses and pleasures. This process involves the transformation of unacceptable impulses to more acceptable ones to deal with anxiety. It is commonly used by patients with OCD and is categorized as an immature defense mechanism. Psychiatrist and thanatologist, Dr. Elizabeth Kubler-Ross, described five stages in the organization of reactions to impending death, which include shock and denial, anger, bargaining, depression, and acceptance. Although clearly identifiable, there is no definite sequence of events applicable to all these patients.

Kaplan HI, Sadock BJ. *Kaplan & Sadock's Synopsis of Psychiatry*. 8th ed. Philadelphia: Lippincott Williams & Wilkins; 1998:66–67, 219–222.

111. Answer: D. The short duration of her illness to date currently excludes schizophrenia and schizophreniform disorder. The bizarre nature of her delusions (in addition to the duration of her illness) rules out delusional disorder. Although she could ultimately be diagnosed with brief psychotic disorder, the duration of her illness must be less than 1 month and she must show eventual full return to her previous level of functioning. Because her psychotic symptoms have lasted for <1 month, but have not yet remitted, her most accurate current diagnosis would be psychotic disorder NOS.

American Psychiatric Association. *Quick Reference to the Diagnostic Criteria from DSM-IV-TR*. Washington, DC: American Psychiatric Association; 2000:153–165.

112. **Answer: E.** Pseudocyesis, a false belief that one is pregnant (associated with objective signs of pregnancy), is classified in the DSM-IV-TR as a somatoform disorder NOS. Endocrine changes may be present in pseudocyesis, but the syndrome cannot be explained by a general medical condition, which causes endocrine changes (e.g., a hormone-secreting tumor).

American Psychiatric Association. *Quick Reference to the Diagnostic Criteria from DSM-IV-TR*. Washington, DC: American Psychiatric Association; 2000:229–236.

113. **Answer: E.** According to the DSM-IV-TR, patients with anorexia nervosa refuse to maintain a minimally normal weight, demonstrate an intense fear of gaining weight or becoming fat, significantly misinterpret their body, and in postmenarchal females, demonstrate the absence of at least three consecutive menstrual cycles. This patient meets almost all of the criteria for anorexia nervosa (with a body weight of approximately 82% of that expected), but has continued to have regular menses without hormone ingestion. Therefore, her diagnosis would be "Eating Disorder NOS".

1. Sadock BJ, Sadock VA. *Kaplan and Sadock's Synopsis of Psychiatry*. 9th ed. Philadelphia: Lippincott Williams & Wilkins; 2003:739.
2. American Psychiatric Association. *Quick Reference to the Diagnostic Criteria from DSM-IV-TR*. Washington, DC: American Psychiatric Association; 2000:263–266.

114. **Answer: A.** Nortriptyline is a tricyclic antidepressant. There exists a curvilinear relationship between clinical response and nortriptyline serum levels. It is one of the few antidepressants with a clear therapeutic window. Response increases with plasma levels and then plateaus in the range of 50 to 150 ng/mL, with a decrease in response at plasma levels >150 ng/mL. Patients with plasma levels of approximately 150 ng/mL, who are not responding to the agent, may respond to a lowering of dosage and hence of plasma levels into the therapeutic window. Therapeutic levels have been described for other drugs, but they do not seem as clear as those described for nortriptyline.

Schatzberg A, Cole J, DeBattista C. *Manual of Clinical Psychopharmacology*. 5th ed. Washington, DC: American Psychiatric Publishing; 2005:103–105.

115. **Answer: B.** Smoking tobacco lowers antipsychotic blood levels. Therefore, when smoking cessation occurs, levels increase and can worsen side effects associated with antipsychotic medications (i.e., extrapyramidal symptoms (EPS)). Phenytoin (enzyme inducer) lowers antipsychotic blood levels, whereas buspirone and sertraline (enzyme inhibitors) increase blood levels. Use of a hallucinogen would worsen hallucinations and not cause EPS.

Stern TA, Herman JB. *Massachusetts General Hospital Psychiatry Update and Board Preparation*. 2nd ed. New York: McGraw-Hill; 2004:338.

116. **Answer: D.** Risperidone is associated with a substantial increase in prolactin compared to the other listed antipsychotic medications. This increase in prolactin is likely secondary to risperidone's high affinity for D2 antagonism and high $5HT_{2A}$ affinity resulting in galactorrhea and menstrual irregularities in women.

1. Haddad P, Dursun SM. Selecting antipsychotics in schizophrenia: lessons from CATIE. *J Psychopharmacol*. 2006;20:332–334.
2. Rosenbaum JF, Arana GW, Hyman SE, et al. *Handbook of Psychiatric Drug Therapy*. 5th ed. Philadelphia: Lippincott Williams & Wilkins; 2005:36.

117. **Answer: C.** Aversion occurs when a noxious consequence (punishment) is presented immediately after a specific behavioral response. This is done with the goal of inhibiting, and eventually extinguishing, the response. Many types of noxious stimuli have been utilized historically in aversion therapy, including electric shocks and substances that induce vomiting. Disulfiram is an aldehyde dehydrogenase inhibitor that interferes with the metabolism of alcohol. While taking disulfiram, the ingestion of even a small amount of alcohol produces a wide array of unpleasant reactions including sweating, nausea, vomiting, headache, hypotension, flushing, thirst, dyspnea, tachycardia, chest pain, vertigo, and blurred vision.

Sadock BJ, Sadock VA. *Kaplan and Sadock's Synopsis of Psychiatry*. 9th ed. Philadelphia: Lippincott Williams & Wilkins; 2003:412–413,953–954,1046.

118. **Answer: B.** The most possible cause of this man's delirium is too much pain medication post operatively. Propoxyphene hydrochloride is a synthetic opioid that has less potency than the naturally occurring opiates like morphine and codeine. One mg PO of codeine is equivalent to 1.5 mg PO of propoxyphene hydrochloride. The patient was taking 130 mg/day of propoxyphene and has now received a total of 210 mg of codeine (equivalent to 315 mg PO of propoxyphene). Even small increases in pain medication can cause delirium in the elderly, especially

during the postoperative period. There is no aspirin withdrawal syndrome and the chance of this patient having had a stroke event with a negative workup is low. Codeine and propoxyphene are metabolized through the cytochrome P450 system and do not influence the metabolism of each other. If anything, delirium can develop due to accumulation of both drugs in the body.

1. Barash PG, Cullen BF, Stoelting RK. *Clinical Anesthesia*. 5th ed. Philadelphia: Lippincott Williams & Wilkins; 2006:1416–1418.
2. Potter JF. The older orthopaedic patient: general considerations. *Clin Orthop Relat Res*. 2004;425:44–49.

119. **Answer: D.** Suicide, according to Edwin Schneidman, is associated with thwarted or unfulfilled needs, feelings of hopelessness and helplessness, ambivalent conflicts between survival and unbearable stress, a narrowing of perceived options, and a need for escape. More than 30,000 people die by suicide each year in the United States, whereas the number of attempted suicides is estimated to be 650,000. Suicide is ranked as the eighth overall cause of death in the United States. It ranks after heart disease, cancer, cerebrovascular disease, chronic obstructive pulmonary disease, accidents, pneumonia and influenza, and diabetes mellitus. Suicide rates have averaged 12.5 per 100,000 in the 20th century. Suicide rates in the United States are at the midpoint of rates for other industrialized countries. Worldwide, the prime suicide site is the Golden Gate Bridge in San Francisco.

Sadock BJ, Sadock VA. *Kaplan and Sadock's Synopsis of Psychiatry*. 9th ed. Philadelphia: Lippincott Williams & Wilkins; 2003:913–922.

120. **Answer: C.** Diffusion weighted MRI is the most sensitive test for detecting an ischemic infarct within the first few hours of the event. The earliest pathological changes seen in cells that are ischemic are the loss of free diffusion of water across their membrane. This is easily detected by the current generation of MRI scanners using diffusion weighted sequences. Although there may be signs of an acute ischemic infarct on CT within the first few hours, the more commonly seen changes from the development of cytotoxic edema in the infarcted territory are not seen in the first few hours on CT. Contrast enhanced head CT, if used for a perfusion imaging protocol, can detect large territorial ischemic infarcts, but are limited to selected regions of the brain and are less sensitive than diffusion-weighted MRI. If contraindications to MRI exist, such as a pacemaker, CT perfusion may be the next best choice. A cerebral angiogram can detect early is-

chemic infarct due to arterial occlusion but is not the study of choice due to its invasive nature. If catheter directed intra-arterial thrombolysis is indicated by the patient's history and MRI findings, a cerebral angiogram may be the next study performed. Carotid ultrasound is of little use in determining if a patient is having an acute stroke but may be useful in the workup after a stroke has occurred to determine if there are significant atherosclerotic plaques in the carotid arteries.

Brant WE, Clyde HA. *Fundamentals of Diagnostic Radiology*. 2nd ed. Philadelphia: Lippincott Williams & Wilkins; 1999:80–81.

121. **Answer: C.** LSD acts as an agonist at the 5-HT2A receptor and is important in the pathophysiology of hallucinations. Atypical antipsychotic medications block the activity of this receptor, which is thought to contribute to their therapeutic effect in patients with psychosis.

Stern TA, Herman, JB. *Massachusetts General Hospital Psychiatry Update and Board Review Preparation*. 2nd ed. New York: McGraw-Hill; 2004:265.

122. **Answer: C.** Velocardiofacial syndrome is a congenital malformation syndrome, most commonly associated with the microdeletion of band 11 on the long arm of chromosome 22. In most cases (85% to 90%), the syndrome appears to be due to a de novo microdeletion of segment on the long arm of chromosome 22; however, an autosomal inheritance has been described as well. The 22q11 microdeletion supposedly affects the migration of the rostral neural crest from the neuroepithelium to the pharyngeal pouches during organogenesis, leading to anomalies in the thymus, the face, the parathyroids, and the branchial arch artery derivatives. The leading test to diagnose these microdeletions is the fluorescent in situ hybridization (FISH).

1. Driscoll DA. Molecular and genetic aspects of DiGeorge/velocardiofacial syndrome. *Methods Mol Med*. 2006;126:43–55.
2. Vogels A, Verhoeven WM, Tuinier S, et al. The psychopathological phenotype of velo-cardio-facial syndrome. *Ann Genet*. 2002;45:89–95.

123. **Answer: D.** MRIs work by placing patients in a magnetic field, which forces the spin axis of protons to be parallel to the magnetic field. In the brain, the signal is detected from protons in water-containing tissue, and the different water content of various brain tissues leads to signals of different intensities. Generally, MRIs can view neuroanatomy in more detail than a CT, including diseases of the white matter (multiple sclerosis and progressive multifocal

leukoencephalopathy). It has several disadvantages or relative contraindications, when compared to the CT. It takes about 40 minutes, and often precipitates a claustrophobic reaction, which often leads to the premature abortion of the procedure. It is no more effective in diagnosing Alzheimer's disease or AIDS dementia. It may not detect lesions with little or no water, such as some meningiomas. Finally, a CT scan can easily and more rapidly detect intracranial blood and should be the first-line test to detect it, particularly when time is limited.

Kaufman DM. *Clinical Neurology for Psychiatrists*. Philadelphia: WB Saunders; 2001:543–549.

124. Answer: A. Patients with peripheral vertigo usually complain of severe and, often, intermittent vertigo. Nystagmus is always present; it tends to be unidirectional and is never vertical. Patients also frequently complain of hearing loss or tinnitus. There are no intrinsic brain stem signs present in the neurological examination of a patient with peripheral vertigo. In contrast, patients with central vertigo typically present with constant mild vertigo. Nystagmus is not always present, and it can be vertical in nature. Patients rarely complain of hearing loss or tinnitus, and they often present with intrinsic brain stem signs on physical examination.

Aminoff MJ, Greenberg DA, Simon RP. *Clinical Neurology*. 6th ed. New York: McGraw-Hill; 2005:94–120.

125. Answer: E. Neurofibromatosis (NF) was first described by von Recklinghausen in 1882 and is one of the most common single-gene disorders of the central nervous system (CNS), with a prevalence of about 1 in 3,000 population. The hallmark of this disorder is the presence of multiple hyperpigmented marks on the skin known as café au lait spot and multiple neurofibromas. There are two forms of the illness. NF-1 is also known as von Recklinghausen disease or peripheral NF. Neurofibromatosis type 2 (NF-2) is also known as central NF or bilateral acoustic neuroma syndrome. Both NF-1 and NF-2 are autosomal-dominant conditions. The penetrance of NF-1 is almost 100%. Mutations account for approximately 50% of new cases. This condition is found worldwide in all racial and ethnic groups with both sexes being affected equally. The café au lait macule is the pathognomonic lesion and is present in almost all patients. If there are six or more café au lait spots >5 mm in diameter before puberty and >15 mm in diameter after puberty, then they are diagnostic. The spots are usually present at birth and increase in size and number during the first decade of life. They involve the trunk and limbs in a random fashion but tend to spare the face. Pigmented iris hamartomas called Lisch nodules seen on slit lamp examination are pathognomonic and consist of small translucent yellow or brown elevations. They are observed only in NF-1 and increase in number with age and are present in almost all patients older than 20 years. Both sexes are affected equally.

1. Kaufman DM. *Clinical Neurology for Psychiatrists*. 5th ed. Philadelphia: WB Saunders; 2001:49, 330–332.
2. Rowland LP. *Merritt's Neurology*. 11th ed. Philadelphia: Lippincott Williams & Wilkins; 2005: 714–718.

126. Answer: C. The patient's history of anticoagulant use makes him more susceptible to intracranial bleeding. The history of progressive symptomatology over weeks suggests the presence of a subdural hematoma. Chronic subdural hematomas are common in elderly patients and those taking anticoagulants. They are often caused after mild trauma and in patients with a tendency to fall. They usually give rise to headaches, changes in personality, and cognitive problems over a period of weeks or months. Treatment is usually by surgical evacuation. Epidural hematomas are usually associated with temporal bone fracture with injury to the underlying middle meningeal artery. They cause sudden onset of symptoms due to compression of the underlying brain by the rapid expansion of blood. Surgery is usually needed to arrest bleeding or this condition is fatal by causing transtentorial herniation of the brain. Subarachnoid hemorrhage (SAH) is caused by the rupture of a berry aneurysm due to exertion or sexual activity. CT or an MRI of the brain shows blood in subarachnoid space or within the ventricles and a lumbar tap will show blood in the CSF. SAH produces severe headache and nuchal rigidity with minimal other physical findings. The subacute clinical presentation makes the likelihood of a brain tumor a less likely explanation for this patient's symptoms.

1. Kaufman DM. *Clinical Neurology for Psychiatrists*. 5th ed. Philadelphia: WB Saunders; 2001:276–277, 581–595.
2. Rowland LP. *Merritt's Neurology*. 11th ed. Philadelphia: Lippincott Williams & Wilkins; 2005: 483–500.

127. Answer: D. This patient has Ataxia-telangiectasia, an illness with autosomal recessive mode of inheritance which is linked to chromosome 11. Patients usually develop symptoms shortly after starting to walk. Some of the most common symptoms include ataxia, dysarthria, intention tremor of the extremities, and sometimes choreoathetosis. Patients with this disorder have a characteristic facies, which is described as "apathetic" or "sad." Median survival is 25 years and life expectancy does not seem to correlate well with the severity of neurological impairment.

1. Crawford TO, Skolasky RL, Fernandez R, et al. Survival probability in ataxia telangiectasia. *Arch Dis Child.* 2006;91:610–611.
2. Goetz C. *Textbook of Clinical Neurology.* 2nd ed. Philadelphia: WB Saunders; 2003:741–756.

128. **Answer: E.** Symptoms of myasthenia gravis develop due to antibodies directed against the acetylcholine receptor (AChR) or against the MuSK. Patients present with fluctuating muscle weakness, which improves with rest. Patients usually present with drooping eyelids, blurred vision, or diplopia after prolonged reading or later on in the day. Ptosis is the presenting symptom in more than 50% of patients with blurring of vision seen in about 15% of patients. Diplopia is seen in 90% to 95% of the patients with myasthenia gravis during the course of their illness. One third of patients may present with dysphagia and dysarthria. Proximal limb weakness is seen in 20% to 30% of patients with 3% of the patients presenting with predominant distal weakness. Head drop due to weakness of the neck extensor muscles is rare, but respiratory failure due to weakness of the diaphragm and accessory muscles of respiration can occur in some patients. Bulbar and or respiratory weakness without ocular involvement is more common in patients with MuSK antibodies. This weakness usually peaks within the first 3 years of the illness. Severe respiratory and bulbar weakness can develop in absence of ocular or extremity weakness. Patients with only mild weakness may respond to anticholinesterase medications and do not need treatment with immunosuppressive or immunomodulating agents.

Samuels MA. *Manual of Neurologic Therapeutics.* 7th ed. Philadelphia: Lippincott Williams & Wilkins; 2004:260–265.

129. **Answer: C.** Pellagra is the late stage of severe niacin or vitamin B_3 deficiency. Pellagra can be either primary or secondary. Primary pellagra results from inadequate nicotinic acid (i.e., niacin) or tryptophan in the diet (long-term parenteral nutrition without appropriate niacin substitution). Secondary pellagra occurs when adequate quantities of niacin are present in the diet, but other diseases or conditions interfere with niacin absorption and/or processing. Examples of these conditions include prolonged diarrhea, chronic alcoholism, chronic dialysis treatment, chronic colitis, particularly ulcerative colitis or regional enteritis, cirrhosis of the liver, tuberculosis of the gastrointestinal (GI) tract, malignant carcinoid tumour, Hartnup syndrome (an inborn error of tryptophan metabolism), anorexia nervosa, HIV, and drug related (e.g., isoniazid, 5-fluorouracil, and aza-

thioprine). The classical symptoms of pellagra are diarrhoea, dementia, and dermatitis. Death can occur if untreated. Dactylitis (inflammation of the digits) is not a feature of pellagra.

Lishman WA. *Organic Psychiatry.* 3rd ed. Boston: Blackwell Science; 1996:573–574.

130. **Answer: B.** Lamotrigine is a newer antiepileptic effective as a first-line treatment for generalized and focal seizures. It is also FDA approved for bipolar depression. It selectively blocks the slow sodium channel, preventing the release of excitatory neurotransmitters. The main limitation is a serious rash in 1% of patients, as well as more minor rashes in 12%. The minor rash is typically maculopapular on the trunk, but more severe rashes can occur, such as Steven's Johnson syndrome. There is a high degree of cross reactivity for this side effect among the aromatic antiepileptics (phenytoin, carbamazepine, phenobarbital, primidone, and lamotrigine). Although most of the rashes are not life threatening, one should switch to an agent from another class. Both gabapentin and valproic acid are *not* aromatic compounds, but only valproic acid is effective as monotherapy for primary generalized epilepsy. One should be cautious in concurrent use of lamotrigine and valproic acid, because valproic acid inhibits the P-450 enzymes that metabolize lamotrigine.

Ropper AH, Brown RH. *Adams and Victor's Principles of Neurology.* 8th ed. New York: McGraw-Hill; 2005:295–296.

131. **Answer: A.** Elder abuse is commonly seen in approximately 10% of elderly Americans. They may take the form of physical, psychological, financial, or material abuse or neglect. The victims are usually very old and frail. The abusers are often financially dependant on and live with the victim. Usually, the abusers and the victims deny or minimize the abuse. Family conflict and other social problems are commonly seen in these situations.

Sadock BJ, Kaplan H. *Synopsis of Psychiatry.* 9th ed. Philadelphia: Lippincott Williams & Wilkins; 2003:1328.

132. **Answer: E.** B-cell and macrophage immune responses are not affected by either sided neocortical lesions. Experiments that were done in the early 1960s showed that lesions of the anterior hypothalamus resulted in decreases in the thymic and splenic cell numbers, splenic mitogen responsiveness, antigen responsiveness, and the natural killer cell activation. Bilateral lesions of the hippocampus and the amygdala resulted in an increase in the thymic and splenic mitogen responsiveness but with no change in thymic or splenic cell number. Left-sided neocortical lesions have been associated with decreases in

splenic T-cell numbers, T-cell mitogen proliferation, T-cell cytotoxicity, and the NKCA. These changes are not associated with or are enhanced by the right-sided lesions.

Sadock BJ, Sadock, VA. *Kaplan and Sadock's Comprehensive Textbook of Psychiatry*. 8th ed. Philadelphia: Lippincott Williams & Wilkins; 2005:148.

133. Answer: A. Suicide no-harm contracts have no legal validity. They are designed to encourage patients to ask for help rather than to commit suicide. They can be oral or written. However, they should never replace an adequate suicide risk assessment for a psychiatric patient. They may be clinically helpful in strengthening the alliance between a patient and his/her psychiatrist. Some patients may refuse to sign a contract to stay longer in the hospital.

Sadock BJ, Sadock VA. *Kaplan and Sadock's Comprehensive Textbook of Psychiatry*. 8th ed. Philadelphia: Lippincott Williams & Wilkins; 2005:3974.

134. Answer: D. The SARS is a scale to assess severity of extrapyramidal side effects. HAM-D, YMRS, BDI, and MADRS are all scales to assess the severity of mood symptoms.

1. Carmody TJ, Rush AJ, Bernstein I, et al. The Montgomery Asberg and the Hamilton ratings of depression: a comparison of measures. *Eur Neuropsychopharmacol*. 2006 Dec;16(8):606–611.
2. Sadock BJ, Sadock VA. *Kaplan and Sadock's Comprehensive Textbook of Psychiatry*. 8th ed. Philadelphia: Lippincott Williams & Wilkins; 2005:931, 943, 945.

135. Answer: A. According to DSM-IV-TR, nightmare disorder is classified as a parasomnia. The category of dyssomnia includes narcolepsy, circadian rhythm sleep disorder, primary insomnia, primary hypersomnia, breathing-related sleep disorder, and dyssomnia NOS. Parasomnias include nightmare disorder, sleep terror disorder, sleepwalking disorder, and parasomnias NOS.

American Psychiatric Association. *Quick Reference to the Diagnostic Criteria from DSM-IV-TR*. Washington, DC: American Psychiatric Association; 2000:267–279.

136. Answer: A. Advancing age (not young age), sensory impairment, family history of delusional disorder, social isolation, and recent immigration are all considered to be risk factors associated with delusional disorder.

Sadock BJ, Sadock VA. *Kaplan and Sadock's Synopsis of Psychiatry*. 9th ed. Philadelphia: Lippincott Williams & Wilkins; 2003:513.

137. Answer: B. Paraphilias are characterized by a significant deviation in the erotic stimulus or activity which is a precondition for sexual excitement and orgasm. However, the sexual response is preserved in these patients. In paraphilias, the sexual excitement is contingent on the acting out of a specific fantasy that is unusual or bizarre. Sigmund Freud initially described paraphilias as "perversions" characterized by a distortion in the sexual aim or object. They are much more commonly seen in men with masochism, sadism, and fetishism being the commonly seen paraphilias in individual psychiatric practices. In clinics that treat sex offenders, the most commonly encountered paraphilias are pedophilia, voyeurism, and exhibitionism. DSM-IV-TR describes the essential features of a paraphilia as recurrent, intense sexually arousing fantasies, sexual urges, or behaviors generally involving nonhuman objects, the suffering or humiliation of oneself, partner, children, or other nonconsenting persons that occur over a period of at least 6 months.

1. American Psychiatric Association. *Quick Reference to the Diagnostic Criteria from DSM-IV-TR*. Washington, DC: American Psychiatric Association; 2000:255–259.
2. Sadock BJ, Sadock VA. *Kaplan and Sadock's Comprehensive Textbook of Psychiatry*. 8th ed. Philadelphia: Lippincott Williams & Wilkins; 2005:1966–1971.

138. Answer: D. The current research criteria for binge eating disorder include all of the above except D. Binge eating is not associated with the regular use of inappropriate compensatory behaviors such as purging, fasting, and inappropriate exercise. Binge eating episodes must also be accompanied by three (or more) of the following: (i) eating much more rapidly than normal, (ii) eating until feeling uncomfortably full, (iii) eating large amounts of food when not feeling physically hungry, (iv) eating alone because of being embarrassed by how much one is eating, and (v) feeling disgusted with oneself, depressed, or very guilty after overeating.

Sadock BJ, Sadock VA. *Kaplan and Sadock's Synopsis of Psychiatry*. 9th ed. Philadelphia: Lippincott Williams & Wilkins; 2003:750.

139. Answer: C. Amitriptyline is a tricyclic antidepressant. It is classified as a tertiary amine, along with imipramine, trimipramine, doxepin, and clomipramine because it has two methyl groups on the nitrogen atom of the side chain. Amitriptyline is one of the most anticholinergic medications in this class. Anticholinergic side effects include dry mouth, constipation, blurred vision, and urinary retention. Severe anticholinergic effects can lead to an anticholinergic syndrome characterized by confusion and delirium. The elderly are more sensitive to possible anticholinergic side effects. This patient has no evidence in her history of alcohol withdrawal. Additionally, her vital signs are stable. Although fentanyl is a psychoactive agent, she has been stable on it for many months. Finally, there is no evidence at this time for occult infection or brain metastases, though both of these could contribute to an altered mental status.

Sadock BJ, Sadock VA. *Kaplan and Sadock's Synopsis of Psychiatry*. 9th ed. Philadelphia: Lippincott Williams & Wilkins; 2002:1127–1128.

140. Answer: E. A single dose of benztropine usually brings relief, however, if even after 20 minutes the dystonia continues to persist, a repeat dose of benztropine should be given. Although dantrolene and baclofen are muscle relaxants, they have not been shown to treat acute dystonic reactions. Lorazepam should be given if the patient does not respond to the second dose of benztropine. Propranolol is not considered a treatment for acute dystonic reactions.

Rosenbaum JF, Arana GW, Hyman SE, et al. *Handbook of Psychiatric Drug Therapy*. 5th ed. Philadelphia: Lippincott Williams & Wilkins; 2005:40–41.

141. Answer: A. Although discontinuation rates for all antipsychotic medications in the CATIE trial were high (74% of the total sample discontinued before 18 months), time to discontinuation for any reason as well as for lack of efficacy was greatest with olanzapine.

Haddad P, Dursun SM. Selecting antipsychotics in schizophrenia: lessons from CATIE. *J Psychopharmacol*. 2006;20:332–334.

142. Answer: D. Partial reinforcement occurs when a response is reinforced only a fraction of the amount of times the behavior occurs. VLTs and slot machines are based upon the concept of partial reinforcement. The individual is kept guessing as to when a payoff will occur. Classical conditioning results from the repeated pairing of a neutral stimulus with one that evokes a response, such that the neutral stimulus eventually comes to evoke the response on its own. Negative reinforcement occurs when a response which leads to the removal of an aversive event is increased. Continuous reinforcement, unlike partial reinforcement, occurs when every response is reinforced, rather than only a fraction of responses. Punishment occurs when an aversive consequence is presented specifically to suppress an undesirable response.

Sadock BJ, Sadock VA. *Kaplan and Sadock's Synopsis of Psychiatry*. 9th ed. Philadelphia: Lippincott Williams & Wilkins; 2003:143–146.

143. Answer: D. Clozapine-induced sialorrhea is a socially stigmatizing side effect, resulting in poor compliance. It develops early in treatment, may be dose related, and is worst during sleep, causing sleep disturbances and, thereby, fatigue. Excessive salivation proximal to the vocal cords can cause dysphonia, and distal to them can cause a chronic cough.

1. Lieberman JA, Safferman AZ. Clinical profile of clozapine: adverse reactions and agranulocytosis. *Psychiatr Q*. 1992;63:51–70.
2. Praharaj SK, Arora M, Gandotra S. Clozapine-induced sialorrhea: pathophysiology and management strategies. *Psychopharmacol (Berl)*. 2006;185:265–273.

144. Answer: B. Anosognosia (ignorance of illness) is part of hemi-inattention, which is due to a lesion involving the nondominant parietal lobe.

Kaufman DM. *Clinical Neurology for Psychiatrists*. 5th ed. Philadelphia: WB Saunders; 2001:187–189.

145. Answer: E. All of the above pairings are correct except for choice E. Cholinergic neurons are located in both the basal forebrain and brainstem. Dopaminergic neurons are located in both the substantia nigra and ventral tegmental area.

Stern TA, Herman JB. *Massachusetts General Hospital Psychiatry Update and Board Review Preparation*. 2nd ed. New York: McGraw-Hill; 2004:265.

146. Answer: C. PET is an imaging technique that introduces a synthetic radionucleotide of potential biological relevance to a person's body. Most compelling, is the ability to provide noninvasive measurements of local neuronal activity, neurochemistry, and pharmacology of the living human brain. PET scans measure the decay of positrons from the radionucleotide. When a positron is ejected from the nucleus, it soon collides with an electron, and in this annihilation, emits two photons that are equivalent in energy and traveling 180 degrees apart. It is the annihilation location that is actually measured. The synthetic radionucleotide can be ingested, inhaled, or injected intravenously, depending on what it is.

Malison RT, Laruelle M, Innis RB. *Positron and Single Photon Emission Tomography. Psychopharmacology: The Fourth Generation of Progress*. New York: Raven Press; 1995:86.

147. Answer: B. Sensory ataxia is secondary to disorders that disturb proprioceptive pathways in peripheral sensory nerves, sensory roots, posterior columns, or medial lemnisci. It usually produces gait disturbances in a symmetric fashion. The arms are usually affected less or not at all. Patients usually do not present with nystagmus, dysarthria, or vertigo. They are frequently able to stand with their feet together while their eyes are open, but become unsteady when asked to close their eyes (Romberg sign). Vibratory and position sense are frequently impaired and ankle reflexes are diminished or absent.

Aminoff MJ, Greenberg DA, Simon RP. *Clinical Neurology.* 6th ed. New York: McGraw-Hill; 2005:94–120.

148. Answer: B. Medical therapy can be helpful in reducing the risk of stroke. For thrombotic stroke, aspirin is probably the most consistently effective treatment, but probably only reduces the risk by 13%. In patients who cannot tolerate aspirin, the platelet aggregate inhibitor clopidogrel or a similar drug (such as ticlopidine or dipyridamole) can be substituted. It is important not to exaggerate the magnitude of their effects. It appears that both dosages are effective and that the addition of dipyridamole further reduces the risk of stroke by a small amount. Ticlopidine and clopidogrel are believed by some, on the basis of clinical trials, to be marginally more effective than aspirin for the prevention of stroke, but they are far more expensive, and ticlopidine is potentially toxic (neutropenia). The cumulative evidence from trials with aspirin alone indicates that a dose of aspirin of at least 30 mg/day reduces by 13%, at most, the progression or recurrence of stroke. The best course of treatment for patients who have lacunar or atherothrombotic strokes while already receiving antiplatelet medications is not clear. Control of blood pressure is recommended. The administration of a lipid lowering drug is advisable, even if lipid levels are normal. The risk of stroke from chronic atrial fibrillation can be reduced by warfarin treatment.

1. Algra A, VanGijn J, Algra A, et al. Secondary prevention after cerebral ischemia of presumed arterial origin: is aspirin still the touchstone? *J Neurol Neurosurg Psychiatry.* 1999;66:557–559.
2. Ropper AH, Brown RH. *Adams and Victor's Principles of Neurology.* 8th ed. New York: McGraw-Hill; 2005:5–296.
3. Singer DE, Nathan DM, Fogel HA, et al. Randomized trials of warfarin for atrial fibrillation. *N Engl J Med.* 1992;327:1451–1453.

149. Answer: E. Approximately 30% to 50% of normally aged individuals show no evidence of neuropathological changes. However, most elderly individuals show some evidence of such changes. Neuritic plaques, neurofibrillary tangles, and cortical atrophy can all be seen in the brains of normal, healthy elderly individuals. When compared to the brains of elderly individuals with dementia, however, these changes are generally much less severe and extensive.

Blazer DG, Steffens DC, Busse EW. *American Psychiatric Publishing Textbook of Geriatric Psychiatry.* 3rd ed. Washington, DC: American Psychiatric Publishing; 2004:69.

150. Answer: C. There is no change in the percentage of natural killer cells (NKC) in chronic stress and major depression. There is also no change in the number of monocytes or the CD4 to CD8 ratio in either chronic stress or major depression. In chronic stress, there is a reduction in the number of B and T lymphocytes, but this change is not seen in major depression.

Sadock BJ, Sadock, VA. *Kaplan and Sadock's Comprehensive Textbook of Psychiatry.* 8th ed. Philadelphia: Lippincott Williams & Wilkins; 2005:149.

151. Answer: A. The Wechsler Adult Intelligence Scale (Third Edition) is considered the gold standard for the assessment of general level of functioning. It can be used in subjects from ages 16 to 89 and it provides a verbal intelligence quotient (VIQ), performance intelligence quotient (PIQ) and a full-scale intelligence quotient (IQ). The Shipley Scale is a brief test that evaluates vocabulary and open ended verbal abstraction. The California Verbal Learning Test evaluates encoding, recognition, immediate, and 30-minute recall. The Delis-Kaplan Test primarily tests for executive functions. The Fuld's Memory Test assesses retrieval, storage, and the ability to benefit from cues.

Sadock BJ, Sadock VA. *Kaplan and Sadock's Comprehensive Textbook of Psychiatry.* 8th ed. Philadelphia: Lippincott Williams & Wilkins; 2005:860–875.

152. Answer: C. The DSM-IV-TR does not define a withdrawal syndrome for caffeine, hallucinogens, inhalants, cannabis, or phencyclidine. All substance classes listed in the DSM-IV-TR have an intoxication syndrome, except for nicotine.

American Psychiatric Association. *Quick Reference to the Diagnostic Criteria from DSM-IV-TR.* Washington, DC: American Psychiatric Association; 2000:105–151.

153. Answer: A. The normal adult sexual response cycle as described by Masters and Johnson (EPOR model) included the following phases: the excitation (E) phase (stimuli from somatogenic or psychogenic sources raise sexual tensions), the plateau (P) phase (sexual tensions intensified), the orgasmic (O) phase (involuntary pleasurable climax), and finally the resolution (R) phase (dissipation of sexual tensions). Helen Kaplan, a New York sex therapist proposed the currently accepted Desire Excitation Orgasmic Resolution (DEOR) model which described the following phases: desire, excitation, orgasmic, and resolution. Males have a refractory period after ejaculation and cannot usually have an erection or another ejaculation until some time has passed. This period varies with age and can last from minutes to days depending on the age of the individual. It is thought to be due to an inhibitory mechanism in the brain. Unlike men, women don't have a refractory period after an orgasm and hence can be multi-orgasmic. Latency is not described as a part of any sexual response cycle model.

Gelder MG, Lopez-Ibor JJ, Andreasen N. *New Oxford Textbook of Psychiatry*. New York: Oxford University Press; 2000:877.

154. Answer: E. All of the above statements are true regarding the diagnosis of factitious disorder using the DSM-IV-TR criteria. The three predominant types of factitious disorders are: (i) with predominantly psychological signs and symptoms, if psychological signs and symptoms predominate in the clinical presentation (300.16); (ii) with predominantly physical signs and symptoms, if physical signs and symptoms predominate the clinical presentation (300.19); and (iii) with combined psychological and physical signs and symptoms, if psychological and physical signs and symptoms are present, but neither predominates the clinical presentation (300.19).

American Psychiatric Association. *Quick Reference to the Diagnostic Criteria from DSM-IV-TR*. Washington, DC: American Psychiatric Association; 2000:237–238.

155. Answer: C. Patients with anorexia nervosa often experience cold, but not heat, intolerance. Numerous medical complications of eating disorders have been identified, including hypothermia, weakness, orthostatic hypotension, acrocyanosis, shortness of breath, arrhythmias, seizures, peripheral neuropathies, edema, muscle cramping, bloating, constipation, parotid hyperplasia, lanugo, xerosis, carotenoderma, dental caries, gingivitis, fertility problems, and osteoporosis.

1. American Psychiatric Association. *Treating Eating Disorders: A Quick Reference Guide & Practice Guideline for the Treatment of Patients with Eating Disorders*. 9th ed. Washington, DC: American Psychiatric Association; 2006:230–235.
2. Sadock BJ, Sadock VA. *Kaplan and Sadock's Synopsis of Psychiatry*. 9th ed. Philadelphia: Lippincott Williams & Wilkins; 2003:741–742.

156. Answer: E. Fluoxetine was the first SSRI approved in the United States, in 1988, and exhibits the longest half-life of all the SSRIs. Since then, it has been FDA approved for the treatment of major depressive disorder, OCD, bulimia nervosa, premenstrual dysphoric disorder (marketed under the trade name Sarafem), panic disorder, and posttraumatic stress disorder. It has not been approved for generalized anxiety disorder. In January 2003, the FDA approved fluoxetine for pediatric use in depression and OCD. Fluoxetine is the only SSRI approved for the treatment of depression in children.

1. Schatzberg A, Cole J, DeBattista C. *Manual of Clinical Psychopharmacology*. 5th ed. Washington, DC: American Psychiatric Publishing; 2005:44–51.
2. U.S. Food and Drug Administration. FDA approves Prozac for pediatric use to treat depression and OCD. *FDA Talk Paper*. Available at http://www.fda.gov/bbs/topics/ANSWERS/2003/ANS01187.html. Accessed August 30, 2006.

157. Answer: B. Carbamazepine is used as a second- or third-line mood stabilizer for the treatment of bipolar and schizoaffective disorders, but its use is often limited by its side effect profile. Specifically, carbamazepine is a CYP450 inducer and will decrease the blood levels of many medications, including haloperidol, which in this patient, caused the return of his auditory hallucinations. Valproate is one of the only anticonvulsants that does not interfere with the CYP450 enzyme system and thus would not decrease the level of haloperidol and worsen psychosis. Although levels of warfarin would be decreased by the concomitant administration of carbamazepine, this would not result in worsening psychosis. Atorvastatin and hydrochlorothiazide would not affect the CYP450 system or psychosis.

Stern TA, Herman, JB. *Massachusetts General Hospital Psychiatry Update and Board Preparation*. 2nd ed. New York: McGraw-Hill; 2004:338.

158. Answer: A. Discontinuation rates due to weight gain and metabolic effects were greatest in patients treated with olanzapine, as compared to other groups (9% vs. 1% to 4%). Weight gain of greater than 7% of baseline was greatest in patients treated with olanzapine compared to other groups (30% vs. 7% to 16%). Patients treated with ziprasidone were least likely to gain weight and experience metabolic effects from antipsychotic medications.

Haddad P, Dursun SM. Selecting antipsychotics in schizophrenia: lessons from CATIE. *J Psychopharmacol*. 2006;20:332–334.

159. Answer: B. Lithium and sodium compete for reabsorption at the level of the proximal convoluted tubule in the kidney. Hydrochlorothiazide blocks the reabsorption of sodium at the distal convoluted tubule resulting in sodium depletion and greater reabsorption of lithium and thus increased potential for lithium toxicity. Any condition resulting in sodium depletion (e.g., dehydration, sodium restricted diet, or use of sodium wasting diuretics) can predispose patients to lithium toxicity. Calcium channel blockers, beta blockers, and angiotensinogen receptor blockers are all acceptable antihypertensive treatments for patients taking lithium.

Rosenbaum JF, Arana GW, Hyman SE, et al. *Handbook of*

Psychiatric Drug Therapy. 5th ed. Philadelphia: Lippincott Williams & Wilkins; 2005:123, 148.

160. Answer: E. To avoid withdrawal symptoms while discontinuing benzodiazepines, a gradual taper is recommended. Choices A through D are all associated with an increased intensity of benzodiazepine withdrawal symptoms. Switching from a short half-life agent to a long half-life agent before tapering may facilitate gradual benzodiazepine discontinuation.

Levenson JL. *Textbook of Psychosomatic Medicine*. Washington, DC: American Psychiatric Publishing; 2005:891.

161. Answer: C. This patient is presenting with symptoms of cerebellar dysfunction which include incoordination, an intention tremor, dysdiadochokinesia (inability to perform rapid alternating movements), ataxic gait, and scanning speech. Scanning speech differs from aphasia in that aphasia is a disorder of speech and language generation and understanding, while scanning speech is a dysarthria which is difficulty in articulating speech. Paresis, an increase in deep tendon reflexes, and a homonymous hemianopsia would not be seen with cerebellar lesions.

Kaufman DM. *Clinical Neurology for Psychiatrists*. 5th ed. Philadelphia: WB Saunders; 2001:20.

162. Answer: A. Biofeedback is the process by which patients learn to control certain involuntary physiological responses such as blood vessel vasoconstriction, cardiac rhythm, and heart rate. Biofeedback and related techniques have been shown to be useful in the management of such conditions as tension headaches, migraines, and Raynaud's disease.

Sadock BJ, Sadock VA. *Kaplan and Sadock's Synopsis of Psychiatry*. 9th ed. Philadelphia: Lippincott Williams & Wilkins; 2003:838, 843.

163. Answer: D. It can be ethically challenging if patients withhold consent to share information that would help a patient's relatives. Huntington's disease is a movement disorder, characterized by choreatic movements, transmitted as an autosomal dominant trait with the affected gene being on the short arm of chromosome 4. The patient's siblings have at least a 25% risk to develop Huntington's disease, and it would be clearly beneficial for the siblings to know, both for their personal health and in family planning. However, opinions in the United States do not support disclosure without permission. The ethical way to proceed would be to educate the patient on Huntington's disease and to discuss the patient's reasons for not wanting to discuss the diagnosis. The patient might be ashamed of the disease, or may not understand the implications of genetic disease. Choice A is

incorrect because it would be unethical to accept the patient's decision at face value, without attempting to understand it. Choice C is incorrect because this is only a potential risk to the patient's siblings. Choice E is premature.

1. Clayton EW. Ethical, legal, and social implications of genomic medicine. *N Engl J Med*. 2003;349:562–569.
2. Williams JK, Skirton H, Masny A. Ethics, policy, and educational issues in genetic testing. *J Nurs Scholarsh*. 2006;38:119–125

164. Answer: B. In general, there is an increase in sympathetic nervous activity in the elderly individual. Higher circulating levels of norepinephrine fill the surface cell receptors of the heart and vascular system, making them less sensitive. This results in a lower maximum heart rate and decreased cardiac contractility. With age, blood vessels become thicker and less distensible, and systolic blood pressure increases. Due to this increase in afterload, as well as the decreased contractility of the heart, there is an overall decline in cardiac output in the elderly individual.

Blazer DG, Steffens DC, Busse EW. *American Psychiatric Publishing Textbook of Geriatric Psychiatry*. 3rd ed. Washington, DC: American Psychiatric Publishing; 2004:39.

165. Answer: A. While thyroid hormone receptor reception dysfunction was once to be implicated in attention deficit and hyperactivity syndrome, subsequent studies have failed to confirm this relationship. Multiple studies have now shown that deficiencies in the dopamine receptor and transporter genes are likely involved in this disorder.

1. Rauch SL, Madras BK, Fischman AJ. Dopamine transporter density in patients with attention deficit hyperactivity disorder. *Lancet*. 1999;354:2132–2133.
2. Sadock BJ, Sadock VA. *Kaplan and Sadock's Comprehensive Textbook of Psychiatry*. 8th ed. Philadelphia: Lippincott Williams & Wilkins; 2005:3184–3185.

166. Answer: E. The Wisconsin Card Sorting Test is designed to test executive functioning, which includes volition, planning, purposive action, and execution. The prefrontal lobes and their connections primarily control these functions. Some of the aspects of language that are usually tested include fluency, comprehension and repetition. Tests such as the Boston Diagnostic Aphasia Examination or the Boston Naming Test are commonly used to evaluate language problems. Retrieval and storage of information are usually tested with tasks that require a multiple-choice format. The Wechsler Memory Scale assesses encoding, retrieval, and recognition of different types of material. Attention is required for almost all areas of functioning. The digit span and the Wechsler Memory Scales evaluate different measures of attention. Visuospatial problems can be seen when there is right or left hemispheric damage. A common test to assess for visuospatial problems is the Rey-Osterreich Complex Figure test, also known as the clock-drawing test.

Sadock BJ, Sadock VA. *Kaplan and Sadock's Comprehensive Textbook of Psychiatry*. 8th ed. Philadelphia: Lippincott Williams & Wilkins; 2005:860–875.

167. **Answer: A.** Their availability, legal status, and low cost have contributed to the current use of inhalants amongst the young and the poor. According to the DSM-IV-TR, inhalant intoxication includes the presence of maladaptive behavioral or psychological changes and two or more physical signs including dizziness, nystagmus, incoordination, slurred speech, unsteady gait, lethargy, depressed reflexes, generalized muscle weakness, and diplopia.

1. American Psychiatric Association. *Quick Reference to the Diagnostic Criteria from DSM-IV-TR*. Washington, DC: American Psychiatric Association; 2000:105–151.
2. Sadock BJ, Sadock VA. *Kaplan and Sadock's Synopsis of Psychiatry*. 9th ed. Philadelphia: Lippincott Williams & Wilkins; 2003:440–442.

168. **Answer: A.** Gender identity is an individual's perception and awareness of being a male or female. Gender role is the group of behaviors that an individual engages in that identifies him or her to others as being a male or female. Sexual orientation is the erotic attraction that is felt by an individual. Biological factors including prenatal hormones that are thought to play a role in the differentiation of the mammalian brain and contribute to the development of gender role behaviors do not appear to contribute to gender identity. Gender identity is generally established by the age of 3 years and it appears to depend on the sex in which an individual is reared. Gender identity, once firmly established, is very resistant to change. Ambiguous physical appearance of the child and inconsistent rearing regarding the actual gender of the child results in confusion regarding their gender identity later in life. Psychoanalytic theory describes the development of gender identity as part of the general identity formation during the separation and individuation phase and is thought to be dependent on the quality of the mother–child dyad. Learning theory describes the development of gender identity when the child imitates or identifies with the same-sex parent and this behavior is reinforced by engaging in the appropriate sex-role behaviors.

Hales RE, Yudofsky SC. *American Psychiatric Publishing Textbook of Clinical Psychiatry*. 4th ed. Washington, DC: American Psychiatric Publishing; 2003.

169. **Answer: E.** Munchausen syndrome represents approximately 10% of all cases of factitious disorder. The term Munchausen syndrome was first used by Richard Asher in 1951. It is also known as chronic factitious disorder with predominantly physical signs and symptoms with the two terms being used interchangeably. Patients with Munchausen syndrome are more severely ill than patients with factitious disorder and have a worse prognosis than these patients. In patients with Munchausen syndrome, the factitious illness has become a behavior, disrupting their regular functioning (i.e., social, occupational, and personal relationships). These patients are constantly seeking medical attention and are often known as hospital hoboes, hospital addicts, or professional patients. Their presentation is usually characterized by pseudological fantastica (i.e., the telling of fascinating but untrue stories) and peregrination (i.e., excessive traveling around).

Sadock BJ, Sadock VA. *Kaplan and Sadock's Comprehensive Textbook of Psychiatry*. 8th ed. Philadelphia: Lippincott Williams & Wilkins; 2005:1829.

170. **Answer: B.** The BMI is a measure which may be used to determine a person's level of obesity. The BMI is traditionally calculated by dividing weight in kilograms by height in meters squared. Alternatively, it may be calculated by dividing weight in pounds by height in inches squared, then multiplying this number by 703. Although there is some debate about the ideal BMI, generally values <18.5 are considered to be underweight, 18.5 to 24.9 healthy weight, 25 to 29.9 overweight, and >30 obese. Generally speaking, increasing weight for a given height reflects increasing obesity (body fat), but not always. Muscular individuals may be "overweight," but not have an excess of body fat. It is also possible for a person to have a "healthy" weight, but have high body fat.

Sadock BJ, Sadock VA. *Kaplan and Sadock's Synopsis of Psychiatry*. 9th ed. Philadelphia: Lippincott Williams & Wilkins; 2003:751.

171. **Answer: D.** Ziprasidone has the shortest half-life (t 1/ 2) among all atypical antipsychotics. Its t 1/2 is about 4 hours compared to olanzapine (t 1/2 = 21 to 50 hours), risperidone (t 1/2 = 3 to 20 hours), quetiapine (t 1/2 = 6 hours), and clozapine (t 1/2 = 11 hours).

Albers LJ, Hahn RK, Reist C. *Handbook of Psychiatric Drugs*. Laguna Hills: Current Clinical Strategies Publishing; 2005:42–48.

172. Answer: D. Antipsychotic medications that are most likely to increase the QTc interval are thioridazine, mesoridazine and pimozide especially when used in combination with medications known to increase the QTc interval, such as quinolone antibiotics.

Rosenbaum JF, Arana GW, Hyman SE, et al. *Handbook of Psychiatric Drug Therapy*. 5th ed. Philadephia: Lippincott Williams & Wilkins; 2005:46–47.

173. Answer: A. The drug in question is gamma hydroxy butyric acid (GHB), which attains peak plasma levels within 40 minutes of oral ingestion and causes rapid loss of consciousness. It also causes respiratory depression, myoclonus, bradycardia, and deep coma. Recovery is usually rapid and uneventful. There is no antidote and management is supportive. Although it is clinically indistinguishable from benzodiazepine overdose or ethanol overdose, the characteristic clinical picture, and the rapid onset of coma following oral ingestion supports the suspicion of GHB overdose. Although physostigmine has been reported to cause reversal of clinical signs, there is no evidence to support its use in overdose treatment.

1. Chin RL, Sporer KA, Cullison B, et al. Clinical course of gammahydroxybutyrate overdose. *Ann Emerg Med*. 1998;31:716–722.
2. Okun MS, Boothby LA, Bartfield RB, et al. GHB: an important pharmacologic and clinical update. *J Pharm Pharm Sci*. 2001;4:167–175.
3. Snead OC 3rd, Gibson KM. Gamma-hydroxybutyric acid. *N Engl J Med*. 2005;352:2721–2732.

174. Answer: A. Diuretics have a paradoxical effect on lithium induced polyuria and result in deceased urine output. Amiloride, a potassium sparing diuretic, can help to decrease urine volume in patients with lithium induced polyuria without adversely effecting lithium or potassium levels. Benztropine has anticholinergic properties and may cause urinary retention; however, it has no role in the reduction of urine output. All other listed treatments also do not have a role in decreasing urine output. Kegel exercises may be helpful for women with urinary stress incontinence. Bladder training is a behavioral technique used to treat people who have stress incontinence, urge incontinence, or a combination of the two. Oxybutynin is an antispasmodic agent and is used in the treatment of urge incontinence.

Rosenbaum JF, Arana GW, Hyman SE, et al. *Handbook of Psychiatric Drug Therapy*. 5th ed. Philadephia: Lippincott Williams & Wilkins; 2005:141.

175. Answer: A. In the elderly, benzodiazepines with long half lives (e.g., diazepam, clonazepam, and flurazepam) should be avoided. Benzodiazepines with acceptable half-lives which do not increase

with age include lorazepam and oxazepam. These anxiolytics have minimal drug interactions and no active metabolites. Lorazepam may be administered orally or intravenously, and is also absorbed well intramuscularly.

Blazer DG, Steffens DC, Busse EW. *American Psychiatric Publishing Textbook of Geriatric Psychiatry*. 3rd ed. Washington, DC: American Psychiatric Publishing; 2004:399–400.

176. Answer: D. Although nonspecific to multiple sclerosis, oligoclonal bands may be found in the cerebrospinal fluid of patients suffering from MS. In the CSF of patients with MS, glucose is typically normal, protein may be normal or slightly elevated, and white blood cells may be normal or slightly elevated.

Neuroland. Multiple sclerosis. Available at http://www.neuroland.com/ms/ms_overview.htm. Accessed September 3, 2006.

177. Answer: E. Relaxation, imagery, hypnosis, and meditation can be utilized as primary or adjunctive treatments for chronic pain. These techniques require motivation on the part of the patient and often, commitment to a daily practice regime. Although the efficacy data for these therapies has been mixed, their use may lessen patients' suffering. Aversion therapy utilizes the pairing of a noxious stimulus with a specific behavioral response, with the aim of inhibiting and eventually extinguishing the unwanted behavior. This technique is not used in the management of chronic pain.

1. Rolak LA. *Neurology Secrets*. 2nd ed. Philadelphia: Hanley & Belfus; 1998:258.
2. Sadock BJ, Sadock VA. *Kaplan and Sadock's Synopsis of Psychiatry*. 9th ed. Philadelphia: Lippincott Williams & Wilkins; 2003:953.

178. Answer: A. Fragile X syndrome is the most common inherited cause of mental retardation. It presents with cognitive deficits and physical symptoms as described above with macroorchidism (postpuberty), hyperextensible joints, and soft skin. It affects males more commonly, but both sexes can be affected. It is caused by an unstable trinucleotide repeat in the FMR-1 gene on the X chromosome, and transmitted by X-linked inheritance. The normal gene is distinguished from the mutation by the number of CGG repeats, approximately divided as follows: normal/intermediate 6 to 60, premutation 61 to 200, full mutation >200. Premutation individuals are almost always unaffected intellectually. Full mutation carrier mothers have a 50% chance of passing the full mutation on to their sons (eliminating choice C). Daughters will inherit one X chromosome from each parent, and will only be carriers if they inherit a normal X chromosome from their father. A male with full mutation cannot pass it on to his son, but his daughters will all be carriers. The transmission pattern is made more complicated by the tendency of the number of repeats in the premutation gene to expand, especially when transmitted from the mother. Expansion during transmission from father to daughter is less likely, as the expansion rate is much less. It is possible that the mother in this case was carrying a premutation that expanded to full mutation in the patient. The brothers may only inherit the premutation. Early intervention education programs are the treatment of choice.

Visootsak J, Warren ST, Anido A, et al. Fragile X syndrome: an update and review for the primary pediatrician. *Clin Pediatr.* 2005;44:371–381.

179. Answer: B. In the ECA study, alcohol abuse or dependence was identified in 13.5% of the study population, which included both community and institutional samples. *Kaplan and Sadock's Synopsis of Psychiatry* lists lifetime prevalence figures as follows: alcohol abuse (10% of women and 20% of men) and alcohol dependence (3% to 5% of women and 10% of men).

1. Reiger DA, Farmer ME, Rae DS, et al. Comorbidity of mental disorders with alcohol and other drug abuse. *JAMA.* 1990;264:2511–2518.
2. Sadock BJ, Sadock VA. *Kaplan and Sadock's Synopsis of Psychiatry.* 9th ed. Philadelphia: Lippincott Williams & Wilkins; 2003:396.

180. Answer: B. Among women with any sexual difficulty, 64% (range:16% to 75%) experienced desire difficulty, 35% (range: 16% to 48%) experienced orgasm difficulty with 31% (range: 12% to 64%) experiencing arousal difficulty, and 26% (range: 7% to 58%) experienced sexual pain. Of the sexual difficulties that occurred for 1 month or more in the previous year, 62% to 89% persisted for at least several months and 25% to 28% persisted for 6 months or more. Between 21% and 67% of women with sexual difficulty were distressed by it.

Hayes RD, Bennett CM, Fairley CK, et al. What can prevalence studies tell us about female sexual difficulty and dysfunction? *J Sex Med.* 2006;3:589–595.

181. Answer: A. Splitting, primitive idealization, projective identification, turning against the self, marked fear of abandonment, impaired object constancy, intense object hunger, unresolved rapprochement subphase of separation-individuation, failure of internal structuralization, and control are all psychodynamic features seen in patients with borderline personality disorder.

Sadock BJ, Sadock VA. *Kaplan and Sadock's Pocket Hand-*

book of Clinical Psychiatry. 3rd ed. Philadelphia: Lippincott Williams & Wilkins; 2001:250.

182. Answer: A. Depression is most commonly comorbid with Anorexia Nervosa (50% to 75% of cases). Bipolar Disorder is generally found in 4% to 6% of cases, but has been quoted as high as 13%. OCD is thought to be comorbid in approximately 25% of cases. Among other anxiety disorders, social phobia is particularly common (approximately 35%). In patients with Anorexia Nervosa, estimates of those with co-morbid substance abuse range from 12% to 18%.

1. American Psychiatric Association. *Practice Guideline for the Treatment of Patients with Eating Disorders.* 3rd ed. Washington, DC: American Psychiatric Association; 2006:70–72.
2. Sadock BJ, Sadock VA. *Kaplan and Sadock's Synopsis of Psychiatry.* 9th ed. Philadelphia: Lippincott Williams & Wilkins; 2003:744.

183. Answer: A. The Human MAO system consists of two isoforms of MAO: MAO-A and MAO-B. MAO-A metabolizes serotonin (5-HT) and norepinephrine (NE). MAO-B metabolizes phenylethylamine and benzylamine. Dopamine and tyramine are metabolized equally by both forms. MAO-A is located in the GI system in much greater concentrations than MAO-B and is therefore primarily responsible for metabolizing dietary tyramine into inactive substances. When peripheral MAO-A is inhibited by at least 80%, tyramine is not metabolized. It can then enter the circulatory system and cause significant release of NE. The result can be a severe hypertensive reaction that typically occurs within 10 minutes and can last up to 2 hours after a meal. At low doses (5 to 10 mg/day), oral selegiline irreversibly and selectively inhibits MAO-B while avoiding inhibition of GI MAO-A. This eliminates the need for dietary restrictions. At higher doses (>20 mg/day), it achieves an antidepressant effect but loses its selectivity for MAO. Animal studies have shown that doses of STS that inhibit activity of both MAO-A and MAO-B in the brain by >90% only partially inhibit GI MAO, with a maximal 40% inhibition of MAO-A and 70% to 75% inhibition of MAO-B. Tyramine challenge studies have demonstrated that STS 6 mg/day is equivalent to oral selegiline 10 mg/day in pressor response. Therefore, STS 6 mg/day does not require any dietary restrictions. However, dietary modifications are required with STS 9 mg/day and 12 mg/day.

Patkar AA, Pae C-U, Masand PS. Transdermal selegiline: the new generation of monoamine oxidase inhibitors. *CNS Spectr.* 2006;11:363–375.

184. Answer: C. Phencyclidine (PCP) is synthesized using piperazine, cyclohexane, and potassium cyanide. It blocks NMDA–type receptors of the excitatory neurotransmitter glutamate. Release of monoamines from storage sites in axon terminals and inhibition of reuptake of monoamines are mechanisms of action of amphetamines and cocaine, respectively. Increasing the flow of chloride ions by binding to the GABA receptor complex is the mechanism of action of benzodiazepines. Phosphodiesterase inhibition is a mechanism of action of caffeine.

Sadock BJ, Sadock VA. *Kaplan and Sadock's Comprehensive Textbook of Psychiatry*. 8th ed. Philadelphia: Lippincott Williams & Wilkins; 2005: 1191, 1203, 1223, 1300–1301.

185. Answer: E. Meprobamate, chloral hydrate, and ethchlorvynol are drugs that have little or no role in modern therapeutics. However, in New York, there is a reported increase in the prescription for these drugs. These older sedative-hypnotics drugs are similar in effect to the barbiturates and lead to tolerance and physiological dependence. Their withdrawal syndrome is also similar to the barbiturate withdrawal syndrome and protocols used for barbiturate withdrawal should be used for the safe withdrawal in patients dependent on these drugs. These drugs should not be used in acute intermittent porphyria as they exacerbate the symptoms. Chlorpromazine is safe to be used in acute intermittent porphyria.

1. Sadock BJ, Sadock VA. *Kaplan and Sadock's Comprehensive Textbook of Psychiatry*. 8th ed. Philadelphia: Lippincott Williams & Wilkins; 2005:1312.
2. Tishler PV. The effect of therapeutic drugs and other pharmacologic agents on activity of porphobilinogen deaminase, the enzyme that is deficient in intermittent acute porphyria. *Life Sci*. 1999;65:207–214.

186. Answer: A. Severe lithium toxicity can result in permanent neurological adverse effects including cerebellar ataxia and anterograde amnesia. Tremor, peripheral neuropathy, downbeat nystagmus, and benign intracranial hypertension are all nontoxic effects from lithium therapy and will abate when lithium therapy is discontinued.

1. Rosenbaum JF, Arana GW, Hyman SE, et al. *Handbook of Psychiatric Drug Therapy*. 5th ed. Philadelphia: Lippincott Williams & Wilkins; 2005:147.
2. Sadock BJ, Sadock VA. *Kaplan & Sadock's Comprehensive Textbook of Psychiatry*. 8th ed. Philadelphia: Lippincott Williams & Wilkins; 2005:31,17.

187. Answer: C. Although the starting dose for the treatment of OCD is the same as the starting dose for the treatment of depression, the maintenance dose required for OCD is generally higher than that required for depression. The onset of response is typically slower in OCD than in depression, with anywhere from 12 to 26 weeks being required to assess whether a response will be seen. Target symptoms do not usually worsen before they improve once an SSRI is initiated. Some patients respond better to one SSRI than to another; if a patient fails to respond to one agent in this class, it may be worth considering a trial of another.

Stahl SM. *Essential Psychopharmacology: Neuroscientific Basis and Practical Applications*. New York: Cambridge University Press; 2000:343–344.

188. Answer: D. Large doses of Pyridoxine (vitamin B_6) can cause a progressive peripheral neuropathy. Deficiency of the other vitamins included above, can cause neuropathy.

Beers MH, Berkow R. *The Merck Manual of Diagnosis and Therapy*. 17th ed. New Jersey: Merck & Co.; 1999:33–50.

189. Answer: B. In patients with Alzheimer's disease (AD), the atrophy of the brain is more pronounced over the temporoparietal junction and the limbic areas, especially in the hippocampus with relative sparing of cortical areas governing motor, sensory, and visual functioning. The plaques and tangles are also more commonly seen in the cortical association areas (temporoparietal junction) and hippocampus.

1. Kaufman DM. *Clinical Neurology for Psychiatrists*. 5th ed. Philadelphia: WB Saunders; 2001:136.
2. Rowland LP. *Merritt's Neurology*. 11th ed. Philadelphia: Lippincott Williams & Wilkins; 2005:772–773.

190. Answer: C. The patient has myasthenia gravis, an autoimmune disease in which antibodies are directed against nicotinic acetylcholine receptors, thus leading to muscular weakness, with effects in particular on ocular and facial muscles. Edrophonium is used to confirm the diagnosis of myasthenia gravis and works by inhibiting acetylcholinesterase, which metabolizes acetylcholine, thus maintaining acetylcholine in the neuromuscular junction.

1. Kaufman DM. *Clinical Neurology for Psychiatrists*. 5th ed. Philadelphia: WB Saunders; 2001:95–97.
2. Zaidat OO, Lerner AJ. *The Little Black Book of Neurology*. 4th ed. St. Louis: Mosby; 2002: 235–236.

191. Answer: B. Motivational interviewing, as described by William Miller and Stephen Rollnick, incorporates four general principles: expressing empathy, developing discrepancy, rolling with resistance, and supporting self-efficacy. Although giving advice is a component of some brief intervention techniques like feedback, responsibility, advice, menu, empathy, and self-efficacy (FRAMES), it is not one of the principles of motivational interviewing.

Miller WR, Rollnick S. *Motivational Interviewing: Preparing People for Change*. 2nd ed. New York: Guilford Press; 2002:36–41.

192. Answer. C. Community samples indicate a current prevalence of 0% to 3% for male orgasmic disorder, 0% to 5% for erectile disorder, and 0% to 3% for male hypoactive sexual desire disorder. Pooling the current and 1-year figures provides a community prevalence estimate of about 4% to 5% for premature ejaculation. Sexual pain disorders are much less common in men with a community sample estimating the prevalence to be approximately 0.2%.

Simons JS, Carey MP. Prevalence of sexual dysfunctions: results from a decade of research. *Arch Sex Behav.* 2001;30:177–219.

193. Answer: C. DSM-IV-TR describes schizotypal personality disorder as being characterized by a pervasive pattern of social and interpersonal deficits marked by acute discomfort with, and reduced capacity for, close relationships as well as by cognitive or perceptual distortions and eccentricities of behavior, beginning by early adulthood and present in a variety of contexts, as indicated by five (or more) of the following: ideas of reference (excluding delusions of reference), odd beliefs or magical thinking that influences behavior and is inconsistent with sub-cultural norms (e.g., being superstitious, belief in clairvoyance, telepathy, or "sixth sense"; in children and adolescents, bizarre fantasies or preoccupations), unusual perceptual experiences, including bodily illusions, odd thinking and speech (e.g., vague, circumstantial, metaphorical, overelaborate, or stereotyped), suspiciousness or paranoid ideation, inappropriate or constricted affect, behavior or appearance that is odd, eccentric, or peculiar, lack of close friends or confidants other than first-degree relatives, excessive social anxiety that does not diminish with familiarity and tends to be associated with paranoid fears rather than negative judgments about self. These should not occur exclusively during the course of Schizophrenia, a Mood Disorder with psychotic features, another psychotic disorder, or a pervasive developmental disorder.

Quick Reference to the Diagnostic Criteria from DSM-IV-TR. Washington DC: American Psychiatric Association, 2000:290–291.

194. Answer: A. Covert video surveillance can record evidence of parent-inflicted harm, or can reveal a very concerned mother transforming into an indifferent one. Reviewing collateral information is another means, although not the gold standard.

Sadock BJ, Sadock VA. *Kaplan and Sadock's Comprehensive Textbook of Psychiatry.* 8th ed. Philadelphia: Lippincott Williams & Wilkins; 2005:1838.

195. Answer: D. Café au lait spots may be found in at least 10% of the population, although more than six spots that are larger than 1.5 centimeters, are strongly suggestive of neurofibromatosis. Lisch nodules, and not individual café au lait spots, are pathognomonic of neurofibromatosis. Neurofibromas are subcutaneous growths along peripheral nerves, and the Lisch nodules are yellow to brown nodules on the iris. NF-1 is inherited in an autosomal dominant pattern, but it can also develop without a prior family history of the disease. Large neurofibromas can compress the spinal cord, nerve roots, or the cauda equina.

Kaufman DM. *Clinical Neurology for Psychiatrists.* 5th ed. Philadelphia: WB Saunders; 2001:330–331.

196. Answer: E. In the neuronal signaling pathway, the generation of cAMP is controlled by the balance between the activity of adenylyl cyclase, its synthetic enzyme and phosphodiesterase, which breaks down cAMP into adenosine monophosphate (AMP), its inactive product. Enzyme, adenylyl cyclase is regulated by adapter proteins called G proteins. These G proteins bind guanosine triphosphate (GTP) when the receptor is activated. The GTP is then converted to guanosine diphosphate (GDP), by GTPase. There are two different classes of G proteins referred to as G_s or G_i, depending on whether they stimulate or inhibit cAMP formation. cAMP-dependent protein kinase is also called as PKA. The transcription regulatory factor that enables elevations in cAMP to regulate gene expression is called cAMP response element binding (CREB) protein. cAMP causes longer-lasting changes in neuronal function as a result of its ability to activate CREB by controlling the expression of specific target genes.

1. Nair A, Vaidya VA. Cyclic AMP response element binding protein and brain-derived neurotrophic factor: molecules that modulate our mood? *J Biosci.* 2006;31:423–434.
2. Sadock BJ, Sadock VA. *Kaplan and Sadock's Comprehensive Textbook of Psychiatry.* 8th ed. Philadelphia: Lippincott Williams & Wilkins; 2005:90.

197. Answer: A. Isoniazid inhibits the metabolism of phenytoin, and so its addition leads to an increase in the level of phenytoin. Therefore, one would want to decrease the dose of phenytoin. Cimetidine also inhibits the metabolism of phenytoin and so it should not be started with the INH. There is no indication for polypharmacy with carbamazepine at this time. When carbamazepine is given with phenytoin, it can induce the metabolism of phenytoin and reduce its blood level.

Katzung, BG. *Basic and Clinical Pharmacology.* 8th ed. New York: McGraw-Hill; 2001:399.

198. Answer: C. This patient is showing signs and symptoms of phenytoin toxicity, which generally occurs with levels >20 mcg/mL. These include ataxia, confusion, weakness, tremor, slurred speech, nystagmus, diplopia, nausea, vomiting, bradycardia, tachycardia, hypotension, lethargy, and coma. Case reports support the potential for fluoxetine to raise phenytoin levels via P450 related inhibition of phenytoin metabolism. Alcohol use increases the metabolism of phenytoin, resulting in decreased levels and increased risk for seizure. The patient's presentation is not typical for a seizure or panic attack. Although drug or alcohol intoxication is less likely in this scenario, these must be ruled out as well.

Ford MD, Delancy KA, Ling LJ. *Clinical Toxicology*. 1st ed. St. Louis: WB Saunders: 2003: 488–489.

199. Answer: A. Use of valproate and other anticonvulsants during pregnancy is classically associated with significantly increased risk of neural tube defects. Other fetal effects include abnormal facies, cleft lip and palate, cognitive deficits. Limb phocomelia or amelia (very short or absent long bones) is associated with intrauterine exposure to thalidomide, which was used in the late 1950s and early 1960s as a seda-

tive and hypnotic. Ebstein's anomaly of the heart has been linked to lithium exposure, yellow or brown staining of the teeth to antibiotic exposure, and uterine abnormalities (as well as clear cell adenocarcinoma of the cervix and vagina) to diethylstilbestrol exposure.

1. Ford MD, Delancy KA, Ling LJ. *Clinical Toxicology*. 1st ed. St. Louis: WB Saunders; 2003:103t.
2. Stenchever MA, Droegemueller W, Herbst AL, Mishell DR. *Comprehensive Gynecology*. 4th ed. St. Louis: Mosby; 2001:407–408.

200. Answer: B. LP is useful in the diagnosis of meningitis. Characteristic CSF profiles can suggest viral versus bacterial etiology. Although the CSF during a multiple sclerosis exacerbation classically shows oligoclonal bands and myelin basic protein, these are not specific findings and may be seen in other central nervous system (CNS) chronic inflammatory illnesses. LP is contraindicated where there is a suspicion of an intracranial mass because of the risk of transtentorial herniation. LP does not have a diagnostic role in Alzheimer's disease or Huntington's disease.

Kaufman DM. *Clinical Neurology for Psychiatrists*. 5th ed. Philadelphia: WB Saunders; 2001:377, 532–533.

Questions

1. A healthy 85-year-old woman without dementia presents to her primary care physician's office for her annual physical exam. Her physician performs a brief cognitive examination. All of the following may be expected findings in the cognitive examination of this patient EXCEPT:
   A. Reduced ability to sustain attention over long periods
   B. Increased time required to learn new information
   C. Decline in short-term, or working, memory
   D. Reduced motor speed and response times
   E. Difficulty performing visuospatial tasks

2. The hydroxylation of tryptophan is the rate limiting step in the production of which neurotransmitter?
   A. Histamine
   B. Epinephrine
   C. Serotonin
   D. Dopamine
   E. Acetylcholine (ACh)

3. Which one of the following is NOT a test of language?
   A. Boston Naming Test (Revised)
   B. Verbal fluency
   C. Token Test
   D. Boston Diagnostic Aphasia Examination
   E. California Verbal Learning Test II

4. Which one of the following statements regarding a psychiatrist's responsibility is NOT TRUE when their patient makes threats of harm toward others?
   A. The psychiatrist only has a duty to warn the concerned parties.
   B. The psychiatrist also has a duty to protect the concerned parties.
   C. There is no national law specifying the psychiatrist's duty to prevent harm to others.
   D. Most state statutes provide immunity for disclosures made to prevent harm to others.
   E. Most state statutes require an actual threat made against a clearly identifiable victim before a psychiatrist can act to prevent harm to others.

5. A 35-year-old patient is performing the Rey–Österreicher Complex Figure Test. When evaluating the patient's drawing, you notice that he is able to draw the global framework of the design, but he forgets to draw the details. Where would you locate the dysfunction?
   A. Right hemisphere
   B. Left hemisphere
   C. Both hemispheres
   D. Amygdala
   E. Putamen

6. A father brings his 11-year-old son to a well-child visit at the child's pediatrician's office. When asked how the child is doing, the father mentions that his son has difficulty finishing his meals, because he spends so much time arranging his food on his plate. The father has also observed the patient clearing his throat many times a day. The patient reports that he has an urge to clear his throat even when he doesn't need to and feels anxious if his food is not exactly the right way. Based on the comorbidity suggested by this history, when doing an assessment, you expect that you would be more likely to hear about all of the following EXCEPT:
   A. The patient always arranges his belongings in order from increasing to decreasing size.
   B. The patient has to chew each bite of his meal 10 times.
   C. The patient is concerned that if he doesn't arrange his food in the right order, his parents might die.
   D. The patient must arrange his vegetables in a way that forms a perfect circle.
   E. The patient must always touch his bedpost many times before falling asleep.

7. You perform an initial evaluation on a 9-year-old boy brought in by his frustrated parents for increasing behavioral problems occurring at home over the past year, which are now occurring in school as well. They complain that their child frequently does not listen to their commands and will not give in when they attempt to negotiate with him. He does not come when called repeatedly for family dinners and breaks other house rules, which he previously kept. When confronted by his parents, he shouts at them. He has never hurt the family cat or other animals, and he has never been in trouble with the law. He gets into verbal fights more frequently with his older sister as he puts the blame on her for not doing her chores. At

times, he persistently teases her until she loses her temper. School teachers recently sent reports home stating that they "miss the old Tommy." Despite his relatively good academic performance, he is more angry and argumentative with teachers, and he gets easily annoyed with his peers. When asked, the child denies that he has been sad, anxious, or acting differently, but says that his parents and teachers have been more "harsh" on him during this school year. What is the best axis I diagnosis for the child at this time?

A. Disruptive Behavior Disorder, Not Otherwise Specified (NOS)
B. Oppositional Defiant Disorder (ODD)
C. Conduct Disorder
D. Attention-Deficit/Hyperactivity Disorder (ADHD)
E. Child antisocial behavior

8. Which one of the following conditions is NOT associated with autism?

A. Huntington's disease
B. Tuberous sclerosis
C. Epilepsy
D. Fragile X syndrome
E. Down syndrome

9. Which one of the following choices represents the most common psychiatric comorbidity in patients with eating disorders?

A. Depression
B. Substance abuse
C. General Anxiety Disorder
D. Obsessive Compulsive Disorder (OCD)
E. Panic Attacks

10. Which of the following statements regarding buspirone is FALSE?

A. It is the single $5HT_{1A}$ agonist approved for the treatment of anxiety.
B. It is not associated with a risk of abuse or dependence.
C. The time to onset of anxiolytic effect is similar to that of antidepressants.
D. It has significant pharmacokinetic drug interactions.
E. It may have a role as an augmenting agent for the treatment of resistant depression.

11. When used in the treatment of alcohol dependence naltrexone is associated with all of the following EXCEPT:

A. Reduced relapse to excessive alcohol use
B. Reduced percentage of days in which alcohol drinking occurs
C. Reduced craving for alcohol

D. Increased abstinence rates
E. Nausea as a major side effect

12. Which one of the following medications is NOT used for the treatment of lithium-induced polyuria or nephrogenic diabetes insipidus (NDI)?

A. Hydrochlorothiazide
B. Amiloride
C. Indomethacin
D. Furosemide
E. Ketoprofen

13. Which one of the following is NOT TRUE of hyperthyroidism and psychiatric disorders?

A. Patients may develop a major depressive episode.
B. In severe cases, psychosis can also occur.
C. Hyperthyroidism occurs seven times more frequently in males than females.
D. In the elderly, it is usually manifested by lethargy, apathy, social withdrawal, and overtly depressed mood.
E. In hyperthyroidism, mania is much less commonly seen than agitated depression.

14. Which one of the following alcohol-dependent patients is the best candidate for disulfiram?

A. A 25-year-old sexually active woman who has missed two menstrual cycles
B. A 40-year-old man with schizophrenia who is hospitalized for acute exacerbation of psychosis
C. A 70-year-old man with renal failure
D. A 35-year-old employed mother with depression who recently relapsed after 5 years of sobriety
E. A 50-year-old man who is of post–myocardial infarction status

15. Which one of the following is the best indicator of increased risk of suicide?

A. Alcohol Dependence
B. Marriage
C. Schizophrenia
D. Previous suicidal behavior
E. Major Depressive Disorder

16. Which one of the following statements regarding the cyclic guanosine monophosphate (cGMP) system is NOT TRUE?

A. Stimulation of the cGMP system is mediated via G-protein coupling.
B. Stimulation of the cGMP system is mediated by calcium via nitric oxide production.
C. One of the main functions of the cGMP system is to mediate the response of photoreceptor cells to light.

D. Light mediates its action on the cGMP system by activation of enzyme phosphodiesterase.

E. Sildenafil (Viagra) exerts its vasodilatory effects by blocking cGMP phosphodiesterase in smooth muscle.

17. Which one of the following statements regarding the noradrenergic system in the brain is NOT TRUE?

A. Norepinephrine-producing neurons are found in the brain at the locus ceruleus (LC) and the lateral tegmental noradrenergic nuclei.

B. The LC provides the major noradrenergic projections to the neocortex, hippocampus, thalamus, and midbrain tectum.

C. The activity of LC neurons is highest when the subject is asleep.

D. Novel and stressful stimuli result in the maximal noradrenergic neuronal firing, and this leads to the disruption of ongoing behavior and reorientation of attention.

E. Projections from lateral tegmental nucleus innervate the amygdala, septum, hypothalamus and lower brainstem, and the spinal cord.

18. Metachromatic Leukodystrophy is classified as a "rare disease." According to the Office of Rare Diseases of the National Institute of Health, which of the following represents the number of people in the U.S. population that a rare disease effects?

A. Less than one person per 50,000
B. Less than one person per 100,000
C. Less than one person per 150,000
D. Less than one person per 200,000
E. Less than one person per 250,000

19. Which of the following is a characteristic of the gait seen in cerebellar ataxia?

A. Patients tend to lift the legs high off the ground.

B. Patients tend to deviate to the opposite side of the lesion when walking in a straight line.

C. Patients often exhibit marked lurching movements without losing balance.

D. Oscillation of the head or trunk is commonly present.

E. Patients usually slap the feet down heavily on the floor when walking.

20. Which one of the following is NOT TRUE of magnetic resonance imaging (MRI) of the brain and spinal cord?

A. MRI is the neuroimaging method of choice for most intracranial and intraspinal abnormalities.

B. It provides better definition of anatomic structures and greater sensitivity to pathologic lesions.

C. Its multiplanar capability displays dimensional information and relationships that are not readily available on computer tomography (CT).

D. It demonstrates physiologic processes, such as blood flow and cerebrospinal fluid (CSF) motion, better than a CT scan.

E. It only requires minimal cooperation from the patient.

21. Which one of the following statements regarding tuberous sclerosis is NOT TRUE?

A. It arises spontaneously and through autosomal recessive inheritance.

B. The mutations arise in chromosomes 9 and 16.

C. Adenoma sebaceum and shagreen patches are unique to this condition.

D. Two thirds of patients have mental retardation ranging from mild to severe retardation.

E. Death is due to seizures, tumors, or renal disease.

22. A 48-year-old man presents to his primary care doctor for an appointment with a complaint that began 1 day ago. On examination, he has loss of his right nasolabial fold and loss of his normal forehead folds on his right side. Which one of the following is TRUE of this condition?

A. Concurrent impairment of taste is rare.
B. Most cases are caused by viral agents.
C. The majority of patients never recover.
D. Acute onset is rare.
E. There are no tests that are helpful in prognosis.

23. The police bring a 52-year-old man into the emergency room (ER) for bizarre behavior. During an interview, the patient claims that God has chosen him for a special mission on Earth. The patient's past history is unknown. Exam reveals hyperactive reflexes, disorientation, inability to do serial sevens, and small irregular pupils. His CSF is clear and shows a protein level of 97 mg/dL, glucose of 60, and 67 lymphocytes/mL. The CSF Venereal Disease Research Laboratory (VDRL) test is negative. What is the most likely diagnosis?

A. Meningococcal meningitis
B. Symptomatic neurosyphilis
C. Bipolar Disorder
D. Alzheimer's disease
E. Wernicke's encephalopathy

24. Which one of the following is the commonest neuropsychiatric manifestation of systemic lupus erythematosus (SLE)?

A. Mild Cognitive Impairment (MCI)
B. Psychosis
C. Depression

D. Anxiety

E. Organic brain syndromes

25. Which one of the following is NOT a typical feature of Parkinson's disease?

    A. Resting tremor
    B. Intention tremor
    C. Bradykinesia
    D. Rigidity
    E. Masked facies

26. A 68-year-old divorced man with a longstanding history of cigarette smoking and hypertension is brought to the emergency department (ED) with profound right-sided weakness and difficulty speaking. He was discovered in this state by his daughter, who is the patient's main social contact and usually visits him at his home once per week. Brain imaging demonstrates infarction of the left hemisphere. He has no significant neurological or psychiatric history. A comprehensive management plan for this patient would likely include all but which of the following?

    A. Physical therapy
    B. Frequent orientation
    C. Repositioning
    D. Cognitive therapy
    E. Speech therapy

27. A 75-year-old man tells his psychotherapist that he is able to look back on his life as a college professor, father, and grandfather with pride and a sense of accomplishment. He is at which stage in Erikson's theory of development across the lifespan?

    A. Industry versus inferiority
    B. Integrity versus despair
    C. Initiative versus guilt
    D. Intimacy versus isolation
    E. Generativity versus stagnation

28. Which subtype of the serotonin receptor is thought to be most responsible for the regulation of mood?

    A. $5\text{-}HT_{1A}$
    B. $5\text{-}HT_{1D}$
    C. $5\text{-}HT_{2A}$
    D. $5\text{-}HT_{2B}$
    E. $5\text{-}HT_{1F}$

29. Which one of the following neuropsychological deficits is NOT seen in left hemispheric damage?

    A. Aphasia
    B. Hemineglect
    C. Right–left disorientation
    D. Finger agnosia
    E. Limb apraxia

30. What is the lifetime prevalence of Alcohol Dependence in the general population?

    A. 1%
    B. 5%
    C. 15%
    D. 40%
    E. 60%

31. Which area of the brain is primarily being tested during the Clock-drawing Test?

    A. Left occipital lobe
    B. Right temporal lobe
    C. Left temporal lobe
    D. Right parietal lobe
    E. Left parietal lobe

32. A 14-year-old girl presents to her primary care physician for a routine annual examination. In the course of the appointment, the patient reveals that she is concerned that she may be developing an eating disorder. She states that over the past month, she has attended several parties at which she has eaten 2 to 3 pieces of pizza and a large piece of cake during the course of the evening. Following each of these parties, the patient has skipped breakfast the next morning and gone for a 30-minute run around her neighborhood. She denies any purging behavior and has regular menstrual periods. The patient is concerned about gaining weight and has a friend who has recently been hospitalized for an eating disorder. At the time of her appointment, the patient is measured at a height of 5'2" and she weighs 120 pounds. Based on this information, what is her most accurate current diagnosis?

    A. Anorexia Nervosa, Restricting Type
    B. Anorexia Nervosa, Binge-Eating/Purging Type
    C. Bulimia Nervosa, Nonpurging type
    D. Eating Disorder NOS
    E. No eating disorder

33. Which of these statements about ADHD is TRUE?

    A. Adults can meet the criteria for adult-onset ADHD if they present with symptoms of hyperactivity, impulsivity, and/or inattention.
    B. A child can meet the criteria for ADHD if he presents with symptoms of hyperactivity, impulsivity, and/or inattention at school only.
    C. A child can meet the criteria for ADHD with significant maladaptive symptoms of inattention only.
    D. A child can meet the criteria for ADHD with significant maladaptive symptoms of impulsivity only.

E. A child can meet the criteria for ADHD with significant maladaptive symptoms of oppositional behavior only.

34. A mother brings her 10-month-old daughter to your office. The baby had a normal prenatal and perinatal history. On examination, you notice that her head circumference has not grown proportional to her age, and she is not babbling as she used to. Which one of the following choices is one of the main criteria for the diagnosis of this disorder?
A. Abnormal breathing patterns
B. Normal head circumference at birth
C. Progressive scoliosis
D. Growth retardation
E. Bruxism

35. A 19-year-old woman is brought to your office for an evaluation. Her mother reports that she has been losing weight and refuses to eat at home. She spends around 2 hours per day at the gym and recently bought a new book about "how to count calories." The patient feels that her weight is normal and thinks her mother is upset because "she comes from a generation when women were fat." Which of the following criteria would make the diagnosis of anorexia nervosa certain?
A. Absence of two consecutive menstrual cycles
B. A body weight 90% of that expected for her age and height
C. Eating in a discrete period of time an amount of food that is larger than what most people would eat
D. Feeling guilty about being underweight
E. Disturbance in the way in which one's body and weight are experienced

36. Which of the following statements regarding first-pass metabolism is TRUE?
A. It describes the metabolism of the drug in the kidneys.
B. After first-pass metabolism has occurred, metabolites are excreted into the urine.
C. When drugs are administered orally, they do not undergo first-pass metabolism.
D. Renal disease affects first-pass metabolism.
E. None of the above.

37. When used in the treatment of alcohol dependence, acamprosate is associated with all of the following EXCEPT:
A. Increased time to first drink
B. No significant drug interactions
C. Reduced craving for alcohol

D. Increased abstinence rates
E. Nausea as a major side effect

38. A review of the most recent data regarding outcomes in couples therapy suggests all of the following EXCEPT:
A. Younger couples have better outcomes.
B. More educated couples have better outcomes.
C. Unemployed couples have worse outcomes.
D. Couples with more severe difficulties have worse outcomes.
E. None of the above.

39. Which one of the following statements is TRUE of the treatment of ADHD in children and adolescents?
A. There are no-head-head studies comparing psychostimulants and atomoxetine in the treatment of ADHD.
B. Methylphenidate immediate-release was found to be better than atomoxetine on the ADHD Rating Scale total score.
C. Tolerability was better for atomoxetine than stimulant medications.
D. Atomoxetine represents an alternative treatment for ADHD and is unlikely to be associated with abuse.
E. All of the above.

40. Which of the following statements about acamprosate is NOT TRUE?
A. In controlled trials, it has shown modest benefit in reducing drinking in alcoholics.
B. Although its exact mechanism of action is unknown, it is hypothesized that acamprosate may stimulate γ-aminobutyric acid (GABA)-ergic neurotransmission.
C. Because acamprosate is excreted unchanged by the kidneys, it is contraindicated in patients with renal failure.
D. Although the medication is generally well-tolerated, gastrointestinal (GI) side effects are the most common side effect.
E. Acamprosate should be initiated following alcohol detoxification and should be stopped if the patient relapses.

41. It has been estimated that more than 50% of psychiatrists and 75% of mental health nurses have experienced an act or threat of violence against them within the past year. Assaults on mental health professionals are typically divided into all of the following categories EXCEPT:
A. Psychological intimidation
B. Physical assault
C. Sexual assault

D. Nonverbal threats/intimidation

E. Verbal assault

42. Which of the following statements regarding second messenger systems is NOT TRUE?

    A. Cyclic adenosine monophosphate (cAMP), cGMP, and phosphoinositide (PI) are second messengers that act as neurotransmitters via diffusion across the synaptic cleft.

    B. All actions of G proteins are mediated by small, diffusible second messengers.

    C. Activation of the receptors linked to the PI system generates diacylglycerol and inositol triphosphate (IP$_3$) as second messengers that affect the cellular processes.

    D. Calcium can act as a second messenger especially when associated with calmodulin.

    E. Lithium played an important role in the discovery of PI as a second messenger system.

43. Which of the following statements regarding the histaminergic system in the brain is TRUE?

    A. Central histaminergic cell bodies are located within the tuberomammillary nucleus region of the posterior hypothalamus.

    B. The activity of tuberomammillary neurons is highest during the waking state.

    C. The activity of tuberomammillary neurons is absent during rapid eye movement (REM) sleep.

    D. The hypothalamus receives the densest histaminergic innervation as it regulates autonomic and neuroendocrine activity.

    E. All of the above.

44. All of the following support a diagnosis of Restless Legs Syndrome (RLS) EXCEPT:

    A. Positive family history

    B. Symptoms begin at rest

    C. An urge to move the legs

    D. Symptoms worsen in the evening

    E. Symptoms worsen with movement

45. Which one of the following statements is NOT TRUE concerning dystonic movements?

    A. They are usually enhanced by emotional stress.

    B. They are present during sleep.

    C. They sometimes only occur during voluntary movements.

    D. They are usually slow and sinuous movements.

    E. They sometimes are only present during specific activities.

46. In which of the following conditions is gadolinium enhancement in the MRI not indicated?

    A. Workup for complex partial seizures

    B. Workup for headaches

    C. Workup for dementia

    D. Workup for psychosis

    E. All of the above

47. A 15-year-old boy experiences severe abdominal pain with vomiting and complains of a painful pins-and-needles sensation in his legs. While obtaining a history with his parents out of the room, you ask him about medications and recreational drug use. He tells you that he has been experimenting with barbiturates with his friends. As you examine him, you realize that he is having difficulty moving his lower extremities. You think that the drug use is incidental and the patient may have Guillain-Barré syndrome; however, you want to be certain that you are not missing other diagnoses and order standard labs, including a urine analysis. While you are completing your workup, you receive a call from the lab. The urine that you sent out was left in the open air for longer than it should have been and has turned a dark color. Which of the following tests is likely to help you the most in order to make the proper diagnosis?

    A. Liver function tests

    B. Thyroid function tests

    C. Serum and urine sodium and osmolality

    D. Urine porphobilinogen and δ-aminolevulinic acid

    E. CSF protein and white cell count

48. A 35-year-old man with new onset depressed mood and irritability has become "fidgety" and demonstrates slowly progressive short-term memory loss. His family history is significant for completed suicide by his father at age 45 years. Which of the following statements is TRUE about his condition?

    A. Children of gene carriers have a 100% chance of inheriting the disease.

    B. Trinucleotide (CAG) repeats of 20 or larger are usually associated with disease expression.

    C. Progressive cognitive deterioration is a rare feature.

    D. CAG repeats of 40 or larger are usually associated with disease expression.

    E. The CAG repeats are found on chromosome 14.

49. A 26-year-old woman traveler from South Africa presents to the ER with nausea, vomiting, and abdominal pain of 4 days duration. Physical examination is unremarkable apart from constipation and white plaques and vesicles over dorsal aspects of her forearms and hands. Her facial complexion is dark compared to the rest of her body. She tells you that she has always had sensitive skin. She also complains of feeling anxious and depressed for the past 3 days. Her medical history is unremarkable apart from

recently commencing trimethoprim for urinary tract infection. She reveals that her mother, a converted Muslim, has similar skin problems and suffers from epileptic fits, which often occur during the month of religious fasting. You suspect a disorder of heme metabolism. Fecal protoporphyrin and coproporphyrin and urinary coproporphyrin are increased. Plasma porphyrins and urinary D-aminolevulinic acid and porphobilinogen are increased. The diagnosis is probably

A. Porphyria cutanea tarda (PCT)
B. Acute intermittent porphyria (AIP)
C. Erythropoietic protoporphyria (EPP)
D. Variegate porphyria (VP)
E. Hereditary coproporphyria (HCP)

50. All of the following drugs can lead to a syndrome resembling lupus EXCEPT:

A. Procainamide
B. Hydralazine
C. Chlorpromazine
D. D-penicillamine
E. Quinine

51. A 70-year-old man is referred to your office for evaluation of 3 months of intermittent confusion and progressive memory loss. He is not currently taking any medications except atenolol and has no diagnosed medical disorders other than hypertension. You notice that he has a unilateral coarse resting tremor and a monotonous voice. He is motorically and cognitively slowed. He also gives a history of a resting tremor for the last 4 years. There is no evidence of any other involuntary movements and his coordination is good. There is no history of neurological disease in his family, including his parents. His clinical presentation is most consistent with which one of the following diagnosis?

A. A side effect of atenolol
B. Huntington's disease
C. Parkinson's disease
D. Cerebellar stroke
E. Hyperthyroidism

52. You are asked to see a patient for a neurology consult. Your patient is a 45-year-old woman who was in a motor vehicle accident and has been in a coma for the past 2 weeks. She has been on pulmonary life support since admission. On examination, you note no posturing or cranial reflexes, but a continued heart beat. The treatment team asks you if you can declare the patient brain dead so that they can have her organs donated. The patient had signed an organ donor card at her last primary care visit.

Under generally accepted practice, what do you tell the treatment team about organ donation?

A. No, because her heart is still beating.
B. No, because an electroencephalogram (EEG) was not performed.
C. No, because the patient is clearly alive.
D. Yes, because the patient is brain dead.
E. Yes, because the patient signed an organ donor card.

53. Lawrence Kohlberg et al. embarked on a long-term longitudinal study of the development of moral judgment in a cohort of boys. The boys were 10, 13, and 16 years of age at the outset and were followed for 20 years. Kohlberg arrived at six discreet stages for the course of moral development. Which statement briefly summarizes stage 3?

A. The child is oriented to obedience and punishment with egocentric deference to authority figures.
B. The child is oriented to be a good person in the eyes of others and oneself with a wish to please and help, but also takes into account the intentions of behavior and interactions with others.
C. The child has a naively egoistic orientation with concern of one's own needs but with some awareness of others' needs. The child is oriented toward exchange and reciprocity and wishes for egalitarianism.
D. The child is oriented to the social order and its maintenance for its own sake and seeks to fulfill agreed duties in conformity to authority.
E. The child is oriented to a sociomoral realm with the recognition of valid universal ethical principles to which a person can choose to commit himself or herself.

54. All of the following molecules may be responsible for the upregulation of the hypothalamic-pituitary axis activity in depression EXCEPT:

A. Serotonin
B. Norepinephrine
C. ACh
D. Corticotrophin Releasing Factor
E. Thyroid Releasing Factor

55. Which one of the following is a test of motor speed?

A. Finger tapping
B. Grooved pegboard
C. Grip strength
D. All the above
E. None of the above

56. All of the following are basic principles of community psychiatry EXCEPT:
  A. Patient and family involvement is an unavoidable component of mental health care strategy.
  B. Primary health care plays a minor role within the greater system of mental health care.
  C. Psychosocial rehabilitation must be considered a fundamental approach, integrating psychopharmacological treatments.
  D. The large majority of patients requiring psychiatric care should have the opportunity to be treated at the community level.
  E. Community psychiatric services should not only be local and accessible, but should also be able to address the multiple needs of individuals.

57. Which one of the following statements correctly describes internal consistency for neuropsychological tests?
  A. The degree to which two equivalent versions of a test give the same result
  B. The degree to which a test will give the same result on two different occasions
  C. The degree to which one test item correlates with all other test items
  D. The probability that two judges will give the same score to a given answer
  E. The degree to which the test measures all the aspects of the quality that is being assessed

58. Which of the following has been established as a positive prognostic factor in anorexia nervosa?
  A. Younger age at onset
  B. Chronicity of illness
  C. Obsessive-Compulsive Personality Traits
  D. Self-induced vomiting
  E. Binge-eating behavior

59. Which of the following statements describing ADHD is FALSE?
  A. ADHD is the most commonly diagnosed childhood psychiatric disorder.
  B. More than 50% of children diagnosed with ADHD also meet the criteria for another disruptive behavior disorder.
  C. Children diagnosed with ADHD have a higher injury rate and are at elevated risk for developing antisocial and criminal behavior, substance abuse, and mood and anxiety disorders.
  D. Children diagnosed with ADHD consume a disproportionate share of resources from the health care system, criminal justice system, schools, and other social service agencies.

  E. Children diagnosed with ADHD often perform better in group situations rather than in one-to-one interactions.

60. Which one of the following is considered a risk factor for Autism?
  A. Month of birth
  B. Parental alcohol use
  C. Weight at birth
  D. Exposure to tetanus vaccine
  E. Low parental age

61. Which one of the following laboratory abnormalities can be found in patients with anorexia nervosa?
  A. Hypercholesterolemia
  B. Leukocytosis
  C. Hypocortisolemia
  D. Hypocarotenemia
  E. Hyperglycemia

62. A patient is referred to your care with a history of refractory atypical depression. You choose to treat this patient with phenelzine. She tolerates this medication well, and there is a significant improvement in the symptoms of depression and her functioning. A few weeks later, you receive a call that your patient has been hospitalized. The clinical picture includes altered mental status, diaphoresis, hyperthermia, hyperactive bowel sounds, tremor, and myoclonus, particularly in the lower extremities. The patient denies a suicide attempt. All of the following drugs could likely have contributed to this presentation EXCEPT:
  A. Meperidine
  B. Diphenhydramine
  C. Dextromethorphan
  D. Methylenedioxymethamphetamine (MDMA)
  E. Selective Serotonin reuptake inhibitor (SSRI)

63. A patient has major depressive disorder coexisting with alcohol dependence and is interested in pharmacological management for his depression. Which one of the following represents the best treatment option for the treatment of his condition?
  A. Naltrexone
  B. Acamprosate
  C. Desipramine
  D. Bupropion
  E. Abstinence for 4 weeks prior to starting an antidepressant

64. A 69-year-old man with a history of diabetes mellitus, hypertension, hyperlipidemia, and an extensive history of untreated depression was started on an antidepressant and subsequently developed racing thoughts, increased energy, and was staying up all night playing online poker. He began to feel that he was becoming a gifted poker player and that his true calling in life was to become a professional gambler. Without further thought, he flew to Las Vegas. After gambling all night and losing his entire retirement savings, he presented to the local ED with chest pain and shortness of breath. An extensive cardiac workup revealed a sick sinus syndrome with multiple areas of old ischemic changes without evidence of an acute myocardial infarction. You are asked to evaluate the patient and recommend psychotropic therapy. Given his cardiac history, which one of the following medications would you avoid prescribing for this patient?

A. Lamotrigine
B. Valproate
C. Gabapentin
D. Olanzapine
E. Lithium carbonate

65. Which of the following is TRUE of day hospital programs and psychiatric patients?

A. Day hospital treatment was feasible for almost all patients who were currently admitted to inpatient hospitals.
B. Patients who attended day hospitals spent less time in the hospital during hospital admissions compared to controls.
C. The readmission rates to the hospital were lower for day hospital patients compared to controls.
D. There was more rapid improvement in the mental state of patients admitted to day hospitals compared to controls.
E. All of the above.

66. Which one of the following statements is TRUE of hyperprolactinemia caused by antipsychotics?

A. It is caused by their effects on the D2 receptors in the mesolimbic system.
B. The antipsychotic potency of the phenothiazines, butyrophenones, and dibenzoxazepines was found to parallel their potency in increasing prolactin levels.
C. The level of elevated prolactin found with the typical antipsychotic medications is usually >100 μg/L.
D. Clozapine is known to cause elevations in prolactin level even higher than those caused by the typical antipsychotics.
E. All of the above.

67. A 43-year-old single white man with a history of bipolar I disorder is brought to the ER by police after creating a disturbance outside a local bar. On examination, he has rapid, continuous speech and is difficult to interrupt. He is extremely agitated, restless, and believes there is a conspiracy afoot against him. What is potentially this patient's greatest risk factor for violence?

A. Diagnosis of Bipolar I Disorder
B. Cocaine Intoxication
C. History of past violence
D. Acute manic state
E. Persecutory delusions

68. Which one of the following statements regarding neuropeptides is NOT TRUE?

A. Neuropeptides can act as neurotransmitters, neuromodulators, or neurohormones.
B. Neuropeptide release is restricted to synapses and axon terminals.
C. The cellular signaling of neuropeptides is mediated by specific neuropeptide receptors.
D. The majority of neuropeptide receptors are G-protein-coupled, seven-transmembrane domain receptors.
E. Each neuropeptide receptor is specifically coupled to one type of G protein.

69. Which one of the following statements is NOT TRUE?

A. ACh is synthesized from acetyl coenzyme A, where there is transfer of an acetyl group to choline and this reaction is mediated by the enzyme choline acetyltransferase (ChAT).
B. Transfer of the acetyl group from acetyl coenzyme A to choline, which is mediated by the enzyme ChAT, is the rate limiting step in the synthesis of ACh.
C. Choline within the brain is transported from the blood and is not synthesized de novo.
D. Following release of ACh into the synaptic cleft, ACh is rapidly broken down by the enzyme acetylcholinesterase.
E. Butyrylcholinesterase is primarily found in the glial cells, liver, and plasma.

70. Approximately what percentage of Tourette's patients have OCD?

A. 15%
B. 30%
C. 50%
D. 70%
E. None of the above

71. During your neurological examination, you notice that a patient is unable to identify a letter traced on

the skin of the palm of his hand. What is this patient presenting with?

A. Abarognosis
B. Astereognosis
C. Apraxia
D. Agraphesthesia
E. Allodynia

72. Which one of the following statements is TRUE of a CT scan of the brain when compared to an MRI?

A. It is a more reliable and unambiguous method for detecting brain parenchymal bleed.
B. It is a more reliable and unambiguous method for detecting subarachnoid bleed.
C. It is superior to the MRI in evaluating the bones of the skull and spine.
D. It is more useful in patients who are uncooperative or claustrophobic.
E. All of the above.

73. Which one of the following is TRUE of multiple sclerosis?

A. Most patients, after the disease begins, experience a steady, unremitting deterioration of their clinical course.
B. MRI findings are typically too nonspecific to be helpful in diagnosing multiple sclerosis.
C. Women with multiple sclerosis are no more likely to have miscarriages than women who do not have this disease.
D. Patients with multiple sclerosis can have internuclear ophthalmoplegia, which is a bitemporal hemianopsia secondary to damage of the medial longitudinal fasciculus.
E. Although patients with multiple sclerosis can experience optic neuritis, they do so rarely.

74. A 22-year-old woman with sickle cell anemia develops fever, headache, and stiffness of neck. Which is the most likely causative organism?

A. Cryptococcus neoformans
B. Streptococcus pneumoniae
C. Haemophilus influenzae
D. Bacteroides
E. Actinomyces

75. One should avoid prescribing one of the following psychotropic medications for psychiatric symptoms of AIP EXCEPT:

A. Tricyclic antidepressants (TCAs)
B. Phenothiazines
C. Monoamine oxidase inhibitors (MAOIs)
D. Carbamazepine
E. Sulpiride

76. A patient suffers from acute stroke, and subsequent to this stroke, he fails to acknowledge that one side of his body is paralyzed. Given this presentation, where is the lesion most likely to be located in his brain?

A. Left parietal lobe
B. Right parietal lobe
C. Bilateral temporo-occipital regions
D. Right subthalamic nucleus
E. Left perisylvian cortex

77. A 55-year-old woman complains of aching pain in her neck for 3 months. She also describes mild weakness of her right hand, pain in her right shoulder, and an electrical sensation down her spine when she coughs or extends her neck. Which of the following signs would support a diagnosis of cervical spondylosis?

A. A positive Babinski sign
B. A positive Hoffman sign
C. Decreased vibration sense in the feet
D. Decreased biceps reflex
E. All of the above

78. A 42-year-old woman comes into your office. She states that she is pregnant and is concerned that she is at risk of having an unhealthy baby. She asks about genetic counseling. Which of the following statements about the definition and goals of genetic counseling is NOT accurate?

A. Help the family comprehend the medical facts about the disorder
B. Discuss how to adjust to the disorder in an affected family member
C. Provide specific advice about what the family should do
D. Educate about the possible role heredity plays in the disorder
E. Provide options about potential management

79. Although Kohlberg's major study was composed only of male subjects, his colleague, Carol Gilligan, interviewed both male and female subjects. From these studies, she developed the idea of fundamental differences between men and women in moral orientation. Which one of the following statements best describes this difference?

A. Men give priority to autonomy and self-determination, whereas women give priority to compromise between individuals.
B. Both men and women agree on the obligation to the law, but men emphasize punishment, whereas women emphasize leniency.
C. Both men and women recognize universal ethical principles, but men emphasize the influence of nation-states over individuals, whereas women

emphasize the influence of communities over individuals.

D. Men give priority to justice and rights, whereas women give priority to care and responsibility.

E. Men give priority to self-regard, whereas women give priority to encouraging others.

80. Which one of the following pairs of homologous dopamine receptors functions through an increase in the production of cAMP?

A. D1 and D2
B. D2 and D3
C. D1 and D5
D. D2 and D5
E. D4 and D5

81. A 60-year-old man presents to a neurology clinic for an evaluation 2 months after a cerebrovascular event and a hospital admission. His family reports that he is doing reasonably well except that he is unable to repeat the instruction that they are giving him. He is otherwise able to comprehend and converse normally. They think that he is stubborn and oppositional. They do not describe any other behavioral problems. Your evaluation indicates that he can read, write, converse, and comprehend, but cannot perform tasks of verbal repetition. The MRI of the brain reveals an infarct in a particular area of the brain. After this evaluation, what should the neurologist tell the patient's family about his condition?

A. He can really repeat, but is faking his presentation.

B. He has Broca's aphasia and the lesion is in the left inferior frontal convolution to the posterior extent of the sylvian fissure.

C. He has conduction aphasia and the lesion is in the arcuate fasciculus.

D. He has Broca's aphasia and the lesion is in the arcuate fasciculus.

E. He has conduction aphasia and the lesion is in the region of left inferior frontal convolution to the posterior extent of the sylvian fissure.

82. Each of the following is an exception to the requirement of informed consent for medical treatment EXCEPT:

A. Unconsciousness in a medical emergency
B. Therapeutic privilege
C. Incompetency
D. Psychosis
E. Patient waiver

83. A 25-year-old man is brought by ambulance to the ED after being found walking on the highway in the middle of the night, talking to himself. He reports

that God has been telling him to save the world by preaching the Bible to strangers. After obtaining collateral information, you find out that he has had several similar episodes after stopping his antipsychotic medications. His urine toxicology screen is negative. If an MRI of the brain is done, you would expect to see which one of the following in this patient?

A. Reduced volume in prefrontal and temporal cortices
B. Increased volume in prefrontal and temporal cortices
C. Only increased volume in prefrontal cortex
D. Only increased volume in temporal cortex
E. Reduced volume in occipital and parietal cortices

84. Which one of the following statements regarding Bipolar Disorder is NOT TRUE?

A. The female:male gender ratio of bipolar disorder (all subtypes combined) is approximately 1:1.
B. Men are over-represented in rapid cycling bipolar disorder illness.
C. Women are over-represented in patients with type II bipolar illness.
D. Women are over-represented in patients with mixed bipolar illness.
E. All of the above.

85. Which one of the following isolated behaviors does not meet a criterion for conduct disorder?

A. An 11-year-old boy often stays out late at night, despite his father's threats of punishment, and twice in the last month he ran away to a friend's house overnight.
B. A 9-year-old boy has attempted to hang his cat. When confronted, he said he wanted to see if the "hangman's noose" really works.
C. A 10-year-old girl easily loses her temper, retorts, and shouts at her teachers when they give her classroom directions.
D. A 13-year-old girl has been caught shoplifting lipstick, cosmetics, and lingerie from expensive department stores over the past year.
E. A 14-year-old boy threatens younger children to give him their lunch money, and, if they refuse, he beats them up.

86. Which one of the following is strongly associated with severity of symptoms in autistic disorder?

A. Intelligence quotient
B. Age of onset
C. Degree of social impairment
D. Severity of stereotyped behaviors
E. Negative family history for psychiatric disorders

87. Which one of the following is considered an indication for immediate medical hospitalization of a patient with anorexia nervosa?
    A. Denial of weight problem
    B. Amenorrhea
    C. Bradycardia
    D. Frequent binge eating
    E. Conflicted family dynamics

88. A 43-year-old man presents for treatment of recurrent depression and Alcohol Dependence. He reports low mood, anhedonia, significant guilt, and impaired appetite for the past 2 months. He denies suicidal ideation, but has made a serious suicide attempt in the past. The patient had been sober for 6 months, but relapsed 2 weeks ago. He has been drinking excessively each day. In addition to an inpatient alcohol detoxification and substance abuse program, you decide to initiate pharmacotherapy. Which one of the following medications is contraindicated?
    A. Acamprosate
    B. Escitalopram
    C. Imipramine
    D. Duloxetine
    E. Lithium

89. Which one of the following treatments is unlikely to be helpful in a patient with acute phencyclidine (PCP) intoxication?
    A. Low-potency antipsychotic
    B. High-potency antipsychotic
    C. Benzodiazepine
    D. Ammonium chloride
    E. Seclusion and restraints

90. Lamotrigine is an effective treatment for bipolar depression; however, its use is somewhat limited by a rare, but potentially fatal, side effect, i.e., Stevens-Johnson syndrome (toxic epidermal necrolysis). Which one of the following patients started on lamotrigine therapy would be LEAST likely to develop Stevens-Johnson syndrome?
    A. A 36-year-old woman with a history of rash secondary to carbamazepine treatment started on 25 mg of lamotrigine with a dose increase of 25 mg every week to a maximum dose of 100 mg.
    B. A 12-year-old boy started on 25 mg of lamotrigine with a dose increase of 25 mg every week to a maximum dose of 100 mg daily.
    C. A 42-year-old man on valproate started on 25 mg of lamotrigine with a dose increase of 25 mg every week to a maximum dose of 100 mg daily.
    D. A 35-year-old woman started on 100 mg of lamotrigine after discontinuing this dose of lamotrigine 1 week ago.

    E. A 60-year-old male on warfarin started on 25 mg of lamotrigine with a dose increase of 25 mg every week to a maximum dose of 100 mg daily.

91. Which one of the following is TRUE of day treatment programs versus outpatient care for psychiatric patients?
    A. There is evidence that a day treatment program is better than outpatient care for clinical outcomes.
    B. There is evidence that a day treatment program is better than outpatient care for a social outcome variable.
    C. There is evidence that a day treatment program is more cost effective than outpatient care.
    D. There is some evidence that transitional day hospital care was superior to outpatient care in keeping patients engaged in treatment.
    E. None of the above.

92. A 44-year-old man comes in to your office with his wife. The wife describes her husband as having a long history of Alcohol Dependence. The patient himself admits to drinking almost every day for 20 years. He agrees to an inpatient detoxification and completes it without incident. During their next visit, the wife voices her fear that her husband will soon "fall off the wagon" and wants her husband to be put on that medication that will "make him sick" when he drinks. You confirm that they are talking about disulfiram. Which one of the following statements about disulfiram is TRUE?
    A. Clinical trial evidence clearly supports its use in most patients.
    B. The disulfiram-ethanol reaction is not dose dependent.
    C. Disulfiram may be useful if special efforts are made to ensure compliance.
    D. Side effects are unlikely to be severe and never life threatening.
    E. A disulfiram-ethanol reaction is unlikely 24 hours after the last dose.

93. Impulsive aggression has been linked to the disruption of which neurotransmitter systems?
    A. Norepinephrine
    B. Serotonin
    C. GABA
    D. Dopamine
    E. ACh

94. Which one of the following choices regarding neuropeptides is NOT TRUE?
    A. Biosynthesis of a neuropeptide involves the transcription of a messenger RNA (mRNA) from a specific gene translation.

B. Neuropeptide genes are composed of multiple exons that encode for a preprohormone.

C. The neuroanatomical localization of neuropeptides is determined mainly by region-specific expression and regulation of its gene.

D. Each neuropeptide gene is expressed in a well-defined population of neurons within the brain.

E. The neuroanatomical pattern of peptide hormone gene expression is determined by the RNA sequences surrounding the gene.

95. Which one of the following statements regarding the GABA neurotransmitter system is NOT TRUE?

A. GABA is formed by the decarboxylation of glutamate by the enzyme glutamate decarboxylase.

B. Vitamin B_6 (pyridoxine) acts as the cofactor for the synthesis of GABA from glutamate.

C. The highest concentrations of GABA are present in the striatum, hypothalamus, temporal lobe, and spinal cord.

D. GABA-A receptor has binding sites for benzodiazepines, barbiturates, alcohol, and flumazenil.

E. GABA-B receptor activity opens up chloride channels which permits the flow of chloride into the cell.

96. All of the following are true statements regarding West Nile Virus (WNV) infection in the United States EXCEPT:

A. Incidence has been rising in recent years.

B. The principal vectors are mosquitos.

C. Birds serve as reservoir hosts.

D. Central nervous system (CNS) infection is rare.

E. None of the above.

97. Which one of the following statements is NOT TRUE regarding an upper motor neuron lesion?

A. They usually present with weakness or paralysis.

B. Patients usually present with spasticity.

C. Superficial abdominal reflexes are increased.

D. There is usually no muscle atrophy.

E. There is an extensor plantar response.

98. A 19-year-old college freshman presents to the health services clinic on campus. He complains of a 2-day history of body aches, headache, rhinorrhea, and fatigue. On examination, his temperature is 39.6°C. He is found to have mild pain upon flexion and extension of his neck, and he had a fine petechial rash on his trunk. Given his complaints and physical findings, he is evaluated for bacterial meningitis. Which one of the following CSF findings is consistent with bacterial meningitis?

A. Opening pressure 120 mm H_2O, protein 30 mg/dL, glucose 70 mg/dL, red blood cells 2, white blood cells 4, differential: 3% neutrophils, 80% lymphocytes, 17% monocytes

B. Opening pressure 130 mm H_2O, protein 25 mg/dL, glucose 200 mg/dL, red blood cells 0, white blood cells 0

C. Opening pressure 240 mm H_2O, protein 200 mg/dL, glucose 20 mg/dL, red blood cells 3, white blood cells 100, differential: 70% neutrophils, 25% lymphocytes, 5% monocytes

D. Opening pressure 210 mm H_2O, protein 60 mg/dL, glucose 70 mg/dL, red blood cells 2, white blood cells 40, differential: 20% neutrophils, 80% lymphocytes

E. Opening pressure 150 mm H_2O, protein 50 mg/dL, glucose 60 mg/dL, red blood cells 100,000, white blood cells 100, differential: 5% neutrophils, 70% lymphocytes, 25% monocytes

99. A 33-year-old man presents to the ER with a complaint of smelling a foul odor. The symptom began 1 month ago, and although he is unsure about the cause, he is beginning to believe that he is being punished for impure thoughts by the devil. What symptom would make a diagnosis of organic olfactory hallucinations unlikely?

A. Cognitive dysfunction

B. Foul smell

C. Ill-defined smell

D. Behavioral disturbances

E. Continuous smell

100. Which one of the following lesions is seen only in neurofibromatosis-1?

A. Pigmented iris hamartomas

B. Meningiomas

C. Six or more *café au lait* spots larger than 5 mm in diameter before puberty

D. Schwannomas

E. Bilateral acoustic neuromas

101. A mother brings her 10-year-old son to your clinic for a psychiatric assessment following concerns over his increasingly aggressive behaviors. The mother reports that he is underachieving at school with reading and writing impediments. He is also impulsive and hyperactive. While taking the history, you notice that his mother has brown nodules over her face. On further enquiry, she reveals that she suffers from epilepsy. Physical examination of the boy reveals several brown spots over his forearms and face. You suspect neurofibromatosis. All of the following should be done in the period immediately following the consultation, EXCEPT:

A. Offer genetic counseling

B. Take an MRI of the brain and cervical spine

C. Investigate for signs of epilepsy
D. Prescribe haloperidol
E. Suggest evaluation of language and speech

102. A previously healthy 67-year-old woman suddenly becomes cognitively impaired, and her cognitive function deteriorates significantly over the next few months. She also becomes mute and loses her ability to walk. She then develops myoclonus and dies in a little less than 6 months after the initial diagnosis was made. Which one of the following represents the most likely diagnosis?

A. Rapidly progressive variant of Alzheimer's disease
B. Lewy body dementia
C. Sporadic form of Creutzfeldt-Jacob disease (CJD)
D. Huntington's chorea
E. Normal Pressure Hydrocephalus

103. An elderly man presents with gait instability and sharp pain in his shoulders for several months. Which one of the following diagnoses would best explain both of his symptoms?

A. Normal Pressure Hydrocephalus
B. Lumbar stenosis
C. Vitamin B_{12} deficiency
D. Cervical spondylosis
E. Friedreich's ataxia

104. A 26-year-old women presents to her physician's office with a history of feeling weak for the last few months. Physical examination reveals blurry vision, unequal ptosis, and fatigue, which is worse later in the day. Which one of the following statements is correct about the proper treatment of this disorder?

A. Surgical procedures are indicated only in intractable cases.
B. Patients rarely respond to anticholinesterases alone.
C. Ocular symptoms generally respond best to corticosteroids.
D. Corticosteroids usually rapidly improve symptoms.
E. Alternative immunosuppressive agents should not be used as monotherapy.

105. Chess and Thomas' conceptualization of "goodness of fit" between parent and child postulates that:

A. A mother provides balanced responses to her child's needs in the context of a holding environment.
B. The expectations and demands of the parents are in consonance with the child's temperament characteristics and capabilities.
C. The expectations and demands of the parents are adapted to fit the child's temperament characteristics and capabilities.
D. The expectations and demands of the parents are in dissonance with the child's temperament characteristics and capabilities.
E. The child's temperament characteristics and capabilities are adapted to fit the expectations and demands of the parents.

106. The anxiolytic effect of benzodiazepines is likely mediated though the modulation of which one of the following neurotransmitters?

A. Serotonin
B. Norepinephrine
C. GABA
D. Glutamate
E. Substance P

107. Which one of the following statements regarding Wernicke's aphasia is NOT TRUE?

A. It is also called sensory aphasia or receptive aphasia.
B. Verbal output in Wernicke's aphasia is either normal or increased.
C. Jargon aphasia can occur in severe cases.
D. Reading out loud and reading comprehension are normal.
E. Writing is abnormal in Wernicke's aphasia.

108. A psychiatrist appears on a weekly radio program where anonymous callers ask general questions about psychiatric illness. Before each show begins, a disclaimer is read that states that no doctor–patient relationship is implied. A female caller receives information about the use of SSRIs for depression. Three weeks later, the caller attempts suicide. Her family attempts to file a malpractice claim against the psychiatrist on the radio program. This lawsuit is unlikely to succeed because which element of a malpractice claim has not been established:

A. Damage to the patient
B. Duty of care
C. Deviation from the standard of care
D. Denial of illness
E. Direct causation

109. Reduction in which area of the brain is seen most consistently during cognitive decline in patients with Alzheimer's disease?

A. Frontal lobes
B. Hippocampus
C. Amygdala
D. Parietal lobes
E. Temporal lobes

110. Risk factors for rapid cycling in bipolar disorder include all of the following EXCEPT:

A. Bipolar type I more frequently than type II
B. Alcohol abuse or caffeine abuse
C. Female gender more frequently than males
D. Temporal lobe dysfunction
E. All of the above

111. A 44-year-old man is referred for treatment by his employer due to difficulties at work. The patient's behavior includes insubordination. He inappropriately strives to maintain his autonomy. He resists situations where he must depend on others, frequently misinterprets his colleagues motives, bears grudges against them and harbors significant anger. When approached by his supervisor to discuss these issues, the patient feels his character is being questioned and is quick to counterattack. During your assessment, the patient blames his colleagues for any problems at work. He also describes making substantial efforts to foil those perceived as trying to humiliate him. He does not report any problems in his personal life, including with his girlfriend and family. Which of the following personality disorders best encapsulates this individual's pathology?

A. Schizoid personality disorder
B. Paranoid personality disorder
C. Histrionic personality disorder
D. Antisocial personality disorder
E. Narcissistic personality disorder

112. Phencyclidine is most closely pharmacologically related to which one of the following substances?

A. Lysergic acid diethylamide (LSD)
B. Cannabis
C. Ketamine
D. Amobarbital
E. Mescaline

113. A 24-year-old woman comes to your office for the first time. She reports that she has been unable to control her weight in the past few months. When she comes home from the office, she occasionally eats a quart of ice cream and cannot stop eating until there is no ice cream left. These episodes occur around twice per month. She then feels so guilty that she does not eat anything until the next day at noon. Although her weight is within a normal range for her age and height, she would like to loose some weight. What is this patient's most likely diagnosis?

A. Bulimia Nervosa, Purging Type
B. Bulimia Nervosa, Nonpurging Type
C. Anorexia Nervosa

D. Body Dysmorphic Disorder
E. Patient does not meet criteria for an eating disorder

114. All of the following statements about psychostimulants are true EXCEPT:

A. They are currently approved for the treatment of narcolepsy and ADHD.
B. Among children with ADHD, longitudinal treatment with stimulants reduces the risk of non-nicotine substance abuse in adolescence and adulthood by half.
C. They are the most frequently prescribed medications in pediatric psychopharmacology.
D. They are an effective treatment in 40% to 50% of children with ADHD and are most successful when combined with educational interventions.
E. Off-label uses include treatment of apathy in the medically ill, potentiation of narcotic analgesics, and antidepressant augmentation.

115. When should bupropion be started, if it is being used in the treatment of smoking cessation?

A. Several months before stopping smoking
B. Several weeks before stopping smoking
C. On the day smoking stops
D. At the first sign of nicotine withdrawal
E. Several weeks after stopping smoking

116. You have been seeing a 32-year-old woman with a diagnosis of bipolar disorder in your outpatient clinic for 1 year. Since starting olanzapine 20 mg daily, her mood has been stable, she is able to work for the first time in "years," and recently has a new romantic relationship. At her last visit, she complained that she has gained weight since starting olanzapine and that diet and exercise have not helped to reduce or even control her weight. On review of her chart, you realize that she has in fact gained 30 pounds since starting olanzapine. After reviewing your patient's medication history and discussing the risks and benefits of alternative treatments as well as the risks and benefits of stopping olanzapine, you and your patient decide to discontinue the olanzapine and start a different medication. You ask that she return to your office in one week. At that visit, she complains of feeling tired throughout the past week. After reviewing her vital signs and completing a physical examination, you check a set of basic labs (results on page 76). Which one of the following medications is most likely to result in this clinical picture?

A. Valproate
B. Gabapentin
C. Lamotrigine

Laboratory data			
Na 145	CL 113	BUN 22	Glu 103
K 4.5	CO2 22	Cr 0.8	Mg 1.5
PH 7.32	Alk Phos 130	ALT 8	AST 15
Total Bili. 0.8	Dir. Bili 0.1	Alb 4.5	Amylase 30, Lipase 10
WBC 7.2	Hg 13.5	HCT 36%	Plat. 250

    D. Topiramate
    E. Quetiapine

117. Which one of the following is TRUE of day hospital care in the elderly?
    A. Day hospitals are better than alternative services, when the odds of death are used as an outcome.
    B. Day hospitals are better than no comprehensive care, when the odds of death are used as an outcome.
    C. Day hospitals are better than alternative services, when disability is used as an outcome.
    D. Day hospitals are better than alternative services, when use of resources is used as an outcome.
    E. All of the above.

118. A 51-year-old man comes into your office with vague complaints of depressed mood. With detailed questioning, you uncover a long history of alcohol dependence. The patient admits to drinking almost every day for 20 years. He agrees to an inpatient detoxification, and completes it without incident. The patient then asks for a medication known to reduce alcohol consumption, and you discuss the use of naltrexone. In educating the patient about the medication, which one of the following is a TRUE statement regarding naltrexone?
    A. Common side effects include hypotension and tachycardia.
    B. The evidence supports the use of naltrexone indefinitely.
    C. The use of depot naltrexone is widely believed to be superior to oral naltrexone.
    D. There is evidence to support the use of nondaily oral naltrexone.
    E. There is no need to question the patient about other illicit substance use.

119. What is the ethical principle underlying the act of performing medical care and research in a way that is both fair and equitable?
    A. Autonomy
    B. Beneficence
    C. Nonmalfeasance
    D. Justice
    E. Temperance

120. Which one of the following cells found in the CNS is responsible for myelin production?
    A. Astrocytes
    B. Oligodendrocytes
    C. Ependymal cells
    D. Microglia
    E. Schwann cells

121. Which one of the following statements regarding the glutamate neurotransmitter system is NOT TRUE?
    A. Glutamate is the most important excitatory neurotransmitter in the brain.
    B. Ionotropic glutamate receptors (iGluR) and G-protein–coupled receptors (GPCRs) are the two general classes of glutamate receptors.
    C. The three iGluR receptors are N-methyl-D-aspartate (NMDA), α-amino-3-hydroxy-5-methylisoxazole-4-propionic acid (AMPA), and kainate (KA).
    D. PCP causes an overactivity of the NMDA calcium channel.
    E. The three metabotropic classes of receptors (mGluR) are quisqualate-, (2R,4R)-aminopyrrolidine-2, 4-dicarboxylate (APDC)-, and L-2-amino-4-phosphonobutanoic acid (L-AP4)–sensitive receptors.

122. All of the following are associated with Wilson's disease EXCEPT:
    A. Liver disease
    B. Corneal deposits
    C. Chromosome 13
    D. Autosomal dominant inheritance
    E. Neurologic disturbance

123. Which one of the following is the LEAST common complication of a lumbar puncture?
    A. Meningitis
    B. Headache
    C. Sixth nerve palsy
    D. Third nerve palsy
    E. Bleeding into meningeal spaces

124. A 42-year-old woman complains of fatigue, which is worse in the later part of the day. She has frequent problems with diplopia and slurred speech when she is fatigued. In the office, she is noted to have bilateral ptosis and weakness of the extraocular muscles with a normal pupillary response to light and accommodation. What finding on blood testing would be helpful in making a correct diagnosis for this patient?

A. Elevated serum calcium
B. Antibodies to the ACh receptor
C. Antinuclear antibodies
D. Elevated thyrotropin (TSH)
E. Low hemoglobin level

125. A 67-year-old man presents with a hoarse voice. On examination, there is left vocal cord palsy. There is no loss of pain or temperature sensation over the left or right face and no palatal weakness. Where is the lesion to the vagal nerve?

A. Intramedullary
B. Extramedullary, but intracranial
C. Posterior lacterocondylar
D. Retroparietal
E. Mediastinum

126. What is the most common site of hemangioblastoma?

A. Spinal cord
B. Area postrema of medulla
C. Paramedian cerebellar hemispheric area
D. Parietal lobe
E. Cerebellar vermis

127. All the following are true of neurofibromatosis EXCEPT:

A. Neurofibromatosis type 2 is carried by the chromosome 22.
B. Lisch nodules are a characteristic feature.
C. Neurofibromas develop in late adolescence.
D. Acoustic neuromas are specific for neurofibromatosis type 1.
E. Café au lait spots develop during early childhood.

128. The facial akinesia of patient's with Parkinson's disease is characterized by all of the following EXCEPT:

A. The appearance of a flat affect
B. Decreased blinking
C. Narrowed palpebral fissures
D. Decreased spontaneous eye movements
E. Decreased head movements

129. A 30-year-old woman presents in clinic for evaluation of "clumsiness" of her right hand. She has been dropping objects frequently and has now developed a blister on her index finger on the right hand. She acquired the blister after touching her curling iron to

test if it was hot enough, and did not have any pain when touching it. Which one of the following choices would best support a diagnosis of type I Chiari malformation?

A. Her age
B. A spinal cord tumor on MRI
C. A normal motor strength in all four extremities
D. Decreased vibration sense on examination
E. All of the above

130. A 28-year-old woman with no significant past medical history presents with weakness and numbness in her left leg. Further history indicates increasing fatigue, intermittent tingling sensations in her extremities, and a several day episode of blurry vision in her right eye that resolved on its own without treatment. A lumbar puncture and MRI support the suspected diagnosis. Which one of the following is a correct statement regarding the pharmacological treatment of this disease with corticosteroids?

A. The majority of patients require large, chronic doses of corticosteroids.
B. Few patients relapse after a taper of their corticosteroids.
C. Steroids significantly alter the course of disease and can prevent recurrences.
D. Controlled trials strongly support the use of corticosteroids in acute cases.
E. If feasible, intravenous steroids are always preferred over oral forms.

131. Chess and Thomas formulated three constellations of temperaments composed of various combinations of nine temperament categories used to evaluate children. The constellations of temperament are easy, difficult, and slow-to-warm-up. Which one of the following is NOT one of the nine temperament categories?

A. Activity level
B. Intensity of reaction
C. Distractibility
D. Feeding behavior
E. Adaptability

132. Drugs, such as donepezil and rivastigmine, are thought to inhibit the progression of Alzheimer's dementia through which of the following actions?

A. Net increase in ACh concentration
B. Net decrease in ACh concentration
C. Excitation of NMDA receptors
D. Inhibition of NMDA receptors
E. None of the above

Study outcome	No true difference exists	True difference exits
Difference found	A	B
No difference found	C	D
Total	A + C	B + D

133. In the above table, which one of the following represents a Type I error?

   A. A
   B. B
   C. C
   D. A + C
   E. B + D

134. Which one of the following structures plays a major role in the processing of fear?

   A. Hippocampus
   B. Prefrontal cortex
   C. Amygdala
   D. Cerebellum
   E. Hypothalamus

135. Which one of the following is NOT TRUE regarding patients with idiopathic insomnia?

   A. These patients do not awaken in response to an auditory tone any more easily than good sleepers.
   B. These patients are excessively sleepy during the daytime as assessed by the multiple sleep latency test (MSLT).
   C. These patients have neurophysiological test results with a pattern of deficits different from that typically seen in sleep deprivation.
   D. These patients do not seem to estimate time differently than good sleepers do.
   E. All of the above.

136. A 44-year-old man is referred for treatment by his employer due to difficulties at work. The patient's behavior has included insubordination, striving inappropriately to maintain his autonomy, resisting situations where he must depend on others, harboring significant anger, and frequently misinterpreting his colleagues' motives and bearing grudges against them. When approached by his supervisor to discuss these issues, the patient feels his character is being questioned, and is quick to counterattack. During your assessment, the patient blames his colleagues for any problems at work. He also describes making substantial efforts to foil those perceived as trying to humiliate him. He does not report any problems in his personal life, including with his girlfriend and family. What would be the most effective psychotherapeutic approach with this patient?

   A. Defend yourself if the patient makes unfounded attacks or accusations.
   B. Put regular group therapy sessions in place as part of the treatment plan.
   C. Challenge cognitive distortions of the patient's interpersonal experiences.
   D. Share your records and notes with the patient if he demands access.
   E. Make an accurate interpretation early on in the therapy to gain respect and trust.

137. Which one of the following patients would be most likely to experience delirium tremens following abrupt stoppage of alcohol consumption?

   A. A healthy 16-year-old male high school student who has been getting drunk with his friends on most weekends over the past year.
   B. A 22-year-old female bank employee who has been drinking two glasses of wine per night since her promotion 6 months ago in order to "calm her nerves."
   C. A 42-year-old male lawyer with hepatitis who has been drinking heavily, particularly during frequent binges, over the past 15 years.
   D. A 70-year-old male retired accountant with arthritis and chronic obstructive pulmonary disease (COPD), newly drinking one to two bottles of beer per night since his wife passed away 3 months ago.
   E. A 28-year-old female graduate student with no history of substance abuse who has been drinking steadily since completing her thesis 10 days ago.

138. Which one of the following mental disorders has the highest mortality rate from both natural and unnatural causes?

   A. Schizophrenia
   B. Anorexia Nervosa
   C. Major Depressive Disorder
   D. Bipolar Disorder
   E. Panic Attacks

139. A 15-year-old boy is brought to the ER by his parents, who found the usually sociable adolescent barricading himself in his room after refusing to attend school. He had not slept the night before. His parents report that they found multiple bottles of prescription medications in his school backpack, none of which belong to him. In the ER, the boy is paranoid, irritable, and restless. Physical exam is notable for blood pressure 160/100 mm HG, heart rate 120 beats/minute, dilated pupils, dry mouth, and bruxism. Which of the following prescription medications found in his backpack has the boy most likely abused?

A. Alprazolam
B. Propranolol
C. Dextroamphetamine
D. Methadone
E. Zolpidem

140. What is the order of switch rate to hypomania or mania for patients with bipolar depression when they are treated with antidepressants?

A. TCA > SNRI (velafaxine) > SSRI > bupropion
B. SSRI > SNRI > bupropion > TCA
C. SSRI > bupropion > TCA > SNRI
D. SNRI > TCA > SSRI > bupropion
E. Bupropion > SNRI > SSRI > TCA

141. A 42-year-old married white woman with three children came to psychiatric attention 2 years ago after being found in the street by the police wandering in the freezing rain dressed only in a t-shirt. Collateral information at that time indicated that over the past 2 years the patient had withdrawn from family and friends. She has showered only upon family insistence, and has believed that her husband and children were dead. She was diagnosed with late onset schizophrenia and started on risperidone. The patient has had very poor insight into her condition and difficulty accepting her diagnosis. She frequently stops taking her medication, resulting in a worsening of her mental state and readmission to the hospital. The decision to start risperidone long-acting injection was made during her most recent admission. How long should the patient continue the oral dose of risperidone after receiving the first injection?

A. Discontinue the oral medication at the time the first injection is given
B. One week
C. Three days
D. Two weeks
E. Three weeks

142. Which of the following is NOT TRUE of caregiving for patients with dementia?

A. It can cause problems only for family-caregivers, but not for professional caregivers.
B. Caregivers who live apart from their patient are more reluctant to admit the person into an institution.
C. There is a low rate of abuse by the demented patients in the community.
D. The move from the community to institutional care in most cases is planned.
E. All of the above.

143. Interpersonal psychotherapy (IPT) is accurately described by all of the following statements EXCEPT:

A. It deals with current, rather than previous relationships.
B. It intervenes in symptom formation rather than addressing aspects of personality.
C. It is time limited.
D. It is structured into three separate phases.
E. IPT therapists offer interpretations to assist patients in better understanding their defense structure.

144. Which one of the following is NOT characteristic of an axonal action potential?

A. All-or-nothing phenomenon
B. Directionally propagated
C. Commences with inflow of potassium ions
D. Consists of depolarization and repolarization phases
E. Includes an absolute refractory period

145. Which one of the following statements regarding the amino acid neurotransmitter glycine is NOT TRUE?

A. Glycine is a major constituent of glutathione.
B. Glycine is more prevalent in the brainstem and spinal cord.
C. Neurons utilizing glycine as a neurotransmitter are small excitatory interneurons.
D. The binding site for glycine exists on the NMDA subtype of glutamate receptors.
E. They often are functionally associated with α-motorneurons.

146. Which one of the following clinical findings is NOT present in myopathies?

A. Proximal weakness
B. Loss of tendon reflexes early in the disease
C. Normal sphincter function
D. Normal sensory function
E. Normal plantar reflexes

147. A 26-year-old woman has had a 6-month history of seizures of many different types, including generalized tonic–clonic, complex partial, and simple motor. MRI of the brain and EEG studies have been unremarkable, and her seizures have not lessened despite treatment with several different anticonvulsants. She was hospitalized for 24-hour video EEG monitoring to help elucidate the cause of her seizures. While hospitalized, she had an apparent generalized tonic–clonic seizure lasting 5 minutes. Although she was not connected to the EEG electrodes at the time of the episode, the seizure was captured on video. Laboratory studies were obtained 15 minutes after the

episode. What laboratory finding might be helpful in determining the cause of her seizures?

A. Normal serum potassium
B. Mild metabolic acidosis
C. Elevated lactic acid
D. Elevated prolactin
E. Mild thrombocytopenia

148. A 28-year-old woman with no significant past medical history presents with weakness and numbness in her left leg. Further history elicits increasing fatigue, intermittent tingling sensations in her extremities, and an episode of blurry vision in her right eye lasting several days that resolved on its own without treatment. A lumbar puncture and MRI support the suspected diagnosis. The patient asks about noncorticosteroid immunomodulatory therapy with either interferon beta or glatiramer acetate. Which one of the following statements is correct about these treatments?

A. Corticosteroids are clearly more effective than these agents in altering the natural history of the disease.
B. Evidence suggests that they can decrease the severity of relapses by almost one-third.
C. All of these treatments must be used daily to be effective.
D. The common side effects include hypertension, hyperglycemia and erratic diabetic control, and osteoporosis.
E. The development of antibody resistance is a nearly inevitable result of treatment.

149. A nearly 3-year-old boy has almost completed toilet training, although he has had occasional accidents at night. When his parents take him to the beach, he often rushes to the water's edge in excitement, and splashes about for a few moments. He then rushes back to the beach blankets where his parents await. He is in which stage of Erik Erikson's Epigenetic model of development?

A. Basic trust versus basic mistrust
B. Preoperational thought
C. Initiative versus guilt
D. Anal phase
E. Autonomy versus shame and doubt

150. The molecular mechanism of which one of the following drugs of abuse is likely to involve increasing the concentration of dopamine transporters on the cell surface?

A. LSD
B. Cannabis
C. Alcohol

D. MDMA
E. Cocaine

151. Abnormality of which one of the following brain structures is commonly found in patients with obsessive-compulsive disorder?

A. Caudate nuclei
B. Frontal cortex
C. Amygdala
D. Cerebellum
E. Striatum

152. Evidence supporting a genetic contribution to depressive disorders includes which one of the following statements?

A. Twin and family epidemiologic studies
B. Linkage analyses of the CREB 1 locus on chromosome 2
C. Locus variants of brain-derived neurotrophic factor (BDNF)
D. Short allele polymorphism (ss) of the serotonin transporter gene
E. All of the above

153. With regard to the "Five-Factor Dimensional Model" (FFM) of borderline personality disorder (BPD), all of the following are true EXCEPT:

A. BPD ranks highest in the neuroticism domain of all the personality disorders.
B. These patients score low in the "trust" and "compliance" facets of the agreeableness domain.
C. These patients score low in the "competence" facet of the conscientiousness domain.
D. A weakness of the FFM is a lack of appreciation for the heterogeneity of BPD pathology.
E. Patients with BPD score highly in all facets of the neuroticism domain except self-consciousness.

154. A 33-year-old construction worker has been using cocaine for 3 years. Over the past year, he has found himself using greater amounts of cocaine than he intends, often in order to achieve a desired effect. He has recently begun to use cocaine shortly before starting his shifts at work, though he believes that he is still able to function competently at his job. He has repeatedly tried to cut down on his use but has been unable to do so, and he has recently called his ex-wife to cancel several scheduled meetings with his 2-year-old daughter. According to the DSM-IV-TR criteria, which aspect of his history would not be used to support a diagnosis of cocaine dependence?

A. Repeated unsuccessful efforts to cut down on his cocaine use
B. Repeated cancellation of meetings with his daughter

C. The use of greater amounts of cocaine than he intends

D. Increased use to achieve a desired effect

E. Recurrent cocaine use prior to his construction shifts

155. Which one of the following is the strongest predictor of mortality in patients with Anorexia Nervosa?

A. Alcohol abuse

B. History of anxiety disorders

C. Age of onset of eating disorder

D. Number of previous hospitalizations

E. Male gender

156. Which one of the following antidepressant medications is approved by the U.S. Food and Drug Administration (FDA) for the treatment of Bulimia Nervosa?

A. Fluoxetine

B. Nortriptyline

C. Valproic acid

D. Sertraline

E. Bupropion

157. Which of the following lamotrigine-associated rashes DOES NOT warrant discontinuation of lamotrigine; possible hospitalization; and/or contraindication to future rechallenge?

A. Purpuric, tender, or papular

B. Fever, malaise, lymphadenopathy, pharyngitis

C. Abnormal complete blood cell (CBC) count, liver function test (LFT), urea, creatinine, urine analysis

D. Pruritic, spotty, or morbilliform

E. Facial involvement (lips, mouth, eyes)

158. A 28-year-old woman with bipolar disorder who has been doing well on valproate for years comes to the perinatal psychiatry clinic. She and her husband want to start a family and she would like to know the risks to her baby associated with continuing to take valproate during her pregnancy. You tell her that although valproate has not been well studied in pregnancy, it is commonly associated with which of the following effects to the fetus?

A. Hemorrhagic pancreatitis

B. Hepatotoxicity

C. Spina bifida

D. Tremor

E. Erythema multiforme

159. Which one of the following is TRUE of cholinesterase inhibitors in the treatment of patients with Alzheimer's disease?

A. For galantamine, higher doses are associated with larger effect on the cognitive tests.

B. The odds of clinical global improvement demonstrated superiority over placebo for each drug with higher doses producing better effects.

C. Dropout rates were lower with galantamine and rivastigmine.

D. There was little difference in dropout rate for each drug at each dose-level, except with high-dose donepezil.

E. All of the above.

160. IPT identifies dysfunction in all of the following domains EXCEPT:

A. Grief

B. Interpersonal role disputes

C. Role transitions

D. Interpersonal deficits

E. Professional conflicts

161. The release of which one of the following neurotransmitters across the neuromuscular junction triggers muscular contraction?

A. ACh

B. Dopamine

C. Serotonin

D. GABA

E. Norepinephrine

162. Which one of the following statements regarding neurons in the brain is NOT TRUE?

A. Neurons are composed of four morphologically identified regions; the cell body (soma), dendrites, the axon, and the axon terminals.

B. Majority of neurons in the human brain are unipolar as they give rise to a single axon with a single dendritic process.

C. Glial cells are at least 10 times more numerous than neurons.

D. Oligodendrocytes form the myelin sheath of the axon.

E. Astrocytes are the most numerous class of glial cells and participate in the formation of the blood-brain barrier.

163. You are called to the ER to evaluate a 50-year-old man for confusion. The available history is limited, but indicates that the man was brought in by police. He smells strongly of alcohol, but serum alcohol is just above the legal limit and vital signs within normal limits. Examination reveals nystagmus, abducens and conjugate gaze palsies, ataxia of gait, and mental confusion. Which one of the following statements is correct about the proper treatment of this patient?

A. The patient should be given cyanobalamin intramuscularly each day for several days.

B. The patient should be given IV fluids with glucose until adequate oral intake is resumed.

C. The patient should be given a benzodiazepine immediately intramuscularly.

D. The patient should be given 1 mg of folic acid intramuscularly immediately.

E. The patient should be given thiamine intravenously immediately.

164. A baby is brought to your office for the first time. During your physical examination, you notice that his arms are more active than his legs, and when lying on his back, he keeps his head to one side. When lifted from the trunk his head falls unless it is supported. When held standing on your examination table, he makes a "walking movement." His mother tells you that he looks at her while being fed. What is this child's age?

A. Newborn
B. 1 week
C. 1 month
D. 3 months
E. 6 months

165. Under what circumstances would serum melatonin levels be most elevated?

A. During the day
B. During the day if it is dark
C. Following exposure to light
D. During the night if it is dark
E. During peak cortisol levels

166. Which one of the following clinical pictures would you most likely expect in a patient with right orbitofrontal pathology on MRI?

A. Anxiety
B. Depression
C. Obsessions
D. Addictions
E. Mania

167. Which one of the following choices about the genetics of alcoholism is NOT TRUE?

A. Cloninger has identified two main forms of alcoholism.
B. Type I is the late-onset form that has low inheritance.
C. Type I is usually associated with stress and anxiety.
D. Type II alcoholism starts at a younger age.
E. Type II alcoholism is as common in males as it is in females.

168. Dialectical behavioral therapy (DBT) is a treatment specifically developed for patients with BPD, as an offshoot of cognitive behavioral therapy.

All of the following are treatment goals of DBT, EXCEPT:

A. Supporting old behaviors for the patient's immediate advantage
B. Reducing suicidal, parasuicidal, and life-threatening behaviors
C. Addressing current problems that impede quality of life for the patient
D. Resolving past issues which are related to post-traumatic stress
E. Reducing behaviors that interfere with therapy

169. A 15-year-old boy in your addictions clinic tests positive for cannabis during routine urine drug testing. Although he previously used cannabis daily over a period of 3 years, he insists that he has not used any marijuana since he began his addictions treatment program 3 weeks ago. Given this patient's history, up to what length of time might you reasonably expect cannabis to be detected in his urine after he achieves abstinence?

A. 24 hours
B. 48 hours
C. 7 days
D. 2 weeks
E. 4 weeks

170. A 24-year-old woman who has been through a series of failed relationships broke up with her boyfriend. Following this incident, she began having command auditory hallucinations instructing her to kill herself. While taking a history, she reveals that a major bone of contention in her past relationships has been her extravagance, disproportionate to her income. She states that most of her boyfriends initially seemed "absolutely perfect" but a few months later, she began to realize that they were "absolute idiots." She also notes that she often binges on food. She has accumulated several tickets for reckless driving in recent months. Which one of the following statements is TRUE regarding this clinical situation?

A. Her command hallucinations almost certainly mark the onset of schizophrenia or a schizophreniform disorder.
B. Parasuicidal behaviors are rarely seen in this condition, and represents an axis II diagnosis.
C. Her binge-eating episodes are completely unrelated to her axis II diagnosis, and they definitely represent an independent eating disorder.
D. The sex ratio for her axis II diagnosis is markedly tilted towards women.
E. Her risk of substance abuse is not significantly higher than that of the normal population.

171. Which one of the following medications has NOT been reported to be effective in reducing binge eating in bulimia nervosa or in binge-eating disorder (BED)?
    A. Fluoxetine
    B. Topiramate
    C. Naltrexone
    D. Sibutramine
    E. Mirtazapine

172. Which one of the following characteristics IS NOT a risk factor for developing a rash due to lamotrigine?
    A. History of another anti-epileptic drug (AED)-related rash
    B. Starting dose and rate of titration above current recommendations
    C. Co-administration with valproate
    D. History of human immunodeficiency virus (HIV), SLE, or concomitant steroid use
    E. Age younger than 13 years

173. A 30-year-old man with a history of bipolar disorder is on a combination of drugs. He presents with fever, headache, and a hacking cough. This progresses to a spreading red rash. Which one of the following combination of drugs is most likely to have caused this condition?
    A. Lamotrigine and valproic acid
    B. Fluoxetine and valproic acid
    C. Lamotrigine and fluoxetine
    D. Lithium and lamotrigine
    E. Lithium and valproic acid

174. Which of the following is TRUE of Narcotics Anonymous (NA)?
    A. It provides residential treatment for addicts.
    B. It follows the "Twelve Steps" program.
    C. It employs professional counselors.
    D. It discourages the use of psychiatric medications.
    E. All of the above.

175. Assigning a formal psychiatric diagnosis to a patient is part of which phase of IPT?
    A. Phase I
    B. Phase II
    C. Phase III
    D. Phase IV
    E. Phase V

176. What is the main component of prions?
    A. RNA
    B. DNA
    C. Myelin
    D. Free radicals
    E. Protein

177. Which one of the following choices is TRUE regarding the development of the neural tube in humans?
    A. In the early stages of human brain development, the neural tube has four primary vesicles.
    B. Prosencephalon gives rise to midbrain structures.
    C. Metencephalon gives rise to the cerebral cortex.
    D. Diencephalon gives rise to the thalamus and the hypothalamus.
    E. Myelencephalon gives rise to the hippocampus and the amygdala.

178. A 57-year-old man presents with weakness in his right side. On further history, you note a 1-month history of erratic behavior, confusion, and dizziness ill-defined, on exam. MRI shows several dense, homogeneous, and enhancing periventricular masses. The patient is diagnosed with an infiltrative tumor most consistent with a primary large-cell lymphoma. Which one of the following is correct about the proper treatment?
    A. This tumor must be surgically resected and is not responsive to chemotherapy.
    B. The side effects to treatment are usually severe.
    C. There is no need for repeated lumbar punctures in the treatment.
    D. The use of corticosteroids is rarely helpful in management.
    E. Median survival is 6 to 12 months.

179. Which one of the following statements regarding the neurochemical activity of MDMA is TRUE?
    A. MDMA use causes a sudden increase in cholinergic effects.
    B. MDMA use causes a sudden increase in serotonergic effects.
    C. MDMA use causes a sudden increase in noradrenergic effects.
    D. MDMA use causes a sudden decrease in serotonergic effects.
    E. MDMA use causes a sudden decrease in dopaminergic effects.

180. A 3-year-old child is brought to the office for an evaluation of new-onset seizures. During your examination, you notice that the boy does not respond when called by his name and can only say a few words. He shows poor eye contact and has not met some of the developmental milestones expected for his age. The mother reports significant behavioral problems, including frequent tantrums and aggression. What is the most likely diagnosis?
    A. Asperger's syndrome
    B. Rett's syndrome

C. Down syndrome
D. Autism
E. Turner syndrome

181. A 75-year-old widow leaves her home for her annual winter vacation in Florida. She forgets to take her prescription medications with her and 2 days later, begins to experience nausea, tremors, sweating, and increased anxiety. She does not use alcohol or street drugs. Cessation of which of the following medications is most likely to be the cause of her symptoms?

A. Lorazepam
B. Lithium
C. Buspirone
D. Trazodone
E. Valproate

182. On questioning a 25-year-old man about history of substance abuse, he states that he has "done mushrooms." On describing his experiences while on the drug, it becomes clear that it is some sort of hallucinogen. Which one of the following is the most likely drug in question?

A. LSD
B. Mescaline
C. Ibogaine
D. Psilocybin
E. Ayahuasca

183. In which of the following patients should bupropion be avoided?

A. A 25-year-old man with major depression and nicotine dependence
B. A 40-year-old woman with dysthymia who has developed sexual dysfunction with fluoxetine
C. A 50-year-old man with bipolar depression who is taking valproic acid
D. An 18-year-old woman with major depression and comorbid bulimia nervosa
E. A 75-year-old man with major depression who is having a partial response to escitalopram

184. Which one of the following rashes is NOT associated with lamotrigine?

A. Erythroderma
B. Stevens-Johnson syndrome
C. Toxic epidermal necrolysis
D. Toxic shock syndrome (TSS)
E. Drug hypersensitivity syndrome (DHS)

185. A 27-year-old woman, who is a concert pianist with juvenile onset diabetes, is prone to attacks of performance anxiety. Her performances are approximately twice a month. Which one of the following is the drug of choice for the treatment of her anxiety disorder?

A. Propranolol
B. Alprazolam
C. Atenolol
D. Citalopram
E. Fluoxetine

186. Which one of the following statements is TRUE of modafinil?

A. It is excreted unchanged via the kidney.
B. It has a half-life of 6 hours.
C. It is classified as a schedule III drug by the FDA.
D. It is not known to effect the sleep architecture.
E. All of the above.

187. Which category of sexual dysfunction in males is most difficult to treat with sex therapy?

A. Problems with sexual desire
B. Problems with arousal
C. Problems with orgasm
D. Problems with fatigue
E. Problems with erectile dysfunction of psychogenic origin

188. Which one of the following statements regarding serotonergic neurons in the brain is NOT TRUE?

A. The majority of the serotonergic innervation of the forebrain arises from the dorsal and median raphe nuclei of the midbrain.
B. Median raphe nucleus provides the majority of the serotonergic innervation of the limbic system, including the hippocampus and septum.
C. The dorsal raphe nucleus provides the primary innervation of the striatum and thalamus.
D. Caudal raphe serotonergic neurons project to the medulla, cerebellum, and spinal cord.
E. MDMA produces a selective loss of the larger beaded projections derived from the median raphe.

189. Which one of the following statements regarding the human brain is NOT TRUE?

A. The cerebral cortex of each hemisphere can be grossly divided into four major regions; the frontal, parietal, temporal, and occipital lobes.
B. The frontal lobe consists of the primary motor, premotor, and prefrontal regions.
C. The inferior portion of the temporal lobe contains the primary auditory cortex and other auditory regions.
D. Primary somatosensory and areas of the brain associated with complex visual and somatosensory functions are located in the parietal lobe.

E. The occipital lobe consists of the primary visual cortex and other visual association areas.

190. A 31-year-old woman presents to your office asking about genetic testing for Huntington's disease. Her mother just died at age 66 after a 15-year battle with the illness. Your patient states she has thought many times about getting tested, but has avoided it until now. Which of the following statements about the genetic testing of Huntington's disease is TRUE?
    A. Studies have found virtually no negative effects of getting tested.
    B. A reported major benefit of testing is relief from not knowing.
    C. The vast majority of at-risk people get tested for carrier status.
    D. The risk of suicide post testing is minimal.
    E. A current history of depression is a contraindication for testing.

191. Which one of the following statements regarding ketamine is NOT TRUE?
    A. It is structurally related to PCP.
    B. It acts via suppression of frontal lobe activity.
    C. It is a potent NMDA antagonist.
    D. It can cause vivid dreams and flashbacks.
    E. It can cause an increase in the intracranial pressure.

192. What is the cardinal feature of Asperger's syndrome?
    A. Repetitive behaviors
    B. Speech impairment
    C. Failure to read social cues
    D. Inability to initiate conversation
    E. Restricted interest

193. Which one of the following personality disorders has the strongest evidence-based support for a genetic contribution?
    A. Avoidant
    B. Histrionic
    C. Antisocial
    D. Dependent
    E. Schizotypal

194. A 40-year-old woman wears a flashy red outfit to a funeral and bursts out into loud uncontrollable sobs on seeing the body of the deceased. She speaks loudly and is dramatic in her behaviors, drawing attention onto herself. Over the years, she has acquired a reputation for such behavior. Which one of the following sets of problems is she most likely to face?
    A. Difficulties in achieving emotional intimacy
    B. Repeated hand washing and somatization

C. Difficulties in achieving emotional intimacy and preoccupation with orderliness
D. Bipolar disorder
E. Eating disorders

195. Which one of the following statements regarding the dopaminergic system in the CNS is NOT TRUE?
    A. Dopaminergic neurons are more widely distributed than other monoamines in the CNS.
    B. Dopaminergic neurons are found in the midbrain substantia nigra and ventral tegmental area, and in the periaqueductal gray, hypothalamus, olfactory bulb, and retina.
    C. Nigrostriatal, mesocorticolimbic, and tuberohypophysial are three important dopamine containing CNS systems.
    D. Motor disturbance of Parkinson's disease is due to the degeneration of the tuberohypophysial system.
    E. Prolonged use of dopaminergic agonist agents can result in abnormal movements or dyskinesia.

196. Which one of the following statements regarding the ventricular system in the brain is NOT TRUE?
    A. It is has two lateral ventricles in the cerebral hemispheres.
    B. The third ventricle is found on the midline of the diencephalons.
    C. The fourth ventricle is found in the pons and the medulla.
    D. The foramina of Monro connect the third ventricle to the fourth ventricle.
    E. Majority of the CSF is produced at the choroid plexus located in the walls of the lateral ventricles and in the roof of both the third and fourth ventricles.

197. Which one of the following statements about malpractice law is TRUE?
    A. Malpractice insurance never covers an intentional tort by a physician.
    B. A specialist is held to a higher standard because of their specialized training.
    C. Damages done to a patient must be economic.
    D. A physician has a duty to consult when the limits of their experience are reached.
    E. Physicians in the same specialty all over the country are held to the same standard.

198. A 21-year-old college senior is brought by ambulance to the ER in a confused state. He has a temperature of 104°F, complains of a severe headache, has photophobia, neck stiffness, and large ecchymoses on his lower extremities. He was reportedly in fine health that morning. Which one of the following statements

is TRUE about the proper treatment of his condition?

A. Treatment in part with a third-generation cephalosporin is reasonable.

B. His college housemates should be given ciprofloxacin daily for 3 weeks.

C. Antibiotic treatment should wait until the organism is isolated.

D. Oral or intramuscular antibiotic treatment will likely be sufficient.

E. Trimethoprim/sulfamethoxazole is an essential part of most regimens.

199. Which one of the following statements about malpractice law is NOT TRUE?

A. Medical malpractice is defined as negligence that causes harm to the patient.

B. Most malpractice cases are decided in favor of the physician.

C. The doctor's actions must have directly caused the injury.

D. Malpractice cases are rarely settled out of court.

E. The injured patient must show that the doctor's care deviated from the norm.

200. A 42-year-old married mother is driving her three children to school when she is rear-ended by a distracted teenage driver. She immediately experiences neck pain which radiates to her shoulders and arms. In subsequent weeks, she also finds that she is fatigued, intermittently dizzy, and inattentive. Imaging studies are negative and the patient is told she has "whiplash injury." Her symptoms persist for several months and she seeks the advice of a local neurologist. A comprehensive management plan to treat this patient may include all of the following EXCEPT:

A. Moderate range of motion exercises

B. Massage

C. Heat

D. "Neck hygiene"

E. Litigation

Answers

1. Answer: C. Although it is often the first cognitive function affected by dementia, short-term memory is generally unaffected in the normal aging individual. The geriatric patient without dementia may exhibit decline in other cognitive areas, such as reduced ability to sustain attention over long periods, decline in motor speed and response times, and difficulty performing visuospatial tasks. A greater amount of time is often required for the elderly to learn new information, and there may be problems accessing data from long-term memory. Cognitive changes with age are not inevitable and may vary from individual to individual.

Blazer DG, Steffens DC, Busse EW. *American Psychiatric Publishing Textbook of Geriatric Psychiatry*. 3rd ed. Washington: American Psychiatric Publishing; 2004:38.

2. Answer: C. Tryptophan is hydroxylated by tryptophan hydroxylase to form serotonin. Tyrosine is the amino acid precursor of epinephrine and dopamine. Histamine is synthesized from histidine. ACh is synthesized by the transfer of an acetyl group from acetyl coenzyme A.

Sadock BJ, Sadock VA. *Kaplan and Sadock's Comprehensive Textbook of Psychiatry*. 8th ed. Philadelphia: Lippincott Williams & Wilkins; 2005:52–53.

3. Answer: E. The California Verbal Learning Test II is a test of memory, which documents encoding, recognition, and immediate recall followed by a 30-minute recall. It tests for possible learning strategies and susceptibility to semantic interference. The Boston Naming Test (Revised), Verbal fluency, Token Test, and Boston Diagnostic Aphasia Examination are all tests for language functioning.

1. Sadock BJ, Sadock VA. *Kaplan and Sadock's Comprehensive Textbook of Psychiatry*. 8th ed. Philadelphia: Lippincott Williams & Wilkins; 2005:869–870.
2. Swiercinsky DP. *NeuropsychTests*. http://www.brainsource.com/nptests.htm. Accessed August 30, 2006.

4. Answer: A. Most state statutes require that the psychiatrist perform some intervention to prevent harm from occurring when their patient threatens harm to others. This duty is not just limited to warning, but to protect the identifiable victim. According to *Tarasoff v Regents of the University of California*, a psychiatrist who treats violent or potentially violent patients may be sued for failure to control aggressive behavior. A psychiatrist is most liable for a lawsuit if he was aware of the patient's violent tendencies and failed to safeguard the public from these tendencies. In *Tarasoff v Regents of the University of California*, the California Supreme Court had ruled that mental health professionals have a duty to protect identifiable third parties from imminent threats of serious harm made by their outpatients. Some states have adopted the Tarasoff ruling, whereas others have accepted this ruling in a limited or modified manner. However, most states expect the mental health professional to act affirmatively to protect an identified third party from their patient's violent or dangerous acts. Although not a federal law, a clinician should consider the Tarasoff duty to be a national standard of care. Most statutes require an actual threat to be made against a clearly identifiable victim before a duty to warn or to protect arises. This duty involves warning the intended victim and the local law enforcement authority.

1. Gutheil TH, Applebaum PS. *Clinical Handbook of Psychiatry and the Law*. 3rd ed. Philadelphia: Lippincott Williams & Wilkins; 2000:12, 68, 148, 187.
2. Sadock BJ, Sadock VA. *Kaplan and Sadock's Comprehensive Textbook of Psychiatry*. 8th ed. Philadelphia: Lippincott Williams & Wilkins; 2005:3975–3977.

5. Answer: B. The Rey-Österreich Complex Figure Test is a helpful tool to assess visuospatial skills. When patients have a lateralized dysfunction to the right hemisphere, they frequently loose the capacity to capture the global features of a design, and they are only able to reproduce isolated details. On the other hand, when there is lateralized damage to the left hemisphere, patients are able to draw the main framework of a design, but they lose the capacity to reproduce details. The amygdala and putamen are not directly involved in visuospatial functions.

Sadock BJ, Sadock VA. *Kaplan and Sadock's Comprehensive Textbook of Psychiatry*. 8th ed. Philadelphia: Lippincott Williams & Wilkins; 2005:860–875.

6. Answer: C. There is an 11% to 26% comorbidity in pediatric OCD and tic disorders. Patients with OCD and Tourette's syndrome in particular are more likely to have the following OCD symptoms: repetitive touching, counting, ordering and arranging, and a need for symmetry, whereas OCD without comorbid tic disorders is more frequently associated with fears of contamination or of harm befalling self or others.

Sadock BJ, Sadock VA. *Kaplan and Sadock's Comprehensive Textbook of Psychiatry*. 8th ed. Philadelphia: Lippincott Williams & Wilkins; 2005:1773–1774, 3229.

7. **Answer: B.** This child meets the criteria for ODD as his behavior, for a period >6 months, has had five of the eight criteria for ODD. From this vignette, these include: arguing with his parents and teachers; actively defying rules and requests from adults; deliberately annoying others (his sister) and often blaming others (his sister) for his mistakes or misbehavior; and finally, being touchy or easily annoyed with others. ODD is often present at home, but may not necessarily manifest at school. The child may not regard himself as having oppositional or defiant behavior. The lack of aggressive behavior to people or animals, destruction of property, deceitfulness, and theft excludes the diagnosis of conduct disorder. Because there are no reports of hyperactivity, inattention and impulsivity, the diagnosis of ADHD is excluded; moreover, onset of some ADHD symptoms must occur before age 7. Disruptive behavior disorder NOS is characterized by conduct or oppositional defiant behaviors that do not meet the criteria for ODD or conduct disorder. Finally, child antisocial behavior is diagnosed when the focus is on antisocial behavior or isolated acts. Also note that the history does not give evidence for a psychotic or mood disorder which also should be excluded from the differential.

American Psychiatric Association. *Diagnostic and Statistical Manual of Mental Disorders*. 4th ed. Washington: American Psychiatric Association; 2000:100–103.

8. **Answer: A.** The following disorders have all been associated with autism: epilepsy, Fragile X syndrome, tuberous sclerosis, cerebral palsy, phenylketonuria, neurofibromatosis, Down syndrome, congenital rubella, and visual and hearing impairments. Huntington's disease has not been associated with pervasive developmental disorders.

Lewis M. *Child and Adolescent Psychiatry*. 2nd ed. Philadelphia: Lippincott and Williams & Wilkins; 1996:587–595.

9. **Answer: A.** Studies have found that the lifetime prevalence of depression in eating disorders is close to 75%. The CNS effects of starvation sometimes confound the diagnosis. Depressed patients with eating disorders present frequently with labile mood and strong neurovegetative symptoms secondary to the starvation. The lifetime prevalence of substance abuse in this population ranges from 17% to 46%. OCD is also common among patients with eating disorders (lifetime prevalence of around 40%). It can sometimes be hard to distinguish OCD from an eating disorder, because a lot of these patients have specific rituals, including exercising and repetitive weighing. General anxiety disorder and panic attacks have similar lifetime prevalence in patients with eating disorders of about 10% each.

Woodside BD, Staab R. Management of psychiatric comorbidity in anorexia nervosa and bulimia nervosa. *CNS Drugs*. 2006;20:655–663.

10. **Answer: D.** Buspirone is the single $5HT_{1A}$ agonist approved for the treatment of anxiety. It is generally well tolerated and has no significant pharmacokinetic drug interactions. It is considered a serotonin partial agonist which, unlike benzodiazepines, is not associated with a risk of abuse/dependence or withdrawal.

Stahl SM. *Essential Psychopharmacology: Neuroscientific Basis and Practical Applications*. New York: Cambridge University Press; 2000:306.

11. **Answer: D.** The euphoric effect of alcohol is related to its ability to increase both dopamine activity and opioid activity in the brain. Alcohol acts to increase the release of endorphins, the body's naturally occurring opiates, and these opiates bind to receptors in the brain. This results in the pleasurable effects of alcohol. Naltrexone is an opioid receptor antagonist. In studies, although it does not typically improve abstinence rates, it helps patients keep one drink from turning into a relapse, where relapse is defined as a man having five or more drinks in one day or a woman having four or more drinks in one day. By blocking the "high" associated with alcohol, naltrexone also reduces craving for alcohol and the percentage of days in which drinking occurs. Its major side effect is nausea. It can also cause vomiting, anorexia, constipation, and abdominal pain. CNS side effects include nervousness, headache, insomnia, and agitation. Joint pain and muscle pain occur in 10% of patients. Finally, it can also cause hepatic enzyme elevation.

1. Schatzberg AF, Cole JO, DeBattista C. *Manual of Clinical Psychopharmacology*. 5th ed. Washington: American Psychiatric Publishing; 2005:498–502.
2. Volpicelli JR. New options for the treatment of alcohol dependence. *Psychiatr Ann*. 2005;35:6:484–491.

12. **Answer: D.** The most prevalent renal effect of lithium is impairment of concentrating ability, estimated to be present in up to 55% of patients on chronic lithium therapy and caused by an unclear

mechanism. This defect may translate into overt polyuria (>3 L per 24 hours) in 20% to 40% of patients on lithium. Polyuria can cause dehydration and significant discomfort. Polyuria usually resolves within 3 weeks of lithium discontinuance, but can also persist beyond a year. Approximately 5% to 20% of patients on lithium will develop NDI. In NDI, the kidney response to vasopressin is impaired. The established treatment for NDI and severe cases of polyuria includes thiazide diuretics. The mechanism by which thiazide diuretics produce the paradoxic antidiuretic effect remains unclear, but it may have to do with upregulation of aquaporin-2, Na-Cl cotransporter. Amiloride works by inhibiting sodium reabsorption in the distal convoluted tubules and collecting ducts in the kidneys. This promotes the loss of sodium and water from the body, but without depleting potassium. Unlike thiazides, amiloride has a weak natriuretic effect and is less likely to increase plasma lithium levels by causing volume contraction. Nonsteroidal anti-inflammatory drugs (NSAIDs) may have a more favorable tolerability and safety profile relative to thiazides and amiloride. Lithium causes excess production of prostaglandins, which decrease the ability of kidneys to reabsorb free water. NSAIDs inhibit prostaglandin synthesis, which is hypothesized to explain their efficacy in treatment of li-induced polyuria. Rehydration must be strictly monitored because of the risk of renal failure connected with NSAIDs. Indomethacin treatment of lithium-induced NDI has preliminary evidence of being efficacious and safe. Intravenous ketoprofen, with its rapid onset of action, may be an effective alternative to indomethacin in the treatment of severe lithium-induced NDI. Furosemide is not used for NDI, because it will exacerbate the renal collecting tubule defect in concentrating capacity and worsen NDI.

1. Boton R, Gaviria M, Batlle DC. Prevalence, pathogenesis, and treatment of renal dysfunction associated with chronic lithium therapy. *Am J Kidney Dis*. 1987;10:329–345.
2. Lam SS, Kjellstrand C. Emergency treatment of lithium-induced diabetes insipidus with nonsteroidal anti-inflammatory drugs. *Ren Fail*. 1997;19:183–188.
3. Movig KL, Baumgarten R, Leufkens HG, et al. Risk factors for the development of lithium-induced polyuria. *Br J Psychiatry*. 2003;182:319–323.

13. Answer: C. Emotional lability, hyperexcitability, inappropriate temper outburst, crying spells or unpredicted euphoric mood, distractibility, impairment of recent memory, and poor attention span can be seen in patients with hyperthyroidism. In severe cases, psychosis can also occur. In many cases, a major depressive episode and generalized anxiety disorder can occur. Hyperthyroidism occurs seven times more frequently in females than males and has a clear familial predisposition. It usually occurs in women in their third and fourth decades of life, whereas in men, the majority of cases occur in the later decades of life. When hyperthyroidism occurs in the elderly, it is usually manifested by lethargy, apathy, social withdrawal, and overtly depressed mood. In subclinical hyperthyroidism, where there is a normal T3 level with elevated T4 levels, some patients develop an agitated form of depression, which is manifested by irritability, intensity, and diminished sleep. Although mania may occur in hyperthyroidism, it is much less common than agitated depression. When hyperthyroidism is medically treated with the return of T3, T4, and TSH levels to normal, most psychiatric symptoms will subside.

Khouzam HR, Weiser PM, Emes R, et al. Thyroid hormones therapy: a review of their effects in the treatment of psychiatric and medical conditions. *Compr Ther*. 2004;30:148–154.

14. Answer: D. Disulfiram is an irreversible inhibitor of aldehyde dehydrogenase, a hepatic enzyme involved in the intermediary metabolism of ethanol. When alcohol is consumed in the presence of this enzyme inhibition, acetaldehyde levels rise five to 10 times higher than normal, resulting in noxious physical symptoms. Five to 10 minutes after consuming alcohol, the patient taking disulfiram experiences whole-body flushing, severe headache, dizziness, nausea, vomiting, and sweating. The symptoms last from 30 minutes to 2 hours, after which time the patient typically sleeps and fully recovers. Disulfiram is recommended only for alcohol-dependent patients who seek total abstinence and are willing and able to comply with the drug. Hence, it is not recommended for use in patients who are psychotic, suicidal, or impulsive. Medical contraindications include pregnancy, renal failure, moderate to severe hepatic dysfunction, and cardiac disease. Although there is no evidence that agents such as disulfiram have any long-term efficacy, the drug may be useful for patients who have a history of sobriety followed by relapse, or for sober patients facing a time of relapse risk (vacation or holidays). Prior to use, patients must be completely detoxified from alcohol. A dose of disulfiram, typically 250 mg/day, results in sensitivity to alcohol for 6 to 14 days. Patients must be advised to avoid alcohol in all forms, including cough syrups and aftershave.

Rosenbaum JF, Arana GW, Hyman SE, et al. *Handbook of Psychiatric Drug Therapy*. 5th ed. Philadelphia: Lippincott Williams & Wilkins, 2005:225–229.

15. Answer: D. More than 30,000 people die by suicide each year in the United States. The number of attempted suicides is estimated to be 650,000. Suicide rates, in the United States, have averaged 12.5 per 100,000 in the 20th century. Suicide is ranked as the eighth overall cause of death in the United States. Marriage reinforced by children is a protective factor and significantly lessens the risk of suicide. The suicide rate is 11 per 100,000 among married persons. Previously married persons, though, have much higher rates than those who have never been married. Previous medical care appears to be a positively correlated risk factor for suicide. Psychiatric patients have an increased risk for suicide that is three to 12 times greater than nonpatients. Among psychiatric outpatients, the period following discharge from an inpatient setting is a time of significantly increased risk. The psychiatric diagnosis with the greatest risk of suicide in both sexes is a mood disorder. The suicide risk in patients with depressive disorders is 15%. Suicide is more common early in the illness than later. Up to 10% of patients with schizophrenia commit suicide. Suicide is also more common during the first few years of the illness. Up to 15% of all alcohol-dependent persons commit suicide. Despite these risk factors, a past suicide attempt is the best indicator that a patient is at increased risk of suicide. Approximately 40% of depressed patients who attempt suicide have made a previous attempt; 19% to 24% of completed suicides occur after a prior attempt. The risk of a second suicide attempt is highest within 3 months of the first attempt.

Sadock BJ, Sadock VA. *Kaplan and Sadock's Synopsis of Psychiatry*. 9th ed. Philadelphia: Lippincott Williams & Wilkins; 2003:913–922.

16. Answer: A. The stimulation of guanylyl cyclase is not mediated via G-protein coupling, but by the elevation in intracellular calcium and increased nitric oxide production. The cGMP system plays an important role in mediating the responses of photoreceptor cells to light. When it is dark, cGMP levels in these cells are high and when it is light, the cGMP are low. Light mediates its effect by the activation of a phosphodiesterase that hydrolyzes cGMP to guanosine monophosphate (GMP). Drugs such as Viagra block the cGMP phosphodiesterase in the smooth muscles and elevate the cGMP levels, thus exerting their vasodilatory effects.

1. Krumenacker JS, Hanafy KA, Murad F. Regulation of nitric oxide and soluble guanylyl cyclase. *Brain Res Bull.* 2004;62:505–515.
2. Sadock BJ, Sadock VA. *Kaplan and Sadock's Comprehensive Textbook of Psychiatry*. 8th ed. Philadelphia: Lippincott Williams & Wilkins; 2005:91.

17. Answer: C. All of the statements regarding the noradrenergic system in the brain are true except that the activity of LC neurons is highest when the subject is most awake.

1. Kaufman DM. *Clinical Neurology for Psychiatrists*. 5th ed. Philadelphia: WB Saunders; 2001:555–557.
2. Sadock BJ, Sadock VA. *Kaplan and Sadock's Comprehensive Textbook of Psychiatry*. 8th ed. Philadelphia: Lippincott Williams & Wilkins; 2005:50–51.

18. Answer: D. According the Office of Rare Diseases of the National Institute of Health, a rare disease is one that affects <1 per 200,000 people in the United States population. Ophanet, who are a consortium of European partners, currently defines a condition rare when if affects 1 person per 2,000.

National Institutes of Health. NIH Web site. http://www.nih.gov/. Published November 25, 2006.

19. Answer: D. Patients with cerebellar ataxia present with a wide-based, staggering gait that is similar to that seen in patients intoxicated with alcohol. Patients oscillate the head and trunk while walking. When there is a cerebellar lesion, patients tend to deviate toward the lesion when walking in a straight line. Tandem gait is always abnormal in patients with cerebellar ataxia. On the other hand, patients with sensory ataxia usually lift the legs high off the ground and slap the feet down heavily on the floor while walking. Gait markedly worsens if patients are asked to close their eyes. Patients that have a conversion disorder or may be malingering sometimes present with marked lurching movements, but don't lose their balance while walking.

Aminoff MJ, Greenberg DA, Simon RP. *Clinical Neurology*. 6th ed. New York: McGraw-Hill; 2005: 94–120.

20. Answer: E. MRI remains the neuroimaging method of choice for most intracranial and intraspinal abnormalities. It has greater soft tissue contrast and provides better definition of anatomic structures and greater sensitivity to pathologic lesions. Its multiplanar capability displays dimensional information and relationships that are not available on a CT scan. It is also better able to demonstrate physiologic processes such as blood flow and CSF motion. It is also better for visualization of the posterior fossa and intraspinal contents. Its lack of ionizing radiation is also an advantage. Disadvantages of the MRI include the need for cooperation from the patient because most individual MRI sequences require several minutes and a complete study may last anywhere between 20 minutes and 60 minutes. Some patients are also claustrophobic inside the conventional MR unit. MRI is contraindicated in patients with some metallic implants, especially cardiac pacemakers, cochlear implants, older-generation aneurysm clips, metallic foreign bodies in the eye, and implanted neurostimulators. Some authorities also consider pregnancy (especially in the first trimester) to be a relative contraindication to MRI, but the safety data is incomplete. To date, no harmful effect of MRI has been demonstrated in pregnant women or fetuses.

Rowland LP. *Merritt's Neurology*. 11th ed. Philadelphia: Lippincott Williams & Wilkins; 2005:72.

21. **Answer: A.** Tuberous sclerosis (epiloia, Bourneville's disease) arises spontaneously in two thirds of patients. In the remaining, it can arise through autosomal dominant inheritance or through gonadal mosaicism (where a portion of one of the parent's gonadal cells contains the defective gene without the other cells of the body being involved). Tuberous sclerosis is caused by mutations, on two genes—TSC1 and TSC2. The TSC1 is on chromosome 9 and produces a protein called hamartin. The TSC2 gene is on chromosome 16 and produces the protein tuberin. The classical picture includes the triad of mental subnormality, epilepsy, and adenoma sebaceum (a misnomer as these are facial angiofibromas). Hypomelanotic macules (ash-leaf spots) are hypopigmented spots seen over the buttocks and trunk, are the most frequent cutaneous manifestation of tuberous sclerosis, and are best seen using a Wood's light. Shagreen patches are areas of thick, leathery, and pebbly skin seen especially over the nape of the neck. Tumors can grow on any organ, but they most commonly occur on the brain, kidneys, heart, lungs, and skin. Malignant tumors are rare, and those that do occur primarily affect the kidneys. Seizures are the most common presenting complaint, which occur in 60% of the individuals with the most commonly described being infantile spasms. However, the full range of seizures may be seen, including complex partial, tonic, and atonic attacks. The earlier the disorder becomes apparent, the more rapid the course. When it declares itself in childhood, the course is usually progressive with death in the second or third decade.

1. Devlin A. Pediatric neurological examination. *Adv Psychiatr Treatment*. 2003;9:125–134.
2. National Institute of Neurological Disorders and Stroke. Tuberous sclerosis fact sheet. Available at: http://www.ninds.nih.gov/disorders/tuberous_sclerosis/detail_tuberous_sclerosis.htm. Accessed September 12, 2007.

22. **Answer: B.** The previously mentioned disorder is called Bell's palsy, which is the most common disease of the facial nerve. There is equal incidence in men and women, and evidence is accumulating that the majority of cases are caused by viral agents.

The onset is typically acute with maximum paralysis achieved in 48 hours in 50% of cases, which is often preceded by pain behind the ear. Early on, most patients have some impairment in taste, indicating involvement above the joining of the motor and chorda tympani fibers. There is evidence that cases with more-pronounced enhancement of the facial nerve have a worse prognosis, and electromyography (EMG) can help determine the degree of denervation. Eighty percent of the patients recover at least partially in one month, and the most favorable prognostic sign is some motor recovery in the first week.

1. Kress B, Griesbeck F, Stippach C, et al. Bell palsy: quantitative analysis of MR imaging data as a method of predicting outcome. *Radiology*. 2004;230:504–509.
2. Murakami S, Honda N, Mizobuchi M, et al. Rapid diagnosis of varicella zoster virus infection in acute facial palsy. *Neurology*. 1998;51:1202–1205.
3. Ropper AH, Brown RH. *Adams and Victor's Principles of Neurology*. 8th ed. New York: McGraw-Hill; 2005:1181–1182.

23. **Answer: B.** This patient has symptomatic neurosyphilis and is showing signs of general paresis. The onset is usually 20 years after infection and indicates widespread parenchymal damage. The abnormalities can be remembered with the acronym paresis personality, affect, reflexes (hyperactive), eye (Argyll Robertson Pupils [ARP] accommodate, but don't react), sensorium (psychosis), intellect (decrease in memory, orientation, calculation, insight, and judgment), and speech.

A positive CSF VDRL provides a definitive diagnosis, but has a high false-negative rate (up to 40%). The diagnosis can also be made from the clinical and CSF (elevated protein >45 and lymphocytosis) profile. Bacterial meningitis would likely have a cloudy CSF with a much higher white count and lower glucose. Bipolar disease would have a normal CSF and a lack of physical findings. Alzheimer's disease would also have a normal CSF and would not have the physical findings. Wernicke's encephalopathy does also present with memory impairments, but would also have nystagmus and occulomotor impairment.

1. Kasper DL. *Harrison's Principles of Internal Medicine*. 16th ed. New York: McGraw-Hill; 2005:980.
2. Kaufman DM. *Clinical Neurology for Psychiatrists*. Philadelphia: WB Saunders; 2001:148, 533.
3. Ropper AH, Brown RH. *Adams and Victor's Principles of Neurology*. 8th ed. New York: McGraw-Hill; 2005:614–618.

24. **Answer: A.** Neuropsychiatric manifestations are seen in up to 60% of patients with SLE. They show a tendency to appear in the later stages. Any region of the brain can be involved in SLE. CNS events often occur when SLE is active in other organs. Mild cognitive

impairment is the most frequent manifestation. Depression and anxiety are common. Seizures may occur. Less often, psychosis, organic brain syndromes, headache, focal infarcts, extrapyramidal disorders, cerebellar dysfunction, hypothalamic dysfunction, subarachnoid hemorrhage, aseptic meningitis, transverse myelitis, cranial nerve palsies, and peripheral sensorimotorneuropathy occur.

1. Isselbacher KJ, Martin JB, Braunwald E, et al. *Harrison's Principles of Internal Medicine*. 13th ed. New York: McGraw-Hill; 1996:1643–1648.
2. Lishman WA.*Organic Psychiatry*. 3rd ed. Oxford: Blackwell Science; 1996:417–422.

25. Answer: B. Tremors at rest are characteristic of Parkinson's disease. Intention tremors can indicate cerebellar disorders. Bradykinesia, rigidity, and masked facies are all features of Parkinson's disease.

Kaufman DM. *Clinical Neurology for Psychiatrists*. 5th ed. Philadelphia: WB Saunders; 2001:446–447.

26. Answer: D. Comprehensive management of the post-stroke patient is multifaceted and often includes physical therapy (to maintain the patient's muscle tone, prevent contractures, and regain mobility), consistent reorientation and explanation, repositioning (to prevent complications such as decubitus ulcers), and speech therapy. Although cognitive interventions (such as cognitive behavioral therapy) may be useful if the patient develops depression, routine cognitive therapy in stroke patients is without proven value.

Kaufman DM. *Clinical Neurology for Psychiatrists*. 5th ed. Philadelphia: WB Saunders; 2001:282.

27. Answer: B. Erik Erikson created a theory of psychological development that occurs in stages across the life cycle. He proposed that the developmental task of late life (defined as about 60 years of age to the time of death) is to reflect upon and find meaning across one's lifespan. In doing so, the goal is to maintain one's integrity rather than despair. The individual at this stage is expected to abandon the wish that important people in his/her life had been different and to accept responsibility for his/her own life. Erikson's psychosocial stages include: trust versus mistrust (birth to 18 months); autonomy versus shame/doubt (18 months to 3 years); initiative versus guilt (3 to 5 years); industry versus inferiority (5 to 13 years); identity versus role confusion (13 to 20 years); intimacy versus isolation (20 to 40 years); generativity versus stagnation (40 to 60 years); and integrity versus despair (60+).

1. Blazer DG, Steffens DC, Busse EW. *American Psychiatric Publishing Textbook of Geriatric Psychiatry*. 3rd ed. Washington: American Psychiatric Publishing; 2004:371.

2. Sadock BJ, Sadock VA. *Kaplan and Sadock's Comprehensive Textbook of Psychiatry*. 8th ed. Philadelphia: Lippincott Williams & Wilkins; 2005:607–615.

28. Answer: A. 5-HT_{1A} has been shown to be involved in the antidepressant action of psychiatric drugs. 5-HT_{2A} is thought to affect psychotic symptoms and interacts with neuroleptics. 5-HT_{1D} and 5-HT_{1F} are involved with migraines. 5-HT_{2B} regulates stomach contraction.

Sadock BJ, Sadock VA. *Kaplan and Sadock's Comprehensive Textbook of Psychiatry*. 8th ed. Philadelphia: Lippincott Williams & Wilkins; 2005:55.

29. Answer: B. Hemineglect is usually seen in right-hemispheric damage compared to the left hemispheric damage. Aphasia, right–left disorientation, finger agnosia, dysgraphia (aphasic), dyscalculia (number alexia), constructional apraxia (details), and limb apraxia are also seen in left hemispheric damage. Visuospatial deficits, dysgraphia (spatial, neglect), dyscalculia (spatial), constructional apraxia (gestalt), dressing apraxia, and anosognosia are all seen in right hemispheric damage.

1. Kaufman DM. *Clinical Neurology for Psychiatrists*. 5th ed. Philadelphia: WB Saunders; 2001:175–201.
2. Sadock BJ, Sadock VA. *Kaplan and Sadock's Comprehensive Textbook of Psychiatry*. 8th ed. Philadelphia: Lippincott Williams & Wilkins; 2005:861.

30. Answer: C. The National Co-morbidity Survey (NCS) was the first national mental health survey to use a structured diagnostic interview to determine the prevalence and correlates of DSM-III disorders. Overall, substance abuse disorders and anxiety disorders were somewhat more prevalent than mood disorders. Approximately one in four persons surveyed reported a lifetime substance abuse disorder. Data from the NCS revealed alcohol dependence to be one of the most common psychiatric disorders with a lifetime prevalence of 14.1%. The lifetime prevalence of alcohol abuse was reported to be 9.4%. The NCS found the following to be correlated with alcoholism: male gender, younger age, being separated or divorced, low educational level, and low occupational level.

Stern TA, Herman JB. *Massachusetts General Hospital Psychiatry Update and Board Preparation*. 2nd ed. New York: McGraw Hill; 2002:484–485.

31. Answer: D. The clock-drawing test is an easy and reliable screening test for dementia. The severity of clock drawing failures progresses over time in Alzheimer's disease, and it correlates with longitudinal changes in cognitive testing. Several neuropsychological functions are tested during this procedure, and they include comprehension, visuospatial tasks, verbal and semantic memory, as well as executive and constructional functions. Functional neuroimaging has shown that the major area activated during this procedure is the right parietal cortex. Other activated areas include the dorsal premotor areas, left ventral prefrontal cortex, and bilateral cerebellum.

1. Ino T, Asada T, Ito J, et al. Parieto-frontal networks for clock drawing revealed with fMRI. *Neurosci Res*. 2003;45: 71–77.
2. Royall DR, Cordes JA, Polk M. CLOX: an executive clock drawing task. *J Neurol Neurosurg Psychiatry*. 1998;64:588–594.

32. Answer: E. This patient does not meet DSM-IV-TR criteria for an eating disorder. She currently has a normal weight for her height, has normal menstrual periods, has not been engaging in purging behavior, and her amount of exercise is not "excessive." Her pattern of food consumption would not be classified as "binge eating." The primary care physician may offer reassurance and information about eating disorders and agree to follow the patient for any changes in her behavior, mental status, and/or physical condition.

American Psychiatric Association. *Quick Reference to the Diagnostic Criteria from DSM-IV-TR*. Washington: American Psychiatric Association; 2000:263–266.

33. Answer: C. This question attempts to reveal the logic of the diagnostic criterion for ADHD. According to the DSM-IV-TR criterion, a child can meet criteria for ADHD solely with inattentive symptoms if he has six out of nine symptoms of inattention: he would be diagnosed with ADHD, predominantly inattentive type. However, a child cannot meet criteria with impulsive symptoms alone, and because there are only three symptoms of impulsivity, this behavior cannot fulfill the criterion of six or more symptoms of hyperactivity and impulsivity for diagnosis. Hyperactive and impulsive symptoms only would indicate the diagnosis, ADHD, predominantly hyperactive-impulsive type. Criterion B requires that impairment for some of the symptoms must have been present before 7 years of age ("adult-onset ADHD" does not exist, although a significant percentage of children continue to experience ADHD symptoms as adults). Criterion C requires that the symptoms be present in two – not just one—settings, often meaning home and school (or work). Finally, oppositional behavior is not a criterion for the diagnosis; however, children with ADHD can exhibit oppositional behavior.

1. American Psychiatric Association. *Diagnostic and Statistical Manual of Mental Disorders*. 4th ed. Washington: American Psychiatric Association; 2000:85–93.

2. Sadock BJ, Sadock VA, Jones RM. *Kaplan & Sadock's Study Guide and Self-Examination Review in Psychiatry*. 7th ed. Philadelphia: Lippincott Williams & Wilkins; 2003:402–407.

34. Answer: B. The Threvatan criteria for the diagnosis of Rett's disorder include eight main criteria and eight supportive criteria for the diagnosis. The following include some of the main criteria included in both the DSM-IV-TR and the Threvatan criteria: normal prenatal and perinatal history, normal psychomotor development for the first 6 months, normal head circumference at birth, postnatal deceleration of head growth in most individuals, loss of purposeful hand skills by the age of 2, hand stereotypes and evolving social withdrawal, communication dysfunction, loss of acquired speech, and cognitive impairment and impairment or deterioration of locomotion. The other problems listed are common in Rett's disorder, but are not necessary to make the diagnosis.

1. American Psychiatric Association. *Quick Reference to the Diagnostic Criteria from DSM-IV-TR*. Washington: American Psychiatric Association; 2000:59–64.
2. Hagberg B, Hanefeld F, Percy A, et al. An update on clinically applicable diagnostic criteria in Rett syndrome. Comment to Rett Syndrome Clinical Criteria Consensus Panel Satellite to European Paediatric Neurology Society Meeting, Baden Baden, Germany. *Eur J Paediatr Neurol*. 2002;6:293–297.
3. Williamson SL, Christodolou J. Rett syndrome: new clinical and molecular insights. *Eur J Hum Gen*. 2006;14:896–903.

35. Answer: E. The four criteria to diagnose anorexia nervosa according to the DSM-IV-TR are the following: refusal to maintain body weight above 85% of that expected; intense fear of gaining weight or becoming fat; disturbance in the way in which one's body and weight are experienced; and the absence of at least three consecutive menstrual cycles. Patients with anorexia nervosa usually feel guilty about being "fat," although they are underweight. Binge eating can be present in anorexia nervosa, but it is more common in bulimia nervosa, and it is not a diagnostic criterion for anorexia.

American Psychiatric Association. *Quick Reference to the Diagnostic Criteria from DSM-IV-TR*. Washington: American Psychiatric Association; 2000:263–266.

36. Answer: E. When a drug is administered orally, it is absorbed in the small bowel and enters the portal circulation to reach the liver. Cytochrome enzymes in the bowel wall and in the liver metabolize a portion of the drug before it reaches the systematic circulation. This metabolism of the drug in the bowel wall and the liver is called first-pass metabolism. This effect can be altered by processes/diseases affecting the bowels and the liver. Transporters in the bowel wall can either increase or decrease the absorption of the drug. Dietary factors, drugs and diseases of the liver like hepatitis, cirrhosis, or congestive heart failure can alter the first-pass metabolism of the drug. Once first-pass metabolism has occurred, metabolites are excreted into the bile and then the small bowel. Lipid soluble metabolites are reabsorbed into the portal circulation and then reach the systemic circulation. Intramuscular or intravenous administration of drugs avoids the first-pass metabolism and the drugs enter the systemic circulation directly. Medical conditions, such as cirrhosis, can cause portacaval shunting, allowing drugs to avoid the first-pass metabolism and enter the systemic circulation directly and, therefore, enhance their effect.

Janicak PG, Davis JM, Preskorn SH. *Principles and Practice of Psychopharmacotherapy*. 3rd ed. Philadelphia: Lippincott Williams & Wilkins; 2001:24.

37. Answer: E. The mechanism of action of acamprosate in the treatment of alcohol dependence is unclear. It is thought, however, that it affects both GABA and glutamate activity. It may help to restore the normal balance between neuronal excitation and inhibition that is altered in chronic alcohol dependence. Although naltrexone generally improves relapse rates and alcohol craving, it has little effect on abstinence rates. Acamprosate, however, produces significant improvements in abstinence rates and increases the time before any drinking occurs. It also reduces alcohol craving. The main side effect is diarrhea, which occurs in approximately 12% of patients. Headache is another common side effect. It has no abuse potential and does not produce any significant drug interactions. The combination of naltrexone and acamprosate may be more effective than either agent alone.

1. Schatzberg AF, Cole JO, DeBattista C. *Manual of Clinical Psychopharmacology*. 5th ed. Washington: American Psychiatric Publishing; 2005:498–502.
2. Volpicelli JR. New options for the treatment of alcohol dependence. *Psychiatr Ann*. 2005;35:6:484–491.

38. Answer: B. In this review, less-educated couples were observed to have better outcomes in therapy. The review also indicted that younger couples have a better outcome and that unemployed couples and couples with more severe difficulties have worse outcomes.

Snyder D, Castellani A, Whisman M. Current status and future directions in couple therapy. *Ann Rev Psychol*. 2006; 57:334–335.

39. Answer: D. In a recent paper, the authors chose to identify, review, and analyze studies comparing ato-

moxetine with psychostimulants with the intent of determining the role of atomoxetine in the pharmacologic management of ADHD. They found five head-to-head trials had compared psychostimulants and atomoxetine in the treatment of ADHD. No significant difference between atomoxetine and methylphenidate immediate-release were found on the ADHD Rating Scale total score. Osmotic oral release system (OROS) methylphenidate showed significantly greater improvement at weeks 1 and 2, and significantly more patients treated with OROS methylphenidate were classified as being responders. Patients on both atomoxetine and mixed amphetamine salts extended-release (MAS XR) showed significant improvements at endpoint over baseline; however, Swanson, Kotkin, Agler, M-Flynn, and Pelham (SKAMP) scores were significantly better with MAS XR. Tolerability was similar between atomoxetine and stimulant medications. Based on available evidence, the authors concluded that psychostimulants are regarded as the first-line pharmacologic treatment for children and adolescents with ADHD, because the efficacy and safety of these agents have been well established based on clinical trials and extensive naturalistic use. Atomoxetine represents an alternative treatment for ADHD and is unlikely to be associated with abuse. However, more long-term safety data are needed to further establish its place in therapy.

Gibson AP, Bettinger TL, Patel NC, et al. Atomoxetine versus stimulants for treatment of attention deficit/hyperactivity disorder. *Ann Pharmacother*. 2006;40:1134–1142.

40. Answer: E. Acamprosate should be started after the patient has been detoxified from alcohol and should *not* be stopped if the patient relapses into drinking. In controlled trials, the medication has shown modest benefit in reducing drinking in alcoholics. Approximately 20% of patients treated with acamprosate maintained abstinence over the course of 1 year compared to 10% of placebo-treated patients. The starting dose is 333 mg three times daily with meals, titrating as tolerated to a dose of 666 mg three times daily. The optimal duration of treatment is not known, but 6 to 12 months of treatment is appropriate when combined with psychosocial treatment. Acamprosate's mechanism of action is not fully understood, but hypotheses include stimulation of GABAergic neurotransmission and antagonism of excitatory amino acids, such as glutamate. Acamprosate is not a sedative and is not habit-forming. Although mild and time-limited, the most common side effects are GI in nature (nausea, diarrhea, flatulence). The medication is contraindicated in pregnancy, renal failure, and in patients with significant liver disease.

Rosenbaum JF, Arana GW, Hyman SE, et al. *Handbook of Psychiatric Drug Therapy*. Philadelphia: Lippincott Williams & Wilkins, 2005:230–232.

41. Answer: A. Unfortunately, it is not uncommon for psychiatrists or mental health providers to be assaulted. It has been estimated that more than 50% of psychiatrists and 75% of mental health nurses have experienced an act or threat of violence within the past year. A 15-year analysis of assaults on staff in a Massachusetts mental health care system divided the acts into four types: physical, sexual, nonverbal threats/intimidation, and verbal assault. Risk factors for violence among psychiatric patients include an individual history of violence; active paranoid delusions; hallucinations associated with negative effects; manic states, neurological abnormalities; alcohol or drug intoxication and withdrawal states; and a history of abuse, family violence, or "rootlessness." A history of past violence is the strongest predictor of future violence in psychiatric patients. The Clinical Antipsychotic Trials of Intervention Effectiveness (CATIE) found an increased risk of violence in patients with positive psychotic symptoms (i.e., in schizophrenic patients with combined low negative and high positive Positive and Negative Syndrome Scale (PANSS) scores). This group of patients was at the highest risk to have caused bodily injury or have harmed someone with a weapon within the past 6 months. On the other hand, there was a decreased risk of violence in patients with predominantly negative symptoms.

1. Battaglia J. Is this patient dangerous? 5 steps to help clinicians prepare for violent behavior and improve safety. *Curr Psychiatry*. 2006;5:11:25–32.
2. Krahn LE, Battaglia J. Protect yourself against patient assault: when to get out of harm's way (interview). *Curr Psychiatry*. 2006;5:11:15–24.

42. Answer: B. All of the statements are true except that most, but not all, of the actions of G proteins are mediated by diffusible second messengers and, in many cases, the G proteins themselves link to neurotransmitter receptors to activate ion channels.

1. Butt AM. Neurotransmitter-mediated calcium signaling in oligodendrocyte physiology and pathology. *Glia*. 2006;54:666–775.
2. Ding D, Greenberg ML. Lithium and valproate decrease the membrane phosphatidylinositol/phosphatidylcholine ratio. *Mol Microbiol*. 2003;47:373–381.
3. Sadock BJ, Sadock VA. *Kaplan and Sadock's Comprehensive Textbook of Psychiatry*. 8th ed. Philadelphia: Lippincott Williams & Wilkins; 2005:91–92.

43. Answer: E. All of the statements regarding the histaminergic system in the brain are true. Histaminergic fibers project diffusely to the hypothalamus, thalamus, hippocampus, amygdala, rostral forebrain, diagonal band, septum, olfactory bulb, midbrain, and spinal cord. These fibers do not make synaptic connections and act as a local hormone at a distant site, away from their original release site.

Sadock BJ, Sadock VA. *Kaplan and Sadock's Comprehensive Textbook of Psychiatry*. 8th ed. Philadelphia: Lippincott Williams & Wilkins; 2005:51.

44. Answer: E. Answer choices B, C, and D are three diagnostic criteria for RLS. The fourth criteria indicates that symptoms improve (not worsen) with movement. Family history supports the diagnosis with more than 50% of the patients with idiopathic RLS endorsing such. Presence of periodic leg movements in sleep and positive response to dopaminergic therapy also support the diagnosis. Current first-line treatment recommendations include dopaminergic agents and gabapentin.

1. Schapira AH. RLS patients: who are they? *Eur J Neuro*. 2006;13(suppl 3):2–7.
2. Vignatelli L, Billiard M, Clarenbach P, et al. EFNS guidelines on management of restless legs syndrome and periodic limb movement disorder in sleep. *Eur J Neurol*. 2006;13:1049–1065.

45. Answer: B. Dystonic movements are abnormal movements that are usually slow and sinuous in nature. They are not present during sleep and are usually exacerbated by emotional stress. These types of movements sometimes only occur during voluntary movement and during specific activities, such as chewing or speaking. Many disorders can present with dystonic movements, including neurological disorders like Parkinson's disease, Wilson's disease, and Huntington's disease, as well as the use of certain medications, such as levodopa, SSRIs, and antipsychotic medications.

Aminoff MJ, Greenberg DA, Simon RP. *Clinical Neurology*. 6th ed. New York: McGraw-Hill; 2005:94–120.

46. Answer: E. Because the use of gadolinium adds to the direct costs of the MRI, increases the imaging time, and also increases the discomfort to the patient from the intravenous needle placement, it should only be used for specific clinical situations in which its efficacy has been demonstrated or compared to where its use may detect significant abnormality as a routine noncontrast MRI. Clinical situations where gadolinium enhanced MRI is not useful, because of relatively few contrast-enhancing lesions, include complex partial seizures, headaches, dementia, head trauma, workup of psychosis, low back or neck pain, and congenital craniospinal anomalies. MRI in these conditions should use special MR pulse sequences directed to detect lesions in the structures of greatest interest.

Rowland LP. *Merritt's Neurology*. 11th ed. Philadelphia: Lippincott Williams & Wilkins; 2005:74.

47. Answer: D. The patient has AIP, an autosomal dominant disease. The attacks can be precipitated by certain drugs, including barbiturates. This disorder often mimics other diseases (e.g., Guillain-Barré syndrome, bowel obstruction, and psychotic disorders) and, for this reason, the diagnosis can be overlooked. The cardinal features which present in different forms include colicky abdominal pain, psychotic symptoms and an ascending paralysis. If the urine is allowed to oxidize, it turns a dark red color secondary to porphobilin, which is an oxidation product of porphobilinogen. Acute intermittent porphyria can be fatal. Depending on the severity, it is treated with intravenous glucose and hematin. (Although one can see syndrome of inappropriate antidiuretic hormones (SIADH) and liver damage, LFTs and serum and urine sodium and osmolality would not be the appropriately specific diagnostic tests. CSF protein would be helpful for diagnosing Guillain-Barré syndrome—where one would expect to see a high protein, but low white blood cell count.)

1. Kaufman DM. *Clinical Neurology for Psychiatrists*. 5th ed. Philadelphia: WB Saunders; 2001:78.
2. Patten J. *Neurological Differential Diagnosis*. 2nd ed. Berlin: Springer-Verlag; 2003:345.
3. Ropper AH, Brown RH. *Adams and Victor's Principles of Neurology*. 7th ed. New York: McGraw-Hill; 2000:1129.

48. Answer: D. Huntington's chorea is a neurodegenerative disorder manifesting in middle age. It is associated with CAG repeat expansions located on chromosome 4. Progressive cognitive impairment is a cardinal feature. It has autosomal dominant inheritance, and the carriers who are heterozygous for the deleterious gene have a 50% chance of transmitting it to their children. CAG repeats of 40 or larger are associated with disease expression, and those with 26 or less repeats are normal.

1. Fragassi NA, Stanzione M, Angelini R, et al. Huntington chorea. Clinical correlations and preliminary neuropsychological data. *Acta Neurol (Napoli)*. 1992;14:530–536.
2. Levin BC, Richie KL, Jakupciak JP. Advances in Huntington's disease diagnostics: development of a standard reference material. *Expert Rev Mol Diagn*. 2006;6:587–596.

49. Answer: D. Porphyrias are a group of disorders relating to heme metabolism. VP is a hepatic porphyria that results from the deficiency of protoporphyrinogen oxidase inherited as an autosomal dominant trait. It frequently occurs in white South Africans with an incidence of 3 in 1,000. Neurovisceral signs and symptoms develop after puberty usually in the third decade. Symptoms are more common in males than in females. VP is clinically indistinguishable from AIP and HCP. The skin lesions are similarly indistinguishable from HCP and PCT by biopsy; these conditions are diagnosed by measurements of porphyrins and porphyrin precursors in blood, urine, and feces. Cutaneous manifestations are present in 80% of the patients usually in light exposed areas. Acute attacks are seen in 50% of the patients and cause neuropsychiatric, GI, and cardiovascular symptoms, which are precipitated by increases in hepatic Aminolevulinic acid synthase (ALA synthase) (e.g., by drugs that increase cytochrome P450, such as sulfonamide antibiotics or by starvation dieting). Other triggers include intercurrent illnesses, alcohol excess, and endocrine influences, such as steroid hormones, menstrual hormonal changes, and estrogens and progesterone. During attacks, symptoms include delirium, colicky abdominal pain, dark urine, axonal neuropathy that can mimic Guillain-Barré syndrome, seizures, coma, tachycardia, and hypertension. Epileptic fits may occur in 20%; status epilepticus may develop. Mental symptoms, such as anxiety, depression, paranoia and hallucinations, delirium, and agitated behaviors, may arise. It may be mistaken for psychiatric illness during attacks, which may be reinforced if a history of unexplained intermittent physical complaints emerges, leading to diagnoses, such as personality disorders and somatoform disorders. In addition to increased fecal protoporphyrin and coproporphyrin and urinary coproporphyrin, the fluorescence emission spectrum of plasma porphyrins is helpful in the diagnosis; the latter especially in differentiating from PCT where there are no CNS signs. The attacks last from a few days to several months. Treatment is with intravenous hematin and avoidance of sun exposure and trigger factors. EPP, the most common of the erythropoietic porphyrias, results from deficiency of ferrochelatase and is transmitted as an autosomal dominant trait. It usually presents in childhood with cutaneous photosensitivity.

1. Endocrine diseases and metabolic disorders. In: Lishman WA, *Organic Psychiatry*. 3rd ed. Oxford: Blackwell Science; 1996:567–569.
2. Isselbacher KJ, Martin JB, Braunwald E, et al. *Harrison's Principles of Internal Medicine*. 13th ed. New York: McGraw-Hill; 1996:2073–2079.

50. Answer: E. Procainamide, hydralazine, chlorpromazine, D-penicillamine, isoniazid, methyldopa, quinidine, alpha interferon, valproate can all cause drug-induced lupus erythematosus, carbamazepine, hydantoins, and ethosuximide. There is genetic predisposition to drug induced lupus, which is partly determined by drug acetylating rates. Most common are systemic complaints and arthralgias. CNS and renal diseases are rare.

1. Isselbacher KJ, Martin JB, Braunwald E, et al. *Harrison's Principles of Internal Medicine*. 13th ed. New York: McGraw-Hill; 1996:1643–1648.
2. Kauffman CL, Lupus Erythematosus, drug induced. http://www.emedicine.com/derm/topic107.htm. Accessed August 28, 2006.

51. Answer: C. Dementia secondary to Parkinson's disease is more common in patients who develop Parkinson's disease after 65 years of age and is not typically an early symptom of this disorder. Patients with Parkinson's disease can have a unilateral tremor for years before it progresses bilaterally. Atenolol can decrease essential tremor and not be a cause for it. There is no evidence of symptoms specific to Huntington's disease, and he has no family history for this disorder. A cerebellar stroke would cause an intention tremor, and hyperthyroidism would likely produce bilateral fine tremors.

Kaufman DM. *Clinical Neurology for Psychiatrists*. 5th ed. Philadelphia: WB Saunders; 2001:447–450.

52. Answer: D. Since 1968, under generally accepted criteria, the criteria for brain death has been irreversible coma with no discernable CNS criteria. Although it has been argued that the diagnosis of brain death fails to correspond to any coherent biological or philosophical understanding of death, and that it is nearly impossible to demonstrate the irreversible cessation of all functions of the entire brain, including the brainstem, brain death continues to be an accepted diagnosis. According to United States law, brain death equals death. After death is declared, it is medically ethical to donate organs. Although the criteria are controversial, brain death can be diagnosed if cardiac function is maintained, there is no spontaneous respiratory functioning, irreversible coma, no posturing, no cranial reflexes, and no evidence of hypothermia. Brain death can be diagnosed in this case, and organ donation is allowable. Choice E is partially correct, but a patient has to be declared dead before donating organs.

1. Potts M, Evans DW. Does it matter that organ donors are not dead? Ethical and policy implications. *J Med Ethics*. 2005;31:406–409.
2. Landmark article Aug 5, 1968: A definition of irreversible coma. Report of the Ad Hoc Committee of the Harvard Medical School to examine the definition of brain death. *JAMA*. 1984;252:677–679.

3. Stead LG, Stead SM, Kaufman MS, et al. *First Aid for the Medical Clerkship*. New York: McGraw-Hill; 2002:100.

53. Answer: B. Statement A describes stage 1; statement C describes stage 2; statement D describes stage 4; and statement E describes stage 6. Stage 5 is of a contractual and legalistic orientation with a sense of obligation to the law, but with the acceptance that people can have a variety of different values; regardless, their individual right takes precedence over the social contract. Colby et al. (1983) grouped these six stages into three levels: level 1 is the premoral (stages 1 and 2); level 2 is the conventional role of conformity (stages 3 and 4); and level 3 (self-accepted moral principles).

Lewis M. *Child and Adolescent Psychiatry: A Comprehensive Textbook*. 3rd ed. Philadelphia: Lippincott Williams & Wilkins; 2002:265–266.

54. Answer: E. Studies in depression have demonstrated that decreased inhibitory tone from serotonin, as well as excitatory effects of norepinephrine, ACh, and corticotrophin-releasing factor, may be responsible for the upregulation of the hypothalamic-pituitary axis, but none have suggested a role for the thyroid releasing factor.

1. Duman RS, Heninger GR, Nestler EJ. A molecular and cellular theory of depression. *Arch Gen Psychiatry*.1997;54:597.
2. Sadock BJ, Sadock VA. *Kaplan and Sadock's Comprehensive Textbook of Psychiatry*. 8th ed. Philadelphia: Lippincott Williams & Wilkins; 2005:55.

55. Answer: D. Finger tapping, grooved pegboard, and grip strength are all tests of motor speed.

1. Sadock BJ, Sadock VA. *Kaplan and Sadock's Comprehensive Textbook of Psychiatry*. 8th ed. Philadelphia: Lippincott Williams & Wilkins; 2005:869–870.
2. Swiercinsky DP. http://www.brainsource.com/nptests.htm. Accessed August 30, 2006.

56. Answer: B. Community-based psychiatry means that the large majority of psychiatric patients should have the opportunity to be treated at the community level. Primary health care is one of the major components of the mental health care system. This basic level of care stands between the general population and psychiatric specialty services. Primary care providers are often the first to see emotional distress, although they may not always recognize it. Another important, unavoidable component of community psychiatry is patient and family involvement. Provision of emotional support and appropriate information (regarding not only psychiatric illness, but also patient rights and resources) to patients and families can reduce individual suffering, illness relapse, and family/caregiver burden. Psychosocial rehabilitation is yet another integral component of community psychiatry. By improving individual competencies and affecting environmental changes, psychosocial rehabilitation allows individuals disabled by mental illness to reach their optimal level of functioning in the community. Community psychiatric services should be local, accessible, and able to address the multiple needs of individuals.

Sadock BJ, Sadock VA. *Kaplan and Sadock's Comprehensive Textbook of Psychiatry*. 7th ed. Philadelphia: Lippincott Williams & Wilkins; 2000:3338–3339.

57. Answer: C. Every test should adhere to a number of statistical and psychometrical principles in order to be helpful. Some of these principles include satisfactory reliability and validity. Internal consistency is the degree to which one test item correlates with all other test items. Parallel-form reliability is the degree to which two equivalent versions of a test give the same result. Test-retest reliability is the degree to which a test will give the same result on two different occasions separated in time. Interrater reliability is the probability that two judges will give the same score to a given answer, rate a given behavior in the same way, or add up the score properly. Content validity is the degree to which a test measures all the aspects of the quality that is being assessed.

Gelder MG, Lopez-Ibor JJ, Andreasen N. *New Oxford Textbook of Psychiatry*. New York: Oxford University Press; 2000:94–100.

58. Answer: A. In patients with anorexia nervosa, a younger age at onset has been consistently associated with better outcomes. Chronicity of illness, obsessive-compulsive personality traits, self-induced vomiting, and binge eating behavior have each been identified as negative prognostic factors in the literature, although their association has been inconsistent across studies. These factors may be more predictive of short-term outcome than longer-term outcome. In general, adolescents have better outcomes than adults, and younger adolescents have better outcomes than older adolescents.

1. American Psychiatric Association. *Practice Guideline for the Treatment of Patients with Eating Disorders*. 3rd ed. Washington: American Psychiatric Association; 2006:70–72.
2. Sadock BJ, Sadock VA. *Kaplan and Sadock's Synopsis of Psychiatry*. 9th ed. Philadelphia: Lippincott Williams & Wilkins; 2003:744.

59. Answer: E. Children with ADHD often perform better in one-to-one interactions as opposed to group interactions. Consequently, this deficit causes them great difficulty in peer relations in a group context such as camps, sports, extra-curricular activities, and group games, leading to unpopularity with peers and siblings. ADHD is the most commonly diagnosed childhood psychiatric disorder and is estimated to occur in 3% to 5% of school-age children. Epidemiological data document prevalence rates ranging from 2% to 12%. Children with ADHD injure themselves more frequently and have an elevated risk of developing other psychiatric and behavioral difficulties in childhood, adolescence, and adulthood, including antisocial/criminal behavior, substance abuse, mood and anxiety disorders, as well as academic and vocational underachievement. This disorder is tremendously costly for society, costing schools over $3 billion annually. Moreover, poor insurance coverage for ADHD can compound the financial burden for families.

1. Lewis M. *Child and Adolescent Psychiatry: A Comprehensive Textbook*. 3rd ed. Philadelphia: Lippincott Williams & Wilkins, 2002: 645–670.
2. Stubbe DE. Attention-deficit/hyperactivity disorder overview: historical perspective, current controversies, and future directions. *Child Adolesc Psychiatr Clin North Am*. 2000:9:469–479.

60. Answer: C. There is a strong association between birth weight and the development of autism. Other risk factors include low Apgar score, gestational age at birth <35 weeks, and parental psychiatric history. Although it was suggested that the month of birth could be associated with the development of autism, larger and more recent studies have not confirmed this association. Parental alcohol use, exposure to the tetanus vaccine, and low parental age have not been associated with autism.

Larsson HJ, Eaton WW, Madsen KM, et al. Risk for autism: perinatal factors, parental psychiatric history, and socioeconomic status. *Am J Epidemiol*. 2005;161:916–925.

61. Answer: A. Patients with anorexia nervosa can present with hypercholesterolemia due to reduced catabolism. Other common laboratory abnormalities include leukopenia with relative leukocytosis, hypercortisolemia, hypercarotenemia, hypoglycemia, abnormal liver function tests, low serum zinc levels, and electrolyte abnormalities. Patients can also have hormonal abnormalities, such as abnormal T4 levels with normal TSH.

American Psychiatric Association. *American Psychiatric Association Practice Guidelines for the Treatment of Psychiatric Disorders: Compendium 2006*. Psychiatry Online: American Psychiatric Association. http://www.psychiatryonline.com/content.aspx?aID=139788. Accessed February 15, 2007.

62. Answer: B. MAOIs may be the treatment of choice in atypical depressive disorders. Their adverse effect profile includes serotonin syndrome (as described in the clinical vignette). There are numerous contributors to serotonin syndrome, including prescription medications, over-the counter (OTC) remedies, drugs of abuse, and dietary supplements. Treatment includes discontinuation of the offending agent, supportive care, 5HT2A antagonists, cyproheptadine or second-generation antipsychotics, control of autonomic instability, and hyperthermia. Diphenhydramine (Benadryl) does not cause this condition. A major complication of diphenhydramine use is anticholinergic syndrome, manifested by hypoactive bowel sounds, dry hot skin, normal reflexes, and urinary retention as well as an altered mental status and other typical symptoms. Malignant hyperthermia would be distinguished by hyporeflexia and rigor mortis-like rigidity.

1. Boyer EW, Shannon M. The Serotonin Syndrome. *N Engl J Med*. 2005;352:1112–1120.
2. Gillman P. A review of serotonin toxicity data: implications for the mechanisms of antidepresssant drug action. *Biol Psych*. 2006;59:1046–1051.
3. Janicak P, Davis J, Preskorn S, et al. *Principles and Practice of Psychopharmacotherapy*. 4th ed. Philadelphia: Lippincott Williams & Wilkins; 2006: 252; 284–285.

63. **Answer: C.** Several studies have shown that fluoxetine and TCAs, such as desipramine, produce significant improvement in depression in active alcoholic patients and decrease alcohol intake simultaneously. In the past, many believed that alcoholic patients should be abstinent for at least 4 weeks (and remain depressed) before starting any antidepressants. However, a 1998 study by Greenfield, et al. found that all alcoholic patients admitted to a hospital for detoxification, who also had a recent diagnosis of major depressive disorder, relapsed into drinking after discharge. None of the patients had been prescribed antidepressants. Given this data, the use of antidepressants in treating depressed alcoholic patients is encouraged even if the patients are likely to still be drinking. Bupropion, although an antidepressant, is contraindicated in conditions that lower the seizure-threshold, such as alcohol withdrawal, and thus would not be an optimal choice in this patient.

1. Greenfield SF, Weiss RD, Muenz LR, et al. The effect of depression on return to drinking: a prospective study. *Arch Gen Psychiatry*. 1998;55:259–265.
2. Schatzberg AF, Cole JO, DeBattista C. *Manual of Clinical Psychopharmacology*. 5th ed. Washington: American Psychiatric Publishing; 2005:498–502.
3. Volpicelli JR. New options for the treatment of alcohol dependence. *Psychiatr Ann*. 2005;35:6:484–491.

64. **Answer: E.** Cardiac arrhythmias have been noted to occur in patients receiving lithium. This side effect, however, almost always occurs in patients with preexisting cardiac disease. The most common types of arrhythmias that occur in patients taking lithium

with preexisting cardiac disease is sinoatrial (SA) node dysfunction (sick sinus syndrome), thus patients with this history should not receive lithium unless a cardiac pacemaker is in place. Before initiating lithium therapy, clinicians should obtain a cardiac history and a baseline electrocardiogram (ECG) in patients over 50 years of age. While a patient is on lithium therapy, cardiac side effects (i.e., palpitations, dizziness, syncope) should be monitored and an ECG should be repeated when clinically indicated. Lamotrigine, valproate, and gabapentin do not have cardiac side effects. QTc prolongation is unlikely to occur with olanzapine and it is safe to use in patients with sick sinus syndrome.

Rosenbaum JF, Arana GW, Hyman SE, et al. *Handbook of Psychiatric Drug Therapy*. 5th ed. Philadelphia: Lippincott Williams & Wilkins; 2005:145.

65. **Answer: D.** In an excellent Cochrane review, the authors assessed the effects of day hospital versus inpatient care for people with acute psychiatric disorders. Combined data suggested that at the most, day hospital treatment was feasible for 23% (CI 21 to 25) of those currently admitted to inpatient care. Individual patient data from three trials showed no difference in the number of days in hospital between day hospital patients and controls (CI 1.32 to 0.55). However, compared to controls, people randomized to day hospital care spent significantly more days in day hospital care (CI 1.97 to 2.70) and significantly fewer days in inpatient care (CI 3.63 to 1.87). There was no significant difference in readmission rates between day hospital patients and controls (RR 0.91, CI 0.72 to 1.15). For patients judged suitable for day hospital care, individual patient data from three trials showed a significant time-treatment interaction, indicating a more rapid improvement in mental state (Chi-squared 9.66, $p = 0.002$), but not social functioning (Chi-squared 0.006, $p = 0.941$) amongst patients treated in the day hospital. Four of five trials found that day hospital care was less expensive than inpatient care (with cost reductions ranging from 20.9% to 36.9%). The authors' concluded that caring for people in an acute day hospital can achieve substantial reductions in the numbers of people needing inpatient care, while also improving patient outcome.

Marshall M, Crowther R, Almaraz-Serrano A, et al. Day hospital versus admission for acute psychiatric disorders. *Cochrane Database Syst Rev*. 2003, Issue 1. Art No.: CD_004026. DOI: 10.1002/14651858.CD00_4026.

66. **Answer: B.** Medications most commonly implicated in causing hyperprolactinemia are antipsychotic (neuroleptic) agents. These drugs are dopamine receptor blockers. Their effects are mediated by D2

receptors in the hypothalamic tuberoinfundibular system and on the lactotrophs. The antipsychotic potency of the older phenothiazines, butyrophenones, and dibenzoxazepine was found to parallel their potency in increasing prolactin levels. The level of prolactin found with these drugs is usually <100 μg/L. Among the atypical antipsychotic medications, risperidone is known to cause elevations in prolactin level even higher than those caused by the typical antipsychotics. In contrast, clozapine, olanzapine, quetiapine, ziprasidone, and aripiprazole are much less likely to elevate prolactin levels. It is believed that the lack of effect of these atypical agents is due to their being only transiently and weakly bound to the D2 receptor or to their having agonist activity as well as antagonist activity at the D2 receptor. Hyperprolactinemia causes decreased libido, erectile dysfunction in men, and galactorrhea and amenorrhea in women.

Molitch ME. Medication-induced hyperprolactinemia. *Mayo Clin Proc*. 2005;80:1050–1057.

67. Answer: C. Unfortunately, it is not uncommon for psychiatrists or mental health providers to be assaulted. It has been estimated that more than 50% of psychiatrists and 75% of mental health nurses have experienced an act or threat of violence within the past year. A 15-year analysis of assaults on staff in a Massachusetts mental health care system divided the acts into four types: physical, sexual, nonverbal threats/intimidation, and verbal assault. Risk factors for violence among psychiatric patients include an individual history of violence; active paranoid delusions; hallucinations associated with anger, sadness, and anxiety; manic states, neurological abnormalities; alcohol or drug intoxication and withdrawal states; and a history of abuse, family violence, or "rootlessness." A history of past violence is the strongest predictor of future violence in psychiatric patients. The diagnosis of bipolar disorder does not in and of itself indicate an increased risk of violence. Psychiatric diagnoses associated with increased risk include schizophrenia, bipolar mania, alcohol and other substance abuse, and personality disorders. Demographic variables associated with higher violence comprise ages 15 to 24, nonwhite race, male gender, poverty, and low educational level. CATIE found an increased risk of violence in patients with positive psychotic symptoms (i.e., in schizophrenic patients with combined low negative and high positive PANSS scores). This group of patients was at the highest risk to have caused bodily injury or have harmed someone with a weapon within the past six months from the time of evaluation. On the other hand, there was a decreased risk

of violence in patients with predominantly negative symptoms.

1. Battaglia J. Is this patient dangerous? 5 steps to help clinicians prepare for violent behavior and improve safety. *Curr Psychiatry*. 2006;5:25–32.
2. Krahn LE, Battaglia J. Protect yourself against patient assault: when to get out of harm's way (interview). *Curr Psychiatry*. 2006;5:11:15–24.

68. Answer: B. Neuropeptides may act as neurotransmitters, neuromodulators, or neurohormones. Although neuropeptides are released into synapses and axon terminals, release may also occur throughout the axon or even from dendrites. Neuropeptides can also diffuse to target cells away from their release site and act as neurohormones. Neuropeptides are usually released by exocytosis of the granules in response to electrical or hormonal stimulation of the neuron. The cellular signaling of neuropeptides is mediated by specific neuropeptide receptors. Most of the neuropeptide receptors are G-protein-coupled, seven-transmembrane domain receptors and each neuropeptide receptor is specifically coupled to one type of G protein.

1. Sadock BJ, Sadock VA. *Kaplan and Sadock's Comprehensive Textbook of Psychiatry*. 8th ed. Philadelphia: Lippincott Williams & Wilkins; 2005:76.
2. Vitetta L, Anton B, Cortizo F, et al. Mind-body medicine: stress and its impact on overall health and longevity. *Ann NY Acad Sci*. 2005;1057:492–505.

69. Answer: B. Choline within the brain is transported from the blood and is taken up into cholinergic neurons by a high-affinity active transport mechanism. This uptake of choline and not the transfer of acetyl group from acetyl coenzyme A to choline, mediated by the enzyme ChAT is the rate limiting step in the synthesis of acetylcholine.

1. Kaufman DM. *Clinical Neurology for Psychiatrists*. 5th ed. Philadelphia: WB Saunders; 2001:558–559.
2. Sadock BJ, Sadock VA. *Kaplan and Sadock's Comprehensive Textbook of Psychiatry*. 8th ed. Philadelphia: Lippincott Williams & Wilkins; 2005:51–52.

70. Answer: C. Approximately 50% of Tourette's patients have comorbid OCD, but <10% of OCD patients have Tourette's.

Sadock BJ, Sadock VA. *Kaplan and Sadock's Comprehensive Textbook of Psychiatry*. 8th ed. Philadelphia: Lippincott Williams & Wilkins; 2005:1774.

71. Answer: D. This patient is presenting with agraphesthesia, which is the inability to identify a number or letter when traced on the palm a patient's hand. Astereognosis is the incapacity to distinguish between different shapes or textures by touch. Abarognosis is the inability to distinguish between different weights. Agraphesthesia, abarognosis, and agraphesthesia imply a lesion in the contralateral parietal lobe. Apraxia is the inability to execute a voluntary motor movement despite having normal muscle function. A patient that interprets a small tactile perception as pain is suffering from allodynia.

Aminoff MJ, Greenberg DA, Simon RP. *Clinical Neurology*. 6th ed. New York: McGraw-Hill; 2005:201–231.

72. Answer: E. CT scan is still widely used in the evaluation of acute strokes, head injury, or acute infections. It is more useful than an MRI in patients who are neurologically or medically unstable, uncooperative, or claustrophobic. It is also better for patients with pacemakers or other metallic implants that may be contraindications for an MRI. CT is better for patients on respirators as respirators will not function in the high magnetic field of the MR scanner. CT is a more reliable and unambiguous method for detecting acute brain parenchymal or subarachnoid hemorrhage. CT is also better in evaluating the bones of the skull and spine.

Rowland LP. *Merritt's Neurology*. 11th ed. Philadelphia: Lippincott Williams & Wilkins; 2005:70.

73. Answer: C. Women with multiple sclerosis (MS), once they conceive, do not have more difficulties than other woman during their pregnancy. In fact, the rate of exacerbations typically is reduced during pregnancy, though they typically have an increased rate postpartum. Only 10% of patients experience primary progressive MS, a steady, deteriorating course. Most have some form of remission during the course of their illness. Although MS is a clinical diagnosis, MRI's are frequently used to help in diagnosis. Internuclear ophthalmoplegia is caused by damage to the medical longitudinal fasciculus (MLF); however, the disruption of the MLF leads to a paralysis of the adducting eye during lateral gazing. Eighty percent of patients with multiple sclerosis will at some point experience optic neuritis.

1. Goetz C. *Textbook of Clinical Neurology*. 2nd ed. Philadelphia: WB Saunders; 2003:1067.
2. Kaufman DM. *Clinical Neurology for Psychiatrists*. 5th ed. Philadelphia: WB Saunders; 2001:370–375.

74. Answer: B. Pneumococcal infections are common in splenectomized patients; hence, they have a higher incidence among sickle cell anemia patients who are autosplenectomized. Cryptococcal meningitis is common in immunosuppressed populations. Bacteroides and actinomyces found in the CSF should raise a strong suspicion of a brain abscess.

1. Jacobs MR. Streptococcus pneumoniae: epidemiology and patterns of resistance. *Am J Med*. 2004;117 (suppl 3A):3S–15S.

2. Lepage P, Dresse MF, Forget P, et al. Infections and antibiotic prophylaxis in sickle cell disease. *Rev Med Liege*. 2004;59:145–148.

75. Answer: B. Attacks in AIP may be triggered by barbiturates, carbamazepine, MAOIs, and TCAs. Sulpiride is contraindicated in porphyria. Phenothiazines, such as chlorpromazine, promazine, and trifluoperazine, may be used safely for emotional disturbance, whereas others such as flupentixol and zuclopenthixol, may be used with caution. Of the atypical antipsychotics, olanzapine may be used safely. Among the anticonvulsants, gabapentin may be used safely; however, sodium valproate and lamotrigine should be used with caution. Fluoxetine and lithium are safe; lithium is excreted exclusively through the kidneys. Benzodiazepines may be used in low doses, especially lorazepam and clonazepam. Diazepam should be used with caution. Chloral hydrate and zopiclone can be safely used as hypnotics. Information about porphyria is not available regarding many drugs.

1. European Porphyria Initiative. Drugs and porphyria. Available at: http://www.porphyria-europe.com/03-drugs/how-to-use-info.asp. Accessed August 28, 2006.
2. Reynolds NC Jr, Miska RM. Safety of anticonvulsants in hepatic porphyrias. *Neurology*. 1981;31:480–484.
3. Larson AW, Wasserstrom WR, Felsher BF, et al. Posttraumatic epilepsy and acute intermittent porphyria: effects of phenytoin, carbamazepine, and clonazepam. *Neurology*. 1978;28:824–828.

76. Answer: B. Middle cerebral artery occlusions involving the right parietal lobe are most likely to be associated with anosognosia, that is, failure to recognize the hemiplegia. These lesions cause left-sided paralysis, anosognosia, and left hemineglect. Bilateral temporo-occipital lesions give rise to prosopagnosia (difficulty in recognizing faces). Lesion of the right subthalamic nucleus will cause left-sided hemiballismus. Lesions of the left perisylvian cortex cause aphasia.

Rowland LP. *Merritt's Neurology*. 11th ed. Philadelphia: Lippincott Williams & Wilkins; 2005:297–299.

77. Answer: E. This patient's symptoms are characteristic of cervical spondylosis, a degenerative condition that can cause progressive damage to the spinal cord. Upper motor neuron signs, such as Babinski and Hoffman, would be positive along with decreased vibration sense, which suggests involvement of the spinal cord. Hyporeflexia is generally indicative of peripheral nervous system lesions, but in cervical spondylosis, there may be decrease in biceps and brachioradialis reflexes, yet hyperreflexia in the triceps reflex.

Victor M, Ropper AH. *Principles of Neurology*. 7th ed. New York: McGraw-Hill; 2001:1322–1324.

78. Answer: C. Prenatal genetic counseling has been available for over three decades. The definition provided by the American Society of Human Genetics states that genetic counseling is a communication process, which deals with the human problems associated with the occurrence or the risk of occurrence in a family. The process involves a genetic counselor helping the family to (i) comprehend the medical facts, including the diagnosis, probable course and the available management, (ii) appreciate the way heredity contributes to the disorder and risk of recurrence in specified relatives, (iii) understand the alternatives for dealing with the risk of recurrence, (iv) choose a course of action that seems to them appropriate in view of their risk, their family goals, and their ethical and religious standards, and act in accordance with those standards, and (v) to make the best possible adjustment to the disorder in an affected family member and/or to the risk of recurrence of the disorder. This model emphasizes the communication process, and shies away from advice giving.

1. Saal HM. Prenatal diagnosis: when the clinician disagrees with the patient's decision. *Cleft Palate J.* 2002;39:174–178.
2. Ad Hoc Commitee. American Society of Human Genetics Ad Hoc Committee on Genetic Counseling. *Am J Hum Genet.* 1975;27:240–242.

79. Answer: D. Carol Gilligan also postulated that hypothetical and real-life moral dilemmas elicit different types of responses. Although her work led to the resurgence considering benevolence in relation to justice, further studies have failed to replicate her findings and cast doubt on her proposition that men and women speak in a "different voice" morally. Other studies, however, have shown that sex differences in early social behavior do occur with girls being more compliant and willing to share more toys, especially with other girls.

Lewis M. *Child and Adolescent Psychiatry: A Comprehensive Textbook.* 3rd ed. Philadelphia: Lippincott Williams & Wilkins; 2002:265–266.

80. Answer: C. Dopamine receptors are divided into two subclasses (type 1 and type 2). Type 1 receptors (D1 and D5) act through an increase in the intracellular cAMP production causing excitatory input, whereas type 2 receptors (D2, D3, and D4) act through a decrease in cAMP production causing inhibitory input.

Sadock BJ, Sadock VA. *Kaplan and Sadock's Comprehensive Textbook of Psychiatry.* 8th ed. Philadelphia: Lippincott Williams & Wilkins; 2005:313.

81. Answer: C. This patient has conduction aphasia and not Broca's aphasia, as he can converse and comprehend speech, but cannot repeat. These patients have relatively intact auditory comprehension and spontaneous speech as the Wernicke's and Broca's areas are unaffected. However, they have trouble repeating words due to damage to the arcuate fasciculus that connects the Wernicke's and Broca's areas. Broca's aphasia (nonfluent or expressive aphasia) is characterized by impaired verbal fluency and repetition, but intact auditory comprehension. Broca's aphasia occurs due to a lesion to the suprasylvian area extending from the Broca's area to the posterior extent of the sylvian fissure.

1. Goetz C. *Textbook of Clinical Neurology.* 2nd ed. Philadelphia: WB Saunders; 2003:88–90.
2. Kaufman DM. *Clinical Neurology for Psychiatrists.* 5th ed. Philadelphia: WB Saunders; 2001:175–201.
3. Sadock BJ, Sadock VA. *Kaplan and Sadock's Comprehensive Textbook of Psychiatry.* 8th ed. Philadelphia: Lippincott Williams & Wilkins; 2005:861–862.

82. Answer: D. Three elements must be satisfied for a patient's consent to be informed: competency, information, and voluntariness. In most cases, competent patients have a right to refuse treatment. Forcing treatment against a competent patient's wishes may result in assault and battery or malpractice. There are important exceptions to the requirement of informed consent for treatment. The most common exception is an *acute, life-threatening crisis* in which an unconscious patient is unable to provide informed consent. Another exception is termed *therapeutic privilege*; that is, a physician determines that disclosing information to the patient would cause significant harm to the patient or prevent rational decision-making. A third exception is the competent patient's right to *waiver*; that is, to decline full disclosure of information. Finally, *incompetency* or incapacity renders a patient unable to fully understand disclosed information; hence, these patients are not able to effectively provide informed consent. In this case, a substitute decision maker is necessary. Because a patient is psychotic does not necessarily mean they lack decision-making capacity.

Sadock BJ, Sadock VA. *Kaplan and Sadock's Comprehensive Textbook of Psychiatry.* 7th ed. Philadelphia: Lippincott Williams & Wilkins; 2000:3284.

83. Answer: A. Structural neuroimaging in schizophrenia has consistently found reductions in prefrontal and temporal cortices, even in first-episode schizophrenia. These abnormalities have also been detected using functional neuroimaging techniques. Other less common abnormalities seen in schizophrenia include smaller total brain volumes and abnormal activation in thalamic and cerebellar areas.

1. Abou-Saleh MT. Neuroimaging in psychiatry: an update. *J Psychosom Res*. 2006;61:289–293.
2. Sadock BJ, Sadock VA. *Kaplan and Sadock's Comprehensive Textbook of Psychiatry*. 8th ed. Philadelphia: Lippincott Williams & Wilkins; 2005:1396–1400.

84. Answer: B. Women are overrepresented among bipolar II patients and in special populations (mixed/dysphoric mania, winter depression, bipolar depression with atypical features, rapid-cycling bipolar disorder). If one looks at the depression-mania continuum, there is a clear trend: the higher the depressive component, the higher the proportion of women.

Sadock BJ, Sadock VA. *Kaplan and Sadock's Comprehensive Textbook of Psychiatry*. 8th ed. Philadelphia: Lippincott Williams & Wilkins; 2005:1578.

85. Answer: C. Often arguing with adults, defying them, and refusing to comply with their direction or rules are criterion for ODD. Conduct disorder is a persistent pattern of behavior in which a person disregards the rights of others and does not follow age-appropriate social norms or rules. The diagnostic criteria fall into four broad categories, including aggression to people and animals, destruction of property, deceitfulness or theft, and serious violations of rules. For diagnosis of the disorder, the child must present with at least three criteria over the past year and at least one over the past 6 months. Staying out late at night and running away overnight (A) meets criterion A 13 and 14. The lack of empathy involved in being physically cruel and endangering the life of the household cat (B) meets criterion A 5. Shoplifting nontrivial items (D) meets criterion A 12. And bullying and threatening others, in addition to initiating physical fights (E), meets criterion A 1 and 2. Note that coding is based on the age of onset. Onset of at least one criterion of conduct disorder prior to age 10 as in answer B qualifies for the subtype: childhood-onset type. Absence of such criteria prior to age 10 is then coded as conduct disorder, adolescent-onset type.

1. American Psychiatric Association. *Diagnostic and Statistical Manual of Mental Disorders*. 4th ed. Washington: American Psychiatric Association; 2000:93–99.
2. Stern TA, Herman JB. *Massachusetts General Hospital Psychiatry Update and Board Preparation*. 2nd ed. New York: McGraw-Hill; 2004:34.

86. Answer: A. Level of intellectual functioning has been strongly associated with severity of symptoms in the three main affected areas in the autistic disorder. Patients with a lower prognostic outcome tend to have a higher association with other medical problems, female gender, and a lower prevalence of family history of psychiatric disorders.

Willemsen-Swinkels SH, Buitelaar JK. The autistic spectrum: subgroups, boundaries, and treatment. *Psychiatr Clin North Am*. 2002;25:811–836.

87. Answer: C. Vital signs are an important indication of the severity of starvation in patients with anorexia nervosa. Some of the indications for immediate hospitalization include marked orthostatic hypotension, bradycardia (heart rate <40 beats/minute), tachycardia (heart rate >110 beats/minute), abnormal body temperature (<97°F), rapid weight loss, and severe dehydration, especially in children. Although amenorrhea is a considerable problem and a marker of nutritional deficiencies, it is not an indication for immediate hospitalization. Denial of a weight problem, binge eating, and family conflicts are commonly seen in patients with eating disorders.

American Psychiatric Association. *Practice Guidelines for the Treatment of Psychiatric Disorders: Compendium 2006*. Psychiatry Online: American Psychiatric Association. Available at: http://www.psychiatryonline.com/content.aspx?aID=138866. Accessed February 15, 2007.

88. Answer: D. Duloxetine (Cymbalta) is associated with a significant dose-dependent increase in liver enzymes (AST, ALT) in some patients. Three patients in clinical trials, additionally, had elevated alk phos and bilirubin levels. All three also had evidence of heavy alcohol use. Thus, the patient package insert discourages dispensing duloxetine to patients with active substantial alcohol use. Acamprosate is FDA approved for maintenance of abstinence in alcohol dependence, and is cleared by the kidneys (not the liver). Lithium is also cleared by the kidneys, and has some evidence of beneficial effect in alcohol dependent patients. It also has been shown to be protective against suicide. "Imipramine is the most extensively studied tricyclic for depressed alcoholics." SSRIs also demonstrate some positive effect in this patient population.

1. Cipriani A, Pretty H, Hawton K, et al. Lithium in the prevention of suicidal behavior and all-cause mortality in patients with mood disorders: a systematic review of randomized trials. *Am J Psychiatry*. 2005;162:1805–1819.
2. Janicak P, Davis J, Preskorn S, et al. *Principles and Practice of Psychopharmacotherapy*. 4th ed. Philadelphia: Lippincott Williams & Wilkins; 2006;273:648–649.
3. Sadock BJ, Sadock VA. *Kaplan and Sadock's Comprehensive Textbook of Psychiatry*. 8th ed. Philadelphia: Lippincott Williams & Wilkins; 2005:2451.

89. Answer: A. PCP enhances dopaminergic transmission and also modulates NMDA and glutamate receptor activity. Acute PCP intoxication can produce behavior that mimics schizophrenia or mania and is also bizarre and violent. Patients who come to the ER are often agitated or violent. They may need seclusion and restraints, because attempting to talk them down is usually unsuccessful. Agitation and violent behavior may also be managed with high-potency antipsychotics, which can be alternated with benzodiazepines. Acidifying the patient's urine with ammonium chloride may facilitate excretion. Low-potency antipsychotics, however, can exacerbate the already significant anticholinergic effects of PCP and are also sometimes associated with delirium in these patients.

Schatzberg AF, Cole JO, DeBattista C. *Manual of Clinical Psychopharmacology*. 5th ed. Washington: American Psychiatric Publishing; 2005:504.

90. **Answer: E.** Stevens-Johnson syndrome is a generalized hypersensitivity reaction that can occur in patients taking lamotrigine. This reaction occurs more frequently in patients with a history of antiepileptic drug related rash (A is incorrect); children younger than 13 years of age (B is incorrect); and when lamotrigine is used in combination with Depakote (C is incorrect). Ideally lamotrigine should be started at 25 mg/day and increased by 25 mg/week. After reaching 100 mg for 1 week, the dose can then be increased by 50 mg/week. Maintenance doses range between 100 to 400 mg daily. Lamotrigine is metabolized by the liver and excreted by the kidney. Its elimination half-life is 24 hours and is altered by hepatic enzyme induction and inhibition. When carbamazepine, an enzyme inducer, is combined with lamotrigine, the elimination half-life of lamotrigine is 12 hours. In contrast, when valproate, an enzyme inhibitor, is combined with lamotrigine, the elimination half-life of lamotrigine rises to 72 to 100 hours. There is no drug-drug interaction between lamotrigine and warfarin.

1. Hirsch LJ, Weintraub DB, Bushsbaum R, et al. Predictors of lamotrigine-associated rash. *Epilepsia*. 2006; 47:318–322.
2. Rosenbaum JF, Arana GW, Hyman SE, et al. *Handbook of Psychiatric Drug Therapy*. 5th ed. Philadelphia: Lippincott Williams & Wilkins; 2005:163–166.

91. **Answer: D.** In a Cochrane review, the authors assessed the effectiveness of day treatment programs versus outpatient care for patients with treatment-refractory disorders; the effectiveness of day care centers versus out-patient care for patients with severe long-term disorders; and the effectiveness of transitional day hospital care for patients who had just been discharged from hospital. The evidence from a trial suggested that day treatment programs were superior to continuing outpatient care for improving psychiatric symptoms. There was no evidence that a day treatment program was better or worse than outpatient care on any other clinical or social outcome variable or on costs. There was no evidence that day care centers were better or worse than outpatient care on any clinical or social outcome variable. There was inconclusive data on costs, which suggested that day care centers might be more expensive than outpatient care. There was also evidence from a trial suggesting that transitional day hospital care was superior to outpatient care in keeping patients engaged in treatment; however, there was insufficient evidence to judge whether it was better or worse on any other clinical or social outcome variable or on costs. The authors concluded that there is only limited evidence to justify the provision of day treatment programs and transitional day hospital care, and there is no evidence yet to support the provision of day care centers.

Marshall M, Crowther R, Almaraz-Serrano AM, et al. Day hospital versus out-patient care for psychiatric disorders. *Cochrane Database Syst Rev*. 2001;3:CD003240.

92. **Answer: C.** Disulfiram is an alcohol-sensitizing agent that makes the ingestion of alcohol unpleasant by irreversibly inhibiting the enzyme, Aldehyde Dehydrogenase (ALDH). Patients can be sensitive to alcohol for up to 2 weeks after stopping disulfiram. The ingestion of alcohol causes a dose dependent reaction, which is characterized by skin flushing, increased heart rate, and decreased blood pressure. Additionally, nausea, vomiting, shortness of breath, dizziness, and confusion are often present. Occasionally, more severe reactions, such as marked tachycardia, congestive heart failure and cardiovascular collapse, occur. Psychotic symptoms can be exacerbated by inhibition of disulfiram dopamine β-hydroxylase, especially at higher doses. The approval of disulfiram predated rigorous testing requirements, and controlled trial evidence is equivocal. With special efforts to ensure compliance, however, several trials have found an improved outcome.

1. Brewer C, Meyers RJ. Does disulfuram help to prevent relapse in alcohol abuse? *CNS Drugs*. 2000;14:329–341.
2. Chick J, Gough K, Falkowski W, et al. Disulfiram treatment of alcoholism. *Br J Psychiatry*. 1992;161:84–89.
3. Kranzler HR, Ciraulo DA. *Clinical Manual of Addiction Psychopharmacology*. Arlington: American Psychiatric Publishing; 2005:19–22.

93. **Answer: B.** Most patients with mental illness are not violent. However, violence can be associated with psychiatric illnesses such as schizophrenia, major depressive disorders, substance abuse, personality disorders (antisocial and borderline), dementia, and traumatic brain injury, in addition to specific states

(e.g., confusion, intoxication, akathisia, fearfulness, agitation, paranoid delusions, and command hallucinations). Aggression and violence can be categorized as either being impulsive, unplanned, and spontaneous behavior that is sometimes explosive, or as premeditated, deliberate behavior that may be predatory (committed for material gain or power), or as pathological, a reaction to misperceptions, hallucinations, or delusions. Biochemically, evidence indicates that impulsive aggression may result from the disruption of serotonin transmission. This leads to loss of inhibitory control of behavior. Low CSF levels of 5-HIAA (low CSF levels of 5-HIAA represent low central serotonin activity) have been found in aggressive psychiatric inpatients, impulsive violent men, aggressive male children and adolescents, victims of violent suicides, and individuals with type 2 alcoholism. Irritable aggression has been linked to catecholamine (norepinephrine and dopamine) neurotransmission. However, only a modest role for catecholamines has been demonstrated in impulsive aggression.

Levenson JL. *The American Psychiatric Publishing Textbook of Psychosomatic Medicine*. Washington: American Psychiatric Publishing; 2005:171–191.

94. Answer: E. All of the statements are true except that the neuroanatomical pattern of peptide hormone gene expression is determined by the DNA sequences and not the RNA sequences surrounding the gene.

Sadock BJ, Sadock VA. *Kaplan and Sadock's Comprehensive Textbook of Psychiatry*. 8th ed. Philadelphia: Lippincott Williams & Wilkins; 2005:74.

95. Answer: E. All the statements are TRUE except that GABA-A and not GABA-B receptor activity opens up chloride channels, causing an influx of chloride ions into the cell. This causes a lowering of the neuronal resting potential and hyperpolarization of the neuronal membrane. This hyperpolarization leads to an inhibitory effect on neuronal activity. GABA acts as a "fast" neurotransmitter in contrast to monoamines, which are considered "slow." The GABA-B receptor is also inhibitory and is G-protein linked to potassium and calcium channels.

1. Kaufman DM. *Clinical Neurology for Psychiatrists*. 5th ed. Philadelphia: WB Saunders; 2001:558–559.
2. Sadock BJ, Sadock VA. *Kaplan and Sadock's Comprehensive Textbook of Psychiatry*. 8th ed. Philadelphia: Lippincott Williams & Wilkins; 2005:60–68.

96. Answer: D. The incidence of WNV infection has been rising with 9,856 cases reported in 2003 and 29% of those manifesting CNS infection. Risk factors include immunocompromise, medical illness, increasing age, and male gender. Common symptoms include fever, flu-like symptoms, lym-

phadenopathy, and rash. More severe cases include GI involvement (pancreatitis or fulminant hepatitis), cardiac involvement (myocarditis), or CNS involvement. Common presentations with CNS involvement include altered mental status (secondary to delirium/encephalitis) or poliomyelitislike effects (flaccid paralysis) among others.

Arciniegas DB, Andersen CA. Viral encephalitis: neuropsychiatric and neurobehavioral aspects. *Curr Psychiatry Rep.* 2004;6:372–379.

97. Answer: C. Patients with an upper motor neuron lesion usually present with spasticity, increased tendon reflexes, and no muscle atrophy. There is muscle weakness or paralysis. Superficial abdominal reflexes are lost and there is an extensor plantar response (positive Babinski sign). Depending on the specific location of the lesion, patients will present with additional clinical findings. If there is a discrete lesion in the cerebral cortex a patient may present with a focal motor deficit; if the lesion is at the level of the internal capsule, patients may present with contralateral hemiparesis. On the other hand, a brainstem lesion usually results in bilateral motor abnormalities, as well as sensory and cranial nerve deficits.

Aminoff MJ, Greenberg DA, Simon RP. *Clinical Neurology*. 6th ed. New York: McGraw-Hill; 2005:154–197.

98. Answer: C. The findings of an elevated opening pressure, elevated protein, low glucose, and elevated white blood cell count with a predominance of neutrophils is characteristic of acute bacterial meningitis. Gram stain of the CSF specimen is also helpful to guide initial antimicrobial therapy until the organism is identified. Choice A represents the findings expected in a normal CSF specimen. In choice B, the elevated glucose is the only abnormality, which reflects elevated serum glucose. The CSF glucose is generally approximately 60% of the serum glucose. Slightly elevated opening pressure and protein, as well as normal glucose and a lymphocytic predominance in the elevated white count suggest viral meningitis, although early in the course of viral infection, the leukocytic infiltration can be primarily neutrophilic. Markedly elevated red blood cells, as seen in choice E, can be seen in the setting of a traumatic tap or in the presence of a subarachnoid hemorrhage. The presence of xanthochromic changes can be helpful in determining the source of the bleed, as can the collection of spinal fluid itself. In a traumatic tap, the spinal fluid should become clear by the collection of the third tube; if not, another source of bleeding should be sought. The white blood cell findings in the presence of the elevated red blood cell count are difficult to interpret. Normal values for spinal fluid: opening pressure: 90 to 180 mm H_2O; protein: 15 to 45 mg/dL; glucose: 50 to 80 mg/dL; lymphocytes: 35% to 80%; monocytes: 20% to 55%; neutrophils: 3% to 10%.

Henry JB, Davey FR, Chester CJ, et al. *Clinical Diagnosis and Management by Laboratory Methods*. 20th ed. Philadelphia: WB Saunders; 2001:426–437.

99. **Answer: E.** Olfactory hallucinations may be a manifestation of partial complex seizures that originate in the medial-inferior surface of the temporal lobe (the uncus). These seizures are characterized by a typically ill defined odor, although any smell is possible. The sensation is superimposed on impaired consciousness and behavioral disturbances. A continuous sensation is unlikely to be caused by a seizure.

Kaufman DM. *Clinical Neurology for Psychiatrists*. Philadelphia: WB Saunders; 2001:35.

100. **Answer: A.** Pigmented iris hamartomas or Lisch nodules are seen only in neurofibromotosis-1 (NF-1) and are pathognomic for the disease. They are seen in almost all patients over the age of 20, and can be observed only under a slit lamp. NF-1 is also characterized by café au lait spots and neurofibromas. NF-2 manifests with bilateral acoustic neuromas. It may also induce neurofibromas, meningiomas, schwannomas, and café au lait spots. Six or more *café au lait* spots larger than 5 mm in diameter before puberty and >15 mm in diameter after puberty are diagnostic of neurofibromatosis.

1. Kordic R, Sabol Z, Cerovski B, et al. Eye disorders in neurofibromatosis (NF1). *Coll Antropol*. 2005;29 (suppl 1):29–31.
2. Lewis RP. *Merritt's Neurology*. 11th ed. Philadelphia: Lippincott Williams & Wilkins; 2005:714–716.

101. **Answer: D.** Neurofibromatosis (Von Recklinghausen's disease) is an autosomal dominant disorder with two major subtypes, NF-1 and NF-2. Here, the mother shows evidence of cutaneous signs of the disorder (i.e., neurofibromas). Epilepsy may arise from cranial neurofibromatosis and signs of epilepsy should be investigated. Considering the autosomal dominant inheritance pattern for neurofibromatosis, genetic counseling should be included in the treatment of all patients affected with this disease. Intellectual impairment is common in patients with NF-1; approximately 25% to 40% have learning disabilities and 5% to 10% are mentally retarded. Mental retardation is thought to be due to cerebral cortex dysplasia. Underachievement is common in affected school children. Language development is delayed with reading and writing difficulties being common. Neuropsychological assessments also have shown problems with visuospatial tasks, memory and sustained attention, organization, and planning. Behavioral disorders are common with hyperactivity, impulsivity, and aggressive tendencies. Remedial class teaching or special schools may be warranted. A multidisciplinary approach is required with the psychologist, educational services, the psychiatrist, and the general practitioner. The American Academy of Pediatrics Committee on Genetics recommends monitoring children with NF-1 by performing annual physical examinations and ophthalmologic evaluations. Audiologic examination should be performed before the child is of school age. A language and speech evaluation should be considered for each child. A behavioral approach is best in attempting to manage the difficult behaviors.

Lishman WA. *Organic Psychiatry*. 3rd ed. Oxford: Blackwell Science; 1996:703–704.

102. **Answer: C.** The patient most likely suffered from the sporadic variant of CJD. CJD exists in one of the following forms: inherited, acquired-variant or iatrogenic, and sporadic. It is a prion disease. It is clinically characterized by rapidly progressive dementia, myoclonus, and akinetic mutism. It has a very rapid clinical course, leading to death in 4 to 6 months from the point of diagnosis. Lewy body dementia is associated with Parkinsonian features and does not progress as rapidly. Huntington's chorea has an earlier age of onset, is associated with involuntary movements, rigidity, and a typical dancing gait with progression, as well as personality changes/behavioral disturbances. Normal pressure hydrocephalus is characterized by urinary incontinence, ataxia, and dementia.

1. Knight R. Creutzfeldt-Jakob disease: a rare cause of dementia in elderly persons. *Clin Infect Dis*. 2006;43:340–346.
2. Meissner B, Kortner K, Bartl M, et al. Creutzfeldt-Jakob disease: magnetic resonance imaging and clinical findings. *Neurology*. 2004;63:450–456.
3. Van Everbroeck B, Michotte A, Sciot R, et al. Increased incidence of sporadic Creutzfeldt-Jakob disease in the age groups between 70 and 90 years in Belgium. *Eur J Epidemiol*. 2006;21:443–447.

103. **Answer: D.** Normal-Pressure Hydrocephalus and vitamin B_{12} deficiency can cause ataxia, but would not explain the sharp shoulder pain. Lumbar stenosis would not affect the shoulders. Friedreich ataxia, also called hereditary spinocerebellar degeneration, usually develops by adolescence. Cervical spondylosis can affect both the upper and lower extremities, and pain is a common symptom in this disorder. The shoulder pain in cervical spondylosis may be sharp or achy in quality.

Victor M, Ropper AH. *Principles of Neurology*. 7th ed. New York: McGraw-Hill; 2001:1322–1326.

104. Answer: C. This patient has myasthenia gravis, a disorder of the neuromuscular junction. It has been associated with tumors of the thymus gland, and thymectomy is considered an appropriate procedure in practically all patients with uncomplicated myasthenia gravis between puberty and 55 years of age, even in cases without tumors. The surgery is performed electively and not during an acute deterioration of myasthenia. The remission rate after thymectomy is approximately 35% provided that the procedure is done in the first year or two after onset of the disease. In patients with myasthenia restricted to the ocular muscles for a year or longer, the prognosis is considered good, so that thymectomy is unnecessary. For mild cases without thymic tumor, for patients in partial remission after thymectomy, and for purely ocular myasthenia, the use of anticholinesterase drugs (neostigmine and pyridostigmine) may be the only form of therapy necessary. In patients with moderate to severe disease incompletely treated by anticholinesterase drugs, long-term corticosteroids are the most effective treatment. Alternative immunosuppressive agents, such as azathioprine or mycophenolate, are a useful adjunct to steroids and can be effective alone in patients who cannot tolerate or fail to respond to prednisone.

Ropper AH, Brown RH. Adams and Victor's Principles of Neurology. 8th ed. New York: McGraw-Hill; 2005:1250, 1254, 1256–1258.

105. Answer: B. "Goodness of fit" describes the consonance of the child's inborn temperament with his or her environment, including the parents' demands and expectations. With such a fit, the potential for the child's optimal development exists. The dissonance between a child's temperament and the parents' expectations (D) describes Chess and Thomas' term of *poorness of fit*. Answer A describes Winnicott's concept of the *good enough mother*. Goodness of fit does not describe the adaptation of the parents or the infant to the other, so answers C and E are wrong.

1. Lewis M. *Child and Adolescent Psychiatry: A Comprehensive Textbook.* 3rd ed. Philadelphia: Lippincott Williams & Wilkins; 2002:220–227.
2. Sadock BJ, Sadock VA, Jones RM. *Kaplan & Sadock's Study Guide and Self-Examination Review in Psychiatry.* 7th ed. Philadelphia: Lippincott Williams & Wilkins; 2003:70.

106. Answer: C. There is evidence that benzodiazepine administration augments the transmission of gamma aminobutyric acid by increasing the sensitivity of the gamma aminobutyric receptor for its substrate.

1. Tasman A, Kay J, Lieberman J. *Psychiatry Therapeutics.* 2nd ed. England: John Wiley and Sons; 2003:316.

2. Tallman JF, Thomas JW, and Gallager DW. GABAergic modulation of benzodiazepine binding site sensitivity. *Nature.* 1978;274:384–385.

107. Answer: D. Reading aloud and reading comprehension are usually abnormal in Wernicke's aphasia. Wernicke's aphasia is also called a sensory aphasia or receptive aphasia. Verbal output in Wernicke's aphasia is either normal or increased. However, sentences have no meaning and convey no information. Paraphasic errors are common. Neologisms, logorrhea, pressured speech, and Jargon aphasia (a severe form of Wernicke's aphasia with incomprehensible rapid speech and frequent paraphasic errors) can be seen. Comprehension of spoken and written language is abnormal in classic Wernicke's aphasia. Repetition, naming, reading out aloud, and writing comprehension are also impaired. Younger patients may erroneously be diagnosed with a psychotic disorder and older patients with dementia, because they present with severe incomprehensible speech without any neurological deficits. Wernicke's aphasia is due to a lesion of the posterosuperior portion of the first temporal gyrus of the left temporal lobe. The outcome and recovery of Wernicke's aphasia is less favorable than Broca's aphasia.

1. Goetz C. *Textbook of Clinical Neurology.* 2nd ed. Philadelphia: WB Saunders; 2003:88–90.
2. Kaufman DM. *Clinical Neurology for Psychiatrists.* 5th ed. Philadelphia: WB Saunders; 2001:175–201.

108. Answer: B. To prove malpractice, this family would have to show evidence of each of the four elements of a malpractice claim (also known as the "4 Ds"). First, there must be an established doctor–patient relationship or a *duty of care*. In the previous vignette, the program clearly stated that no doctor–patient relationship was implied between the callers and the psychiatrist. Second, there must be evidence that the physician *deviated from the standard of care*. Third, there must be *damage to the patient*, and fourth, this damage must be *directly caused* by the physician's deviation.

Sadock BJ, Sadock VA. Kaplan and Sadock's Comprehensive Textbook of Psychiatry. 7th ed. Philadelphia: Lippincott Williams & Wilkins; 2000:3272.

109. Answer: B. Brain imaging in patients with Alzheimer's disease shows reductions in total brain volume and in specific areas, such as the temporal lobes, hippocampus and amygdala. Hippocampal reductions correlate best with cognitive impairment. Left hippocampal reductions are associated with delayed verbal recall, whereas right hippocampal reductions are associated with delayed non-verbal memory performance. Other studies have shown that hippocampal atrophy usually progresses with time and can even be a predictor of subsequent conversion to Alzheimer's disease in subjects with mild cognitive impairment.

Sadock BJ, Sadock VA. *Kaplan and Sadock's Comprehensive Textbook of Psychiatry*. 8th ed. Philadelphia: Lippincott Williams & Wilkins; 2005:3607–3648.

110. **Answer: A.** Rapid cycling is defined as the occurrence of at least four episodes of depression and hypomania (or mania)-per year. Risk factors include: female gender; borderline hypothyroidism; menopause; temporal lobe dysrhythmias; alcohol, minor tranquilizer, stimulant, or caffeine abuse; and long-term, aggressive use of antidepressant medications.

1. American Psychiatric Association. *Diagnostic and Statistical Manual of Mental Disorders*. 4th ed. Washington: American Psychiatric Association; 2000:427–428.
2. Sadock BJ, Sadock VA. *Kaplan and Sadock's Comprehensive Textbook of Psychiatry*. 8th ed. Philadelphia: Lippincott Williams & Wilkins; 2005:1639.

111. **Answer: B.** DSM-IV-TR criteria for Paranoid Personality Disorder include suspiciousness, unjustified doubts, misinterpreting benign remarks/events, bearing grudges, perceiving attacks, reacting angrily, and suspiciousness of infidelity. Themes associated with this disorder include externalizing blame, difficulty with authority figures, "making mountains out of molehills," "missing the forest for the trees," inability to relax, projection of envy/jealousy or anger/hostility, and seeking autonomy. These patients also display a substantial degree of narcissism. However, Narcissistic Personality Disorder is contrasted by its themes of need for admiration, grandiosity, and lack of empathy. Narcissists desire attention, admiration, affirmation of their being special, and they can exploit others for their personal gain. A schizoid patient would avoid any interaction with others (e.g., the patient would be unlikely to have a girlfriend). An antisocial individual would be involved in criminal activity without remorse. Histrionic individuals can be provocative, display shallow expressions of emotion, impressionistic speech, theatricality, and suggestibility.

1. American Psychiatric Association. *Diagnostic and Statistical Manual of Mental Disorders*, 4th ed. Washington: American Psychiatric Association; 2000:690–694.
2. Gabbard G. *Psychodynamic Psychiatry in Clinical Practice*. 4th ed. Washington: American Psychiatric Association; 2005:401–412.
3. Robinson D. *Disordered Personalities*. 3rd ed. Port Huron: Rapid Psychler Press; 2005:94–124.

112. **Answer: C.** Phencyclidine (PCP) is also known as "angel dust." It was originally developed as an anesthetic, but is no longer used for this purpose because of its association with disorientation, agitation, and hallucinations. It is closely pharmacologically related to ketamine ("Special K"), which is still used as a human anesthetic in the United States. Although the effects of PCP are similar to hallucinogens, such as LSD, it is significantly different pharmacologically and is therefore classified separately in the DSM-IV-TR.

Sadock BJ, Sadock VA. *Kaplan and Sadock's Synopsis of Psychiatry*. 9th ed. Philadelphia: Lippincott Williams & Wilkins; 2003:456.

113. **Answer: E.** This patient does not meet criteria for a specific eating disorder. Although her concerns about weight and occasional episodes of over-eating put her at risk for developing an eating disorder, she does not meet criteria for one at the current time. To make the diagnosis of bulimia nervosa, a patient must have episodes of binge eating and compensatory behaviors, such as excessive exercise, fasting, vomiting or misuse of medications, at least twice a week for 3 months. Patients with anorexia nervosa refuse to keep at or above a minimally normal weight for age and weight.

American Psychiatric Association. *Quick Reference to the Diagnostic Criteria from DSM-IV-TR*. Washington: American Psychiatric Association; 2000:263–266.

114. **Answer: D.** Psychostimulants, including dextroamphetamine, mixed amphetamine salts, and methylphenidate, are effective in 70% to 80% of children with ADHD. They increase attention and decrease hyperactivity/impulsivity, and they are most successful when combined with behavioral, educational, and/or cognitive interventions. They are the most frequently prescribed medications in pediatric psychopharmacology. Meta-analytic data of children with ADHD followed through adolescence and adulthood show a decrease in the risk of non-nicotine substance abuse among those treated with stimulants. Psychostimulants are FDA-approved for the treatment of narcolepsy and ADHD, though they also have many off-label uses. Such uses include the treatment of apathy in the medically ill and elderly, potentiation of narcotic analgesics, antidepressant augmentation, and treatment of SSRI-induced fatigue, sexual side effects, and apathy.

Rosenbaum JF, Arana GW, Hyman SE. *Handbook of Psychiatric Drug Therapy*. 5th ed. Philadelphia: Lippincott Williams & Wilkins; 2005:280–285.

115. **Answer: B.** Unlike nicotine replacement therapy (which should start the day the patient stops smoking), the smoker should begin taking bupropion several weeks before stopping smoking. Bupropion SR is well studied for this indication, although

bupropion immediate release is also effective. With bupropion SR, the patient can start at 150 mg daily and then after 1 week increase to 150 mg BID (*bis in die* which means twice-daily dosage). Some patients may require up to 450 mg/day. After the patient has been on bupropion for 2 to 3 weeks and not suffered any adverse reactions, the patient can stop smoking.

Rosenbaum JF, Arana GW, Hyman SE, et al. *Handbook of Psychiatric Drug Therapy*. 5th ed. Philadelphia: Lippincott Williams & Wilkins; 2005:240–241.

116. Answer: D. This patient is showing signs of a hyperchloremic, nonanion gap metabolic acidosis. Topiramate can cause hyperchloremic, nonanion gap metabolic acidosis by inhibiting carbonic anhydrase and thus decreasing production of bicarbonate (similar to acetazolamide). This is an uncommon, but important side effect of topiramate. Anion gap (AG) is the difference between calculated serum anions and cations. It is calculated by the formula, AG = (serum sodium) – (serum chloride + serum bicarbonate). The normal anion gap is $12 +/- 2$ meq/L. The normal blood pH is tightly regulated between 7.35 and 7.45. A normal blood sodium level is between 135 to 145 meq/L. The normal blood potassium level is between 3.5 to 5.0 meq/L. The normal serum range for chloride is 98 to 108 meq/L. The normal serum range for bicarbonate is 22 to 30 meq/L. Using this formula, we can calculate that this patient has a normal anion gap of 10 meq/L, but with an elevated chloride level and a low blood pH (metabolic acidosis). The most common side effects of topiramate are a change in taste and feelings of pins and needles in the head and extremities. Less common side effects include cognitive deficiency (particularly word-finding difficulty); lethargy; renal stones; impairment of fine motor skills; vision abnormality and transient or permanent vision loss; weight loss; breast pain; abdominal pain; menstrual disorder; taste changes; pharyngitis; sinusitis; diplopia; rash; leukopenia; fatigue; dizziness; insomnia; anxiety; depression; paresthesia; diarrhea; nausea; dyspepsia; constipation; and dry mouth. Despite its lack of efficacy as a monotherapeutic mood stabilizer, topiramate is often used in clinical practice as an adjunctive agent because of its weight loss potential, especially in patients who have gained weight from atypical antipsychotic medications.

1. Chengappa KN, Rathore D, Levine J, et al. Topiramate as add-on treatment for patients with bipolar mania. *Bipolar Disord*. 1999;1:42–53.
2. Health Canada. Important drug safety information: Topamax is associated with metabolic acidosis. Available at: http://www.napra.ca/pdfs/advisories/topamax_prof.pdf. Accessed September 4, 2006.
3. Wikipedia. Topiramate. Available at: http://en.wikipedia.org/wiki/Topiramate. Accessed September 4, 2006.

117. Answer: B. In a study examining the effectiveness of day hospital attendance in prolonging independent living for elderly people, the researchers reviewed controlled clinical trials comparing day hospital care with comprehensive care (five trials), domiciliary care (four trials), or no comprehensive care (three trials). Overall, there was no significant difference between day hospitals and alternative services for death, disability, or use of resources. However, when compared to subjects receiving no comprehensive care, patients attending day hospitals had lower odds of death or "poor" outcome (0.72, 95% CI, 0.53 to 0.99; $p <0.05$) and functional deterioration (0.61, 0.38 to 0.97; $p <0.05$). The day hospital group also showed trends toward reductions in hospital bed use and placement in institutional care. Of the eight trials reporting treatment costs, six reported that day hospital attendance was more expensive than other care, although only two analyses took into account cost of long-term care. The researchers concluded that day hospital care seems to be an effective service for elderly people who need rehabilitation, but may have no clear advantage over other comprehensive care.

1. Forster A, Young J, Langhorne P. Systematic review of day hospital care for elderly people. The Day Hospital Group. *BMJ*. 1999;318:837–841.
2. Forster A, Young J, Langhorne P. Medical day hospital care for the elderly versus alternative forms of care. *Cochrane Database Syst Rev*. 2000;2:CD001730.

118. Answer: D. Naltrexone is an opiate antagonist approved for both alcohol and opiate dependence. Common side effects include nausea, abdominal pain, and diarrhea. Transaminasemia is sometimes found in higher doses. There are no known cardiovascular or pulmonary side effects. Patients should be questioned about other substance use, because the concurrent use of opiates is a contraindication and naltrexone may precipitate a severe withdrawal with delirium, hallucinations, and stupor. Most of the evidence supports the effectiveness of oral naltrexone use for 12 weeks, although there is growing evidence to support use for longer periods in the depot form. Several studies support the targeted use of naltrexone. Several studies also have supported the nondaily use of naltrexone, during periods of high craving, although this remains experimental.

1. Kranzler HR, Ciraulo DA. *Clinical Manual of Addiction Psychopharmacology*. Arlington: American Psychiatric Publishing; 2005:22–28.

2. Heinala P, Alho H, Kiianmaa K, et al. Targeted use of naltrexone without prior detoxification in the treatment of alcohol dependence: a factorial double blind, placebo-controlled trial. *J Clin Psychopharmacol*. 2001: 2001 Jun; 21(3):287–292.
3. Rosenbaum JF, Arana GW, Hyman SE, et al. *Handbook of Psychiatric Drug Therapy*. 5th ed. Philadelphia: Lippincott Williams & Wilkins; 2005:222–225.

119. **Answer: D.** Moral considerations guide ethical inquiry in medicine according to four general principles of biomedical ethics. The first principle is autonomy. This principle requires that professionals recognize the right of competent adults to make their own decisions about health care or participation in research. Next, beneficence directs health care professionals to promote the well-being and health of patients by offering competent medical care. Nonmalfeasance involves avoiding harming patients or research subjects. Together, beneficence and non-malfeasance require practitioners to assess risk-benefit ratios for all patient care and research interventions. Finally, justice requires that medical care and research be performed fairly and equitably. Temperance is not an ethical principle. It refers to moderation in all things. Complex medical problems are rarely solved by the single application of one of these principles. They usually involve carefully weighing each principle in the context of both the patient and his or her situation. This process is referred to as ethical inquiry.

Levenson JL. *The American Psychiatric Publishing Textbook of Psychosomatic Medicine*. Washington: American Psychiatric Publishing; 2005:55–65.

120. **Answer: B.** Oligodendrocytes are myelin-forming glial cells found in the CNS. Myelin in the peripheral nervous system (PNS) is produced by Schwann cells. (Oligodendrocytes are to Schwann cells as the CNS is to the PNS.) Astrocytes are large glial cells which stabilize extracellular potassium concentrations and limit the accumulation of extracellular glutamate. They proliferate in response to many CNS insults and may release growth factors and form barriers to the spread of infection. Ependymal cells are neuroepithelial cells that line the ventricular system, choroid plexus, and central canal of the spinal cord. Microglia are phagocytic cells that become reactive in degenerative diseases and demyelinating disorders, and also in more acute CNS insults.

1. Kaufman DM. *Clinical Neurology for Psychiatrists*. 5th ed. Philadelphia: WB Saunders; 2001:75.
2. Rolak LA. *Neurology Secrets*. 2nd ed. Philadelphia: Hanley & Belfus; 1998:1.

121. **Answer: D.** All the statements are true except that when PCP binds to the NMDA receptor, it prevents glutamate from activating the receptor. This binding also prevents the normal influx of calcium into the cell.

1. Sadock BJ, Sadock VA. *Kaplan and Sadock's Comprehensive Textbook of Psychiatry*. 8th ed. Philadelphia: Lippincott Williams & Wilkins; 2005:51–52.
2. Kaufman DM. *Clinical Neurology for Psychiatrists*. 5th ed. Philadelphia: WB Saunders; 2001:561–563.

122. **Answer: D.** Wilson's disease is inherited via autosomal recessive transmission. Copper accumulates causing lesions in the brain, liver, cornea, and other organs. The disorder is also called "Hepatolenticular degeneration," referring to the lenticular nuclei in the brain (putamen and globus pallidus).

1. Kaufman DM. *Clinical Neurology for Psychiatrists*. 5th ed. Philadelphia: WB Saunders; 2001:443, 466.
2. Kitzberger R, Madl C, Ferenci P. Wilson disease. *Metab Brain Dis*. 2005;20:295–302.

123. **Answer: D.** Postlumbar puncture headache is a common complication thought to be secondary to a drop in the intracranial pressure due to leakage of CSF into the paravertebral muscles. It appears in approximately one third of patients that have a lumbar puncture. It can last from days to weeks and usually worsens when the patient is standing and improves while lying down. Some patients may present with neck stiffness, nausea, and vomiting. Sixth nerve palsy has been associated with lumbar puncture with or without the occurrence of headache. Meningitis is also a serious complication of a lumbar puncture. Bleeding into meningeal spaces can occur in patients who are taking anticoagulants or have an abnormal platelet function. Third nerve palsy has been very rarely associated with a lumbar puncture procedure.

Aminoff MJ, Greenberg DA, Simon RP. *Clinical Neurology*. 6th ed. New York: McGraw–Hill; 2005:12–20.

124. **Answer: B.** Myasthenia gravis is mediated by autoantibody-mediated attack on the ACh receptor. ACh receptors are found in the postsynaptic membranes of skeletal muscle fibers, and bind ACh released from nerve endings, which cause a muscle contraction when a threshold level of ACh has been released.

Ropper AH, Brown RH. *Adams and Victor's Principles of Neurology*. 8th ed. New York: McGraw-Hill; 2005:1536–1553.

125. **Answer: E.** The vagus nerve travels a long course from the brain to the mediastinum. If the lesion is intramedullary, there are usually ipsilateral cerebellar signs, loss of pain and temperature sensation over the ipsilateral face and contralateral arm and leg, and an ipsilateral Bernard-Horner syndrome. If the lesion is extramedullary, but intracranial, the

glossopharyngeal and spinal accessory nerves are frequently involved as well. If extracranial in the posterior lacterocondylar or retroparotid space, there may be a combination of ninth, tenth, eleventh, and twelfth cranial nerve palsies and a Bernard-Horner syndrome. If there is no palatal weakness and no pharyngeal or palatal sensory loss, the lesion is below the origin of the pharyngeal branches, which leave the vagus nerve high in the cervical region. The usual site of disease is then the mediastinum. This presentation should provoke an evaluation for lung carcinoma.

Ropper AH, Brown RH. *Adams and Victor's Principles of Neurology*. 8th ed. New York: McGraw-Hill; 2005: 1186.

126. **Answer: C.** The most common site of hemangioblastoma is in the paramedian cerebellar hemispheric area; the second site where it is seen most frequently is the spinal cord. Hemangioblastomas also occur in the area postrema of the medulla. The clinical manifestations are those of cerebellar masses which include headaches, ataxia, and papilledema.

Lewis RP. *Merritt's Neurology*. 11th ed. Philadelphia: Lippincott Williams & Wilkins; 2005:458.

127. **Answer: D.** Neurofibromatosis type 1 is carried by chromosome 17 and encodes for a protein called *neurofibromin*, which acts as a tumour suppressor. *Café au lait* spots, lisch nodules, and neurofibromas are characteristic features of neurofibromatosis. *Café au lait spots* develop during the first 3 years of life. Neurofibromas develop in late adolescence. The plexiform subtype is specific for NF-1. Axillary (Crowe sign) and inguinal freckling develop in early puberty. This disease can involve various body systems over time. The disorder may be associated with other tumors of the CNS, such as optic glioma, glioblastoma, and meningioma. It may be associated rarely with phaeochromocytoma through multiple endocrine neoplasia syndromes. Accoustic neuromas are specific for neurofibromatosis type 2. The mortality rate is higher than that of the healthy population, because of the increased potential for malignant transformation of diseased tissues and the development of neurofibrosarcoma. Patients with NF-1 have an estimated 3% to 15% additional risk of malignant disease in their lifetime.

1. Isselbacher KJ, Martin JB, Braunwald E, et al. *Harrison's Principles of Internal Medicine*.13th ed. New York: McGraw-Hill; 1996:2339.
2. Lishman WA. *Organic Psychiatry*. 3rd ed. Oxford: Blackwell Science; 1996:703–704.
3. Kam JR. Neruofibromatosis. eMedicine. Available at: http://www.emedicine.com/derm/topic287.htm. Accessed August 30, 2006.

128. **Answer: C.** Patients who suffer from Parkinson's disease are typically described as having a "masked face." This includes showing little or no emotion through facial expression, decreased blinking and eye movements, decreased head movements, and widened palpebral fissures. Many times, patients with Parkinson's disease are erroneously labeled as depressed because of these symptoms.

Kaufman DM. *Clinical Neurology for Psychiatrists*. 5th ed. Philadelphia: WB Saunders; 2001:446.

129. **Answer: A.** Type I Chiari malformation is an idiopathic or developmental syringomyelia that affects males and females equally. The symptoms of type I Chiari malformation usually begin around ages of 20 to 40 years. Type III Chiari malformation is syringomyelia associated with another disorder of the spinal cord, such as a tumor, trauma, infection, or another abnormality. Weakness and atrophy of the hands are also typical features of syringomyelia. In syringomyelia, patients have decreased pain and temperature sense, but vibration sense and proprioception remain intact.

Victor M, Ropper AH. *Principles of Neurology*. 7th ed. New York: McGraw-Hill; 2001:1337–1338.

130. **Answer: D.** This patient likely has multiple sclerosis (MS). It presents with weakness and numbness, sometimes both, in one or more limbs and as the initial symptom in approximately 50% of patients. Symptoms of tingling of the extremities and tight bandlike sensations around the trunk or limbs are common and are probably the result of involvement of the posterior columns of the spinal cord. The symptoms generally appear over a period of hours or days, at times being so trifling that they are ignored, and less often, coming on so suddenly and prominently as to bring the patient to immediate medical care. Corticosteroids appear to hasten recovery from an acute attack, including an attack of optic neuritis. However, a substantial group of patients with acute exacerbations fail to respond, and there is limited evidence that steroids have a significant effect on the ultimate course of this disease or that they prevent recurrences. The Optic Neuritis Treatment Trial cautioned against the use of oral prednisone in the treatment of acute optic neuritis. In this study, it was found that the use of intravenous methylprednisolone followed by oral prednisone did indeed speed the recovery from visual loss, although at 6 months there was little difference between the patients treated in this way and those treated with placebo. There is limited evidence for daily steroid treatment over a period of many months or years except in those infrequent cases where

withdrawal of the medication consistently leads to relapse (alternative diagnoses should be considered in this event). A randomized trial comparing oral and intravenous methylprednisolone in acute relapses of MS has demonstrated no clear advantage of the intravenous regimen.

1. Barnes D, Hughes RA, Morris RW, et al. Randomised trial of oral and intravenous methylprednisolone in acute relapses of multiple sclerosis. *Lancet*. 1997;349:902–906.
2. Beck RW, Cleary PA, Anderson MM Jr, et al. A randomized, controlled trial of corticosteroids in the treatment of acute optic neuritis. The Optic Neuritis Study Group. *N Engl J Med*. 1992;326:581–588.
3. Ropper AH, Brown RH. *Adams and Victor's Principles of Neurology*. 8th ed. New York: McGraw-Hill; 2005:777, 787–788.

131. Answer: D. Via qualitative analysis, supplemented by factor analyses, Chess and Thomas formulated the three constellations of temperament composed of various combinations of nine temperament categories. These categories are: activity level, the motor component of a child's functioning; rhythmicity or regularity, as in the predictability/unpredictability of the sleep/wake cycle, hunger, feeding pattern, or elimination pattern; approach or withdrawal, the nature of the response to a novel stimulus; adaptability, responses to new or altered situations; threshold of responsiveness, the intensity level of stimulation needed to evoke a discernible response; intensity of reaction, the energy level of response; quality of mood, the amount of pleasant behavior in contrast to unpleasant behavior; distractibility, the effectiveness of extraneous environmental stimuli in distracting the infant; and attention span and persistence, the length of time a particular activity is pursued and the continuation of an activity in the face of obstacles, respectively.

Lewis M. *Child and Adolescent Psychiatry: A Comprehensive Textbook*. 3rd ed. Philadelphia: Lippincott Williams & Wilkins; 2002:220–227.

132. Answer: A. Donepezil and rivastigmine are acetylcholinesterase inhibitors, and aim to correct the profound deficit of acetyl choline in patients with Alzheimer's dementia. Memantine targets the NMDA receptor and consequently decreases calcium induced neuronal damage.

1. Ringman JM, Cummings JL. Current and emerging pharmacological treatment options for dementia. *Behav Neurol*. 2006;17: 5–16.
2. Tasman A, Kay J, Lieberman J. *Psychiatry Therapeutics*. 2nd ed. England: John Wiley and Sons; 2003:870.

133. Answer: A. When there is no true difference between the experimental and control treatments, but the test by chance alone finds a statistically significant difference, it represents a false positive result in a diagnostic test or in statistical terms a type I error (probability =alfa). Usually the threshold is set that the type I error occurs <5% of the time. In statistical terms, it is represented as alfa = 0.05.

Gray GE. *Evidence-Based Psychiatry*. Washington: American Psychiatric Publishing; 2004:61.

134. Answer: C. The amygdala plays a major role in the learning and processing of fear and anxiety. Studies have shown that the amygdala is a likely facilitator of potentially threatening stimuli in the environment. Other structures interact with the amygdala during fear learning and include mesotemporal cortical structures, the sensory thalamus and cortex, orbital and medial prefrontal cortex, anterior insula, hypothalamus, and multiple brainstem nuclei.

1. Larson CL, Schaefer HS, Siegle GJ, et al. Fear is fast in phobic individuals: amygdala activation in response to fear-relevant stimuli. *Biol Psychiatry*. 2006;60:410–417.
2. Sadock BJ, Sadock VA. *Kaplan and Sadock's Comprehensive Textbook of Psychiatry*. 8th ed. Philadelphia: Lippincott Williams & Wilkins; 2005:1749–1757.

135. Answer: B. Patients diagnosed with idiopathic insomnia are usually not excessively sleepy during the day; they may even tend to be hyper-aroused. These patients do not appear to have a conditioned sleep disorder or dissociation between subjective experience and polygraphic data.

Sadock BJ, Sadock VA. *Kaplan and Sadock's Comprehensive Textbook of Psychiatry*. 8th ed. Philadelphia: Lippincott Williams & Wilkins; 2005:2024.

136. Answer: D. This patient has paranoid personality disorder. When working with such patients, "agree to disagree" instead of confronting or colluding with them. Accept blame without admitting to any transgression. "Analyze the resistance before content"; provide straightforward answers in a spirit of openness and sincerity. Even share your notes and records if a paranoid patient asks. Paranoid patients typically use defenses, such as denial, projective identification, reaction formation, and splitting. Avoid displaying strong reactions; "act as a container" for the patient's anger/hatred/hostility. These patients often have low self-esteem, causing them to find fault in others. Also, keep in mind that paranoid patients have a significantly increased risk of violence.

1. Gabbard G. *Psychodynamic Psychiatry in Clinical Practice*. 4th ed. Washington: American Psychiatric Association; 2005:401–412.
2. Robinson D. *Disordered Personalities*. 3rd ed. Port Huron: Rapid Psychler Press; 2005:94–124.

137. Answer: C. Episodes of delirium tremens (DTs) usually begin in a patient's 30s or 40s after 5 to 15 years of heavy drinking, typically of the binge type. Concurrent physical illnesses, such as hepatitis or pancreatitis, predispose an individual to delirium tremens. A patient in good physical health will rarely experience DTs during alcohol withdrawal.

Sadock BJ, Sadock VA. *Kaplan and Sadock's Synopsis of Psychiatry.* 9th ed. Philadelphia: Lippincott Williams & Wilkins; 2003:405.

138. Answer: B. Anorexia nervosa and substance abuse have the highest risk of death from both natural and unnatural causes. The risk of death from unnatural causes is also elevated in psychotic disorders and affective disorders. Among patients with anorexia, two of the most common causes of death include suicide and the direct effects of starvation.

Harris EC, Barraclough B. Excess mortality of mental disorder. *Br J Psychiatry.* 1998;173:11–53.

139. Answer: C. Because of their potential for abuse and dependence, psychostimulants (including methylphenidate, dextroamphetamine, and mixed amphetamine salts) are classified as schedule II drugs by the FDA. Pemoline is the only stimulant medication classified as schedule IV, though its utility is limited because of its potential for hepatotoxicity. Abuse of psychostimulants often results in mood lability, insomnia, restlessness, formication, bruxism, and paranoia. Physical exam findings of amphetamine intoxication result from sympathetic hyperactivity, and include elevated blood pressure, increased heart rate, dilated pupils, and dry mouth. Overdose of stimulants can lead to death as a result of arrhythmias, hypertension, hyperthermia, or uncontrolled seizures.

Intoxication with benzodiazepines (A) results in sedation, ataxia, slurred speech, hypotension, hypotonia, and hyporeflexia. Abuse of beta-blockers (A) would likely lead to bradycardia, hypotension, and bronchospasm. Opiate intoxication (D) results in CNS depression, bradycardia, hypotension, and pupillary constriction. Overdose on hypnotics (E) results in sedation, dizziness, and ataxia.

1. Rosenbaum JF, Arana GW, Hyman SE. *Handbook of Psychiatric Drug Therapy.* 5th ed. Philadelphia: Lippincott Williams & Wilkins; 2005:289–290.
2. Sadock BJ, Sadock VA. *Kaplan and Sadock's Synopsis of Psychiatry.* 9th ed. Philadelphia: Lippincott Williams & Wilkins; 2003:984–988.

140. Answer: A. A recent meta-analysis of 12 randomized, controlled trials (with a total of 1,088 assigned patients) that tested the efficacy and safety of antidepressants in the short-term treatment of bipolar depression showed that antidepressants overall did NOT induce more switching to mania (the event rate for antidepressants was 3.8% and for placebo, it was 4.7%). Six trials allowed comparison between two antidepressants. However, the rate of switching for TCAs was 10%, which was significantly greater than the rate for all other antidepressants combined, 3.2%. This result confirmed the well-accepted tenet that TCAs are the greatest culprits of antidepressant-induced switch. This study also demonstrated that SSRIs may not have a greater switch risk than placebo. One randomized study suggested that the noradrenergic-active drug desipramine showed a much higher incidence of manic switches during long-term continuation and prophylactic therapy. This raises the question of whether some inherent component of the TCAs or the noradrenergic selectivity of desipramine accounts for the greater switch liability. Two recent randomized studies have indicated a higher switch rate on venlafaxine compared with bupropion, sertraline, or paroxetine. These data suggest that it is the noradrenergic component of the dual actions of venlafaxine that account for the greater switch liability. Although bupropion is believed to have a lower switch rate than SSRIs, there is not enough evidence to support this belief. There is not enough evidence to estimate the switch rate of MAOIs, although some believe them to have higher switch rates than SSRIs.

1. Gijsman HJ, Geddes JR, Rendell JM, et al. Antidepressants for bipolar depression: a systematic review of randomized, controlled trials. *Am J Psychiatry.* 2004;161:1537–1547.
2. Sadock BJ, Sadock VA. *Kaplan and Sadock's Comprehensive Textbook of Psychiatry.* 8th ed. Philadelphia: Lippincott Williams & Wilkins; 2005:1683.

141. Answer: E. Risperidone long-acting injection is a long acting antipsychotic medication that is administered by injection every 2 weeks. Peak concentration is reached in 3 weeks of the initial injection. Thus, when starting the medication, two injections are given 2 weeks apart and simultaneously oral medication is continued for 3 weeks. Risperidone long-acting injection is a water-based suspension, in contrast to the oil-based preparations of haloperidol decanoate and fluphenazine hydrochloride. The water-based suspension is encapsulated by a carbohydrate polymer and is slowly released similar to dissolving sutures.

Rosenbaum JF, Arana GW, Hyman SE, et al. *Handbook of Psychiatric Drug Therapy.* 5th ed. Philadelphia: Lippincott Williams & Wilkins; 2005:33.

142. Answer: E. It is now recognized that caregiving can create difficulties for both professional and family caregivers of patients with dementia. Caregivers have high rates of physical and mental disorders. Live-in caregivers are far more reluctant to admit the patient into an institution, and more likely to be depressed than caregivers who live apart from their patient. Results from various studies indicate that there is a high rate of abuse both of and by demented patients. Although institutionalization is a solution, it is not always the best one for caregiver stress, as it creates guilt, exclusion from decision-making and care, financial burden, and difficulties in maintaining relationships. Even now, the move from the community to institutional care in most cases is poorly planned and often a response to a crisis. Behavioral disorder and functional loss, mainly aggression and incontinence, are the main determinants of institutionalization rather than cognitive deterioration. Alternative approaches include models of care that bring the institution closer to the community and involve family caregivers within the professional care setting.

Ritchie K, Lovestone S. The dementias. *Lancet*. 2002;360: 1759–1766.

143. Answer: E. IPT is a time-limited, noninterpretive therapy used in the treatment of depressive spectrum syndromes. It is usually divided into three phases (gathering of information and diagnosis, implementation of strategies identified, and termination phase), and operates on the assumption that the patients immediate social context is pivotal in the development of depressive symptoms.

1. Feijo de Mello M, de Jesus Mali J, Bacaltchuk J, et al. A systematic review of research findings on the efficacy of interpersonal therapy for depressive disorders. *Eur Arch Psychiatry Clin Neurosci*. 2005;255:75–82.
2. Sadock BJ, Sadock VA. *Kaplan and Sadock's Comprehensive Textbook of Psychiatry*. 8th ed. Philadelphia: Lippincott Williams & Wilkins; 2005:2610–2618.

144. Answer: C. An action potential is an all-or-nothing, regenerative, directionally propagated, depolarizing nerve impulse. In axons, the rising (depolarization) phase of the action potential is mediated by the activation of voltage-dependent sodium currents. Initial inflow of sodium ions depolarizes the membrane and initiates an action potential, which propagates itself along the membrane by sequentially triggering adjacent voltage-gated sodium channels. Calcium channels open next, allowing the positively charged calcium ions to enter the neuron and further contribute to the spike of the action potential. Calcium ion entry activates ion channels that carry an outflow of potassium ions which are involved in arresting the action

potential. Repolarization is influenced by inactivation of sodium currents and the activation of potassium currents. When sodium currents are largely inactivated, a new action potential cannot be initiated (absolute refractory period).

1. Rolak LA. *Neurology Secrets*. 2nd ed. Philadelphia: Hanley & Belfus; 1998:2.
2. Sadock BJ, Sadock VA. *Kaplan and Sadock's Synopsis of Psychiatry*. 9th ed. Philadelphia: Lippincott Williams & Wilkins; 2003:89–90.

145. Answer: C. All the statements regarding amino acid neurotransmitter glycine are true except that neurons utilizing glycine as a neurotransmitter are small inhibitory interneurons and not excitatory interneurons.

Sadock BJ, Sadock VA. *Kaplan and Sadock's Comprehensive Textbook of Psychiatry*. 8th ed. Philadelphia: Lippincott Williams & Wilkins; 2005:63.

146. Answer: B. Myopathies can be both inherited or acquired. Some examples of myopathies include muscular dystrophies, inflammatory myopathies (such as polymyositis and dermatomyositis), and metabolic myopathies. Patients present with weakness that is more marked proximally than distally. No muscle wasting or diminished tendon reflexes occurs until late stages of the illness. Abdominal and plantar reflexes are normal. Patients do not present with sensory loss or sphincter disturbances. Many of the myopathies have a progressive course and can be fatal.

Aminoff MJ, Greenberg DA, Simon RP. *Clinical Neurology*. 6th ed. New York: McGraw-Hill; 2005:187–200.

147. Answer: D. After generalized tonic–clonic seizures, and some types of complex partial seizures, prolactin becomes transiently elevated for 15 to 30 minutes. Not all seizures cause a rise in prolactin, and vasovagal syncopal attacks can cause elevations in prolactin, but serum prolactin measurements can be useful in distinguishing pseudoseizures or nonepileptic seizures from epileptic seizures. The routine measurement of prolactin after seizures is unnecessary.

Lusic I, Pintaric I, Hozo I, et al. Serum prolactin levels after seizure and syncopal attacks. *Seizure*. 1999;8:218–222.

148. Answer: B. This patient has multiple sclerosis. For years, corticosteroids were the only treatment available, but controlled evidence suggests that they do little to alter the natural course of the illness. Immunomodulatory therapy with interferon beta and glatiramer acetate, however, can modestly alter the natural history of the disease. Several trials have now shown that the subcutaneous injection of IFN-β-1b every second day for up to 5 years decreases the frequency and severity of relapses by almost one-third, and also decreases the number of new or enlarging lesions (lesion burden) in serial MRIs. The treatment of relapsing-remitting MS with IFN-β-1a is equally effective and has the advantage that it may be taken once weekly as an intramuscular injection. Glatiramer acetate, which was synthesized to mimic the actions of myelin basic protein, a putative autoantigen in MS, is given daily in subcutaneous doses. More recent changes in the preparation of interferon have led to reported rates of interferon antibody production of only 2% after 1 year of use. There is some evidence that the presence of these antidrug antibodies diminishes the effectiveness of interferons. Antibodies do not develop to glatiramer acetate, and this has been emphasized as a relative advantage of the latter drug. Overall, the side effects of these interferon agents are modest, consisting mainly of flu-like symptoms, sweating, and malaise beginning several hours after the injection and persisting for up to 14 hours; they are reduced by pre- and posttreatment several hours later with NSAIDs and tend to abate with continued use of the agents.

1. Arnason BG. Interferon beta in multiple sclerosis. *Neurology*. 1993;43:641–643.
2. Ropper AH, Brown RH. *Adams and Victor's Principles of Neurology*. 8th ed. New York: McGraw-Hill; 2005:777, 787–788.

149. **Answer: E.** In Erikson's second stage—autonomy versus shame and doubt—the child's sense of self is based upon his success at controlling his bodily functions such as anal sphincter regulation while undergoing toilet-training. He is able to explore and separate from his parents for brief periods without experiencing significant distress if he succeeds at establishing basic trust, the positive outcome of the first stage (basic trust vs. basic mistrust). According to Piaget's model of cognitive development, he is in the age range for the preoperational, or prelogical, stage in which symbolic functions, egocentric, and magical thinking predominates. Freud described the anal phase for this age in his psychosexual model of development. When this child develops into the next of Erikson's epigenetic stages, he will be struggling with issues of initiative versus guilt.

Stern TA, Herman JB. *Massachusetts General Hospital Psychiatry Update and Board Preparation*. 2nd ed. New York: McGraw-Hill; 2004:29.

150. **Answer: E.** Research has demonstrated in vitro increases in plasma membrane concentrations of dopamine transporters in response to both cocaine and amphetamines. The hallucinogenic effects of LSD are likely mediated via serotonin receptors. Cannabis interacts with the G-protein coupled cannabinoid receptors. Alcohol appears to interact with a variety of receptors including opioidergic, GABAergic, serotonergic and glutamatergic. MDMA (ecstasy) directly causes a release of serotonin from nerve endings.

1. Daws LC, Callaghan PD, Morón JA, et al. Cocaine increases dopamine uptake and cell surface expression of dopamine transporters. *Biochem Biophys Res Comm*. 2002;290:1545–1550.
2. Tasman A, Kay J, Lieberman J. *Psychiatry Therapeutics*. 2nd ed. England: John Wiley and Sons; 2003:939, 995, 1046, 1056.

151. **Answer: A.** Structural imaging studies have shown decreased basal ganglia volumes and increased thalamic volumes in patients with OCD, although there has been significant variability in findings among different studies. The area that has been most consistently implicated in OCD is the caudate nucleus, which is a main component of the basal ganglia. The thalamus also seems to play a major role in this illness. Some studies have shown that abnormalities in the thalamus can be associated with symptom severity and treatment response. The frontal cortex, cerebellum, amygdala, and striatum have also been linked to OCD, but not as strongly as the caudate nucleus.

1. Friedlander L, Desrocher M. Neuroimaging studies of obsessive-compulsive disorder in adults and children. *Clin Psychol Rev*. 2006;26:32–49.
2. Sadock BJ, Sadock VA. *Kaplan and Sadock's Comprehensive Textbook of Psychiatry*. 8th ed. Philadelphia: Lippincott Williams & Wilkins; 2005:3281–3286.

152. **Answer: E.** All of the statements support the evidence for a genetic contribution to depressive disorders.

1. Janicak P, Davis J, Preskorn S, et al. *Principles and Practice of Psychopharmacotherapy*. 4th ed. Philadephia: Lippincott Williams & Wilkins; 2006:207.
2. Sadock BJ, Sadock VA. *Kaplan and Sadock's Comprehensive Textbook of Psychiatry*. 8th ed. Philadelphia: Lippincott Williams & Wilkins; 2005:1571,1592.

153. **Answer: D.** The FFM approach to personality disorders accounts for the heterogeneity observed in BPD. There is much interest in dimensional models of psychopathology and psychiatric diagnosis. DSM-IV-TR mentions dimensional models (including the FFM specifically) and identifies them as an area of active investigation. The dimensional FFM is an alternative approach to the categorical model employed in DSM. "The FFM is a hierarchical model of personality traits." (Costa, 5). Traits are defined as enduring dispositions, as opposed to more variable or

transient "states." The five dimensions of the FFM are: (i) neuroticism, (ii) extraversion, (iii) openness to experience, (iv) agreeableness, and (v) conscientiousness. Neuroticism (N) refers to the chronic level of emotional adjustment and instability. Extraversion (E) refers to quality and intensity of preferred interpersonal interactions, activity level, need for stimulation, and capacity for joy. Openness to experience (O) involves the active seeking and appreciation of experiences for their own sake. Agreeableness (A) refers to the kind of interactions a person prefers along a continuum from compassion to antagonism. Conscientiousness (C) assesses the degree of organization, persistence, control, and motivation in goal-directed behavior. The "NEO-PI-R" (NEO Personality Inventory Revised) is an instrument used to evaluate these five factors or domains, which are further divided into six "facet scales" each. In the case of neuroticism, the six facets are: (i) anxiety, (ii) anger/hostility, (iii) depression, (iv) self-consciousness, (v) impulsiveness, and (vi) vulnerability. BPD is thought to score highly in all six of these facets except self-consciousness.

1. American Psychiatric Association. *Diagnostic and Statistical Manual of Mental Disorders*. 4th ed. Washington: American Psychiatric Association; 2000:689–690.
2. Costa P, Jr. Widiger T. *Personality Disorders and the Five-Factor Model of Personality*. 2nd ed. Washington: American Psychological Association; 2005:5–7, 90, 93–94.

154. Answer: E. As defined in the DSM-IV-TR, substance dependence is a maladaptive pattern of substance use leading to clinically significant impairment or distress, as manifested by three or more of the following criteria: (i) tolerance, (ii) withdrawal, (iii) the substance being taken in larger amounts or over a longer period than intended, (iv) a persistent desire or unsuccessful efforts to cut down/control substance use, (v) a great deal of time being spent in activities surrounding substance use, (vi) important activities being reduced or given up because of substance use, and (vii) continued substance use despite associated physical or psychological problems. Criteria (i), (iii), (iv), and (vi) are described in this case scenario. In isolation, the fact that the patient has been using cocaine prior to his construction shifts could be appropriately cited in support of substance abuse, rather than dependence ("recurrent substance use in situations in which it is physically hazardous"). However, given that he meets criteria for cocaine dependence, he should be given a diagnosis of "dependence," rather than "abuse."

American Psychiatric Association. *Quick Reference to the Diagnostic Criteria from DSM-IV-TR*. Washington: American Psychiatric Association; 2000:105–151.

155. Answer: A. A prospective longitudinal study assessed different predictors of mortality in patients with anorexia nervosa and found that the strongest predictor was comorbid alcohol abuse. Other studies have found the following variables to be associated with higher mortality rates in anorexia nervosa: lower weight, low psychosocial functioning, and older age at first psychiatric hospitalization. History of anxiety disorders, age of onset of eating disorders, number of previous hospitalizations, and gender differences have not been associated with a higher mortality rate.

1. Keel PK, Dorer DJ, Eddy KT, et al. Predictors of mortality in eating disorders. *Arch Gen Psychiatry*. 2003;60:179–183.
2. Moller-Madsen S, Nystrup J, Nielsen S. Mortality in anorexia nervosa in Denmark during the period 1970–1987. *Acta Psychiatr Scand*. 1996;94:454–459.
3. Patton GC. Mortality in eating disorders. *Psychol Med*. 1988;18:947–951.

156. Answer: A. Antidepressants are the most widely-studied class of medication for the treatment of eating disorders. All antidepressants appear to work equally effectively; however, the SSRIs are generally better tolerated than TCAs and MAOIs. Only fluoxetine is FDA-approved for the treatment of bulimia nervosa.

Levenson JL. *Textbook of Psychosomatic Medicine*. Washington: American Psychiatric Publishing; 2005:327.

157. Answer: D. Lamotrigine is approved by the FDA for maintenance therapy in patients with bipolar I disorder. Its most serious potential side effect is a rash. Rashes associated with lamotrigine typically occur between day 5 and week 8 after the start of lamotrigine. Most rashes associated with lamotrigine are simple, benign, morbilliform (both pruritic and not) and occur at a rate of 5% to 15%, which is slightly higher than placebo associated rashes; 5% to 10%. A morbilliform rash resembles measles and consists of macular lesions that are red and 2–10 mm in diameter. A minority of patients, however, may develop a serious cutaneous reaction to lamotrigine, such as Stevens-Johnson syndrome, toxic epidermal necrolysis, or DHS at a rate of 0.1% to 0.2%. A rash occurring in the first 5 days of therapy is probably nondrug related. The patient should hold the next dose and contact their physician. The rash is most likely benign if it has the following characteristics: peaks within days, resolves in 10 to 14 days, or is spotty, nonconfluent, or nontender. Benign rashes also often have no systemic features, and CBC count, LFTs, urea, creatinine, and urine analysis values within normal limits. In these cases, the lamotrigine dose should be reduced or no further dosage increases be made. If the rash is pruritic, antihistamines or topical corticosteroids may be prescribed. The patient should be monitored closely and should be ready to discontinue lamotrigine if the rash worsens or new symptoms emerge. The patient may be rechallenged at a lower dose of 5 to 12.5 mg/day and with slower titration.

A rash occurring between 5 days and 8 weeks is probably lamotrigine related. The patient should hold the next dose and contact their physician. The rash is likely to be serious if it has the following characteristics: confluent and widespread, purpuric, tender, associated fever, malaise, pharyngitis, lymphadenopathy, anorexia, abnormal laboratory test values (see previous text), and any involvement of the eyes, lips, mouth, and other mucous membranes, as well as prominent involvement of the neck or upper trunk. In such cases, lamotrigine should be stopped and the patient should be monitored closely for internal organ involvement and possible hospitalization. The patient should not be rechallenged in the future.

1. Calabrese JR, Sullivan JR, Bowden CL, et al. Rash in multicenter trials of lamotrigine in mood disorders: clinical relevance and management. *J Clin Psychiatry.* 2002;63:1012–1019.
2. Sadock BJ, Sadock VA. *Kaplan and Sadock's Comprehensive Textbook of Psychiatry.* 8th ed. Philadelphia: Lippincott Williams & Wilkins; 2005:1689.

158. Answer: C. Valproate is known to cause congenital malformations especially when taken during the first trimester. The most common congenital malformation is spina bifida which occurs in approximately 5% of the cases of women taking valproate during pregnancy. This rate does not appear to be altered by concomitant use of folic acid. All other answers are adverse effects associated with the use of valproate in patients and have not been shown to occur in fetuses. Alternative treatments for mania include electroconvulsive therapy (ECT) and high-potency antipsychotic drugs. Currently, all mood stabilizers carry some risk in pregnancy; therefore, the risk benefit ratio of continuing therapy versus discontinuation of therapy for the mother and fetus needs to be weighed.

Rosenbaum JF, Arana GW, Hyman SE, et al. *Handbook of Psychiatric Drug Therapy.* 5th ed. Philadelphia: Lippincott Williams & Wilkins; 2005:151–152.

159. Answer: D. A recent meta-analysis examined the effect of cholinesterase drugs on clinical outcomes and completion rates in trials of patients with Alzheimer's disease. Regression analyses compared the effect of dose on clinical outcomes and completion rates, using 10 donepezil, 6 galantamine, and 5 rivastigmine articles. All three drugs showed beneficial effects on cognitive tests when compared to placebo. For donepezil and rivastigmine, larger doses were associated with larger effect. This was not the case with galantamine. The odds of clinical global improvement demonstrated superiority over placebo for each drug, with no dose effects noted. Dropout rates were greater with galantamine and rivastigmine. There was little difference in dropout rate for each drug at each dose-level, except with high-dose donepezil. This was accounted for by the high dropout rate in two 52-week studies using larger doses. In summary, all three drugs had similar cognitive efficacy, with donepezil and rivastigmine showing a dose effect across the dosing levels studied. However, both galantamine and rivastigmine were associated with a greater risk of trial dropout than placebo, especially at higher dosing levels.

Ritchie CW, Ames D, Clayton T, et al. Metaanalysis of randomized trials of the efficacy and safety of donepezil, galantamine, and rivastigmine for the treatment of Alzheimer disease. *Am J Geriatr Psychiatry.* 2004;12:358–369.

160. Answer: E. IPT identifies dysfunction in the domains of grief, interpersonal role disputes, role transitions, and interpersonal deficits. These domains are addressed in order to treat maladaptive relational patterns that contribute to pathology.

Sadock BJ, Sadock VA. *Kaplan and Sadock's Comprehensive Textbook of Psychiatry.* 8th ed. Philadelphia: Lippincott Williams & Wilkins; 2005:2610–2618.

161. Answer: A. In normal neuromuscular transmission, discrete amounts (packets or quanta) of ACh are released across the neuromuscular junction to trigger a muscle contraction. The ACh packets cross the synaptic cleft of the neuromuscular junction to reach numerous deep ACh receptor binding sites. ACh-receptor interactions open cation channels which induce an end-plate potential. If the potential is large enough, it will trigger an action potential along the muscle fiber. Action potentials open calcium storage sites and this produces muscle contraction. Afterward, acetylcholinesterase enzymes or cholinesterases inactivate ACh.

Kaufman DM. *Clinical Neurology for Psychiatrists.* 5th ed. Philadelphia: WB Saunders; 2001:94–95.

162. Answer: B. All of the statements regarding neurons are true, except that the majority of neurons in the human brain are multipolar as they give rise to a single axon with multiple dendritic processes. Astrocytes also help in the removal of certain neurotransmitters from the synaptic cleft, buffer the extracellular potassium concentration, and provide nutrition to the nerve cells. Microglia, the third class of glial cells, function as scavengers and eliminate neuronal debris.

Sadock BJ, Sadock VA. *Kaplan and Sadock's Comprehensive Textbook of Psychiatry*. 8th ed. Philadelphia: Lippincott Williams & Wilkins; 2005:4–5.

163. **Answer: E.** Wernicke's disease is characterized by nystagmus, abducens/conjugate gaze palsies, ataxia of gait, and mental confusion. These symptoms develop acutely or subacutely and may occur singly or, more often, in various combinations. Wernicke's disease is due specifically to a deficiency of thiamine and is observed mainly but not only in alcoholics. It represents a medical emergency; its recognition (or even the suspicion of its presence) demands the immediate administration of thiamine. Prompt use of thiamine prevents progression of the disease and reverses those lesions that have not yet progressed to the point of fixed structural change. Although small doses of oral thiamine may be sufficient to modify the ocular signs, much larger doses are needed to sustain improvement and replenish the depleted thiamine stores—50 mg intravenously and 50 mg intramuscularly—the latter dose being repeated each day until the patient resumes a normal diet. Additionally, in order to avoid precipitating Wernicke's disease, it is standard practice to administer thiamine if intravenous fluids that contain glucose are given. Cyanobalamin, or vitamin B-12, is used to treat pernicious anemia, which is characterized by megaloblastic anemia and peripheral neuropathy. Benzodiazepines would be used to treat acute alcohol withdrawal, which is a strong potential in this patient, but is not indicated immediately. Folic acid is not typically given intramuscularly and its deficiency is characterized by megaloblastic anemia.

Ropper AH, Brown RH. *Adams and Victor's Principles of Neurology*. 8th ed. New York: McGraw-Hill; 2005: 984, 987–988, 992, 996–997.

164. **Answer: C.** A 1-month-old baby usually keeps his head to one side when lying down, the arms tend to be more active than legs, and he keeps his hands closed most of the time. He would not have head support when lifted and shows a "walking" reflex when he is held standing on a hard surface. At around the third week babies are able to look at familiar faces when being fed. A 3-month-old baby usually keeps his head in midline when lying down and has very little head lag when pulled to sit. A 6-month-old baby is able to raise his head up to look at his feet when lying down and has complete head support.

Sheridan MB. *From Birth to Five Years. Children's Developmental Progress*. London: Routledge; 1997:1–43.

165. **Answer: D.** Serum melatonin levels are elevated at night. Serum levels return to baseline during the day. Exposure to light suppresses melatonin levels. Darkness during the day does not stimulate melatonin secretion. Cortisol levels peak in the morning, when melatonin levels approach baseline.

Sadock BJ, Sadock VA. *Kaplan and Sadock's Comprehensive Textbook of Psychiatry*. 8th ed. Philadelphia: Lippincott Williams & Wilkins; 2005:161–169, 284.

166. **Answer: E.** Right-sided frontal lesions have been associated with the development of mania. Recent studies have shown that manic patients have decreased right rostral and orbital prefrontal cortex activation using functional neuroimaging techniques. Other studies have suggested that a functional imbalance between right and left orbitofrontal cortices may be important in the development of mania.

1. Blumberg HP, Stern D, Martinez S, et al. Increased anterior cingulated and caudate activity in bipolar mania. *Biol Psychiatry*. 2000;48:1045–1052.
2. Mimura M, Nakagome K, Hirashima N, et al. Left frontotemporal hyperperfusion in a patient with post-stroke mania. *Psychiatry Res*. 2005;139:263–267.

167. **Answer: E.** The genetics of alcohol abuse and its relationship with personality is an important area of research. Scandinavian adoption studies have found that the risk of alcoholism in male children of male alcoholics is the same regardless of whether the child is reared by the alcoholic father or by a non-drinking adoptive family. Using this data, Cloninger has described two main forms of alcoholism. Type I is the late-onset form which has low inheritance and is usually associated with stress and anxiety. In this form, subjects use alcohol in binges to relieve the stress. Type II alcoholism is the more severe form of the illness where subjects start abusing alcohol at a younger age. In this form, the alcohol use is regular and heavy and is usually associated with impulsivity, antisocial personality traits, and criminality. This form is limited to males and is associated with abnormalities in the brain 5-hydroxytryptamine system. Studies have demonstrated genetic polymorphisms of the 5-hydroxytryptamine receptors.

Gelder MG, Lopez-Ibor JJ, Andreasen N. *New Oxford Textbook of Psychiatry*. 1st ed. New York: Oxford University Press; 2000:473.

168. **Answer: A.** DBT was developed by Marsha Linehan. It mainly pertains to extinguishing maladaptive behaviors in BPD, to helping patients change, and reinforcing good behaviors. The therapist and patient enter into a 1-year contract, which is renewable, but not automatically. Patients must comply

with the contract and there are consequences (such as non-renewal or discharge from treatment) for transgressions (including prolonged or repeated absences). A primary goal of DBT is extinguishing suicidal, parasuicidal, and life-threatening behaviors. Answer choices C, D, and E are additional treatment goals, as well as "stabilization of behavioral skills learned," and "achieving broad based self-respect and self-validation." Four components to DBT are (i) individual outpatient therapy, (ii) skills training, (iii) supportive group therapy, and (iv) telephone consultation.

1. Linehan M. *Cognitive Behavioral Treatment of Borderline Personality Disorder*. New York: Guilford Press; 1993.
2. Robinson D. *Disordered Personalities*. 3rd ed. Port Huron: Rapid Psychler Press; 2005:297–299.

169. **Answer: E.** Cannabis may continue to be detected in urine drug testing up to 4 weeks following cessation of use, depending on the patient's pattern of use. Given this patient's daily pattern of heavy use for the past 3 years, it is likely that he may continue to test positive for approximately 4 weeks following stoppage of use. He, therefore, may have been abstinent over the previous 3 weeks, despite the positive drug test.

Sadock BJ, Sadock VA. *Kaplan and Sadock's Synopsis of Psychiatry*. 9th ed. Philadelphia: Lippincott Williams & Wilkins; 2003:268, 427.

170. **Answer: D.** The most likely axis II diagnosis in this situation is BPD, characterized by affective instability, a pattern of unstable interpersonal relationships, unstable self-image, an imagined fear of abandonment in relationships, and frequent suicidal behavior or deliberate self harm. These patients commonly exhibit the defense mechanism of "splitting"; that is, idealization and devaluation, or seeing phenomena/people as being either singularly good or completely bad. They exhibit impulsivity in at least two, sometimes several, areas. These may be reckless driving, overspending, substance abuse, binge eating, or sexual promiscuity. Eating disorders are more commonly seen in patients with BPD; however binge eating as an isolated symptom is very likely part of the pattern of impulsivity seen in this disorder. People with this disorder can have episodes of "micropsychosis," characterized by hallucinations, paranoid ideation, and ideas of reference in response to stress. These phenomena are usually brief in duration (lasting for a few hours or a maximum of a few days) and are usually not associated with loss of insight. BPD is far more commonly diagnosed in women.

1. Paris J. Borderline personality disorder. *Can Med Assoc J*. 2005;172:1579–1583.

2. Sadock BJ, Sadock VA. *Kaplan and Sadock's Comprehensive Textbook of Psychiatry*. 8th ed. Philadelphia: Lippincott Williams & Wilkins; 2005:2085.

171. **Answer: E.** Mirtazapine is more often associated with increased appetite and weight gain than with reduction in binge eating or weight loss. SSRIs, including fluoxetine and fluvoxamine, have been reported to reduce binge-eating episodes in both bulimia nervosa and BED. The anticonvulsant topiramate has been found to reduce binge-eating episodes in patients with BED, and has also been known to cause weight loss in obese patients. Naltrexone has been shown to reduce binge eating, suggesting that opiate blockade may be considered in the treatment of BED. Sibutramine, which blocks reuptake of serotonin and norepinephrine, has also been found to be more effective than placebo in reducing the frequency of binge eating in obese patients with BED.

1. Kruger S, Kennedy SH. Pharmacotherapy of anorexia nervosa, bulimia nervosa, and binge-eating disorder. *J Psychiatry Neurosci*. 2000;25:497–508.
2. Levenson JL. *Textbook of Psychosomatic Medicine*. Washington: American Psychiatric Publishing; 2005: 327.

172. **Answer: E.** All the choices except a history of HIV, SLE, or concomitant steroid use are risk factors for the development of a lamotrigine-associated rash. Children younger than age 13 years are also at risk for developing lamotrigine-associated rash. Stevens-Johnson syndrome associated with lamotrigine occurs more frequently in children than in adults, affecting approximately 2 in 10,000 adults versus 4 in 10,000 children.

1. Calabrese JR, Sullivan JR, Bowden CL, et al. Rash in multicenter trials of lamotrigine in mood disorders: clinical relevance and management. *J Clin Psychiatry*. 2002;63:1012–1019.
2. Sadock BJ, Sadock VA. *Kaplan and Sadock's Comprehensive Textbook of Psychiatry*. 8th ed. Philadelphia: Lippincott Williams & Wilkins; 2005:1689.

173. **Answer: A.** Stevens-Johnson syndrome is characterized by fever, body aches, redness and tearing of the eyes, and the blistering of oral, vaginal, urethral mucous membranes, as well as the spread of red rash over the body. These symptoms may be preceded by symptoms of an upper respiratory respiration. Concomitant use of lamotrigine and valproic acid is associated with the development of Stevens-Johnson syndrome. Valproate increases the serum levels of lamotrigine, thereby increasing the risk of Stevens-Johnson syndrome. All the other drug combinations are less likely to produce this condition.

1. Famularo G, De Simone C, Minisola G. Stevens-Johnson syndrome associated with single high dose of lamotrigine

in a patient taking valproate. *Dermatol Online J.* 2005;11:25.

2. Habif. *Clinical Dermatology*. 4th ed. St Louis: Mosby; 2004:630.

3. Yalcin B, Karaduman A. Stevens-Johnson syndrome associated with concomitant use of lamotrigine and valproic acid. *J Am Acad Dermatol*. 2000;43:898–899.

174. Answer: B. NA started in the late 1940s with meetings first emerging in the Los Angeles area of California. The NA program movement has grown into one of the largest organizations of its type. Membership is open to all drug addicts, regardless of the particular drug or combination of drugs used. There are no social, religious, economic, racial, ethnic, national, gender, or class-status membership restrictions. There are no dues or fees for membership. NA provides a recovery process and support network inextricably linked together. One of the keys to NA's success is the therapeutic value of addicts working with other addicts. Members share their successes and challenges in overcoming active addiction and living drug-free productive lives through the application of the principles contained within the Twelve Steps and Twelve Traditions of NA. These principles are the core of the NA recovery program. Principles incorporated within the steps include: (i) admitting there is a problem, (ii) seeking help, (iii) engaging in a thorough self-examination, (iv) confidential self-disclosure, (v) making amends for harm done, and (vi) helping other drug addicts who want to recover. Central to the NA program is its emphasis on practicing spiritual principles. NA itself is nonreligious, and each member is encouraged to cultivate an individual understanding—religious or not—of this "spiritual awakening." NA is not affiliated with other organizations, including other twelve step programs, treatment centers, or correctional facilities. As an organization, NA does not employ professional counselors or therapists nor does it provide residential facilities or clinics. Additionally, the fellowship does not provide vocational, legal, financial, psychiatric, or medical services. NA's only mission is to provide an environment in which addicts can help one another stop using drugs and find a new way to live. In NA, members are encouraged to comply with complete abstinence from all drugs including alcohol. It has been the experience of NA members that complete and continuous abstinence provides the best foundation for recovery and personal growth. NA as a whole has no opinion on outside issues, including prescribed medications. The use of psychiatric medications and other medically indicated drugs prescribed by a physician and taken under medical

supervision is not seen as compromising a person's recovery in NA.

Narcotics Anonymous. Information about NA. Available at: http://www.na.org/basic.htm. Accessed April 9, 2007.

175. Answer: A. IPT consists of three phases (I, II, III). Phase I involves assigning a name to the patient's diagnosis and educating the patient about his/her condition. Phase II involves implementing strategies to address relational problems identified. Phase III involves discussion of termination issues.

Sadock BJ, Sadock VA. *Kaplan and Sadock's Comprehensive Textbook of Psychiatry*. 8th ed. Philadelphia: Lippincott Williams & Wilkins; 2005:2610–2618.

176. Answer: E. Prions (proteinaceous infective agents) are composed totally or almost totally of protein. They lack DNA and RNA. Prions are transmissible agents, but differ from viruses in that they lack nucleic acid. They are generated from the human prion protein gene (PrP), which is located on the short arm of chromosome 20. PrP mutates into a disease-related isoform, PrP-Super-C, which has the ability to replicate and possesses infectious properties.

1. Kaufman DM. *Clinical Neurology for Psychiatrists*. 5th ed. Philadelphia: WB Saunders; 2001:149.

2. Sadock BJ, Sadock VA. *Kaplan and Sadock's Synopsis of Psychiatry*. 9th ed. Philadelphia: Lippincott Williams & Wilkins; 2003:364.

177. Answer: D. In the early stages of brain development, the neural tube has three primary vesicles. These three vesicles are called the prosencephalon, the mesencephalon, and the rhombencephalon. The prosencephalon divides to become the telencephalon and the diencephalon. The telencephalon gives rise to the cerebral cortex, hippocampus, the amygdala, and some components of the basal ganglia. The diencephalon gives rise to the thalamus and hypothalamus. The mesencephalon develops into the midbrain structures. The rhombencephalon further divides into the metencephalon and the myelencephalon. The metencephalon develops into the pons and the cerebellum with the myelencephalon giving rise to the medulla.

Sadock BJ, Sadock VA. *Kaplan and Sadock's Comprehensive Textbook of Psychiatry*. 8th ed. Philadelphia: Lippincott Williams & Wilkins; 2005:7.

178. Answer: C. CNS lymphoma has assumed increasing significance in the last two decades because of its frequency in acquired immunodeficiency syndrome (AIDS) and other immunosuppressed states. However, for unexplained reasons, it is also occurring with increased frequency in immunocompetent persons. It is more common in men, with the peak incidence in the fifth through seventh decades, or in the third and fourth decades in patients with AIDS. Behavior/personality changes, confusion, dizziness, and focal cerebral signs predominate over headache and other signs of increased intracranial pressure as presenting manifestations. Seizures may occur but are less common. Because the tumors are deep and often multicentric, surgical resection is ineffective except in rare instances. Until recently the median survival of patients has been 10 to 18 months, but less in those with AIDS or in individuals who are otherwise immunocompromised. More recent regimen consists of several cycles of intravenous methotrexate and citrovorum, administered at 2- to 3-week intervals and at times continued indefinitely if tolerated. The side effects of these treatments are modest and there is no need for repeated lumbar punctures or the placement of a permanent reservoir. Most patients do not develop mucositis or any of the other of the usual side effects of this type of chemotherapy. Corticosteroids are added at any point as needed to control prominent neurological symptoms. The median survival time has been in the range of 3.5 years with intravenous methotrexate alone and 4 years or more if radiation is given subsequently. Some patients are still alive at 10 years.

Ropper AH, Brown RH. *Adams and Victor's Principles of Neurology*. 8th ed. New York: McGraw-Hill; 2005: 560–562.

179. Answer: B. MDMA use results in a sudden increase in the brain serotonergic effects by causing the calcium-dependent release of serotonin from nerve terminals. When taken orally, its onset of action begins after 30 to 60 minutes, and peaks by 90 and 120 minutes. Its effect persists for about 6 to 12 hours. It is primarily metabolized by demethylation by the hepatic cytochrome P-450 enzyme, debrisoquine hydroxylase coded for by CYP 2D6. There are two phenotypes of this enzyme and 9% are poor metabolizers of the drug. The drug is abused intranasally, rectally, and intravenously. As it is related to both amphetamine and mescaline, MDMA possesses both stimulant and hallucinogenic properties. Concurrent use of cocaine and amphetamines potentiate the stimulant effects of MDMA and can cause hyperthermic and cardiac problems. Hepatocellular failure, arterial aneurysms, and cerebral hemorrhages may also be seen with the use of MDMA. Concurrent consumption of SSRIs and MAOIs may potentiate the harmful neurochemical and behavioral effects of MDMA.

Gelder MG, Lopez-Ibor JJ, Andreasen N. *New Oxford Textbook of Psychiatry*. 1st ed. New York: Oxford University Press; 2000:543–544.

180. Answer: D. This patient is exhibiting the classic symptoms of autism. According to DSM-IV-TR criteria, a child must exhibit impairments before the age of 3 in the following areas: social interactions, communication, and behavior. Autistic children have a very limited vocabulary (or cannot speak at all) and do not use compensatory mechanisms to communicate. They do not develop peer relationships appropriate to their age, are not interested in shared games, tend to adhere to specific routines, and have repetitive stereotyped behaviors. Approximately 25% of children with autism develop seizures in a bimodal fashion (either earlier in life or in their teenage years). Children with Asperger's syndrome present with social impairments, but usually do not have difficulties in their speech development. In Rett's disorder, patients have a short period of normal development followed by head deceleration and severe psychomotor retardation. Patients with autistic disorder may have mental retardation, but in children with only mental retardation the adaptive functioning measures are consistent with their IQ. In Down syndrome, patients exhibit characteristic facies and symptomatology at birth.

1. American Psychiatric Association. *Quick Reference to the Diagnostic Criteria from DSM-IV-TR*. Washington: American Psychiatric Association; 2000:59–64.
2. Lewis M. *Child and Adolescent Psychiatry*. 2nd ed. Philadelphia: Lippincott and Williams & Wilkins; 1996:587–595.
3. Scahill L. Diagnosis and evaluation of pervasive developmental disorders. *J Clin Psychiatry*. 2005;66 (suppl 10):19–25.

181. Answer: A. Her symptoms have most likely been caused by the abrupt cessation of a benzodiazepine, such as lorazepam. The withdrawal syndrome associated with cessation of regular benzodiazepine use may include sweating, increased heart rate, tremors, insomnia, nausea/vomiting, hallucinations, agitation, anxiety, and seizures. The onset of withdrawal usually occurs 2 to 3 days after cessation of use, but may demonstrate an increased latency in the case of longer-acting benzodiazepines. Predictable and circumscribed withdrawal syndromes have not been described for the other medications listed above.

1. American Psychiatric Association. *Quick Reference to the Diagnostic Criteria from DSM-IV-TR*. Washington: American Psychiatric Association; 2000:105–151.
2. Sadock BJ, Sadock VA. *Kaplan and Sadock's Synopsis of Psychiatry*. 9th ed. Philadelphia: Lippincott Williams & Wilkins; 2003:462.

182. Answer: D. The drug psilocybin is largely ingested as mushrooms. Psilocybin is commonly found in mushrooms of the genus Psilocybe. It is cultivated on a large scale in Florida and Texas in the United States. The hallucinogenic active ingredient is indolethylamine, or tryptamine. Mescaline is the active hallucinogenic alkaloid in peyote "buttons," picked from small blue-green cacti *Lophophora williamsii* and *Lophophora diffusa*. LSD, commonly called "acid" or "blotter's acid" is distributed as tablets, liquids, gelatin squares, or powder, and produces symptoms similar to psilocybin and mescaline, although it is much more potent. Ibogaine is an alkaloid found in the African shrub *Tabernanthe iboga*. It is not popularly used as a hallucinogenic due to its somatic side effects, but there have been claims regarding its therapeutic value in the pharmacotherapy of heroin addiction. Ayahuasca, originally referred to a South American drink, is made by boiling parts of a Western Amazonian vine, which contains the alkaloids harmine and harmaline–both of these have hallucinogenic properties. It now refers to any drink which is a mixture of two hallucinogens.

1. Halpern JH. Hallucinogens and dissociative agents naturally growing in the United States. *Pharmacol Ther*. 2004;102:131–138.
2. Sadock BJ, Sadock VA. *Kaplan and Sadock's Comprehensive Textbook of Psychiatry*. 8th ed. Philadelphia: Lippincott Williams & Wilkins; 2005:1242–1243.

183. Answer: D. Bupropion should be avoided in patients at high risk for seizures, including those with eating disorders and those with a history of seizures. With bupropion sustained release, the rate of seizures is 0.1% at doses up to 300 mg/day, a rate similar to other antidepressants. Because of the risk of seizures, the total daily dose of bupropion is not recommended to be >450 mg/day. Bupropion is indicated for the treatment of major depressive disorder and for use in combination with behavioral modification for smoking cessation. Unlike SSRIs, bupropion is known for decreased incidence of sexual side effects; some patients taking this medication may actually experience increased sexual responsiveness.

Rosenbaum JF, Arana GW, Hyman SE. *Handbook of Psychiatric Drug Therapy*. 5th ed. Philadelphia: Lippincott Williams & Wilkins; 2005:96–97.

184. Answer: D. The rash associated with lamotrigine typically occurs between day 5 and week 8 after the start of therapy. Most rashes associated with lamotrigine are simple benign morbilliform (both pruritic and not) and occur at a rate of 5% to 15%, slightly higher than placebo associated rash: 5% to 10%. A minority of patients, however, may develop a serious cutaneous reaction to lamotrigine–Stevens-Johnson syndrome, toxic epidermal necrolysis, or DHS at a rate

of 0.1% to 0.01% of patients on lamotrigine. Stevens-Johnson syndrome is characterized by a high fever, ulceration of mucous membranes, skin blistering or crusting, and malaise. It is associated with 5% mortality. It occurs in approximately 2 in 10,000 adults and 4 in 10,000 children. Toxic epidermal necrolysis presents similarly to Stevens-Johnson syndrome, but is more rapidly progressive (over 1 to 5 days), with widespread skin detachment and erythema that involves more than 30% of the body surface area. It is associated with 25% to 30% mortality. DHS presents with fever, internal organ involvement, rash, and typically without mucous membrane involvement. The rash usually begins with patchy macular erythema that may become papular and pruritic. It can evolve to erythroderma (an abnormal redness of the skin over extensive areas of the body), with prominent desquamation and occasionally pustules. The face, upper trunk, and upper extremities are usually affected early in the course of eruption. Internal organ changes associated with lamotrigine-induced DHS include hepatitis, nephritis, pneumonitis, colitis, meningitis/encephalitis, and lymphadenopathy. Hematologic abnormalities include hemolytic anemia, thrombocytopenia, neutropenia, agranulocytosis, and eosinophilia. TSS is characterized by sudden onset of fever, chills, vomiting, diarrhea, muscle aches, and rash. It can rapidly progress to severe and intractable hypotension and multisystem dysfunction. Desquamation, particularly on the palms and soles, can occur 1 to 2 weeks after onset of the illness. Etiologic agent is usually an exotoxin-producing strain of *Staphylococcus aureus*. In the United States, the annual incidence is 1 to 2 per 100,000 women 15 to 44 years of age. Five percent of all cases are fatal. *S. aureus* commonly colonizes skin and mucous membranes in humans. TSS has been associated with use of tampons and intravaginal contraceptive devices in women and occurs as a complication of skin abscesses or surgery.

1. Calabrese JR, Sullivan JR, Bowden CL, et al. Rash in multicenter trials of lamotrigine in mood disorders: clinical relevance and management. *J Clin Psychiatry*. 2002;63:1012–1019.
2. Centers for Disease Control and Prevention. Toxic shock syndrome. Available at: http://www.cdc.gov/ncidod/dbmd/diseaseinfo/toxicshock_t.htm. Accessed September 17, 2006.
3. Sadock BJ, Sadock VA. *Kaplan and Sadock's Comprehensive Textbook of Psychiatry*. 8th ed. Philadelphia: Lippincott Williams & Wilkins; 2005:1683.

185. Answer: B. In predictable, occasional situations, the best drugs to treat anxiety are short or intermediate acting benzodiazepines such as lorazepam or alpra-zolam. Beta-blockers may also be helpful in such sit-uations, but their use is contraindicated in bronchial asthma, COPD, diabetes mellitus, heart blocks, bradyarrhythmias, angle-closure glaucoma, cardio-genic shock, and congestive cardiac failure. They are also contraindicated in patients receiving clonidine, pregnancy, peripheral vascular disease, and in renal impairment. In patients with type-I diabetes, hypo-glycemic response may be exacerbated or prolonged by the beta-blockers as they inhibit glycogenolysis. SSRIs are indicated for chronic recurrent anxiety or anxiety in unpredictable situations.

Sadock BJ, Sadock VA. *Kaplan and Sadock's Comprehen-sive Textbook of Psychiatry*. 8th ed. Philadelphia: Lippincott Williams & Wilkins; 2005:1782–1783.

186. **Answer: D.** Modafinil is a novel wake-promoting agent that has FDA approval for narcolepsy and shift work sleep disorder and as adjunctive treatment of ob-structive sleep apnea/hypopnea syndrome. Modafinil has a novel mechanism of action and is theorized to work in a localized manner, utilizing hypocretin, histamine, epinephrine, GABA, and glutamate. It is a well-tolerated medication with low propensity for abuse and is frequently used for off-label indications. Ninety percent of modafinil is metabolized in the liver via the cytochrome P-450–3A4 system and ex-creted via the kidney. It has a t1/2 of 15 hours and is used in doses of 100 mg to 400 mg/day. It is desig-nated as a category C drug for pregnancy and sched-ule IV drug by the FDA. It is not known to affect the sleep architecture. Most common side effects include headache, nausea, diarrhea, and anorexia.

1. Albers LJ, Hahn RK, Reist C. *Handbook of Psychiatric Drugs*. Laguna Hills: Current Clinical Strategies Publish-ing; 2005:92–93.
2. Ballon JS, Feifel D. A systematic review of modafinil: po-tential clinical uses and mechanisms of action. *J Clin Psy-chiatry*. 2006;67:554–566.

187. **Answer: A.** Sexual dysfunction is usually divided into disorders of four types: (i) sexual desire, (ii) arousal, (iii) orgasm, and (iv) other problems not included in the first three categories. Although variable rates of success of sex therapy have been reported for differ-ent etiologies, data indicate that it is particularly dif-ficult to address decreased sexual desire in the male partner.

Hawton K. Treatment of sexual dysfunctions by sex ther-apy and other approaches. *Br J Psychiatry*. 1995;167:307–314.

188. **Answer: E.** All of the statements are true except that MDMA produces a selective loss of fine axons, while

sparing the larger beaded projections derived from the median raphe.

1. Kaufman DM. *Clinical Neurology for Psychiatrists*. 5th ed. Philadelphia: WB Saunders; 2001:557–558.
2. Sadock BJ, Sadock VA. *Kaplan and Sadock's Comprehen-sive Textbook of Psychiatry*. 8th ed. Philadelphia: Lippin-cott Williams & Wilkins; 2005:49–50.

189. **Answer: C.** The cerebral cortex of each hemisphere can be divided into four major areas: the frontal lobe, parietal lobe, temporal lobe, and the occipital lobe. The frontal lobe is located anterior to the central sul-cus and consists of the primary motor area, premo-tor area, and the prefrontal cortex. The primary so-matosensory cortex and the cortical regions related to complex visual and somatosensory functions are located in the anterior and posterior parietal lobes respectively. The primary auditory cortex and other auditory regions are present in the superior portion of the temporal lobe with the inferior portion con-taining regions associated with complex visual func-tions. The occipital lobe is associated with primary visual cortex and other visual association areas.

Sadock BJ, Sadock VA. *Kaplan and Sadock's Comprehen-sive Textbook of Psychiatry*. 8th ed. Philadelphia: Lippincott Williams & Wilkins; 2005:7.

190. **Answer: B.** Huntington's disease is an autosomal dom-inant genetic disease characterized by chorea, cog-nitive decline, and dementia. It manifests in midlife, and has no cure or effective treatment. Predictive testing became available in the mid-1980s. However, testing for an incurable illness is somewhat con-troversial. Testing can have both positive and neg-ative consequences, regardless of outcome. The ma-jor benefit reported was relief from the uncertainty of not knowing, and negative consequences for noncar-riers has included psychological distress and guilt. Possibly because of this, only 3% to 21% of at risk patients get tested worldwide. A significant percent-age of patients have suicidal thoughts after testing for Huntington's disease. Studies have found that a history of depression, hopelessness, and suicidal tendencies are associated with an increased risk of suicide. These risk factors are not contraindications for testing, but do require increased counseling and careful follow-up.

1. Codori AM, Brandt J. Psychological costs and benefits for predictive testing of Huntington's disease. *Am J Med Genet*. 1994;54:174–184.
2. Robins-Wahlin TB. To know or not to know: a review of behaviour and suicidal ideation in preclinical Hunting-ton's disease. *Patient Educ Couns*. 2006; in press.

191. **Answer B.** Ketamine is an anesthetic and analgesic agent that is structurally related to PCP. It works

via the suppression of the reticular activating system which then causes a functional and electrophysiological dissociation between the thalamocortical and limbic systems. This results in higher brain centers being prevented from perceiving auditory, visual, and painful stimuli. Ketamine is a potent NMDA receptor antagonist. It is abused orally and intranasally. After oral ingestion, the effects appear within 30 minutes and lasts for about 3 hours. It can cause vivid dreams, flashbacks, hallucinations, synesthesia, psychosis, delirium, and memory impairments. Physical effects include tachycardia, hypertension, GI disturbances, hypersalivation, nystagmus, numbness, ataxia, slurred speech, and raised intracranial pressure.

Gelder MG, Lopez-Ibor JJ, Andreasen N. *New Oxford Textbook of Psychiatry*. 1st ed. New York: Oxford University Press; 2000:544–545.

192. Answer: E. Patients with Asperger's syndrome usually have one focus of interest (e.g., dinosaurs, a specific episode in history, etc.) and they tend to accumulate an enormous amount of information on that subject. When approached with another topic, they soon lose interest and do not engage in conversation. A distinct difference between autism and Asperger's syndrome is that patients with the latter usually have a normal verbal development. In Asperger's syndrome patients can also show repetitive behaviors, an inability to read or respond to social cues, and a lack of interest in initiating a conversation. However, the distinct feature of this syndrome is the restricted range of interests.

1. Lewis M. *Child and Adolescent Psychiatry*. 2nd ed. Philadelphia: Lippincott and Williams & Wilkins; 1996: 587–595.
2. Scahill L. Diagnosis and evaluation of pervasive developmental disorders. *J Clin Psychiatry*. 2005;66 (suppl 10):19–25.

193. Answer: E. Antisocial, schizotypal, avoidant, and dependent personality disorders all show evidence of genetic transmission in family risk studies. However, only schizotypal disorder demonstrates genetic transmission in twin and molecular risk studies as well. There is a substantial body of literature linking schizotypal PD to schizophrenia, suggesting it may be "a muted form of schizophrenia." A recent Chinese twin study of 324 pairs reported no observed genetic effect with histrionic personality disorder, but did report significant effects with schizotypal, dependent, and narcissistic personality disorders.

1. Gabbard G. *Psychodynamic Psychiatry in Clinical Practice*. 4th ed. Washington: American Psychiatric Press; 2005:413.
2. Hilty D, Bourgeois J, Hales R, et al. *Study Guide to Clinical Psychiatry*. 4th ed. Washington: American Psychiatric Press; 2006:75–76.
3. Ji W, Hu Y, Huang Y, et al. A twin study of personality disorder heritability. *Zhonghua Liu Xing Bing Xue Za Zhi*. 2006;27:137–141.

194. Answer: A. Histrionic personality disorder is associated with excessive dramatization and attention-seeking behavior. It is more commonly seen in women and may be associated with seductive gestures/behavior. Interpersonal relationships tend to be shallow, and marital problems abound owing to failure to achieve emotional intimacy. There is an increased risk of somatization disorder, conversion disorder, and major depression. However, there is no association with obsessive-compulsive traits, bipolar disorder, or eating disorders.

Sadock BJ, Sadock VA. *Kaplan and Sadock's Comprehensive Textbook of Psychiatry*. 8th ed. Philadelphia: Lippincott Williams & Wilkins; 2005:2084.

195. Answer: D. All of the statements regarding the dopaminergic system in the CNS are true, except that the motor disturbance of Parkinson's disease is due to the degeneration of the nigrostriatal system and not the tuberohypophysial system.

1. Kaufman DM. *Clinical Neurology for Psychiatrists*. 5th ed. Philadelphia: WB Saunders; 2001:552–555.
2. Sadock BJ, Sadock VA. *Kaplan and Sadock's Comprehensive Textbook of Psychiatry*. 8th ed. Philadelphia: Lippincott Williams & Wilkins; 2005:50.

196. Answer: D. All the statements are true except that the foramina of Monro or the intraventricular foramina are two apertures that connect the two lateral ventricles with the third ventricle. The cerebral aqueduct connects the third ventricle with the fourth ventricle. The ventricular system is filled with CSF. The choroid plexus is a complex of ependyma, pia, and capillaries that invaginate the ventricle and 70% of the CSF is produced at the choroid plexus located in the walls of the lateral ventricles and in the roof of both the third and fourth ventricles.

Sadock BJ, Sadock VA. *Kaplan and Sadock's Comprehensive Textbook of Psychiatry*. 8th ed. Philadelphia: Lippincott Williams & Wilkins; 2005:8.

197. Answer: D. Malpractice cases are part of the general field of tort (a civil wrong) law. Most claims are because of unintentional torts or negligence. An intentional tort (sexual misconduct, fraud, or physical assault) is rarely covered by insurance, except when the act is part of normally accepted practice (restraint of a patient for medical or behavioral reasons). The injured party (the patient or their estate) must prove the four D's: **Dereliction** of **Duty Directly** caused **Damages**. Physicians are held to the same standard as respectable, average physicians in the same or similar community. Specialists, however, are held to a higher standard if they hold themselves out to the community as an expert, regardless of actual training. Physicians also have a duty to consult when the limits of their expertise have been reached. Lastly, damages can be economic, physical, or in the form of emotional pain and suffering.

Stern TA, Herman JB. *Massachusetts General Hospital Psychiatry Update & Board Preparation*. 2nd ed. New York: McGraw-Hill; 2004:503.

198. Answer: A. This patient is presenting with the classic signs of meningitis, specifically meningococcal meningitis (*Neisseria meningitidis*). It should be suspected when the evolution is extremely rapid (delirium and stupor may supervene in a matter of hours), when the onset is associated with a petechial rash or by large ecchymoses and lividity of the skin of the lower parts of the body, when there is circulatory shock, and especially during local outbreaks of meningitis. All household contacts of patients with meningococcal meningitis should be given prophylactic antibiotics. The risk of secondary cases is small for adolescents and adults, and if 2 weeks or more have elapsed since the initial case was found, no prophylaxis is needed. Treatment should begin while awaiting the results of diagnostic tests and may be altered later in accordance with the laboratory findings. In children and adults, third-generation cephalosporins are probably the best initial therapy for the three major types of community-acquired meningitides. In areas with penicillin-resistant pneumococci, consideration should be given to adding vancomycin and rifampin until the susceptibility of the organism is established. Most cases should be treated for about 2 weeks, except when there is a persistent parameningeal focus of infection (otitic or sinus origin). Antibiotics should be administered in full doses parenterally (preferably intravenously) throughout the period of treatment. First-line treatment for meningococcal meningitis is penicillin G or ampicillin.

Ropper AH, Brown RH. *Adams and Victor's Principles of Neurology*. 8th ed. New York: McGraw-Hill; 2005: 595–600.

199. Answer: D. Medical malpractice is defined as negligence resulting in harm to the patient. Negligence alone is not sufficient to bring a malpractice claim. A claim must meet the four Ds (**Dereliction** of **Duty Directly** caused **Damages**) and show that the physician fell below the standard of care set by reasonable physicians of the community. Many claims are settled out of court, and most that are tried are decided in favor of the physician.

Stern TA, Herman JB. *Massachusetts General Hospital Psychiatry Update & Board Preparation*. 2nd ed. New York: McGraw-Hill; 2004:503, 633, 663.

200. Answer: E. Treatment of whiplash injury remains largely empirical and variable. The majority of patients improve with minimal or no treatment. Patients with persistent symptoms usually respond to range of motion exercises, massage, and heat. Vigorous cervical manipulation should be avoided. Whiplash patients are likely to benefit from "neck hygiene." Patients should not cradle phones in their neck, should elevate computer keyboards and monitors to comfortable levels, only use one pillow, and curtail sports which strain the neck. Although legal issues should be acknowledged, effects of litigation are controversial. Litigating and nonlitigating patients have been found to have similar recovery rates, and most patients involved in litigation are not cured by its resolution.

Kaufman DM. *Clinical Neurology for Psychiatrists*. 5th ed. Philadelphia: WB Saunders; 2001:593–594.

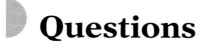

Questions

1. A girl is brought to your office for a routine check-up. While you talk to her parents she is sitting unsupported on the floor and is able to lean over to grab some toys. She is able to pull herself up, but needs help to come back to the floor and is not able to walk yet. She babbles loudly and likes to put everything in her mouth. Given this information, how old do you think this child is at present?

   A. 6 months
   B. 9 months
   C. 12 months
   D. 15 months
   E. 24 months

2. What are common electroencephalogram (EEG) findings in stage II sleep?

   A. High amplitude slow waves occupying >50% of epoch
   B. Alpha activity
   C. K complexes
   D. Theta activity
   E. High amplitude slow waves occupying 20% to 50% of epoch

3. A 75-year-old man suffers from an infarction of the left watershed area (large border zone between the middle, anterior, and posterior cerebral arteries) due to recent prolonged cardiac arrest. He is not able to participate in any conversation, follow requests, or name objects, but he involuntarily and often compulsively repeats long and complex sentences with ease. He also echoes what people say to him in a parrot-like manner (echolalia). Which one of the following choices best identifies the pattern of speech deficit seen in this patient?

   A. Anomia
   B. Conduction aphasia
   C. Isolation aphasia
   D. Sensory aphasia
   E. Motor aphasia

4. In the following 2 × 2 table, which one of the choices represents a type II error?

Study outcome	No true difference exists	True difference exists
Difference found	A	B
No difference found	C	D
Total	A+C	B+D

   A. A
   B. B
   C. C
   D. D
   E. A+C

5. All of the following changes seen on a magnetic resonance imaging (MRI) scan can be associated with the normal process of aging EXCEPT:

   A. Increase in whole brain cerebrospinal fluid (CSF) volume
   B. Increase in high-intensity lesion volumes
   C. Decreased cerebral hemisphere volume
   D. Increase ventricular volume
   E. Pronounced decrease in hippocampal volume

6. Cassandra Perkins is a 21-year-old woman who loses her entire family in an earthquake. However, she manages to escape with minor injuries. She had tried to save her family members when they were caught under debris, but she did not succeed. A few days later, she disappears from the rehabilitation camp. Several days later she is found in a neighboring town. She has no memory of the earthquake or the rehabilitation camp. She did not find the name Cassandra Perkins familiar and gave her name as "Dana Smith." Given her presentation, which one of the following choices is the most likely diagnosis?

   A. Dissociative amnesia
   B. Dissociative fugue
   C. Dissociative disorder, not otherwise specified (NOS)
   D. Dissociative trance
   E. Dissociative identity disorder

7. Which one of the following is the strongest risk factor for developing Posttraumatic Stress Disorder (PTSD) after being exposed to a traumatic event?
   A. Age when exposed to traumatic event
   B. Male gender
   C. Higher levels of anxiety in the peri-event period
   D. Substance abuse
   E. Loss of consciousness during traumatic event

8. A 16-year-old girl is brought to your office for an initial consultation. Since her parent's divorce 2 months ago, she has been irritable and has had problems keeping up with her grades in school. She spends most of the time at home and does not want to engage in social activities. She denies any change in her appetite or weight, reports being able to sleep well, and denies any feelings of helplessness or hopelessness. What would be the best initial treatment for this patient?
   A. A trial of Citalopram
   B. A trial of Sertraline
   C. Supportive psychotherapy
   D. Long-term psychodynamic psychotherapy
   E. Inpatient admission to a psychiatric unit

9. Which one of the following choices is TRUE regarding the prognosis of elderly patients with bipolar disorder?
   A. They have a worse prognosis than their younger counterparts.
   B. They often have incomplete response to treatments, recurrent episodes of the illness, and higher mortality rates than in the younger population.
   C. They have higher incidence of cognitive deficits, even when they are well.
   D. Mortality rate for patients with late life bipolar disorder is higher than that of the general population.
   E. All of the above.

10. All of the following factors suggest suitability for sex therapy as a treatment for sexual dysfunction EXCEPT:
    A. The dysfunction has been present for at least several months.
    B. Neither partner has psychiatric symptoms or active substance abuse.
    C. The couple has other relationship problems not related to sexual function.
    D. The couple is motivated for therapy.
    E. The female partner is not pregnant.

11. Which one of the following statements is NOT TRUE regarding N-acetyl cysteine?
    A. It is used as an antidote in poisoning by acetaminophen.

B. It is converted into a substrate for the glutamate/cystine antiporter, which is located on glial cells.
C. It causes glial cells to release glutamate into the extrasynaptic space, eventually causing reduced synaptic release of glutamate.
D. It inhibits glial release of glutamate into the extrasynaptic space, thereby causing reduced synaptic release of glutamate.
E. It stimulates metabotropic glumatergic receptors on nerve terminals.

12. Who was/were the first to induce therapeutic seizures in humans using electricity?
    A. Kenneth Kesey
    B. Ugo Cerletti and Lucio Bini
    C. Sigmund Freud
    D. Ladislas Joseph von Meduna
    E. Carl Jung

13. Which one of the following is not a focus area for Interpersonal therapy (IPT)?
    A. Grief/bereavement
    B. Early childhood relationships
    C. Unresolved disputes
    D. Role transitions
    E. Interpersonal deficits

14. Which agent is the drug of choice for the treatment of trigeminal neuralgia (tic douloureux)?
    A. Carbamazepine
    B. Clonazepam
    C. Morphine sulfate
    D. Nortriptyline
    E. Phenytoin

15. All of the following are basic exceptions to obtaining informed consent EXCEPT:
    A. Emergencies
    B. Incompetence
    C. Therapeutic privilege
    D. Waiver
    E. Mental retardation

16. Which one of the following statements regarding the ventricular system in the brain and cerebrospinal fluid (CSF) is NOT TRUE?
    A. The CSF is finally absorbed by the arachnoid villi and released into the superior sagittal sinus.
    B. Interruption to the flow CSF usually causes hydrocephalus.
    C. CSF is a colorless liquid containing relatively low concentrations of sodium and chloride and high concentrations of protein, glucose, and potassium.
    D. CSF serves to cushion the brain against trauma.
    E. CSF also controls the extracellular environment and transport endocrine hormones in the brain.

17. Monocular quadrantanopsia occurs due to a lesion of which one of the following structures?
    A. Optic nerve
    B. Optic chiasm
    C. Optic tract
    D. Occipital cortex
    E. None of the above

18. All of the following have been associated with an increased risk of Parkinson's disease EXCEPT:
    A. Cigarette smoking
    B. Pesticide exposure
    C. Family history of Parkinson's disease
    D. Increasing age
    E. Perinatal infections

19. A 12-year-old boy was an unrestrained front seat passenger in a motor vehicle accident. He struck his head on the windshield of the car during the accident. He was found to be unconscious on the scene of the accident, and was transported to the hospital and placed in the pediatric intensive care unit. He had emergent surgery to evacuate an intracranial hemorrhage but did not regain consciousness after 5 days postoperative. Which one of the following tests might provide useful information in deciding his continued care?
    A. Repeat computed tomography (CT) scan of the brain
    B. Brainstem auditory evoked potentials
    C. Visual evoked potentials
    D. Electromyography
    E. Somatosensory evoked potentials

20. Which of the following is a current clinical application of blood-oxygen-level-dependent functional MRI (BOLD fMRI), which evaluates regional changes in oxygen utilization and cerebral blood flow in the context of activation of different brain regions?
    A. It is not useful clinically and is used only for research purposes at this time.
    B. Its main use is to diagnose cerebrovascular accidents.
    C. Its main use is to evaluate and diagnose cerebral palsy.
    D. It can be used to evaluate changes in the brain postoperatively.
    E. It is used to map localization of important brain functions prior to neurosurgery.

21. A 60-year-old man presents with neck stiffness, unilateral leg weakness, and upper arm pain. These symptoms started a year ago and are progressively worsening. Which of the following statements is NOT TRUE regarding his condition?
    A. The presence of arm and neck pain are not characteristic of spinal multiple sclerosis.

    B. A MRI of the spinal cord is indicated.
    C. Imaging studies may show spinal cord compression and obliteration of the subarachnoid space.
    D. His cluster of symptoms suggests a diagnosis of amyotrophic lateral sclerosis.
    E. A cervical spine x-ray may show calcification and radiologic changes that are similar to osteoarthritis.

22. A 29-year-old man suffers from sudden onset of diarrhea and fever. A few days following this episode, he develops diplopia and difficulty walking. On serology, his anti-G1Qb antibodies are positive. What is the classic triad of neurological symptoms seen in patients with this diagnosis?
    A. Ataxia, confusion, opthalmoplegia
    B. Ataxia, opthalmoplegia, areflexia
    C. Ataxia, confusion, areflexia
    D. Ataxia, urinary incontinence, dementia
    E. Ataxia, opthalmoplegia, urinary incontinence

23. Neuropathies associated with diabetes mellitus include all of the following EXCEPT?
    A. Polyneuropathy
    B. Mononeuropathy multiplex
    C. Syringomyelia
    D. Plexopathy
    E. Mononeuropathy simplex

24. A 39-year-old man with newly diagnosed diabetes mellitus presents with frontal baldness, bilateral ptosis, and wasting of the temporalis and facial muscles. Given this information, what is the most likely diagnosis?
    A. Myotonic dystrophy
    B. Thomsen's disease
    C. Inclusion body myositis
    D. Duchenne's dystrophy
    E. Paramyotonia congenita

25. You are asked to see an 84-year-old woman at a short-term rehabilitation facility. She had a stroke 1 month ago, which resulted in right upper and lower extremity hemiparesis and aphasia. The staff describes her as "underachieving" in her rehabilitation program and is asking for recommendations to assist in her recovery. Given the patient's age as well as functional and language disability, you suspect that she is also suffering from post-stroke depression (Mood Disorder Due to a General Medical Condition). What percentage of patients can develop depression following a stroke?
    A. 5% to 20%
    B. 30% to 50%
    C. 50% to 65%
    D. 70% to 85%
    E. 100%

26. A 30-year-old security guard is working the night-shift, patrolling a large site currently undergoing construction. He accidentally trips and falls into a deep hole, sustaining a traumatic brain injury. In the following months, he engages in a comprehensive re-habilitation program. Which of the following scales will likely be used to measure his functional recovery?

    A. Glasgow Coma Scale
    B. Glasgow Outcome Scale
    C. Global Assessment of Functioning
    D. Scale for the Assessment of Negative Symptoms
    E. Scale for the Assessment of Positive Symptoms

27. A child is brought to your office for his routine im-munizations. He is running around your office and is able to stop without falling. He is able to climb onto a chair by himself and his mother tells you that he started throwing a ball overhead. He likes to sit on a tricycle, but is unable to use the pedals. He likes look-ing at books and is able to build a six-block tower. He uses around 50 words and is able to form simple sen-tences. He likes to play near his sister but does not play with her. How old is this child?

    A. 15 months
    B. 24 months
    C. 36 months
    D. 42 months
    E. 48 months

28. Which of the following is a characteristic of the phasic component of rapid eye movement (REM) sleep?

    A. Extraocular muscle atonia
    B. Muscle twitches
    C. Theta activity on EEG
    D. Diaphragm atonia
    E. An EEG similar to stage I sleep

29. Which of the following scenarios depicts negative re-inforcement?

    A. A child is sent to his room after hitting his younger sibling; the child no longer hits his sibling.
    B. A teenager is given money by his parents for im-provement on his report card; he achieves straight A's the next two semesters.
    C. A shy college student sits in the back of the class-room and does not get called on by the professor; she begins sitting in the back of the classroom ev-ery day.
    D. A mother stops attending to her child's crying after being put to bed; over time the cries diminish.
    E. A child cleans her room and is given praise and affection from her parents; she begins cleaning her room more frequently.

30. In the following 2 × 2 table, which one of the choices represents the power of the study?

Study outcome	No true difference exists	True difference exists
Difference found	A	B
No difference found	C	D
Total	A+C	B+D

    A. A
    B. B
    C. C
    D. D
    E. A+C

31. Which one of the following is TRUE of the Rorschach test?

    A. It is a projective test.
    B. Its results are highly reliable among most clini-cians.
    C. It involves showing pictures of recognizable scenes (e.g., a family in a kitchen) and asking the patient to interpret the scenes.
    D. The way the patient responds to the colors in the scenes can be viewed as a marker of an individual's intellectual capabilities.
    E. It is a test of organic brain dysfunction.

32. A 35-year-old man experiences intermittent episodes of depersonalization over a period of 6 months. He is found to have a fasting blood sugar of 60 mg%. In the course of his workup, a CT scan of his abdomen is done, and it shows a mass on the uncinate process of the pancreas. Which of the following statements regarding this clinical situation is most likely to be TRUE?

    A. He does not have a Depersonalization Disorder, but the mass bears absolutely no relation to his depersonalization episodes.
    B. He does not have depersonalization disorder, and on complete surgical excision of the mass, his symptoms are likely to resolve completely.
    C. He has Depersonalization Disorder, and the mass is an "incidentaloma," which should be ignored.
    D. He has Dissociative Disorder NOS.
    E. He has Depersonalization Disorder, despite the fact that his depersonalization episodes may be related to the mass.

33. A 44-year-old woman was raped by a stranger at a friend's house. Although she reports having been ter-rified during the event, she felt "detached" from what was happening. Later on in the police station, she

couldn't recall many details surrounding the event. After the event, she spent most of her time at home and avoided seeing friends or family members. She had nightmares and flashbacks about the rape several times per week and was very alert if someone passed close to her when walking in the streets. Her symptoms gradually improved and by the third week after the event she was able to go back to her full work schedule and continue with most of her social activities. Although she would occasionally have nightmares about the event, they seemed to be less intense and did not provoke the same amount of fear. Given this history, what is this patient's most likely diagnosis?

A. PTSD
B. Generalized Aanxiety Disorder
C. Acute Stress Disorder
D. Adjustment Disorder
E. Bereavement

34. A 44-year-old man comes to your office complaining of insomnia and poor concentration since he was fired from his job a few weeks ago. He reports being hopeful that he will find a new job soon and has sought out the support of his family and friends through this difficult time. However, he has found it difficult to pursue some of his daily activities, such as going to the gym. He has also noticed that he feels very tired during the day, which he attributes to poor sleep. Given this history, what is this patient's most likely diagnosis?

A. Acute Stress Disorder
B. Major Depressive Disorder
C. Dysthimia
D. Cyclothymia
E. Adjustment Disorder

35. Which one of the following statements regarding the treatment algorithm for elderly patients with bipolar disorder is NOT TRUE?

A. Available evidence indicates that carbamazepine is a first-line drug for the treatment of a manic episode.
B. Elderly patients need slower titration of mood stabilizers, a more conservative dosage regimen, and closer monitoring of their medication regimens for side effects.
C. Those patients with comorbid brain disease may require even lower doses of anticonvulsants.
D. Carbamazepine causes more hematological toxicity and drug interactions than divalproex sodium.
E. Although there are no specific treatment guidelines, clinical experience indicates that an initial trial should last at least 3 to 4 weeks.

36. Which one of the following medications used for the treatment of opioid dependence is a partial opioid agonist with agonist effects at mu receptors and antagonist effects at kappa receptors?

A. Methadone
B. Clonidine
C. Naltrexone
D. Levomethadylacetate (LAAM)
E. Buprenorphine

37. Which one of the following treatments was not used in level 2 of the Sequenced Treatment Alternatives to Relieve Depression (STAR*D) trial as a switch strategy after nonremission to the Selective Serotonin Reuptake Inhibitor (SSRI) used in level 1?

A. Venlafaxine
B. Mirtazapine
C. Cognitive therapy
D. Bupropion
E. Sertraline

38. Which one of the following would be an appropriate indication for electroconvulsive therapy (ECT)?

A. Delusional depression with suicidal ideation
B. Depression of bipolar disorder with marked psychomotor retardation
C. Mania non-responsive to pharmacotherapy
D. Schizophrenia with a strong patient preference for ECT
E. All of the above

39. A 37-year-old man with a diagnosis of schizoaffective disorder develops an alteration in his level of consciousness, marked muscle rigidity, mild fever, hypertension, leukocytosis [white blood cell (WBC) count 21,000/mm^3], and elevated creatinine phosphokinase (CPK 19,700 U/mL). He is transferred to the intensive care unit for acute renal failure. A recent change in which one of the following medications is most likely responsible for this presentation?

A. Lithium
B. Citalopram
C. Fluphenazine
D. Clonazepam
E. Benztropine

40. Moderate evidence exists for tricyclic antidepressants in the treatment of all of the following conditions EXCEPT:

A. Migraine headaches
B. Cluster headaches
C. Diabetic neuropathy
D. Cocaine abuse
E. Low back pain

41. A 75-year-old married white man with a history of prostate cancer, in remission, is admitted to the medicine floor after presenting with anemia, occult blood loss, and altered bowel habits. He is diagnosed with colon cancer and scheduled to begin chemotherapy. The patient, however, is unsure about starting the treatment. The medicine team is concerned that he may lack decision-making capacity, because he has seemed depressed since learning of his diagnosis. A psychiatry consult is requested. At bedside, the patient appears hopeless, helpless, and tearful regarding his recent diagnosis. Which of the following statements regarding major depression in the medically ill is NOT TRUE?

A. Depression may influence a patient's ability to tolerate uncomfortable symptoms and maintain hope.

B. Untreated depression has been linked to poor compliance with medical care and increased pain and disability.

C. A refusal of life-saving treatment by a depressed patient often constitutes suicidal feelings and/or a lack of decision-making capacity.

D. Untreated depressed patients have a greater likelihood of considering euthanasia and physician-assisted suicide.

E. Depression may influence a patient's ability to assess a treatment's risk-benefit ratio.

42. Which one of the following statements regarding the thalamus in the brain is TRUE?

A. Thalamus is the smallest portion of the diencephalon.

B. Thalamus acts as a major synaptic relay station for information reaching the brain stem.

C. On an anatomical basis, thalamic nuclei can be divided into ten groups.

D. The medial geniculate nuclei receive afferents from inferior colliculus and project to the visual cortex.

E. Lateral geniculate nuclei receive afferents from the sensory nuclei of the trigeminal nerve and project to the somatosensory cortex.

43. Injury to which one of the following brain structures produces homonymous quadrantanopsia and hemianopsia?

A. Optic nerve
B. Optic chiasm
C. Optic tract
D. Occipital cortex
E. None of the above

44. A 14-year-old girl is seen in consultation with her parents. When she was 11 years of age, she began to walk into furniture and doorways, and trip frequently, which was initially attributed to poor attention. Shortly after this, she began having slurred speech and lower extremity weakness. Her parents then sought neurologic evaluation, and she was diagnosed with Friedreich's ataxia. She is currently followed yearly to monitor hypertrophic cardiomyopathy associated with her disorder and receives regular vision and hearing screenings. What is the likelihood that her 8-year-old brother will also be affected by this disorder?

A. Zero, this disorder is a sequelae of a viral infection.

B. 100%, this disorder is X-linked.

C. 50%, this disorder has an autosomal dominant inheritance.

D. 25%, this disorder has an autosomal recessive inheritance.

E. Zero, this disorder is always due to a sporadic mutation.

45. A 29-year-old man, previously healthy, begins having generalized tonic-clonic seizures, witnessed by others on more than one occasion. An MRI of the brain and laboratory test results are unremarkable. His initial EEG did not show any epileptiform discharges (EDs). Which of the strategies below might be tried to increase the probability of an informative EEG?

A. Sleep deprivation
B. Photic stimulation
C. Hyperventilation
D. Obtain while sleeping
E. All of the above

46. All of the following are true of the Minnesota Multiphasic Personality Inventory (MMPI) EXCEPT:

A. Although an important instrument in personality assessment, it is rarely used.

B. It is an objective test.

C. Variables such as socioeconomic, educational, and religious backgrounds are or may be important in the consideration of its results.

D. It contains validity scales.

E. Although developed in 1937, the test has been updated based on a contemporary sample.

47. The manager of the local shelter brings in an approximately 50-year-old man for increased confusion. The patient is mostly uncooperative with interview, and the manager believes that the patient abuses alcohol. When asked to hold his hands out, he is noted to have intermittent flapping of his wrists. Which of the following is NOT characteristic of the diagnosis and treatment of this disorder?

A. EEG likely would show paroxysms of bilaterally synchronous slow or triphasic waves in the delta range.

B. The concentrations of blood ammonia (NH_3) would usually be well in excess of 200 mg/dL.

C. It is always associated with overt clinical signs of liver failure (mainly jaundice and ascites).

D. The most plausible hypothesis relates to an abnormality of nitrogen metabolism.

E. Definitive treatment involves surgery and lifestyle changes.

48. A 14-year-old boy presents with ataxia, tremor, and drooling. His serum shows low ceruloplasmin and copper levels. What is the common mode of inheritance for his condition?

A. Autosomal dominant
B. Autosomal recessive
C. Mitochondrial inheritance
D. X-linked dominant
E. X-linked recessive

49. A 32-year-old woman had a week-long episode of watery diarrhea. She now complains of bilateral leg weakness, which has progressed over the last several days. She also has paresthesias and numbness of her toes and feet. There is no disturbance of bladder, bowel, or sexual function. On physical exam, she has bilateral symmetrical weakness and decreased sensation to vibration and pinprick in her lower extremities. Deep tendon reflexes (DTRs) are absent in her lower extremities. What is the most likely diagnosis for this patient's condition?

A. Multiple sclerosis
B. Poliomyelitis
C. Friedreich's ataxia
D. Peroneal nerve lesion
E. Guillain-Barré syndrome

50. A 33-year-old single white woman has a history of insomnia, fatigue, muscle pain, and mildly depressed mood. She uses a prescribed dietary supplement nightly for insomnia. Both her mother and her sister have been diagnosed with Major Depressive Disorder and take antidepressant medication. The patient's physical exam is within normal limits. Complete blood count shows elevated eosinophils, but no other abnormalities. Given this history, what is the most likely diagnosis for her condition?

A. Major depressive disorder
B. Fibromyalgia
C. Chronic Fatigue Syndrome
D. Depressive Disorder NOS
E. Eosinophilia-Myalgia Syndrome

51. Which one of the following signs is not typically seen in disorders of the basal ganglia?

A. Athetosis
B. Chorea
C. Spasticity
D. Rigidity
E. Tremors

52. A 28-year-old woman with a history of bipolar disorder, seizure disorder, and noncompliance with medications is sent to your office from a colleague for a psychopharmacological consultation. When discussing the issue of noncompliance with this patient, you realize that her inability to take her medications as prescribed is secondary to having to remember to take multiple medications scheduled throughout the day. You decide to simplify her regimen by treating both her mood disorder and seizure disorder with one medication. In considering the available options and side effect profiles of various medications, you are careful to avoid which one of the following medications considering that she is also taking oral birth control?

A. Divalproex
B. Gabapentin
C. Topiramate
D. Lamotrigine
E. Tiagabine

53. You are evaluating a child in your office. She is able to walk on a narrow line and run and skip on alternate feet. She is able to bend and touch her feet without bending the knees. She is able to copy a square and can write some letters by herself. She can construct elaborate models. She is now able to dress and undress on her own, tie her own shoelaces, and can wash her face and hands, but needs help with the rest. She likes to play with other friends and is able to follow rules. What is this child's age?

A. 24 months
B. 36 months
C. 3 1/2 years
D. 4 years
E. 5 years

54. A young healthy adult spends approximately 50% of sleep time in which one of the following sleep stages?

A. Stage I
B. Stage II
C. Stage III
D. Stage IV
E. REM

55. Which one the following statements regarding memory systems of the brain is TRUE?
    A. Implicit memory is an emotional, behavioral, and perceptual form of memory.
    B. Implicit memory is also known as declarative memory.
    C. Explicit memory is present from birth.
    D. Implicit memory requires conscious attention.
    E. Explicit memory cannot be expressed in words.

56. Which one of the following choices about standard deviation for a normal distribution is NOT TRUE?
    A. The standard deviation of a probability distribution is defined as the square of the variance.
    B. It is the most common measure of statistical dispersion.
    C. If all the data values are equal, then the standard deviation is zero.
    D. In a group of repeated measurements, it gives the precision of those measurements.
    E. About 99.7% of the values lie within 3 standard deviations of the mean.

57. Which of the following are not present in the Salpetriere Retardation Scale to measure psychomotor retardation?
    A. Slumped posture with downcast gaze
    B. Increased fatigue
    C. Decreased latency of responses
    D. Reduced concentration
    E. Indecisiveness

58. Which of the following disorders is not included as a specific dissociative disorder in the DSM-IV-TR?
    A. Dissociative Fugue
    B. Dissociative Amnesia
    C. Derealization Disorder
    D. Depersonalization Disorder
    E. Dissociative Identity Disorder

59. Which one of the following is most common in chronic anxiety states?
    A. Decreased locus ceruleus firing
    B. Increased locus ceruleus firing
    C. Increased raphe nucleus firing
    D. Decreased raphe nucleus firing
    E. Baseline firing at the locus ceruleus and raphe nucleus

60. You are asked to see a 56-year-old woman who was recently admitted to the medical ward and was diagnosed with cancer. What is the likelihood of this patient developing an adjustment disorder in the near future?

    A. Less than 5%
    B. Between 10% and 20%
    C. Between 30% and 40%
    D. Between 50% and 60%
    E. More than 70%

61. Which one of the following is the most common anxiety disorder in the elderly?
    A. Generalized anxiety disorder (GAD)
    B. Phobias
    C. Panic Disorder
    D. Obsessive Compulsive Disorder (OCD)
    E. PTSD

62. Which of the following statements regarding cholinesterase inhibitors is TRUE?
    A. There is no clear evidence that donepezil alters the course of Alzheimer's disease, and over time, the efficacy of the medication could diminish.
    B. Galantamine reversibly inhibits two enzymes that regulate acetylcholine in the brain, acetylcholinesterase and butyrylcholinesterase.
    C. Due to severe gastrointestinal (GI) side effects, donepezil may not be as well-tolerated as galantamine and rivastigmine.
    D. Tacrine has been associated with renal failure, and hence, should not be used in patients with significant renal impairment.
    E. Memantine is a new cholinesterase inhibitor which is indicated for the treatment of moderate to severe Alzheimer's disease.

63. A 48-year-old woman presents with a 30-year history of smoking a pack of cigarettes a day. She has recently developed a cough, and after years of pressure from her husband and children, she is finally ready to quit. She asks for a medication that will help her quit. She wants a pill that does not contain any nicotine, and you both agree that buproprion is the right medication for her. Which of the following statements is correct about this medication?
    A. Bupropion should not be used in combination with nicotine replacement treatment.
    B. Bupropion is more effective for smoking cessation for depressed patients.
    C. Bupropion is better tolerated in depressed patients.
    D. The mechanism of action is well understood.
    E. The patient should wait for several weeks after treatment begins to quit smoking.

64. Which one of the following is/are not a common side effect associated with ECT?
    A. Temporary confusion
    B. Head and muscle aches

C. Nausea

D. Diarrhea

E. Anterograde and retrograde amnesia

65. Which one of the following is the least typical symptom of neuroleptic malignant syndrome (NMS)?

A. Muscular rigidity

B. Autonomic instability

C. Myoclonus

D. Elevated creatinine phosphokinase

E. Leukocytosis

66. What is the relative weight gain risk of anticonvulsant drugs used in the treatment of bipolar illness?

A. Depakote and lithium > carbamazepine > oxcarbazepine, lamotrigine, levetiracetam > topiramate and zonisamide

B. Depakote and lithium > oxcarbazepine, lamotrigine, levetiracetam > carbamazepine > topiramate and zonisamide

C. Carbamazepine > depakote and lithium > oxcarbazepine, lamotrigine, levetiracetam > topiramate and zonisamide

D. Topiramate and zonisamide > depakote and lithium > oxcarbazepine, lamotrigine, levetiracetam > carbamazepine

E. Topiramate and zonisamide > oxcarbazepine, lamotrigine, levetiracetam > carbamazepine > depakote and lithium

67. What percentage of patients with schizophrenia commit suicide?

A. 5%

B. 10%

C. 15%

D. 20%

E. 25%

68. Which one of the following statements regarding the cerebral cortex is NOT TRUE?

A. Neocortex forms over 90% of the cerebral cortical area.

B. Neocortex can be further subdivided into paleocortex and archicortex.

C. Allocortex, forms roughly 10% of the cerebral cortical area.

D. Pyramidal cells constitute about 70% of all neocortical neurons.

E. Nonpyramidal cells are small and are involved only in local circuits.

69. You are asked to evaluate a patient who had a cerebrovascular accident 3 months ago. During the examination, you notice that he is selectively neglecting all stimuli given to the left side of his body. He even fails to make normal compensatory exploratory eye or limb movements on the left side. Given this important finding, you order an MRI scan of the brain. This MRI scan would show a lesion in which one of the following brain structures?

A. Dominant frontal lobe

B. Nondominant frontal lobe

C. Dominant parietal lobe

D. Nondominant parietal lobe

E. Dominant occipital lobe

70. Iatrogenic Creutzfeldt-Jakob disease (CJD) has been associated with which of the following?

A. Treatment with human growth hormone derived from cadaveric pituitary extracts

B. Dura mater grafts

C. Blood transfusions

D. Neurosurgical instruments

E. All of the above

71. An 8-year-old girl is referred from her pediatrician for a neurological evaluation. She has been having a difficult time at school and her grades are worsening. Her teachers have said that although she has not been disruptive in class, she frequently "zones out" and doesn't pay attention to instructions. Her parents have noticed the same behavior. A trial of methylphenidate was unsuccessful. While in the pediatrician's office, she was noted to have a discrete episode of "zoning out," which her parents said was "exactly what she does." On an EEG recording, which one of the following patterns would you expect to find?

A. Hypsarrhythmia

B. A normal electroencephalograph

C. Generalized slowing

D. Three-per-second spike and wave complexes simultaneously in all leads

E. Focal EDs from the left temporal lobe

72. All of the following are true of projective tests EXCEPT:

A. The interpretation of projective tests is typically not based on a conception of what counts as a correct or incorrect answer.

B. Herman Rorschach developed a projective test.

C. Such tests typically present stimuli with ambiguous meanings.

D. The MMPI is a projective test.

E. The Thematic Apperception Test is a projective test.

73. Which one of the following statements is TRUE regarding Broca's aphasia?

A. Writing to dictation is not possible.
B. In its classic form, the lesion is restricted to Brodmann's areas 44 and 45.
C. The frontoparietal operculum is never involved.
D. Speech is correct in phrasing and inflections.
E. The patient is apparently unaware of the deficit.

74. A 45-year-old woman with diabetes mellitus presents with a 4-week history of tingling and numbness in her right hand. Her thumb and index fingers are affected the most with occasional pain involving her forearm and upper arm. The symptoms are worse at night and often awaken her from sleep. On physical examination, she has a positive Phalen's maneuver. Given her history, which one of the following is the most likely cause of her symptoms?

   A. Interdigital neuropathy
   B. Ulnar nerve dysfunction
   C. Thoracic outlet syndrome
   D. Median nerve compression
   E. Radial nerve compression

75. What is the most common polyneuropathy associated with human immunodeficiency virus (HIV)-1 infection?

   A. Sensorimotor polyneuropathy
   B. Inflammatory demyelinating polyneuropathy
   C. Lumbosacral polyradiculopathy
   D. Mononeuropathy multiplex
   E. Mononeuropathy simplex

76. A patient had a normal early development, but now exhibits poor growth, generalized seizures, and recurrent acute episodes, which resemble strokes or prolonged transient ischemic attacks. The patient also suffers from episodic lactic acidosis. What is the most common mode of inheritance for this disorder?

   A. Autosomal dominant
   B. Autosomal recessive
   C. Mitochondrial
   D. X-linked recessive
   E. Polygenetic

77. Which one of the following symptoms, if present, is considered a late finding in Parkinson's disease?

   A. Dementia
   B. Resting tremor
   C. Bradykinesia
   D. Facial akinesia
   E. Gait impairment

78. A 19-year-old female college student comes to see you for an evaluation because she thinks she may be depressed. She reports having difficulty concentrating in her classes and describes periods of "spacing out" during lectures. Although you think she may be depressed, included in your differential diagnosis is absence-seizures. You send her for an EEG that reveals an excessive amount of beta activity even during periods of eye closure with relaxation. Given this history, which of the following drugs is she most likely to be using?

   A. St. John's Wart
   B. Clonazepam
   C. Amphetamine
   D. Methylphenidate
   E. Atomoxetine

79. What percentage of children are victims of being bullied during their childhood?

   A. 5%
   B. 10%
   C. 30%
   D. 50%
   E. 80%

80. Which one of the following pairs of homologous dopamine receptors functions through an increase in the production of cyclic adenosine monophosphate (cAMP)?

   A. D1 and D2
   B. D2 and D3
   C. D1 and D5
   D. D2 and D5
   E. D4 and D5

81. Each one of the following statements regarding Freud's topographic model of the mind is true EXCEPT?

   A. The model divides the mind into three regions: the conscious, the unconscious, and the preconscious.
   B. The model divides the mind into three regions: the id, the ego, and the superego.
   C. The topographic theory operates under the assumption that there exists unconscious psychological processes.
   D. The topographic theory hypothesizes that neurotic symptoms are related to unconscious conflicts.
   E. The topographic model of the mind was discussed by Freud in the 1900s in *Interpretation of Dreams*.

82. Which one of the following statements about confidence intervals (CI) is NOT TRUE?

   A. P value is less informative that CI.
   B. CI gives a measure of precision or uncertainty of the study results.
   C. CI is always calculated so that this percentage is 95%.
   D. The wider the confidence interval, the less precise we are about the unknown parameter.

E. A very wide interval may indicate that more data needs to be collected before a definite inference can be made about the parameter.

83. Which one of the following represents the principal distinguishing feature between akathisia and pseudoakathisia?

   A. Marching in one place is seen in akathisia and not seen in pseudoakathisia.
   B. Pacing is seen in akathisia and not seen in pseudoakathisia.
   C. Subjective complaint of inner agitation is seen in akathisia and not in pseudoakathisia.
   D. Fidgety movements are seen more than 50% of the time in akathisia and less than 50% of the time in pseudoakathisia.
   E. Shifting weight from one foot to the other foot is observed in akathisia and not observed in pseudoakathisia.

84. Which one of the following statements regarding Ganser syndrome is NOT TRUE?

   A. It was classified as a factitious disorder prior to DSM-III.
   B. Paralogia is a characteristic feature.
   C. Vorbeireden is a hallmark of this syndrome.
   D. "Hysterical stigmata" are found on neurological examination.
   E. Visual and auditory hallucinations are rarely observed.

85. Which one of the following has been found to be a poor prognostic factor in OCD?

   A. Female gender
   B. Male gender
   C. Comorbid psychiatric illness
   D. Age of diagnosis
   E. Initial response to SSRIs

86. Which one of the following statements is TRUE about Mood Disorder due to a General Medical Condition with depressive features?

   A. Women are affected more than men.
   B. Men and women are affected equally.
   C. Post-stroke patients rarely have depression.
   D. Men are affected more than women.
   E. Suicide risk is low among patients with terminal illness.

87. Which one of the following statements regarding the comorbidity of depression and anxiety in the elderly is TRUE?

   A. Thirty-five percent of elderly patients with depressive disorder had at least one lifetime anxiety disorder diagnosis.
   B. Twenty-three percent of elderly patients with depressive disorder had a current anxiety disorder diagnosis.
   C. The most common current comorbid anxiety disorder with depression is Generalized Anxiety Disorder (GAD).
   D. Presence of a comorbid anxiety disorder is associated with poorer social functioning and higher level of somatic symptoms.
   E. All of the above.

88. A 37-year-old woman with severe bipolar I disorder whom you have been treating with lithium comes to your office because she has recently discovered that she is pregnant. She states that she wants to remain pregnant. Which one of the following statements is NOT TRUE regarding the use of lithium in this patient?

   A. Exposure of the fetus to lithium in the first trimester of pregnancy is associated with an increased risk of Ebstein's anomaly.
   B. The first-line treatment for this patient, if she experiences a severe manic episode, would be ECT.
   C. Given that lithium is secreted in breast milk, it is recommended that patients on lithium not breast-feed.
   D. Women should never take lithium during pregnancy.
   E. Although there is an increased risk of Ebstein's anomaly in the first trimester for patients taking lithium, the risk does not justify a recommendation that patients on lithium receive a therapeutic abortion.

89. A 32-year-old man presents to the emergency room (ER) asking for a detoxification from heroin. He is admitted to the substance disorders unit of your hospital, whose policy is to perform a methadone detoxification if there are no precautions. Which of the following is not a relative contraindication for the use of methadone?

   A. Chronic obstructive pulmonary disease
   B. History of myocardial infarction
   C. Alcohol intoxication
   D. Volume depletion
   E. Acute abdominal pain

90. Which one of the following may be a particularly favorable prognostic sign for the use of ECT?

   A. Severe personality disorder
   B. Refractoriness to pharmacologic treatment
   C. Acute catatonic symptoms
   D. Nonresponse to prior ECT trials
   E. Depression due to a medical condition

91. A week after treatment with an intramuscular injection of haloperidol decanoate a 26-year-old woman with schizophrenia develops confusion, fever, elevated WBC count, muscle rigidity, and dark urine. Which of the following is the least appropriate course of action?
   A. Prescribe antibiotics for the presumed infection at the injection site.
   B. Consider a trial of dantrolene or bromocriptine.
   C. Discontinue medications.
   D. Closely monitor vital signs and renal function.
   E. Medical admission, fluids, and symptomatic treatment.

92. Which one of the following antidepressants has an FDA indication for the treatment of seasonal affective disorder (SAD)?
   A. Fluoxetine
   B. Bupropion
   C. Sertraline
   D. Venlafaxine
   E. Paroxetine

93. Which of the following is not a specific risk factor for suicide among schizophrenic patients?
   A. Female gender
   B. Less than 45 years of age
   C. Being unemployed
   D. A recent hospital discharge
   E. Feelings of hopelessness

94. Disruption to the basal ganglia pathways results in all of the following clinical signs EXCEPT:
   A. Chorea
   B. Athetosis
   C. Bradykinesia
   D. Hypotonia
   E. Tremors

95. A 75-year-old white man with a recent cerebrovascular accident (CVA) is seen in a neurology clinic for a follow-up. Examination of the visual field indicates that he has lost his vision in the left temporal and right nasal fields. A repeat MRI scan of the brain would show a lesion in which one of the following structures?
   A. Optic chiasm
   B. Right optic tract
   C. Left optic tract
   D. Right occipital lobe
   E. Left occipital lobe

96. The parents of a 6-year-old boy are awakened by him screaming. Upon entering his room, they find him getting out of his bed and still crying, but not answering any questions or responding to them. He cannot be consoled. After a few minutes, he calms down, and they are able to get him back into bed. In the morning, he does not remember the event and denies having a nightmare. He has similar episodes three to four times a month for the next year. Which of the following statements are TRUE of this condition?
   A. They are associated with REM sleep.
   B. The peak incidence is in children between the ages of 4 and 10 years.
   C. They are typically recurrent.
   D. Night terrors always persist into adulthood.
   E. There is no available treatment.

97. A 38-year-old man with a history of migraine headaches presented to the emergency department complaining of "the worst headache" he'd ever had, which was not responding to his typically effective abortive therapy, sumatriptan. Given that the headache was worse than his typical headache and not responding to previously effective therapy, the physician in the emergency department decides to order an imaging study to rule out an aneurysm. Which one of the following imaging studies would be most useful in detecting an aneurysm?
   A. Computed tomography with contrast
   B. Plain skull films
   C. Magnetic resonance angiography (MRA)
   D. Ultrasonography
   E. MRI

98. Which of the following is TRUE about the intelligence quotient (IQ)?
   A. IQ = chronological age/mental age × 100.
   B. Mental retardation per the DSM-IV-TR is an IQ < 90.
   C. Superior intelligence per the DSM-IV-TR is an IQ above 100.
   D. Borderline intelligence occurs below an IQ of 90.
   E. Approximately 1 out of every 50 people in the general population has an IQ in the mild to severe mental retardation range.

99. A 65-year-old woman who recently underwent a renal transplant and post transplant corticosteroid treatment develops proptosis, opthalmoplegia, decreased vision, and increased intraocular pressure in her right eye. She is febrile and has severe rhinorrhoea and a headache. She is a diabetic and within a few days, she develops proptosis and hemiplegia. What is the most likely cause of her symptoms?
   A. Cryptococcal infection
   B. Cerebral mucormycosis
   C. Cerebral myiasis
   D. Candidiasis
   E. Aspergillosis

100. A 38-year-old African American woman with diabetes mellitus develops weakness of her left wrist and thumb extensors and pain on the dorsum of her hand. She has a history of right lower extremity foot drop and was diagnosed several months ago with carpal tunnel syndrome. What is the most likely cause of her symptoms?

A. Mononeuropathy simplex
B. Mononeuropathy multiplex
C. Axonal polyneuropathy
D. Acute idiopathic polyneuropathy
E. Amyotrophic lateral sclerosis

101. A 6-year-old boy has a waddling gait and is unable to run. On physical examination, he has pronounced weakness in his proximal lower extremities and is incapable of rising from a supine position without using his arms to climb up his body. Which statement about the pathogenesis of this disorder is correct?

A. The genetic defect responsible for this disorder is located on the short arm of the X chromosome and codes for the protein dystrophin.
B. This disorder is dominantly inherited and is caused by an expanded trinucleotide (CTG) repeat.
C. It is inherited as a dominant trait that relates to a mutation on chromosome 7q35.
D. The etiology suggests a T-cell mediated myocytotoxicity and multifactorial genetic susceptibility.
E. It is likely related to heavy binge drinking.

102. A 35-year-old single white man frequently inhales nitrous oxide from cartridges used to make whipped cream at home in order to experience the euphoric effects of the gas. He has no other significant past medical or psychiatric history. Aside from the risk of neuropathy, what else is the patient at risk of developing?

A. Vitamin B_{12} deficiency
B. Pellagra
C. Acute intermittent porphyria
D. Solvent-induced encephalopathy
E. Wernicke-Korsakoff syndrome

103. Which of the following is a characteristic histopathologic finding on brain autopsy in patients with Parkinson's disease?

A. Beta amyloid plaques
B. Neurofibrillary tangles
C. Tau proteins
D. Lewy bodies
E. Copper deposition

104. A 30-year-old man with a history of heroin dependence who is now on methadone maintenance is admitted to the hospital following several seizures. Given that he is on methadone maintenance, which of the following anti-epileptic medications would you avoid in this patient?

A. Phenytoin
B. Divalproex
C. Ethosuximide
D. Lamotrigine
E. Topiramate

105. A 7-year-old boy is brought to your office because his mother is concerned about his health. About 2 months ago, he started developing severe stomachaches that would resolve during the weekends. He has been having nightmares about his parents dying in a car accident, and he wants to sleep in his parent's room. He is usually a good student but his family recently moved to a new neighborhood and he has been attending a new school for the past 8 weeks. He has missed several classes due to his stomachaches and his refusal to go to school. What is this child's most likely diagnosis?

A. Irritable Bowel Syndrome
B. Acute Stress Disorder
C. Generalized Anxiety Disorder
D. Separation Anxiety Disorder
E. Panic Attacks

106. Which of the following sleep patterns is most common?

A. A 65-year-old who is difficult to arouse at the beginning of the sleep period
B. A 15-year-old who spends 16 to 18 hours per day asleep
C. A 35-year-old with sleep-wake cycles of 3 or 4 hours
D. Prolonged latency to sleep onset in a 70-year-old
E. A 5-month-old with increased sleep arousals

107. Each one of the following is a mature defense mechanism EXCEPT:

A. Humor
B. Suppression
C. Sublimation
D. Altruism
E. Rationalization

108. A biotechnology company has developed a new ELISA test to diagnose HIV infections. Serum from 1,000 patients, which was positive by Western Blot (the gold standard assay), was tested with this new test and 999 of them were found to be positive. The manufacturer then used this new test to check the serum of 1,000 nuns who denied any risk factor for HIV infection. Nine hundred and ninety-nine of these samples were negative with one positive result compared to all negative by the Western Blot. Given this information, what is the sensitivity of this new ELISA test?

A. 99.9%
B. 9.99%
C. 10.0%
D. 1.0%
E. 90.0%

109. Which one of the following is a self-administered rating scale in psychiatry?

A. Montgomery Asberg Depression Rating Scale (MADRS)
B. Hamilton Rating Scale for Depression (HAM-D)
C. Hamilton Rating Scale for Anxiety
D. Beck Depression Inventory (BDI)
E. Clinical Global Impression of Change (CGI)

110. Which one of the following choices is NOT an autohypnotic symptom of Dissociative Identity Disorder?

A. Trance logic
B. Spontaneous age regression
C. Made feelings from alter identity
D. Negative hallucinations
E. Deep enthrallment

111. A 10-year-old boy was brought in to his pediatrician's office after the sudden development of what his parents described as "strange behavior." He was noticed to be extremely worried about washing his hands and would spend an excessive amount of time washing them every morning. During the day he would avoid touching any surface that he thought could be "contaminated" and refused to play during school break because of being afraid of "getting germs on himself." He was also noticed to be blinking frequently and has been markedly hyperactive. The mother recalls that he was complaining of a sore throat a few days before the appearance of the symptoms. What would be the most expected course of illness in this patient?

A. Early complete remission
B. Gradual worsening of symptoms
C. Chronic stable course
D. Chronic course with periods of exacerbation
E. Fatal outcome

112. A 45-year-old woman presents to a psychiatric clinic with symptoms of depressed mood, passive suicidal thoughts, fatigue, and cold intolerance for the past 2 months. She is also complaining of weight gain and having a very dry skin. She has no family or personal history of a psychiatric illness. What should be the next step in the management of this patient's symptoms?

A. Inpatient psychiatric hospitalization
B. Start the patient on an SSRI
C. Check the patient's labs, including thyroid stimulating hormone
D. Refer her for outpatient psychotherapy
E. Refer for ECT

113. Which one of the following symptoms indicates a delirium rather than dementia?

A. Insidious onset
B. Progressive course
C. Impaired attention
D. Clear consciousness
E. Persistent deficits

114. A 17-year-old girl who has been diagnosed with bipolar disorder and has been treated with lithium develops psoriasis. Which of the following is TRUE regarding the relationship between psoriasis and lithium?

A. Psoriasis is not a side effect of lithium treatment.
B. Psoriasis can be a side effect of lithium and, when it is a side effect, it will most likely improve with treatment with ultraviolet light and coal tar.
C. Psoriasis can be a side effect of lithium, and it often improves if the lithium is stopped.
D. Pre-existing psoriasis is an absolute contraindication to lithium use.
E. Patients who have psoriasis before taking lithium are unlikely to experience a worsening of their condition.

115. You are relieving a colleague from call at the psychiatric ER. It was a slow night, and when you arrive, he is deeply involved in a debate with the medical ER attending on the relative merits of lorazepam versus diazepam for alcohol withdrawal. Your colleague immediately asks you for your opinion. Which of the following would NOT be a true statement about this issue?

A. When you use lorazepam, you have to worry about active metabolites.
B. You definitely want to use lorazepam if the person has significant hepatic impairment.
C. When you use lorazepam, you will probably have to dose more often.
D. Diazepam is more likely to have less fluctuation in plasma concentration.
E. When you use lorazepam, you will have finer control of symptoms.

116. Which of the following is/are potential major medical complications of ECT?

A. Transient neurological deficits
B. Arrhythmia or other cardiovascular event

C. Prolonged seizure or status epilepticus
D. Prolonged apnea
E. All of the above are potential complications

117. Each one of the following medications has a primary mechanism of action that involves affecting dopamine potentiation or dopamine metabolism except:

A. Cocaine
B. Methylphenidate
C. Modafinil
D. Bupropion
E. Dextroamphetamine

118. Which one of the following is NOT TRUE of methadone?

A. Methadone can block N-methyl-D-aspartate (NMDA) receptors and monoaminergic reuptake transporters.
B. Methadone has weaker analgesia than morphine in equivalent daily doses.
C. When using methadone as an analgesic agent, it should be administered at intervals of no more than 8 hours.
D. Tolerance and physical dependence usually develop more slowly with methadone than with morphine.
E. Withdrawal signs and symptoms occurring after the abrupt discontinuance of methadone are milder, but more prolonged than those of morphine.

119. Which of the following suggests the greatest risk for completed suicide?

A. Older age, significantly socially isolated, and diagnosis of alcohol abuse
B. Diagnosis of alcohol abuse and borderline personality disorder
C. Married woman with two children and prior serious suicide attempt
D. Diagnosis of pancreatic cancer in a homeless man
E. Adolescent diagnosed with bipolar disorder

120. Which one of the following structures is not thought to be part of the limbic system?

A. Cingulate gyrus
B. Hippocampus
C. Parahippocampal gyrus
D. Anterior thalamus
E. Internal capsule

121. Injury to the sympathetic innervation of eye muscles results in which of the following?

A. Ptosis
B. Miosis

C. Anhydrosis
D. All of the above
E. None of the above

122. A 52-year-old man was referred for neurologic evaluation after new onset of seizures. Reviewing his history, he reported an insidious onset of memory loss, and a month-long history of daily headache associated with nausea, which he had assumed was a worsening of his migraines. The first seizure occurred 1 week ago and was observed to have started with jerking movements of his left hand, before becoming a generalized tonic-clonic seizure. Gadolinium enhanced MRI showed a contrast-enhancing lesion in the right frontal lobe with an area of central necrosis, suggestive of a glioblastoma. Stereotactic biopsy confirmed the diagnosis. Which one of the following statements about gliomas is NOT TRUE?

A. Approximately 18,000 cases of new primary malignant brain and central nervous system (CNS) tumors occur each year in the United States.
B. Two-year survival for patients with glioblastoma is very low.
C. Gliomas are more common in women than men.
D. Exposure to high-dose or therapeutic radiation has been associated with an increased risk of developing a glioma.
E. Some genetic syndromes are associated with a higher incidence of gliomas.

123. Firemen and emergency medicine technicians (EMTs) responded to a 911 call placed by a neighbor, reporting smoke seeping under the door of an apartment across the hall. When they arrived on the scene, they found a pan on the stove, with burning food in the bottom, and an elderly man lying prone in the living room, unconscious. He was found to be hypertensive with a blood pressure of 180/110 mm HG, but all other vital signs were normal. His blood glucose was 64 mg% and he was responsive to painful stimulation. In his medicine cabinet, they found metoprolol, metformin, atorvastatin, Coumadin, and acetaminophen with codeine. The EMTs stabilized his cervical spine for transport, and he was brought to the emergency department. After reassessment of his airway, breathing, and circulation, what imaging study would be most helpful to rule out intracranial pathology?

A. Noncontrast CT scan
B. MRI scan
C. Plain skull films
D. Magnetic Resonance Angiography (MRA)
E. No imaging studies are needed

124. Which of the following disparities on the Weschler Adult Intelligence Scale is associated with Attention-Deficit/Hyperactivity Disorder (ADHD)?

    A. A disparity between the personality IQ and the full-scale IQ
    B. A disparity between the verbal IQ and the full-scale IQ
    C. A disparity between the full-scale IQ and the performance IQ
    D. A disparity between the verbal IQ and the performance IQ
    E. A disparity between the personality IQ and the performance IQ

125. In December of 1995, the 43-year-old editor-in-chief of Elle France magazine, Jean-Dominique Bauby, suffered from a stroke and lapsed into a coma. He awoke a few weeks later, only to find that he had lost control over all motor activity with the exception of some movement of his left eye. Apart from being able to blink his left eyelid, he could not move at all. Owing to his resilient spirit and positive outlook on life, he wrote a memoir of his condition. He painstakingly communicated what he wanted to write by blinking his left eyelid in response to the frequency-ordered alphabet recited by an amanuensis. What is the most likely area of the brain that was affected in his condition?

    A. Lateral medulla
    B. Medial medulla
    C. Ventral pons
    D. Tegmental pons
    E. Central pons

126. A patient presents with weakness in his quadriceps muscle. He also has decreased sensation over the medial part of his leg below the knee. His knee jerk is also noted to be decreased on physical examination. Involvement of which nerve root is most likely the cause of these symptoms?

    A. C7
    B. C8
    C. L4
    D. L5
    E. S1

127. Which of the following statements about polymyositis is NOT TRUE?

    A. Polymyositis is characterized by destruction of muscle fibers and inflammatory infiltration of muscles.
    B. It leads to weakness and wasting, especially of the proximal limb and girdle muscles.
    C. Raynaud's phenomenon, arthralgia, and malaise are associated with polymyositis.
    D. Polymyositis has been reported in association with autoimmune disorders, including lupus erythematosus and rheumatoid arthritis.
    E. There is a definite correlation between adult-onset polymyositis and cancer.

128. A 76-year-old man is brought to your outpatient clinic by his daughter, because she is concerned that her father might be depressed. She states that her father is uninterested in his usual hobbies and indifferent to his grandchildren. She describes a gradual decline in his ability to manage his finances and frequently getting lost while driving around their neighborhood. Physical examination reveals hyperrelexia and weakness in both upper and lower right extremities and dysarthria. After completing your workup and evaluation, which of the following provides the most reliable evidence to support the diagnosis of vascular dementia versus Alzheimer's disease?

    A. Focal physical findings
    B. Apathy
    C. Memory loss
    D. Atrophy of the brain seen on an MRI
    E. Stepwise deterioration of symptoms

129. A 70-year-old man is brought to your clinic by his wife. She states that over the past 6 months her husband has looked depressed but has always insisted that he was in a good mood. He continues to be able to handle their finances, but she no longer allows him to write checks because his handwriting is now illegible. In addition, he often falls and when he calls her for help, she cannot always hear him. The patient denies feeling depressed, but does agree with the rest of what his wife has said. Given this history, which is the most likely diagnosis for his condition?

    A. Major Depressive Disorder
    B. Diffuse Lewy Body Disease
    C. Normal Pressure Hydrocephalus
    D. Alzheimer's disease
    E. Parkinson's disease

130. Most antiepileptic medications (AED) are dosed to a therapeutic response and monitored by blood draws to assure that the drug levels are not in a toxic range. Based on the clinical history and physical examination, you can often determine if the dose of an antiepileptic drug is in the toxic range. Signs and symptoms of antiepileptic medication toxicity include all of the following EXCEPT:

    A. Lethargy
    B. Nystagmus
    C. Dysarthria
    D. Tremor
    E. Hemiparesis

131. Which of the following factors make it more stressful for a first-born child to adjust to having a new sibling?

A. Being less than 24 months of age
B. Being more than 24 months of age
C. New sibling's gender
D. Firstborn's gender
E. Parental age

132. Which of the following is an effect of total sleep deprivation?

A. Cognitive impairment
B. Decreased peripheral metabolic rate
C. Decreased cortisol levels
D. Increased glucose tolerance
E. Increased brain metabolic rate

133. A biotechnology company has developed a new ELISA test to diagnose HIV infections. Serum from 1,000 patients which was positive by Western Blot (the gold standard assay) was tested with this new test and 999 were found to be positive. The manufacturer then used this new test to check the serum of 1,000 nuns who denied any risk factor for HIV infection. Nine hundred and ninety-nine of these samples were negative with one positive result compared to all negative by the Western Blot. Given this information, what is the specificity of this new ELISA test?

A. 99.9%
B. 9.99%
C. 10.0%
D. 1.0%
E. 90.0%

134. Which one of the following findings can be consistently seen on a Positron emission tomography (PET) or Single photon emission computed tomography (SPECT) scan of a patient with "pure" OCD with no other comorbidities in a resting state when compared to controls?

A. Reduced metabolism or regional blood flow to the head of caudate nucleus
B. Reduced metabolism or regional blood flow to the orbitofrontal cortex
C. Reduced metabolism or regional blood flow to the thalamus
D. Reduced metabolism or regional blood flow to the anterior cingulate
E. None of the above

135. A 45-year-old man never delegates work to any of his subordinates, because he does not believe they can do the work the way it needs to be done. He spends an excessive amount of time trying to complete each task, because he believes that "everything should be done perfectly or not attempted at all." His favorite catchphrase is "God is in the details." Which of the following statements is TRUE regarding his personality disorder?

A. It is a Cluster A Personality Disorder.
B. It is a Cluster B Personality Disorder.
C. It is a Cluster C Personality Disorder.
D. It is now considered a variant of OCD.
E. This condition was included for the first time in DSM-IV.

136. Which of the following statements regarding the demographics of psychiatric disorders is FALSE?

A. The number of older adults with psychiatric disorder is estimated to be 7 million.
B. By the year 2030, the number of older adults with psychiatric illness would double.
C. The National Institute of Mental Health (NIMH) Epidemiological and Catchment Area (ECA) survey data suggest that the prevalence of bipolar disorder decreases with age.
D. There are reports suggesting that up to 1% of older adults may have bipolar disorder.
E. None of the above.

137. A 50-year-old man with a history significant only for Huntington's disease is admitted to the hospital for anorexia. He states his family is trying to poison him. Therefore, he refuses to eat. He is awake and scores 30/30 on the Folstein Mini-Mental State Examination (MMSE). His family denies a family history of mental illness, and his medical workup, including a urine drug screen, is negative. He has had no changes in his medications in the recent past. Given his history and presentation, what is his most likely diagnosis for his presentation?

A. Psychotic disorder due to Huntington's disease
B. Schizophrenia
C. Substance-Induced Psychosis
D. Delirium-related psychosis
E. Paranoid Personality Disorder

138. Which one of the following statements regarding the Confusion Assessment Method (CAM) developed by Inouye et al. is NOT TRUE?

A. It is the most commonly used tool to detect delirium.
B. It measures 3 main symptoms to detect the presence of delirium.
C. It has a positive predictive value of 91% to 94%.
D. It has a sensitivity of 94% to 100%.
E. It has a specificity of 90% to 95%.

139. An 18-year-old man diagnosed with schizophrenia two years ago is referred to you, because his previous psychiatrist has moved away. When you meet him, you notice that he smacks his lips and that, on occasion, he seems to be pushing his tongue against his cheeks. After an unsuccessful trial with several atypical antipsychotics and clozapine, his previous psychiatrist started him on haloperidol a year ago with good effect. The patient has not noticed the lip smacking and tongue movements, but his parents do mention that they have noticed them within the last month. In informing the patient about this condition, it is reasonable to tell him which one of the following statements?

A. His age makes him particularly vulnerable to this condition.
B. This condition can be effectively treated with an anticholinergic drug, such as benztropine.
C. This condition can be effectively treated with propanolol.
D. His lip smacking and pushing his tongue against his cheek are often the earlier signs to occur in his condition.
E. Given that this is a first generation antipsychotic and has caused this condition, it is clear that the patient should switch to another medication.

140. During treatment with ECT, which one of the following medications will not lower the seizure threshold or prolong seizures?

A. Clozapine
B. Fluoxetine
C. Theophylline
D. Bupropion
E. Phenobarbital

141. A 34-year-old woman has a history of recurrent episodes of moderate depression for each of the last three autumns with worsening of symptoms in the winter. She has not responded to adequate trials of fluoxetine and sertraline and has multiple questions about side effects. A trial of which one of the following treatment modalities would be most appropriate at the present time?

A. Paroxetine
B. Dawn phototherapy at 10,000 lux for 30 minutes daily
C. Clonazepam
D. Quetiapine
E. ECT

142. An 11-year-old boy is being treated for behavioral difficulties at school and at home. He has been skipping class and often comes home smelling of cigarette smoke. A drug screen is negative for nonprescribed substances of abuse. His parents report he has developed sudden facial twitches and makes more frequent repetitive guttural sounds, especially since

starting a new medication. Which of the following is the most likely cause of his facial twitches and guttural sounds?

A. Guanfacine
B. Nicotine
C. Bupropion
D. Venlafaxine
E. Dextroamphetamine

143. Which of the following has not been responsible for the improved safety of ECT?

A. Improved anesthetic agents
B. Adoption of brief pulse stimulus machine
C. Introduction of electroencephalographic and cardiopulmonary monitoring devices
D. Healthier patient population
E. All of the above

144. During a neurological examination, you ask the patient to wave goodbye to an imaginary friend. The patient is unable to perform this simple task despite having clearly understood your request. This inability to convert an idea into action is due to a lesion in which one of the following brain structures?

A. Left frontal lobe
B. Right frontal lobe
C. Left temporal lobe
D. Right temporal lobe
E. Right parietal lobe

145. Which one of the following statements regarding senile neuritic plaques in the brain of patients with Alzheimer's disease is NOT TRUE?

A. These plaques are spherical microscopic lesions with a core of extracellular $A\beta$ surrounded by enlarged axonal endings or neurites.
B. The $A\beta$ peptide is derived from the amyloid precursor protein (APP), a transmembrane protein present in most tissues.
C. APP is cleaved by a group of protease enzymes called secreatases α, β, and γ.
D. When cleaved by β secretase, a soluble peptide derivative of amyloid is formed.
E. These plaques are less well correlated with Alzheimer's disease than neurofibrillary tangles (NFT).

146. Which one of the following is the TRUE principle behind the functioning of an MRI machine?

A. Injection of radioactive glucose (^{18}F-deoxyglucose) and study of differential utilization of glucose in diseased areas of the brain versus normal brain structures
B. Study of the changes in cerebral oxygenation in different parts of the brain by examining

signal intensity changes in the obtained digital image

C. Detection of echo signals from sound waves transmitted into the brain

D. Infusion of contrast media into the vascular structures of the brain to look for filling defects or aneurysm

E. A change in hydrogen protons spin position in relation to a radiofrequency pulse applied externally

147. A 20-year-old college student presents to the ER complaining of severe headache, nausea, and vomiting. Physical examination is notable for fever and nuchal rigidity. A lumbar puncture (LP) is performed. Which of the following CSF findings would support a diagnosis of bacterial meningitis?

A. Clear fluid, 0 WBC/mm, protein 30 mg/100 mL, glucose 80 mg/100 mL

B. Turbid fluid, 350 WBC/mm (mostly polymorphonuclear cells), protein 100 mg/100 mL, glucose 20 mg/100 mL

C. Clear fluid, 5 WBC/mm, protein 200 mg/100 mL, glucose 80 mg/mL

D. Turbid fluid, 100 WBC/mm (mostly lymphocytes), protein 100 mg/100 mL, glucose 40 mg/100 mL

E. Bloody fluid, 45 WBC/mm, protein 100 mg/100 mL

148. A 39-year-old man presents to an ER after a generalized seizure. The patient had no prior history of seizures and upon imaging, a hypodense mass in the temporal lobe with relatively well-defined borders is seen. Pathology shows a small round nucleus and a halo of unstained cytoplasm ("fried egg" appearance). Which of the following statements is TRUE about the treatment for this disorder?

A. Surgical excision and radiation is the first-line treatment in all cases.

B. Genetic testing can be used to predict chemoresponsivity.

C. Intravenous methotrexate is generally effective.

D. Palliative care with corticosteroids is the only option.

E. These tumors are too infrequent to make clinical recommendations.

149. Erik Erikson was one of the major advocates of adult developmental theory. According to his work, the specific phase during which contacts with others are made, intimate relationships develop, and when commitment to another person occurs is characterized by which of the following conflicts?

A. Initiative versus guilt

B. Industry versus inferiority

C. Identity versus role confusion

D. Intimacy versus isolation

E. Generativity versus stagnation

150. Which of the following statements about the function and anatomy of the hypothalamus is FALSE?

A. A lesion to it can lead to anorexia or hyperphagia.

B. A lesion to it can cause dysregulation of the thyroid and adrenal glands.

C. A lesion to it can cause aversion to water and adipsia.

D. A lesion to it can cause loss of day-night cycle.

E. A lesion to it can cause dysfunctional expression of emotion.

151. Structural MRI of the brain in patients with schizophrenia shows which one of the following findings?

A. Reduction in the volume of prefrontal cortex

B. Increase in the volume of prefrontal cortex

C. Reduction in the volume of parietal cortex

D. Increase in the volume of the parietal cortex

E. None of the above

152. According to the DSM-IV-TR, which one of the following symptoms is NOT representative of the "persistent avoidance of stimuli associated with the trauma and numbing of general responsiveness (not present before the trauma)"?

A. Restricted range of affect

B. Sense of a foreshortened future

C. Feeling of estrangement from others

D. Hypervigilance

E. Inability to recall an important aspect of the trauma

153. A 19-year-old woman of African descent presents with symptoms of depression during her third trimester of pregnancy. Upon evaluation, you are told that she may have been sexually molested as a child. Additionally, her mother and grandmother have history of bipolar disorder. Which one of the following is TRUE of this patient's condition?

A. Thirty percent of women may evidence depressive symptoms during pregnancy and 4% meet criteria for Major Depressive Disorder.

B. Studies suggest that supportive therapy may be more efficacious than group therapy [educational, transactional, and Cognitive Behavioral Therapy (CBT)] as an alternative to pharmacology.

C. Animal and human studies show that although prenatal stress may affect growth, it has no effect on cognitive function of offspring.

D. Given this patient's family history, a mood stabilizer may be a more appropriate therapeutic option at this time.

E. None of the above.

154. A 20-year-old woman with no prior psychiatric history presents with sweating, headache, difficulty breathing, and an overwhelming feeling that she is going to die. She also reports that other members in her family also suffer from a similar problem. A 24-hour urine specimen indicates that she has elevated urine catecholamines. What is the most likely diagnosis for this patient?
   A. Panic Attack
   B. PTSD
   C. GAD
   D. Anxiety disorder due to pheochromocytoma, with Panic Attacks
   E. Alcohol Withdrawal

155. Which of the following statements regarding behavioral disturbances in dementia is TRUE?
   A. They are seen in about 40% to 65% of elderly demented patients living in the community.
   B. They are seen in about 45% to 90% of elderly demented patients living in nursing homes.
   C. These behaviors are often chronic with different symptoms emerging as the illness progresses.
   D. They also fluctuate with psychomotor agitation being the most persistent.
   E. All of the above.

156. Which one of the statements regarding object-relations oriented couples' therapy is NOT TRUE?
   A. A common initial resistance exists where both partners expect the therapist to "fix" their spouse.
   B. Each partner is encouraged to appreciate their own internal conflicts being played out within the couple rather than "marital conflicts."
   C. Resistance to change arises in the couple as the therapist tries to alter the "unconscious contract," which binds their system of behavior.
   D. To overcome the couple's resistance, the therapist must exert increasing effort toward facilitating positive change.
   E. The therapist may make progress by openly identifying the couple's "unconscious contract," which is impeding change.

157. During treatment with ECT, which one of the following medications is least likely to significantly shorten seizure duration or interfere with seizure expression?
   A. Pentobarbital
   B. Diazepam
   C. Nortriptyline
   D. Phenytoin
   E. Valproic acid

158. Which one of the following describes the use of biofeedback principles in the treatment of primary insomnia?
   A. The patient learns to progressively relax different muscles to control sleep initiation.
   B. The patient gives feedback on sensations of various organ systems as he or she falls asleep.
   C. The patient learns to make environmental changes that affect his or her sleep patterns.
   D. The patient learns to affect physiologic parameters with the help of electronic equipment.
   E. The patient learns to self-induce a meditative trance to induce sleep.

159. An 8-year-old boy who is in treatment for difficult to control ADHD develops severe nausea, light colored stools, and upon laboratory testing has a transaminitis. Which of the following do you suspect may be responsible for his transminitis?
   A. Methylphenidate
   B. Bupropion
   C. Magnesium pemoline
   D. Clonidine
   E. Desipramine

160. Which one of the following statements is NOT TRUE regarding response to ECT?
   A. Increasing age is a negative predictor of response.
   B. The presence of psychotic features in a major depressive episode is a positive predictor of response.
   C. The presence of catatonic symptoms in a major depressive episode may be a positive predictor of response.
   D. Patients with longer episodes of depression are less likely to show a response than those with shorter episodes.
   E. The presence of a personality disorder is a positive predictive factor of response.

161. During an MMSE, you ask a 75-year-old man to take a piece of paper from the table with his left hand, fold it into half, and place it back on the table. He says that he understood your instruction, but is unable to proceed beyond taking the piece of paper with his left hand. This inability to perform a sequence of steps that requires a plan and continued monitoring is due to the lesion in which one of the following brain structures?
   A. Frontal lobes
   B. Parietal lobes
   C. Temporal lobes
   D. Occipital lobes
   E. Basal ganglia

162. Which one of the following statements regarding NFT is NOT TRUE?

   A. They are intracytoplasmic structures found inside the neurons.
   B. They are better visualized using silver impregnation techniques like Bielschowsky or the Bodian stain.
   C. In patients with Alzheimer's disease, NFTs are commonly found in the neurons of the hippocampus and amygdala.
   D. They are mainly composed of abnormally-phosphorylated tau protein.
   E. They are unique to Alzheimer's disease.

163. A 67-year-old man presents to the neurology clinic with a left-sided tremor, three falls in the past month, and a feeling of being slowed down. Upon examination, you note bradykinesia, a left-sided tremor at rest, and a slow shuffling gait. The patient asked about newer advances in pharmacological treatment for his condition. Which of the following statements about the nonergot dopamine agonists are TRUE for the treatment of this patient's condition?

   A. They are generally accepted as first-line treatment.
   B. They can be easily started at the full dose.
   C. These medications are clearly neuroprotective.
   D. They should not be used in combination with L-dopa.
   E. They are never associated with dyskinetic movements.

164. In Mary Ainsworth's description of strange situation, when children are exposed to brief separations from their mother, they react in all of the following ways EXCEPT:

   A. Securely attached
   B. Anxious-avoidantly attached
   C. Anxious-ambivalently attached
   D. Anxious-dependently attached
   E. Disorganized/disoriented

165. Lithium toxicity can lead to which one of the following EEG abnormalities?

   A. Triphasic waves
   B. Diffuse slowing
   C. Spikes with sharp waves
   D. Spikes with burst suppression
   E. Frontal intermittent rhythmic delta activity (FIRDA)

166. Which one of the following findings is most consistently seen on structural neuroimaging studies of patients with mood disorder?

   A. Smaller third ventricle
   B. Larger cerebellum
   C. Smaller thalamus
   D. Increase in white matter and periventricular hyperintensities
   E. Smaller hippocampus

167. A young man comes to your office because he just started college and has had a difficult time making friends. He feels very embarrassed when he meets new people and experiences increased sweating, tachycardia, trembling, and stuttering. His fear that others will notice his anxiety has made him avoid most social activities around campus. Which of the following factors would predict a better chance of recovery for this patient?

   A. Number of feared situations
   B. Age at onset
   C. Severity of symptoms
   D. Absence of an affective disorder
   E. Age at first encounter with psychiatrist

168. Which one of the following statements is TRUE regarding the use of antidepressant therapy during pregnancy?

   A. The rate of major malformations in the general population is lower than that associated with antidepressant therapy.
   B. The rate of major malformations is so high that pharmacologic intervention is not recommended.
   C. Studies indicate that malformation rate associated with antidepressant therapy is no greater than that associated with the general population.
   D. All of the above.
   E. None of the above.

169. Which of the following may indicate sexual dysfunction due to a general medical condition?

   A. Diminished interest in sex with age
   B. Elevated fasting blood glucose
   C. Depressed mood
   D. Avoidant personality disorder
   E. Treatment with an SSRI

170. Which one of the following statements regarding the use of EEG in the diagnosis of cognitive impairment in the elderly is TRUE?

   A. It has limited utility in the diagnosis of dementia.
   B. In delirium, it shows a triphasic periodic burst pattern.
   C. In Creutzfeldt-Jakob Disease (CJD), it shows generalized slow wave activity.
   D. In hepatic encephalopathy, it shows a triphasic wave pattern.
   E. None of the above.

171. Which of the following treatments for OCD does not have data from controlled studies?
    A. Intravenous clomipramine
    B. Cognitive-Behavioral Group Therapy (CBGT)
    C. Venlafaxine
    D. ECT
    E. Inositol

172. Which one of the following comorbid medical conditions is a contraindication to treatment with ECT?
    A. Coronary artery disease
    B. Space occupying brain tumor
    C. Pregnancy
    D. History of strokes
    E. None of the above

173. Which one of the following statements best distinguishes the characteristics of IPT and cognitive behavioral therapy (CBT) in treatment of depression?
    A. IPT focuses almost exclusively on the therapist-patient relationship, whereas CBT pays little attention to this relationship.
    B. IPT is not manualized, but CBT is manualized.
    C. IPT approaches depression from the medical model, and CBT involves homework.
    D. IPT does not involve psychoeducation, although CBT does.
    E. IPT focuses only on the patient's feelings and relationships, whereas CBT focuses only on the patient's thoughts and beliefs.

174. Patients presenting with alcohol withdrawal who have a history of alcohol withdrawal seizures, delirium tremens, complicated withdrawals, or serious medical conditions are best managed with which one of the following regimens?
    A. Symptom-triggered medication regimens
    B. Structured, or fixed-schedule, medication regimens
    C. Either symptom-triggered or fixed-schedule treatment regimens
    D. Outpatient detoxification
    E. Ethanol administration

175. In the administration of ECT, electrode placement has been found to be an important determinant in the therapeutic outcome and adverse effects. Which of the following is TRUE of the location of the electrode during administration of ECT?
    A. The stimulus should be substantially above convulsive threshold to ensure efficacy with right unilateral electrode placement.
    B. The stimulus should not be excessively above the convulsive threshold to avoid undue memory loss when bilateral placement is deployed.

    C. Studies have shown that the convulsive threshold has significant variability in large patient samples.
    D. All of the above.
    E. None of the above.

176. A 70-year-old woman is being evaluated in a neurology clinic, 1 month after a CVA. This examination reveals that she is unable to read, write, or calculate. Further testing indicates that she cannot identify fingers correctly and is confused about the left and right side of her body. An MRI of the brain with and without contrast will show a lesion in which one of the following brain areas?
    A. Dominant frontal lobe
    B. Nondominant frontal lobe
    C. Dominant parietal lobe
    D. Nondominant parietal lobe
    E. Dominant occipital lobe

177. Which one of the following statements regarding alpha-synuclein is NOT TRUE?
    A. Alfa-synuclein is an abnormal protein found in the brain.
    B. It is predominantly a presynaptic neuronal protein, but can also be found in glial cells.
    C. It can aggregate to form insoluble fibrils in pathological conditions characterized by Lewy bodies.
    D. Alpha-synuclein fragments are also found in amyloid plaques in Alzheimer's disease.
    E. Antibodies against alpha-synuclein have replaced antibodies against ubiquitin as the gold standard for immunostaining of Lewy bodies.

178. Which one of the following is TRUE about the serum levels of anticonvulsants?
    A. The ideal serum level is drawn just before bedtime ("trough levels").
    B. Higher serum levels are needed for the treatment of partial seizures than for tonic-clonic seizures.
    C. It is extremely dangerous to medicate a patient outside the therapeutic range.
    D. Malnourished or chronically ill patients generally need higher serum levels.
    E. It is important to track the serum levels of levetiracetam and topiramate.

179. A 45-year-old woman comes to your office because she has been having problems at work. She has a hard time focusing on her job because she is constantly thinking about having to pay the bills on time, making sure she put enough food in her children's lunch boxes, and wondering if there is anything she forgot to do at home before leaving for work. During her free time at home, she worries about what her boss thinks about her productivity and finds it hard

to go to sleep due to concerns about not waking up on time. According to the DSM-IV-TR, which of the following is considered an associated symptom to make a diagnosis of GAD?

A. Sleep disturbances
B. Headaches
C. Weight loss
D. Low self-esteem
E. Problems with peers

180. A 25-year-old woman, two-weeks postpartum, is referred to the acute psychiatric service of an inner city hospital for an evaluation. The history obtained indicates that she only slept 3 hours in 4 days, and she says everything is "glorious" and proclaims herself "Queen of Norway." Her speech is also rapid and pressured. Given this information, which one of the following statements regarding this presentation is TRUE?

A. This patient's risk for infanticidal behavior is no more or less than the general population.
B. A family history of bipolar disorder, onset of psychosis soon after childbirth, and a childhood history of sexual abuse may be risk factors for postpartum mood disorder.
C. Contacting the child protection service department is probably not warranted and carries a risk of being sued as no harm has been done.
D. Breast feeding is probably not an important factor to consider in planning therapy, because unlike antidepressants, mood stabilizers are not secreted in breast milk.
E. Breast feeding history is not relevant at this point as she is too ill and the risks posed by secretion of mood stabilizers in breast milk is probably worth the expected benefits.

181. Elderly patients with depression commonly present with each of the following symptoms EXCEPT:

A. Irritability/anxiety
B. Apathy
C. Weight loss
D. Feelings of guilt
E. Homicidal ideation

182. Which one of the following statements regarding inappropriate sexual behaviors in the demented elderly is NOT TRUE?

A. There are very few studies looking at the prevalence rates for these behaviors.
B. The best estimate is that 7% to 25% of demented patients exhibit these behaviors.
C. The elderly are thought to be involved in 5.5% of all reported sex crimes.

D. These behaviors are more common in females than in males.
E. There are four main kinds of inappropriate sexual behaviors seen in elderly demented patients.

183. Which one of the following neonatal outcomes has been associated with use of SSRIs in the treatment of maternal depression during pregnancy?

A. Intussusception
B. Respiratory distress
C. Meconium aspiration syndrome
D. Preterm delivery
E. Bowel obstruction

184. Which one of the following is not a concern for the concurrent use of lithium and ECT?

A. Worsening mood disorder
B. Increased risk of cognitive deficits
C. Encephalopathy or delirium
D. Prolongation of succinylcholine's neuromuscular blockade
E. Spontaneous and prolonged seizures

185. Who is generally credited with developing structured IPT?

A. Victor Frankl
B. Gerald Klerman
C. Aaron T. Beck
D. B.F. Skinner
E. Marsha Linehan

186. Of the anticonvulsants, valproic acid is the most commonly used agent in the prophylaxis of migraine headaches. Valproic acid has been shown to be effective in the prophylactic treatment of migraines in:

A. Up to one third of the patients
B. Between one third and one half of the patients
C. About one half of the patients
D. Between one half and two thirds of the patients
E. Over two thirds of the patients

187. Which one of the following statements is NOT TRUE?

A. The negative image regarding cognitive deficit associated with ECT may be an important factor determining availability in certain areas.
B. Electrode placement, frequency of sessions, and the intensity of electrical stimuli are determinants of severity of cognitive sequelae.
C. Memory loss associated with ECT is usually retrograde.
D. Memory loss associated with ECT may be anterograde and retrograde.
E. In a few patients, retrograde memory loss may be permanent.

188. A 65-year-old music teacher suffers from a CVA. Two months after the CVA, she returns to work at the local school. To their surprise, her colleagues note that she is unable to sing despite being able to repeat the lyrics of various songs. She also speaks without inflections or style and is unable to discern between the various emotions from the tone of others' voices. Given this history, she most probably suffered from a CVA of which of the following brain areas?

A. Dominant cerebral hemisphere
B. Nondominant hemisphere
C. Basal ganglia
D. Limbic system
E. Cerebellum

189. A 70-year-old man with a history of hypertension and diabetes is brought to the ER because of sudden onset of pain in the back of the head, vomiting, and inability to walk. His speech is slurred and he is unable to look towards the right. However, he is awake, aware of his surroundings, moving all his limbs and does not indicate any sensory loss. An MRI of the brain with and without contrast is ordered and would show a lesion in which one of the following structures?

A. Cerebral cortex
B. Midbrain
C. Basal ganglia
D. Cerebellum
E. Brainstem

190. A 27-year-old woman with a long history of epilepsy, well controlled on anticonvulsant therapy, reports to her neurologist that she is pregnant. Which of the following is TRUE about the proper management of seizures during pregnancy?

A. The anticonvulsant should be immediately tapered off.
B. Polypharmacy may increase the risk of teratogenicity.
C. Approximately 15% of exposed infants have major congenital defects.
D. The best choice of anticonvulsants during pregnancy is magnesium.
E. Serum drug levels are typically higher in pregnancy.

191. Which one of the following patients has the highest risk of developing Panic Disorder?

A. A 52-year-old man with history of opiate and cannabis abuse
B. A 19-year-old woman with history of sexual abuse and alcohol abuse
C. A 19-year-old woman with history of tension-type headaches

D. A 32-year-old man with pheocromocytoma
E. A 44-year-old man with history of borderline personality disorder

192. Which one of the following statements regarding Mixed Episodes in Bipolar Disorder (BPD) is TRUE?

A. When using the DSM-IV-TR criteria for diagnosis, these episodes constitutes about 20% to 30% of all episodes of BPD.
B. Studies have shown that lithium may be more effective than divalproex sodium in the treatment of these episodes.
C. The long-term prognosis of these episodes is similar to the other episodes of BPD.
D. Antidepressants are considered to be central in the management of these episodes.
E. In therapeutic trials, antipsychotic agents and divalproex have demonstrated superior efficacy to lithium in the treatment of these episodes.

193. What percent of elderly patients develop depressive symptoms after a stroke?

A. 40% to 50%
B. 10% to 15%
C. 15% to 20%
D. 20% to 30%
E. 30% to 40%

194. Which one of the following statements was NOT MADE by the FDA on the issue of increased mortality due to the use of atypical antipsychotic agents in the treatment of behavioral disturbances in dementia?

A. Seventeen placebo-controlled trials, which enrolled a total of 5,106 patients, were reviewed with olanzapine (Zyprexa), aripiprazole (Abilify), risperidone (Risperdal), or quetiapine (Seroquel) in the treatment of elderly demented patients with behavioral disturbances.
B. Fifteen of these trials showed numerical increase in mortality (1.6 to 1.7 fold) in the drug-treated group compared to the placebo-treated patients.
C. Examination of the specific causes of these deaths revealed that most deaths were either due to heart related events (e.g., heart failure, sudden death) or infections (mostly pneumonia).
D. The agency also extended the warning to older, typical antipsychotic agents used in the treatment of these behaviors.
E. The warning is also extended to atypical antipsychotic medications including clozapine (Clozaril), ziprasidone (Geodon), and Symbyax, a combination product containing olanzapine and fluoxetine, approved for the treatment of depressive episodes associated with bipolar disorder.

195. Which one of the following structures is not part of the basal ganglia in the brain?
    A. Caudate nucleus
    B. Corpus striatum
    C. Subthalamic nucleus
    D. Thalamus
    E. Substantia nigra

196. A 50-year-old man is brought to a neurology clinic for an evaluation. His wife reports that he is frequently bumping into things that appear to be in his peripheral field of vision. She is concerned that he has premature cataracts, but his primary care doctor thinks that he has a brain lesion. They want to confirm this opinion with a neurologist. On neurological examination, the patient is found to have bitemporal hemianopsia without any other deficits. You order an MRI of the brain to confirm the presence of a space-occupying lesion pressing on which one of the following structures?
    A. Right optic nerve
    B. Left optic nerve
    C. Optic chiasm
    D. Optic tracts
    E. Occipital lobes

197. In a patient with migraine headaches and comorbid depression, which of the following treatments is most likely to be effective in treating both conditions?
    A. Tricyclic antidepressants (TCAs)
    B. SSRIs
    C. Divalproex
    D. Beta blockers
    E. Non Steroidal Analgesic Agents (NSAIDs)

198. Which one of the following statements regarding the surgical treatment of partial complex seizures is NOT TRUE?
    A. Surgery is indicated when seizures are refractory to antiepileptic drugs.
    B. Only about 20% of patients experience near or complete cessation of seizures.
    C. Candidates should have a single, clearly identifiable frontal or temporal lesion.
    D. Less than 8% of patients experience behavioral or cognitive decline related to surgery.
    E. Severe comorbid medical illness or progressive neurological disorder may serve as relative contraindications.

199. Which one of the following best describes the mechanism of action of carbidopa in the treatment of Parkinson's disease?
    A. Inhibits catechol-O-methyltransferase
    B. Inhibits CNS dopa decarboxylase only
    C. Inhibits peripheral dopa decarboxylase only
    D. Inhibits both peripheral and CNS dopa decarboxylase
    E. Inhibits tyrosine hydroxylase

200. A 78-year-old man with an 8-year history of Parkinson's disease presents to his neurologist. He reports that he has been experiencing nausea, involuntary pursing of his lips, and jerking movements of his arms. Which medication is most likely responsible for these symptoms?
    A. Entacapone
    B. Selegiline
    C. L-dopa
    D. Amantadine
    E. Vitamin E

Test 3

Answers

1. Answer: B. This child is 9 months old. Nine-month-old children should be very attentive to people and things around them. They are able to point at things and are able to pick things up between their finger and thumb. They can sit unsupported, and some of them start crawling. They usually babble and shout and clearly distinguish people they know from strangers. They are able to pull themselves up, but cannot lower themselves without help. A 6-month-old child is unable to pull himself up. A 12-month-old child can pull himself up and sit down.

Sheridan MB. *From Birth to Five Years. Children's Developmental Progress*. London: Routledge; 1997:1–43.

2. Answer: C. K complexes are negative sharp waves followed by positive slow waves found on EEG in stage II sleep. High amplitude slow waves, or delta waves, occupying >50% of epoch are found in stage IV sleep. Alpha activity is seen in wakefulness when the patient's eyes are closed. Slow alpha activity is seen in REM sleep. Theta activity is seen in stage I and REM sleep. High amplitude slow waves, or delta waves, occupying 20% to 50% of epoch are seen in stage III sleep.

Sadock BJ, Sadock VA. *Kaplan and Sadock's Comprehensive Textbook of Psychiatry*. 8th ed. Philadelphia: Lippincott Williams & Wilkins; 2005:282.

3. Answer: C. This patient is exhibiting mixed transcortical aphasia or isolation aphasia. The pattern of speech is equivalent to global aphasia with preserved repetition. These patients do not speak unless spoken to and show classic echolalia. Their ability to name objects, read out loud, and to comprehend reading and writing are severely impaired. Damage to both the anterior and posterior vascular borderzone cortical areas (watershed area) of the left hemisphere is responsible for this pattern of speech impairment. It occurs in its pure form in individuals with acute left internal carotid occlusion, residuals of severe cerebral edema, or prolonged hypoxia due to cardiac or respiratory arrest. Anomia is the inability to name objects and it can be seen in small strokes or dementias. Conduction aphasia is due to a lesion of the arcuate fasciculus, which connects the Wernicke's and Broca's areas. Wernicke's aphasia, also called sensory aphasia or receptive aphasia, is due to a lesion of the posterosuperior portion of the first temporal gyrus of the left temporal lobe. Broca's aphasia occurs due to a lesion to the suprasylvian area extending from the Broca's area to the posterior extent of the sylvian fissure.

1. Goetz C. *Textbook of Clinical Neurology*. 2nd ed. Philadelphia: WB Saunders; 2003:88–90.
2. Kaufman DM. *Clinical Neurology for Psychiatrists*. 5th ed. Philadelphia: WB Saunders; 2001:175–201.

4. Answer: D. Type II error occurs when there is a true difference between the two groups, regardless of how small the difference. The test does not detect this difference, because this difference does not exceed the threshold for statistical significance. In a diagnostic test, a type II error would be considered to be equivalent to a false negative result. Type II error is also known as a beta error.

Gray GE. *Evidence-Based Psychiatry*. Washington: American Psychiatric Publishing; 2004:61.

5. Answer: E. Although increases in CSF volume, ventricular volume, and high-intensity lesion volume, as well as decreases in cerebral hemisphere volume, have been seen in healthy control subjects, it has been shown that hippocampal volume is diminished in patients with Alzheimer's disease, and not normal aging.

1. Csernanski JG, Hamstra J, Wang L, et al. Correlations between antemortem hippocampal volume and postmortem neuropathology in Alzheimer's disease subjects. *Alzheimer Dis Assoc Disord*. 2004;18:190–195.
2. Sadock BJ, Sadock VA. *Kaplan and Sadock's Comprehensive Textbook of Psychiatry*. 8th ed. Philadelphia: Lippincott Williams & Wilkins; 2005:3640–3641.

6. Answer: B. Dissociative fugue is characterized by purposeful travel away from home or the usual place of stay/operations with an inability to recall the past, either partially or completely. There are three types of fugue: fugue with awareness of loss of personal identity, fugue with change in personal identity, and fugue with retrograde amnesia. Fugue usually occurs in the wake of a traumatic episode, such as rape, childhood sexual abuse, natural disasters, wars/combat situations, and social dislocations, which results in the urge to flee.

Sadock BJ, Sadock VA. *Kaplan and Sadock's Comprehensive Textbook of Psychiatry*. 8th ed. Philadelphia: Lippincott Williams & Wilkins; 2005:1873–1874.

7. Answer: C. Several studies have tried to find different risk factors associated to PTSD to try to intervene as early as possible in susceptible individuals. Some of the risk factors found to date include higher levels of anxiety in the peri-event period, female gender, being involved in litigation, previous psychiatric history, autonomic hyperarousal, acute stress symptoms, and persistent medical problems. Previous substance abuse has not been associated with a higher risk of developing PTSD.

1. Mason S, Turpin G, Woods D, et al. Risk factors for psychological distress following injury. *Br J Clin Psychol.* 2006;45:217–230.
2. McFarlane AC. Posttraumatic stress disorder: a model of the longitudinal course and the role of risk factors. *J Clin Psychiatry.* 2000;61 (suppl 5): 15–20, 21–23 (discussion).

8. Answer: C. This patient is presenting with symptoms consistent with an adjustment disorder. The most recommended treatment for an acute adjustment disorder (less than 6 months) is supportive psychotherapy. Pharmacological options, such as SSRIs, have been tried empirically in patients with adjustment disorders, but there is little evidence for their use when a patient does not meet criteria for major depressive disorders. Long-term psychodynamic psychotherapy could be considered if the patient's symptoms did not improve gradually, but it should not be considered as the best initial approach. This patient does not meet criteria for inpatient psychiatric admission at this point.

1. American Psychiatric Association. *Quick Reference to the Diagnostic Criteria from DSM-IV-TR.* Washington: American Psychiatric Association; 2000:285–286.
2. Sadock BJ, Sadock VA. *Kaplan and Sadock's Comprehensive Textbook of Psychiatry.* 8th ed. Philadelphia: Lippincott Williams & Wilkins; 2005:2061

9. Answer: E. All the statements regarding the prognosis of elderly patients with bipolar disorder are true.

Depp CA, Jeste DV. Bipolar disorder in older adults: a critical review. *Bipolar Disord.* 2004;6:343–367.

10. Answer: C. Sex therapy as a treatment modality for sexual dysfunction typically requires a supportive and healthy relationship to best allow for collaborative work by both members of the couple.

Hawton K. Treatment of sexual dysfunctions by sex therapy and other approaches. *Br J Psychiatry.* 1995;167:307–314.

11. Answer: D. N-acetyl cysteine is an antioxidant. It is used in the treatment of acetaminophen toxicity. It exerts glutamate-modulating properties by its conversion to cystine, which is a substrate for the glutamate/cystine antiporter that is located on glial cells. The uptake of cystine by glia corresponds to increased release of glutamate into the extrasynaptic space, resulting in stimulation of metabotropic receptors that are inhibitory in nature. It is proposed that N-acetyl cysteine improves clearance of synaptic glutamate by glial cells. N-acetyl cysteine is hence a promising drug for use in treatment-resistant OCD, because glutamatergic dysfunction has been suggested to be a significant neurobiological correlate of OCD.

1. Lafleur DL, Pittenger C, Kelmendi B, et al. N-acetylcysteine augmentation in serotonin reuptake inhibitor refractory obsessive-compulsive disorder. *Psychopharmacology (Berl).* 2006 Jan; 184(2): 254–256.
2. Pittenger C, Krystal JH, Coric V. Glutamate-modulating drugs as novel pharmacotherapeutic agents in the treatment of obsessive-compulsive disorder. *NeuroRx.* 2006 Jan; 3(1):69–81.

12. Answer: B. In 1938, Cerletti and Bini induced seizures in a human patient with electricity. Prior to that, Meduna had used pentylenetetrazol (Metrazol) and intramuscular camphor to induce therapeutic seizures chemically. Freud developed psychoanalysis, and Jung was his contemporary. Kesey, of course, wrote the book *One Flew Over the Cuckoo's Nest*, which was made into a movie that portrayed ECT harshly.

Abrams R. *Electroconvulsive Therapy.* 4th ed. New York: Oxford University Press; 2002:3–16.

13. Answer: B. IPT focuses on life events that occur after early childhood. The others are the four main problem areas generally cited as areas for focus with IPT.

1. Hales RE, Yudofsky SC. *Textbook of Clinical Psychiatry.* 4th ed. Washington: American Psychiatric Publishing; 2003:1201–1222.
2. Levenson H, Butler SF, Powers TA, et al. *Concise Guide to Brief Dynamic and Interpersonal Psychotherapy.* 2nd ed. Washington: American Psychiatric Publishing; 2002:55–75.

14. Answer: A. The symptoms of trigeminal neuralgia (tic douloureux) include persistent burning, unprovoked paroxysms of lancinating pain, and dysesthesias. Even innocuous stimuli applied to the affected region may produce severe pain (allodynia) at times. Carbamazepine is the drug of choice for the treatment of trigeminal neuralgia (tic douloureux). It is more effective for this condition than phenytoin, which is also an effective treatment. Clonazepam may have a role in neuropathic pain. Tricyclic antidepressants have shown effectiveness in the treatment of chronic pain, especially neuropathic pain. The use of opioids for neuropathic pain remains controversial, because studies have been small, have yielded equivocal results, and have not established the long-term risk-benefit ratio of this treatment.

1. Arana GW, Rosenbaum JF. *Handbook of Psychiatric Drug Therapy*. 4th ed. Philadelphia: Lippincott Williams & Wilkins; 2000:152–153.
2. Eisenberg E, McNicol ED, Carr DB. Efficacy and safety of opioid agonists in the treatment of neuropathic pain of nonmalignant origin: systematic review and meta-analysis of randomized controlled trials. *JAMA*. 2005;293:3043–3052.

15. Answer: E. The main purpose of informed consent is to promote individual autonomy. There are three essential ingredients to informed consent. They are competency, information, and volition. Competency refers to the clinician's determination whether or not to accept the patient's treatment decision. The patient must be given adequate information regarding the treatment proposed. The patient must voluntarily either consent to or refuse the proposed therapy. There are four basic exceptions to obtaining informed consent. They are emergencies, incompetence, therapeutic privilege, and waiver. When emergency treatment is necessary to save a life or prevent imminent serious harm and it is impossible to obtain the patient's consent, the law will presume consent is granted. This exception does not apply if the patient is competent and refusing treatment (e.g., in the case of blood transfusion in a Jehovah's Witness). Under the condition that someone lacks sufficient capacity to provide consent or has been judged legally incompetent, then consent is obtained from a substitute decision-maker. Therapeutic privilege is the most difficult to apply. Essentially, the exception allows that informed consent may not be required if a psychiatrist determines that a complete disclosure of possible risks and alternatives may have a negative impact on the patient's health and welfare. Waiver constitutes that a physician need not disclose the risks of treatment when the patient has competently, knowingly, and voluntarily waived his or her right for information. Finally, mental retardation does not create a general exception to obtaining informed consent. There are different degrees of mental retardation, ranging from mild to profound, and patients may or may not be able to provide consent depending upon the extent of the patient's illness and the specific situation in question.

Levenson JL. *The American Psychiatric Publishing Textbook of Psychosomatic Medicine*. Washington: American Psychiatric Publishing; 2005:38–40.

16. Answer: C. The ventricular system is filled with CSF, which is a colorless liquid containing low concen-

trations of protein, glucose, and potassium and relatively high concentrations of sodium and chloride. The CSF circulates through the lateral ventricles to the third ventricle and then to the fourth ventricle. It then flows through the medial and lateral apertures to the cisterna magna and pontine cistern to travel over the cerebral hemispheres and is then absorbed by the arachnoid villi to be released into the superior sagittal sinus. Interruption to the flow of CSF causes hydrocephalus. CSF acts to cushion the brain against trauma, to maintain the extracellular environment of the brain, and to transport the endocrine hormones.

Sadock BJ, Sadock VA. *Kaplan and Sadock's Comprehensive Textbook of Psychiatry*. 8th ed. Philadelphia: Lippincott Williams & Wilkins; 2005:8.

17. Answer: A. Monocular quadrantanopsia, hemianopsias, scotomas, and blindness occur due to an injury to the optic nerve.

1. Kaufman DM. *Clinical Neurology for Psychiatrists*. 5th ed. Philadelphia: WB Saunders; 2001:302–303.
2. Rowland LP. *Merritt's Neurology*. 11th ed. Philadelphia: Lippincott Williams & Wilkins; 2005: 38–40.

18. Answer: A. The pattern of development of Parkinson's disease is consistent with a multifactorial etiology. Although no clear cause has been found, multiple studies have found that cigarette smoking and coffee drinking are protective.

In the 1980s, a group of young opiate abusers developed acute Parkinsonian symptoms after intravenous injection of MPTP (1-methyl-4-phenyl-1,2,3,6-tetrahydropyridine), a meperidine derivative. MPTP was found to have a direct toxic effect on the cells of the substania nigra with depletion of dopaminergic neurons. In animal studies, the neuronal changes predate the onset of clinical symptoms, so it was theorized that early exposure to viral infection or toxins, such as pesticides, would kill dopaminergic neurons until a certain threshold of loss had been reached, resulting in the disease state in genetically vulnerable individuals. This was thought to implicate an interplay of genetic and environmental causes.

Logroscino G. The role of early life environmental risk factors in Parkinson's disease: what is the evidence? *Environ Health Perspect*. 2005;113:1234–1238.

19. Answer: B. Brainstem auditory evoked potentials (BAER) will help us decide on continued care for this unfortunate child. An abnormal brainstem auditory evoked response is indicative of brainstem damage and can be used for prognostic purposes in patients with head trauma. In a BAER, a series of clicks sequentially activates cranial nerve VIII, the cochlear nucleus, the superior olivary nucleus, the lateral lemniscus, and the inferior colliculus. Interpretation of the BAER is based on the time interval between the initial waves and the interpeak latencies. The BAER can also be used to evaluate hearing in patients unable to cooperate with behaviorally based hearing tests (infants).

Menkes JH, Sarnat HB, Maria BL. *Child Neurology*. 7th ed. Philadelphia: Lippincott Williams & Wilkins; 2006:16–20.

20. **Answer: E.** Although much of the use of BOLD fMRI has been in research involving changes in cerebral blood flow during language, motor, and cognitive activation, it has proven very useful in presurgical mapping of these same pathways, aiding in more precision and preservation of as much intact functioning as possible after neurosurgical intervention.

Rowland LP. *Merritt's Neurology*. 11th ed. Philadelphia: Lippincott Williams & Wilkins; 2005:74–75.

21. **Answer: D.** This patient's symptoms are characteristic of cervical spondylosis, in which degenerative changes of the annulus fibrosus can eventually lead to compression of the spinal cord or nerve roots. An MRI is often helpful in visualizing the compression of the spinal cord and narrowing or absence of the CSF space surrounding the spinal cord. Neck and arm pain are not typical features of multiple sclerosis. Calcification and narrowed disc space can occur in both cervical spondylosis and osteoarthritis. Amyotrophic lateral sclerosis is purely a motor disease and usually presents with muscle weakness and atrophy and not sensory symptoms like pain.

Victor M, Ropper AH. *Principles of Neurology*. 7th ed. New York: McGraw-Hill; 2001:1323–1325.

22. **Answer: B.** The most likely diagnosis is the Miller-Fischer syndrome, a variant of Guillain-Barré syndrome. Anti-G1Qb antibodies are found in the serum in over 90% of the cases. The classic triad of Miller Fisher syndrome is ataxia, opthalmoplegia, and areflexia. Ataxia, confusion, and opthalmoplegia is the triad of Wernicke's encephalopathy. Ataxia, urinary incontinence, and dementia constitute the triad of normal pressure hydrocephalus.

Overell JR, Willison HJ. Recent developments in Miller Fisher syndrome and related disorders. *Curr Opin Neurol*. 2005;18:562–566.

23. **Answer: C.** Peripheral nerve involvement is common in diabetes mellitus. It may be characterized by polyneuropathy which is mixed (sensory, motor, and autonomic) in 70% of cases or predominantly sensory in the remaining 30%. Polyneuropathy is generally symmetric with greater involvement of the distal lower extremities than the upper limbs. It often manifests as impaired vibratory sense in the legs along with depressed tendon reflexes. Mononeuropathy multiplex occurs in a mixed distribution. Mononeuropathy simplex can involve the peripheral nerves (i.e., ulnar, median, radial, lateral femoral cutaneous, sciatic, peroneal, and others, or the cranial nerves, (CN), CNIII > CNVI > CNVII). Diabetic amyotrophy is due to plexopathy or polyradiculoneuropathy. Pain, weakness, and atrophy of the pelvic girdle and thigh muscles are characteristic. Quadriceps reflexes are absent and there is little sensory loss. The distribution is asymmetric and proximal. Diabetes is not associated with syringomyelia, cavitation of the spinal cord, in which there is usually sensory loss and wasting of the muscles at the level of the lesion.

Greenberg DA, Aminoff MJ, Simon RP. *Clinical Neurology*. 5th ed. New York: McGraw-Hill; 2002:214, 224.

24. **Answer: A.** Myotonic dystrophy is a dominantly inherited disorder. It is caused by a CTG repeat. There is weakness and wasting of the facial, sternocleidomastoid, and distal limb muscles. Patients may have cataracts, frontal baldness, testicular atrophy, diabetes mellitus, cardiac abnormalities, and intellectual changes. The disorder usually becomes apparent in the third or fourth decade, although it may occur earlier. Myotonia congentia (Thomsen's disease) is inherited as a dominant trait. It is caused by a mutation on chromosome 7q35. Symptoms may not develop until early childhood and include muscle hypertrophy and muscle stiffness, which is enhanced by cold and inactivity and relieved by exercise. Inclusion body myositis is more common in men. It has an insidious onset and usually begins after age 50. There is painless proximal weakness of the lower and then the upper extremities. The course is progressive. The etiology suggests T-cell mediated myocytotoxicity and multifactorial genetic susceptibility. Duchenne's dystrophy is an X-linked recessive disorder. Symptoms begin by age 5. Early signs include impaired toe walking, waddling gait, and inability to run. Weakness is pronounced in the proximal lower extremities. Patients with this disorder may be incapable of rising from a supine position without using their arms to climb up their body, Gower's sign. Pseudohypertrophy of the calves caused by fatty infiltration of muscle occurs commonly. The genetic defect responsible for Duchenne's dystrophy is located on the short arm of the X chromosome. It codes for the protein dystrophin, which is absent or reduced in the muscle of patients with this disorder. Paramyotonia congenita is dominantly inherited and involves mutation of the SCN4A

gene. Weakness and myotonia (i.e., an abnormality of muscle fiber membranes, which leads to muscle stiffness) are provoked by cold and worsened by exercise. Attacks of hyperkalemic periodic paralysis may also occur.

Greenberg DA, Aminoff MJ, Simon RP. *Clinical Neurology*. 5th ed. New York: McGraw-Hill; 2002:187–194.

25. Answer: B. On average, 30% to 50% of patients develop depression following a stroke. The involvement of the frontal lobe was once thought to be a correlate for depression; however, recent studies have challenged this claim. Older age, functional disability, aphasia, cognitive impairment, and a slower recovery than expected, given the deficits, are all associated with post-stroke depression.

Kaufman DM. *Clinical Neurology for Psychiatrists*. 5th ed. Philadelphia: WB Saunders; 2001:278–279.

26. Answer: B. Functional recovery from traumatic brain injury is usually measured on the Glasgow Outcome Scale, which ranges from "good recovery" to "death." The Glasgow Coma Scale measures a patient's level of consciousness based on readily apparent neurological functions including eye opening, best verbal response, and best motor response. The Global Assessment of Functioning is recorded on axis V of a DSM-IV-TR diagnosis and is considered a composite of three major areas: social, occupational, and psychological functioning. The Scales for the Assessment of Negative and Positive Symptoms were developed by Dr. Nancy Andreason to evaluate symptoms of schizophrenia.

1. Kaufman DM. *Clinical Neurology for Psychiatrists*. 5th ed. Philadelphia: WB Saunders; 2001:583–585.
2. Sadock BJ, Sadock VA. *Kaplan and Sadock's Synopsis of Psychiatry*. 9th ed. Philadelphia: Lippincott Williams & Wilkins; 2003:290, 303–304.

27. Answer: B. This child is approximately 24 months old. Children at this age run and are able to start and stop without major problems. They squat and climb on furniture. They can go up and down the stairs holding onto the rail, and can throw a ball forwards. They are not able to use pedals yet. They can build a tower of six blocks and are able to hold a pencil. They usually use around 50 words and can form simple sentences and can carry out simple instructions. They can feed themselves with a spoon and like parallel play. A 15-month-old child is unable to run yet. A child 36 months or older is able to use pedals, can throw and catch a ball, and builds a tower of at least nine cubes.

Sheridan MB. *From Birth to Five Years. Children's Developmental Progress*. London: Routledge; 1997:1–43.

28. Answer: B. Muscle twitches are characteristic of the phasic (episodic) component of REM sleep. Theta activity and an activated EEG similar to stage I sleep are characteristics of the tonic (persistent) phase of REM sleep. Extraocular muscle atonia is not seen in REM sleep. Diaphragmatic atonia during sleep is not compatible with life.

Sadock BJ, Sadock VA. *Kaplan and Sadock's Comprehensive Textbook of Psychiatry*. 8th ed. Philadelphia: Lippincott Williams & Wilkins; 2005: 282.

29. Answer: C. Each of the scenarios depicts examples of operant conditioning. Operant conditioning, elaborated upon by B.F. Skinner, describes a form of learning in which behavior is either increased or decreased via the application of positive and negative consequences. In *negative reinforcement* (scenario C), behavior (sitting in the back of class) is increased because the behavior removes an aversive consequence (being called upon in class). Scenario A depicts *punishment*, whereby an aversive consequence (being sent to his room) leads to a reduction in the child's behavior (hitting the sibling). Scenarios B and E depict *positive reinforcement*: positive reinforcers (money and praise, respectively) result in an increase in behavior (achieving good grades and cleaning the room, respectively). Finally, scenario D depicts *extinction*, where the removal of a positive reinforcer (mother's attention) results in a reduction in behavior (child's crying).

Sadock BJ, Sadock VA. *Kaplan and Sadock's Comprehensive Textbook of Psychiatry*. 7th ed. Philadelphia: Lippincott Williams & Wilkins; 2000:413–420.

30. Answer: B. *Power* is the term given to a study's ability to detect a true difference when such a difference truly exists. In a diagnostic test, the power is equivalent to a true-positive result. In general, a large number of subjects are usually required for the power of the study to be able to detect a real difference between the groups.

Gray GE. *Evidence-Based Psychiatry*. Washington: American Psychiatric Publishing; 2004:61–62.

31. Answer: A. The Rorschach test is a projective personality test as opposed to an objective one in the sense that, rather than lending itself to numerical analysis, it forces the test takers to impute their own meanings onto the test object. The Rorschach involves showing patients inkblots and evaluating their responses to, for example, form, color, and shading. The way patients respond to the color of an inkblot, for example, is viewed as reflecting their emotional responses. Only among highly skilled clinicians are its results reliable. It is not a test of organic brain function.

Kaplan HI, Sadock BJ. *Kaplan & Sadock's Synopsis of Psychiatry*. 8th ed. Philadelphia: Lippincott Williams & Wilkins; 1998:193–197.

32. **Answer: B.** This patient is most likely to have an insulinoma, a tumor of the islet cells of the pancreas, which results in a triad of symptoms: hypoglycemia, central nervous system (CNS) dysfunction and a reversal of CNS dysfunction on glucose administration. This insulinoma is possibly causing episodes of hypoglycemia and the feelings of depersonalization. Depersonalization is a symptom that may be observed in a variety of conditions, which may be neurological (such as epilepsy, migraine, etc.), toxic and metabolic (hypoglycemia, hypothyroidism, hypoparathyroidism, carbon monoxide poisoning, etc.), psychiatric (schizophrenia, anxiety disorders, etc.), in normal people (in conditions such as exhaustion or emotional shock), and hemidepersonalization (usually in right parietal lobe lesions). To diagnose a Depersonalization Disorder (according to DSM-IV-TR), these episodes of depersonalization should not be due to a general medical condition. In this case, depersonalization is a symptom and not a disorder given that the patient has an insulinoma that is causing hypoglycemia resulting in depersonalization. It should subside following complete surgical resection of the tumor. According to the DSM-IV-TR, derealization unaccompanied by depersonalization in adults is classified as a "Dissociative Disorder NOS"

1. Sadock BJ, Sadock VA. *Kaplan and Sadock's Comprehensive Textbook of Psychiatry*. 8th ed. Philadelphia: Lippincott Williams & Wilkins, 2005:1870–1873.
2. Service FJ. Recurrent hyperinsulinemic hypoglycemia caused by an insulin-secreting insulinoma. *Clin Pract Endocrinol Metab*. 2006 Aug;2(8):467–70.
3. *Quick Reference to the Diagnostic Criteria from DSM-IV-TR*. Washington DC: American Psychiatric Association, 2000:239–241.

33. **Answer: C.** This patient is experiencing an acute stress disorder, which is characterized by the development of anxiety and specific symptoms within 4 weeks after being exposed to a traumatic event. The prevalence ranges from 14% to 33% in persons exposed to severe trauma. Patients feel numb or detached during the event and may have dissociative amnesia. They usually re-experience the event through thoughts, dreams, or flashbacks and tend to avoid situations that can trigger memories of the event. The disturbance must cause significant distress or impairment in the patient's functioning, and it must last between 2 days and 4 weeks in order to be considered an acute stress disorder. PTSD stress disorder requires the presence of symptoms for more than a month. In generalized anxiety disorder, patients have usually not been exposed to a traumatic event and tend to worry about situations that should usually not cause such stress. Although a stressor also triggers adjustment disorder, the stressor does not have to be as extreme as the one in acute stress disorder and it can involve a wide array of possible symptoms, which are not as specific as the ones for acute stress disorder.

1. American Psychiatric Association. *Quick Reference to the Diagnostic Criteria from DSM-IV-TR*. Washington: American Psychiatric Association; 2000:218–222.
2. Bryant RA, Panasetis P. The role of panic in acute dissociative reactions following trauma. *Br J Clin Psychol*. 2005; 44:489–494.

34. **Answer: E.** This patient is presenting with symptoms of an adjustment disorder. Adjustment disorders are characterized by an emotional response to a stressful event, such as a break-up, medical, or financial problems. Patients develop unspecific symptoms that do not fit the criteria for any other axis I diagnosis and that cause some impairment in social or emotional functioning. An acute stress disorder is characterized by the presence of a life-threatening or very disturbing events such as a natural disaster or abuse, and it includes very specific symptoms, such as hyperarousal and nightmares. This patient does not meet criteria for major depressive disorder. Dysthimia is a chronic disorder that is characterized by minor depressive symptoms that are present more often than not for at least 2 years. In cyclothymic disorder, the patient presents with fluctuating mood with separate episodes of hypomanic and depressive symptoms for a 2-year period.

1. American Psychiatric Association. *Quick Reference to the Diagnostic Criteria from DSM-IV-TR*. Washington: American Psychiatric Association; 2000:285–286.
2. Sadock BJ, Sadock V. *Kaplan and Sadock's Comprehensive Review of Psychiatry*. 8th ed. Philadelphia: Lippincott Williams & Wilkins; 2005:2061.

35. **Answer: A.** All the statements are true except that carbamazepine is a second line drug for the treatment of a manic episode in the elderly. Lithium and divalproex sodium are the first-line drugs for the treatment of a manic episode.

Young RC. Evidence-based pharmacological treatment of geriatric bipolar disorder. *Psychiatr Clin North Am*. 2005;28:837–869.

36. **Answer: E.** Buprenorphine is a partial opioid agonist approved for use as replacement therapy in the

treatment of opioid dependence. It is a schedule III narcotic, which may only be prescribed by physicians who meet certain qualifying requirements. It is available in sublingual and injectable forms, and its long half life allows for dosing once a day or every other day. Methadone is a long-acting synthetic opioid with agonist effects at mu receptors, which is used for abstinence in opioid-addicted patients. It prevents opioid withdrawal symptoms while having minimal euphoric effects. Unlike buprenorphine, methadone is only prescribed by specialized treatment centers. LAAM is an mu-receptor agonist very similar to methadone, but with a longer half life (it may be dosed 3 times per week). Clonidine is an alpha-2 agonist that is frequently used for the treatment of acute opioid withdrawal. Naltrexone is a semisynthetic opioid antagonist at mu receptors used for the treatment of both alcohol and opioid dependence.

Rosenbaum JF, Arana GW, Hyman SE, et al. *Handbook of Psychiatric Drug Therapy*. Philadelphia: Lippincott Williams & Wilkins; 2005:230–232.

37. **Answer: B.** The treatment modalities used in the different levels of the STAR*D trial are as follows:

Level 1: Citalopram

Level 2: Nonresponders of level 1 either:

Switch to one among: bupropion, venlafaxine, sertraline, cognitive therapy

Augment to one among: buspirone, bupropion, cognitive therapy

Level 2A: nonresponders to cognitive therapy switch to either venlafaxine, or bupropion

Level 3: Either:

Switch to one among: nortryptyline or mirtazapine

Augment to one among: Li or T3

Level 4: Switch to one among: tranylcypromine or venlafaxine + mirtazapine.

Hence, mirtazapine was used in level 3 and level 4, but not in level 2.

1. Rush AJ, Fava M, Wisniewski SR, et al. Sequenced treatment alternatives to relieve depression (STAR*D): rationale and design. *Control Clin Trials*. 2004 Feb;25(1):119–142
2. Rush AJ, Trivedi MH, Wisniewski SR, et al. Bupropion-SR, sertraline, or venlafaxine-XR after failure of SSRIs for depression. *N Engl J Med*. 2006;354:1231–1242.

38. **Answer: E.** All of the statements are indications for ECT, especially mood disorders, disorders refractory to pharmacotherapy, and conditions requiring a rapid response, when there is a strong preference or a history of response to ECT. ECT should

not always be considered merely a treatment of last resort.

1. American Psychiatric Association Committee on Electroconvulsive Therapy. *The Practice of Electroconvulsive Therapy: Recommendations for Treatment, Training, and Privileging*. 2nd ed. Washington: American Psychiatric Association; 2001:5–22.
2. Hales RE, Yudofsky SC. *Textbook of Clinical Psychiatry*. 4th ed. Washington: American Psychiatric Publishing; 2003:1123.

39. **Answer: C.** This patient has developed NMS, and a dose change in typical high-potency antipsychotics is usually antecedent, although other antipsychotics may also be causative. Concurrent lithium use increases the risk for NMS and may cause leukocytosis, but is usually not causative for the full presentation of NMS. Serotonin syndrome from citalopram would have a different presentation with prominent hyperthermia, hypertonicity, and myoclonus. Clonazepam or benztropine intoxication may cause delirium, and benzodiazepine withdrawal can be associated with hypertension, but neither is known to cause the symptom pattern mentioned.

Hales RE, Yudofsky SC. *Textbook of Clinical Psychiatry*. 4th ed. Washington: American Psychiatric Publishing; 2003:1091–1092.

40. **Answer: E.** Antidepressants have shown efficacy in the treatment of a number of medical disorders. With regard to TCAs, amitriptyline has been used in the treatment of migraine and cluster headaches. Amitriptyline and doxepin may be more effective for diabetic neuropathy than serotonin reuptake inhibitors. TCAs also may be useful in facial pain, fibrositis, and arthritis. However, they have not been useful in the treatment of low back pain and cancer pain. Desipramine has also been used in the treatment of cocaine craving. Protriptyline may be helpful in the treatment of sleep apnea. Uncommon uses include the treatment of peptic ulcer disease, because many tricyclics are potent histamine blockers, particularly doxepin and amytriptyline. Finally, their quinidine-like effect makes them plausible antiarrhythmic agents.

Tasman A, Kay J, Lieberman JA. *Psychiatry Therapeutics*. 2nd ed. London: John Wiley and Sons; 2003:300–302.

41. **Answer: C.** Major depression in the medically ill does not typically cause a patient to be unable to render medical decisions. Depression may influence a patient's ability to tolerate uncomfortable symptoms, maintain hope, and assess a treatment's risk-benefit ratio. Untreated depression has been linked to poor compliance with medical care, increased pain and

disability, and a greater likelihood of considering euthanasia and physician-assisted suicide. However, refusal of life-saving treatment by a depressed patient should not be assumed to constitute suicidality and/or lack of decision-making capacity. Depressed patients should be encouraged to begin treatment for their depression. Decisions overriding refusal of medical treatment should be based on whether or not the patient lacks decision making capacity and not solely on their depressed mood.

Levenson JL. *The American Psychiatric Publishing Textbook of Psychosomatic Medicine*. Washington: American Psychiatric Publishing; 2005:60–61.

42. Answer: D. The thalamus is the largest portion of the diencephalon which is located medial to the basal ganglia and serves as a major synaptic relay station for the information reaching the cerebral cortex. It can be divided on an anatomical basis into six groups of nuclei: anterior, medial, lateral, reticular, intralaminar, and midline nuclei. The myelinated fibers of the internal medullary lamina divide the anterior, medial, and lateral groups of nuclei. The lateral group of nuclei is covered by the myelinated fibers of the external medullary lamina. In between the external medullary lamina and the internal capsule are a group of neurons that form the reticular nucleus of the thalamus. The medial geniculate nuclei receive afferents from inferior colliculus and project to the visual cortex. Lateral geniculate nuclei receive afferents from the optic tract and project to the visual cortex. The ventral posterior medial nuclei of the thalamus receive the afferents from the sensory nuclei of the trigeminal nerve and project to the somatosensory cortex.

Sadock BJ, Sadock VA. *Kaplan and Sadock's Comprehensive Textbook of Psychiatry*. 8th ed. Philadelphia: Lippincott Williams & Wilkins; 2005:9–10.

43. Answer: C. Injury to the optic tract between the optic chiasm and occipital cortex produces homonymous quadrantanopsia and hemianopsia. It is most commonly associated with middle cerebral artery infarction, where it also produces hemisensory loss and hemiparesis.

Kaufman DM. *Clinical Neurology for Psychiatrists*. 5th ed. Philadelphia: WB Saunders; 2001:41.

44. Answer: D. Friedreich's ataxia has an autosomal recessive inheritance, with greater than 96% of affected individuals found to have a GAA triplet-repeat expansion in the FXN gene on chromosome 9. Onset of symptoms is generally between ages 10 to 15, although there can be a wide range of onset. The initial presenting symptoms are usually gait ataxia,

followed by slurring of speech, and arm ataxia with later lower extremity weakness and loss of position and vibration sense. Two thirds of the affected individuals also have scoliosis and/or hypertrophic cardiomyopathy. Diabetes mellitus, visual deficits, and hearing deficits may also occur. The life span of affected children used to be in the mid-thirties, but with improved treatment and physical mobility, and greater monitoring of cardiac problems, life expectancy has increased.

Bidichandani SI, Delatycki MB, Ashizawa T. Friedreich Ataxia. *GeneReviews* [serial online]. http://www.geneclinics.org. Published February 18, 2007.

45. Answer: E. When epilepsy is suspected, an EEG is the most useful diagnostic test to obtain. The presence of characteristic interictal EDs are diagnostic, although their absence does not exclude the diagnosis of epilepsy. In patients with epilepsy, only 30% to 50% have EEGs with EDs on the first study. Of patients with epilepsy, 60% to 90% will have documented EDs by the third EEG; further EEGs after this time have not been shown to increase the yield of the test. To improve the likelihood of interictal discharges being detected on EEG, obtaining the study under sleeping or sleep-deprived conditions, while the patient is hyperventilating, and during exposure to photic stimulation have been successfully employed. Even with these measures, 10% to 40% of individuals with epilepsy will have negative interictal EEGs.

Rowland LP. *Merritt's Neurology*. 11th ed. Philadelphia: Lippincott Williams & Wilkins; 2005:79–82.

46. Answer: A. The MMPI is an extensively researched and widely used personality assessment test. It is an objective personality test and has the distinctive feature of validity scales, which assess the test taker's disposition while taking the test. In part, because it takes into account the complexities of such variables as social and educational backgrounds and may incorporate racial and religious variables, it requires significant experience to interpret the results. Although developed in 1937, the test has been updated based on a contemporary sample.

Kaplan HI, Sadock BJ. *Kaplan & Sadock's Synopsis of Psychiatry*. 8th ed. Philadelphia: Lippincott Williams & Wilkins; 1998:195–196.

47. Answer: C. This patient has hepatic encephalopathy, a syndrome remarkably diverse in its course and evolution. It usually appears over a period of days to weeks and may terminate fatally. With appropriate treatment, the symptoms may regress completely or fluctuate in severity for several weeks or months. The

EEG is a sensitive and reliable indicator of impending coma, becoming abnormal during the earliest phases of the disordered mental state. The concentrations of blood ammonia usually are in excess of 200 mg/dL, and the severity of the neurologic and EEG disorders roughly parallels to the ammonia levels. With treatment, a fall in the ammonia levels precedes clinical improvement. The few effective means of treating this disorder include restriction of dietary protein; reduction of bowel flora by oral administration of neomycin or kanamycin, which suppresses the urease-producing organisms in the bowel; and the use of enemas. Definitive treatment, however, is liver transplantation.

Ropper AH, Brown RH. *Adams and Victor's Principles of Neurology*. 8th ed. New York: McGraw-Hill; 2005:967–969.

48. Answer: B. The boy is suffering from Wilson's disease or hepatolenticular degeneration. This is characterized by low serum levels of copper and ceruloplasmin. It is coupled with abnormally elevated levels of hepatic copper and increased 24-hour urinary copper excretion. There are two possible presentations: the hepatic and the neurological. The most common symptom in neurological presentation is difficulty in speech and swallowing, along with drooling. In the hepatic presentation, there may be jaundice, ascites, hematemesis, and melena. This condition has an autosomal recessive mode of inheritance.

1. Das SK, Ray K. Wilson's disease: an update. *Nat Clin Pract Neurol*. 2006;2:482–493.
2. Leggio L, Addolorato G, Abenavoli L, et al. Wilson's disease: clinical, genetic and pharmacological findings. *Int J Immunopathol Pharmacol*. 2005;18:7–14.

49. Answer: E. These symptoms described are consistent with a diagnosis of Guillain-Barré syndrome (GBS). This syndrome typically follows an upper respiratory or gastrointestinal illness and is an acute inflammatory demyelinating polyradiculopathy of the peripheral nervous system. Cases following a week's episode of watery diarrhea are often due to *Campylobacter jejuni* infection. GBS occasionally complicates mononucleosis, Lyme disease, hepatitis, cytomegalovirus (CMV), or HIV. Symptoms include progressive weakness of more than one limb, distal areflexia with proximal areflexia or hyporeflexia, relatively symmetric deficits, mild sensory involvement, autonomic dysfunction, increased CSF protein after 1 week, CSF WBC count <10/mm, and nerve conduction slowing or block by several weeks. Symptoms stop progressing by about 4 weeks into the illness. It can become life-threatening if the muscles of respiration or swallowing are affected. In GBS, as in most other peripheral neuropathies other than dia-

betic neuropathy, bladder, bowel, and sexual function are preserved. Friedreich's ataxia is caused in many cases by a triplet repeat expansion and has an autosomal recessive inheritance. Ataxic gait, clumsiness of the hands, and other signs of cerebellar dysfunction develop. Peroneal nerve lesions occur secondary to the trauma or pressure around the knee at the head of the fibula. They result in weakness or paralysis of the foot and toe extension. They are accompanied by impaired sensation over the dorsum of the foot and lower anterior leg. The ankle reflex is preserved. Poliomyelitis is a viral infection of the anterior horn (motor neuron) cells of the spinal cord and lower brainstem. It presents with lower motor neuron (LMN) signs such as asymmetric paresis, muscle fasciculations, and absent DTRs. Sensation is not affected. Multiple sclerosis is a chronic illness in which the myelin sheaths, white matter of the nerves in the central nervous system are demyelinated, as opposed to GBS which involves demyelination of peripheral nerves. Symptoms include paresis, sensory disturbances, ataxia, ocular impairments, bladder dysfunction, and psychiatric disturbances.

1. Greenberg DA, Aminoff MJ, Simon RP. *Clinical Neurology*. 5th ed. New York: McGraw-Hill; 2002:212–213, 220, 222.
2. Kaufman DM. *Clinical Neurology for Psychiatrists*. 5th ed. Philadelphia: WB Saunders; 2001:73–75, 81, 369–371.

50. Answer: E. For many years, people took tryptophan pill to treat insomnia and depression. Tryptophan is an amino acid, which is converted in the brain into serotonin. However, in 1989, the Food and Drug Administration (FDA) banned all sales of over-the-counter tryptophan because of an outbreak of Eosinophilia-Myalgia Syndrome among thousands of people taking the pill. Eosinophilia-myalgia syndrome results from tryptophan or tryptophan-containing products. Patients may develop several days of severe myalgias. They may also develop fatigue, rash, neuropathy, cardiopulmonary impairments, and mild depression. On laboratory tests, they may have an elevated number and proportion of eosinophils in the blood. These patients are often in danger of being mislabeled with chronic fatigue syndrome, because of their variable symptoms and lack of objective findings, except for eosinophilia. Chronic Fatigue Syndrome results in a generalized sense of weakness, sometimes preceded by flu-like symptoms with myalgias. Many patients also complain of impaired memory and poor concentration. Symptoms are variable and unaccompanied by objective findings. Fibromyalgia is characterized by pain and stiffness of muscles, ligaments, and tendons. There are local areas of tenderness known as "trigger points." Pain must be present for 3 months and be widespread. Digital palpation must elicit pain in at least 11 of 18 possible tender-point sites. The illness is more common in women. The etiology is unknown, but is often precipitated by stress. There are no pathognomonic laboratory findings, and it is a diagnosis of exclusion. Fibromyalgia is often present in depressive disorders and Chronic Fatigue Syndrome. The patient's symptoms of depression appear to be related primarily to a general medical condition, and so diagnoses of depressive disorder NOS or major depressive disorder would not be warranted at this time.

1. Kaufman DM. *Clinical Neurology for Psychiatrists*. 5th ed. Philadelphia: WB Saunders; 2001:94–100.
2. Sadock BJ, Sadock VA. *Kaplan and Sadock's Synopsis of Psychiatry*. 9th ed. Philadelphia: Lippincott Williams & Wilkins; 2003:837.

51. **Answer: C.** Athetosis, chorea, rigidity, and tremors are all involuntary movements that result from varying disorders of the basal ganglia. Spasticity results from damage to the corticospinal (pyramidal) tract.

Kaufman DM. *Clinical Neurology for Psychiatrists*. 5th ed. Philadelphia: WB Saunders; 2001:14–15.

52. **Answer: C.** Topiramate should not be used in patients taking oral birth-control (OBC). Topiramate is a cytochrome inducer and will reduce the efficacy of OBC. Other medications listed will not reduce the efficacy of OBC. Other anti-epileptic medications that should be avoided when taking OBC include carbamazepine, phenytoin, and phenobarbital.

Kaufman DM. *Clinical Neurology for Psychiatrists*. 5th ed. Philadelphia: WB Saunders; 2001:244.

53. **Answer: E.** This child is around 5 years of age. Children at that age can walk on a narrow line, run easily, and skip on alternate feet. They have a strong grip and can bend to touch their toes without flexing their knees. They can follow rules, like to play with playmates, and can engage in all types of ball games. They can draw a recognizable man, copy a square, and by 5 1/2 years of age, they can copy a triangle. Children younger than 5 years of age are still trying to master their skills in ball games and are not able to walk on a narrow line; they are also not able to copy a square and still have problems with elaborate models. They need more help with dressing and are unable to tie their shoelaces. They enjoy playmates, but they are still unable to follow rules.

Sheridan MB. *From Birth to Five Years. Children's Developmental Progress*. London: Routledge; 1997:1–43.

54. **Answer: B.** A young healthy adult spends about 50% of the sleep period in stage II. Five percent of the sleep period is spent in stage I. Stages III, IV, and REM each comprise approximately 20% to 25% of the sleep period.

Sadock BJ, Sadock VA. *Kaplan and Sadock's Comprehensive Textbook of Psychiatry*. 8th ed. Philadelphia: Lippincott Williams & Wilkins; 2005: 282.

55. **Answer: A.** The brain has two main forms of memory: implicit and explicit. *Implicit memory* is an emotional, behavioral, and perceptual form of memory, which is present from birth and remains active throughout the lifespan. Implicit memory is also known as early, procedural, or nondeclarative memory. It cannot be expressed in words and does not require conscious attention. This form of memory lacks the subjective internal experience of recalling something from the past. An example of implicit memory is riding a bicycle; while riding, one is not aware of recalling the memory of how to ride. Neural circuits hypothesized to be involved in implicit memory include those of the basal ganglia, limbic system, and sensory cortices. *Explicit memory*, also known as late, semantic, or declarative memory, involves a subjective sense of recalling something from the past. Examples of explicit memory are factual and autobiographical information. It may be expressed in words and, as such, may be shared with others. Autobiographical recall requires the maturation of the hippocampus and orbitofrontal cortex, which does not occur until after the first 2 years of life.

Sadock BJ, Sadock VA. *Kaplan and Sadock's Comprehensive Textbook of Psychiatry*. 7th ed. Philadelphia: Lippincott Williams & Wilkins; 2000:389.

56. **Answer: A.** The term *standard deviation* was introduced to statistics by Karl Pearson in 1894. It is defined as the square root of the variance. Standard deviation is the most common measure of statistical dispersion, which measures the spread of the values in a data set when compared to its mean. The mean and the standard deviation are usually reported together. The standard deviation is measured in the same units as the value of the data set. Approximately 95% of the values having a normal distribution are within two standard deviations away from the mean. The standard deviation is the root mean square (RMS) deviation of the values from their arithmetic mean. If the data points are all close to the mean, then the standard deviation is close to zero. If the data points are far from the mean, then the standard deviation is far from zero. If all the data values are equal, then the standard deviation is zero. Standard deviation may also serve as

a measure of uncertainty and the standard deviation of a group of repeated measurements gives the precision of those measurements. In normally distributed data, about 68% of the values are within one standard deviation of the mean, about 95% of the values are within two standard deviations, and about 99.7% lie within three standard deviations. This is known as the "68–95-99.7 rule." For a normal distribution, the two points of the curve, which are one standard deviation from the mean are also the inflection points.

http://en.wikipedia.org/wiki/Standard_deviation. Published September 12, 2006.

57. Answer: C. The Salpetriere Retardation Scale was developed by Daniel Widlocher and his colleagues. It is a scale to measure psychomotor retardation with precision. It includes several symptoms, but lays special stress on all of the following:

1. Reduced spontaneous movements
2. Slumped posture with downcast gaze
3. Tremendous fatigue
4. Reduction in flow and amplitude of speech, increased latency of responses giving rise to monosyllablic speech
5. The feeling that time is slowing down or that time has stopped
6. Reduced concentration and forgetfulness
7. Ruminating on unpleasant topics
8. Indecisiveness

1. Dantchev N, Widlocher DJ. The measurement of retardation in depression. *J Clin Psychiatry*. 1998;59 (suppl 14):19–25.
2. Sadock BJ, Sadock VA. *Kaplan and Sadock's Comprehensive Textbook of Psychiatry*. 8th ed. Philadelphia: Lippincott Williams & Wilkins; 2005:1616.
3. Widlocher DJ. Psychomotor retardation: clinical, theoretical, and psychometric aspects. *Psychiatr Clin North Am*. 1983;6:27–40.

58. Answer: C. According to the DSM-IV-TR, derealization unaccompanied by depersonalization in adults is classified as a Dissociative Disorder NOS. The specific dissociative disorders recognized by the DSM-IV-TR are: Dissociative Amnesia, Dissociative Fugue, Depersonalization Disorder, and Dissociative Identity Disorder. The category of "Dissociative Disorders NOS" includes: clinical presentations similar to dissociative identity disorder in which the criteria for dissociative identity disorder are not met, derealization unaccompanied by depersonalization, dissociative states in persons subjected to prolonged and intensive coercive persuasion (e.g., brainwashing), dissociative trance disorder, including culture-bound syndromes, such as Amok (Indonesia) and Possession (India), loss of consciousness/stupor/coma that cannot be attributed to a general medical condition (due to "nonorganic" causes) and Ganser syndrome.

1. American Psychiatric Association. *Quick Reference to the Diagnostic Criteria from DSM-IV-TR*. Washington: American Psychiatric Association; 2000:239–243.
2. Sadock BJ, Sadock VA. *Kaplan and Sadock's Comprehensive Textbook of Psychiatry*. 8th ed. Philadelphia: Lippincott Williams & Wilkins; 2005:1892–1893.

59. Answer: B. Chronic anxiety symptoms such as panic attacks, startle, hyperarousal, and insomnia are secondary to increased noradrenergic function. Some patients with chronic anxiety report improvement in their symptoms with the use of depressant drugs, such as alcohol, benzodiazepines and opiates, which typically decrease locus ceruleus firing. Different studies have shown elevated plasma norepinephrine (NE) levels in subjects with anxiety disorders, such as PTSD. Some theories speculate that different 5-hydroxytryptamine (5HT/serotonin) receptors may be involved in the development of chronic anxiety, but a clear pattern of abnormal functioning of serotonin receptors has not been established yet.

Sadock BJ, Sadock VA. *Kaplan and Sadock's Comprehensive Textbook of Psychiatry*. 8th ed. Philadelphia: Lippincott Williams & Wilkins; 2005:1740–1743.

60. Answer: B. The most common psychiatric diagnosis in patients with cancer includes adjustment disorders and a Major Depressive Disorder. In a recent study, the prevalence of psychiatric disorders among terminally ill cancer patients was 14% for depression and 14% for adjustment disorders. Another study showed prevalence rates for adjustment disorder of 16% in a similar population. Lower performance status, concern about being a burden to others, and lower satisfaction with social support were significantly associated with the presence of an adjustment disorder. These finding suggests that patients with cancer should have a routine screening for adjustment and affective disorders to improve their quality of life and general care.

1. Akechi T, Okuyama T, Sugawara Y, et al. Major depression, adjustment disorders, and post-traumatic stress disorder in terminally ill cancer patients: associated and predictive factors. *J Clin Oncol*. 2004;22:1957–1965.
2. Kelly BJ, Pelusi D, Burnett PC, et al. The prevalence of psychiatric disorder and the wish to hasten death among terminally ill cancer patients. *Palliat Support Care*. 2004;2:163–169.

61. Answer: B. Phobias are the most common anxiety disorder in the elderly, affecting 3% to 10% of the elderly. GAD is the next most common (3% to 7%) followed by PTSD (2%), Panic Disorder (0.1% to 1%) and OCD (0.6% to 0.8%).

Blazer DG, Steffens DC, Busse EW. *The American Psychiatric Publishing Textbook of Geriatric Psychiatry*. 3rd ed. Washington: American Psychiatric Publishing; 2004:283–293.

62. **Answer: A.** Currently available cholinesterase inhibitors approved for the treatment of Alzheimer's disease include donepezil, galantamine, and rivastigmine. These medications have been shown to improve cognitive performance and activities of daily living in patients with Alzheimer's disease compared to placebo, but do not alter the course of the disease. With progression of the disease, these medications may lose efficacy. All of these medications inhibit acetylcholinesterase; galantamine additionally modulates nicotinic acetylcholine receptors, while rivastigmine also inhibits butyrylcholinesterase. No one medication in this class has been proven to be more efficacious than the others. Gastrointestinal side effects such as nausea, vomiting, and diarrhea are not uncommon with this class of medications and are the main reason these medications require titration. Most side effects are mild and time-limited. Rivastigmine, not donepezil, may be less well-tolerated than the others due to significant GI side effects. Tacrine is associated with hepatic toxicity, not renal failure, and hence is not considered a first-line treatment. Memantine is not a cholinesterase inhibitor, but is an NMDA-receptor antagonist, which is indicated for the treatment of moderate to severe Alzheimer's disease.

Rosenbaum JF, Arana GW, Hyman SE, et al. *Handbook of Psychiatric Drug Therapy*. Philadelphia: Lippincott Williams & Wilkins; 2005:269–275.

63. **Answer: E.** Unlike nicotine replacement treatment, the patient should wait for 2 to 3 weeks before quitting smoking. Bupropion is one of the most effective smoking cessation treatments and might be more effective in combination with nicotine replacement treatment. The mechanism of action in smoking cessation is unknown. It appears to be effective in both depressed and nondepressed patients, and side effects might be less in nondepressed patients.

Rosenbaum JF, Arana GW, Hyman SE, et al. *Handbook of Psychiatric Drug Therapy*: 5th ed. Philadelphia: Lippincott Williams & Wilkins; 2005:240–241.

64. **Answer: D.** Although diarrhea may occur, it is not a common side effect of ECT. Temporary confusion, headaches, muscle aches, and both anterograde and retrograde memory loss are common side effects of ECT.

1. American Psychiatric Association Committee on Electroconvulsive Therapy. *The Practice of Electroconvulsive Therapy: Recommendations for Treatment, Training, and Privileging*. 2nd ed. Washington: American Psychiatric Association; 2001:62–73.
2. Hales RE, Yudofsky SC. *Textbook of Clinical Psychiatry*. 4th ed. Washington: American Psychiatric Publishing; 2003:1125.

65. **Answer: C.** Myoclonus is more typical of serotonin syndrome than of NMS. Each of the other symptoms is typical of NMS, although they may overlap with other syndromes.

Hales RE, Yudofsky SC. *Textbook of Clinical Psychiatry*. 4th ed. Washington: American Psychiatric Publishing; 2003:1091–1092.

66. **Answer: A.** The weight gain associated with lithium ranges from 5 to 15 kg in 20% to 60% of patients who take lithium. Of the three randomized placebo-controlled trials (RCTs) of lithium done as of 2003, in two of these studies, mean weight gain among lithium-treated patients over 1 year was 4 kg and significantly greater than placebo. Two studies reported that most weight gain occurred during the first and second years of treatment and then stabilized. In one RCT that analyzed the use of depakote to treat bipolar disorder, weight gain >5 kg occurred in 21% of the patients receiving depakote and in 7% of patients receiving placebo in one year. In another RCT, mean weight gain was 1 kg per approximately 1 year of follow-up. According to the epilepsy and migraine prophylaxis studies of depakote, 20% to 60% of the patients report weight gain. In two RCTs of carbamazepine in bipolar disorder, mean weight change ranged from 2 kg gain in one study to 3 kg loss in the other one. According to the epilepsy trials, carbamazepine is associated with 2% to 14% average weight gain. Oxcarbazepine and levetiracetam have an improved obesity side effect profile relative to carbamazepine according to epilepsy trials data. In three RCTs that analyzed the use of lamotrigine to treat bipolar disorder, mean weight change ranged from 1 kg gain to 2 kg loss per 0.5 to 1.5 years of follow-up. There are no RCTs of topiramate in bipolar disorder. However, available open-label trials all support mean weight loss of 1 to 6 kg during 1 month to 1 year of follow-up.

1. Aronne LJ, Segal KR. Weight gain in the treatment of mood disorders. *J Clin Psychiatry*. 2003;64 (suppl 8):22–29.
2. Keck PE, McElroy SL. Bipolar disorder, obesity, and pharmacotherapy-associated weight gain. *J Clin Psychiatry*. 2003;64:1426–1435.

3. Sadock BJ, Sadock VA. *Kaplan and Sadock's Comprehensive Textbook of Psychiatry*. 8th ed. Philadelphia: Lippincott Williams & Wilkins; 2005:1673.

67. Answer: B. Approximately 10% of patients with schizophrenia commit suicide. However, a greater number, between 20% and 40%, make at least one attempt over the course of the illness. The risk for suicide remains high over the whole lifespan, but the risk is elevated during postpsychotic periods. Specific risk factors for suicide include male gender, being under 45 years of age, depressive symptoms, feelings of hopelessness, being unemployed, and a recent hospital discharge. Men successfully complete suicide more often than women, but both groups are at increased risk relative to the general population.

American Psychiatric Association. *Diagnostic and Statistical Manual of Mental Disorders American Psychiatric Association*. 4th ed. Washington: American Psychiatric Association; 2000. http://www.psychiatryonline.com/content.aspx?aID=8939. Accessed January 9, 2007.

68. Answer: B. Cerebral cortex is made up of laminated sheets of neurons that cover the cerebral hemispheres. The cortex can be divided into neocortex and allocortex of which the neocortex constitutes 90% of the area. The allocortex can be further subdivided into paleocortex and archicortex which are restricted to the base of telencephalon and hippocampal formation respectively. Pyramidal neurons are the most common type of cortical neurons, constituting about 70% of all neurons in the cortex. Pyramidal neurons are also called stellate neurons and have a single axon that ascends to the cortical surface. Nonpyramidal neurons are small and are involved in local circuits. Most pyramidal cell projections are thought to be excitatory whereas nonpyramidal neurons are considered inhibitory.

Sadock BJ, Sadock VA. *Kaplan and Sadock's Comprehensive Textbook of Psychiatry*. 8th ed. Philadelphia: Lippincott Williams & Wilkins; 2005:10–11.

69. Answer: D. This patient is presenting with a condition known as hemi-spatial neglect or hemi-attention, a condition that usually arises from a lesion/stroke of the nondominant parietal lobe, the underlying thalamus, and reticular activating system. In this condition, patients ignore all stimuli arising from their left side. Unlike patients with homonymous hemianopsia, these patients are unaware of their deficits and do not make any compensatory eye or limb movements to preserve the objects in their visual fields. In the extreme form of this condition called *alien hand syndrome*, the left hand moves by itself and performs simple motor tasks without the awareness of the patient.

1. Kaufman DM. *Clinical Neurology for Psychiatrists*. 5th ed. Philadelphia: WB Saunders; 2001:187–188.
2. Scepkowski LA, Cronin-Golomb A. The alien hand: cases, categorizations, and anatomical correlates. *Behav Cogn Neurosci Rev*. 2003;2:261–277.

70. Answer: E. All of the statements are true. In the late 1980s, CJD infections began to be identified after corneal transplants, treatment with cadaveric human growth hormone, and dura mater grafts, and the number of infections reached its peak in the 1990s. Improved donor screening is partly responsible for the decrease in new cases, and the introduction of recombinant human growth hormone in 1985 was also a major contributor in the decline. The transfusion-related cases of CJD transmission were recent events, however, leading to concerns about future transmission of CJD and also leading to restrictions on blood donor eligibility in the United States for individuals who have spent a significant amount of time in regions where CJD or variant CJD is prevalent.

1. Brown P, Brandel JP, Preece M, et al. Iatrogenic Creutzfeldt-Jakob disease: the waning of an era. *Neurology*. 2006;67:389–393.
2. Brown P, Preece M, Brandel JP, et al. Iatrogenic Creutzfeldt-Jakob disease at the millennium. *Neurology*. 2000;55:1075–1081.
3. http://www.fda.gov/cber/guidelines.htm. Accessed February 18, 2007. ?TeX \vspace*{-1pt}?>

71. Answer: D. Three-per-second spike and wave complexes that arise simultaneously in all leads are pathognomonic for absence seizures. The initiating focus of the seizures is unknown, but theorized to be in the thalamus. Absence seizures are easily provoked by hyperventilation, so the likelihood of capturing a typical EEG is quite high. The presentation of this seizure type is very typical of the previously described scenario with children having school difficulty and frequently "zoning out" until the condition is diagnosed, and often being diagnosed with ADHD, inattentive type, that is not responsive to medication. Hypsarrhythmia is a characteristic EEG finding of a severe type of childhood epilepsy, infantile spasm. Generalized slowing is found in brain insult, such as metabolic disease and anoxic brain injury. A focal ED can indicate the site of a lesion, such as a localized area of scarring or a mass.

Ropper AH, Brown RH. *Adams and Victor's Principles of Neurology*. 8th ed. New York: McGraw-Hill; 2005:334–335.

72. Answer: D. Projective tests are unstructured tests and typically present ambiguous stimuli to tease out qualities such as defenses, needs, and other characteristics. Because of their nature, they are typically not interpreted by reference to a set of correct and incorrect answers. Two important examples of projective test are the Rorschach test, designed by Herman Rorschach, and the Thematic Apperception Test. The MMPI is an objective test.

Kaplan HI, Sadock BJ. *Kaplan & Sadock's Synopsis of Psychiatry*. 8th ed. Philadelphia: Lippincott Williams & Wilkins; 1998:193, 195, 196–199.

73. Answer: A. The lesion in the classic form of Broca's aphasia involves the inferior frontal gyrus, adjacent white matter, the head of the caudate nucleus and putamen, the anterior insula, frontoparietal operculum, and adjacent cerebrum. This implies that the lesion in Broca's aphasia extends well beyond the so-called Broca's area (Brodmann's areas 44 and 45). In these patients, speech is sparse, as it is a motor aphasia. Writing is also impaired with wrong spellings and malformed words and sentences, and writing to dictation is not possible. Dysgraphia is thus present to varying extents. The patient is aware of the deficit, unlike Wernicke's aphasia and is often extremely saddened and frustrated with his condition.

Ropper AH, Brown RH. *Adams & Victor's Principles of Neurology*. 8th ed. New York: McGraw-Hill; 2005:417–419.

74. Answer: D. Carpal tunnel syndrome results from entrapment of the median nerve in the carpal tunnel of the wrist. The median nerve may be injured by repetitive stresses from keyboarding or assembly line work. Carpal tunnel syndrome is common in pregnancy due to fluid retention. It may also occur as a complication of diabetes mellitus, trauma, degenerative arthritis, tenosynovitis, myxedema, or acromegaly. Symptoms are characteristically worse at night and include paresthesias and pain which shoot from the wrist to the palm, thumb, second, third, and the lateral half of the fourth fingers. There may also be pain in the forearm and, in some patients, even in the upper arm, shoulder, and neck. Prolonged median nerve entrapment leads to thenar muscle weakness and atrophy. Deep tendon reflexes (DTRs) are not affected. Upon physical examination, the Tinel's sign may be elicited by percussing the wrist leading to the generation of electric sensations, which shoot into the palm and fingers. The Phalen's maneuver, flexion of the wrist for 1 minute that exacerbates or reproduces symptoms, may be positive. Interdigital neuropathy is an entrapment neuropathy, which leads to pain in one or two fingers. Ulnar nerve dysfunction is characterized by paresthesias, hyperesthesia, and nocturnal pain in the fifth digit and ulnar border of the hand. There can also

be weakness of the deep flexor muscles and intrinsic muscles of the hand. Radial nerve compression affects sensation on the dorsum of the hand; the wrist and thumb extensors; and the brachioradialis reflex. In thoracic outlet syndrome, the C8 or T1 roots may be compressed by a cervical rib. This leads to wasting of the intrinsic hand muscles, especially those in the thenar eminence, accompanied by pain and numbness in the affected dermatomes.

1. Greenberg DA, Aminoff MJ, Simon RP. *Clinical Neurology*. 5th ed. New York: McGraw-Hill; 2002:180, 221–222.
2. Kaufman DM. *Clinical Neurology for Psychiatrists*. 5th ed. Philadelphia: WB Saunders; 2001:70–72.

75. Answer: A. Neuropathy is a common complication of HIV-1. Involvement of peripheral nerves is seen in up to 40% of patients with AIDS at autopsy. Distal symmetric sensorimotor polyneuropathy is the most common neuropathy associated with HIV-1. Axons are affected. Sensory symptoms predominate and include pain and paresthesias in the feet especially. Weakness is a minor feature. Ankle and knee reflexes are absent sometimes. The course is progressive and no treatment is available at this time. Inflammatory demyelinating polyneuropathy is characterized by proximal and sometimes distal weakness, less pronounced sensory deficits, and areflexia or hyporeflexia. Lumbosacral polyradiculopathy occurs late in the illness, usually in patients with prior opportunistic infections. Cytomegalovirus infection is thought to be the cause in many cases. There can be diffuse, progressive leg weakness, back pain, painful paresthesias of the feet, lower extremity areflexia, and urinary retention. Mononeuropathy multiplex affects two or more peripheral and/or cranial nerves. It results in focal weakness and sensory loss. Mononeuropathy simplex involves a single peripheral or cranial nerve.

Greenberg DA, Aminoff MJ, Simon RP. *Clinical Neurology*. 5th ed. New York: McGraw-Hill; 2002: 215–216.

76. Answer: C. Muscle disorders in general are characterized by proximal weakness or paresis. The muscles themselves are sometimes tender or dystrophic. DTRs are normal or hypoactive. The Babinski reflex is negative, and there is typically no sensory loss. Chromosomal DNA is derived equally from both parents, while mitochondrial DNA is ring-shaped and derived entirely from the mother. Mitochondrial DNA abnormalities produce mitochondrial myopathies. These disorders are maternally inherited and involve combinations of impaired muscle metabolism, abnormal lipid storage, and brain damage. There are usually numerous misshapen mitochondria present. They may be filled with ragged red fibers. The disorder described in the vignette is mitochondrial myopathy, encephalopy, lactic acidosis, and stroke-like episodes (MELAS). Patients have normal early development, followed by poor growth, focal or generalized seizures, and recurrent acute episodes which resemble strokes or prolonged transient ischemic attacks. Stroke deficits improve, but can lead to progressive encephalopathy. Patients also suffer from episodic lactic acidosis and repetitive vomiting. Some have hemicranial headaches. Focal seizures often herald a stroke. Most patients have ragged red fibers, but weakness and exercise intolerance are not typical features. Other mitochondrial myopathies include: progressive external ophthalmoplegia (PEO); Leigh disease (subacute necrotizing encephalomyelopathy); neuropathy, ataxia, retinitis pigmentosa syndrome (NARP); and myoclonic epilepsy with ragged red fiber myopathy (MERRF).

1. Kaufman DM. *Clinical Neurology for Psychiatrists*. 5th ed. Philadelphia: WB Saunders; 2001:94–107.
2. Ropper AH, Brown RH. *Adams and Victor's Principles of Neurology*. 8th ed. New York: McGraw-Hill; 2005:841–845.

77. Answer: A. Patients with Parkinson's disease typically present with bradykinesia, facial akinesia, rigidity, gait impairment, and a tremor at rest. Dementia can occur in patients with Parkinson's disease, but this is typically a later finding.

Kaufman DM. *Clinical Neurology for Psychiatrists*. 5th ed. Philadelphia: WB Saunders; 2001:447–448.

78. Answer: B. Psychotropic medications can potentially confound EEG results mostly intermittent or continuous background slowing with theta or even delta activity. In particular, benzodiazepines and barbiturates produce beta waves. Phenothiazines and tricyclic antidepressants (at therapeutic doses) and lithium (at toxic doses) produce spikes and sharp waves.

Kaufman DM. *Clinical Neurology for Psychiatrists*. 5th ed. Philadelphia: WB Saunders; 2001: 232.

79. Answer: C. Approximately 30% of children report being victims of being bullied at some point in their lives, and around 5% to 10% are bullied on a regular basis. Being bullied has been associated with anxiety, depression, and low self-esteem. The most negative outcome seems to be present in children who felt little or no social support during the time when they were being bullied. Bullying is more prevalent with younger children, although it frequently prevails until adolescence. Among elementary school-age children, those who are psychologically distressed are prone to engage in some form of bullying, whereas those who have academic problems tend to be more often victims of being bullied.

1. Anonymous. Bullying among elementary school children. *Child Health Alert*. 2006;24:1–2.
2. Newman ML, Holden GW, von Delville Y. Isolation and the stress of being bullied. *J Adolesc*. 2005;28:343–357.

80. Answer: C. Dopamine receptors are divided into two subclasses (type 1 and type 2). Type 1 receptors (D1 and D5) act through an increase in the intracellular cAMP production causing excitatory input, whereas type 2 receptors (D2, D3, and D4) act through a decrease in cAMP production causing inhibitory input.

Sadock BJ, Sadock VA. *Kaplan and Sadock's Comprehensive Textbook of Psychiatry*. 8th ed. Philadelphia: Lippincott Williams & Wilkins; 2005:313.

81. Answer: B. Freud's topographical model of the mind divides the mind into three regions: the conscious, the unconscious, and the preconscious. (It is Freud's structural model of the mind that divides the psyche into the id, the ego, and the superego.) The conscious system is the part of the mind in which internal or external perceptions are brought into conscious awareness. The unconscious system holds primitive wishes and desires seeking fulfillment, which are kept from conscious awareness. The preconscious region of the mind interfaces with the conscious and the unconscious. It is the preconscious which can deliberately bring that which is unconscious into conscious awareness. Alternately, the preconscious has the ability to repress and censor those unconscious wishes/desires which are deemed unacceptable. Topographic theory assumes that neurotic symptoms are the result of these unconscious psychological conflicts. Freud elaborated on his topographic model of the mind in the 1900s in *Interpretation of Dreams*.

Sadock BJ, Sadock VA. *Kaplan and Sadock's Comprehensive Textbook of Psychiatry*. 7th ed. Philadelphia: Lippincott Williams & Wilkins; 2000:572.

82. Answer: C. Confidence interval gives a measure of precision or uncertainty of the study results, for making any inference about the population under study. A correct CI will contain the true population value and it places an emphasis on the quantification of the effect. The CI is based on the idea that the same study carried out on different samples of patients would not yield identical results, but the results would be spread around the true but unknown value. Confidence intervals are usually calculated so that this percentage is 95%, but this is arbitrary and results can be generated with 90%, 99%, and 99.9% confidence intervals for the unknown parameter. The wider the confidence interval, the less precise we are about the unknown parameter. A very wide interval may indicate that more data needs to be collected before a definite inference can be made about the parameter. Confidence intervals are more informative than hypothesis tests (P value), because they provide a range of plausible values for the unknown parameter. Confidence limits are the lower and upper values that define the range of a confidence interval. The major drawback of CI is that it is not designed to incorporate the impact of losses to follow, poor compliance to treatments, imprecise outcome measures, and the lack of blinding.

1. Strauss SE, Richardson WS, Glasziou P, et al. *Evidence-Based Medicine. How to Practice and Teach EBM*. 3rd ed. Edinburgh: Elsevier Churchill Livingstone; 2005: 263–277.
2. http://www.cas.lancs.ac.uk/glossary_v1.1/confint.html#confinterval. Accessed September 13, 2006.

83. Answer: C. Akathisia is characterized by subjective complaints (feeling of inner restlessness or agitation), and objective symptoms (fidgety movements, marching, pacing, shifting weight from one foot to the other). In pseudoakathisia, the subjective inner restlessness/agitation is absent, however the movements typical of akathisia are seen. Barnes Akathisia Rating Scale (BARS) is commonly used to rate akathisia.

1. Havaki-Kontaxaki BJ, Kontaxakis VP, Christodoulou GN. Prevalence and characteristics of patients with pseudoakathisia. *Eur Neuropsychopharmacol.* 2000;10:333–336.
2. Mattoo SK, Singh G, Vikas A. Akathisia–diagnostic dilemma and behavioral treatment. *Neurol India.* 2003;51:254–256.
3. Rapoport A, Stein D, Grinshpoon A, et al. Akathisia and pseudoakathisia: clinical observations and accelerometric recordings. *J Clin Psychiatry.* 1994 Nov;55(11):473–477.

84. Answer: E. Visual and auditory hallucinations are seen in nearly 50% of the cases of Ganser syndrome. In DSM-III, the classification of Ganser syndrome changed from that of a factitious disorder to a dissociative disorder. It is primarily characterized by clouding of consciousness and paralogia, which means giving approximate answers. Vorbeireden is the name given to the symptom of "passing over" the correct answer, but giving a related but incorrect answer. As conversion and somatoform symptoms are commonly associated, neurological examination can reveal "hysterical stigmata" (a phrase coined by Ganser himself), referring to non-neurological analgesia or shifting hyperalgesia.

1. American Psychiatric Association. *Quick Reference to the Diagnostic Criteria from DSM-IV-TR.* Washington: American Psychiatric Association; 2000:243.
2. Andersen HS, Sestoft D, Lillebaek T. Ganser syndrome after solitary confinement in prison: a short review and a case report. *Nord J Psychiatry.* 2001;55:199–201.
3. Sadock BJ, Sadock VA. *Kaplan and Sadock's Comprehensive Textbook of Psychiatry.* 8th ed. Philadelphia: Lippincott Williams & Wilkins; 2005:1897.

85. Answer: C. Few studies have been published that evaluate the presence of both risk and prognostic factors in OCD. A recent meta-analysis found that comorbid psychiatric illness was a predictor of severity, persistence, and lower global functioning in patients with OCD. Earlier age at onset, previous inpatient admissions, and longer OCD duration at ascertainment were predictive of longer persistence of OCD symptoms. On the other hand, gender and age at diagnosis were not found to be predictive factors in OCD.

Stewart SE, Geller DA, Jenike M, et al. Long-term outcome of pediatric obsessive-compulsive disorders: a meta-analysis and qualitative review of the literature. *Acta Psychiatr Scand.* 2005;8:6.

86. Answer: B. Unlike Major Depressive Disorder, which affects more women than men, Mood Disorder due to a General Medical Condition seems to affect men and women equally. Nearly half of all post-stroke patients develop depressive illness. Patients with terminal illness and depression have the highest risk of suicide.

Sadock BJ, Sadock VA. *Kaplan and Sadock's Comprehensive Textbook of Psychiatry.* 8th ed. Philadelphia: Lippincott Williams & Wilkins; 2005:1120.

87. Answer: E. All of the statements are true. The most common current co-morbid anxiety disorders with depression in the elderly are GAD (27.5%), Panic Disorder (9.3%), Specific Phobia (8.8%), and Social Phobia (6.6%).

1. Blazer DG, Steffens DC, Busse EW. *The American Psychiatric Publishing Textbook of Geriatric Psychiatry.* 3rd ed. Washington: American Psychiatric Publishing; 2004:283–293.
2. Lenze EJ. Comorbidity of depression and anxiety in the elderly. *Curr Psychiatry Rep.* 2003;5:62–67.

88. Answer: D. Use of lithium during the first trimester is associated with an increased risk of a fetus' developing Ebstein's anomaly. Given that the occurrence of Ebstein's anomaly is estimated at 1 in 2,000 exposures to lithium, lithium use alone does not clearly indicate a need to terminate a pregnancy. Because of the teratogenic risks of mood stabilizers, ECT is generally the first-line treatment for severe manic episodes. Lithium is secreted in breast milk; hence, it is recommended that women who take lithium refrain from breastfeeding. Despite the risks, continued lithium use, after a weighing of costs and benefits, may still be an option for some women during pregnancy.

Rosenbaum JF, Arana GW, Hyman SE, et al. *Handbook of Psychiatric Drug Therapy*. 5th ed. Philadelphia: Lippincott Williams & Wilkins; 2005:138–139.

89. Answer: B. History of myocardial infarction is not a relative contraindication for the use of methadone. Additional relative contraindications are asthma, respiratory depression, hypercapnia, hypoxia, concurrent use of drugs with alpha 1 blockade or CNS depressants, or traumatic brain injury.

Rosenbaum JF, Arana GW, Hyman SE, et al. *Handbook of Psychiatric Drug Therapy*. 5th ed. Philadelphia: Lippincott Williams & Wilkins; 2005:208–210.

90. Answer: C. Acute catatonic symptoms may be a particularly favorable sign for response to ECT. Pharmacotherapy refractory patients are often referred for ECT and do not have a more favorable prognosis, but perhaps a less favorable one. Severe personality disorders are neither an indication nor a good prognostic sign for ECT. Nonresponse to prior ECT trials is not a favorable prognostic sign. Depression due to a general medical condition responds less well to ECT than do primary depressions.

1. American Psychiatric Association Committee on Electroconvulsive Therapy. *The Practice of Electroconvulsive Therapy: Recommendations for Treatment, Training, and Privileging*. 2nd ed. Washington: American Psychiatric Association; 2001:13.
2. Coffey CE. *The Clinical Science of Electroconvulsive Therapy*. Washington American Psychiatric Press; 1993:53–71.
3. Hales RE, Yudofsky SC. *Textbook of Clinical Psychiatry*. 4th ed. Washington: American Psychiatric Publishing; 2003:1123–1124.

91. Answer: A. This patient most likely has NMS. Treatments includes medical admission, often to the intensive care unit (ICU), close monitoring of vital signs and laboratories, and symptomatic treatment with fluids, antipyretics, and/or cooling blankets. Elevated creatinine phosphokinase may lead to renal failure. Both dantrolene and bromocriptine have been studied in NMS, and the risk:benefit ratio may favor a trial. Discontinuation of medications, especially potentially offending antipsychotics, should be routine treatment. Choosing to simply prescribe antibiotics could result in missing a potentially lethal diagnosis of NMS.

1. Hales RE, Yudofsky SC. *Textbook of Clinical Psychiatry*. 4th ed. Washington: American Psychiatric Publishing; 2003: 1091–1092.

92. Answer: B. Although phototherapy is the main thrust of treatment in patients with seasonal affective disorder, there is increasing interest in psychopharmacologic intervention. There are studies suggesting that bupropion has superior efficacy versus a placebo. The relative rate of prevention for patients taking bupropion was 40% versus a placebo. The Food and Drug Administration recently approved bupropion (Wellbutrin XL) for the treatment of SAD.

1. http://www.fda.gov/bbs/topics/NEWS/2006/NEW01388.html. Accessed on November 21, 2006.
2. Modell JG, Rosenthal NE, Harriett AE et al. Seasonal affective disorder and its prevention by anticipatory treatment with bupropion XL. *Biol Psychiatry*. 2005;58:658–667.

93. Answer: A. Male not female gender is a specific risk factor for suicide. Approximately 10% of patients with schizophrenia commit suicide with greater numbers (i.e., 20% to 40%) making at least one attempt over the course of the illness. The risk for suicide remains high over the whole lifespan, but risk is elevated during postpsychotic periods. Specific risk factors for suicide include male gender, being under 45 years of age, depressive symptoms, feelings of hopelessness, being unemployed, and a recent hospital discharge. Men successfully complete suicide more often than women, but both groups are at increased risk relative to the general population.

American Psychiatric Association. *Diagnostic and Statistical Manual of Mental Disorders American Psychiatric Association*. 4th ed. Washington: American Psychiatric Association; 2000. http://www.psychiatryonline.com/content.aspx?aID=8939. Accessed on January 9, 2007.

94. Answer: D. The basal ganglia consists of nuclei that are grouped together on the basis of their interconnections. These nuclei play an important role in regulating movement and muscle tone. Disruptions to the pathways of the basal ganglia result in dyskinesias, which include jerky chorea (jerky movements), athetosis (writhing movements), tremors (rhythmic movements), muscular rigidity, shuffling gait, and bradykinesia. Hypotonia is usually produced by cerebellar lesions, lower motor neuron lesions, and lesions of the neuromuscular junctions.

1. Kaufman DM. *Clinical Neurology for Psychiatrists*. 5th ed. Philadelphia: WB Saunders; 2001:8–9, 16–25.

2. Sadock BJ, Sadock VA. *Kaplan and Sadock's Comprehensive Textbook of Psychiatry.* 8th ed. Philadelphia: Lippincott Williams & Wilkins; 2005:23–27.

95. Answer: D. Homonymous hemianopia results from a retrochiasmal lesion. This gentleman has left homonymous hemianopsia, which is usually produced by a lesion of right (contralateral) occipital lobe. It can present with or without macular sparing. Other associated deficits can include left hemiattention and anosognosia.

1. Kaufman DM. *Clinical Neurology for Psychiatrists.* 5th ed. Philadelphia: WB Saunders; 2001:303.
2. Rowland LP. *Merritt's Neurology.* 11th ed. Philadelphia: Lippincott Williams & Wilkins; 2005:41–42, 404.

96. Answer: B. Night terrors, or sleep terrors, are a non-REM associated parasomnia that has a peak incidence in children 4 to 10 years of age, but adult onset can occur. Episodes typically occur in the first third of the night during stage 3 or 4 sleep and are not associated with dreaming. In severe episodes, the individual may try to get out of bed or leave the room. The child is not responsive, and is inconsolable, and efforts to console the child may prolong the episode. Amnesia for the event the next day is the norm. Episodes decrease in frequency and severity with age, and are usually gone by adolescence. If the episodes are very severe, disruptive to the family, or injury has occurred, treatment including rigorous maintenance of good sleep hygiene and behavioral strategies, as well as pharmacologic management with imipramine, diazepam, or clonazepam may be indicated.

Goetz CG. *Textbook of Clinical Neurology.* 2nd ed. Philadelphia: WB Saunders; 2003:1220.

97. Answer: C. Magnetic resonance angiography (MRA) is a noninvasive tool that can detect aneurysms before rupture. The sensitivity of MRA to detect aneurysms 5 mm or greater in size is approximately 90%. The gold standard for detection of aneurysms is still traditional angiography, particularly for preoperative planning, but MRA provides a useful noninvasive screening tool.

Goetz CG. *Textbook of Clinical Neurology.* 2nd ed. Philadelphia: WB Saunders; 2003:432–457.

98. Answer: E. IQ = mental age/chronological age × 100. Borderline intelligence occurs when IQ is between 70 and 79, and mental retardation occurs below that. It is the case that 2.2% of the population has an IQ of less than 70. Superior intelligence is an IQ of 120 to 130.

1. Kaplan HI, Sadock BJ. *Kaplan & Sadock's Synopsis of Psychiatry.* 8th ed. Philadelphia: Lippincott Williams & Wilkins; 1998:193–195.

2. *Quick Reference to the Diagnostic Criteria from DSM-IV-TR.*™ Washington DC: American Psychiatric Association; 2000:52.

99. Answer: B. Cerebral mucormycosis is caused by the fungus rhizopus, which belongs to the phycomycetes class. It is observed clinically in immunosuppression, diabetes mellitus, or a blood dyscrasia. In the clinical vignette outlined previously, the patient has two risk factors: diabetes mellitus and use of corticosteroids postrenal transplant surgery. She develops sinusitis, and through the orbital walls and venous channels, the infection spreads to the orbit, resulting in orbital cellulitis. This then extends to the internal carotid artery through penetration, resulting in proptosis and hemiplegia. Cryptococcal infection usually presents as subacute meningitis or encephalitis. Myiasis is the infestation of tissue with fly larvae (maggots). Cerebral myiasis is extremely rare, and there have only been a few isolated case reports. Candidal CNS infection presents as meningitis and not as the picture outlined previously. Aspergillosis is a diagnostic possibility given the vascular penetration, and the setting of renal transplant. However, it is less likely in the previous clinical scenario than mucormycosis.

1. Georgiev VS. *Opportunistic Infections: Treatment and Prophylaxis.* Totowa: Humana Press; 2003.
2. Rowland LP. *Merritt's Neurology.* 11th ed. Philadelphia: Lippincott Williams & Wilkins; 2005:229–231.

100. Answer: B. The patient's current symptoms are consistent with left radial neuropathy. She also has a history of carpal tunnel syndrome and foot drop. Her course is suggestive of mononeuropathy multiplex. In this disorder, several individual nerves are affected usually at random and at different points in time. It is typically the result of systemic illnesses such as diabetes mellitus, vasculitis (systemic lupus erythematosus or polyarteritis), lead toxicity, or leprosy. Mononeuropathy simplex signifies the involvement of a single peripheral nerve. Polyneuropathy denotes a disorder in which the function of numerous peripheral nerves is affected at the same time. In most polyneuropathies, the axon is the principle pathologic target, although some, such as acute idiopathic polyneuropathy (Guillain-Barré syndrome), may involve the myelin sheath surrounding the axon. Guillain-Barré syndrome is characterized by ascending symmetric weakness beginning in the legs, which can become life-threatening if the muscles of respiration or swallowing become involved. Last, a third type of polyneuropathy, neuronopathy, principally affects nerve cell bodies in the anterior horn of the spinal cord or dorsal root ganglion is seen with Type 2 Charcot-Marie-Tooth hereditary motor and sensory neuropathy is an example. Amyotrophic lateral sclerosis is a motor neuron disease involving both upper and lower motor neurons.

1. Greenberg DA, Aminoff MJ, Simon RP. *Clinical Neurology*. 5th ed. New York: McGraw-Hill; 2002:180, 208–213.
2. Kaufman DM. *Clinical Neurology for Psychiatrists*. 5th ed. Philadelphia: WB Saunders; 2001:72, 79.

101. **Answer: A.** This boy has Duchenne's dystrophy, an X-linked recessive disorder where symptoms begin by the age of 5 years. Patients are often disabled by adolescence with death occurring in the third decade. Early symptoms include impaired toe walking, waddling gait, and inability to run. Weakness is pronounced in the proximal lower extremities. Patients with this disorder may be incapable of rising from a supine position without using their arms to climb up their body, called the Gower's sign. Pseudohypertrophy of the calves caused by fatty infiltration of muscle occurs commonly. The genetic defect responsible for Duchenne's dystrophy is located on the short arm of the X chromosome. It codes for the protein dystrophin, which is absent or reduced in the muscle of patients with this disorder. Myotonic dystrophy type 1 is dominantly inherited and caused by an CTG repeat. There is weakness and wasting of the facial, sternomastoid, and distal limb muscles. Patients may have cataracts, frontal baldness, testicular atrophy, diabetes mellitus, cardiac abnormalities, and intellectual changes. The disorder usually becomes apparent in the third or fourth decade. Myotonia congenita (Thomsen's disease) is inherited as a dominant trait that relates to a mutation on chromosome 7q35. Symptoms may not develop until early childhood. Muscle stiffness is enhanced by cold and inactivity and relieved by exercise. Muscle hypertrophy also occurs. Inclusion body myositis is more common in men. It has an insidious onset and usually begins after age 50. There is painless proximal weakness of the lower and then the upper extremities. The course is progressive. The etiology suggests T-cell mediated myocytotoxicity and multifactorial genetic susceptibility. Finally, heavy binge drinking may result in an acute necrotizing myopathy that develops over 1 to 2 days. Symptoms include muscle pain, weakness, and occasionally dysphagia. Weakness is proximal and may be asymmetric or focal. Because hypokalemia and hypophosphatemia can produce similar symptoms, they should be ruled out in the differential diagnosis.

Greenberg DA, Aminoff MJ, Simon RP. *Clinical Neurology*. 5th ed. New York: McGraw-Hill; 2002:187–194.

102. **Answer: A.** Nitrous oxide is often abused to produce periods of brief euphoria. Its abuse is an occupational hazard for dentists. Nurses are also subject to the risk of nitrous oxide neurotoxicity. It is also available as the gas in cartridges used to make whipped cream at home. Its inhalation may produce a neuropathy, and even brief exposures to nitrous oxide can cause vitamin B_{12} deficiency. A deficiency of thiamine, vitamin B_1, is responsible for Wernicke-Korsakoff syndrome. It is characterized by amnesia, dementia, and cerebellar degeneration. Pellagra is caused by niacin deficiency. It is characterized by dementia, diarrhea, and dermatitis. Solvent-induced encephalopathy is caused by industrial solvents such as ethylene oxide and carbon disulfide. These solvents can affect both the peripheral nervous system (PNS) and the CNS. Symptoms include cognitive impairment, personality changes, inattention, depression, headaches, and fatigue. Acute intermittent porphyria is an autosomal dominant genetic disorder of porphyrin metabolism. Patients develop attacks of colicky abdominal pain, psychosis, and quadriparesis. During an acute attack, the urine turns red because it contains porphyrins.

1. Kaufman DM. *Clinical Neurology for Psychiatrists*. 5th ed. Philadelphia: WB Saunders; 2001:77–79.
2. Ropper AH, Brown RH. *Adams and Victor's Principles of Neurology*. 8th ed. New York: McGraw-Hill; 2005:1132–1133.

103. **Answer: D.** Lewy bodies are eosinophilic intracytoplasmic neuronal inclusions that are seen in brain autopsy results of patients suffering from Parkinson's disease. Beta amyloid plaques, neurofibrillary tangles and tau proteins are typical autopsy findings in brain specimens taken from patients with Alzheimer's disease but also may be seen in other disorders. Copper deposition is characteristic of Wilson's disease.

Beers MH, Berkow R. *The Merck Manual of Diagnosis and Therapy*. 17th ed. New Jersey: Merck & Co; 1999:1395–1399.

104. **Answer: A.** Phenytoin will decrease methadone level in the blood and precipitate severe opioid withdrawal symptoms. In patients on methadone who are inadvertently started on phenytoin and experience opiate withdrawal, doubling the methadone dose can be done to attenuate the withdrawal symptoms. However, it is best to avoid the use of phenytoin in patients on methadone maintenance.

Kaufman DM. *Clinical Neurology for Psychiatrists*. 5th ed. Philadelphia: WB Saunders; 2001:260.

105. Answer: D. The child has separation anxiety disorder. This disorder involves persistent problems attending activities away from home because of fear of separation. This fear usually causes significant interference with activities of daily living (such as going to school). The onset is before 18 years, and it has a minimal duration of 4 weeks. Peak age at onset is 7 to 9 years of age. It can have an acute or insidious onset and it can be precipitated by a major life event. This child might have an underlying gastrointestinal condition that needs to be ruled out; however, the clinical picture and the fact that his symptoms are worse on school days make separation anxiety disorder a most likely diagnosis. Generalized Anxiety Disorder is characterized by excessive anxiety and worry for at least 6 months about a number of events or activities. Acute Stress Disorder is the development of anxiety and dissociative symptoms that occurs within 1 month after exposure to an extreme traumatic event. Panic Attacks are discrete periods of intense fear or discomfort in the absence of real danger that is accompanied by somatic symptoms.

1. American Psychiatric Association. *Quick Reference to the Diagnostic Criteria from DSM-IV-TR*. Washington: American Psychiatric Association; 2000:76–77.
2. Hanna GL, Fischer DJ, Fluent TE. Separation anxiety disorder and school refusal in children and adolescents. *Pediatr Rev.* 2006;27:56–63.

106. Answer: D. Sleep in older adulthood is characterized by prolonged latency to sleep onset and increased sleep arousals. Newborn infants spend 16 to 18 hours per day asleep with short sleep-wake cycles of 3 to 4 hours. Young children have the highest percentage of slow wave sleep (stages III and IV), which makes them difficult to arouse at the beginning of the sleep period.

Sadock BJ, Sadock VA. *Kaplan and Sadock's Comprehensive Textbook of Psychiatry*. 8th ed. Philadelphia: Lippincott Williams & Wilkins; 2005:283.

107. Answer: E. Freud classified defenses according to severity of psychopathology. According to him, *mature* defense mechanisms include humor, suppression, sublimation, and altruism. *Humor* involves the use of comedy to express feelings in a way that avoids distressing self or others. *Suppression* is a defense whereby attention to painful feelings is temporarily postponed, but not avoided. *Sublimation* is a mature defense mechanism which refers to gratifying one's impulses and instincts by acknowledging them, modifying them, and directing them toward socially acceptable channels. *Altruism* involves the use of service toward others to undergo a vicarious experience which is internally gratifying. Rationalization is a neurotic defense in which one utilizes rational explanations to justify attitudes or behaviors which may be considered to be unacceptable.

Sadock BJ, Sadock VA. *Kaplan and Sadock's Comprehensive Textbook of Psychiatry*. 7th ed. Philadelphia: Lippincott Williams & Wilkins; 2000:582–585.

108. Answer: A. The sensitivity refers to the proportion of patients with the disease (as assessed by the gold standard), who are detected by the diagnostic test as having the disease. A highly sensitive test detects most cases of the disease. In this case the possible results of the diagnostic test can be represented in the following 2 × 2 table.

Test result outcome	Disease present	Disease absent	Total
Positive	999	1	1,000
Negative	1	999	1,000
Total	1,000	1,000	

Sensitivity of the test would be the number of true positives (patients who have the disease and are tested positive) divided by the total number of patients with the disease. In this case, it would be 999/1000; 99.9%.

1. Gray GE. *Evidence-Based Psychiatry*. Washington: American Psychiatric Publishing; 2004:123–125.
2. http://www.musc.edu/dc/icrebm/sensitivity.html. Accessed on September 16, 2006.

109. Answer: D. Except for BDI, all of the other rating scales are administered by a clinician. The BDI was created by Dr. Aaron T. Beck as a 21-question multiple choice self-report inventory and is one of the most widely used instruments for measuring the severity of depression. The questionnaire is designed for adults aged 17 to 80 years. It takes a few minutes to complete. The original BDI consists of 21 questions about how the subject has been feeling in the last week. Each question has a set of at least four possible answer choices that range in intensity. The test is scored on a scale of 0 to 3 for each answer, and then the total score is compared to a key to determine the depression's severity. The standard cut-offs are: 0 to 9 indicates that a person is not depressed, 10 to 18 indicates mild-moderate depression, 19 to 29 indicates moderate-severe depression, and 30 to 63 indicates severe depression. Higher total scores indicate more severe depressive symptoms. Limitations of BDI include the subjective nature of reporting symptoms where the symptoms can be exaggerated or minimized by the person completing the inventory, and the reliance on physical symptoms, such as fatigue, that might artificially inflate scores due to symptoms of a physical illness rather than of depression.

1. Sadock BJ, Sadock VA. *Kaplan and Sadock's Comprehensive Textbook of Psychiatry*. 8th ed. Philadelphia: Lippincott Williams & Wilkins; 2005:929–959.
2. http://en.wikipedia.org/wiki/Beck_Depression_Inventory. Accessed December 19, 2006.

110. Answer: C. "Made feelings from alter identity" is a Dissociative Identity Disorder process symptom. The rest of the choices indicate autohypnotic symptoms of Dissociative Identity Disorder.

Sadock BJ, Sadock VA. *Kaplan and Sadock's Comprehensive Textbook of Psychiatry*. 8th ed. Philadelphia: Lippincott Williams & Wilkins; 2005:1879.

111. Answer: D. Patients with pediatric autoimmune neuropsychiatric disorders associated with streptococcal infection (PANDAS) usually have an abrupt onset of symptoms followed by dramatic exacerbations that are related to infection with group A B-hemolytic streptococcus. Age of onset is usually between 3 years of age and puberty, and patients have an abnormal neurological exam (hyperactivity, choreiform movements, tics). PANDAS are believed to be caused by an autoimmune process similar to the one seen in Sydenham's chorea and rheumatic fever. Autoimmune activation should lead to inflammation of basal ganglia and disruption of cortical-striato and thalamo-cortical functions. Some studies also suggest that antineuronal antibodies might be involved in the development of PANDAS.

1. Kurlan R, Kaplan EL. The pediatric autoimmune neuropsychiatric disorders associated with streptococcal infection (PANDAS) etiology for tics and obsessive-compulsive symptoms: hypothesis or entity? Practical considerations for the clinician. *Pediatrics*. 2004;113:883–886.
2. Sadock BJ, Sadock VA. *Kaplan and Sadock's Comprehensive Textbook of Psychiatry*. 8th ed. Philadelphia: Lippincott Williams & Wilkins; 2005:3280–3285.
3. Snider LA, Swedo SE. PANDAS: current status and directions for research. *Mol Psychiatry*. 2004;9:900–907.

112. Answer: C. This patient likely has a mood disorder with depressive features due to hypothyroidism. The next step in her management would be to confirm the diagnosis with thyroid studies and initiate hormone replacement. A temporal relationship between the onsets of mood symptoms and medical symptoms is common in mood disorders due to a medical condition. The prognosis for mood symptoms is best when the underlying medical condition is treated. If the patient's symptoms do not improve with thyroid hormone replacement, formal psychiatric treatment is recommended.

Sadock BJ, Sadock VA. *Kaplan and Sadock's Comprehensive Textbook of Psychiatry*. 8th ed. Philadelphia: Lippincott Williams & Wilkins; 2005:1122.

113. Answer: C. Impaired attention is indicative of a delirium rather than a dementia. Other features that distinguish delirium from a dementia include all of the following: abrupt onset, brief duration, reduced consciousness, incoherent or disorganized speech, and a fluctuating course.

1. American Psychiatric Association. *Quick Reference to the Diagnostic Criteria from DSM-IV-TR*. Washington: American Psychiatric Association; 2000:83–98.
2. Hanley C. Delirium in the acute care setting. *Medsurg Nurs*. 2004;13:217–225.

114. Answer: C. Psoriasis can be a side effect of lithium treatment and often is resistant to treatment, but often improves when lithium is stopped. Although some patients with pre-existing psoriasis have a worsening of their condition, not all do, and pre-existing psoriasis is not an absolute contraindication to lithium use.

1. Kasper DL, Fauci AS, Longo DL, et al. *Harrison's Principles of Internal Medicine*. 16th ed. New York: McGraw-Hill; 2005:292.
2. Rosenbaum JF, Arana GW, Hyman SE, et al. *Handbook of Psychiatric Drug Therapy*. 5th ed. Philadelphia: Lippincott Williams & Wilkins; 2005:146.

115. Answer: A. Benzodiazepines are the mainstay of alcohol withdrawal treatment. Virtually any benzodiazepine can be safely used, but the different properties of each necessitate knowledge of the individual pharmacology of each. Lorazepam has a half-life of 10 to 20 hours, but can be dosed every 2 to 6 hours for acute withdrawal. There are no active metabolites for lorazepam. Diazepam, on the other hand, has a half-life of up to several days, and has an active metabolite with an even longer half-life. Lorazepam's advantages include this short half-life, no active metabolites, and being safe in hepatic impairment. It should be used when finer control is needed. Disadvantages are a more varied symptom presentation, as there can be re-emergence of symptoms as the plasma concentration drops below a therapeutic level. Diazepam, with its longer half-life, provides a longer, slower taper with less fluctuation in plasma concentration. The disadvantages include the potential build up of metabolites with aggressive dosing, leading to excessive sedation and cognitive impairment, which can be difficult to distinguish from withdrawal symptoms and delirium.

Rosenbaum JF, Arana GW, Hyman SE, et al. *Handbook of Psychiatric Drug Therapy*. 5th ed. Philadelphia: Lippincott Williams & Wilkins; 2005:219–220.

116. **Answer: E.** Potential major medical complications of ECT include: transient neurological deficits, arrhythmias, myocardial infarctions, prolonged seizures, status epilepticus, and prolonged apneas from anesthesia. Another serious major complication is patient recall of a failed seizure attempt.

1. Abrams R. *Electroconvulsive Therapy*. 4th ed. New York: Oxford University Press; 2002:161–169.
2. American Psychiatric Association Committee on Electroconvulsive Therapy. *The Practice of Electroconvulsive Therapy: Recommendations for Treatment, Training, and Privileging*. 2nd ed. Washington: American Psychiatric Association; 2001:59–74.

117. **Answer: C.** Modafinil (Provigil) is a wake-promoting agent with an unclear mechanism of action. Amphetamines stimulate the release of catecholamines (including dopamine) from presynaptic neurons. Cocaine and methylphenidate block dopamine reuptake at the synaptic cleft. Bupropion works largely via affecting dopamine function.

Sadock BJ, Sadock VA. *Kaplan & Sadock's Comprehensive Textbook of Psychiatry*. 7th ed. Philadelphia: Lippincott Williams & Wilkins; 2000:973–974.

118. **Answer: B.** Methadone is not only a potent opioid-receptor agonist, but it can also block both NMDA receptors and monoaminergic reuptake transporters. These properties help explain its ability to relieve neuropathic and cancer pain especially when a previous trial of morphine has failed. When tolerance or intolerable side effects have developed with the use of higher doses of morphine or hydromorphone, "opioid rotation" to methadone has provided superior analgesia at 10% to 20% of the morphine-equivalent daily dose. Using methadone as an analgesic agent requires administration at intervals of no more than 8 hours. However, given its highly variable pharmacokinetics and long half-life (25 to 52 hours), the initial administration should be closely monitored to avoid respiratory depression. Methadone is used in the treatment of opioid dependence. Tolerance and physical dependence usually develop more slowly with methadone than with morphine. Withdrawal signs and symptoms occurring after the abrupt discontinuance of methadone are milder, but more prolonged than those of morphine. These properties make methadone a useful drug for detoxification and for maintenance of the chronic relapsing heroin addict.

Katzung BG. *Basic and Clinical Pharmacology*. 10th ed. Access Medicine: McGraw-Hill; 2007. http://www.accessmedicine.com/content.aspx?aID=2506170. Accessed April 25, 2007.

119. **Answer: C.** A prior suicide attempt, especially within the last three months, is considered the most significant risk factor for completed suicide. Approximately 30% to 50% of suicide completers have had a prior attempt. The other scenarios also suggest increased risk; a priori, however, the greatest risk is for the person with a past suicide attempt and it should raise significant concern, even if other factors (such as marriage and having young children) are protective. Major risk factors, besides prior attempt, also include older adult, substance use, history of violence, isolation, and male gender. Lesser risk factors include white race, socially isolated, Jewish or Protestant, psychosis, professional, chronic illness, low job satisfaction, and financial distress.

Fadem B. *Behavioral Science in Medicine*. Philadelphia: Lippincott Williams & Wilkins; 2004:213.

120. **Answer: E.** The term *limbic system* was coined by Paul MacLean. It is thought to consist of cingulate gyrus, hippocampus, parahippocampal gyri, amygdala, mammillary body, anterior thalamus, septal area, and hypothalamus. These structures are involved in mediating emotional behavior and cognition. Internal capsule is not part of the limbic system.

Sadock BJ, Sadock VA. *Kaplan and Sadock's Comprehensive Textbook of Psychiatry*. 8th ed. Philadelphia: Lippincott Williams & Wilkins; 2005:27–31.

121. **Answer: D.** Injury to the sympathetic innervation of the eye muscles results in Horner's syndrome which presents with ptosis (drooping eyelids), miosis (small pupil), and anhidrosis (lack of sweating). As the sympathetic tract has a long course, it can be injured in a variety of conditions. Some common conditions that can cause sympathetic tract lesions are lateral medullary syndrome of Wallenberg, cervical spinal cord injuries, apical lung tumors, carotid artery abnormality, and cluster headaches. Horner's syndrome is distinguished from oculomor nerve injury by the presence of miosis and anhidrosis.

1. Kaufman DM. *Clinical Neurology for Psychiatrists*. 5th ed. Philadelphia: WB Saunders; 2001:309–310.
2. Rowland LP. *Merritt's Neurology*. 11th ed. Philadelphia: Lippincott Williams & Wilkins; 2005:299.

122. **Answer: C.** Gliomas, tumors of glial cell origin, account for almost 80% of primary malignant brain

tumors in adults, comprised of glioblastomas, astrocytomas, anaplastic astrocytomas, anaplastic oligodendrogliomas, oligodendrogliomas, and malignant glioma NOS. Between 1998 and 2002 in the United States, the average annual age-adjusted incidence of these tumors was 9 per 100,000 person-years with approximately 13,000 deaths per year. The gliomas are more common in men. Glioblastoma multiforme, the highest grade of the tumors, has the highest median age at diagnosis and has the lowest mean 2-year survival rate, which ranges from about 2% to 30%, depending on age at diagnosis. The only definitive associated risk is exposure to high-dose radiation, which was usually administered to treat an earlier primary cancer. Some genetic syndromes, including neurofibromatosis 1 and 2, tuberous sclerosis, retinoblastoma, and Li-Fraumeni syndrome, are also associated with a higher incidence of gliomas.

Schwartzbaum JA, Fisher JL, Aldape KD, et al. Epidemiology and molecular pathology of glioma. *Nat Clin Pract Neurol.* 2006;2:494–503.

123. Answer: A. A noncontrast CT would be the best imaging modality in this case, as the patient is an elderly man on multiple medications, including blood thinners. A noncontrast CT would be a very quick, effective way to evaluate for the presence of an intracranial hemorrhage, either as a result of trauma, or secondary to a hemorrhagic stroke. A relatively mild trauma might be sufficient to cause an intracranial hemorrhage in an elderly person on coumadin, so that possibility should always be included in the differential. Additionally, a CT scan is also a good screen for the evaluation of possible skull fractures. Plain skull films may detect a fracture, but are less likely to detect intracranial hemorrhage.

Rowland LP. *Merritt's Neurology.* 11th ed. Philadelphia: Lippincott Williams & Wilkins; 2005:70–71.

124. Answer: D. The Weschler Adult Intelligence Scale (WAIS) consists of 11 subtests whose results are reflected in scores for verbal IQ, performance IQ, and full-scale IQ. There is no personality IQ. A significant disparity between the verbal and performance IQs is associated with, among other disorders, ADHD.

Kaplan HI, Sadock BJ. *Kaplan & Sadock's Synopsis of Psychiatry.* 8th ed. Philadelphia: Lippincott Williams & Wilkins; 1998:194–195.

125. Answer: C. The syndrome depicted in the previous scenario is called "Locked-In Syndrome" and is characterized by total/near total motor paralysis with intact consciousness. There is selective differentiation. The

patient can possibly communicate with the environment using eye-controlled technology. There are few chances of complete motor recovery. Acute ventral pontine lesions constitute the most common cause. Lateral medullary vascular lesions due to occlusion of the posterior inferior cerebellar artery cause "Wallenberg's Syndrome," consisting of ataxia, numbness to pain and temperature of ipsilateral face and contralateral body, ipsilateral hoarseness, dysphagia, diminished gag reflex, vestibular dysfunction, and ipsilateral Horner's syndrome. Medial medullary vascular lesions cause ipsilateral hypoglossal nerve palsy and contralateral hemiparesis and loss of deep touch. Tegmental pontine lesions are associated with mild motor deficits, sensory symptoms, and vestibular symptoms. Central pontine myelinolysis is one of the causes of "Locked-In Syndrome", although not the most common.

1. Bauby JD. *The Diving Bell and the Butterfly.* New York: Vintage Books; 1997.
2. Gan R, Noronha A. The medullary vascular syndromes revisited. *J Neurol.*1995;242:195–202.
3. Laureys S, Pellas F, Van Eeckhout P, et al. The locked-in syndrome: what is it like to be conscious but paralyzed and voiceless? *Prog Brain Res.* 2005;150:495–511.

126. Answer: C. Radiculopathy refers to the involvement of nerve roots. The most common patterns of weakness, sensory symptoms, and reflex changes in nerve root lesions are:

C7:
Motor deficit: triceps and wrist extensors
Sensation: second, third, and fourth digits
Reflexes: triceps

C8:
Motor deficit: finger extensors plus abductors of the first and fifth digits
Sensation: fifth digit
Reflexes: none

L4:
Motor deficit: quadriceps
Sensation: medial shin
Reflexes: knee

L5:
Motor deficit: great toe extension
Sensation: medial foot, great toe
Reflexes: none

S1:
Motor deficit: plantar flexion ("get up on toes")
Sensation: lateral foot, small toe
Reflexes: ankle

Greenberg DA, Aminoff MJ, Simon RP. *Clinical Neurology.* 5th ed. New York: McGraw-Hill; 2002:180, 205.

127. Answer: E. Polymyositis is an inflammatory myopathy. It is characterized by destruction of muscle fibers and inflammatory infiltration of muscles. It can occur at any age and leads to weakness and wasting, especially of the proximal limb and girdle muscles. It is often associated with muscle pain, tenderness, dysphagia, and difficulty with respiration. Raynaud's phenomenon, arthralgia, malaise, weight loss, and low-grade fever can also complicate the picture. Polymyositis has been reported in association with autoimmune disorders, including lupus erythematosus, rheumatoid arthritis, scleroderma, and Sjögren's syndrome. There is a correlation between adult-onset dermatomyositis and cancer; however, polymyositis has not been associated with cancer. Serum CK is generally elevated in polymyositis. On EEG, short, low-amplitude, polyphasic motor unit potentials are found, similar to most myopathies. However, abnormal spontaneous muscle activity is often present as well.

Greenberg DA, Aminoff MJ, Simon RP. *Clinical Neurology.* 5th ed. New York: McGraw-Hill; 2002:191.

128. Answer: A. Physical manifestations of infarction to the CNS are the most reliable characteristics in the diagnosis of vascular dementia. Although a stepwise deterioration is common in vascular dementia it is no longer a requirement for the diagnosis. Apathy, memory loss, and atrophy seen on MRI are common to both Alzheimer's disease and vascular dementia.

Kaufman DM. *Clinical Neurology for Psychiatrists.* 5th ed. Philadelphia: WB Saunders; 2001:277–278.

129. Answer: E. This patient is presenting with micrograhia and hypophonia, which are common in Parkinson's disease patients. In addition, he appears depressed due to the facial akinesia of Parkinson's disease and not actually depression. He has frequent falls which are common in Parkinson's patients due to impaired postural reflexes. With Alzheimer's disease and diffuse Lewy Body Disease, dementia would be a presenting complaint. In Normal Pressure Hydrocephalus, presenting symptoms would include gait disturbance, incontinence, and dementia.

1. Kaufman DM. *Clinical Neurology for Psychiatrists.* 5th ed. Philadelphia: WB Saunders; 2001:446.
2. Stern TA, Herman JB. *Massachusetts General Hospital Psychiatry Update and Board Preparation.* 2nd ed. New York: McGraw-Hill; 2004:315.

130. Answer: E. Signs and symptoms of AED intoxication include lethargy, stupor, and dysarthria as well as cerebellum dysfunction which includes dysmetria on heel to shin testing, tremor on finger to nose testing, gait ataxia, and nystagmus.

Kaufman DM. *Clinical Neurology for Psychiatrists.* 5th ed. Philadelphia: WB Saunders; 2001:246.

131. Answer: B. It has been shown that firstborn children tend to show a significant decrease in their attachment to their mothers after a second child is born. This change is more marked in children who are 24 months or older, since the ability to feel threatened by a new baby requires more sophisticated social and cognitive skills. The baby's gender has not been found to be a consistent predictor of the impact of a newborn in the firstborn's attachment to a mother. The mother's marital harmony and affective involvement with firstborns was a protective factor for the strength of a firstborn attachment after a new baby was born. Other studies have shown that mothers tend to have more positive face-to-face interactions with their second born children most likely due to a feeling of greater competence and ease in the role of parenting.

1. Moore GA, Cohn JF, Campbell SB. Mother's affective behavior with infant siblings: stability and change. *Dev Psychol.* 1997;33:856–860.
2. Teti DM, Sakin JW, Kucera E, et al. And baby makes four: predictors of attachment security among preschool-age firstborns during the transition to siblinghood. *Child Dev.* 1996;67:579–596.

132. Answer: A. Cognitive impairment is one of the most prominent effects of total sleep deprivation. Brain metabolic rate decreases, but peripheral metabolic rate increases. Cortisol levels increase in sleep deprivation. Glucose tolerance decreases.

Sadock BJ, Sadock VA. *Kaplan and Sadock's Comprehensive Textbook of Psychiatry.* 8th ed. Philadelphia: Lippincott Williams & Wilkins; 2005:289.

133. Answer: A. The specificity refers to the proportion of patients without the disease (as assessed by the gold standard) who are identified by the diagnostic test as not having the disease. A highly specific test is one that does not misidentify healthy individuals as having the disease. In this case, the possible results of the diagnostic test can be represented in the following 2 × 2 table.

Test result outcome	Disease present	Disease absent	Total
Positive	999	1	1,000
Negative	1	999	1,000
Total	1,000	1,000	

Specificity of the test would be the number of true negatives (patients who don't have the disease and are tested negative) divided by the total number of patients without the disease. In this case, that would be 999/1000; 99.9%.

1. Gray GE. *Evidence-Based Psychiatry*. Washington: American Psychiatric Publishing; 2004:123–125.
2. http://www.musc.edu/dc/icrebm/sensitivity.html. Published September 16, 2006.

134. Answer: E. Resting-state studies that used PET or SPECT to examine the basal brain metabolism or cerebral blood flow (CBF) in "pure" OCD patients, compared to controls, have shown an increase in metabolism or blood flow in the orbitofrontal cortex, striatum, and thalamus, anterior cingulate and dorsolateral prefrontal cortices. However, a recent meta-analysis of resting-state studies found that the only consistent findings were increased metabolism and regional blood flow in the orbitofrontal cortex and head of the caudate nucleus in patients compared to controls. In OCD patients with comorbid major depression, lower metabolism in the hippocampus, caudate nucleus, and thalamus has been found in one study, when compared to "pure" OCD patients and healthy controls.

Mitterschiffthaler MT, Ettinger U, Mehta MA, et al. Applications of functional magnetic resonance imaging in psychiatry. *J Magn Reson Imaging*. 2006;23:851–861.

135. Answer: C. Obsessive-compulsive personality disorder (OCPD) is a Cluster C personality disorder. Studies have shown that 80% of individuals with OCPD do not have OCD, and about 75% of the patients with OCD do not have OCPD. This condition was first included in DSM-II. In DSM-III, it was called compulsive personality, and in DSM-IV, it was again referred to as OCPD. Cluster A personality disorders are: paranoid, schizoid, schizotypal personality disorders. Cluster B personality disorders are: antisocial, narcissistic, histrionic, borderline personality disorders. Cluster C personality disorders are: avoidant, dependent, obsessive-compulsive personality disorders.

1. Mancebo MC, Eisen JL, Grant JE, et al. Obsessive compulsive personality disorder and obsessive compulsive disorder: clinical characteristics, diagnostic difficulties, and treatment. *Ann Clin Psychiatry*. 2005;17:197–204.
2. Sadock BJ, Sadock VA. *Kaplan and Sadock's Comprehensive Textbook of Psychiatry*. 8th ed. Philadelphia: Lippincott Williams & Wilkins; 2005:2081–2087.

136. Answer: D. The population of the elderly is growing rapidly. In tandem with this growth, there is also an increase in the number of those with psychiatric disorders. It is estimated that the number of people age 65 years and older with psychiatric disorder will more than double from 7 million to 15 million by 2030. Although the NIMH ECA has estimated the prevalence of bipolar disorder to be 0.1, 0.4, and 1.4 in the elderly, 45 to 65, and 18 to 45 years, respectively, some studies estimate a prevalence of up to 0.5 in older adults. The prevalence of bipolar disorder across all age groups has been estimated to be 1%.

1. Hischfeld RM, Simon G, Calabrese JR, et al. Screening for bipolar disorder in the community. *J Clin Psychiatry*. 2003;64:53–59.
2. Kyonmen HH. The impact of elderly patients with bipolar disorder on the health care system. Paper presented at: American Psychiatric Association 159th Annual Meeting; May 20–25, 2006; Toronto, Ontario, Canada.

137. Answer: A. Psychotic disorders due to a general medical condition are often seen in neurological diseases like Huntington's disease. Atypical features, such as onset at >45 years of age and no prior psychotic symptoms, are common in psychotic disorders due to a generally medical condition. Late onset of psychotic symptoms and no personal or family history of mental illness is uncommon in schizophrenia and paranoid personality disorder. This patient has no disturbance in consciousness or cognition, which would characterize the acute, fluctuating course of delirium-induced psychosis. A substance-induced psychosis is unlikely as the patient has a negative drug screen.

Sadock BJ, Sadock VA. *Kaplan and Sadock's Comprehensive Textbook of Psychiatry*. 8th ed. Philadelphia: Lippincott Williams & Wilkins; 2005:1123.

138. Answer: B. CAM, the most common tool used to detect delirium, measures four symptoms to diagnose delirium. These four items are: (i) acute onset and fluctuating course; (ii) inattention; (iii) disorganized thinking, and (iv) altered level of consciousness. To make a diagnosis of delirium, you need to have (i) and (ii) and (iii) or (iv). It has a sensitivity of 94% to 100%; specificity of 90% to 95%; positive predictive value of between 91% to 94%; and a negative predictive value of 90% to 100%.

1. Adamis D, Treloar A, MacDonald AJ, et al. Concurrent validity of two instruments (the Confusion Assessment Method and the Delirium Rating Scale) in the detection of delirium among older medical inpatients. *Age Ageing*. 2005;34:72–75.
2. Inouye SK, van Dyck CH, Alessi CA, et al. Clarifying confusion: the confusion assessment method. A new method for detection of delirium. *Ann Intern Med*. 1990;113:941–948.

139. Answer: D. The patient has tardive dyskinesia (TD) of which buccolingual-masticatory movements are frequently early manifestations. People over 50 years of age have an increased risk of developing tardive dyskinesia, and so the patient's age does not make him particularly vulnerable. Because the symptoms do not seem to be causing this patient great distress, and he has had an unsuccessful trial with atypicals and clozapine, and has been stable on haloperidol, a justification can be made to maintain him on haloperidol despite his tardive dyskinesia. No reliable treatments exist for tardive dyskinesia.

Rosenbaum JF, Arana GW, Hyman SE, et al. *Handbook of Psychiatric Drug Therapy*. 5th ed. Philadelphia: Lippincott Williams & Wilkins; 2005:44–46.

140. Answer: E. As a barbiturate and an anticonvulsant, phenobarbital will raise the seizure threshold. Most antipsychotics, typical and atypical, lower the seizure threshold. Most serotonin re-uptake inhibitors, such as fluoxetine, and other antidepressants will lower the seizure threshold. Theophylline increases seizure duration and increases the risk of prolonged seizures. Bupropion has been associated with spontaneous seizures, and lowers the seizure threshold.

American Psychiatric Association Committee on Electroconvulsive Therapy. *The Practice of Electroconvulsive Therapy: Recommendations for Treatment, Training, and Privileging*. 2nd ed. Washington: American Psychiatric Association; 2001:83–93.

141. Answer: B. Light therapy can be a safe and effective treatment for Seasonal Affective Disorder (SAD). Usual effective doses range from 2,500 lux at 2 hours daily to 10,000 lux at 30 minutes daily. Light therapy may also have a modest benefit for non-seasonal depression. Although antidepressants can be useful adjuncts, the patient has already failed adequate trials of two other serotonin re-uptake inhibitors, such as paroxetine. There is no good evidence that benzodiazepines or atypical antipsychotics are indicated for SAD. ECT may help, but is fraught with potential complications and side effects for this patient with mild to moderate depression.

1. Golden RN, Gaynes BN, Ekstrom RD, et al. The efficacy of light therapy in the treatment of mood disorders: a review and meta-analysis of the evidence. *Am J Psychiatry*. 2005;162:656–662.
2. Hales RE, Yudofsky SC. *Textbook of Clinical Psychiatry*. 4th ed. Washington: American Psychiatric Publishing; 2003:1127.

142. Answer: E. Stimulants such as amphetamines and methylphenidate may exacerbate or produce tics as common side effects in children treated for attention deficit disorders. Nicotine is unlikely to cause

tics. Guanfacine (Tenex) in an alpha-adrenergic receptor agonist unlikely to produce tics. Bupropion and venlafaxine are not the cause of tics as frequently as stimulants.

1. Sadock BJ, Sadock VA. *Kaplan & Sadock's Comprehensive Textbook of Psychiatry*. 7th ed. Philadelphia: Lippincott Williams & Wilkins; 2000:2686.
2. Task Force on DSM-IV. *Diagnostic and Statistical Manual of Mental Disorders, DSM-IV-TR*. Washington: American Psychiatric Publishing; 2000:108–111.

143. Answer: D. The introduction of sophisticated electroenchalographic and cardiopulmonary monitoring, advent of brief pulse stimulus machine, and adoption of improved anesthetic agents have resulted in a remarkable improvement in ECT safety. The health of the population at large has no direct impact on the safety of ECT.

UK ECT Review Group. Efficacy and safety of electroconvulsive therapy in depressive disorders: a systemic review and meta-analysis. *Lancet*. 2003;361:799–808.

144. Answer: A. Inability to convert ideas into action is called ideomotor apraxia. It is due to the disconnection of cognitive regions from motor regions of the brain and is usually associated with nonfluent aphasia. The lesion is usually seen in the left frontal or parietal lobes. Ideomotor apraxia can be further subdivided into buccofacial apraxia where patients are unable to use buccofacial muscles to perform actions, such as blowing out a match and sucking on a straw, and limb apraxia where patients are unable to use their limbs on command (i.e., they cannot pretend to brush their teeth, turn a key, and kick a ball).

1. Kaufman DM. *Clinical Neurology for Psychiatrists*. 5th ed. Philadelphia: WB Saunders; 2001:186–187.
2. Rowland LP. *Merritt's Neurology*. 11th ed. Philadelphia: Lippincott Williams & Wilkins; 2005:11, 12.

145. Answer: D. Senile neuritic plaques are spherical microscopic lesions with a core of extracellular $A\beta$ surrounded by enlarged axonal endings (neurites). $A\beta$ peptide is derived from the APP, a transmembrane protein that is present in most tissues. Secretases (α, β, and γ) are a group of protease enzymes that are responsible for cleavage of APP. When cleaved by a secretase, a soluble peptide derivative of amyloid is formed, but when cut by β secretase first, γ secretase generates two peptides, $A\beta40$ and $A\beta42$. The $A\beta$ peptide monomer binds other peptides, forming oligomers, ultimately leading to the accumulation of amyloid in all forms of the disease. In Alzheimer's disease, the amyloid is deposited around meningeal and cerebral vessels and in gray matter. The gray matter deposits are multifocal and are called plaques. Aβ plaques are distributed in the brain in a characteristic fashion. Senile neurotic plaques are also less well correlated with Alzheimer's disease than NFT.

1. Kaufman DM. *Clinical Neurology for Psychiatrists*. 5th ed. Philadelphia: WB Saunders; 2001:136.
2. Rowland LP. *Merritt's Neurology*. 11th ed. Philadelphia: Lippincott Williams & Wilkins; 2005:773.

146. Answer: E. The principle behind MRI is based on the propensity of hydrogen protons in tissue water to align parallel to an externally applied magnetic field. The hydrogen protons in effect act as small bar magnets in the tissue. However, not all of the protons align parallel to the magnetic field, and a small net magnetic vector is produced, which then forms the basis of images produced. When a radiofrequency pulse is applied, the high-energy proton "spins" to a relaxed state, which releases energy and produces a detectable signal. Tissues with a greater water content, such as CSF or blood, will therefore have a brighter signal, depending on the detection window used in the image capture.

147. Answer: B. CSF can reveal characteristic abnormalities in several neurologic disorders. The findings of a normal CSF profile are seen in (A). In infectious or inflammatory diseases, pleocytosis (increase in WBC count) is commonly seen. In bacterial meningitis (B), this pleocytosis includes mostly polymorphonuclear cells; in viral meningitis (D), primarily lymphocytes are present. In both instances, CSF is turbid with an increase in protein and a decrease in glucose. In the case of a subarachnoid hemorrhage (E), one would expect to see bloody CSF with mild elevation of WBCs and elevated protein. The centrifuged supernatant would be xanthochromic. Guillain-Barré syndrome (C) is one neurologic disorder in which the CSF does not show pleocytosis. In this case, CSF is typically clear with few WBCs and elevated protein.

Kaufman DM. *Clinical Neurology for Psychiatrists*. 5th ed. Philadelphia: WB Saunders; 2001:532–533.

148. Answer: B. This patient has an oligodendroglioma. It occurs most often in the third and fourth decades,

T1 Weighted Image	Intensity	T2 Weighted Image	Intensity
Fat Intracellular methemoglobin Extracellular methomoglobin Contrast media Complex calcifications Entry slice Melanin Flow in vessels	**Increased**	Extracellular methemoglobin **CSF** Edema Neoplasms Demyelination Dysmyelination Acute/subacute infarcts Abcess	**Increased**
Bone **CSF** Air Ligaments Calcifications Deoxyhemoglobin Hemosiderin Flow void in vessels Acute/subacute infarcts	**Decreased**	**Bone** Ligaments Air Calcifications Deoxyhemoglobin Intracellular methemoglobin Hemosiderin Flow void in vessels Fat	**Decreased**

T1 refers to the amount of time it takes for a proton to recover 63% of its longitudinal magnetization, also known as *spin-lattice time*. T2 refers to the amount of time it takes a proton to lose 63% of it transverse magnetization, also known as *spin-spin relaxation time*. You can always identify the T2 weighted image by its bright CSF signal.

Goetz CG. *Textbook of Clinical Neurology*. 2nd ed. Philadelphia: WB Saunders; 2003:437–447.

with an earlier peak at 6 to 12 years. It is uncommon, and males outnumber females 2:1. The neoplastic oligodendrocyte has a small round nucleus and a halo of unstained cytoplasm ("fried egg" appearance). The most common sites of this tumor are the frontal and temporal lobes (40% to 70%), often deep in the white matter, with one or more streaks of calcium but little or no surrounding edema. The presenting symptom is a focal or generalized seizure in greater than 50% of patients. The most typical appearance on diagnostic imaging is a hypodense mass near the cortical surface with relatively well-defined borders. Calcium is seen in CT scans in more than half the cases and is a helpful diagnostic sign. Many oligodendrogliomas, especially anaplastic ones, respond impressively to chemotherapeutic agents, and genetic markers (chromosomes 1p and 19q) predict a remarkable chemoresponsivity and prolonged survival. Surgical excision used to be the first-line treatment. Intravenous methotrexate is a treatment for CNS lymphomas.

Ropper AH, Brown RH. *Adams and Victor's Principles of Neurology*. 8th ed. New York: McGraw-Hill; 2005:557–558.

149. Answer: D. Erik Erikson drew on Freudian psychology but added to it by concluding that human personality is determined not only by childhood experiences but also by those of adulthood. His theory of human development encompassed the entire human life span. He emphasized that the development of the ego, while the result of inner psychic energies, was also related to the environment and social relationships. His eight psychosocial stages are points along development which trigger internal crises. They are trust versus mistrust (birth–), autonomy versus shame and doubt (18 months–), initiative versus guilt (3 years–), industry versus inferiority (5 years–), identity versus role confusion (13 years–), intimacy versus isolation (20s–), generativity versus stagnation (40s–), and integrity versus despair (60s–). Young adults must navigate the crisis posed by the sixth stage (i.e., intimacy versus isolation). Intimacy in the young adult is the ability to make and honor commitments even when they require sacrifice and compromise. The person who cannot tolerate the fear of ego loss arising out of experiences of self-abandonment (e.g., moments of intensity in friendships, aggression, inspiration, or intuition) is at risk for becoming deeply isolated and self-absorbed.

Sadock BJ, Sadock VA. *Kaplan and Sadock's Synopsis of Psychiatry*. 9th ed. Philadelphia: Lippincott Williams & Wilkins; 2002:211–217.

150. Answer: C. The hypothalamus only represents 0.3% of the total mass of the brain, but is extremely important in function. This question covers some of these important functions. The supraoptic nucleus, located in the anteromedial hypothalamus, contains osmoreceptors that monitor the osmorality of the blood, stimulating the release of vasopressin. A lesion to this section would cause diabetes insipidus, characterized by polyuria and polydipsia. The other choices are correct. The lateral

hypothalamus contains a tonically active eating center, which can be inhibited by high blood glucose in the satiety center in the ventromedial nucleus. The hypothalamus secretes various hormones that regulate the pituitary, which in turn regulate various endocrine organs, including the thyroid, adrenals, and gonads. The suprachiasmatic nucleus, also contained within in the hypothalamus, functions as an intrinsic clock for the body. It receives light input from the retinosuprachiasmatic pathway, which synchronizes the body to the environment. Loss of the nucleus means loss of circadian cycles. Finally, the hypothalamus is involved in expression of rage, fear, and pleasure, and lesions have led to rage attacks.

Waxman SG. *Correlative Neuroanatomy*. 24th ed. New York: McGraw-Hill; 2000:129–133.

151. Answer: A. Studies using structural MRI of the brain in patients with schizophrenia, including those patients experiencing their first episode, have conclusively demonstrated a reduction in the volume of prefrontal and medial temporal cortex. Twin studies have also demonstrated structural abnormalities in the twin with the disorder, but not in the healthy twin. Studies using function MRI (fMRI) have also demonstrated reduced activation in the prefrontal cortex and medial temporal cortex in patients with schizophrenia. A study by Abou-Saleh, et al. using SPECT scan in Arab patients with schizophrenia reported greater right CBF than normal controls in all cerebral regions except in the right and left anterior frontal regions. Patients showed a reversed left-to-right laterality in the anterior frontal regions only. Several symptom scores were predicted by the CBF: delusions of control by greater left temporo-occipital CBF and longer duration of illness by greater left midfrontal, left temporal, right midfrontal, and right perisylvian CBF. These results were suggestive of generalized cerebral activation in patients with schizophrenia.

Abou-Saleh MT. Neuroimaging in psychiatry: An update. *J Psychosom Res*. 2006;61:289–293.

152. Answer: D. Hypervigilance is considered to be symptomatic of "increased arousal (not present before the trauma)". The symptoms falling under the category of "persistent avoidance of stimuli associated with the trauma and numbing of general responsiveness (not present before the trauma)" are:

1. Efforts to avoid thoughts / feelings/ conversations associated with the trauma
2. Efforts to avoid activities/places/people arousing recollections of the trauma

3. Inability to recall an important aspect of the trauma
4. Markedly diminished interest/participation in significant activities
5. Feeling of detachment/estrangement from others
6. Restricted range of affect
7. Sense of a foreshortened future

Three or more of the above should be present in a patient with PTSD.

The symptoms of increased arousal (not present before the trauma) are:

1. Difficulty falling/staying asleep
2. Irritability/outbursts of anger
3. Difficulty in concentrating
4. Hypervigilance
5. Exaggerated startle response

Two or more of the above should be present in a patient with PTSD.

The symptoms of persistent re-experiencing of the trauma are:

1. Recurrent and intrusive distressing recollection of events including images, thoughts, or perceptions
2. Recurrent distressing dreams of the event
3. Acting or feeling as if the traumatic event were recurring
4. Intense psychological distress at exposure to internal or external cues that symbolize or resemble an aspect of the traumatic event
5. Physiological reactivity on exposure to internal or external cues that symbolize or resemble an aspect of the traumatic event

One or more of the above should be present in a patient with PTSD.

American Psychiatric Association. *Quick Reference to the Diagnostic Criteria from DSM-IV-TR*. Washington: American Psychiatric Association; 2000:243.

153. Answer: E. None of the statements are true. Contrary to a widely held view that pregnancy is a period of emotional tranquility, up to 70% of women may have depressive symptoms and 16% meet criteria for Major Depressive Disorder. Sexual molestations are grossly under-reported. In children, it is often perpetuated by a family member or "friend of the family." It may be complicated by depression or PTSD. In some cases the latter may go unrecognized for years; the initial manifestation may be reenactments in the form of physiological and psychological reactivity upon exposure to cues of initial trauma as in this case.

1. Bloch M, Rotenberg N, Koren D, et al. Risk factors for early postpartum depressive symptoms. *Gen Hosp Psychiatry*. 2006;28:3–8.

2. Evans J, Heron J, Francomb H, et al. Cohort study of depressed mood during pregnancy and after child birth. *BMJ*. 2001;323:257–260.
3. Weissman MM, Olfson M. Depression in women: implications for health care research. *Science*. 1995;269:799–801.

154. Answer: D. A catecholamine-secreting tumor of the adrenal gland, or pheochromocytoma, can produce panic attacks in addition to headache, tachycardia, and hypertension. A common diagnostic test for pheochromocytoma is a 24-hour urine collection for urinary catecholamines. Increased catecholamine production would not be seen in primary panic attacks, generalized anxiety disorder, PTSD, or alcohol withdrawal.

Sadock BJ, Sadock VA. *Kaplan and Sadock's Comprehensive Textbook of Psychiatry*. 8th ed. Philadelphia: Lippincott Williams & Wilkins; 2005:1126.

155. Answer: E. All of the statements regarding behavioral disturbances seen in dementia are true.

Lawlor B. Managing behavioural and psychological symptoms in dementia. *Br J Psychiatry*. 2002;181:463–465.

156. Answer: D. Transition from seeing the problem as marital conflict to perceiving it as an internal conflict played out within the couple is a difficult task for each partner. Projective identification in the marital dyad requires a continued state of conflict, which is the polarization inherent in the splitting process which maintains the stable balance. The need for the spouse to be the "bad object" may be so compelling that all therapeutic efforts may not lead to any benefits. Sometimes, the more the therapist pushes for change, the more the couple is likely to resist.

Gabbard G. *Psychodynamic Psychiatry in Clinical Practice*. 4th ed. Washington: American Psychiatric Publishing; 2005:140.

157. Answer: C. Anticonvulsants such as barbiturates, valproic acid, and phenytoin raise seizure threshold and interfere with seizure expression. Benzodiazepines reduce seizure duration in a dose-dependent fashion and likely interfere with seizure expression. Tricyclic antidepressants, such as nortriptyline, may lower seizure threshold and potentially prolong seizures.

American Psychiatric Association Committee on Electroconvulsive Therapy. *The Practice of Electroconvulsive Therapy: Recommendations for Treatment, Training, and Privileging*. 2nd ed. Washington: American Psychiatric Association; 2001:84–93.

158. Answer: D. Biofeedback is a technique where the patient learns to affect physiologic parameters with the help of electronic equipment. It can be particularly helpful in the treatment of insomnia and pain disorders. Sleep hygiene, hypnosis, meditation, and progressive relaxation are each helpful with insomnia, but utilize different underlying principles.

Hales RE, Yudofsky SC. *Textbook of Clinical Psychiatry*. 4th ed. Washington: American Psychiatric Publishing; 2003:981.

159. Answer: C. Patients on magnesium pemoline (Cylert) have a 2% to 3% rate of developing hepatitis. Multiple cases of hepatic failure have been reported with pemoline treatment, mostly in patients under 10-years taking additional medications. Almost any medication may produce hepatitis, but magnesium pemoline is more likely to produce this effect. Liver function tests should be checked as frequently as every 2 weeks while on pemoline.

1. Janicak PG, Davis JM, Preskorn SH, et al. *Principles and Practice of Pharmacotherapy*. 3rd ed. Philadelphia: Lippincott Williams & Wilkins; 2001:567–573.
2. Sadock BJ, Sadock VA. *Kaplan and Sadock's Comprehensive Textbook of Psychiatry*. 7th ed. Philadelphia: Lippincott Williams & Wilkins; 2000;2691.

160. Answer: E. Possible positive predictors of response to ECT are increasing age, presence of psychotic and catatonic symptoms in mood disorders. Potentially negative predictors include presence of dysthymic disorder, comorbid personality disorder, and prolonged depressive episodes.

1. O'Connor MK, Knapp R, Husain M, et al. The influence of age on the response of major depression to electroconvulsive therapy: a C.O.R.E. report. *Am J Geriatr Psychiatry*. 2001;9:382–390.
2. Parker G, Roy K, Wilhelm K, et al. Assessing the comparative effectiveness of antidepressant therapies: a prospective clinical practice study. *J Clin Psychiatry*. 2001;62: 117–125.

161. Answer: A. Inability to perform a sequence of steps that require a plan and continued monitoring is called ideational apraxia. It is usually seen in demented patients who have frontal lobe lesions. It may, however, be seen in patients with dementia who also have extensive cerebral disease. Unlike ideomotor apraxia, these patients do not have nonfluent aphasia.

1. Kaufman DM. *Clinical Neurology for Psychiatrists*. 5th ed. Philadelphia: WB Saunders; 2001:187.
2. Rowland LP. *Merritt's Neurology*. 11th ed. Philadelphia: Lippincott Williams & Wilkins; 2005:11–12.

162. Answer: E. Neurofibrillary tangles are intracytoplasmic structures found inside the neurons. Although NFTs can be seen in microscopic sections stained with hematoxylin and eosin, they are better visualized using silver impregnation techniques (e.g., Bielschowsky or the Bodian stain). They can also be stained with Congo red or with the fluorescent dye thioflavine-S. In patients with Alzheimer's disease, NFTs are commonly found in the neurons of the cerebral cortex and are most common in the hippocampus and amygdala. They consist of paired 10-nanometer diameter filaments twisted around one another in a helical fashion and are composed mainly of abnormally phosphorylated tau protein. Tau is a neuron-specific phosphoprotein that is the major constituent of neuronal microtubules. Neurofibrillary tangles are not unique to Alzheimer's disease and can be found in a variety of other neurologic disorders. They are seen in the substantia nigra neurons in postencephalitic Parkinsonism, throughout the nervous system in the Parkinsonism-dementia-Amyotrophic lateral sclerosis (ALS) complex disorder, in the cerebral cortex in dementia pugilistica ("punch-drunk syndrome"), and in the brain stem and thalamus in Steele-Richardson-Olszewski progressive supranuclear palsy (PSP).

1. http://w3.uokhsc.edu/pathology/DeptLabs/Alzheimer/neurofibrillary_tangles.htm. Accessed November 11, 2006.
2. Kaufman DM. *Clinical Neurology for Psychiatrists*. 5th ed. Philadelphia: WB Saunders; 2001:136.
3. Rowland LP. *Merritt's Neurology*. 11th ed. Philadelphia: Lippincott Williams & Wilkins; 2005:773.

163. Answer: A. The nonergot dopamine agonists ropinirole and pramipexole directly stimulate striatal neurons, and partially bypass the depleted nigral neurons, and have become the first-line treatment in early Parkinson's disease. They are associated with fewer, but not zero, dyskinetic motor complications. Dopamine agonists, however, are consistently less potent than L-dopa in managing the main features of Parkinson disease and produce similar side effects in higher doses. All these drugs should be introduced cautiously, because of the potential of a prolonged episode of hypotension. These medications are also useful in diminishing side effects of L-dopa, especially dyskinesias. The neuroprotective properties of these medications remains controversial.

Ropper AH, Brown RH. *Adams and Victor's Principles of Neurology*. 8th ed. New York: McGraw-Hill; 2005:922–923.

164. Answer: D. Attachment theory places importance on a child's real experiences. Bowlby, one of the early developers of attachment theory, believed the entire system of behavior on the part of the child was designed to maintain nearness to the mother. The strange situation was developed by Mary Ainsworth to assess the quality and security of an infant's attachment. It consists of seven steps. First, the parent and infant are introduced to the experimental room. Next, an unfamiliar adult stranger joins the pair. The parent leaves inconspicuously while the stranger remains behind. This results in the first separation episode. The parent, then, returns while the stranger leaves. After that, the parent leaves again, leaving the infant alone this time. This is the second separation episode. Subsequently, the stranger returns. Finally, the parent enters and greets the infant, while the stranger leaves the room. When exposed to brief separations from the mother, children react in four different ways. These include: (i) securely attached, (ii) anxious-avoidantly attached, (iii) anxious-ambivalently attached, and (iv) disorganized/disoriented. According to Ainsworth, 65% of infants are securely attached by 2 years of age.

1. Gabbard GO. *Long-Term Psychodynamic Psychotherapy: A Basic Text*. Washington: American Psychiatric Publishing; 2004:8–9.
2. Sadock BJ, Sadock VA. *Kaplan and Sadock's Synopsis of Psychiatry*. 9th ed. Philadelphia: Lippincott Williams & Wilkins; 2002:141.

165. Answer: B. Lithium toxicity can result in diffuse slowing on EEG. In addition, widening of the frequency spectrum and potentiation and disorganization of the background rhythm can occur. Triphasic waves can be seen in patients with metabolic encephalopathy. Spikes with sharp waves are characteristically seen in patients with seizures. Spikes with burst suppression can result from a bilateral hemisphere insult, such as an hypoxic injury which may occur post-operatively or after a myocardial infarction for example. FIRDA typically occurs with encephalopathy but can also be a non-specific abnormality in the elderly.

1. http://www.mentalhealth.com/drug/p30-l02.html. Accessed September 5, 2006.
2. http://www.rxlist.com/cgi/generic/lithium_ad.htm. Accessed September 5, 2006.

166. Answer: D. The structural neuroimaging finding best replicated in patients with mood disorder is increased rate of white matter and periventricular hyperintensities. Smaller frontal lobe, cerebellum, caudate, and putamen are present in unipolar depression. A larger third ventricle, smaller cerebellum, and perhaps smaller temporal lobe appear to be present in patients with bipolar disorder. These structural changes involve regions of the brain that may be critical to the pathogenesis of mood disorders.

Abou-Saleh MT. Neuroimaging in psychiatry: an update. *J Psychosom Res*. 2006;61:289–293.

167. Answer: D. Social phobia is characterized by marked fear of social or performance situations in which embarrassment could occur. When patients are exposed to feared situations, their response may take the formed of a panic attack. Recent studies have looked into the predictors of recovery in social phobia. Recovery has not been associated with any intrinsic characteristics of the disorder (e.g., functional impairment, severity of social phobia, number of feared situations, and age at onset). Factors associated with recovery included the following: absence of an affective disorder, less psychopathology, being employed, and less anxiety sensitivity.

1. American Psychiatric Association. *Quick Reference to the Diagnostic Criteria from DSM-IV-TR*. Washington: American Psychiatric Association; 2000:215–216.
2. Vriends N, Becker ES, Meyer A, et al. Recovery from social phobia in the community and its predictors: data from longitudinal epidemiological study. *J Anxiety Disord*. 2007;21(3):320–337.

168. Answers: C. A recent meta-analysis of prospective comparative cohort studies to quantify the relationship between maternal exposure to the antidepressants and major malformations comparing outcomes in first trimester exposures to citalopram, escitalopram, fluoxetine, fluvoxamine, paroxetine, sertraline, reboxetine, venlafaxine, nefazodone, trazodone, mirtazapine, and bupropion to those of non-exposed mothers indicated that the relative risk was 1.01 (95% CI: 0.57 to 1.80). The study also found that as a group, the newer antidepressants are not associated with an increased risk of major malformations above the baseline of 1% to 3%. The data currently available indicate that it is prudent to imperative to treat depression during pregnancy as the risks of untreated depression far outweighs that of exposure to the available antidepressants.

1. Blier P. Pregnancy, depression, antidepressants and breast-feeding. *J Psychiatry Neurosci*. 2006;31:226–228.
2. Einarson TR, Einarson A. Newer antidepressants in pregnancy and rates of major malformations: a meta-analysis of prospective comparative studies. *Pharmacoepidemiol Drug Saf*. 2005;14:823–827.

169. Answer: B. Diabetes mellitus, as evidenced by elevated fasting blood glucose, may cause sexual dysfunction. Sexual dysfunction may have psychiatric etiologies as well, such as is seen in depression and some personality disorders. Treatment with medications such as SSRIs may cause or exacerbate sexual dysfunction. Diminished interest in sex with aging is not classified as sexual dysfunction due to a medical condition.

Sadock BJ, Sadock VA. *Kaplan and Sadock's Comprehensive Textbook of Psychiatry*. 8th ed. Philadelphia: Lippincott Williams & Wilkins; 2005:1130.

170. Answer: A. EEG has limited utility in the diagnosis of dementia. In delirium, the EEG shows generalized slow wave activity. In CJD, it shows a triphasic, periodic burst pattern with triphasic waves being seen in hepatic encephalopathy.

Kaufman DM. *Clinical Neurology for Psychiatrists.* Philadelphia: WB Saunders; 2001:134–135, 230–231.

171. Answer: D. There are a few case studies and retrospective studies that have reported the beneficial use of ECT in OCD. However, there are no controlled studies for the use of ECT in patients with OCD. Placebo-controlled trials of rapid pulse loading of intravenous clomipramine have shown significant decrease in OCD symptoms in patients who are nonresponders/intolerant to oral therapy. Treatment-refractory patients have been shown to improve better with intravenous clomipramine than with oral clomipramine. There has been a placebo-controlled trial involving 30 patients, which showed that venlafaxine was not more effective than placebo, however, the dose of venlafaxine in this trial was theorized to be insufficient, and the duration of the trial (8 weeks) was thought to be too small as compared to an adequate length of around 12 weeks. Controlled studies have demonstrated the efficacy of CBGT as compared to SSRIs. There has been one double blind, controlled crossover trial of inositol versus placebo in which inositol significantly reduced OCD scores compared with placebo.

1. Schruers K, Koning K, Luermans J, et al. Obsessive-compulsive disorder: a critical review of therapeutic perspectives. *Acta Psychiatr Scand.* 2005;111:261–271.
2. Sousa MB, Isolan L, Oliveira RR, et al. A randomized clinical trial of cognitive-behavioral group therapy and sertraline in the treatment of obsessive-compulsive disorder. *J Clin Psychiatry.* 2006;67:1133–1139.

172. Answer: E. There are no absolute contraindications to ECT, although relatively riskier conditions exist. A recent myocardial infarction or arrhythmia may increase the risk for cardiovascular complications, but CAD is not a contraindication. Intracerebral lesions and space-occupying masses may increase the risk of ECT, but potential benefit must be balanced against alternatives. With proper precautions, ECT may be performed safely in pregnant patients (usually with obstetrical consultation and fetal monitoring). Careful medical evaluation for modifiable risk factors should always be carried out prior to ECT.

1. Abrams R. *Electroconvulsive Therapy.* 4th ed. New York: Oxford University Press; 2002:72–100.
2. American Psychiatric Association Committee on Electroconvulsive Therapy. *The Practice of Electroconvulsive Therapy: Recommendations for Treatment, Training, and Privileging.* 2nd ed. Washington: American Psychiatric Association; 2001:27–30, 32–37, 46–51.
3. Hales RE, Yudofsky SC. *Textbook of Clinical Psychiatry.* 4th ed. Washington: American Psychiatric Publishing; 2003:1124.

173. Answer: C. IPT treats depression in the "medical model" as a medical illness that is treatable and not the patient's fault. CBT does involve homework, whereas IPT typically does not. Both IPT and CBT are manualized, pay attention to the therapeutic dyad, involve psychoeducation, and also focus on relationships and affect, but CBT does have a particular focus on how thoughts impact affect. Both treatments are usually time-limited.

1. Cutler JL, Goldyne A, Markowitz JC, et al. Comparing cognitive behavior therapy, interpersonal psychotherapy, and psychodynamic psychotherapy. *Am J Psychiatry.* 2004;161:1567–1573.
2. Hales RE, Yudofsky SC. *Textbook of Clinical Psychiatry.* 4th ed. Washington: American Psychiatric Publishing; 2003:1207–1222.
3. Levenson H, Butler SF, Powers TA, et al. *Concise Guide to Brief Dynamic and Interpersonal Psychotherapy.* 2nd ed. Washington: American Psychiatric Publishing; 2002:55–75.

174. Answer: B. For routine detoxifications, symptom-triggered, or as needed, treatment has been found to be as safe and effective as fixed-schedule protocols. However, patients who have a history of alcohol withdrawal seizures, delirium tremens, complicated withdrawals, or serious medical conditions should not be treated with symptom-triggered therapy but instead require a full detoxification protocol, which includes structured, or fixed-schedule, medication regimens. Safe detoxification occurs when autonomic signs and symptoms are well controlled. Benzodiazepines are used for the treatment and prevention of withdrawal symptoms. Sedation is a clinically useful indicator of adequate treatment in early withdrawal. Use of ethanol for alcohol detoxification is not the standard of treatment. Despite this, the practice continues in some hospitals, primarily among surgeons.

Levenson JL. *The American Psychiatric Publishing Textbook of Psychosomatic Medicine.* Washington DC: American Psychiatric Publishing; 2005:398.

175. Answer: D. The potency of electrical energy delivered during ECT administration is determined and directly related to cognitive deficits resulting from the procedure. One of the several factors affecting potency is electrode placement during the procedure. While ECT administration using bilateral electrode placement is more potent than unilateral placement, it is also associated with more cognitive deficits. The need to balance potency with minimal cognitive deficits in clinical practice informs guild line of deploying stimulus that are substantially above the seizure threshold when using the unilateral electrodes and applying stimulus marginally above seizure threshold when patients are treated with bilateral electrodes. Convulsive threshold is highly variable across age, gender, race electrode placement, and cranial dimensions lines. Some studies have documented convulsive threshold variability by a factor of 40.

1. McCall WV, Roboussin D, Weiner RD, et al. Titrated moderately suprathreshold vs fixed high-dose right unilateral electroconvulsive therapy: acute antidepressant and cognitive effects. *Arch Gen Psychiatry*. 2000;57:438–444.
2. Sackeim HA, Prudic J, Devanand DP, et al. Effects of stimulus intensity and electrode placement on the efficacy and cognitive effects of electroconvulsive therapy. *N Engl J Med*. 1993;328:839–846.

176. Answer: C. This patient is presenting with the classic picture of Gerstmann's syndrome where the subjects have alexia (inability to read), agraphia (inability to write), acalculia (inability to calculate), finger agnosia (unable to identify fingers), and left/right confusion. The lesion for this syndrome is thought to occur in the angular or supramarginal gyri of the dominant parietal lobe. Although the status of Gershmann's syndrome as a distict clinical entity has been questioned, as it is rare for all the components to present at the same time, they are important to distinguish in adults with stroke and during evaluation of children with learning disability.

1. Kaufman DM. *Clinical Neurology for Psychiatrists*. 5th ed. Philadelphia: WB Saunders; 2001:185–186.
2. Rowland LP. *Merritt's Neurology*. 11th ed. Philadelphia: Lippincott Williams & Wilkins; 2005:297.

177. Answer: A. Alpha-synuclein is a normal protein found in the brain. It is predominantly a presynaptic neuronal protein without any known function, but can also be found in glial cells. It is normally an unstructured soluble protein, but can aggregate to form insoluble fibrils in pathological conditions characterized by Lewy bodies, such as Parkinson's disease, dementia with Lewy bodies, and multiple system atrophy. Alpha-synuclein is the primary structural component of Lewy body fibrils. Alpha-synuclein fragment, known as the non-Abeta component (NAC) can also be found in amyloid plaques in Alzheimer's disease. In familial forms of Parkinson's disease, mutations in the gene coding for alpha-synuclein has been found. Three point mutations and triplication of the gene appears to be the cause of Parkinson's disease in another lineage. Antibod-

ies against alpha-synuclein have replaced antibodies against ubiquitin as the gold standard for immunostaining of Lewy bodies.

1. http://en.wikipedia.org/wiki/Alpha-synuclein. Accessed November 11, 2006.
2. Blazer DG, Steffens DC, Busse EW. *Textbook of Geriatric Psychiatry*. Washington: American Psychiatric Publishing; 2004:73–75.

178. Answer: B. Anticonvulsant drug measurements are helpful in regulating dosage, detecting irregular drug intake, identifying the toxic agent in patients on multiple medications, and monitoring adherence. Serum levels are ideally drawn in the morning before breakfast and the morning dose ("trough levels"), which assures uniformity in the measurement of drug concentrations. The upper and lower levels of the "therapeutic range" are not to be regarded as absolute limits, as some patients' seizures are controlled at serum levels below the therapeutic range; in others, the seizures continue despite serum values within this range. In general, higher serum concentrations of drugs are necessary for the control of simple or complex partial seizures than for the control of tonic-clonic seizures alone. The serum level is not an exact measure of the amount of drug entering the brain, because laboratory measurements only detect the protein-bound fraction, which does not cross the blood brain barrier. In patients who are malnourished or chronically ill or who have a constitutional reduction in proteins, this may lead to intoxication at low total serum levels. Common anticonvulsants for which serum levels are not easily available include levetiracetam, topiramate, tiagabine, and gabapentin.

Ropper AH, Brown RH. *Adams and Victor's Principles of Neurology*. 8th ed. New York: McGraw-Hill; 2005:293–294.

179. Answer: A. Generalized Anxiety Disorder is characterized by excessive anxiety and worry about a number of situations occurring more days than not for at least 6 months. The intensity of the worry is out of proportion to the actual likelihood or impact of the feared situation. The DSM-IV-TR lists six associated symptoms that include the following: restlessness or feeling keyed up or on edge, being easily fatigued, difficulty concentrating or mind going blank, irritability, muscle tension, and sleep disturbances (difficulty falling or staying asleep, or restless unsatisfying sleep). A patient must have at least three to make the diagnosis of general anxiety disorder.

American Psychiatric Association. *Quick Reference to the Diagnostic Criteria from DSM-IV-TR*. Washington: American Psychiatric Association; 2000:222–223.

180. Answer: B. Peri-partum mood disorders including bipolar disorder are associated with increased risk of dangerous behaviors, probably driven by psychosis and poor insight and judgment. A family history of bipolar disorder, onset of psychosis soon after childbirth and childhood history of sexual abuse are all for the development of post-partum bipolar disorder. The clinician has an obligation to protect his patient's potential victim. If the potential victim is a child or elderly, there exists an obligation to report to the appropriate authorities. Failure to report these potential abuses may be grounds for disciplinary actions by the state medical board. The obligation to report comes with immunity from possible legal reprisal even if the allegations are not proven. All psychotropic medications are secreted in breast milk. Preterm infants and neonates with hepatic impairment are more vulnerable to the side effects of secreted psychotropic medications. Lithium has the potential to rapidly accumulate in breast fed infants to very high levels. Owing to the substantial risk of lithium toxicity in infants, use of lithium during nursing is not recommended. Other mood stabilizers pose varying and often slightly less risk to the nursing infants and risk benefit analysis needs careful analysis; if the decision is made to initiate cabarmazepine or divalproex therapy, careful regular laboratory monitoring with a complete blood and liver function test is recommended, because these medications are associated with blood dyscrasias and hepatotoxicity.

1. Henshaw C. Mood disturbance in the early puerperium: a review. *Arch Womens Ment Health*. 2003;6 (suppl 2):S33-S42.
2. Chaudron LH, Pies RW. The relationship between postpartum psychosis and bipolar disorder: a review. *J Clin Psychiatry*. 2003;64:1284–1292.
3. Grover S, Avasthi A, Sharma Y. Psychotropics in pregnancy: weighing the risks. *Indian J Med Res*. 2006;123: 497–512.

181. Answer: E. Elderly patients with depression commonly present with all of these symptoms except homicidal ideation. They usually present with more suicidal ideation than their younger counterparts. Hypochondriasis, psychotic symptoms, and executive dysfunction are also more common in the elderly depressed than younger patients with depression.

Blazer DG. Depression in late life: review and commentary. *J Gerontol A Biol Sci Med Sci*. 2003;58:249–265.

182. Answer: D. Inappropriate sexual behaviors are much more common is men than in women. Although there are very few studies looking at the prevalence of these behaviors, the available studies indicate that about 7% to 25% of all demented patients exhibit these behaviors and that 5.5% of all reported sex crimes are committed by the elderly. The four common kinds of inappropriate sexual behaviors seen in demented patients include; sexual talks, sexual acts, implied sexual acts, and false sexual allegations.

Black B, Muralee S, Tampi RR. Inappropriate sexual behaviors in dementia. *J Geriatr Psychiatry Neurol*. 2005;18:155–162.

183. Answer: B. The use of SSRIs during pregnancy has been associated with respiratory distress and low birth weight, two outcomes that were significant in a retrospective cohort study, despite propensity score matching to account for differences in severity of maternal depression. A case-control study found an association between use of SSRIs in late pregnancy and Persistent Pulmonary Hypertension of the Newborn. However, these studies cannot recommend whether or not SSRI use is advisable during pregnancy. This clinical decision has to be made on a case-by-case basis; however, use of SSRIs in pregnancy in maternal depression is not without risk of certain adverse neonatal outcomes, respiratory distress being one of them.

1. Chambers CD, Hernandez-Diaz S, Van Marter LJ, et al. Selective serotonin-reuptake inhibitors and risk of persistent pulmonary hypertension of the newborn. *N Engl J Med*. 2006;354:579–587.
2. Oberlander TF, Warburton W, Misri S, et al. Neonatal outcomes after prenatal exposure to selective serotonin reuptake inhibitor antidepressants and maternal depression using population-based linked health data. *Arch Gen Psychiatry*. 2006;63:898–906.

184. Answer: A. Views of lithium use during ECT vary, but there is no evidence that lithium use worsens mood, and some experts advocate for its potential to control mood and prevent relapse in seriously ill patients undergoing ECT. Concurrent use of lithium and ECT has been reported to cause cognitive deficits, delirium, encephalopathy, and spontaneous and prolonged seizures, as well as prolongations of the neuromuscular blockade of succinylcholine.

American Psychiatric Association Committee on Electroconvulsive Therapy. *The Practice of Electroconvulsive Therapy: Recommendations for Treatment, Training, and Privileging*. 2nd ed. Washington: American Psychiatric Association; 2001:83–84.

185. Answer: B. Gerald Klerman and Marna Weissman developed IPT in the course of the Boston-New Haven Collaborative Depression Project in the 1970s. Harry Stack Sullivan developed an interpersonal theory of psychiatry, but is generally not credited with the development of IPT. Beck developed cognitive behavioral therapy (CBT). Skinner was a behaviorist. Frankl developed Logotherapy. Linehan developed dialectical behavioral therapy (DBT).

Hales RE, Yudofsky SC. *Textbook of Clinical Psychiatry*. 4th ed. Washington: American Psychiatric Publishing; 2003:1207–1222.

186. Answer: E. Anticonvulsants are effective for the treatment of trigeminal neuralgia, diabetic neuropathy, postherpetic neuralgia, and migraine recurrence. The number needed to treat (NNT) ranges from less than two to four anticonvulsants. There is some evidence that drug levels lower than those for seizures may be effective in decreasing pain. Valproate is an effective prophylactic treatment in over two thirds of the patients with migraines and almost three quarters of those with cluster headaches. Improvement occurs in the frequency of headaches, duration of headache days per month, intensity of headaches, use of other medications for acute treatment of headaches, the patient's opinion of the treatment, and ratings of depression and anxiety.

Levenson JL. *The American Psychiatric Publishing Textbook of Psychosomatic Medicine*. Washington DC: American Psychiatric Publishing; 2005:845.

187. Answer C. One of the most controversial aspects of ECT administration is its cognitive adverse effect. It is an important determinant of availability and utility in several areas. Memory deficits associated with ECT are anterograde and retrograde, more prominent around the time of treatment, and reversible in the vast majority of recipients, although in a very small proportion of patients retrograde amnesia may be enduring. Studies indicate that several factors affecting severity of cognitive deficits: advancing age, presence of pre-existing medical illness and brain injury or cognitive deficits, frequency of treatment, and electrode placement.

American Psychiatric Association Task Force on Electroconvulsive Therapy. *The Practice of Electroconvulsive Therapy: Recommendations for Treatment, Training and Privileging. Task Force Reports on ECT*. Washington DC: American Psychiatric Association; 2001:1–355.

188. Answer: B. This patient has *aprosody*, which is the term used to describe a person's inability to appreciate or endow speech with emotional or affective qualities. It is caused by a nondominant hemispheric lesion and is usually accompanied by the loss of nonverbal communication called paralinguistic components of speech (body language), such as facial expression or body movements.

1. Kaufman DM. *Clinical Neurology for Psychiatrists*. 5th ed. Philadelphia: WB Saunders; 2001:189–190.

2. Williamson JB, Harrison DW, Shenal BV, et al. Quantitative EEG diagnostic confirmation of expressive aprosodia. *Appl Neuropsychol*. 2003;10:176–181.

189. Answer: D. Cerebellar hemorrhage usually presents with sudden onset of occipital headache, vomiting, and severe ataxia, which usually prevents the patient from standing or walking. It may be associated with dysarthria due to the involvement of the adjacent cranial nerve, mostly the sixth and seventh nerves. The involvement of the sixth cranial nerve also may result in paralysis of conjugate lateral gaze to the affected side. This finding may mislead clinicians into thinking the disease is primarily in the brainstem. Lack of changes in the level of consciousness and lack of focal weakness or sensory loss indicates a cerebellar origin. Coma happens when there is enlargement of the mass with associated brainstem compression. After the patient is comatose, no intervention can help the patient. As there is a small margin of time between the alert and comatose state, prompt diagnosis using a CT scan or MRI should be carried out, and surgery should be performed. It is important especially for all larger hemorrhages, which are defined as those seen on three CT sections or those of a mass larger than 3 cm.

1. Kaufman DM. *Clinical Neurology for Psychiatrists*. 5th ed. Philadelphia: WB Saunders; 2001:277–278.
2. Rowland LP. *Merritt's Neurology*. 11th ed. Philadelphia: Lippincott Williams & Wilkins; 2005:303–305.

190. Answer: B. Seizures represent a clear danger to the fetus, and anticonvulsant medications should not be discontinued or arbitrarily reduced, particularly if there have been recent seizures. The conventional drugs (phenytoin, carbamazepine, phenobarbital, valproate) are all appropriately tolerated in pregnancy. Serum levels of most anticonvulsants, both the free and protein-bound fractions, fall slightly in pregnancy and are cleared more rapidly from the blood. The most common recorded teratogenic effects have been cleft lip and cleft palate, but the risk of major congenital defects is low. Most studies show a doubling of the risk to about 5% in women taking anticonvulsants during pregnancy. This is compared to 2% to 3% in the overall population of pregnant women. These risks are higher with polypharmacy. When lamotrigine is combined with valproate the risk of major congenital defects is close to 12%. If a woman with epilepsy has been off medications before pregnancy and seizes during the pregnancy, the drug of choice is probably phenytoin. Eclamptic seizures are best managed by infusion of magnesium.

Ropper AH, Brown RH. *Adams and Victor's Principles of Neurology*. 8th ed. New York: McGraw-Hill; 2005:296.

191. Answer: B. Panic Disorder is more common in women and has a bimodal distribution in the age at onset, with one peak in late adolescence and another one in the mid-30s. Patients with first-degree relatives with Panic Disorder have a significantly higher risk of developing this disorder. Other conditions associated with panic disorder include Major Depression, General Anxiety Disorder, Agoraphobia, PTSD, Bipolar Disorder, and Alcohol Abuse. Patients with medically unexplained syndromes (irritable bowel syndrome, palpitations and labile hypertension with negative tests for pheocromocytoma, negative chest pain) have higher rates of panic disorder than patients with documented medical disorders.

1. American Psychiatric Association. *Quick Reference to the Diagnostic Criteria from DSM-IV-TR*. Washington: American Psychiatric Association; 2000:209–213.
2. Katon WL. Clinical practice. Panic disorder. *N Engl J Med*. 2006;354:2360–2367.

192. Answer E. Using the narrow DSM-IV-TR definition of a mixed episode of bipolar disorder (BPD) (the concomitant presence of manic and major depressive episodes occurring in one or more weeks), 10% of the patients with BPD will meet criteria for mixed state. However, a broader definition (including dysphoric mania and agitated depression) puts this figure closer to 30%. Both randomized and observational studies have found no benefit with the use of antidepressants in patients with mixed episode and in some cases symptoms have been known to worsen. Although lithium has demonstrated clear efficacy in several phases of Bipolar Disorder, divalproex and antipsychotic agents are increasingly being recognized as drugs of choice in patients with Mixed Episodes.

1. Cassidy F, Murry E, Forest K, et al. Signs and symptoms of mania in pure and mixed episodes. *J Affect Disord*. 1998;50:187–201.
2. Goldberg JF, Truman CJ. Anti-depressant-induced mania: overview of current or no adverse controversies. *Bipolar Disorder*. 2003;5(6):407–420.
3. Tohen M, Greil W, Calabrese JR, et al. Olanzapine versus lithium in the maintenance treatment of bipolar disorder: a 12 month, randomized, double blind, controlled clinical trial. *Am J Psych*. 2005;162:1281–1290.

193. Answer: A. Depressive symptoms develop in about 40% to 50% of elderly patients after a stroke. Major depressive disorder is less common and develops in about 25% of these patients.

Williams LS. Depression and stroke: cause or consequence? *Semin Neurol*. 2005;25:396–409.

194. Answer: D. All of the statements were made by the FDA except statement D. The agency was considering

adding a similar warning to the labeling for older antipsychotic medications, but they have not yet done so at the present time.

http://www.fda.gov/bbs/topics/ANSWERS/2005/ANS01350. html. Accessed September 10, 2006.

195. Answer: D. Basal ganglia consists of the caudate nucleus, putamen, globus pallidus, subthalamic nucleus, and the substantia nigra. Striatum is the term used to describe the caudate nucleus and the putamen together. *Corpus striatum* refers to the caudate nucleus, the putamen, and the globus pallidus and the term *lentiform nucleus* refers to the putamen and the globus pallidus together.

Sadock BJ, Sadock VA. *Kaplan and Sadock's Comprehensive Textbook of Psychiatry*. 8th ed. Philadelphia: Lippincott Williams & Wilkins; 2005:23–25.

196. Answer: C. Loss of vision in the temporal aspect of the visual field bilaterally (bitemporal hemianopsias), are caused by lesions that compress the optic chiasm. Visual field abnormalities are caused by compression of the crossing fibers in the optic chiasm. Initially this compression presents as bitemporal superior quandrantanopia, but as the lesion enlarges, the visual field cut extends to bitemporal hemianopsia. Most of these tumors are pituitary macroadenoma that may present with panhypopituitarism when the normal pituitary gland is destroyed. Headaches resulting from stretching of the diaphragma sellae and adjacent dural structures that transmit sensation through the first branch of the trigeminal nerve may also be seen.

1. Kaufman DM. *Clinical Neurology for Psychiatrists*. 5th ed. Philadelphia: WB Saunders; 2001:303.
2. Rowland LP. *Merritt's Neurology*. 11th ed. Philadelphia: Lippincott Williams & Wilkins; 2005:404, 421–422.

197. Answer: A. Treatment of migraines consists of abortive and prophylactic therapy. NSAIDs may be used as abortive treatment, while TCAs, SSRIs, divalproex, and beta blockers may be used for prophylaxis. Of the above choices, only TCAs and SSRIs are useful in the treatment of depression, and beta blockers may actually contribute to depression. SSRIs are equal to or less effective than TCAs in the treatment of migraines, and their use with serotonin agonists like sumatriptan may precipitate serotonin syndrome.

Kaufman DM. *Clinical Neurology for Psychiatrists*. 5th ed. Philadelphia: WB Saunders; 2001:209.

198. Answer: B. Surgery may be indicated when seizures are refractory to optimal medical treatment and disrupt quality of life. Generally surgery may be considered after two trials of high dose monotherapy and one trial of combination therapy. After the procedure, seizures completely or nearly cease in about two thirds of the patients with another one fourth experiencing significant reduction. Often a Wada test or other determination of dominance is performed prior to surgery to predict possible postop complications. Focal resection is the most common type of epilepsy surgery.

1. Kaufman DM. *Clinical Neurology for Psychiatrists*. 5th ed. Philadelphia: WB Saunders; 2001:247.
2. Rowland, LP. *Merritt's Neurology*. 11th ed. Philadelphia: Lippincott Williams & Wilkins; 2005:1007–1008.

199. Answer: C. Carbidopa is combined with L-dopa in the initial treatment of Parkinson's disease. Carbidopa inactivates dopa decarboxylase, but does not cross the blood brain barrier in any significant amount. This leaves more L-dopa intact to be converted to dopamine in the nigrostriatal tract. This also helps to reduce the systemic side effects of dopamine.

Kaufman DM. *Clinical Neurology for Psychiatrists*. 5th ed. Philadelphia: WB Saunders; 2001:455–456.

200. Answer: C. L-dopa and dopamine agonists cause a variety of side effects. Nausea is likely the result of stimulation of the emesis center in the medulla. Postural hypotension, sleep disturbance, hallucinations, and mental status changes may also result. Dyskinesias from the use of L-dopa and dopamine agonists include buccal-lingual movements, chorea, akathisia, dystonia, and rocking.

Kaufman DM. *Clinical Neurology for Psychiatrists*. 5th ed. Philadelphia: WB Saunders; 2001:255, 457.

Test 4

Questions

1. Rates of divorce are highest in couples who:
   A. Marry as teenagers
   B. Come from different socioeconomic backgrounds
   C. Experience the accidental death of a child
   D. Grapple with sexual difficulties
   E. Suffer severe financial losses

2. All the following statements are TRUE of neurotransmission through G-protein receptors EXCEPT:
   A. Their action is linked to the binding of guanyl nucleotides.
   B. They consist of six transmembrane-spanning proteins, the largest of which interacts with the G-protein.
   C. The G-protein has three subunits (alpha, beta, and gamma).
   D. The alpha unit contains GTP-ase activity.
   E. The G-protein mechanism can either be inhibitory or excitatory.

3. A 45-year-old executive is at the office preparing for an important company presentation when she learns that her ill grandmother has passed away. Although saddened by the news, she decides she must complete her presentation, which is scheduled for that afternoon. She makes an effort to put the news of her grandmother's death temporarily out of her mind while focusing on her work project. Later that evening at home, she grieves privately for the loss of her grandmother. This is an example of which of the following defense mechanisms?
   A. Repression
   B. Sublimation
   C. Dissociation
   D. Suppression
   E. Regression

4. A biotechnology company has developed a new enzyme-linked immunosorbent assay (ELISA) test to diagnose human immunodeficiency virus (HIV) infections. The serum from 1,000 patients, which was positive by Western blot (the gold standard assay), was tested with this new test and 999 were found to be positive. The manufacturer then used this new test to check the serum of 1,000 nuns who denied any risk factor for HIV infection. Nine hundred and ninety-nine of these samples were negative with one positive result, compared to all negative by the Western blot.

Given this information, what is the positive predictive value (PPV) of this new ELISA test?
   A. 99.9%
   B. 9.99%
   C. 10.0%
   D. 1.0%
   E. 90.0%

5. Which one of the following tests would be most helpful in identifying a patient with a posterior right-hemisphere lesion, assuming that the patient failed the test?
   A. Boston Diagnostic Aphasia Examination
   B. Facial Recognition Test
   C. Rorschach Test
   D. Thematic Apperception Test
   E. Wisconsin Card Sorting Test

6. Which one of the statements is TRUE regarding lamotrigine therapy for bipolar disorder?
   A. It has been found to be empirically useful, but is yet to be approved by the Food and Drug Administration (FDA) for the treatment of bipolar disorder.
   B. It has proven to have better efficacy for the treatment of mania than prevention of depressive relapses.
   C. Although it has demonstrated efficacy in the treatment of bipolar disorder, a few studies have questioned its efficacy.
   D. Lamotrigine-induced rash is not dose dependent.
   E. All rashes associated with lamotrigine should be evaluated carefully as this is a clear indication for discontinuation of therapy without exception and patients who develop such rashes should never again be exposed to lamotrigine.

7. A 35-year-old woman is brought to the emergency department by police after accusing her 8-year-old daughter of attempted poisoning. The patient believes that she is the target of a multi-organizational plot, which has recently culminated in attempts on her life. In the emergency department, she insists that the CIA has implanted a monitoring device into her abdomen. Her acute presentation has been preceded by 8 months of gradual functional decline, social isolation, and odd beliefs. She is admitted to the hospital, given an organic workup, diagnosed with

schizophrenia, and treated with antipsychotic medication. Upon improvement of her psychiatric condition, she asks about the likelihood that her daughter will later develop schizophrenia. Given the patient's diagnosis of schizophrenia and assuming no additional family history, her daughter's lifetime risk of developing schizophrenia is approximately:

A. 1%
B. 5%
C. 12%
D. 25%
E. 40%

8. A 25-year-old man presents to the emergency room (ER) with a chief complaint of chest pain and an impending sense that he is going to die. His blood pressure is 190/120 and his heart rate is 110 beats per minutes. He also endorses numbness and tingling, as well as a headache and palpitations. Of the following, which would be the most appropriate approach?

A. Perform an electrocardiogram (EKG) and, if it is negative, send the patient home with a referral to a psychiatrist
B. Perform an EKG and obtain cardiac enzymes and, if they are negative, send the patient home with a referral to a psychiatrist
C. Obtain a 24-hour plasma collection
D. Obtain a 24-hour urine collection
E. Obtain an EKG, routine labs, and thyroid function tests and, if they are negative, start the patient on paroxetine and send him home with a referral to a psychiatrist

9. You are asked to evaluate an 18-year-old woman who recently set fire to her porch "accidentally." She smiles as she describes the pleasurable feelings she has when witnessing fires. She reports that she has burned many other items, which upsets her mother, but she has never before been in any legal trouble. She has nothing apparent to gain by these actions. She is not psychotic and does not abuse substances. Her parents divorced and she was raised as an only child by her mother, who has depression. There is no history of childhood abuse. Given her history what is the most possible diagnosis for her condition?

A. Conduct Disorder
B. Manic Episode
C. Impulse Control Disorder, Not Otherwise Specified (NOS)
D. Antisocial Personality Disorder
E. Posttraumatic Stress Disorder (PTSD)

10. Systematic desensitization, as developed by Joseph Wolpe, incorporates all of the following EXCEPT:

A. Relaxation training
B. Implosion
C. Hierarchy construction
D. Desensitization
E. Reciprocal inhibition

11. Which one of the following statements is NOT TRUE regarding the selegiline patch?

A. Randomized controlled trials in patients with major depressive disorder have shown it to be efficacious, as compared to placebo.
B. Randomized controlled trials have shown it to be devoid of side effects such as hypertensive crisis.
C. It offers the advantage of reduced/minimal dietary restriction.
D. It preferentially inhibits gastrointestinal monoamine oxidase (MAO)-A, in addition to brain MAO-B.
E. In the randomized controlled trials, application site reactions appear to be a common side effect.

12. Which one of the following benzodiazepines has the longest half life?

A. Alprazolam
B. Lorazepam
C. Diazepam
D. Chlordiazepoxide
E. Oxazepam

13. Which one of the following statements is correct when considering electroconvulsive therapy (ECT)?

A. Atropine is administered to lower the seizure threshold.
B. Etomidate is a muscle relaxant.
C. Succinylcholine is administered to reduce secretions.
D. Beta blockers are contraindicated.
E. If succinylcholine is contraindicated, mivacurium can be used.

14. Which of the following is NOT a principle used in motivational interviewing for patients with substance use disorders?

A. Rolling with resistance
B. Establish personal goals
C. Develop discrepancy
D. Support self-efficacy
E. Develop confrontational interviewing strategies

15. Which finding regarding 5-hydroxyindolacetic acid (5-HIAA) and homovanillic acid (HVA) in the cerebrospinal fluid (CSF) of suicide attempters is accurate?

A. Levels of 5-HIAA and HVA are both decreased.
B. Levels of 5-HIAA are increased and levels of HVA are decreased.
C. Levels of 5-HIAA are decreased and levels of HVA are increased.

D. Levels of 5-HIAA are decreased and levels of HVA are normal.

E. Levels of 5-HIAA are decreased and there is no HVA in the cerebrospinal fluid (CSF).

16. Which one of the following would not be seen as part of a cerebral hemisphere injury?

A. Lower facial weakness on the contralateral side

B. Weakness of the contralateral trunk, arm, and leg

C. Hypoactive deep tendon reflexes in the contralateral arm and leg

D. Spasticity of the the contralateral trunk, arm, and leg

E. Babinskis sign

17. Acquired immunodeficiency syndrome (AIDS) has a widespread effect on both the peripheral and central nervous system (CNS). Which of the following is the most common peripheral nervous system (PNS) manifestation of AIDS?

A. Neuropathy

B. Guillain-Barré syndrome

C. Mononeuritis multiplex

D. Mononeuropathy

E. Myelopathy

18. A 9-year-old boy is brought for evaluation of seizures. He began having seizures at the age of 4, which were initially well controlled with phenytoin; at this time, his seizures have become refractory to treatment. His father noted that some of the seizures appear to start in his left foot, but quickly generalize. The child has not had any head imaging. He is noted to have a hypopigmented area on his back, as well as several erythematous maculas around his nose, which are similar in appearance to some lesions his father has on his forehead. A more detailed family history reveals many individuals in the paternal lineage with skin lesions and epilepsy, as well as a cousin that was recently diagnosed with autism. Which of the following disorders is a diagnostic possiblity?

A. Rett syndrome

B. Tuberous sclerosis (TS)

C. Fragile X syndrome

D. Juvenile myoclonic epilepsy

E. None of the above

19. Which of the following findings would NOT be expected in a 45-year-old woman with internuclear ophthalmoplegia, spastic paraparesis, incontinence, and scanning speech?

A. Increased rate of synthesis of CSF IgG

B. The presence of CSF oligoclonal bands

C. The presence of CSF myelin basic protein

D. Xanthochromic supernatant

E. Normal CSF protein concentration

20. A 68-year-old alcoholic patient is brought to the ER because his wife found him to be behaving bizarrely. He has a history of alcohol-induced cirrhosis and on examination he is agitated, disoriented and speaking nonsensically. Blood draw reveals an ammonia level of 90 mg/dL. On an electroencephalogram (EEG) recording, which one of the following would be the most characteristic finding in this patient?

A. A fully flat EEG recording

B. Increased high frequency alpha waves

C. Normal frequency and amplitude

D. Triphasic delta waves

E. Almost entirely theta wave activity

21. Which of the following is the rate limiting step in the synthesis of dopamine?

A. Conversion of tyrosine to L-dihydroxyphenylalanine (L-dopa) by tyrosine decarboxylase

B. Conversion of L-dopa to dopamine by dopa decarboxylase

C. Conversion of phenylalanine to tyrosine by phenylalanine hydroxylase

D. Conversion of tyrosine to L-dopa by tyrosine hydroxylase

E. Conversion of L-dopa to dopamine by tyrosine hydroxylase

22. A 47-year-old man, who recently arrived from Bangladesh, presents with complaints of skin lesions and peripheral neuropathy. He notes insidious onset of numbness and tingling in his toes and fingertips, which has progressed slowly to symmetrically involve his feet and hands. He has difficulty gripping objects. Upon examination, he has a skin rash with hyperpigmentation and hyperkeratosis. He has diminished proprioception in his hands and feet, with a hyperesthetic response to pinprick sensation on the soles of his feet. There is slight bilateral muscular weakness in the dorsiflexors of his toes and ankles, wrist extensors, and intrinsic muscles of the hand. Reflexes are absent at the ankles and 1+ in the knees. Laboratory studies indicate anemia and leukopenia. He is likely suffering from toxicity of which agent?

A. Arsenic

B. Thallium

C. Toluene

D. Radon

E. Lead

23. Which of the following tracts does NOT carry sensory information?

A. Corticospinal tract

B. Lateral spinothalamic tract

C. Anterior spinothalamic tract

D. Spinocerebellar tract

E. Posterior columns

24. Which of the following is NOT TRUE of Horner's syndrome (lesion of the hypothalamospinal tract)?

A. Ptosis

B. Miosis

C. Anhidrosis

D. Signs are ipsilateral to the side of the lesion

E. Signs are contralateral to the side of the lesion

25. A 35-year-old man complains that he has a headache which is causing him excruciating pain. He has suffered from these headaches many times before, and they have been so great that, at times in the past, he has strongly considered suicide. He distrusts doctors, but his friend, witnessing his suffering, has finally convinced him to seek help. He tends to have several of these headaches at one time over the span of a couple of days after which they remit, often for months, and then recur. He describes the pain as sharp and often feels like an ice pick is boring into his left eye. He also endorses mild rhinorrhea. To help relieve his suffering and hopefully improve his trust in doctors, your next step is to:

A. Admit him immediately to the psychiatric ER.

B. Administer 100% oxygen as an abortive treatment.

C. Give lithium as an abortive treatment and prescribe home oxygen treatments for prophylaxis.

D. Administer 100% oxygen and amitriptyline.

E. Prescribe amitriptyline alone.

26. A 54-year-old man developed aphasia after a recent stroke. His neurologist has referred him for speech therapy. What is one of the most important factors that the therapist needs to consider to help this patient?

A. Determine the patient's premorbid functioning.

B. Set specific goals with the patient.

C. Keep a rigid schedule in the therapy to provide structure.

D. Identify patient's areas of strength to use for compensatory purposes.

E. Explain to patient that there is no treatment for post-stroke aphasia.

27. According to Erik Erikson, in middle adulthood, if a person does not have any impulses to steer the new generation or to nurture and guide children, then they are suffering from a crisis of which one of the following?

A. Generativity

B. Stagnation

C. Isolation

D. Identity

E. Role confusion

28. All of the following are examples of G-protein receptors EXCEPT:

A. Dopamine receptors

B. Noradrenaline receptors

C. Most serotonin receptors

D. Nicotinic receptors

E. Muscarinic receptors

29. Each one of the following statements regarding object relations theory is correct EXCEPT:

A. It originated in the work of Melanie Klein, DW Winnicott, and WRD Fairbairn.

B. It stresses that all drives emerge in the context of the mother-infant relationship.

C. It is a theory which involves the unconscious transformation of interpersonal relationships into internalized structures.

D. It regards conflict as a struggle between wishes and desires, or between intrapsychic agencies.

E. Character is viewed as heavily influenced by the presence of self-representations and object-representations deriving from introjections.

30. A biotechnology company has developed a new ELISA test to diagnose HIV infections. The serum from 1,000 patients which was positive by Western blot (the gold standard assay) was tested with this new test and 999 were found to be positive. The manufacturer then used this new test to check the serum of 1,000 nuns who denied any risk factor for HIV infection. Nine hundred and ninety-nine of these samples were negative with one positive result, compared to all negative by the Western blot. Given this information, what is the negative predictive value (NPV) of this new ELISA test?

A. 99.9%

B. 9.99%

C. 10.0%

D. 1.0%

E. 90.0%

31. The Bender Visual Motor Gestalt Test would be the most appropriate screening tool for which of the following conditions:

A. Damage to frontal lobes or caudate

B. Dominant, or left, hemisphere lesion

C. Korsakoff's syndrome

D. Short-term memory loss

E. Signs of organic dysfunction

32. A 45-year-old man on lamotrigine therapy develops a spotty, nontender, and nonconfluent rash on the right forearm 3 days after you initiate lamotrigine therapy for bipolar disorder. Which of the following is TRUE of this presentation?

A. This patient has Stevens-Johnson syndrome and lamotrigine should be discontinued immediately and patient should never be re-challenged with this medication.

B. This rash may resolve in 120 days.

C. Antihistamine is unlikely to affect this rash, because it is a hypersentivity reaction.

D. Upon resolution of this rash, therapy may be re-initiated at the previously highest effective dose.

E. Rashes occurring within 5 days of initiating lamotrigine therapy may be benign.

33. Schizophrenia, Catatonic Type, as defined in the DSM-IV-TR, is a type of Schizophrenia in which the clinical picture is dominated by at least two specific clinical features. Which of the following is NOT included in the DSM-IV-TR criteria for this condition?

A. Stupor

B. Affective flattening

C. Excessive motor activity

D. Echopraxia

E. Prominent grimacing

34. In the DSM-IV-TR definition of Schizophrenia, which one of the following is NOT included as a characteristic symptom?

A. Delusions

B. Affective flattening

C. Alogia

D. Anhedonia

E. Avolition

35. Which one of the following statements is NOT TRUE in people with a diagnosis of Pathological Gambling?

A. Greater than 60% have a history of a comorbid substance abuse disorder in their lifetime.

B. The reported suicide rate is between 17% and 24%.

C. More than 50% develop a subsequent affective disorder.

D. As many as 90% may meet criteria for a personality disorder.

E. None, all of the above are true.

36. Which of the following strategies has demonstrated the greatest success with respect to smoking cessation?

A. Physician advice

B. Over-the-counter gum

C. Over-the-counter patch

D. Behavior therapy

E. Self-help books

37. A 37-year-old man presents to your clinic asking for a detoxification from heroin. The patient is having mild withdrawal symptoms, and asks about buprenorphine maintenance. Which of the following statements is correct about this medication?

A. It has clear benefit over methadone in maintaining sobriety.

B. It can safely be given every other day.

C. It has no known drug-to-drug interactions.

D. Symptomatic hyperthyroidism is a relative contraindication.

E. It has only minimal abuse potential.

38. Which one of the following statements is TRUE regarding the treatment of sleep-related disturbances in PTSD?

A. Selective Serotonin Reuptake Inhibitors (SSRIs) have a high success rate in the treatment of sleep-related disturbances in PTSD.

B. Nightmares are particularly resistant to pharmacological treatment in PTSD.

C. Trazodone is contraindicated in the treatment of sleep-related disturbances in PTSD.

D. Benzodiazepines are the treatment of choice for sleep-related disturbances in PTSD.

E. Cyproheptadine is contraindicated in the treatment of sleep-related disturbances in PTSD.

39. Which one of the following approaches is used to reduce cognitive side-effects in ECT?

A. Using sine wave form stimulation

B. Placing electrodes bilaterally

C. Inducing three seizures per session

D. Using brief pulse stimulation

E. Increasing the lithium dose for patients on lithium

40. Which one of the following is NOT a stage in the transtheoretical model of behavior change?

A. Precontemplation stage

B. Meditation stage

C. Preparation stage

D. Action stage

E. Maintenance stage

41. Since 1994 the rate of suicide rates among those aged 15 to 24 years and those aged 80 or older has:

A. Increased for the elderly and decreased for the young

B. Increased for both age groups

C. Remained the same for both age groups

D. Decreased for both age groups

E. Has decreased for the elderly and increased for the young

42. Presence of muscle flaccidity, atrophy, and hypoactive deep tendon reflexes indicates which of the following conditions?
    A. Peripheral nerve lesion
    B. Injury to the anterior horn cell of the spinal cord
    C. Motor neuron disease
    D. All of the following conditions
    E. None of the following conditions

43. A frantic mother brings her 14-year-old son into the ER after finding him in their garage, confused, unable to walk, and having difficulty seeing. She reports that over the past year her son's grades have gone from A's to D's, he is no longer interested in athletics, and spends an excessive amount of time sleeping. Given his change in mental status, ataxia, and confusion, a head computed tomography (CT) followed by a magnetic resonance imaging (MRI) are completed. The MRI shows cerebral demyelination. Which of the following properties enable volatile substances, such as n-hexane and toluene to be toxic to the CNS?
    A. Promote free radical generation
    B. Lipophilia
    C. Hydrophilia
    D. Easily enter the blood stream
    E. Block neurotransmitter action

44. Which of the following features are characteristic of a mitochondrial inheritance pattern?
    A. Transmission through women only
    B. Recurrent miscarriages in a family
    C. Earlier onset or worsening of the genetic condition over successive generations
    D. Appearance of the disorder in offspring of a consanguineous union
    E. New onset of the disorder in a family

45. A 75-year-old man is brought in to the physician's office for evaluation of urinary incontinence. On examination he is noted to have cognitive impairment and gait apraxia. CT of the brain reveals dilatation of the ventricles, particularly the temporal horns. Which of the following statements regarding this patient's illness is TRUE?
    A. CSF pressure will be elevated.
    B. CSF glucose will be decreased.
    C. EEG would be helpful in the diagnosis of this illness.
    D. Removal of CSF will always improve the cognitive impairment.
    E. Improvement in gait after removal of CSF is helpful in the diagnosis of this illness.

46. A 65-year-old woman is admitted to the medical intensive care for respiratory support following an anoxic brain injury. The family would like to speak with the team regarding the likelihood that the patient will make any significant recovery. To better inform this discussion, an EEG is obtained and it reveals continued high voltage delta activity. What does this finding tell you about the patient's prognosis?
    A. Such a finding is nondiagnostic in a patient who is being mechanically ventilated.
    B. It is a poor prognostic finding, usually present only in later stages of coma.
    C. It is a good prognostic finding, and likely predicts a high degree of recovery of function.
    D. It is almost always associated with toxic encephalopathies, and so clearance of this toxin should result in good recovery.
    E. All patients with anoxic brain injury would have continuous high voltage delta activity, and so no prognostic conclusions can be made.

47. The L-dopa/Carbidopa (Sinemet) combination is beneficial in Parkinson's disease for which of the following reasons?
    A. Carbidopa inhibits tyrosine hydroxylase peripherally
    B. Carbidopa inhibits tyrosine hydroxylase centrally
    C. Carbidopa inhibits dopa decarboxylase peripherally
    D. Carbidopa inhibits dopa decarboxylase centrally
    E. Carbidopa inhibits tyrosine hydroxylase both centrally and peripherally

48. When compared to children, adults with lead poisoning are more likely to develop which one of the following?
    A. Mononeuropathies
    B. Mental retardation
    C. Poor work performance
    D. Acute encephalopathy
    E. Mees lines

49. Following a motor vehicle accident, a patient presents with paresis and loss of position sense of his right leg. Babinski sign and increased deep tendon reflexes are also present on the right side. In addition, he has decreased sensation of his left leg. This clinical presentation is most likely due to an acute injury in which of the following areas?
    A. Spinal cord left side
    B. Spinal cord right side
    C. Left frontal lobe
    D. Fractured right hip
    E. Right cerebellum

50. Vitamin B_{12} deficiency can result in damage to which part of the spinal cord?
   A. The dorsal column
   B. The lateral corticospinal tract
   C. The spinocerebellar tract
   D. All of the above
   E. None of the above

51. Which of the following is TRUE of cluster headaches?
   A. They occur predominantly in women.
   B. They are typically associated with auras.
   C. They can never be aborted with indomethacin.
   D. They frequently occur at night.
   E. They typically are bilateral in nature.

52. A 64-year-old man was admitted to the hospital after a left-sided stroke that caused him to be paraplegic. After a week of hospitalization, the patient is sent to a rehabilitation facility to receive physical therapy. Before his discharge, the patient asks what his chances are of walking again. What would be the most accurate answer to this patient's question?
   A. He will most likely be able to walk to some extent within 2 weeks.
   B. He will most likely never be able to walk.
   C. There is a 10% chance of him walking again to some extent in 3 to 6 months.
   D. Most hemiplegic patients are able to walk to some extent after 3 to 6 months.
   E. There is a 20% chance of him walking again to some extent in 3 to 6 months.

53. By what age are women supposed to reach their sexual prime?
   A. Mid-teens
   B. Mid-20s
   C. Mid-30s
   D. Mid-40s
   E. Mid-50s

54. Which one of the following statements is TRUE of the ion channel linked receptors?
   A. They are also called ionotropic receptors.
   B. They are concerned with fast neurotransmission.
   C. Binding of the transmitter to the receptor opens the channel to specific ions.
   D. Glutamate (NMDA and AMPA receptors) γ-aminobutyric acid (GABA)-A and nicotinic receptors are examples of ionotropic receptors.
   E. They contain about 18 transmembrane segments which are arranged to form a central channel.

55. Which of the following statements about reinforcement schedules in operant conditioning is TRUE?
   A. In a fixed-ratio schedule, there is usually a rapid rate of response.
   B. In a variable-ratio schedule, there is a fairly constant rate of response.
   C. In a fixed-interval schedule, the rate of response drops to near zero after reinforcement.
   D. In a variable-rate schedule, there is a fairly constant rate of response.
   E. All of the above.

56. In a recent study, 34 participants age 60 and older, with a DSM-IV anxiety disorder [mainly generalized anxiety disorder (GAD)], and a Hamilton Anxiety Rating Scale score of 17 or higher were randomly assigned under double-blind conditions to either citalopram or placebo. Response was defined as a score of 1 (very much improved) or 2 (much improved) on the Clinical Global Improvement Scale or a 50% reduction in the Hamilton Anxiety Rating Scale score. Response and side effects with citalopram and placebo were compared by using Chi-square tests and linear modeling. Eleven (65%) of the 17 citalopram-treated participants responded by 8 weeks versus four (24%) of the 17 placebo-treated participants. In this study, what is the relative risk (RR) for patients taking citalopram to continue having anxiety compared to patients taking placebo?
   A. 2.70
   B. 2.17
   C. 0.46
   D. 0.36
   E. 3.16

57. Which one of the following statements is TRUE of the Wechsler Adult Intelligence Scale (WAIS)?
   A. A disparity between the verbal test and the performance test on the WAIS may indicate a personality disorder.
   B. Although the WAIS is a very good intelligence test, the Stanford-Binet test is more widely used.
   C. Because the reliability of the WAIS is very high, the Intelligent Quotient (IQ) is a measure of future potential.
   D. The average or normal range of IQ is 80 to 110, which is based on the assumption that intellectual abilities are normally distributed throughout the population.
   E. The validity of the WAIS is high in identifying mental retardation and in predicting future school performance.

58. A 45-year-old man on lamotrigine therapy develops a spotty, nontender, and nonconfluent rash on the right forearm 3 days after you initiate lamotrigine therapy for bipolar disorder. His rash resolves, but another rash erupts on his neck 2 weeks later. Which one of the following statements is TRUE about this rash?

A. Inquire about fever, malaise, and pharyngitis, because these may be part of the clinical picture at this time and consider having him come in for further evaluation.

B. Reassure him that since this rash began several days following initiation of therapy, it is the "benign type" and warrants no further intervention.

C. Tell him that laboratory tests may be helpful but if they show abnormalities in liver, blood count or urine, it would be highly unusual.

D. Tell him that the severity of this rash is independent of the anatomic area that is affected.

E. None of the above.

59. A 34-year-old woman with a history of depression and PTSD related to severe childhood physical and sexual abuse reports the following distressing incident to her therapist. Over the weekend, the patient was in a shopping mall with her husband, when she was approached by a strange man whom she did not recognize. The man, who appeared irritated, called her by a name that was not her own, and insisted, despite her protests, that the two of them had met in a bar several weeks ago and had made plans to meet again. Now, the patient's husband has accused her of having an affair and her marriage is in jeopardy. The patient continues to assert that she never met the man before that day. Further questioning reveals that the patient's family and friends sometimes refer to conversations or events for which she has no memory and describe her as having spoken or behaved unlike her usual self. Which one of the following is the most likely diagnosis for this woman's presentation?

A. Dissociative Fugue
B. Depersonalization
C. Dissociative Identity Disorder
D. Delirium
E. Schizophrenia

60. A 19-year-old man is brought in by his parents because during the last month they have noticed that he has appeared to be talking to himself. He has become increasingly socially withdrawn and 7 months ago dropped out of school. A medical student interviews the patient, who tells her that he hears two male voices talking about him. The medical student diagnoses him with schizophrenia based on the criteria of the patient's having auditory hallucinations,

evidence of social/occupational dysfunction, and reports by the parents that he has not seemed to want to do anything and has spoken little for almost a year. She believes that she has done so correctly based on the DSM-IV-TR criteria. Which one of the following statements is TRUE regarding this patient's diagnosis?

A. One needs at least three of the characteristic symptoms (delusions, hallucinations, disorganized speech, disorganized behavior, or negative symptoms) to diagnose schizophrenia according to the DSM-IV-TR.

B. Patients must have characteristic symptoms for at least 3 months and less than 6 months to diagnose a patient with schizophreniform disorder.

C. As a rule, one needs to have at least one of the characteristic symptoms as a requirement to diagnose schizophrenia.

D. Given the nature of the auditory hallucinations the patient is experiencing, this one characteristic symptom is sufficient for fulfilling the number of characteristic symptoms needed for a diagnosis of schizophrenia.

E. Patients must have signs consistent with schizophrenia for less than 6 weeks to receive a diagnosis of a brief psychotic disorder.

61. A 19-year-old single woman is referred to you for evaluation by a dermatologist. She has several patches of scalp with hair of various lengths or missing entirely. Her father says this has happened before and he sees her picking at her scalp more often in the evening. Her mother had a recent medical hospitalization for emergent surgery. The woman says that she has the urge to pull her hair and she feels better afterwards. She is not psychotic and denies feeling sad, though she is upset by how this affects her appearance. There is no history of any medical problems or substance abuse. Given her presentation, what is the most likely diagnosis for her condition?

A. Alopecia areata
B. Trichotillomania
C. Tricho-bezoar
D. Adjustment Disorder
E. Tinea capitis infection

62. Which of the following drugs is most suitable to manage infrequent Panic Attacks, in a patient with bronchial asthma?

A. Propranolol
B. Labetalol
C. Pindolol
D. Carvedilol
E. Bisoprolol

63. A 25-year-old man with a history of bipolar disorder who was recently admitted to the hospital for a manic episode is becoming increasingly more agitated and is refusing to take any oral medications. After threatening to punch a staff member and throwing a chair across the room, the patient received 10 mg of intramuscular (IM) haloperidol and 1 mg of IM lorazepam and was placed in 4-point restraints. After approximately 3 hours the patient has received a total of 15 mg of IM haloperidol, but continues to be very agitated, keeps screaming, and trying desperately to get out from the restraints. What will be the next best treatment option for this patient?

    A. Haloperidol 10 mg IM
    B. Haloperidol 5 mg IM
    C. No further medications are necessary since he is already on restraints.
    D. Lorazepam 2 mg IM
    E. Benztropine 1 mg IM

64. Which one of the following statement is TRUE regarding pregabalin?

    A. Pregabalin is a GABA-A receptor agonist.
    B. Pregabalin has been shown to be effective for the treatment of GAD.
    C. Pregabalin is a serotonin receptor agonist.
    D. Pregabalin has a longer onset of action when compared to benzodiazepines.
    E. Pregabalin is associated with significant and serious withdrawal symptoms.

65. Which one of the following neurophysiological changes is theorized to occur with ECT?

    A. Neurogenesis in the hippocampus
    B. Neurogenesis in the anterior cingulate gyrus
    C. Apoptosis in the orbital-frontal cortex
    D. Apoptosis in the prefrontal cortex
    E. Neurogenesis in the right parietal lobe

66. What percentage of patients with Substance Abuse disorders relapse within the first 3 months after initial treatment?

    A. Over 10% of patients
    B. Over 20% of patients
    C. Over 40% of patients
    D. Over 50% of patients
    E. Over 70% of patients

67. Dilemma that arises when choosing the distribution of scarce medical resources falls under which one of the following ethical principles?

    A. Justice
    B. Nonmaleficence
    C. Beneficence
    D. Autonomy
    E. Paternalism

68. Which one of the following statements regarding plaques in the CNS of a patient with multiple sclerosis (MS) is NOT TRUE?

    A. Plaques are sharply circumscribed lesions that are diffusely scattered throughout the brain and spinal cord.
    B. Plaques in the brain tend to be grouped around the lateral and third ventricles.
    C. Plaques of varying size may be found in the optic nerves, chiasm, or tracts.
    D. Plaques in the corpus callosum are not uncommon.
    E. Plaques in the brain stem are rare.

69. You are asked as a consultant to evaluate a patient on the neurology service for new onset psychosis. The patient is a 30-year-old woman with diabetes mellitus with a 3-year history of painful peripheral neuropathy. Her husband states that his wife has not been herself since starting pain medications to treat her condition and that she is often forgetful and irritable. In addition to her personality and cognitive changes, she has recently developed difficulty walking thus was admitted to the neurology service. Upon initial evaluation, it is determined that she has been experiencing auditory hallucinations. Physical examination reveals hyperreflexia and spasticity. You recommend an MRI and checking for which one of the following enzyme deficiencies?

    A. Glucose-6-phosphate dehydrogenase
    B. Phosphofructokinase enzyme
    C. Alpha-1-antitrypsin
    D. Alpha-galactosidase A
    E. Arylsulfatase A

70. The parents of a 1-week old infant are contacted by the state newborn screening program and informed that their child has an elevated blood phenylalanine on his newborn screening test. They bring the infant for follow-up at their pediatrician's office, where they are advised to institute a formula low in phenylalanine immediately, and that the child will need a diet low in phenylalanine indefinitely to avoid cognitive impairment. A mutation in which enzyme is responsible for the elevated serum amino acid level?

    A. Aromatic amino acid decarboxylase
    B. Tryptophan hydroxlase
    C. Phenylalanine hydroxylase
    D. Serine hydroxylmethyltransferase
    E. Cystathionine beta-synthase

71. A 30-year-old man with a history of cocaine and heroin dependence is hospitalized for persistent cough with a fever of unknown origin. A friend of the patient tells the staff that for the past several months,

the patient has been increasingly forgetful, disorganized, and has even gotten lost on his way home from work. The patient states he also feels more clumsy than usual and has had an increasingly difficult time with his hobby of putting together small model cars. The patient admits to relapsing and using heroin regularly in the past year. Which of the following tests would be most useful in diagnosis for this case?

A. CD4 count
B. CT head
C. EEG
D. Liver function tests
E. Serum drug toxicology screen

72. Which of the following is NOT an indication for continuous video EEG (VEEG) monitoring?

A. Classification of seizure type
B. Diagnosis of seizure disorder
C. Evaluation of precipitating factors
D. Surgical localization
E. Initial evaluation of seizure activity

73. A 55-year-old man presents with intermittent, excruciating pain in the lower half of the right side of his face. He states that it has been going on for several weeks and is precipitated by the slightest touch to a certain area of his face. Which of the following is correct about this disorder?

A. Sensory and motor examination is likely to be normal.
B. The cause of the pain is likely psychosomatic.
C. The cause is always idiopathic.
D. This disorder is most commonly found in young men.
E. The treatment of choice is analgesics and antidepressants.

74. A 35-year-old man presents with a history of recurrent nosebleeds over the last several months. He notes becoming easily fatigued at work; he works as a diesel mechanic. He also has noticed bruising on his arms along with weight loss. What is the most likely diagnosis for his symptoms?

A. Lead toxicity
B. Arsenic poisoning
C. Thallium poisoning
D. Benzene toxicity
E. Vitamin K deficiency

75. Which one of the following is NOT a sign of lower motor neuron (LMN) lesion?

A. Atrophy
B. Flexor plantar response
C. Flaccidity
D. Weakness
E. Spasticity

76. Which one of the following is NOT TRUE of CNS tumors?

A. Personality changes are associated with frontal lobe tumors.
B. In adults, they are most commonly a manifestation of metastases.
C. Metastatic tumors are one of the tumors most likely to hemorrhage.
D. Meningiomas and oligodendrogliomas are tumors prone to calcification.
E. A headache associated with a brain tumor will be bilateral.

77. A 56-year-old man presents with blurry vision, and careful evaluation of the eyes reveals only an impairment of the left eye to move laterally. Which one of the following statements is TRUE regarding the proper evaluation of this patient?

A. Bilateral findings should promote an examination of the nasopharynx.
B. An immediate serum sodium should be ordered.
C. This condition is unlikely to be associated with eye pain.
D. Head trauma is the most common cause of this clinical scenario.
E. Diagnostic imaging is unlikely to be helpful.

78. A 65-year-old man is being transferred to a rehabilitation facility for forced-use therapy after having a stroke. The patient would like to have more information about this modality. Which of the following statements regarding forced-use therapy in stroke is NOT TRUE?

A. It involves restraining the unaffected limb.
B. Patients need to train approximately 6 hours per day.
C. This therapy has shown to produce cortical reorganization in stroke patients.
D. The therapy usually lasts approximately 15 days.
E. The main goal of this intervention is to improve patient's balance.

79. According to Erik Erikson, which developmental crisis faces a 50-year-old woman, and with which virtue, or strength, is it associated?

A. Industry versus inferiority; fidelity
B. Generativity versus stagnation; care
C. Autonomy versus shame and doubt; will
D. Intimacy versus isolation; wisdom
E. Integrity versus despair; purpose

80. All of the following are neurotransmitters that are associated with anxiety disorders EXCEPT:

A. Noradrenaline
B. Neuropeptide Y

C. GABA
D. Cholecystokinin
E. Corticotropin-releasing factor

81. Which one of the following definitions in learning theories is NOT CORRECT?

   A. Classical conditioning describes a form of learning where the occurrence of behaviors are changed via the application of positive and negative consequences.
   B. Conditioned stimulus is described in the classical conditioning theory as the original neutral stimulus that becomes associated with an unconditioned stimulus to elicit a conditioned response.
   C. Unconditioned stimulus is described in the classical conditioning theory as a stimulus that produces a specific response without any previous training.
   D. Unconditioned response is described in the classical conditioning theory as a spontaneous response that occurs to the unconditioned stimulus.
   E. Habituation is a simple form of learning in which response lessens over time, if a stimulus is repeatedly presented.

82. In a recent study, 34 participants age 60 and older, with a DSM-IV anxiety disorder (mainly GAD), and a Hamilton Anxiety Rating Scale score of 17 or higher were randomly assigned under double-blind conditions to either citalopram or placebo. Response was defined as a score of 1 (very much improved) or 2 (much improved) on the Clinical Global Improvement Scale or a 50% reduction in the Hamilton Anxiety Rating Scale score. Response and side effects with citalopram and placebo were compared by using Chi-square tests and linear modeling. Eleven (65%) of the 17 citalopram-treated participants responded by 8 weeks versus four (24%) of the 17 placebo-treated participants. In this study, what is the RR reduction in anxiety in patients taking citalopram compared to patients taking placebo?

   A. 0.53
   B. 0.46
   C. 0.36
   D. 3.16
   E. 2.17

83. Impairment of all the following types of memory is common in aging EXCEPT:

   A. Episodic memory
   B. Immediate memory
   C. Recent memory
   D. Remote memory
   E. Semantic memory

84. A 45-year-old man on lamotrigine therapy develops a spotty, non-tender, and non-confluent rash on the right forearm 3 days after you initiate lamotrigine therapy for bipolar disorder. He calls you up to discuss this rash and during this conversation, he mentions in passing that his "out of town physician friend" had prescribed divalproex to "prevent his one sided headaches." Given this information, which one of the following statements is TRUE?

   A. This is a distraction; it has no relevance to this patient's treatment.
   B. Divalproex may increase the blood levels of lamotrigine and may have contributed to the rash.
   C. Divalproex may affect blood levels of lamotrigine, but there is no indication for changing treatment strategy at this time.
   D. Divalproex does not affect lamotrigine blood levels.
   E. When initiating lamotrigine therapy in a patient already being treated with divalproex you should escalate lamotrigine dose more rapidly.

85. Which of the following is required in order to make a diagnosis of Dissociative Amnesia?

   A. Recent history of trauma
   B. Inability to recall important personal information
   C. Memory loss is limited to a few hours or days
   D. Distress over the lost memory
   E. All of the above

86. Who coined the term *Dementia Praecox*?

   A. Emil Kraepelin
   B. Karl Jaspers
   C. Adolf Meyer
   D. Eugen Bleuler
   E. Harry Stack Sullivan

87. A 17-year-old woman is brought to the ER after passing out at home. She appears pale and somewhat thin on exam, though her body-mass index is in the normal range. She is found to be dehydrated, and the labs reveal anemia and a metabolic acidosis. The patient reluctantly admits that she used laxatives earlier today, after consuming a large package of cookies. Further questioning reveals that the patient has been using laxatives on a regular basis over the past year, generally after she has been "bad" and eaten too much. She states she has tried repeatedly to diet, but cannot seem to stop herself from eating. This has escalated to a nearly daily pattern over the past 4 months, which she relates to increased stress over college applications. The patient has also self-induced vomiting on occasion and exercises for about an hour a day because of concerns over her

weight. Based on this history, what is the most appropriate diagnosis for this patient at this time?

A. Bulimia Nervosa, Purging Type
B. Bulimia Nervosa, Nonpurging Type
C. Anorexia Nervosa, Restricting Type
D. Anorexia Nervosa, Binge-Eating/Purging Type
E. Eating Disorder NOS

88. A 48-year-old man is brought into the ER with a long history of Alcohol Dependence. The patient admits to drinking almost every day for 25 years. The patient agrees to an inpatient detoxification and completes it without incident. He asks to go on a medication that will help him stay abstinent. After discussing the options, he agrees to begin acamprosate. Which of the following statements about acamprosate is correct?

A. Acamprosate dramatically improves the chances of remission.
B. Nausea and diarrhea are the most common side effects.
C. It is generally effective in once a day dosing.
D. Use for more than a month is not recommended.
E. Renal failure is not a contraindication for use.

89. A 54-year-old man is brought to the emergency department due to assaultive and agitated behavior in the context of Alcohol Intoxication. The psychiatry resident on-call is asked to evaluate the patient for escalating and threatening behavior. The patient has an extensive medical history and the resident is concerned about the cardiac side effects of antipsychotic agents. Which of the following is NOT considered to be a risk factor for the development of QTc prolongation with the use of typical and atypical antipsychotics?

A. Obesity
B. Hypothyroidism
C. Alcoholism
D. Congestive heart failure (CHF)
E. Young age

90. The acute management of alcohol withdrawal may include any of the following medications EXCEPT:

A. Naltrexone
B. Chlordiazepoxide
C. Propranolol
D. Clonidine
E. Haloperidol

91. A 40-year-old woman with Major Depressive Disorder, recurrent with seasonal pattern, presents to your office and inquires about phototherapy. She is unsure what type of light box to buy and how to use it. Which one of the following would you recommend?

A. 5,000 lux of light for at least 30 minutes daily on awakening

B. 50,000 lux of light for at least 30 minutes daily on awakening
C. 10,000 lux of light for at least 30 minutes daily on awakening
D. 100,000 lux of light for at least 30 minutes daily on awakening
E. 10,000 lux of light for at least 10 minutes daily on awakening

92. Which of the following is the strongest long-term predictor of being able to work in patients with Schizophrenia?

A. Absence of hallucinations
B. Absence of negative symptoms
C. Cognitive function
D. Absence of delusions
E. Degree of anxiety

93. In a patient with a sudden change in mental status, a lumbar puncture is indicated. The psychiatrist evaluating the patient decides to perform the lumbar puncture himself. From an ethical perspective, which of the following principles is most closely related to the psychiatrist performing the lumbar puncture?

A. Competency
B. Autonomy
C. Informed consent
D. Exploitation
E. Confidentiality

94. Which one of the following statements regarding the lesion in Marchiafava-Bignami disease is NOT TRUE?

A. The classical lesion is a necrosis of the medial zone of the corpus callosum.
B. Lesions also commonly occur in the internal capsule, corona radiata, and subgyral arcuate fibers.
C. The gray matter is not grossly affected.
D. There is loss of myelin, but relative preservation of axis cylinders in the periphery of the lesions.
E. There is usually no evidence of inflammation aside from a few perivascular lymphocytes.

95. Which of the following areas, when disturbed, is thought to cause an inability to learn new information (anterograde amnesia) or recall recently acquired memories (retrograde amnesia) in patients with Korsakoff's syndrome?

A. Mammillary bodies
B. Cingulate gyrus
C. Thalamus
D. Hippocampus
E. Fornix

96. Approximately what percentage of Tourette's patients has comorbid Obsessive Compulsive Disorder (OCD)?

A. 15%
B. 30%
C. 50%
D. 70%
E. None of the above

97. A 17-year-old woman is admitted to the hospital with somnolence and bizarre behavior. She has a history of Polysubstance Dependence and a bottle of lorazepam was found on her person by the police. She appears to have a toxic encephalopathy. Which of the following findings would be seen on an EEG performed on this patient?

A. Increased frequency and increased beta activity
B. Decreased frequency and increased beta activity
C. Increased frequency and decreased beta activity
D. Decreased frequency and decreased beta activity
E. No abnormalities are likely to be seen

98. A 37-year-old woman comes to your neurology clinic reporting episodes of left arm tingling followed by paralysis. These episodes have occurred episodically, and seem to have begun following a cerebrovascular accident that patient had 1 year earlier. If the left arm symptoms are indeed seizure activity, what EEG finding would be most likely seen on a routing ambulatory EEG in this patient?

A. Spikes, sharp waves, and spike-and-slow wave complexes
B. Generalized slowing
C. A higher frequency of theta and delta waves
D. Uniform alpha wave activity
E. A normal EEG

99. A 35-year-old man with no significant medical history other than chronic, recurrent headache presents to the ER after a grand mal seizure. A systolic bruit is heard over the carotid in the neck and over the mastoid process, in addition, an MRI of the brain shows a small focal area of new hemorrhage, consistent with an arteriovenous malformation. Given this information, which of the following is TRUE of this disorder?

A. Systolic blood pressure is almost certainly elevated above 200 mm Hg.
B. This patient has a 50% chance of dying in the next 2 years.
C. This disorder rarely occurs in subsequent generations.
D. Seventy-five percent of patients with this disorder have migraine headaches
E. Future development of a focal neurological deficit is very unlikely.

100. Which of the following spinal pathways transmits temperature and pain sensation?

A. Corticospinal tract
B. Lateral spinothalamic tract
C. Anterior spinothalamic tract
D. Spinocerebellar tract
E. Posterior columns tract

101. Which of the following statements are TRUE about Tardive Dyskinesia (TD)?

A. It is a syndrome of repetitive, involuntary movements.
B. It can involve the face and trunk.
C. Antipsychotic medications are a common cause of tardive dyskinesia.
D. Metoclopramide, an antiemetic, can cause tardive dyskinesia.
E. All of the above.

102. Which of the following is NOT TRUE of paraneoplastic syndromes?

A. Lambert-Eaton syndrome is not a paraneoplastic syndrome.
B. Myasthenia gravis is not a paraneoplastic syndrome.
C. Neurologic symptoms from paraneoplastic syndromes precede the diagnosis of the underlying cancer in most cases.
D. Limbic encephalitis is a paraneoplastic syndrome associated with memory difficulties.
E. Paraneoplastic syndromes are autoimmune disorders whose etiologies are tumors.

103. While you were traveling in Peru, as the only doctor available at the time, you are asked to evaluate two young men who have fallen very sick after having taken a direct flight from the seashore of Lima to the high altitude of Lake Titicaca, many thousand feet above sea level. These patients had been in excellent physical health prior to their flight. They are now presenting with sudden onset of headache, anorexia, nausea and vomiting, weakness, and insomnia. Given this history, which one of the following statements is TRUE regarding their condition?

A. Psychotic symptoms are extremely uncommon.
B. A mild sedative can improve these symptoms.
C. The development of retinal hemorrhages is common.
D. Fatal cerebral edema is common.
E. Symptoms are diminished during sleep.

104. Which of the following factors is considered to be a poor predictive factor to being able to return to work after a stroke?

A. White-collar work
B. Right hemisphere damage

C. Young age

D. Aphasia

E. Level of visuomotor speed

105. A 36-year-old man lives alone in a small apartment and works as a computer programmer. He prefers to work from home and has chosen jobs that allow him to do so. He enjoys his work and such hobbies as reading and watching movies. He has few friends and has avoided romantic relationships. With which one of Erik Erikson's psychosocial stages is this man's condition associated with?

A. Trust versus mistrust

B. Identity versus role confusion

C. Intimacy versus isolation

D. Autonomy versus shame and doubt

E. Initiative versus guilt

106. All of the following are true regarding the organization of psychopharmacologically important transmitters EXCEPT:

A. The long ascending and descending axonal pathways arise from discrete neuronal cell groups located within specific brain nuclei.

B. The long ascending and descending axonal pathways are seen with glutamate and GABA pathways.

C. The long and short axonal pathways arise from neuronal cell bodies widely spread throughout the brain and are associated with the major excitatory and inhibitory pathways.

D. The long and short axonal pathways lack the very precise organizational structures of the amine pathways.

E. The short intraregional pathways including interneurons are associated with neuropeptides and GABA inhibition.

107. Which one of the following choices is part of the preoperational period of intellectual development as postulated by Jean Piaget?

A. Combinatorial system

B. Conservation of quantity

C. Object permanence

D. Reciprocity

E. Symbolic play

108. In a recent study, 34 participants age 60 and older with a DSM-IV anxiety disorder (mainly GAD) and a Hamilton Anxiety Rating Scale score of 17 or higher were randomly assigned under double-blind conditions to either citalopram or placebo. Response was defined as a score of 1 (very much improved) or 2 (much improved) on the Clinical Global Improvement Scale or a 50% reduction in the Hamil-

ton Anxiety Rating Scale score. Response and side effects with citalopram and placebo were compared by using Chi-square tests and linear modeling. Eleven (65%) of the 17 citalopram-treated participants responded by 8 weeks versus four (24%) of the 17 placebo-treated participants. In this study, what is the absolute risk reduction in anxiety in patients taking citalopram compared to patients taking placebo?

A. 41%

B. 24%

C. 65%

D. 35%

E. 76%

109. Impairment in which of the following types of memory is often the first sign of beginning cerebral disease?

A. Implicit memory

B. Recent past memory

C. Remote memory

D. Semantic memory

E. Short-term memory

110. Regarding concomitant carbamazepine and lamotrigine therapy, which one of the following is TRUE?

A. Carbamazepine increases the blood level of lamotrigine, but dose adjustment is not necessary.

B. Carbamazepine decreases the blood level of larmotrigine, but dose adjustment is not necessary.

C. Lamotrigine increases the blood level of carbamazepine, and the dose of carbamazepine should be lowered.

D. Lamotrigine increases the blood levels of carbamazepine, and its dose should be increased.

E. Carbamazepine inhibits the metabolism of lamotrigine, and the dose of lamotrigine should be increased.

111. Which one of the following physical signs is NOT commonly associated with Anorexia Nervosa?

A. Bradycardia

B. Hypothermia

C. Constipation

D. Fine body hair

E. Heat intolerance

112. A 7-year-old girl is brought to your office by her parents who are concerned because she often wakes up in the middle of the night screaming. Assuming that she is having nightmares, they often try to calm her by asking her about them, but she never remembers them. The next morning she usually cannot recall that she woke up in the middle of the night. Which

of the following statements is NOT TRUE about her condition?

A. It is associated with non-rapid eye movement (REM) sleep.
B. These episodes are most frequently seen in children.
C. Sleepwalking is associated with this disorder.
D. Stimulant use is associated with the disorder.
E. When these episodes occur in children, they are likely to be a manifestation of psychopathology.

113. Which one of the following metabolic dysregulations is most characteristic of patients with Bulimia Nervosa who engage in frequent self-induced vomiting?

A. Hyperkalemic, hyperchloremic metabolic alkalosis
B. Hypokalemic, hypochloremic metabolic acidosis
C. Hyperkalemic, hyperchloremic metabolic acidosis
D. Hyperkalemic, hypochloremic metabolic alkalosis
E. Hypokalemic, hypochloremic metabolic alkalosis

114. A 46-year-old woman in the inpatient unit begins to develop diarrhea and a fever. She also begins to manifest alterations in her gait. She gradually becomes extremely confused and disoriented. She is currently on fluoxetine and phenelzine for severe depression. The use of which of the following measures is contraindicated in the treatment of her condition?

A. Discontinuation of fluoxetine and phenelzine
B. Use of cyproheptadine
C. Use of IM chlorpomazine
D. Use of vecuronium
E. Use of succinylcholine

115. Which one of the following is the most common complication with the use of seclusion in patients who are acutely agitated?

A. Patient injury
B. Increased harmful behavior
C. Patient's escape from seclusion
D. Vomiting
E. Psychological harm

116. Which one of the following drugs use in the management of acute opioid intoxication and has a relatively short half-life?

A. Nalmefene
B. Buprenorphine
C. Naloxone
D. Levomethadyl acetate (LAAM)
E. Promethazine

117. You diagnose a patient with Circadian Rhythm Sleep Disorder (CRSD), Delayed-Sleep-Phase Type, based on the DSM-IV-TR criteria. Given this diagnosis, which one of the following would you recommend?

A. Delay his normal bedtime by 3 hours each day until he has cycled through to a new, earlier bedtime.
B. Wake each morning at the same time, regardless of his sleep onset time.
C. Take trazodone 50 mg qhs for 7 to 14 days.
D. Go to bed 3 hours earlier than his desired bedtime for at least 7 days; this resets his internal clock so that he will experience fatigue at his desired bedtime.
E. Eliminate or drastically reduce coffee and other caffeinated beverages.

118. In Cognitive Therapy, which one of the following is an automatic thought?

A. "I guess I was trying to suppress my embarrassment."
B. "I felt embarrassed when I saw him."
C. "I think that I am afraid of my own aggression."
D. "I am such a loser."
E. "I think I was feeling that the people at the party would not like me if they knew what I was really like."

119. Which of the following best captures the principle of informed consent?

A. Agreement with the physician's recommendations
B. Right to refuse interventions
C. Choice among alternatives
D. Shared decision making
E. Enhancement of autonomy

120. What is the term used to describe brain herniation that occurs when unilateral or asymmetric expansion of the cerebral hemisphere displaces the cingulate gyrus under the falx cerebri?

A. Subfalcine herniation
B. Uncal herniation
C. Mesial temporal herniation
D. Transtentorial herniation
E. Tonsillar herniation

121. Ninety percent of the population is thought to be right-handed with left hemisphere language dominance. Given that information, which one of the following is considered to be a dominant hemispheric language function?

A. Inflection in voice
B. Speaking obscenities
C. Sign language
D. Prosody
E. Rhythm

122. Which one of the following is NOT crucial for the diagnosis of a mitochondrial disease?
    A. Recognition of an appropriate clinical syndrome
    B. Presence of lactic acidosis in blood or CSF
    C. Detection of ragged-red fibers (RRF) in the muscle biopsy
    D. Mutations transmitted by Mendelian inheritance
    E. Identification of a pathogenic mutation in mitochondrial DNA (mtDNA) or in nucleus DNA (nDNA)

123. The major difference between EEG recordings collected using the referential, or monopolar, method and the bipolar method is which of the following?
    A. The bipolar method records electrical activity between various electrodes and an electrically neutral point, usually an ear.
    B. The bipolar method, as opposed to the monopolar method, records activity between pairs of electrodes.
    C. The monopolar method only records amplitude of wave activity, whereas the bipolar method records both amplitude and frequency.
    D. The monpolar method only records wave activity on one brain hemisphere.
    E. The monopolar method is most useful in the waking patient, whereas the monopolar method should be used for the sleeping patient.

124. Which one of the following is NOT TRUE of a positron emission tomography (PET) scan?
    A. PET image is basically a density map of radioactivity in a slice of tissue viewed in two dimensions.
    B. The most commonly used PET radionuclides is 2-fluoro-2-deoxy-D-glucose (FDG).
    C. PET scanning is severely limited by its need for close proximity to a cyclotron.
    D. The spatial resolution of PET scan is not as good as that of a functional MRI (fMRI) or single photon emission computed tomography (SPECT) scan.
    E. Hypermetabolism due to increased blood flow can be seen in tumors, infections, or seizure foci.

125. Which one of the following is the initial manifestation of Normal Pressure Hydrocephalus (NPH)?
    A. Aphasia
    B. Gait disturbance
    C. Impaired executive function
    D. Urinary incontinence
    E. Memory loss

126. Which of the following spinal tracts transmit position and vibratory sensation?
    A. Corticospinal

B. Lateral spinothalamic
C. Anterior spinothalamic
D. Spinocerebellar
E. Posterior columns

127. Huntington's disease results from which one of the following?
    A. A loss of dopaminergic neurons in the striatum
    B. An overabundance of GABA in the substantia nigra
    C. An overabundance of GABA in the striatum
    D. Increased cholinergic activity in the caudate
    E. None of the above

128. A 45-year-old man has noticed that he has been having increasing difficulty with his hearing and ringing in his ears. His neurologist performs an MRI of the brain as well as other diagnostic tests and tells the patient that he has an acoustic neuroma. Which of the following is TRUE of acoustic neuromas?
    A. They are highly malignant.
    B. They are associated with tuberous sclerosis.
    C. They are associated with neurofibromatosis II.
    D. They are associated with neurofibromatosis I.
    E. They represent a proliferation of Schwann cells covering the eighth cranial nerve and are unlikely to involve any other cranial nerves.

129. A 78-year-old man is in the neurological intensive care unit recovering from a subarachnoid hemorrhage. A nurse calls you to the patient's bedside saying that he appears more lethargic from the morning. On review of morning labs, the serum sodium is recorded at 119 mmol/l and you note that the patient's urine is hypertonic relative to his serum. Given this history, which of the following statements is TRUE regarding his condition?
    A. The more slowly that the condition developed, the worse the prognosis.
    B. A specific type of intravenous fluid should be immediately administered.
    C. Central pontine myelinolysis is the end result of this disorder when untreated.
    D. This condition is almost always fatal if not caught within the first few days.
    E. In more severe cases, a diuretic like furosemide needs to be given.

130. Which of the following factors does NOT play an important role in cortical reorganization after a stroke?
    A. Letting the affected extremity rest so that it can recover strength
    B. Intensive practice sessions
    C. Forcing the patient to use the affected extremity

D. Progressive increase of the complexity of the motor tasks
E. Practice sessions with repetitive exercises

131. Which of the following statements regarding Daniel Levinson's developmental periods are TRUE?
A. It outlined stages in adulthood.
B. It included transitional phases.
C. It applies to men and women.
D. All the statements are TRUE.
E. None of the statements are TRUE.

132. Which one of the following statements is TRUE regarding the limbic system?
A. There is unanimity about what structures belong in it.
B. The sole purpose of all the structures is in emotional regulation.
C. The medial forebrain bundle is the principle output of the limbic system.
D. The entorhinal cortex is the principle source of inputs to the amygdale.
E. The CA1 axons project to the CA3 cells in hippocampus.

133. In a recent study, 34 participants age 60 and older, with a DSM-IV anxiety disorder (mainly GAD), and a Hamilton Anxiety Rating Scale score of 17 or higher were randomly assigned under double-blind conditions to either citalopram or placebo. Response was defined as a score of 1 (very much improved) or 2 (much improved) on the Clinical Global Improvement Scale or a 50% reduction in the Hamilton Anxiety Rating Scale score. Response and side effects with citalopram and placebo were compared by using Chi-square tests and linear modeling. Eleven (65%) of the 17 citalopram-treated participants responded by 8 weeks versus four (24%) of the 17 placebo-treated participants. In this study, what is the number needed to treat (NNT) for citalopram?
A. 3.0
B. 2.0
C. 4.0
D. 1.0
E. 5.0

134. Which of the following is NOT part of the usual mental status examination?
A. Description of the patient's attitude
B. Description of the patient's emotions
C. Description of the patient's marital status
D. Description of the patient's reliability
E. Description of the patient's visuospatial ability

135. Symptoms of alcohol withdrawal include all of the following EXCEPT:
A. Craving
B. Autonomic hyperactivity
C. Nystagmus
D. Sensory distortions
E. Insomnia

136. Which one of the following statements about Anorexia Nervosa is NOT TRUE?
A. Psychodynamic theories emphasize a lack of autonomy and sense of self as important in the development of the disorder.
B. A primary consideration when starting treatment is restoring the patient's nutritional status.
C. SSRIs are well studied and proven to be effective in the treatment of anorexia nervosa.
D. Patients are preoccupied with the fear of gaining weight and becoming fat, despite evidence to the contrary.
E. Mortality rates for anorexia nervosa have been found to range between 5% and 18%.

137. A 60-year-old woman calls your office to make an appointment for marital therapy with her husband. She indicates they have participated in therapy at her initiative in the past and that she has taken "every effort" to improve the relationship. She reports that she has "significantly changed," but she sees no such improvement in her husband. She wants "him to change too." She advises that her husband probably needs medications; although she would never consider taking medications herself, as she "refuses to endure any side effects." The patient states she maintains an "immaculate home" all by herself, and that she is a dutiful and considerate wife. In return, her husband is reportedly "verbally abusive and cruel." He apparently labels the patient as "too set in her ways" and "controlling." Her husband is annoyed that the patient won't accept a cleaning service for the home. The patient reports "my father was also a strict disciplinarian when I was a child, I can't take that anymore!" Given this history, what is the most likely personality type exhibited by this woman?
A. Histrionic
B. Borderline
C. Dependent
D. Schizotypal
E. Obsessive-Compulsive

138. A 20-year-old man with a 5-year history of anorexia nervosa is hospitalized for severe and ongoing weight loss, despite intensive outpatient treatment. He is found to be at 75% of his ideal body weight, and a strict and monitored refeeding program is initiated.

Which of the following is/are potential complications of refeeding in severely malnourished individuals?

A. Hypophosphatemia
B. Edema
C. CHF
D. Abdominal distress
E. All of the above

139. Which of the following best represents the tasks of treatment/outcome goals of treatment in stage I of Dialectical Behavioral Therapy for Borderline Personality Disorder (BPD)?

A. Expanded awareness, spiritual fulfillment
B. Understanding and reducing the sequelae of early trauma
C. Achieving self-control, stability and control of action
D. Achieving the capacity for sustained joy
E. Addressing self-respect and self-trust as primary goals

140. A 46-year-old man with a past medical history of asthma and hypertension has been treated for social anxiety disorder with a combination of sertraline and clonazepam for the past 3 months. The patient asks to come for an appointment with a 2-month history of anorgasmia. A month ago, his outpatient psychiatrist tapered him off the sertraline, but he has not noticed any significant improvement in his sexual functioning. What is the most likely cause of his complaint?

A. His anorgasmia is most likely a permanent side effect from SSRI use.
B. His anorgasmia is most likely secondary to chronic hypertension.
C. His anorgasmia is most likely secondary to his advancing age.
D. His anorgasmia is most likely secondary to medications used for asthma.
E. His anorgasmia is most likely secondary to benzodiazepine use.

141. Which one of the following is the first-line treatment for acute hallucinogen intoxication?

A. Diazepam administered intravenously
B. Diazepam administered orally
C. Lorazepam administered parenterally
D. Lorazepam administered orally
E. The provision of supportive measures

142. Which of the following statements is TRUE regarding motivational enhancement therapy for alcohol dependence?

A. The therapist uses confrontation as a key intervention.

B. The focus is in identifying high-risk situations.
C. It aims to mobilize energy in the patient to change.
D. It is usually a long-term therapy.
E. The therapist frequently suggests solutions.

143. In the Beck model of cognitive behavior therapy, which of the following is NOT TRUE of core beliefs?

A. One of the broad categories they fall into is that associated with a sense of helplessness.
B. One of the broad categories they fall into is that associated with a sense of hopelessness.
C. One of the broad categories they fall into is that associated with a sense of unlovability.
D. They are thought to originate in childhood.
E. Therapists hypothesize about the content of core beliefs early in the treatment.

144. Acute bacterial meningitis with *Listeria monocytogenes* is usually associated with in which of the following patient population?

A. Neonates
B. Children
C. Adolescents
D. Young adults
E. Elderly

145. Imaging studies have found that there is symmetry between the left and right cerebral hemispheres except in the dominant temporal lobe. The superior surface of the dominant temporal lobe has more cortical area compared to the rest of the cortex due it its larger gyri and deeper sulci. This finding however, is absent in which of the following conditions?

A. Chronic Schizophrenia
B. Bipolar Disorder
C. Major Depressive Disorder
D. Dementia
E. GAD

146. The most prominent wave observed on a normal EEG in a waking adult is which of the following?

A. Alpha
B. Theta
C. Beta
D. Delta
E. Lambda

147. Which of the following is an advantage of SPECT scan over a PET scan?

A. It is much cheaper to obtain than a PET scan.
B. It has the ability to evaluate glucose metabolism and perfusion simultaneously.
C. It also produces relatively lower levels of radiation exposure from the injected radionuclides.

D. Multiple studies are possible with little increase in distress to the patient.

E. All of the above.

148. A 84-year-old man with a history of severe Alzheimer's disease was admitted to the psychiatric ward due to increased agitation. After a week in the hospital, the patient started thinking that he was still a train driver and would give commands to other patients and staff, to "keep everybody safe on the train." Which would be the best approach for staff members in the unit?

A. Tell the patient that he is not in a train and escort him to his room.

B. Ignore the patient's behavior.

C. Give the patient a sedating medication and wait until it has an effect.

D. Explain to the patient that the train has arrived and that he should rest now.

E. Call a code since the patient is bothering other patients.

149. Which one of the following statements regarding George Vaillant's longitudinal study of Harvard male undergraduate students is TRUE?

A. There is no correlation between mental and physical health.

B. A close relationship to a sibling does not correlate with later emotional well-being.

C. Stability in the family during childhood years does not correlate with psychological health as an adult.

D. Tranquilizer use before the age of 50 was a strong predictor of physical health at age 65.

E. One's childhood environment does not affect physical health as an adult.

150. Which one of the statements about serotonin is NOT TRUE?

A. Stress leads to increased serotonin release.

B. Serotonin has neurotrophic factor-like effects.

C. Serotonin is not involved in pain perception.

D. Altering function of the serotonin system results in changes of appetite, sleep, sexual function, and circadian rhythms.

E. All of the above.

151. Which one of the following is TRUE of a mental status examination?

A. Delusions can be described as mood-congruent or mood-incongruent.

B. Depersonalization and derealization are disturbances in thought processes.

C. Intellectual insight is the highest level of insight.

D. Neologisms and word salad are disturbances in speech characteristics.

E. Thought blocking is assumed to occur when a patient does not want to talk.

152. Which one of the following is the approximate lifetime prevalence of either Alcohol Abuse or Dependence?

A. 0.1%

B. 1%

C. 5%

D. 15%

E. 30%

153. Which one of the following disorders is most often comorbid with anorexia nervosa?

A. Depression

B. OCD

C. Social Phobia

D. Schizophrenia

E. Avoidant Personality Disorder

154. Roger MacKinnon and Robert Michels characterize the central conflict within obsessive-personality patients as which one of the following?

A. Initiative versus guilt

B. Obedience versus defiance

C. Industry versus inferiority

D. Identity versus role confusion

E. Generativity versus stagnation

155. What are the effects of depression and alcohol on sleep architecture?

A. Depression and alcohol both increase stage III and IV sleep.

B. Depression and alcohol both decrease stage III and IV sleep.

C. Depression increases and alcohol decreases stage III and IV sleep.

D. Depression decreases and alcohol increases stage III and IV sleep.

E. Depression decreases stage III and alcohol increases stage IV sleep.

156. You are called as an expert witness to give your opinion regarding the unfortunate death of a gentleman with Chronic Paranoid Schizophrenia. The 43-year-old white man had been taking clozapine for the past several years. You are asked to comment on the FDA black box warnings for this medication which include all of the following EXCEPT:

A. Agranulocytosis

B. Seizures

C. Hypotension

D. Myocarditis

E. Thrombocytopenia

157. Which one of the following is NOT considered a poor prognostic factor for a positive response to an SSRI in the treatment of Social Anxiety Disorder?
    A. Female gender
    B. History of excessive alcohol use
    C. Patients with passive-dependent personality disorder
    D. Patients with higher systolic blood pressure
    E. Patient with higher heart rate

158. Which of the following agents and corresponding dose might prove most useful when treating a patient with cannabis dependence?
    A. Olanzapine 2.5 mg PO qhs
    B. Fluoxetine 20 mg PO qhs
    C. Buspirone 60 mg PO daily
    D. Gabapentin 600 mg PO TID
    E. Seroquel 300 mg PO qhs

159. Which one of the following statements is NOT TRUE regarding Alcoholics Anonymous?
    A. It offers peer support.
    B. It encourages role modeling.
    C. It involves a twelve-step program.
    D. It is offered to members for a small fee.
    E. It is not a professionally delivered treatment.

160. A 30-year-old man with chronic paranoid schizophrenia has been treated with a combination of quetiapine and haloperidol for 5 years. You decide to perform the Abnormal Involuntary Movement Scale (AIMS) examination. While doing the examination, which one of the following would you NOT do as a procedure?
    A. Ask him to open his mouth twice.
    B. Ask him to rapidly alternate each of his hands on the ipsilateral thigh.
    C. Observe him at rest when he is unaware.
    D. Ask him to tap his thumb with each finger rapidly on each hand.
    E. Ask him to protrude his tongue twice.

161. A patient is diagnosed with rabies after exposure to bats while spelunking. Upon microscopic examination, what is the pathognomonic finding associated with this disease?
    A. JC virus
    B. Negri bodies
    C. Kuru plaques
    D. Hirano bodies
    E. Lewy bodies

162. As a consult liaison psychiatrist you are asked to evaluate a 26-year-old man who was brought to the ER by an ambulance after being found unresponsive at home. On-site emergency medical services personnel indicate that the patient was in and out of ventricular fibrillation requiring cardiac defibrillation and resuscitation. Family members suspect a possible suicide attempt via overdose. Laboratory data is positive for heroin overdose. During the first week of the hospitalization, the patient is awake and alert, but is unresponsive to requests. The following week, he will only repeat phrases heard on TV or from his medical team. He is unable to carry a conversation, follow commands, or name objects. The language impairment seen in this man would be classified as which one of the following?
    A. Transcortical or isolation aphasia
    B. Anomia
    C. Interruption of the Perisylvian Arc
    D. Nonfluent aphasia
    E. Global aphasia

163. Which of the following factors does NOT play a major role in the development of aggression in patients with dementia?
    A. Delusional thinking
    B. Coexistence of depressive symptoms
    C. Poor communication between patient and caregiver
    D. Premorbid history of substance abuse
    E. Patient's perception of being threatened

164. Which one of the statements regarding the superego is TRUE?
    A. It includes parental values internalized by a child
    B. It is mostly conscious
    C. It is part of the topographical model of the psyche
    D. It functions primarily under the reality principle
    E. It operates using defense mechanisms

165. A 24-year-old woman presents with a worsening headache. A CT scan of the head is done and it indicates hydrocephalus. Which one of the following statements is TRUE of the ventricular system and hydrocephalus?
    A. The majority of CSF is usually in the ventricular system of the brain.
    B. Communicating and noncommunicating hydrocephalus have fundamentally dissimilar causes.
    C. Hydrocephalus is often caused by obstruction of the central canal of the medulla and spinal cord.
    D. The lateral ventricle provides the main outflow of the CSF out of the ventricular system.
    E. Stenosis of the cerebral aqueduct or both the interventricular foramina causes noncommunicating hydrocephalus.

166. While briefly scanning a report of a patient's disturbances in perception on a mental status examination, which of the following types of hallucinations would generally be considered the least pathologic?
    A. Auditory
    B. Haptic
    C. Hypnogogic
    D. Olfactory
    E. Visual

167. A 24-year-old man enters the ER with altered mental status. Subjectively he reports a "feeling of warmth" as well as an itchy face. Upon exam, he demonstrates facial flushing and pupillary constriction. His blood pressure is 90/60 mm Hg. He is most likely to be intoxicated with which one of the following substances?
    A. Heroine
    B. Cocaine
    C. Alcohol
    D. Cannabis
    E. Lorazepam

168. A 65-year-old man with a long history of Alcohol Dependence presents to the psychiatrist with his wife, who complains of her husband's memory impairment. She reports he has virtually no ability to retain recent events, though his recall for things in the distant past is good. His activities of daily living are intact, though his memory disturbance recently led to his dismissal from his job. During the interview, the patient is alert, pleasant, and cooperative. He introduces himself to the psychiatrist, though he is unable to recall the psychiatrist's name later in the interview. His general cognitive examination is notable for significant deficits in short-term memory, although other cognitive domains such as language, praxis, attention, and executive functioning are relatively intact. Neurological examination is unremarkable. Which of the following is the MOST likely diagnosis?
    A. Alcohol-Induced Persisting Dementia
    B. Alcohol-Induced Persisting Amnestic Disorder
    C. Wernicke's Encephalopathy
    D. Dementia of the Alzheimer's type
    E. Delirium

169. Which one of the following is the most frequently observed behavioral and psychological symptom in Alzheimer's disease?
    A. Delusions
    B. Depressive symptoms
    C. Hallucinations
    D. Apathy
    E. Disinhibition

170. What is the estimated constitutional predisposition for the development of a mood disorder in the presence of severe stressors and in the absence of protective factors?
    A. 5%
    B. 15%
    C. 30%
    D. 45%
    E. 60%

171. A 26-year-old woman with bipolar disorder, who has been doing well on divalproex 500 mg twice a day, comes to see you at her regularly scheduled follow-up visit. She has just come from an appointment with her gynecologist and is terribly upset and sobbing. She has been compliant with her medication and feeling well but just learned that she is 11-weeks pregnant. She has read that divalproex can have untoward effects on her unborn child and asks, what are the chances that her baby will be harmed by this medication? After explaining about neural tube defects, you inform her that the risk of these defects in pregnant women taking divalproex is about what percent?
    A. Less than 0.5%
    B. 1% to 2%
    C. 4% to 5%
    D. 6% to 8%
    E. 10%

172. Which one of the following statements is TRUE regarding the use of antipsychotic medications in PTSD?
    A. Antipsychotic medications are considered a first-line treatment for PTSD.
    B. Antipsychotic medications have only been found to be helpful for the treatment of hallucinations in PTSD.
    C. There is some evidence suggesting that antipsychotic medications can improve the core symptoms in PTSD.
    D. Antipsychotic medications are contraindicated in the treatment of PTSD.
    E. Antipsychotic medications have been associated with increased hyperarousal in PTSD.

173. Which of the following pharmacological agents is most effective for smoking cessation?
    A. Nicotine gum
    B. Nicotine patch
    C. Nicotine lozenge
    D. Nicotine nasal spray
    E. They are all equally effective

174. Which one of the following statements is NOT TRUE regarding Respite Care in the United States?

A. It can reduce homeless patients' utilization of in-patient services.

B. It requires homeless people to vacate the center during the day.

C. It encourages patients to comply with post-hospital rehabilitation.

D. It reduced homeless patient's future hospitalizations after hospital discharge.

E. It usually offers a range of social services.

175. A 45-year-old woman with an acute exacerbation of Schizophrenia is being treated on an inpatient unit. She has been receiving haloperidol in increasing doses for the two weeks while being treated in the unit. She now complains to her doctor that her muscles feel stiff and she is drooling. When her doctor examines her, he notices that the patient has cogwheel rigidity in her upper limbs and that she shuffles when she walks. These findings are different from how she had presented at the admitting physical examination. Given her history, all of the following are reasonable treatments for her physical symptoms EXCEPT:

A. Benztropine

B. Trihexphenidyl

C. Bromocriptine

D. Diphenhydramine

E. Amantadine

176. What is the usual composition of the neurofibrillary tangles associated with Alzheimer's disease?

A. $A\beta$; a peptide of 40 to 43 amino acid residues derived from amyloid precursor protein

B. Paired helical filaments of hyperphosphorylated forms of the protein tau

C. Ubiquitin and alpha–synuclein

D. Sulfatides

E. Paracrystalline arrays of beaded filaments, with actin as the major component

177. Although the majority of the children who are left-handed are found to be of normal intelligence, left-handedness is overrepresented among children with certain impairments. Which one of the following conditions is not more common in children who are left-handed as compared to children who are right-handed?

A. Epilepsy

B. Mental Retardation

C. Autism

D. Dyslexia

E. Attention-deficit/hyperactivity disorder (ADHD)

178. A 32-year-old man was being treated in the hospital with high doses of opioid analgesics for severe pain after a surgery. After his third day in the hospital, he developed intractable seizures. The patient was immediately treated with naloxone with no response. Given this history, which analgesic was this patient most likely receiving?

A. Ketorolac

B. Codeine

C. Morphine

D. Meperidine

E. Methadone

179. Use of cocaine can cause all of the following EXCEPT:

A. Decreased testosterone synthesis

B. Nasal ulceration

C. Chronic sore throat

D. Rhabdomyolysis

E. Pulmonary edema

180. All of the following are recommended in the routine assessment of cognitive impairment in late life EXCEPT:

A. Complete blood count

B. Urinalysis

C. Neuroimaging (CT or MRI)

D. EEG

E. Serum B_{12} level

181. A 23-year-old man has been experiencing episodes of violent aggression in response to minor stressors, which has gotten him into minor legal trouble. He has no history of psychiatric care, no medical problems, no history of trauma, takes no medications, does not abuse drugs, had a normal childhood, has an unremarkable family history, and has no psychotic symptoms or mood disturbance between episodes. Which one of the following is the most likely diagnosis for his condition?

A. Antisocial Personality Disorder

B. Bipolar Disorder, Type II

C. Seizure Disorder

D. Intermittent Explosive Disorder

E. Attention Deficit Disorder

182. What is the percent weight change that satisfies the minimum DSM-IV-TR criteria for weight loss or gain for a major depression disorder?

A. 5%

B. 10%

C. 15%

D. 20%

E. 25%

183. You are evaluating a 36-year-old woman in your mood disorders research clinic. Based on the Structured Clinical Interview for Diagnosis, you establish five discrete major mood episodes over the past 12 months. You assign your patient a diagnosis of Bipolar I Disorder with rapid cycling and suggest starting divalproex for the treatment of her mood disorder. Before starting this medication, you counsel the patient regarding all of the possible adverse effects of this medication EXCEPT:

    A. Hepatic failure
    B. Hemorrhagic pancreatitis
    C. Thrombocytopenia
    D. Fetal neural tube defects
    E. Hypothyroidism

184. What is the mechanism of action of buspirone?

    A. 5-HT1a antagonist
    B. 5-HT1a partial agonist
    C. 5-HT2 antagonist
    D. 5-HT2 partial agonist
    E. GABA-A receptor blocker

185. Each of the following is an indication for ECT EXCEPT:

    A. Major depressive disorder with psychotic features
    B. Parkinson's disease
    C. Neuroleptic malignant syndrome
    D. MS
    E. Intractable seizure disorder

186. Which one of the following is NOT a principle of Integrated Dual Disorder Treatment (IDDT)?

    A. Mental health and substance abuse treatment should be integrated.
    B. Treatment should focus on one specific therapeutic modality.
    C. Treatment should be provided in a stage-wise, flexible manner.
    D. Treatment is offered in a long-term format.
    E. Each treatment is individualized for the patient's needs.

187. Which one of the following best describes the mechanism of action of benztropine?

    A. It blocks muscarinic receptors.
    B. It works as a partial agonist at D2 receptors.
    C. It increases the synthesis of dopamine.
    D. It inhibits the reuptake of dopamine.
    E. It inhibits the reuptake of serotonin.

188. Which chromosome and gene pairing is matched correctly in the genetic contributors to Alzheimer's disease?

    A. Chromosome 19 and Presenilin-1
    B. Chromosome 19 and Presenilin-2

    C. Chromosome 14 and Amyloid precursor protein
    D. Chromosome 21 and Apolipoprotein E
    E. Chromosome 19 and Apolipoprotein E

189. Gerstmann's syndrome is thought to result from damage to the angular gyrus of the dominant parietal lobe. It usually presents with four neurological/cognitive deficits. Which one of the following deficits is NOT seen in Gerstmann's syndrome?

    A. Agraphia
    B. Acalculia
    C. Finger agnosia
    D. Left-right confusion
    E. Anomia

190. A 25-year-old patient was admitted to the hospital after a motor vehicle accident. After undergoing surgery for several fractures, he was brought to the postoperative unit for monitoring. He received an initial dose of 10 mg of oxycodone, but after 3 hours, the patient is still complaining of intense pain. The patient is alert and oriented and there are no signs of sedation. What should be your next step in the treatment of this patient's condition?

    A. Discontinue opioid analgesics, because the patient is most likely addicted to opioids.
    B. Give the patient an additional dose.
    C. Increase the patient's fluid intake.
    D. Wait until the patient's next scheduled dose of opioid analgesics.
    E. Ask for a pain management consultation.

191. Eugen Bleuler identified several "primary" symptoms of Schizophrenia. These included all of the following EXCEPT:

    A. Associational disturbances
    B. Autism
    C. Ambivalence
    D. Audible thoughts
    E. Affective disturbances

192. A consultation psychiatrist is asked to evaluate a 58-year-old woman hospitalized following a recent seizure. The woman's family reports a rapid decline in cognitive and functional abilities over the prior 5 months. There is no prior psychiatric history and no family history of dementia. Mental status examination reveals severe cognitive impairment with mutism. Neurological examination reveals myoclonus, extrapyramidal signs, and cerebellar signs. All of the following regarding this woman's illness are true EXCEPT:

    A. Light microscopy of brain tissue will reveal spongiform changes.
    B. The disorder typically affects people between the ages of 55 and 70 years.

C. The disorder is transmitted by a virus.

D. Prognosis is poor; the illness is rapidly fatal.

E. Detection of 14–3-3 protein in the CSF has a sensitivity and specificity of 90% for the sporadic variant of the disease.

193. A popular 34-year-old actress has recently been caught stealing clothes at a department store. For years she has repeatedly had the impulse to steal items that she could easily afford. She reports a sense of relief and gratification upon completing the act. She is aware of her actions, and is remorseful, but says she cannot control herself. She has chronic dysphoria, has a remote history of abusing alcohol, and a pattern of disturbed sexual relationships. She has no history of psychosis. Given this history, what is the most likely diagnosis for her condition?

A. Bipolar Disorder, Type II

B. Antisocial Personality Disorder

C. Impulse Control Disorder NOS

D. Obsessive Compulsive Disorder (OCD)

E. Narcissistic Personality Disorder

194. Which one of the following is TRUE of tricyclic antidepressant (TCAs) medications?

A. In general, there is a linear relationship between increasing blood levels and effectiveness.

B. The tertiary amines have better side effect profiles than the secondary amines.

C. The tertiary amines are metabolites of the secondary amines.

D. Only nortriptyline has a therapeutic serum level.

E. All of the above.

195. Which area of the brain is the most susceptible to the effects of irreversible global cerebral ischemia?

A. Pyramidal cells of the hippocampus

B. Purkinje cells of the cerebellum

C. Neurons of the substantia nigra

D. Stellate cells of the cerebral cortex

E. Pyramidal neurons of the neocortex

196. A 69-year-old man with a history of diabetes mellitus, hypertension, and hyperlipidemia presents with right arm weakness and slurred speech. During the physical examination you note that he responds appropriately to commands but is unable to repeat a phrase or name objects. His speech is slow and he is only able to utter a few words. When describing the case to the attending physician, how would you classify his aphasia?

A. Fluent aphasia

B. Global aphasia

C. Nonfluent aphasia

D. Anomia

E. Interruption of the Perisylvain Arc

197. Which of the following painful conditions does NOT respond to tricyclic antidepressants?

A. Diabetic neuropathy

B. Tension headache

C. Acute muscular pain

D. Chronic back pain

E. Migraine headache

198. A 54-year-old man comes to your office for an initial visit. He reports excruciating "shocks" of pain in his lower lip, gums, and cheek that come in clusters and only last for a few seconds. The pain episodes seem to be triggered by specific movements, such as chewing or washing his teeth. Which of the following would NOT be a recommended treatment for this patient's condition?

A. Carbamazepine

B. Baclofen

C. Phenytoin

D. Rhizotomy

E. Ibuprofen

199. A 55-year-old man comes for an initial visit due to chronic and severe lower back pain. He has had several surgeries, but continues to suffer from severe, chronic, and disabling back pain. He has failed several trials of nonsteroidal anti-inflammatory drugs (NSAIDs) and acetaminophen. The rest of the patient's medical history is unremarkable. There is no history of alcohol or illicit substance abuse. Which should be your next step to alleviate this patient's pain?

A. Prescribe higher doses of NSAIDs

B. Stop all analgesics and recommend chiropractic manipulation

C. Prescribe standing doses of oxycodone

D. Prescribe a fentanyl patch

E. Prescribe meperidine

200. A 38-year-old man with intractable bilateral frontal seizures undergoes commissurotomy. Which of the following is often a complication of this surgery?

A. Cognitive impairment

B. Lethargy

C. Bone marrow suppression

D. Dysarthria

E. Split-brain syndrome

Answers

1. Answer: C. Divorce tends to run in families and rates are highest in couples who marry as teenagers or are from different socioeconomic backgrounds. Problems regarding sex, money, or unrealistic expectations can be other causes of marital distress. However, the parenting experience places the greatest strain on a marriage. Couples without children report gaining more pleasure from their partner than those with children. Illness in a child creates the greatest strain of all in a marriage. More than 50% of marriages in which a child has died through accident or illness end in divorce.

Sadock BJ, Sadock VA. *Kaplan and Sadock's Synopsis of Psychiatry*. 9th ed. Philadelphia: Lippincott Williams & Wilkins; 2003:49–50.

2. Answer: B. Receptors for neurotransmitters can either be ion-channel linked, G-protein linked, membrane-kinase linked (insulin, growth factors) or may mediate their effects through gene transcription (steroids). G-protein receptors, also called metabotropic receptors, are coupled to an intracellular second messenger system via a G-protein. They are responsible for slow neurotransmission. When the transmitter binds to the receptor, alpha-guanyl triphosphate is released, which then either activates or inhibits the adenylate cyclase/cAMP pathway or the phospholipase C/inositol triphosphate (IP_3)/diacylglycerol (DAG) pathway.

Anderson IM, Reid IC. *Fundamentals of Clinical Psychopharmacology*. London: Taylor & Francis Group; 2004:7–9.

3. Answer: D. The executive is using the mature defense mechanism of *suppression*. She is consciously postponing attention to her internal discomfort. Her discomfort is acknowledged, but temporarily minimized (not completely avoided). On the contrary, *repression* is a neurotic defense which involves the unconscious expulsion of unwanted ideas or feelings from conscious awareness. Another neurotic defense mechanism is *dissociation*, which involves the temporary, drastic modification of one's sense of personal identity (as in a fugue state or Dissociative Identity Disorder [DID]). *Sublimation* is a mature defense mechanism which refers to gratifying one's impulses and instincts by acknowledging them, modifying them, and directing them toward socially acceptable channels. Finally, *regression* is an immature defense mechanism in which one reverts to an earlier stage of development in order to avoid the tension or conflict of the present stage.

Sadock BJ, Sadock VA. *Kaplan and Sadock's Comprehensive Textbook of Psychiatry*. 7th ed. Philadelphia: Lippincott Williams & Wilkins; 2000:584–585.

4. Answer: A. The PPV refers to the proportion of positive test results that is true positives. PPV indicates the probability that an individual with a positive result has the disease. PPV is dependant on the prevalence of the disease in the population being tested. Because it is dependant on the disease prevalence, screening for diseases in low prevalence populations yields only a few true positive test results regardless of the sensitivity and specificity of the test. In this case, the possible results of the diagnostic test can be represented in the following 2 × 2 table.

Test result outcome	Disease present	Disease absent	Total
Positive	999	1	1,000
Negative	1	999	1,000
Total	1,000	1,000	

PPV would be the number of true positives (patients who have the disease and are tested positive) divided by the total number of patients who are tested positive. In this case, that would be 999/1000; 99.9%.

1. Gray GE. *Evidence-Based Psychiatry*. Washington: American Psychiatric Publishing; 2004:123–125.
2. http://www.musc.edu/dc/icrebm/sensitivity.html. Published September 16, 2006.

5. Answer: B. Although the inability to recognize familiar faces is an uncommon disorder, defective discrimination of unfamiliar faces is a common finding in patients with right-hemisphere lesions. The Facial Recognition Test is a test requiring identifying a photograph of a face originally presented in a front view when it is included in various displays (i.e., side view, front view with shadows) and produces a high frequency of failure in patients with posterior right-hemisphere lesions. An abnormal response to the Wisconsin Card Sorting Test appears in people with damage to the frontal lobes or to the caudate and in some people with schizophrenia. Patients with left-hemisphere lesions tend to perform within normal range in visuospatial tests, but may have defects in the use of language, which can be tested via an aphasia exam. The Rorschach and Thematic Apperception Tests are types of Projective Personality Assessments.

Kaplan HI, Sadock BJ. *Kaplan & Sadock's Synopsis of Psychiatry*. 8th ed. Philadelphia: Lippincott Williams & Wilkins; 1998:197–203.

6. **Answer: C.** Although lamotrigine was approved by the FDA in 2003 for the maintenance treatment of bipolar I disorder, it has been found to have better efficacy for prevention of depression relapse than for the treatment of mania and data supporting its utility appear mixed. The most serious side effect of lamotrigine is rash which may occur in up to 40% of patients and may culminate in Stevens-Johnson syndrome. It is important to determine if lamotrigine associated rash is benign or malignant. A benign rash begins within 5 days of initiating lamotrigine therapy; it is spotty, nontender, nonconfluent, not associated with laboratory abnormalities, and usually resolves in 10 to 14 days. Given that the immune system requires several days to mount a true hypersensitivity reaction, most rashes occurring within a few days of lamotrigine therapy are likely to be benign. The management of lamotrigine induced benign rash includes halting dose escalation temporarily or discontinuing medication while the rash is monitored. The patient is instructed to call should the rash worsen or should new symptoms emerge. Antihistamine or topical steroids may also be prescribed to manage itching. Upon resolution of the rash, lamotrigine therapy may be reinitiated at a much lower dose than recommended: 5 mg to 12.5 mg. A rash occurring more than 5 days following the initiation of lamotrigine therapy is more likely to be drug related. Such rashes are tender, confluent, itchy, widespread, and are usually prominent in the upper trunk and neck areas. It is recommended that lamotrigine be discontinued immediately and permanently if a serious rash occurs. The likelihood of developing lamotrigine induced rash increases with rapid dose escalation or blood level elevations. The latter makes lamotrigine drug-drug interactions pertinent. Gradual titration of lamotrigine is recommended to reduce the potential for rash: beginning at 25 mg daily during week 2, 50 mg per day at weeks 3 and 4, 100 mg per day at week 5, and 200 mg per day at week 6.

1. http://www.fda.gov/cder/drug/InfoSheets/patient/lamotriginePIS.pdf. Published November 25, 2006.
2. Calabrese JR, Bowden CL, Sachs G, et al. A placebo-controlled 18-month trial of lamotrigine and lithium maintenance treatment in recently manic or hypomanic patients with bipolar I disorder. *Arch Gen Psychiatry*. 2003;60:392–400.
3. Calabrese JR, Suppes T, Bowden CL, et al. A double-blind, placebo-controlled, prophylaxis study of lamotrigine in rapid-cycling bipolar disorder. Lamictal 614 Study Group. *J Clin Psychiatry*. 2000;61:841–850.
4. Dunner DL. Safety and tolerability of emerging pharmacological treatments for bipolar disorder. *Bipolar Disord*. 2005;7:307–325.

7. **Answer: C.** The prevalence of Schizophrenia in children who have one parent with Schizophrenia is approximately 12%. Schizophrenia affects approximately 1% of the general population. The likelihood of any given person being diagnosed with Schizophrenia is correlated with the closeness of their genetic relationship to an affected patient. The following prevalence rates have been shown: non-twin siblings (8%), dizygotic twins (12%), children with 2 schizophrenic parents (40%), and monozygotic twins (47%).

Sadock BJ, Sadock VA. *Kaplan and Sadock's Synopsis of Psychiatry*. 9th ed. Philadelphia: Lippincott Williams & Wilkins; 2003:482.

8. **Answer: D.** Although the patient's chest pain, palpitations, and sense that he is going to die are consistent with a simple panic attack, the associated elevated blood pressure in particular suggests that he may have a pheochromocytoma. One would initially do a 24-hour urine collection of vanillylmandelic acid, metanephrines, and unconjugated catecholamines to diagnose a pheochromocytoma; though, if the results were equivocal, one might then consider a plasma collection. Performing an EKG and obtaining routine labs and thyroid function tests are often part of an evaluation for panic disorder; however, elevated blood pressure is not a typical feature of a simple panic attack.

Kasper DL, Fauci AS, Longo DL, et al. *Harrison's Principles of Internal Medicine*. 16th ed. New York: McGraw-Hill; 2005:2148–2151, 2547–2548.

9. **Answer: C.** Pyromania is the purposeful setting of a fire, which happens more than once, is preceded by tension, and followed by fascination, relief, or pleasure. Fire setting is not performed for another motive or as a result of impaired judgment; nor is it better accounted for by mania, Conduct Disorder, or Antisocial Personality Disorder. This patient has no clear history of trauma or mood disturbance. She has never been in trouble and is not maliciously setting fires for secondary gain, as in conduct disorder or antisocial personality. Pyromaniacs often have a history of absent fathers, depressed mothers, or distant relationships.

1. American Psychiatric Association. *Quick Reference to the Diagnostic Criteria from DSM-IV-TR*. Washington: American Psychiatric Association; 2000:282–283.

2. Hales RE, Yudofsky SC. *Textbook of Clinical Psychiatry*. 4th ed. Washington: American Psychiatric Publishing; 2003:788–790.

10. **Answer: B.** Systematic desensitization is based on the behavioral principle of counter-conditioning, whereby a patient overcomes maladaptive anxiety by approaching a feared stimulus gradually, in a psychophysiological state that inhibits anxiety. In systematic desensitization, patients attain a state of relaxation (through relaxation training) and are then exposed to an anxiety-provoking stimulus. The negative reaction of anxiety is inhibited by the relaxed state, a process known as reciprocal inhibition. Rather than use actual situations or objects that elicit fear, a graded list or hierarchy of anxiety-provoking scenes is constructed. The learned relaxation and anxiety-provoking scenes are systematically paired in treatment. This results in gradual desensitization of the stimulus and extinguishing of the fear response. Implosion, or flooding, differs from systematic desensitization in that it involves exposing the patient to a feared object in vivo and does not make use of a hierarchy.

Sadock BJ, Sadock VA. *Kaplan and Sadock's Synopsis of Psychiatry*. 9th ed. Philadelphia: Lippincott Williams & Wilkins; 2003:951–952.

11. **Answer: D.** Transdermal selegiline has been marketed as the EMSAM patch. Randomized controlled trials in patients with major depressive disorder have shown it to have efficacy, as compared to placebo. Selegiline is a selective MAO-B inhibitor, but at doses showing maximal MAO-B inhibition in the brain, it also produces a dose and time dependent inhibition of MAO-A in the brain. At doses producing maximal MAO-A inhibition in the brain, it produces 30% to 40% inhibition of gastrointestinal MAO-A. It is owing to this preferential inhibition of brain MAO-A over gastrointestinal MAO-A, which the patch is devoid of side effects with tyramine-rich foods. In the placebo-controlled trials, there were no adverse reactions such as hypertensive crisis even in the absence of dietary restrictions. Application site reactions appear to be commonly seen with the use of the patch.

1. Amsterdam JD. A double-blind, placebo-controlled trial of the safety and efficacy of selegiline transdermal system without dietary restrictions in patients with major depressive disorder. *J Clin Psychiatry*. 2003;64:208–214.
2. Feiger AD, Rickels K, Rynn MA, et al. Selegiline transdermal system for the treatment of major depressive disorder: an 8-week, double-blind, placebo-controlled, flexible-dose titration trial. *J Clin Psychiatry*. 2006;67:1354–1361.
3. Wecker L, James S, Copeland N, et al. Transdermal selegiline: targeted effects on monoamine oxidases in the brain. *Biol Psychiatry*. 2003;54:1099–1104.

12. **Answer: C.** Benzodiazepines are commonly used for the treatment of anxiety disorders. It is important to know the half life of these medications to prevent oversedation and excessive drug accumulation. Oxazepam has a half life of 5 to 15 hours, alprazolam has a half-life of 8 to 15 hours, lorazepam has a half-life of 10 to 20 hours, Diazepam has a half-life of 20 to 70 hours and chlordiazepoxide has a half-life of 10 to 20 hours. However, some benzodiazepines with long half lives may have a shorter duration of action than other benzodiazepines due to extensive distribution.

Janicak PG, Davis JM, Preskorn SH, et al. *Principles and Practices of Psychopharmacotherapy*. 4th ed. Philadelphia: Lippincott Williams & Wilkins; 2006:465–475.

13. **Answer: E.** Anticholinergic agents, such as atropine and glycopyrrolate, are administered to reduce secretions and to decrease the bradycardia, which develops after the electrical stimulus. General anesthetics, used to induce consciousness, include etomidate, thiopental, methohexital, propofol, and ketamine. Succinylcholine is a depolarizing muscle relaxant. If its use is contraindicated by pseudocholinesterase deficiency, a nondepolarizing agent such as mivacurium can be used. Beta-blockers are not contraindicated and are routinely used to address tachycardia or severe hypertension.

Sadock BJ, Sadock VA. *Kaplan and Sadock's Comprehensive Textbook of Psychiatry*. 8th ed. Philadelphia: Lippincott Williams & Wilkins; 2005:2977.

14. **Answer: E.** Motivational interviewing is being widely used in the treatment of substance use disorders. Some of the core principles in this technique include establishing personal goals, developing discrepancy, rolling with resistance, and supporting self-efficacy. The interviewer or clinician tends to avoid confrontation and works on expressing empathy.

Brunette MF, Mueser KT. Psychosocial interventions for the long-term management of patients with severe mental illness and co-occurring substance use disorder. *J Clin Psychiatry*. 2006;67 (suppl 7):10–17.

15. **Answer: D.** Levels of 5-HIAA are decreased in the CSF of suicide attempters. Some studies have also shown that low 5-HIAA levels predict suicidal behavior. A relationship between suicide attempt and levels of HVA has not been substantiated.

Gelder MG, López-Ibor JJ, Andreasen N. *New Oxford Textbook of Psychiatry*. 1st ed. Philadelphia: Lippincott Williams & Wilkins; 2000:1047.

16. **Answer: C.** Cerebral hemispheric injury leads to contralateral hemiparesis, where there is weakness and spasticity of the muscles of the lower part of the face, trunk, arm, and leg on the opposite side of the lesion.

These patients also have hyperactive deep tendon reflexes on the contralateral side along with upgoing plantar reflex (Babinski sign). These symptoms result from an injury to the corticospinal tract and are known as upper motor neuron (UMN) lesion. Hypoactive deep tendon reflexes are seen in injury to peripheral nerve or anterior horn cell.

Kaufman DM. *Clinical Neurology for Psychiatrists.* 5th ed. Philadelphia: WB Saunders; 2001:8–9.

17. Answer: A. Neuropathy is the most common PNS manifestation of AIDS. Guillain-Barré syndrome and mononeuritis multiplex can occur as a result of AIDS but are uncommon. Of note, antiretroviral medications [i.e., ddI (dideoxyinosine/Videx) and ddC (dideoxycytidine/Hivid)] are known to also cause peripheral neuropathy. Myelopathy refers to the spinal cord, and thus is not part of the PNS.

Kaufman DM. *Clinical Neurology for Psychiatrists.* 5th ed. Philadelphia: WB Saunders; 2001:78.

18. Answer: B. TS is an autosomal dominant disorder that exhibits a wide spectrum of manifestations, ranging from no symptoms to profound neurologic disability. Neurological manifestations may include mental retardation, seizure disorders ranging from simple partial seizures to infantile spasms, and autism associated with the growth of cortical tubers during embryogenesis. Almost all individuals with TS (approximately 90%) have an associated skin finding. Hypopigmented macules ("ash leaf spots") are best viewed with a Wood's lamp and are generally present by early childhood, while shagreen patches are more prominent after age 5. Facial angiofibromas (adenoma sebaceum), erythematous lesions that typically appear on the face during late childhood and adolescence, may resemble severe acne. Ungual fibromas may also develop. TS can also be associated with cardiac rhabdomyomas, renal angiomyolipomas and cysts, pulmonary lymphangiomyomatosis, and subependymal giant cell tumors of the brain. This disorder results from mutations in one of the two genes, TSC1 (hamartin) or TSC2 (tuberin).

Crino PB, Nathanson KL, Henske EP. The tuberous sclerosis complex. *N Engl J Med.* 2006;355:1345–1356.

19. Answer: D. When analyzed during an attack of MS, CSF typically has a normal or slightly elevated protein concentration, with an elevated gamma globulin portion (nonspecific finding). Findings typically noted in the CSF of a patient suffering an attack of MS include the presence of myelin basic protein (a myelin breakdown product), oligoclonal bands (an IgG antibody), and an increased rate of synthesis of CSF IgG. It should be noted that these findings are not specific for MS; they may also be found in other chronic inflammatory conditions such as sarcoidosis, Lyme disease, and neurosyphilis. Xanthochromic supernatant is typical of CSF withdrawn from a patient with subarachnoid hemorrhage.

Kaufman DM. *Clinical Neurology for Psychiatrists.* 5th ed. Philadelphia: WB Saunders; 2001:377.

20. Answer: D. The most characteristic finding of hepatic encephalopathy is the triphasic delta wave, also known as the liver wave. They are delta waves (2 to 3 Hz) with a high amplitude positive wave in between two lower amplitude negative waves.

1. Husain AM. Electroencephalographic assessment of coma. *J Clin Neurophysiol.* 2006;23:208–220.
2. Khoshbin H. Clinical neurophysiology. *UpToDate 2006.* http://www.uptodateonline.com/utd/content/topic.do?topicKey=neuropat/4649&type=A&selectedTitle=1~71. Accessed January 23, 2007.

21. Answer: D. Conversion of tyrosine to L-dopa by tyrosine hydroxylase is the rate limiting step in the synthesis of tyrosine to dopamine. Phenylalanine is converted to tyrosine by phenylalanine hydroxylase. Tyrosine is then converted to L-dopa by tyrosine hydroxylase. This is the rate limiting step. Finally, L-dopa is converted to dopamine by dopa decarboxylase.

1. Kaufman DM. *Clinical Neurology for Psychiatrists.* 5th ed. Philadelphia: WB Saunders; 2001:552.
2. Messer WS: Chemistry of the Brain. http://www.neurosci.pharm.utoledo.edu/MBC3320/dopamine.htm. Accessed December 3, 2006.

22. Answer: A. Skin lesions and peripheral neuropathy are the hallmarks of arsenic ingestion. Chronic arsenic poisoning occurs from drinking groundwater contaminated with arsenic over a long period of time. This has become a problem in many third world countries, including Bangladesh. Sensorimotor polyneuropathy can occur insidiously. Skin lesions are characterized by hyperpigmentation and hyperkeratosis. Mees lines (transverse white lines) on the nails are occasionally noted. Patients may also have multisystemic involvement including anemia, leukopenia, skin changes, or elevated liver function tests. Anemia often accompanies skin lesions in patients chronically poisoned by arsenic. Lung cancer and skin cancer are serious long-term concerns. Toluene is a solvent. Repeated high-dose exposures can result in progressive memory loss, fatigue, poor concentration, irritability, persistent headaches, and signs and symptoms of cerebellar dysfunction. Muscular weakness has been noted in patients who develop renal-tubular acidosis. Thallium may result in a scaly rash, hair loss, and sensorimotor polyneuropathy. Sensory symptoms are often the first sign of polyneuropathy. They are followed by symmetric motor impairment, which is greater distally than proximally and occurs in the legs rather than the arms. Lead toxicity in adults manifests with peripheral neuropathies, which are mainly motor and greater in the arms than in the legs. They typically affect the radial nerves, causing wrist drop, or the peroneal nerves, causing foot drop. Systemic manifestations include anemia, constipation, colicky abdominal pain, gum discoloration, and nephropathy. Lead toxicity is common in persons involved in the manufacture or repair of storage batteries, the ship breaking industry, the smelting of lead or lead containing ores, or from the consumption of homemade alcohol made in lead containing pipes. Radon exposure causes no acute or subacute health effects. The only established human health effect associated with residential radon exposure is lung cancer.

1. Case studies in environmental medicine. http://www.atsdr.cdc.gov/HEC/CSEM/csem.html. Published Decmber 14, 2006.
2. Greenberg DA, Aminoff MJ, Simon RP. *Clinical Neurology*. 5th ed. New York: McGraw-Hill; 2002:182–183.

23. Answer: A. The corticospinal tract contains motor axons only. The rest of the choices carry sensory information. The lateral spinothalamic tracts transmit pain and temperature sensations to the thalamus. The anterior spinothalamic tracts carry light touch to the thalamus. The spinocerebellar tracts convey joint position sense to the cerebellum. The posterior columns of the spinal cord transmit position and vibratory sensations to the thalamus.

1. Burt AM. *Textbook of Neuroanatomy*. Philadelphia: WB Saunders; 1993:329.
2. Kaufman DM. *Clinical Neurology for Psychiatrists*. 5th ed. Philadelphia: WB Saunders; 2001: 21.

24. Answer: E. All the signs listed are found in Horner's syndrome and are found on the same side of the lesion (ipsilateral).

Fix JD. *High-Yield Neuroanatomy*. Baltimore: Williams & Wilkins; 1995:34.

25. Answer: B. The patient has cluster headaches, which are severe unilateral headaches, that often present with significant frequency during a single period and then remitting for months or even years. Patients often describe them as sharp pains boring into one eye. The pain is so excruciating that patients can feel suicidal. Although the patient reports having been suicidal in the past, it is not clear that he is suicidal during this visit and, before one would want to admit him to the psychiatric ER, one would want to assess whether he is currently suicidal and try to treat his symptoms, which would be the likely cause of suicidal ideation. Oxygen inhalation treatment is considered an effective form of abortive treatment for cluster headaches. Lithium is indeed used to treat cluster headaches, although prophylactically. Amitriptyline is a treatment for trigeminal neuralgia.

1. Kaufman DM. *Clinical Neurology for Psychiatrists*. 5th ed. Philadelphia: WB Saunders; 2001:213–214.
2. Zaidat OO, Lerner AJ. *The Little Black Book of Neurology*. 4th ed. St Louis: Mosby; 2002:161, 367.

26. Answer: D. Speech therapy is an important part of the cognitive rehabilitation of patients with aphasia. One of the main goals of the therapist is to identify different areas of receptive and expressive weaknesses and strengths, which can then be used for compensatory purposes. The therapy has to be tailored for each patient, taking into consideration the severity of the patient's symptoms, other areas of weakness besides speech, and premorbid functioning.

Rowland LP. *Merritt's Neurology*. 11th ed. Philadelphia: Lippincott Williams & Wilkins; 2005:1196–1199.

27. Answer: B. Erik Erikson developed eight psychosocial stages, which are points along development that trigger internal crises. They are trust versus mistrust (birth-), autonomy versus shame and doubt (18 months-), initiative versus guilt (3 years-), industry versus inferiority (5 years-), identity versus role confusion (13 years-), intimacy versus isolation (20s-), generativity versus stagnation (40s-), and integrity versus despair (60s-). The major conflict of middle adulthood is between generativity and stagnation. Generativity is the process by which persons guide the oncoming generation or society. This stage includes having and raising children, but having children does not guarantee generativity. To be stagnant means a person stops developing. For Erikson, stagnation also referred to adults without any impulses to guide the new generation or to those who produce children without caring for them.

Sadock BJ, Sadock VA. *Kaplan and Sadock's Synopsis of Psychiatry*. 9th ed. Philadelphia: Lippincott Williams & Wilkins; 2002:46, 214.

28. Answer: D. Nicotinic receptors are ion channel-linked receptors. Most serotonin receptors are G-protein receptors except 5 HT3 receptors which are directly coupled to ion channels.

Anderson IM, Reid IC. *Fundamentals of Clinical Psychopharmacology*. London: Taylor & Francis Group; 2004:7.

29. Answer: D. Object relations, along with ego psychology and self psychology, is one of the three major theoretical frameworks used by psychoanalytic clinicians today. Object relations theory originated in the work of Melanie Klein, DW Winnicott, and WRD Fairbairn. It involves the unconscious transformation of interpersonal relationships into internalized structures. In this psychoanalytic theory, object relations always involve an interface between a self and an object with an affect. Unlike ego psychology, which views drives as primary and object relations as secondary, object relations theory views all drives as emerging from the context of the mother-infant relationship. In object relations theory, conflict is seen as a struggle between different "self-object-affect units," each of which wants primary psychic attention. It is ego psychology which regards conflict as a struggle between wishes/desires or between intrapsychic agencies (i.e., the id and the superego). In object relations theory, character is viewed as heavily influenced by the presence of self-representations and object-representations deriving from introjections and identifications. Introjection is a process where one internalizes an object that functions as it does externally (e.g., a soothing mother or critical father). Identification occurs when one adapts oneself to take on attributes of an internalized object which functions as a role model.

Sadock BJ, Sadock VA. *Kaplan and Sadock's Comprehensive Textbook of Psychiatry*. 7th ed. Philadelphia: Lippincott Williams & Wilkins; 2000:587–589.

30. Answer: A. The NPV refers to the probability that an individual with a negative test result does not have the disease. NPV is dependant on the prevalence of the disease in the population being tested. In this case, the possible results of the diagnostic test can be represented in the following 2 × 2 table.

Test result outcome	Disease present	Disease absent	Total
Positive	999	1	1,000
Negative	1	999	1,000
Total	1,000	1,000	

The NPV of the test would be the number of true negatives (patients who don't have the disease and are tested negative) divided by the total number of patients tested negative by the diagnostic test. In this case, that would be 999/1,000; 99.9%.

1. Gray GE. *Evidence-Based Psychiatry*. Washington: American Psychiatric Publishing; 2004:123–125.
2. http://www.musc.edu/dc/icrebm/sensitivity.html. Accessed September 16, 2006.

31. Answer: E. The Bender Visual Motor Gestalt Test is a test of visuomotor coordination that is useful for both children and adults, and in the latter, is used more frequently as a screening device for signs of organic dysfunction. The Wisconsin Card Sorting Test assesses a person's abstract reasoning ability and flexibility in problem solving, which can reveal damage to the frontal lobes or caudate. The Wechsler Memory Scale screens for verbal and visual memory and can reveal amnestic conditions such as Korsakoff's syndrome. Language tests, like the Boston Diagnostic Aphasia Exam, can reveal left-hemisphere lesions, if it is the dominant hemisphere. The Benton Visual Retention Test is sensitive to short-term memory loss.

Kaplan HI, Sadock BJ. *Kaplan & Sadock's Synopsis of Psychiatry*. 8th ed. Philadelphia: Lippincott Williams & Wilkins; 1998:200–203.

32. Answer: E. The most serious side effect of lamotrigine is rash which may occur in up to 40% of patients and may culminate in Stevens-Johnson syndrome. It is important to determine if lamotrigine associated rash is benign or malignant. A benign rash begins within 5 days of initiating lamotrigine therapy; it is spotty, nontender, nonconfluent, not associated with laboratory abnormalities, and usually resolves in 10 to 14 days. The management of lamotrigine induced benign rash includes halting dose escalation temporarily or discontinuing medication while the rash is monitored. The patient is instructed to call should the rash worsen or should new symptoms emerge. Antihistamine or topical steroids may also be prescribed to manage itching. Upon resolution of the rash, lamotrigine therapy may be re-initiated at a much lower dose than recommended: 5 mg to 12.5 mg. A rash occurring more than 5 days following the initiation of lamotrigine therapy is more likely to be drug related. Such rashes are tender, confluent, itchy, and widespread and are usually prominent in the upper trunk and neck areas. A poor prognostic sign is involvement of eye, lips, and mouth. There may be accompanying systemic signs and symptoms: fever, malaise, anorexia, sore throat, lymph node enlargement, and laboratory abnormalities (complete blood count, liver function and basic metabolic panel). It is recommended that lamotrigine be discontinued immediately and permanently if a serious rash occurs.

1. www.fda.gov/cder/drug/InfoSheets/patient/lamotriginePIS.pdf. Published November 25, 2006.
2. Dunner DL. Safety and tolerability of emerging pharmacological treatments for bipolar disorder. *Bipolar Disord*. 2005;7:307–325.

33. Answer: B. Affective flattening is considered a negative symptom of schizophrenia, and is not included in the clinical features of catatonia. The Catatonic type of Schizophrenia is diagnosed when a patient's clinical picture is dominated by at least two of: (i) motoric immobility as evidenced by catalepsy or stupor; (ii) excessive motor activity; (iii) extreme negativism or mutism; (iv) peculiarities of voluntary movement as evidenced by posturing, stereotyped movements, prominent mannerisms, or prominent grimacing; or (v) echolalia or echopraxia.

1. American Psychiatric Association. *Quick Reference to the Diagnostic Criteria from DSM-IV-TR.* Washington: American Psychiatric Association; 2000:153–165.
2. Sadock BJ, Sadock VA. *Kaplan and Sadock's Synopsis of Psychiatry.* 9th ed. Philadelphia: Lippincott Williams & Wilkins; 2003:487.

34. Answer: D. Delusions are positive characteristic symptoms of Schizophrenia and affective flattening, alogia, and avolition are the negative characteristic symptoms. The others are hallucinations, disorganized speech, and grossly disorganized or catatonic behavior. Although anhedonia is a symptom which can occur as part of Schizophrenia, it is not included in the definition.

American Psychiatric Association. *Quick Reference to the Diagnostic Criteria from DSM-IV-TR.* Washington: American Psychiatric Association; 2000:153–154.

35. Answer: E. In the DSM-IV-TR, Pathological Gambling falls under the category of impulse control disorders NOS. Many of the criteria resemble those of substance abuse/dependence. The main exclusionary criteria is that behavior is not better accounted for by a manic episode. Otherwise, comorbidity is the nature of the illness, as reflected in the answers.

1. American Psychiatric Association. *Quick Reference to the Diagnostic Criteria from DSM-IV-TR.* Washington: American Psychiatric Association; 2000:283–284.
2. Hales RE, Yudofsky SC. *Textbook of Clinical Psychiatry.* 4th ed. Washington: American Psychiatric Publishing; 2003:790–793.

36. Answer: D. Typical quit rates for smoking cessation strategies include the following: self-quit (5%), self-help books (10%), physician advice (10%), over-the-counter patch or gum (15%), medication plus advice (20%), behavior therapy alone (20%), and medication plus behavior therapy (30%). Behavior therapy is the most widely accepted and well-proven psychological therapy utilized in smoking cessation. In behavior therapy, skills training and relapse prevention identify high-risk situations in addition to planning and practicing coping skills for these situations. Stimulus control involves eliminating cues for smoking in the environment. Several studies have shown that combining nicotine replacement and behavior therapy increases quit rates over either therapy alone.

Sadock BJ, Sadock VA. *Kaplan and Sadock's Synopsis of Psychiatry.* 9th ed. Philadelphia: Lippincott Williams & Wilkins; 2003:446–448.

37. Answer: B. Buprenorphine, a partial opioid agonist, is an alternative choice to methadone for long-term opioid replacement therapy. Although it has some advantages in that it can be prescribed in a traditional office based practice instead of a methadone clinic, no studies have shown any advantage over methadone in maintaining sobriety. It is usually combined with naltrexone to reduce the chance of abuse (the combination reduces the effectiveness of grinding and taking nasally or intravenously), and can be given 16 mg daily or 32 mg 3 times a week. It is metabolized by the 3A4 cytochrome, and drugs that inhibit this enzyme (ketoconazole and fluvoxamine) can raise the serum level and cause increased sedation. When used in combination with other sedatives, it can lead to respiratory depression. It should be used with severe caution in patients with impaired respiration, increased intracranial pressure, symptomatic hypothyroidism, prostatic hypertrophy, CHF, and liver disease.

Rosenbaum JF, Arana GW, Hyman SE, et al. *Handbook of Psychiatric Drug Therapy.* 5th ed. Philadelphia: Lippincott Williams & Wilkins; 2005:213–215.

38. Answer: B. Approximately 70% to 87% of patients with PTSD report sleep disruption. Sleep problems in PTSD have a high impact in the quality of life and symptom-severity in PTSD. Nightmares are frequently reported and are also particularly resistant to pharmacotherapy. SSRIs have been reported to have a positive, but small, effect on sleep problems in PTSD, especially for insomnia. However, occasionally these medications can produce insomnia as a side effect. In the Expert Consensus Guidelines for PTSD, trazodone was considered to be a first-line hypnotic and was rated as the most effective and best-tolerated hypnotic for the treatment of sleep disturbances in this patient population. There are a few studies showing that it might even have a positive effect in the treatment of nightmares. Benzodiazepines are helpful in inducing sleep, but they have not been shown to improve the rate of sleep disruption or frequency of nightmares. These medications should be used with caution, because they can cause dependence, serious withdrawal symptoms, and cognitive impairment after prolonged use. A few case reports have reported that the antihistamine cyproheptadine might be helpful in the treatment of nightmares and other disturbances in PTSD, but there is limited data to support this notion.

Maher MJ, Rego SA, Asnis GM. Sleep disturbances in patients with post-traumatic stress disorder: epidemiology, impact and approaches to management. *CNS Drugs*. 2006;20:567–590.

39. **Answer: D.** Brief pulse stimulation has replaced sine wave forms. The following help minimize cognitive side effects: (i) placing electrodes unilaterally on the right; (ii) administering one seizure per session; (iii) reducing the dosage of lithium, antipsychotics and sedatives; and (iv) reducing the total number of sessions and frequency of sessions.

Sadock BJ, Sadock VA. *Kaplan and Sadock's Comprehensive Textbook of Psychiatry*. 8th ed. Philadelphia: Lippincott Williams and Wilkins; 2005:2981.

40. **Answer: B.** The transtheoretical model of behavior change is commonly used for the treatment of substance abuse disorders. It consists of five different stages, starting with a precontemplation stage, where patients are still not aware of the negative consequences of their behavior. This stage is followed by the contemplation and preparation stages, where making a change is contemplated, as well as the action and maintenance stages, where the change is made and sustained. Meditation is not a formal stage in this psychosocial intervention.

Peterson PL, Baer JS, Wells EA, et al. Short-term effects of a brief motivational intervention to reduce alcohol and drug risk among homeless adolescents. *Psychol Addict Behav*. 2006;20:254–264.

41. **Answer: D.** The rate of suicide (per 100,000 population) from 1994 to 2004 decreased from 13.8 to 10.4 for those aged 15 to 24 years, and from 21.9 to 16.6 for those aged 80+ years. The rate among men is four times that of women and the rate among whites is twice that of non-whites. Firearm suicides account for 54%, suffocation 21%, poisoning 17%, cutting 2%, and drowning 1% (not all methods are included). In 2004, the last year in which the CDC updated its data, 82-year-olds had the distinction of having the highest suicide rate per 100,000 with 20.2.

1. American Association of Suicidology. *U.S.A. Suicide: 2003 Official Final Data*. http://www.suicidology.org/associations/1045/files/2003data.pdf. Published December 10, 2006.
2. Center for Disease Control and Prevention. *National Center for Injury Prevention and Control. Web-based Injury Statistics Query and Reporting System (WISQARSTM™)*. http://www.cdc.gov/ncipc/wisqars/. Published December 10, 2006.

42. **Answer: D.** Muscle flaccidity, atrophy, hypoactive deep tendon reflexes, and absence of plantar reflex (Babinski's sign) indicates LMN lesion. Common causes of LMN lesion are peripheral nerve lesions, injury to the anterior horn cell of the spinal cord, and motor neuron disease.

Kaufman DM. *Clinical Neurology for Psychiatrists*. 5th ed. Philadelphia: WB Saunders; 2001:8–9.

43. **Answer: B.** The lipophilic nature of solvents is what allows them to easily permeate the CNS. Solvents affect both the PNS and CNS via demyelination. CNS changes include cerebral demyelination, optic nerve damage, pyramidal, and cerebellar injury resulting in cognitive impairment, personality changes, inattention, ataxia, depression, fatigue, and headaches. Chronic exposure to solvents such as toluene can result in dementia that is proportional to cerebral myelin injury.

Kaufman DM. *Clinical Neurology for Psychiatrists*. 5th ed. Philadelphia: WB Saunders; 2001:79.

44. **Answer: A.** The hallmark characteristic of mitochondrial inheritance is transmission through female parents only, with male and female offspring affected. There can be a wide range of expression of the disease. The manifestations of mitochondrial diseases can involve a single organ system, as in Leber's hereditary optic neuropathy, or involve multiple organ systems. The genes in the mitochondria encode for many of the components of the respiratory transport chain and are responsible for the cell's energy metabolism, so myopathies, cardiomyopathy, and neurologic problems are typical sequelae of these mutations. Some disorders found to be associated with mitochondrial inheritance patterns are Leber's hereditary optic neuropathy (midlife sudden central vision loss with cardiac conduction defects and cerebellar dysfunction), myoclonic epilepsy with RRF (ataxia, myoclonic seizures, sensioneural hearing loss, diabetes, short stature, and lactic acidosis), and Kearns-Sayres syndrome (ophthalmoplegia and retinal degeneration, usually before 20 years, ataxia, deafness, diabetes, short stature, and lactic acidosis).

1. Zeviani M. Mitochondrial disorders. *Suppl Clin Neurophysiol*. 2004;57:304–312.
2. Zeviani M, Carelli V. Mitochondrial disorders. *Curr Opin Neurol*. 2003;16:585–594.

45. **Answer: E.** NPH is commonly considered a "reversible" form of dementia. The classic triad of symptoms includes cognitive impairment, urinary incontinence, and gait apraxia (usually the first and most prominent symptom of NPH). Common diagnostic tests include withdrawal of 30 mL of CSF by lumbar

puncture or a series of three lumbar punctures, which, theoretically, would reduce hydrocephalus temporarily. CSF pressure, glucose, and protein are all normal. Improvement in the patient's gait following CSF removal is indicative of the diagnosis of NPH and predicts benefit from shunt installment to permanently drain the CSF. Improvement in cognitive impairment following CSF removal is not necessarily seen. In theory, shunting of CSF from the ventricles to the abdominal cavity can relieve NPH. Unfortunately, shunting produces a clinically beneficial response in only 50% of patients whose NPH has an established cause (such as a subarachnoid hemorrhage) and in only 15% of patients with idiopathic NPH. EEG is not helpful in the diagnosis of NPH.

Kaufman DM. *Clinical Neurology for Psychiatrists*. 5th ed. Philadelphia: WB Saunders; 2001:146–147.

46. Answer: B. Continuous high voltage delta wave activity is an EEG finding usually seen in patients with subcortical white matter, but it can also be seen in metabolic encephalopathies. It is associated with a poorer outcome than the intermittent rhythmic delta wave activity or the triphasic delta wave activity seen in earlier stages of coma.

Husain AM. Electroencephalographic assessment of coma. *J Clin Neurophysiol*. 2006;23:208–220.

47. Answer: C. L-dopa is converted to dopamine by DOPA decarboxylase. Carbidopa inhibits DOPA decarboxylase peripherally allowing more L-Dopa to penetrate the CNS. This allows a greater conversion of L-dopa to dopamine in the CNS at a lower overall L-dopa dose thereby also reducing side effects.

Kaufman DM. *Clinical Neurology for Psychiatrists*. 5th ed. Philadelphia: WB Saunders; 2001:552–553.

48. Answer: A. Lead can produce both CNS and PNS dysfunction. Children often develop lead poisoning by craving unnatural foods (pica) or eating lead-pigment paint chips from decaying tenement walls. In children, mental retardation and poor school performance may develop. Acute encephalopathy can be the major neurological feature. In contrast, because lead has a different effect on a mature nervous system, adults most often develop mononeuropathies, such as foot drop (peroneal nerve) or wrist drop (radial nerve). There may be loss of or depression of deep tendon reflexes. Adults can develop lead poisoning through the manufacture or repair of storage batteries, the ship breaking industry, the smelting of lead or lead containing ores, or the consumption of home-made alcohol. Other manifestations of lead poisoning include anemia, constipation, colicky abdominal pain, gum discoloration, and

nephropathy. Mees lines are horizontal lines of discoloration which occur on the nails of fingers and toes after an episode of poisoning with arsenic, thallium, or other heavy metals.

1. Greenberg DA, Aminoff MJ, Simon RP. *Clinical Neurology*. 5th ed. New York: McGraw-Hill; 2002:182–183.
2. Kaufman DM. *Clinical Neurology for Psychiatrists*. 5th ed. Philadelphia: WB Saunders; 2001:76.

49. Answer: B. This patient is presenting with Brown-Sequard syndrome, which is due to hemisection of the spinal cord. Patients present with ipsilateral paralysis due to transection of the corticospinal tract, ipsilateral loss of proprioception and vibratory sense due to transection of the posterior columns, and contralateral loss of pain and temperature due to transection of the spinothalamic tract.

Kaufman DM. *Clinical Neurology for Psychiatrists*. 5th ed. Philadelphia: WB Saunders; 2001:22.

50. Answer: D. Vitamin B_{12} deficiency can cause neuropathy and affect all of the listed parts of the spinal cord. Damage to the dorsal column can lead to loss of tactile discrimination, vibration sense, and position. Damage to the lateral corticospinal tract can result in spastic paresis and spinocerebellar tract damage can result in abnormalities of arm and leg movements.

Fix JD. *High-Yield Neuroanatomy*. Baltimore: Williams & Wilkins; 1995:38.

51. Answer: D. Cluster headaches are severe unilateral headaches often presenting with significant frequency during a single period and then remitting for months or even years. They occur most commonly in men and are not associated with auras. One hundred percent oxygen or sumatriptan injections are treatments for cluster headaches. They often occur with regularity during REM sleep. Chronic paroxysmal hemicrania is a type of cluster headache which can be aborted with indomethacin.

1. Kaufman DM. *Clinical Neurology for Psychiatrists*. 5th ed. Philadelphia: WB Saunders; 2001:213–214.
2. Zaidat OO, Lerner AJ. *The Little Black Book of Neurology*. 4th ed. St Louis: Mosby; 2002:161.

52. Answer: D. Nearly all hemiplegic patients are able to walk to some extent within 3 to 6 months after their stroke. There is research suggesting that more intensive physical therapies are more helpful in helping patients to walk again. Some authors suggest that adding specific focal physical therapy to the affected leg, after the traditional physical therapy for walking, is especially helpful for this goal.

http://dissertations.ub.rug.nl/FILES/faculties/medicine/2004/r.b.huitema/c1.pdf. Accessed February 15, 2006.

53. Answer: C. Women do not reach their sexual prime until their mid-30s. They have a greater capacity for orgasm in middle adulthood than in young adulthood. However, as they lose their youthful appearance, they may feel less sexually desirable. As a consequence, declines in sexual functioning in middle-aged women are usually related to psychological rather than physical causes.

Sadock BJ, Sadock VA. *Kaplan and Sadock's Synopsis of Psychiatry*. 9th ed. Philadelphia: Lippincott Williams & Wilkins; 2002:47.

54. Answer: E. Ionotropic receptors are directly coupled to an ion channel. These receptors are protein structures containing about 20 transmembrane segments. The ion channel opening occurs in milliseconds, leading to rapid excitatory or inhibitory effects, depending on the ion the channel is permeable to.

Anderson IM, Reid IC. *Fundamentals of Clinical Psychopharmacology*. London: Taylor & Francis Group; 2004:7.

55. Answer: E. Reinforcement schedules define how a behavior is influenced by the thought of a reward. In a fixed-ratio schedule, there is a rapid rate of response to obtain the greatest number of rewards. In a variable-ratio schedule, because the probability of reinforcement remains relatively stable, there is a fairly constant rate of response. Because the reinforcement occurs at regular intervals in a fixed-interval schedule, the rate of responding drops to near zero after reinforcement and then increases rapidly as the expected time of reward is anticipated. In a variable-rate schedule, there is a fairly constant response, because reinforcement occurs at random intervals, which is similar to variable-ratio schedule. Partial reinforcement, where reinforcement only occurs occasionally to a particular behavior, maintains that behavior at full strength and they are particularly resistant to extinction.

1. Lattal K, Reilly M, Kohn J. Response persistence under ratio and interval reinforcement schedules. *J Exp Anal Behav*. 1998;70:165–183.
2. Sadock BJ, Sadock VA. *Kaplan and Sadock's Comprehensive Textbook of Psychiatry*. 8th ed. Philadelphia: Lippincott Williams & Wilkins; 2005:546.

56. Answer: C. The responses in this study, as represented in a 2 × 2 table, showed that 76% of patients on placebo continued to have anxiety compared to 35% in the citalopram group. Given this information, the RR of continued anxiety in the citalopram group as compared to the placebo group can be reported: anxiety in the citalopram group/anxiety in the placebo group: 35%/76% = 0.46.

Treatment	Not responding (%)	Responding (%)
Placebo	76	24
Citalopram	35	65

More effective treatments provide greater reduction in the risk of negative outcome. The RR for effective treatments vary between 0 and 1 with smaller values indicating a more effective treatment.

1. Gray GE. *Evidence-Based Psychiatry*. Washington: American Psychiatric Publishing; 2004:64–68.
2. Lenze EJ, Mulsant BH, Shear MK, et al. Efficacy and tolerability of citalopram in the treatment of late-life anxiety disorders: results from an 8-week randomized, placebo-controlled trial. *Am J Psychiatry*. 2005;162:146–150.

57. Answer: E. The WAIS is the best standardized and most widely used intelligence test (Answer B) and comprises 11 subtests made up of verbal and performance subtests which yield a verbal IQ, a performance IQ, and a combined or full-scale IQ. A disparity between the verbal test and the performance test may indicate psychopathology, such as ADHD, and has nothing to do with identifying personality disorders (Answer A). Although the reliability of the WAIS is very high, the IQ is a measure of present functioning ability, not of future potential (Answer C), and the average or normal range of IQ is 90 to 110 (Answer D), where an IQ of 100 corresponds to the 50th percentile in intellectual ability for the general population (based on the assumption that intellectual abilities are normally distributed throughout the population). Under ordinary circumstances, the IQ is stable throughout life, but there is no certainty about its predictive properties. According to DSM-IV, mental retardation is defined as an IQ of 70 or below, which is found in the lowest 2.2% of the population and the validity of the WAIS is high in identifying MR and in predicting future school performance.

Kaplan HI, Sadock BJ. *Kaplan & Sadock's Synopsis of Psychiatry*. 8th ed. Philadelphia: Lippincott Williams & Wilkins; 1998:193–195.

58. Answer: A. The most serious side effect of lamotrigine is rash which may occur in up to 40% of patients and may culminate in Stevens-Johnson syndrome. It is important to determine if lamotrigine associated rash is benign or malignant. A benign rash begins within 5 days of initiating lamotrigine therapy. The rash is spotty, nontender, nonconfluent, not associated with laboratory abnormalities, and usually resolves in 10 to 14 days. Given that the immune system requires several days to mount a true hypersensitivity reaction, most rashes occurring within a few days of lamotrigine therapy are likely to be benign. A rash occurring more than 5 days following the initiation of lamotrigine therapy is more likely to be drug related. Such rashes are tender, confluent, itchy, and widespread and are usually prominent in the upper trunk and neck areas. A poor prognostic sign is involvement of eye, lips, and mouth. There may be accompanying systemic signs and symptoms: fever, malaise, anorexia, sore throat and lymph node enlargement, and laboratory abnormalities (complete blood count, liver function, and basic metabolic panel). It is recommended that lamotrigine be discontinued immediately and permanently if a serious rash occurs.

1. http://www.fda.gov/cder/drug/InfoSheets/patient/lamotriginePIS.pdf. Accessed November 25, 2006.
2. Dunner DL. Safety and tolerability of emerging pharmacological treatments for bipolar disorder. *Bipolar Disord.* 2005;7:307–325.

59. Answer: C. DID is a chronic disorder in which two or more distinct personalities exist within the same individual, with at least two of the personalities alternately controlling the individual's behavior. The median number of personalities is between five and ten. Most often, one personality cannot recall what occurred when another personality was dominant. The personalities may differ significantly in terms of behavior, mannerisms, speech, etc. Switches between personalities can be quite sudden, but are often so rare that they are difficult to pick up on without prolonged treatment. The mean age at diagnosis is 30 years, although the disorder likely begins earlier, in childhood or adolescence. Although female:male ratios of 5 to 9 : 1 have been reported, men may be under diagnosed. Almost all individuals with DID have a history of trauma, most often childhood sexual abuse. Common symptoms include losing time, being recognized by strangers, finding oneself suddenly in an unexpected place or with objects for which one cannot account, and voices coming from within. Treatment may focus on integrating the various personalities, to help the individual gain better control over their behavior.

1. American Psychiatric Association. *Quick Reference to the Diagnostic Criteria from DSM-IV-TR.* Washington: American Psychiatric Association; 2000:239–243.
2. Sadock, BJ, Sadock VA. *Kaplan and Sadock's Synopsis of Psychiatry.* 9th ed. Philadelphia: Lippincott Williams & Wilkins; 2003:676–691.

60. Answer: D. To receive a diagnosis of Schizophrenia, patients must have at least two of the "characteristic" symptoms (delusions, hallucinations, disorganized speech, disorganized behavior, or negative symptoms) for at least a month and attenuated signs of the disease for at least 6 months. One of the exceptions to the requirement that the patient have at least two of the characteristic symptoms occurs when the auditory hallucinations consist of two or more voices conversing (as well as a voice containing running commentary or bizarre delusions). A diagnosis of Schizophreniform Disorder requires the presence of characteristic symptoms for at least 1 month but less than 6 months, and a Brief Psychotic Disorder requires the presence of characteristic symptoms for at least 1 day but less than 1 month.

American Psychiatric Association. *Quick Reference to the Diagnostic Criteria from DSM-IV-TR.* Washington: American Psychiatric Association; 2000:153–165.

61. Answer: B. Trichotillomania is recurrent hair pulling with noticeable hair loss. Pulling is preceded by tension and followed by relief or gratification. Pulling is not better accounted for by another mental or medical disorder, and causes significant distress or impairment. It may be more common in females than males, and is most common in pre-adolescents. Diurnal variation and premenstrual exacerbations frequently occur. Stress often triggers or worsens symptoms. Comorbidity is common, especially with OCD, Mental Retardation (MR), Schizophrenia, Depression, and Borderline Personality Disorders. Trichophagia is common and may result in a bezoar. Alopecia areata or tinea capitis would have been diagnosed by the referring dermatologist.

1. American Psychiatric Association. *Quick Reference to the Diagnostic Criteria from DSM-IV-TR.* Washington: American Psychiatric Association; 2000:284.
2. Hales RE, Yudofsky SC. *Textbook of Clinical Psychiatry.* 4th ed. Washington: American Psychiatric Publishing; 2003:793–797.

62. Answer: E. The receptors present in the respiratory tract are beta-subtype-2 receptors, whereas those present in the heart are beta-subtype-1 receptors. The cardioselective (or beta-1-receptor selective) agents are most suitable for patients with chronic obstructive pulmonary disease (COPD) and bronchial asthma. Of all the drugs listed only bisoprolol is beta-1 selective.

Ashrafian H, Violaris AG. Beta-blocker therapy of cardiovascular diseases in patients with bronchial asthma or COPD: the pro viewpoint. *Prim Care Respir J.* 2005;14:236–241.

63. Answer: D. When a patient is acutely agitated, the most important factor is to maintain the patient's safety and to prevent anyone around him from getting hurt. The patient's behavior must be controlled by physical restraints when other alternatives fail.

Patients that are very agitated can get hurt even while restrained, either through self-inflicted behaviors or through aspiration or limb ischemia. Studies have shown that intramuscular haloperidol has a sigmoidal dose-effect curve between 2.5 mg and 15 mg given within the first 4 hours of treatment. Doses greater than 15 mg have not shown to be more efficacious, and can even provide lesser degrees of improvement and higher risks of side effects. Benzodiazepines, and in particular lorazepam, have proven to be efficacious and fast acting for the treatment of acute agitation, alone, or in combination with antipsychotics. Benztropine is helpful to treat extrapyramidal symptoms, but it does not seem to have a therapeutic effect in the treatment of agitation.

Rund DA, Ewing JD, Mitzel K, et al. The use of intramuscular benzodiazepines and antipsychotic agents in the treatment of acute agitation or violence in the emergency department. *J Emerg Med*. 2006;31:317–324.

64. **Answer: B.** Pregabalin has demonstrated efficacy in the treatment of general anxiety disorder with efficacy rates similar to those of benzodiazepines, and it is generally well tolerated. Although its mechanism of action is still unclear, pregabalin binds selectively and with high affinity to voltage-gated calcium channels in CNS tissues and acts as a presynaptic modulator of the excessive release of excitatory neurotransmitters. Despite being structurally similar to GABA, pregabalin does not interact with GABA-A, GABA-B orbenzodiazepine receptors, or to presynaptic or postsynaptic serotonin receptors. The onset of action of pregabalin has been shown to be similar to that of alprazolam, with improvements seen 1 week after starting treatment. In contrast to benzodiazepines, pregabalin has not been associated with rebound anxiety or severe withdrawal symptoms.

1. Frampton JE, Foster RH. Pregabalin: in the treatment of generalized anxiety disorder. *CNS Drugs*. 2006;20:685–693.
2. Rickels K, Pollack MH, Feltner DE, et al. Pregabalin for treatment of generalized anxiety disorder: a 4-week, multicenter, double-blind, placebo-controlled trial of pregabalin and alprazolam. *Arch Gen Psychiatry*. 2005;62:1022–1030.

65. **Answer: A.** The mechanism of action of ECT remains unknown, but animal studies have suggested that neurogenesis and other changes occur in the hippocampus.

Sadock BJ, Sadock VA. *Kaplan and Sadock's Comprehensive Textbook of Psychiatry*. 8th ed. Philadelphia: Lippincott Williams & Wilkins; 2005:2971.

66. **Answer: D.** Over 50% of patients who received initial treatment for substance use disorder relapsed within 3 months. During this period, called early recovery period, craving is at its peak and remains significantly strong for months. Although this number is not very encouraging, 10% to 20% of treated patients never relapse after their first treatment, and approximately 2% to 3% achieve sobriety after each additional year of attempted abstinence.

Gitlow S. *Substance Use Disorders: A Practical Guide*. Philadelphia: Lippincott Williams & Wilkins; 2001:179–184.

67. **Answer: A.** Justice in medical ethics concerns itself with the issues of reward and punishment and the equitable distribution of social benefits. Nonmalfeasance is an issue of *primum non nocere* or *first do no harm*. Beneficence is promoting the well-being of individuals and society. Autonomy describes a person acting as she determines best for herself, given the risk and benefits of all reasonable options. In paternalism, a physician acts how she perceives to be in the patient's best interest without sufficiently collaborating with the patient.

Sadock BJ, Sadock VA. *Kaplan and Sadock's Comprehensive Textbook of Psychiatry*. 8th ed. Philadelphia: Lippincott Williams & Wilkins; 2005:3991–3992.

68. **Answer: E.** Plaques present as sharply circumscribed lesions that are diffusely scattered throughout the brain and spinal cord. In the brain they tend to be grouped around the lateral and third ventricles. These plaques in the cerebral hemispheres vary from the size and small lesions may be found in the gray white matter interphase. Plaques of varying size may also be seen in the optic nerves, chiasm, or tracts. Plaques in the corpus callosum are not uncommon. Numerous plaques are also present in the brain stem and when stained by the Weigert method, they have the characteristic Holstein cow appearance.

1. Kaufman DM. *Clinical Neurology for Psychiatrists*. 5th ed. Philadelphia: WB Saunders; 2001:378–379.
2. Rowland LP. *Merritt's Neurology*. 11th ed. Philadelphia: Lippincott Williams & Wilkins; 2005:945–946.

69. **Answer: E.** The clinical vignette is most consistent with Metachromatic Leukodystrophy (MLD). This autosomal recessive disorder is diagnosed in children or young adults. The symptoms include progressive personality changes, cognitive impairment, and psychosis as well as signs of peripheral neuropathy and CNS demyelination, such as spasticity and ataxia. In addition to CNS white matter demyelination seen on MRI and the multisystem accumulation of metachromatic granules that can be seen in biopsy of peripheral nerves, patients with MLD

also have markedly decreased Arylsulfatase A activity. Although the pathophysiology of MLD is well described, there are no available treatments to arrest the disease.

Kaufman DM. *Clinical Neurology for Psychiatrists*. 5th ed. Philadelphia: WB Saunders; 2001:78–79.

70. Answer: C. Phenylketonuria (PKU) is an autosomal recessive defect in amino acid metabolism that results in mental retardation, if untreated. Phenylalanine hydroxylase is the enzyme responsible for the conversion of phenylalanine to tyrosine in the liver, and the resultant tyrosine is then used to make dopamine. The inability to convert phenylalanine to tyrosine results in excess phenylalanine in the blood, which gets converted to phenylketones that are excreted in the urine. The phenylketones are not responsible for the brain damage in PKU; the elevated phenylalanine is toxic to brain tissue. As soon as the disorder is diagnosed, transition to a low phenylalanine diet prevents major neurologic sequelae. Current guidelines recommend maintaining a low phenylalanine diet indefinitely to avoid any loss of cognitive function. Newborn screening programs obtain a sample of the infant's blood via a dried blood spot on a filter paper at 24 to 48 hours of life, giving time for the infant to have digested a sufficient quantity of protein to yield an unambiguous result.

1. Behrman RE, Kliegman RM, Jenson HB. *Nelson Textbook of Pediatrics*. 17th ed. Philadelphia: WB Saunders; 2004:399–401.
2. Kahler SG, Fahey MC. Metabolic disorders and mental retardation. *Am J Med Genet C Semin Med Genet*. 2003;117:31–41.

71. Answer: A. The patient described uses IV drugs and has a presentation consistent with an HIV-associated cognitive disorder/dementia caused by the direct toxic effect of the HIV virus on the brain. A low CD4 count (less than 200) is usually associated with HIV dementia and would be the most useful diagnostic test in this case. Low CD4 count in HIV patients is also associated with increased risk for opportunistic infections and could account for his fever of unknown origin. Cognitive decline and motor slowing are the predominant characteristics of HIV dementia. Cognitive changes tend to occur gradually over several months. Therefore, patients often maintain insight into the nature of the decline and difficulty concentrating and memory impairment are frequent complaints. Motor deficits are usually symmetrical, affect the extremities, and may include weakness, ataxia, and loss of fine motor coordination. Behavioral changes and depressed mood may also occur, although psychotic symptoms are rare. In later stages of the disease, an individual may progress to mutism, incontinence, or paraplegia.

Sadock BJ, Sadock VA. *Kaplan and Sadock's Comprehensive Textbook of Psychiatry*. 8th ed. Philadelphia: Lippincott Williams & Wilkins; 2005:1088.

72. Answer: E. Continued VEEG monitoring should not be used as part of the intial evaluation of patients presenting with seizure activity. For these patients, a routine EEG is usually sufficient. However, when diagnosis or classification of a seizure disorder is not settled by routine EEG, VEEG can be helpful. It is also used to evaluate precipitating factors and to localize seizure focus for the purpose of surgical intervention.

Cascino GD. Clinical indications and diagnostic yield of video-electroencephalographic monitoring in patients with seizures and spells. *Mayo Clin Proc*. 2002;77:1111–1120.

73. Answer: A. This patient has a classic case of trigeminal neuralgia, the most frequent, and at the same time the most elusive disease of the fifth nerve from the standpoint of its pathologic basis. The overall incidence rate for both sexes combined is 4.3 per 100,000 persons per year, but it is higher for women than for men (in a ratio of 3 : 2) and is much higher in the elderly. The mean age of onset is 52 to 58 years for the idiopathic form. Recently, it has been noted that a proportion of cases is due to compression of trigeminal nerve rootlets by small branches of the basilar artery with this compression causing demyelination of the proximal nerve root. The paroxysmal nature of the facial pain, its unilaterality and tendency to involve the second and third divisions of the trigeminal nerve, an intensity that makes the patient grimace or wince (tic), the presence of an initiating or trigger point, the lack of demonstrable sensory or motor deficit, and its response in more than half of the cases to anticonvulsants are characteristic.

Ropper AH, Brown RH. *Adams and Victor's Principles of Neurology*. 8th ed. New York: McGraw-Hill; 2005:1178–1179.

74. Answer: D. Acute benzene toxicity is characterized by CNS depression. Symptoms can progress from light headedness, headache, and euphoria to respiratory depression, apnea, coma, and death. Other symptoms include bronchial and laryngeal irritation after inhalation along with pulmonary edema. After ingestion, patients may experience substernal chest pain, cough, hoarseness, and burning of the mouth, pharynx, and esophagus. Benzene can cause stomach pain, nausea, and vomiting. Symptoms of chronic benzene exposure may be nonspecific. They include fever, bleeding, fatigue, and anorexia.

Conditions that first bring a patient to medical attention are typically either fever due to infection or manifestations of thrombocytopenia (e.g., a hemorrhagic diathesis with bleeding from the gums, nose, skin, gastrointestinal tract, or elsewhere). Fatigue and anorexia may also prompt an evaluation. Hematological abnormalities are the primary concern in benzene exposure. In terms of risk, workers employed in industries using or producing benzene such as petrochemical companies; petroleum refining and coke and coal chemical manufacturing; rubber tire manufacturing; and companies involved in the storage or transport of benzene and petroleum products containing benzene have the greatest likelihood of exposure. Lead toxicity in adults is characterized by mononeuropathies, such as foot drop (peroneal nerve) or wrist drop (radial nerve). Skin lesions and sensorimotor polyneuropathy are the hallmarks of arsenic ingestion. The skin lesions are characterized by hyperpigmentation and hyperkeratosis. Thallium may result in scaly rash, hair loss, and sensorimotor polyneuropathy. Bleeding and easy bruisability, in response to minor trauma, is the major symptom of vitamin K deficiency. Any site can be involved, including mucosal and subcutaneous bleeding. Patients may develop epistaxis, hematoma, gastrointestinal bleeding, menorrhagia, hematuria, gum bleeding, and oozing from venipuncture sites. Fatigue and weight loss are not symptoms of vitamin K deficiency.

1. Case studies in environmental medicine. http://www. atsdr.cdc.gov/HEC/CSEM/csem.html. Accessed December 14, 2006.
2. Greenberg DA, Aminoff MJ, Simon RP. *Clinical Neurology.* 5th ed. New York: McGraw-Hill; 2002:182–183.

75. Answer: E. Signs of a LMN lesion include atrophy, hypoactive deep tendon reflexes, flaccidity, weakness, and a flexor plantar response (Babinski sign absent). Spasticity would be a characteristic of a UMN lesion.

Kaufman DM. *Clinical Neurology for Psychiatrists.* 5th ed. Philadelphia: WB Saunders; 2001:5.

76. Answer: E. Most adult CNS tumors are metastatic. Metastatic tumors (particularly those due to renal cell cancer, melanomas, and choricarcinomas) and glioblastoma multiforme are the tumors most likely to hemorrhage. Meningiomas and oligodendrogliomas are more likely to have calcifications. Headaches associated with brain tumors are not of one type. They can, for example, mimic tension or migraine headaches, although most are unilateral and ipsilateral to the tumor location. Frontal lobe tumors can produce personality changes.

Zaidat OO, Lerner AJ. *The Little Black Book of Neurology.* 4th ed. St Louis: Mosby; 2002:369–373.

77. Answer: A. This patient has isolated sixth nerve palsy. The sixth nerve (abducens) arises at the level of the lower pons from cells in the floor of the fourth ventricle, adjacent to the midline. Isolated sixth nerve palsy with global headache, especially when the palsy is bilateral, is often caused by neoplasm. The most common tumor involving the sixth nerve is a metastatic tumor arising from the nasopharynx. It is therefore essential that the nasopharynx be examined carefully in every case of unexplained sixth nerve palsy, particularly if it is accompanied by sensory symptoms on the side of the face. Infarction of the sixth nerve is another common cause of sixth nerve palsy in diabetics, usually accompanied by pain near the outer canthus of the eye. It would therefore make sense to check a serum glucose, as well as a CT or MRI, to evaluate for infarction. A very common cause of fourth nerve palsy is head trauma.

Ropper AH, Brown RH. *Adams and Victor's Principles of Neurology.* 8th ed. New York: McGraw-Hill; 2005:233.

78. Answer: E. Forced-use or constraint-induced movement therapy (CI) is becoming a popular rehabilitative intervention for post-stroke patients. In this therapy, the uninvolved extremity is restrained, while the affected limb undergoes intensive training for up to 6 hours per day, for 10 to 15 days. Outside of the therapy, the uninvolved extremity is restrained for 90% of the day, to "force" the patient to use the affected extremity as much as possible. This therapy has shown to improve clinical outcomes and to produce cortical reorganization in stroke patients. The main goal of this therapy is to improve the strength and functional capacity of the affected limb, as well as to produce cortical reorganization, with more cortical representation of the affected leg.

Dombovy ML. Understanding stroke recovery and rehabilitation: current and emerging approaches. *Curr Neurol Neurosci Rep.* 2004;4:31–35.

79. Answer: B. Erik Erikson proposed eight stages of ego development, each associated with a particular internal crisis whose successful resolution leads to development of a particular virtue. The stages and virtues are as follows:

1. Birth to 18 months, trust versus mistrust, hope
2. 18 months to 3 years, autonomy versus shame and doubt, will
3. 3 years to 5 years, initiative versus guilt, purpose
4. 5 years to 13 years, industry versus inferiority, competence
5. 13 years to 21 years, identity versus role confusion, fidelity
6. 21 years to 40 years, intimacy versus isolation, love

7. 40 years to 60 years, generativity versus stagnation, care

8. 60 years to death, integrity versus despair, wisdom

Sadock BJ, Sadock VA. *Kaplan and Sadock's Synopsis of Psychiatry*. 9th ed. Philadelphia: Lippincott Williams & Wilkins; 2003:211–217.

80. Answer: B. Neuropeptide Y is associated with feeding disorders and blood pressure and not anxiety. Cholecystokinin administration can induce panic attacks.

Anderson IM, Reid IC. *Fundamentals of Clinical Psychopharmacology*. London: Taylor & Francis Group; 2004:5.

81. Answer: A. Classical conditioning describes the process of association between a neutral stimulus and an unconditioned stimulus, such that the neutral stimulus now elicits a response similar to that originally elicited by the unconditioned stimulus. Operant conditioning on the other hand, describes a form of learning where the occurrence of behaviors are changed via the application of positive and negative consequences. All the other choices are correct in their description.

Sadock BJ, Sadock VA. *Kaplan and Sadock's Comprehensive Textbook of Psychiatry*. 8th ed. Philadelphia: Lippincott Williams & Wilkins; 2005:542–543.

82. Answer: A. In this study, the responses can be represented in a 2 × 2 table as the following; 76% of the patients on placebo continue to have anxiety compared to 35% in the citalopram group. Given this information, the RR reduction of anxiety in the citalopram group compared to the placebo group can be reported as: (anxiety in the placebo group to anxiety in the citalopram group)/anxiety in the placebo group: 76%–35%/76% = 0.53.

Treatment	Not responding (%)	Responding (%)
Placebo	76	24
Citalopram	35	65

More effective treatments provide greater reduction in the risk of negative outcome. The RR reduction for effective treatments varies between 0 and 1. Unlike RR, where smaller values indicate more effective treatment, in RR reduction, larger values indicate a more effective treatment.

1. Gray GE. *Evidence-Based Psychiatry*. Washington: American Psychiatric Publishing; 2004:64–68.
2. Lenze EJ, Mulsant BH, Shear MK, et al. Efficacy and tolerability of citalopram in the treatment of late-life anxiety disorders: results from an 8-week randomized, placebo-controlled trial. *Am J Psychiatry*. 2005;162:146–150.

83. Answer: E. Semantic memory is for knowledge and facts (i.e., the capital of a state), and this typically does not decline with age. Impairment of various types of memory, most notably short-term and recent memory, is a prominent behavioral deficit in patients with brain damage, and is often the first sign of cerebral disease and of aging. Immediate memory is memory after 5 seconds, and recent memory is also known as short-term memory and concerns events over the past few hours or days. Remote memory is also known as long-term memory and consists of childhood data and events in the distant past; although it is commonly believed that remote memory is well-preserved in senile patients, on close exam, there are usually gaps and inconsistencies in their recitals. Episodic memory involves retention of specific events that may be recent or remote (i.e., a telephone message).

Kaplan HI, Sadock BJ. *Kaplan & Sadock's Synopsis of Psychiatry*. 8th ed. Philadelphia: Lippincott Williams & Wilkins; 1998:200.

84. Answer: B. Divalproex inhibits lamotrigine's metabolism (increases blood levels) and carbamazepine induces elimination (decreases blood levels). Gradual titration of lamotrigine is recommended to reduce the potential for rash: beginning at 25 mg daily during week 2, 50 mg per day at weeks 3 and 4, 100 mg per day at week 5, and 200 mg per day at week 6. The dose of lamotrigine should be cut in half when used in conjunction with divalproex and doubled when used with carbamazepine.

1. http://www.fda.gov/cder/drug/InfoSheets/patient/lamotriginePIS.pdf. Accessed November 25, 2006.
2. Dunner DL. Safety and tolerability of emerging pharmacological treatments for bipolar disorder. *Bipolar Disord*. 2005;7:307–325.

85. Answer: B. The key feature of dissociative amnesia, according to DSM-IV-TR criteria, is "one or more episodes of inability to recall important personal information, usually of a traumatic or stressful nature, that is too extensive to be explained by ordinary forgetfulness." Although dissociative amnesia is most commonly seen after a precipitating trauma, rare spontaneous cases have occurred. Affected individuals generally remain alert, often remember general, but not personal information, and are able to learn new information. Patients are usually aware that they have lost memory, but may be undisturbed by this fact. Dissociative amnesia may be localized to events over a short period of time, generalized to a lifetime of events, or selective to only certain events over a short period of time. Most patients recover suddenly and completely.

1. American Psychiatric Association. *Quick Reference to the Diagnostic Criteria from DSM-IV-TR*. Washington: American Psychiatric Association; 2000:239–243.

2. Sadock BJ, Sadock VA. *Kaplan and Sadock's Synopsis of Psychiatry*. 9th ed. Philadelphia: Lippincott Williams & Wilkins; 2003:676–691.

86. Answer: A. Emil Kraepelin coined the term to describe what was later termed *Schizophrenia* by Eugen Bleuler. Kraepelin's term emphasized the cognitive nature of the disease (dementia) as well as the observation that the disease has an early onset (praecox) (although we now know that the disease does not always have an early onset). Meyer, Jaspers, and Stack Sullivan are also important figures in the history of the understanding of schizophrenia.

Kaplan HI, Sadock BJ. *Kaplan & Sadock's Synopsis of Psychiatry*. 8th ed. Philadelphia: Lippincott Williams & Wilkins; 1998:456–457.

87. Answer: A. This patient meets DSM-IV-TR criteria for Bulimia Nervosa, Purging Type. She regularly (at least twice a week for 3 months) eats larger than normal amounts of food, feels out of control about eating, engages in recurrent inappropriate compensatory behaviors, and unduly values body shape and weight. Because of her regular laxative use, she is in the purging subtype. She does not meet criteria for anorexia nervosa because her weight is within normal range. Consequences of laxative abuse, especially stimulant laxatives, include diarrhea, electrolyte abnormalities, and dehydration. Chronic stimulant laxative abuse may lead to colon dysfunction and constipation, GI blood loss, steatorrhea, osteomalacia, hypocalcemia, and hypomagnesemia.

1. Sadock BJ, Sadock VA. *Kaplan and Sadock's Synopsis of Psychiatry*. 9th ed. Philadelphia: Lippincott Williams & Wilkins; 2003:746–750.
2. Schneider M. Bulimia nervosa and binge-eating disorder in adolescents. *Adolesc Med*. 2003;14:119–131.

88. Answer: B. Acamprosate was recently approved by the FDA for use in Alcohol Dependence, although it was in use for several years in Europe prior. It has modest, but clear benefit over placebo in prolonging abstinence. Studies have shown benefit for at least a year. It is generally well tolerated; the most common side effects are gastrointestinal (nausea/diarrhea). It is excreted unchanged by the kidney, making use in renal failure contraindicated. The dosing is somewhat cumbersome, starting at 333 mg TID, and the effective dose is generally 1,333 mg to 1,998 mg daily.

1. Kranzler HR, Ciraulo DA. *Clinical Manual of Addiction Psychopharmacology*. Arlington: American Psychiatric Publishing; 2005:28–29.
2. Rosenbaum JF, Arana GW, Hyman SE, et al. *Handbook of Psychiatric Drug Therapy*. 5th ed. Philadelphia: Lippincott Williams & Wilkins; 2005:230–232.

89. Answer: E. The use of typical and atypical antipsychotics has been associated with the development of QTc prolongation and *torsade de pointes*, although this seems to be an uncommon occurrence (a recent study showed an incidence of QTc prolongation of 3% in patients treated with typical and atypical antipsychotics). Some of the risk factors associated with the development of QTc prolongation include: obesity, hypothyroidism, alcoholism, advanced age, CHF, athletic training, hypoglycemia, bradycardia, hypokalemia, hypomagnesemia, cardiac dysrhythmias, and polypharmacy.

1. Mackin P, Young AH. QTc interval measurement and metabolic parameters in psychiatric patients taking typical or atypical antipsychotic drugs: a preliminary study. *J Clin Psychiatry*. 2005;66:1386–1391.
2. Rund DA, Ewing JD, Mitzel K, et al. The use of intramuscular benzodiazepines and antipsychotic agents in the treatment of acute agitation or violence in the emergency department. *J Emerg Med*. 2006;31:317–324.

90. Answer: A. Naltrexone is used in maintenance treatment for Alcohol Dependence. Benzodiazepines are the indicated class of medications for alcohol withdrawal symptoms, along with the barbiturates, although these have a lower margin of safety. Propranolol and clonidine have also been used to help manage withdrawal symptoms as has haloperidol; haloperidol has a relatively low seizure risk, but its use is still a concern when managing a patient at risk for having a seizure.

Sadock BJ, Sadock VA. *Kaplan and Sadock's Comprehensive Textbook of Psychiatry*. 8th ed. Philadelphia: Lippincott Williams & Wilkins; 2005:1185–1187.

91. Answer: C. The recommended treatment is 10,000 lux of light for at least 30 minutes daily on awakening, although it can be as long as two hours. One study showed that 250 lux for 90 minutes was better than a placebo dawn. Major Depressive Disorder, recurrent with seasonal pattern (the proper, DSM definition for seasonal affective disorder) has a mean age of onset of 40 years.

Sadock BJ, Sadock VA. *Kaplan and Sadock's Comprehensive Textbook of Psychiatry*. 8th ed. Philadelphia: Lippincott Williams & Wilkins; 2005:2991.

92. Answer: C. Cognitive function has been shown to be the strongest predictor of obtaining and keeping a job in patients with Schizophrenia. Although the severity of illness and the presence of both positive and negative symptoms are important factors that affect the patient's social skills and quality of life, they do not have such a strong prediction of work as cognitive function. Supported employment seems to improve work functioning partly by helping patients find jobs that are matched to their cognitive skills.

McGurk SR, Mueser KT. Cognitive and clinical predictors of work outcomes in clients with schizophrenia receiving supported employment services: 4-year follow-up. *Adm Policy Ment Health.* 2006;33:598–606.

93. **Answer: A.** Competency. The primary ethical concern is whether or not the psychiatrist is competent to perform the procedure. Section 1 of the APA ethics guidelines states "[A] physician shall be dedicated to providing competent medical service with compassion and respect for human dignity." Section 1-L states that a psychiatrist can perform a nonpsychiatric medical procedure if he or she is competent to do so. The psychiatrist of course must discuss the risks and benefits to allow the patient, or his proxy, to make the best decision for himself (autonomy), needs to obtain informed consent, must not perform the lumbar puncture simply for his own gain or pleasure (exploitation), and must maintain confidentiality.

American Psychiatric Association. Opinions of the Ethics Committee on the principles of medical ethics with annotations especially applicable to psychiatry. 2001 ed. http://www.psych.org/psych_pract/ethics/ethics_opinions 53101.cfm. Published December 11, 2006.

94. **Answer: B.** Marchiafava-Bignami disease is caused by demyelination of the corpus callosum without inflammation. It was first described by Marchiafava and Bignami in 1903. Although this disease was first noted in middle-aged and elderly Italian men who consumed red wine, the definitive cause is still not known. The classical lesion is the necrosis of the medial zone of the corpus callosum with sparing of the dorsal and ventral rims. Bilaterally symmetrical degeneration of the anterior commissure, posterior commissure, centrum semiovale, subcortical white matter, long association bundles, and middle cerebellar peduncles may also be seen. Internal capsule, corona radiata, and subgyral arcuate fibers, and the gray matter are not grossly affected. The lesion shows demyelination, but relative preservation of axis cylinders in the periphery of the lesions. There is usually no evidence of inflammation except for a few perivascular lymphocytes. Fat-filled phagocytes and capillary endothelial proliferation may be present in the affected area without the presence of a thrombus.

1. Kaufman DM. *Clinical Neurology for Psychiatrists.* 5th ed. Philadelphia: WB Saunders; 2001:383.
2. Rowland LP. *Merritt's Neurology.* 11th ed. Philadelphia: Lippincott Williams & Wilkins; 2005:963–964.

95. **Answer: A.** In Korsakoff's syndrome, demyelination of nerve fibers in multiple brain structures disrupts the Papez circuit and leads to disturbances in episodic memories in chronic alcoholics with poor nutrition. In Korsakoff's syndrome, demyelination occurs primarily in the mammillary bodies and the dorsomedial and laterodorsal thalamic nuclei and thus interrupts the Papez circuit. This interruption leads to anterograde amnesia and retrograde amnesia. The Papez circuit includes the hippocampus, fornix, mammillary bodies, anterior nucleus of the thalamus, cingulate gyrus, and presubiculum.

Budson AE, Price BH. *Memory: Clinical Disorders. Encyclopedia of Life Sciences.* London: Macmillan Publishers; 2001:1–3.

96. **Answer: C.** Approximately 50% of Tourette's patients have comorbid OCD, but less than 10% of OCD patients have Tourette's.

Sadock BJ, Sadock VA. *Kaplan and Sadock's Comprehensive Textbook of Psychiatry.* 8th ed. Philadelphia: Lippincott Williams & Wilkins; 2005:1774.

97. **Answer: B.** Generally speaking, encephalopathies usually produce increased theta and delta activity on EEG. Metabolic encephalopathies are frequently accompanied by slowing with high wave amplitude. Sedative drug use, as is likely the case in this patient, typically produces slowing with increased beta activity.

Khoshbin H. Clinical neurophysiology. *UpToDate 2006.* http://www.uptodateonline.com/utd/content/topic. do?topicKey=neuropat/4649&type=A&selectedTitle= 1~71. Published January 23, 2007.

98. **Answer: A.** The spike, sharp wave, and spike-and-slow wave complexes are the three types of interictal epileptiform discharges (IEDs). These IEDs are the most diagnostic EEG findings for an epileptogenic brain. Generalized slowing and increased frequency of theta and delta waves are often seen in encephalopathy. Alpha activity is normally seen in the healthy waking adult EEG.

Khoshbin H. Clinical neurophysiology. *UpToDate 2006.* http://www.uptodateonline.com/utd/content/topic. do?topicKey=neuropat/4649&type=A&selectedTitle= 1~71. Published January 23, 2007.

99. **Answer: C.** Arteriovenous malformations (AVM) consist of a tangle of dilated vessels that form an abnormal communication between the arterial and venous systems, really an arteriovenous fistula. Arteriovenous malformations are about equally frequent in males and females. Rarely, AVMs occur in more than one member of a family in the same generation or successive ones. Bleeding or seizures are the

main modes of presentation. Most AVMs are clinically silent for a long time, but sooner or later they bleed. The rate of hemorrhage in untreated patients is established to be 2% to 4% per year, far lower than for aneurysms. The mortality rate in two major series has been 1% to 2% per year, but as high as 6% to 9% in the immediate year following a first hemorrhage. Before rupture, chronic, recurrent headache may be a complaint; usually the headache is of a nondescript type, but a classic migraine with or without neurologic accompaniment occurs in about 10% of patients—probably with greater frequency than it does in the general population. A systolic bruit heard over the carotid in the neck or over the mastoid process or the eyeballs in a young adult is almost pathognomonic of an AVM. However, such bruits have been heard in fewer than 25% of patients. The blood pressure may be elevated or normal; but the occurrence of intracranial bleeding with a previously normal blood pressure should raise the suspicion of an AVM, but also of ruptured saccular aneurysm, bleeding diathesis, cerebral vessel amyloidosis, or hemorrhage into a tumor. Ninety-five percent of AVMs are disclosed by CT scans if enhanced, with an even larger number being detected by an MRI. Magnetic susceptibility MRI shows small areas of previous bleeding around AVMs.

Ropper AH, Brown RH. *Adams and Victor's Principles of Neurology.* 8th ed. New York: McGraw-Hill; 2005:722–723.

100. Answer: B. The lateral spinothalamic tracts transmit pain and temperature sensations to the thalamus.

Kaufman DM. *Clinical Neurology for Psychiatrists.* 5th ed. Philadelphia: WB Saunders; 2001:21.

101. Answer: E. Tardive dyskinesia is typically seen in the context of long-term use of antidopaminergic medications, such as antipsychotic medications or antiemetics like metoclopramide. It causes involuntary choreic movements and can be monitored with an AIMS.

Fix JD. *High-Yield Neuroanatomy.* Baltimore: Williams & Wilkins; 1995:94.

102. Answer: A. Paraneoplastic syndromes are autoimmune disorders which are remote effects of cancers. Lambert-Eaton syndrome is one such syndrome associated with small cell lung cancer. It resembles myasthenia gravis, which is not a paraneoplastic syndrome—in contrast to myasthenia gravis, there is impaired release of acetycholine from presynaptic membranes, rather than antibodies against ACh antibodies and, among other differences, increased strength with repetitive exertion as compared to increased weakness in myasthenia. Symptoms from paraneoplastic syndromes, in most cases, precede the diagnosis of the cancer. Limbic encephalitis is a paraneoplastic syndrome associated with small cell cancer of the lung and testicular cancer. People with the disorder develop difficulty with memory alone or in combination with other neuropsychiatric symptoms.

1. Kaufman DM. *Clinical Neurology for Psychiatrists.* 5th ed. Philadelphia: WB Saunders; 2001:97–98, 515–516.
2. Zaidat OO, Lerner AJ. *The Little Black Book of Neurology.* 4th ed. St Louis: Mosby; 2002:20–21, 288–289.

103. Answer: C. These two patients have acute high-altitude (mountain) sickness, a special form of cerebral hypoxia. It occurs when a sea-level inhabitant abruptly ascends to a high altitude. Headache, anorexia, nausea and vomiting, weakness, and insomnia appear at altitudes above 8,000 feet; at higher altitudes, there may be ataxia, tremor, drowsiness, mild confusion, and hallucinations. At 16,000 feet, 50% of individuals develop asymptomatic retinal hemorrhages. Extreme altitude sickness may result in fatal cerebral edema. Hypoxemia at high altitude is intensified during sleep, because ventilation normally diminishes. Sedatives, alcohol, and a slightly elevated PCO_2 in the blood all reduce one's tolerance to high altitude.

Ropper AH, Brown RH. *Adams and Victor's Principles of Neurology.* 8th ed. New York: McGraw-Hill; 2005:964.

104. Answer: D. Stroke is a common cause of disability for many patients. Studies have shown that neurological impairment and aphasia are poor predictive factors for return to work. The following factors were found to be good predictive factors for patients to be able to return to work after a stroke: white-collar job, right-hemisphere damage, young age, good activities of daily living at discharge, good attentional ability, visuomotor speed, and communicative abilities.

Hofgren C, Bjorkdahl A, Esbjornsson E, et al. Recovery after stroke: cognition, ADL function and return to work. *Acta Neurol Scand.* 2007;115:73–80.

105. Answer: C. Erik Erikson formulated eight stages of development of the ego, which span the life cycle. These are, in order, trust versus mistrust, autonomy versus shame and doubt, initiative versus guilt, industry versus inferiority, identity versus role confusion, intimacy versus isolation, generativity versus stagnation, and integrity versus despair. The stage of intimacy versus isolation spans approximately age 21 to age 40. Successful navigation of this stage is tied to the virtue of fidelity—the ability to make and honor concrete commitments. Difficulty with this stage can lead to schizoid personality and *distantiation*, which is Erikson's term for the desire to distance oneself from anyone or anything that might seem threatening.

Sadock BJ, Sadock VA. *Kaplan and Sadock's Synopsis of Psychiatry*. 9th ed. Philadelphia: Lippincott Williams & Wilkins; 2003:211–217.

106. Answer: B. The major neurotransmitter pathways that are important from the psychopharmacological point of view are the long ascending and descending axonal pathways, the long and short axonal pathways, and the short intraregional pathways. The long ascending and descending axonal pathways are seen with dopamine, noradrenaline, serotonin, and acetylcholine pathways. The long and short axonal pathways arise from neuronal cell bodies widely spread throughout the brain and are associated with the major excitatory (glutamate) and inhibitory (GABA) pathways.

Anderson IM, Reid IC. *Fundamentals of Clinical Psychopharmacology*. London: Taylor & Francis Group; 2004:6.

107. Answer: E. Jean Piaget was genetic epistemologist who first described four stages of cognitive development in children. These four stages constitute a structured whole that can be defined by a set of criteria. These are named as sensorimotor, preoperational, concrete operational, and formal operational stages. Each of the four stages is briefly described below:

(i) The sensiromotor stage which occurs between 0 and 2 years is characterized by primary circular reaction, secondary circular reaction, teritiary circular reaction, egocentrism, insight, and object permanence.

(ii) The preoperational stage which occurs between 2 and 7 years is characterized by deferred imitation, symbolic play, graphic imagery, mental imagery, and language.

(iii) The concrete operations stage occurs between the ages of 7 and 11 years and is characterized by conservation of quantity, weight, volume, length, time, reversibility by inversion or reciprocity, class inclusion, and seriation.

(iv) The formal operations stage occurs between the ages of 11 years and the end of adolescence and is characterized by a combinatorial system where all variables are isolated and all possible combinations are examined and hypothetical-deductive thinking is initiated.

1. Sadock BJ, Sadock VA. *Kaplan and Sadock's Comprehensive Textbook of Psychiatry*. 8th ed. Philadelphia: Lippincott Williams & Wilkins; 2005:528–534.
2. Greenspan S, Curry JF. Expanding Jean Piaget's Approach to Intellectual Functioning. http://www.ship.edu/~cgboeree/piaget. html. Accessed December 10, 2006.

108. Answer: A. In this study, the responses can be represented in a 2 × 2 table as the following: 76% of the

Treatment	Not responding (%)	Responding (%)
Placebo	76	24
Citalopram	35	65

patients on the placebo continue to have anxiety as compared to 35% in the citalopram group. Given this information, the absolute risk reduction of anxiety in the citalopram group compared to the placebo group can be reported as; anxiety in the placebo group to anxiety in the citalopram group: 76%–35% = 41%.

Because absolute risk reduction is an absolute, not relative value, it can be used to determine the percentage of patients undergoing treatment who benefit from the medication compared to placebo. The ARR varies from 0% to 100% or 0 and 1, if not expressed as a percentage, with larger values indicating more effective treatments.

1. Gray GE. *Evidence-Based Psychiatry*. Washington: American Psychiatric Publishing; 2004:64–68.
2. Lenze EJ, Mulsant BH, Shear MK, et al. Efficacy and tolerability of citalopram in the treatment of late-life anxiety disorders: results from an 8-week randomized, placebo-controlled trial. *Am J Psychiatry*. 2005;162:146–150.

109. Answer: E. Impairment of various types of memory, most notably short-term and recent memory, is a prominent behavioral deficit in patients with brain damage, and is often the first sign of beginning cerebral disease and of aging. Short-term memory is also known as immediate memory (memory after 5 seconds), or of recent memory, which concerns events over the past few hours or days. Recent past memory concerns the retention of information over the past few months (i.e., current events). Remote memory is also known as long-term memory and consists of childhood data and events in the distant past. Semantic memory is for knowledge and facts, and implicit memory is for automatic skills (i.e., driving a car); these do not decline with age, and people continue to accumulate information over a lifetime.

Kaplan HI, Sadock BJ. *Kaplan & Sadock's Synopsis of Psychiatry*. 8th ed. Philadelphia: Lippincott Williams & Wilkins; 1998: 200.

110. Answer: E. Divalproex inhibits lamotrigine's metabolism (increases blood levels) and carbamazepine induces elimination (decreases blood levels). Gradual titration of lamotrigine is recommended to reduce the potential for rash: beginning at 25 mg daily during week 1 and 2, 50 mg per day at weeks 3 and 4, 100 mg per day at week 5, and 200 mg per day at week 6. The dose of lamotrigine should be cut in half when used in conjunction with divalproex and doubled when used with carbamazepine.

1. http://www.fda.gov/cder/drug/InfoSheets/patient/lamotriginePIS.pdf. Accessed November 25, 2006.
2. Dunner DL. Safety and tolerability of emerging pharmacological treatments for bipolar disorder. *Bipolar Disord.* 2005;7:307–325.

111. Answer: E. The weight loss that is characteristic of anorexia nervosa carries many medical complications. Among these are reduced thyroid metabolism, cold intolerance, hypothermia, cardiac arrhythmias and bradycardia, delayed gastric emptying, abdominal pain, constipation, amenorrhea, fine (lanugo) downy hair covering body, leukopenia, and osteoporosis.

Sadock BJ, Sadock VA. *Kaplan and Sadock's Synopsis of Psychiatry.* 9th ed. Philadelphia: Lippincott Williams & Wilkins; 2003:742.

112. Answer: E. The patient has Sleep Terror Disorder. Although the disorder can occur in adults, it is more frequently seen in children and, in childhood, it is not associated with any psychopathology. It occurs during sleep stages 3 and 4, and the night terrors often become sleepwalking episodes. Patients typically do not remember the episodes. Stimulants can lead to these episodes (as well as neuroleptics, sedative-hypnotics, and antihistamines), and their use should be evaluated during the evaluation of a sleep-terror disorder.

1. Mason T, Pac A. Sleep terrors in childhood. *J Pediatr.* 2005;147:388–392.
2. Sadock BJ, Sadock VA. *Kaplan and Sadock's Comprehensive Textbook of Psychiatry.* 8th ed. Philadelphia: Lippincott Williams & Wilkins; 2005:2033.

113. Answer: E. Hypokalemic, hypochloremic metabolic alkalosis is the classic metabolic derangement seen in excessive vomiting. Other complications of frequent purging include dehydration, erosion of tooth enamel, calluses on the back of the hand (known as Russell's sign), parotid enlargement, hyperamylasemia, acute pancreatitis, gastroesophogeal irritation, reflux and bleeding, and Mallory-Weiss tears.

Schneider M. Bulimia nervosa and binge-eating disorder in adolescents. *Adolesc Med.* 2003;14:119–131.

114. Answer: E. This patient appears to have developed serotonin syndrome, which is characterized by cognitive alterations, autonomic dysfunction, behavioral disturbances, and alterations in neuromuscular activity. Symptoms observed include confusion, irritability, agitation, unresponsiveness, myoclonus, hy-perreflexia, rigidity, ataxia, hyperthermia, sweating, and tachypnoea. This is caused by the excessive accumulation of serotonin. It has been documented due to the following drug combinations: phenelzine and SSRIs; phenelzine and meperidine; tranylcypromine and imipramine; paroxetine and buspirone; linezolide and citalopram; moclobemide and SSRIs; tramadol, venlafaxine, and mirtazapine. The treatment of serotonin syndrome includes the discontinuation of the offending drug/drugs, supportive care, control of agitation using benzodiazepines and control of hyperthermia using benzodiazepines. In severe hyperthermia, with temperatures up to and exceeding 41°C, paralysis should be induced using nondepolarizing agents, such as vecuronium, followed by orotracheal intubation, and ventilation. Succinylcholine is not recommended for this purpose, because there is a high risk of developing arrhythmias owing to the hyperkalemia that results due to rhabdomyolysis. Anti-serotonergic agents, such as cyproheptadine or chlorpromazine in intramuscular form, may be used in severe cases.

1. Boyer EW, Shannon M. The serotonin syndrome. *N Engl J Med.* 2005;352:1112–1120.
2. Martin TG. Serotonin syndrome. *Ann Emerg Med.* 1996;28:520–526.

115. Answer: C. Seclusion is a common intervention used in the treatment of acutely agitated patients. A recent survey of the medical directors of emergency departments across the United States showed that the use of seclusion was associated with several complications. The most common complication with the use of restraints was patient's escape from the seclusion room (30.1%), followed by staff injury (29.2%), patient injury (19.8%), increased harmful behavior (11.3%), and psychological harm (2.8%).

1. Marder SR. A review of agitation in mental illness: treatment guidelines and current therapies. *J Clin Psychiatry.* 2006;67 (suppl 10):13–21.
2. Zun LS, Downey L. The use of seclusion in emergency medicine. *Gen Hosp Psychiatry.* 2005;27:365–371.

116. Answer: C. Naloxone has a half-life of 60 to 90 minutes and thus requires repeated dosing in opioid overdose. Nalmefene can also be used in opioid overdose but has a much longer half life, which is approximately 10 hours. Buprenorphine can be used for treatment of withdrawal and for maintenance treatment of opioid dependence. LAAM is used for maintenance treatment of dependence. Promethazine is used for symptoms of nausea.

Sadock BJ, Sadock VA. *Kaplan and Sadock's Comprehensive Textbook of Psychiatry.* 8th ed. Philadelphia: Lippincott Williams & Wilkins; 2005:1279.

117. **Answer: A.** CRSD, Delayed-Sleep-Phase Type, is treated using chronotherapy, which consists of delaying the normal bedtime and wake time progressively each night until the patient has cycled through the clock to an earlier bedtime. An alternative treatment is bright light therapy which consists of bright light in the morning to help reset the internal clock; however, relapse is frequent once treatment ends. Recommending a regular waking time can often be helpful for patients with insomnia, but is not an approach generally effective for CRSD. Using trazodone may also seem reasonable clinically, but this is not the treatment for CRSD, and there is no evidence a 7- to 14-day course would eliminate the problem. The elimination of caffeinated beverages is reasonable, but this disorder is not secondary to the use of caffeinated beverages.

1. American Psychiatric Association, American Psychiatric Association Task Force on DSM-IV. *Diagnostic and Statistical Manual of Mental Disorders: DSM-IV-TR.* 4th ed. Washington: American Psychiatric Association; 2000. http://www.med.yale.edu/library/. Accessed December 9, 2006.
2. Sinton CM, McCarley RW. Neurophysiology and neuropsychiatry of sleep and sleep disorders. In: Schiffer RB, Rao SM, Fogel BS. *Neuropsychiatry.* 2nd ed. Philadelphia: Lippincott Williams & Wilkins; 2003:378–379.

118. **Answer: D.** According to Judith Beck, automatic thoughts are "a stream of thinking" thoughts and are thoughts that are evaluated "according to their validity and utility." "I am such a loser" can readily be evaluated as true or untrue and can be evaluated as useful or not in terms of what it does, for example, to a person's mood. Choices A, C, and E are interpretations in the sense that they are not the actual thoughts going through the person's mind but interpretations of motivations, feelings, and thoughts. Choice B is an expression of an emotion. (In cognitive therapy, automatic thoughts are conceived as having a causal relationship to emotions.)

Beck JS. *Cognitive Therapy: Basics and Beyond.* New York: Guilford; 1995:75–77, 88–89, 94–97.

119. **Answer: D.** Shared decision making is the most comprehensive view of informed consent among the options listed. In the process of informed consent, the patient may agree with the physician's recommendations, may refuse the intervention proposed, and chooses among alternatives after considering risks and benefits. However, it is shared decision making that underlies the process of informed consent.

Lo B. *Resolving Ethical Dilemmas: A Guide For Clinicians.* 3rd ed. Philadelphia: Lippincott Williams & Wilkins; 2005:17–18.

120. **Answer: A.** Raised intracranial pressure is defined as an increase of mean CSF pressure above 200 mm water while recumbent. Most cases are associated with mass effect which is either diffuse, as in generalized brain edema, or focal, as with tumors, abscesses, or hemorrhages. Although the cranial vault is subdivided by rigid dural folds (falx and tentorium), expansion of brain structures causes them to be displaced in relation to these structures. Subfalcine (cingulate gyrus) herniation occurs when unilateral or asymmetric expansion of the cerebral hemisphere displaces the cingulate gyrus under the falx cerebri. Branches of the anterior cerebral artery may be compressed. Transentorial (uncal or mesial temporal) herniation occurs when the medial temporal lobe is compressed against the tentorium cerebelli. As displacement of the temporal lobe progresses, the third cranial nerve becomes compressed, resulting in pupillary dilation and impairment of ocular movements on the side of the lesion. The posterior cerebral artery is also frequently compressed. Progression of the herniation is often accompanied by hemorrhagic lesions in the pons and midbrain. Finally, tonsillar herniation involves the displacement of the cerebellar tonsils through the foramen magnum. This herniation is life-threatening, as it causes brain stem compression that affects respiratory centers in the medulla oblongata.

Cotran RS, Kumar V, Collins T. *Robbins Pathologic Basis of Disease.* 6th ed. Philadelphia: WB Saunders; 1999:1298.

121. **Answer: C.** Sign language is considered to a dominant hemisphere function. A middle cerebral artery occlusion in the dominant hemisphere in deaf individuals results in aphasia of sign language. Inflection, obscenities, prosody, rhythm as well as tone, a second language acquired as an adult, and the average persons' ability to process music are all considered to be nondominant hemisphere functions.

Kaufman DM. *Clinical Neurology for Psychiatrists.* 5th ed. Philadelphia: WB Saunders; 2001:175–176.

122. **Answer: D.** Diagnosis of a mitochondrial disease is based on five major elements. These are the recognition of an appropriate clinical syndrome, the presence of lactic acidosis in blood or CSF, detection of RRF in the muscle biopsy, documentation of impaired respiration in biochemical assays of muscle extracts or isolated mitochondria, and identification of a pathogenic mutation in mtDNA (or in nDNA). However, not all of them need necessarily be present in an individual syndrome to make the diagnosis. Mitochondrial functions are under the control of two genomes—their own (mtDNA) and that of the

nucleus (nDNA). Mitochondrial diseases caused by nDNA mutations are transmitted by Mendelian inheritance.

Rowland LP. *Merritt's Neurology.* 11th ed. Philadelphia: Lippincott Williams & Wilkins; 2005:697–698.

123. Answer: B. The main difference between EEGs obtained with the monopolar and bipolar method is that monopolar EEGs are obtained by measuring electrical activity between various points on the skull and a point that is considered to be electrically neutral (usually an ear). Bipolar EEGs measure electrical activity between pairs of brain electrodes. Both methods allow measurement of both amplitude and frequency of wave activity over both hemispheres.

Khoshbin H. Clinical Neurophysiology. *UpToDate 2006.* http://www.uptodateonline.com/utd/content/topic.do?topicKey=neuropat/4649&type=A&selectedTitle=1~71. Published January 23, 2007.

124. Answer: D. PET scan is a direct measure of metabolic activity in the body and the PET image is basically a density map of radioactivity in a slice of tissue viewed in two dimensions. The radionuclides used in the PET scans are designed to target areas of high metabolic activity. The most common PET radionuclides used is FDG. PET scanning is severely limited by its need for close proximity to a cyclotron (because of the very short half life of the artificially produced unstable nuclei), the expense of dedicated PET scanners, and the expense of positron emitting radiopharmaceuticals. The spatial resolution of PET has been the best when compared to the other functional modalities like fMRI or SPECT scan. The spatial resolution for PET scanners has been shown to be approximately 4 or 5 mm. Generalized hypometabolism can be seen in anoxia, degenerative disease, trauma, and aging or a focal hypometabolism. Hypermetabolism due to increased blood flow can be seen in tumors, infections, or seizure foci.

1. http://www.brainmattersinc.com/functional_imaging.html. Accessed January 28, 2007.
2. Goetz CG. *Textbook of Clinical Neurology.* 2nd ed. Philadelphia: WB Saunders; 2003. http://home.mdconsult.com/das/book/66246566–2/view/1158. Published January 28, 2007.

125. Answer: B. NPH is characterized by the clinical triad of dementia, gait apraxia, and urinary incontinence. It often follows meningitis or a subarachnoid hemorrhage. However, most often it results from an unknown injury. These insults impair CSF absorption from the arachnoid granulations in the subarachnoid space over the convexity of the cerebral hemispheres. NPH is also sometimes called communicating or nonobstructive hydrocephalus. It is communicating because the lateral, third, and fourth ventricles remain in communication. It is nonobstructing because the flow of CSF between the ventricles is not blocked. Clinically, it develops over weeks to months. Gait disorder is often the initial manifestation and also the first symptom to resolve. It is characterized by failure to alternate leg movements and shift weight to the forward foot. When the patient's weight remains on the foot they are trying to lift, the foot can appear stuck or glued to the floor. The apraxia is most pronounced when patients begin walking or start a turn. Urinary incontinence is a later development. It initially consists of frequency and urgency but may progress to total incontinence. Patients usually do not develop fecal incontinence. Urinary incontinence and gait abnormality present at the onset of dementia help to distinguish NPH from Alzheimer's disease.

1. Greenberg DA, Aminoff MJ, Simon RP. *Clinical Neurology.* 5th ed. New York: McGraw-Hill; 2002:52–55.
2. Kaufman DM. *Clinical Neurology for Psychiatrists.* 5th ed. Philadelphia: WB Saunders; 2001:145–147.

126. Answer: E. The posterior columns of the spinal cord transmit position and vibratory sensations to the thalamus.

Kaufman DM. *Clinical Neurology for Psychiatrists.* 5th ed. Philadelphia: WB Saunders; 2001:21.

127. Answer: E. Huntington's disease results from a loss of cholinergic and GABA-ergic neurons in the striatum.

Fix JD. *High-Yield Neuroanatomy.* Baltimore: Williams & Wilkins; 1995:100.

128. Answer: C. Acoustic neuromas are, in fact, a proliferation of Schwann cells over cranial nerve VIII. They are fairly benign tumors; however, they can extend to adjacent structures, often impinging on cranial nerves V and VII. Symptoms from these tumors include hearing loss, tinnitus, and vertigo from eighth nerve compression and facial sensory loss and/or weakness (if the fifth and/or seventh nerves are compressed). They are associated with the neurocutaneous syndrome neurofibromatosis II, an autosomal dominant disease.

1. Kaufman DM. *Clinical Neurology for Psychiatrists.* 5th ed. Philadelphia: WB Saunders; 2001:520.
2. Zaidat OO, Lerner AJ. *The Little Black Book of Neurology.* 4th ed. St Louis: Mosby; 2002:255–256.

129. Answer: E. This patient has hyponatremia, most likely due to the syndrome of inappropriate antidiuretic hormone secretion (SIADH). It complicates many neurologic diseases: head trauma, bacterial meningitis and encephalitis, cerebral infarction, subarachnoid hemorrhage, neoplasm, and Guillain-Barré syndrome. The diagnosis of SIADH should be suspected in any critically ill neurologic or neurosurgical patient who excretes urine that is hypertonic relative to the plasma. As the hyponatremia develops, there is a decrease in alertness, which progresses through stages of confusion to coma, often with convulsions. The severity of the clinical effect is related to the rapidity of decline in serum Na. Administration of sodium chloride (NaCl) intravenously must be done cautiously, because in most of these patients the intravascular volume is already expanded and there is a risk of CHF. There is also the danger of provoking central pontine myelinolysis and related brainstem, cerebellar, and cerebral lesions (extrapontine myelinolysis). Most cases respond to the restriction of fluid intake, but in extreme cases of hyponatremia with stupor or seizures, infusion of NaCl is necessary. If hypertonic saline is administered, it is usually necessary to simultaneously reduce intravascular volume with furosemide. Although the syndrome of SIADH is usually self-limiting, it may continue for weeks or months, depending on the type of associated brain disease.

Ropper AH, Brown RH. *Adams and Victor's Principles of Neurology.* 8th ed. New York: McGraw-Hill; 2005:971–975.

130. Answer: A. Recent studies have shown that cortical reorganization after a stroke is activity dependent. There is more functional recovery and cortical reorganization, when patients are forced to use the affected extremity with intensive and repetitive sessions. The complexity of the tasks should be increased gradually, and the approach should be task-specific and repetitive. Not using the affected limb does not lead to functional recovery or cortical reorganization.

Dombovy ML. Understanding stroke recovery and rehabilitation: current and emerging approaches. *Curr Neurol Neurosci Rep.* 2004;4:31–35.

131. Answer: D. Levinson's developmental model for adulthood includes early, middle and late adulthood stages with transitions before and after each stage. His model applies to both genders.

Sadock BJ, Kaplan H. *Synopsis of Psychiatry.* 9th ed. Philadelphia: Lippincott Williams & Wilkins; 2003:41–42.

132. Answer: C. The limbic lobe was first described in detail in 1878 by Broca and was initially thought to be primarily involved with the sense of smell. Sub-

sequent neuroanatomists recognized its connection with drive related and emotional behavior, but this is not the sole purpose of all the structures. There is no universal agreement for the total list of structures in it, but the vast majority include the cingulate and parahippocampal gyri, the hippocampus, the amygdala, and the septal nuclei. The hippocampus and the amygdala represent the major subsystems with their principal output being the medial forebrain bundle. The hippocampus is important in memory and has a role in mood. The entorhinal cortex is its principal input, and the fornix is the principal output. The connections of the hippocampus have been mapped in detail, with CA3 projecting to CA2, and in subsequently to CA1, to the subiculum and out of the hippocampus.

Notle J. *The Human Brain: An Introduction to Its Functional Anatomy.* 4th ed. St Louis: Mosby; 1999:547–560.

133. Answer: A. In this study, the responses can be represented in a 2 × 2 table as the following; 76% of patients on placebo continue to have anxiety

Treatment	Not responding (%)	Responding (%)
Placebo	76	24
Citalopram	35	65

compared to 35% in the citalopram group. Given this information, the absolute risk reduction of anxiety in the citalopram group compared to the placebo group can be reported as: anxiety in the placebo group to anxiety in the citalopram group; 76%–35% = 41% or 0.41. The NNT is the reciprocal of ARR. In this case, it would be 1/0.41 = 2.43 or 3 (taken to the next whole number). An NNT of 3 means that for every three patients treated with citalopram, there will be one less case of nonresponse than if all patients had received placebo **OR** for every three patients treated with citalopram, there is one additional patient who responds to medication who would not have responded to the placebo.

Clinical epidemiologists state that the NNT is the most useful and least misleading clinical measure of treatment effectiveness. Most psychotropic medications have the NNTs in the range of 3 to 6, which means that for every three to six patients treated, there is one good outcome that would not otherwise have occurred.

1. Gray GE. *Evidence-Based Psychiatry.* Washington: American Psychiatric Publishing; 2004:64–68.
2. Lenze EJ, Mulsant BH, Shear MK, et al. Efficacy and tolerability of citalopram in the treatment of late-life anxiety disorders: results from an 8-week randomized, placebo-controlled trial. *Am J Psychiatry.* 2005;162:146–150.

134. Answer: C. A description of the patient's marital status is not part of a mental status examination; it is part of the identifying data detailed during the first part of the interview when obtaining a psychiatric history. The mental status examination is the part of the clinical assessment that describes the observations and impressions of a patient at that particular time of the interview and is subject to change (unlike a patient's history which remains stable). This includes descriptions of a patient's appearance, attitude, actions, feelings, thoughts, cognitive abilities, and reliability during an interview. Visuospatial ability is tested by asking the patient to copy a figure. The mental status part of the report often concludes with the interviewer's impressions of the patient's reliability and capacity to report his or her situation accurately.

Kaplan HI, Sadock BJ. *Kaplan & Sadock's Synopsis of Psychiatry*. 8th ed. Philadelphia: Lippincott Williams & Wilkins; 1998:245, 250–254.

135. Answer: C. Although craving, increased blood pressure and heart rate, delirium with hallucinations, and insomnia are all symptoms seen in alcohol withdrawal syndromes, nystagmus is normally seen during alcohol intoxication.

Ebert M, Loosen P, Nurcombe B. *Current Diagnosis and Treatment in Psychiatry*. Access Medicine: McGraw Hill; 2000: www.accessmedicine.com/content.aspx?a1D=27152. Accessed October 24, 2007.

136. Answer: C. SSRIs, though often used, have not been definitely shown to be effective in the treatment of Anorexia Nervosa. The other statements are true. Psychodynamic theory suggests that through control of food intake and body size, patients are attempting to exert a sense of separateness and uniqueness in the face of an overly enmeshed relationship with the mother and/or family system. The medical stability and nutritional status of the patient are of primary concern. Fear of gaining weight and becoming fat is a core feature of the illness. Anorexia nervosa is associated with a high rate of morbidity and mortality.

1. Claudino AM, Hay P, Lima MS, et al. Antidepressants for anorexia nervosa. *Cochrane Database Systematic Rev*. 2006;1:CD004365.
2. Gabbard GO. *Psychodynamic Psychiatry in Clinical Practice*. 3rd ed. Washington: American Psychiatric Press; 2000:342–345.
3. Sadock BJ, Sadock VA. *Kaplan and Sadock's Synopsis of Psychiatry*. 9th ed. Philadelphia: Lippincott Williams & Wilkins; 2003:739–746.

137. Answer: E. This patient displays characteristics attributed to obsessive-compulsive personality. She exhibits control issues (with her husband, with refusal of medication), is very orderly ("immaculate home"), can't delegate the cleaning job, and there is a theme of perfectionism. Her husband's comments further reflect her inflexibility ("too set in her ways"), in addition to her controlling nature. One possible etiology of OCD is exposure to rigid, controlling, disciplinary parents as a child; perhaps there were problems during Freud's anal phase of development (a second possible etiology). Classic analytic thinking regards difficulty with expressing aggression related to toilet training, with stubbornness also possibly arising from this stage. Obsessive orderliness may be a reaction formation against a wish to engage in anal messiness. OCD patients find anger and dependency consciously unacceptable. A punitive superego displays defense mechanisms such as isolation of affect, intellectualization, reaction formation, undoing, and displacement. Contemporary thinking on OCD includes issues pertaining to self-esteem, anger/dependency, cognitive style, problems with balancing work and emotional relationships, and impulsive aggression. Obsessive-compulsive personality disorder (OCPD) is thought to be more common in men than women, but can occur with either gender.

1. Gabbard G. *Psychodynamic Psychiatry in Clinical Practice*. 4th ed. Washington: American Psychiatric Publishing; 2005:571–577.
2. Villemarette-Pittman NR, Stanford MS, et al. Obsessive-compulsive personality disorder and behavioral disinhibition. *J Psychol*. 2004;138:5–22.

138. Answer: E. All the choices represent potential complications seen in refeeding after a prolonged period of malnutrition. During refeeding, carbohydrate intake causes insulin release. Phosphorous, which is needed for glucose metabolism and protein synthesis, moves into the cells, causing extracellular levels to drop. Consequences include muscle weakness, paresthesias, seizure, coma, cardiopulmonary failure, and death. The release of insulin in refeeding also leads to increased renal water and sodium reabsorption, which can lead to fluid overload and edema. The weakened heart, which loses muscle mass and functional capacity during starvation, may be unable to manage the increased volume, leading to CHF. Starvation also causes disturbances of gastrointestinal (GI) motility, which can cause abdominal distress during early refeeding.

1. Feldman M, Friedman LS, Sleisenger MH. *Sleisenger and Fordtran's Gastrointestinal and Liver Disease*. 7th ed. Philadelphia: WB Saunders; 2003:277–278.
2. Sigman GS. Eating disorders in children and adolescents. *Pediatr Clin North Am*. 2003;50:1139–1177.

139. Answer: C. The stage-wise goals in Dialectical Behavior Therapy for Borderline Personality Disorder can be outlined as follows:

Stage I: Achieving reasonable self-control and a reasonable immediate life expectancy (getting client in control of himself/herself and his/her life), reducing high-risk suicidal behaviors, reducing seriously self-damaging behavioral patterns, and reducing client and therapist behaviors that interfere with therapy.

Stage II: Understanding and reducing the sequelae of early trauma, particularly neglect and physical and sexual assaults. This involves focused exposure (e.g., using recall, imagery, role-playing) to events, persons, and activities associated with childhood traumas.

Stage III: Addressing residual problematic patterns, which interfere with the achievement of other important goals. Self-respect and self-trust become of paramount importance during this stage.

Stage IV: Resolution of the residual sense of incompleteness and achievement of the capacity for sustained joy.

1. Bohus M, Haaf B, Simms T, et al. Effectiveness of inpatient dialectical behavioral therapy for borderline personality disorder: a controlled trial. *Behav Res Ther*. 2004;42:487–499.
2. Linehan MM. An illustration of dialectical behavior therapy in session. *Psychother Pract*. 1998;4:21–44.
3. Rizvi SL, Linehan MM. Dialectical behavior therapy for personality disorders. *Curr Psychiatry Rep*. 2001;3:64–69.

140. Answer: E. Although many clinicians are aware of the potential for sexual dysfunction associated with the use of SSRIs and other antidepressants, it is sometimes forgotten that clonazepam has also been associated with a substantial percentage of sexual side effects. Studies have reported a 23% to 42% rate of sexual dysfunction in patients treated with clonazepam. Although hypertension and advancing age have been associated with sexual dysfunction, clonazepam-induced sexual dysfunction should be ruled out first in a patient who reports recent onset of anorgasmia after being started on clonazepam.

1. Davidson JR. Pharmacotherapy of social anxiety disorder: what does the evidence tell us? *J Clin Psychiatry*. 2006;67 (suppl 12):20–26.
2. Fossey MD, Hamner MB. Clonazepam-related sexual dysfunction in male veterans with PTSD. *Anxiety*. 1994;1:233–236.

141. Answer: E. Benzodiazepines—administered orally or parenterally—may be given for the rapid relief of anxiety; however, hallucinogen intoxication does not require specific pharmacologic measures. The passage of time in a calm, supportive environment generally suffices. Anti-psychotics may worsen symptoms.

Sadock BJ, Sadock VA. *Kaplan and Sadock's Comprehensive Textbook of Psychiatry*. 8th ed. Philadelphia: Lippincott Williams & Wilkins; 2005:1244.

142. Answer: C. Motivational Enhancement Therapy is based on mobilizing energy in the patient to change and to highlight the discrepancies between their current and their desired level of functioning. It is usually brief, and the therapist maintains an empathic and nonconfrontational attitude during the sessions. The therapist focuses on developing self-efficacy and tries to allow patients to generate their own solutions. Cognitive Behavioral Therapy for substance abuse focuses on identifying high-risk situations and developing skills to minimize the chances of relapse.

Weiss RD, Kueppenbender KD. Combining psychosocial treatment with pharmacotherapy for alcohol dependence. *J Clin Psychopharmacol*. 2006;26(suppl 1):S37–S42.

143. Answer: B. According to the Beck's model, core beliefs are "one's most central ideas about the self." They are beliefs that develop based on childhood experience and are often not as easily articulated as are automatic thoughts. Such beliefs in this model fall into two broad categories—that pertaining to helplessness (e.g., "I am inadequate," "I am needy," "I am ineffective," etc.) and that pertaining to unlovability [e.g., "I am unworthy," "I am bad," "I am not good enough (to be loved by others)"]. The therapist from early on in the therapy hypothesizes about the patient's core beliefs and, with care, eventually shares that information with the patient and helps the patient to modify them.

Beck JS. *Cognitive Therapy: Basics and Beyond*. New York: Guilford; 1995:166–170.

144. Answer: E. Microorganisms which cause acute bacterial meningitis vary with the age of the patient. They include: neonates—*Escherichia coli* and group B streptococci; infants and children—*Haemophilus influenzae*; young adults—*Neisseria meningitidis*; and the elderly—*Streptococcus pneumoniae* and *L. monocytogenes*. Symptoms of meningitis include headache, photophobia, irritability, clouding of consciousness, and neck stiffness. CSF may be cloudy or purulent. There is also increased CSF pressure, raised protein level, significantly reduced glucose content, and many neutrophils. Untreated, it can be fatal.

Cotran RS, Kumar V, Collins T. *Robbins Pathologic Basis of Disease*. 6th ed. Philadelphia: WB Saunders; 1999:1314–1315.

145. Answer: A. Imaging studies suggest that patients with chronic Schizophrenia differ from the general population in that the dominant temporal lobe is similar in size to the nondominant temporal lobe. This finding is also seen in patients with autism and dyslexia.

Kaufman DM. *Clinical Neurology for Psychiatrists*. 5th ed. Philadelphia: WB Saunders; 2001:176.

146. Answer: A. The alpha wave is the most prominent wave observed in the normal EEG of a waking adult. It is most pronounced over the posterior part of the head. Anteriorly, there are often some low voltage beta waves. In the fronto-central and temporal regions, low voltage theta activity can also be seen.

Khoshbin H. Clinical neurophysiology. *UpToDate 2006*. http://www.uptodateonline.com/utd/content/topic.do?topicKey=neuropat/4649&type=A&selectedTitle=1~71. Published January 23, 2007.

147. Answer: E. Like PET, SPECT measures the spatial concentration of injected radionuclides over time. Whereas PET uses positrons to localize the target, SPECT uses gamma rays. However, they both rely on the correlation between local changes in neuronal activity, metabolism, and blood flow to create functional maps of areas of the brain. SPECT measures blood flow and brain metabolism by monitoring photons emitted by iodine-labeled monoamine and diamine tracers carried in the blood to the brain. SPECT also has the advantage over PET as it has the ability of simultaneously imaging two isotopes, which are at different energy levels. These two isotope imaging methods allows SPECT to be used to evaluate glucose metabolism in addition to perfusion. SPECT also has a relatively low radiation exposure from the injected radionuclides which allows for multiple studies to be possible with little increase in distress to the patient. The SPECT scan is also much cheaper than PET, because it does not rely on artificially produced unstable nuclei, the expense of dedicated PET scanners, and the expense of positron-emitting radiopharmaceuticals. However, the sensitivity of the SPECT system to radiotracers and, hence its intrinsic-spatial resolution, continues to be lower than that of PET.

1. http://www.brainmattersinc.com/functional_imaging.html. Accessed January 28, 2007.
2. Goetz CG. *Textbook of Clinical Neurology*. 2nd ed. Philadelphia: WB Saunders; 2003. http://home.mdconsult.com/das/book/66246566-2/view/1158. Accessed January 28, 2007.

148. Answer: D. Patients with dementia have episodes of reliving the past that can be sometimes hard to manage. Reorientation is usually not a helpful intervention, because most patients become more anxious and agitated and continue to believe that they are still in the past. The best approach is to enter the patient's world and find an intervention that responds to their needs. Pharmacological interventions and the use of restraints should be left until other alternatives have failed.

Yuhas N, McGowan B, Fontaine T, et al. Psychosocial interventions for disruptive symptoms of dementia. *J Psychosoc Nurs Ment Health Serv*. 2006;44:34–42.

149. Answer: D. Vaillant's study spanned decades and found that mental and physical health are correlated in multiple ways. Poor psychological adjustment in college was associated with poor physical health in middle age. He also found that a close relationship with a sibling correlated with emotional well-being later in life, stability in the family during childhood correlates with emotional adjustment as an adult, and a warm childhood environment positively effects physical health as an adult. Tranquilizer use before age 50 years was a strong predictor of poor physical health at age 65.

1. Sadock BJ, Kaplan H. *Synopsis of Psychiatry*. 9th ed. Philadelphia: Lippincott Williams & Wilkins; 2003:46–47.
2. Vaillant GE, Vaillant CO. Natural history of male psychological health, XII: a 45-year study of predictors of successful aging at age 65. *Am J Psychiatry*. 1990;147:31–37.

150. Answer: C. The serotonin system is the largest cohesive neurotransmitter system in the brain and serotonin neurons innervate all areas of the brain. The system has two major subdivisions: the ascending and descending arms. The descending arm of the serotonin system projects to the spinal cord and is involved in pain perception. Serotonin release is increased in many brain areas of laboratory animals with physical stress, such as foot shock, immobilization, forced swimming, and nonphysical stress paradigms. Preclinical studies in laboratory animals showed that altering the function of the serotonin system alters many of the behaviors and somatic functions that form the core symptoms of clinical depression, including appetite, sleep, sexual function, pain sensitivity, and circadian rhythms. Serotonin may play an important role in maintaining synaptic connections in several brain regions, such as the hippocampus. When serotonin input to the adult rat hippocampus is disrupted, loss of neuronal synapses occurs within 10 to 14 days. On the other hand, stimulation of 5-HT1A receptors leads to restoration of lost synapses and to an increase in dendritic growth. Stimulation of 5-HT1A receptors results in release of a neurotrophic factor, S100β, from astrocytes and glial cells. This data supports the role of serotonin as a neurotriphic-like factor.

1. Duman RS. Depression: a case of neuronal life and death? *Biol Psychiatry*. 2004;56:140–145.
2. Stein DJ, Kupfer DJ, Schatzberg AF. *American Psychiatric Association Textbook of Mood Disorders*. Washington: American Psychiatric Publishing; 2006:102–103.

151. Answer: A. Delusions are fixed, false beliefs out of keeping with the patient's cultural background and are disturbances in content of thought. They may be described as mood-congruent or mood-incongruent and may be bizarre or have themes that are persecutory or paranoid, grandiose, jealous, somatic, guilty, nihilistic, or erotic. Depersonalization and derealization are examples of disturbances in perceptions and not thought processes, which are also described as form of thinking. Intellectual insight is present when patients can admit that they are ill and acknowledge that their failures to adapt are partly due to their own irrational feelings, yet they are unable to apply their knowledge to alter future experiences. This is one level below the highest of insight, known as true emotional insight, which is present when patients' awareness of their own motives and feelings leads to a change in their behaviors. Neologisms and word salad are examples of impairments in thought processes rather than speech characteristics that are described in terms of their physical qualities, including quantity, tone, volume, rate, and rhythm or prosody. Thought blocking occurs when there is an interruption in the train of thought before an idea has been completed and is not assumed to be volitional.

Kaplan HI, Sadock BJ. *Kaplan & Sadock's Synopsis of Psychiatry*. 8th ed. Philadelphia: Lippincott Williams & Wilkins; 1998: 250–254.

152. Answer: D. The lifetime prevalence of Alcohol Dependence or Abuse is 16.7%. The lifetime prevalence for abuse/dependence of other drugs is: marijuana 4.3%, cocaine 0.2%, opioid 0.7%, and amphetamine 1.7%.

Regier DA, Farmer ME, Rae DS, et al. Comorbidity of mental disorders with alcohol and other drug abuse. Results from the Epidemiologic Catchment Area (ECA) Study. *JAMA*. 1990;264:2511–2518.

153. Answer: A. Anorexia Nervosa is associated with depression in approximately 65% of cases, with OCD in approximately 26% to 35% of cases, social phobia in approximately 34% of cases. Moderate overlap has been shown between Avoidant Personality Disorder and Anorexia Nervosa. Anorexia Nervosa has

not been shown to be significantly comorbid with schizophrenia.

1. Sadock BJ, Sadock VA. *Kaplan and Sadock's Synopsis of Psychiatry*. 9th ed. Philadelphia: Lippincott Williams & Wilkins, 2003:739–746.
2. Steiner H, Lock J. Anorexia nervosa and bulimia nervosa in children and adolescents: a review of the past 10 years. *J Am Acad Child Adolesc Psychiatry*. 1998;37:352–359.

154. Answer: B. Obsessive individuals are involved in a conflict between obedience and defiance. This leads to a continuing alternation between the emotions of fear and rage—fear that he will be caught at his naughtiness and punished for it and rage at relinquishing his desires and submitting to authority. This fear stemming from defiance leads to obedience, while the rage, derived from obedience, leads back again to defiance. Thus, there is a vicious cycle that these individuals play out internally. This conflict appears to have its origins in childhood experiences, and punctuality, conscientiousness, tidiness, orderliness, and reliability are derived from this fear of authority. For the obsessive individual such behavior is not motivated by mature, healthy, constructive forces, but stems from unrealistic fear. These contradictory traits are not only essential features in the obsessive individual, but they even appear in the same person at the same time. The most relevant epigenetic stage relating to MacKinnon and Michels' theories noted previously would be Erikson's second stage: autonomy versus shame and doubt, which also correlates with Freud's "anal" stage.

MacKinnon R, Michels R. *The Psychiatric Interview in Clinical Practice*. Philadelphia: WB Saunders; 1971:89–91.

155. Answer: B. Depression is often characterized by multiple sleep disturbances—including delayed falling asleep, midnight and early morning awakenings, and nonrestorative sleep. Frequent awakenings and painful arousal of depression result in decreased time spent in deep stages of sleep—stages III and IV, or slow wave sleep. Depressed patients may resort to alcohol to decrease time falling asleep or number of awakenings. Alcohol does decrease time falling asleep and number of awakenings. However, it has the same effect on sleep as depression; it further decreases sleep time in stages III and IV, while increasing the time spent in less restorative or light sleep. Even though alcohol works in the short-term, the time spent in deep stages of sleep continues to decrease, which in turn is hypothesized to exacerbate and prolong depression.

1. Feige B, Gann H, Brueck R, et al. Alcohol on polysomnographically recorded sleep in healthy subjects. *Alcohol Clin Exp Res*. 2006;30:1527–1537.

2. Sadock BJ, Sadock VA. *Kaplan and Sadock's Comprehensive Textbook of Psychiatry*. 8th ed. Philadelphia: Lippincott Williams & Wilkins; 2005:1619.

156. Answer: E. The FDA has issued black box warnings for clozapine for all of the listed items except for E. In addition to agranulocytosis, seizures, hypotension, and myocarditis, there is also a black box warning regarding the use of clozapine in dementia related psychosis secondary to the increased risk of cerebral vascular events.

Prescribing information. *Physicians' Desk Reference®*. 59th ed. Montvale: Medical Economics; 2005.

157. Answer: A. SSRIs are considered the pharmacological treatment of choice for patients with social anxiety disorder. Many studies have shown a significant reduction in symptoms or remission of symptoms with the use of SSRIs when compared to placebo in social anxiety disorder. Although improvement in symptoms can be seen in 4 to 6 weeks, it might take months to see the full efficacy of pharmacological treatment. Factors that have been associated with a poor response to SSRIs include a history of excessive alcohol use, passive dependent personality disorder, higher systolic blood pressure and heart rate, and a family history of social phobia. Female gender has not been associated with a decreased response to treatment with SSRIs.

Davidson JR. Pharmacotherapy of social anxiety disorder: what does the evidence tell us? *J Clin Psychiatry*. 2006;67 (suppl 12):20–26.

158. Answer: B. Depressive disorders along with anxiety are often comorbid with cannabis dependence. Focus of treatment is on maintaining abstinence; however, anti-depressants may be indicated.

Sadock BJ, Sadock VA. *Kaplan and Sadock's Comprehensive Textbook of Psychiatry*. 8th ed. Philadelphia: Lippincott Williams & Wilkins; 2005:1219.

159. Answer: D. Alcoholics Anonymous is a self-help group that offers support, structure, role modeling, problem-solving advice, a social network, and sober activity. It is widely available and it is offered free of charge. It is a twelve-step program that focuses on self-growth. It is also the most frequently recommended intervention for alcohol-dependent patients.

Weiss RD, Kueppenbender KD. Combining psychosocial treatment with pharmacotherapy for alcohol dependence. *J Clin Psychopharmacol*. 2006;26(suppl 1):S37–S42.

160. Answer: B. The AIMS exam is a test administered every 3 to 6 months for patients taking neuroleptic drugs in order to diagnose tardive dyskinesia.

The test includes observing patients unobtrusively when they are at rest, asking them to open their mouths and asking them to protrude their tongues, observing their facial and leg movements while distracting them by asking them to tap their thumbs against each finger, as well as other tasks. It does not involve asking them to perform rapidly alternating hand movements.

Kaplan HI, Sadock BJ. *Kaplan & Sadock's Synopsis of Psychiatry*. 8th ed. Philadelphia: Lippincott Williams & Wilkins; 1998:960.

161. Answer: B. Rabies virus enters the CNS by ascending along the peripheral nerves from the wound site. The incubation period may be between 1 and 3 months. The disease manifests with nonspecific symptoms of malaise, headache, and fever. The conjunction of these symptoms with local paresthesias around the wound is diagnostic. In advanced cases, the patient has CNS excitability with extreme pain to touch and violent motor responses progressing to convulsions. Periods of alternating mania and stupor progress to coma and death from respiratory failure. On microscopic examination, the pathognomonic finding associated with this disease is Negri bodies. These are cytoplasmic, eosinophilic inclusions. They can be found in the hippocampus and cerebellum. Progressive multifocal encephalopathy is caused by the JC virus. It usually occurs in immunosuppressed individuals. Kuru plaques are extracellular deposits of aggregated abnormal protein. They occur in the cerebellum in cases of Gerstmann-Sträussler-Scheinker syndrome and in the cerebral cortex in cases of variant Creutzfeldt-Jakob disease. Hirano bodies are found in Alzheimer's disease in hippocampal cells. Lewy bodies are associated with Parkinson's disease and are demonstrable by immunohistochemistry for ubiquitin and α–synuclein.

Cotran RS, Kumar V, Collins T. *Robbins Pathologic Basis of Disease*. 6th ed. Philadelphia: WB Saunders; 1999:1319.

162. Answer: A. Transcortical or isolation aphasias are a result of preservation of the Perisylvian arc (Wernicke's area, arcuate fasiculous, and Broca's area) with destruction of the surrounding cortex. Although the language center is intact, it is unable to communicate with the rest of the damaged cortex. These injuries are commonly caused by watershed infarctions during states of decreased cerebral perfusion (i.e., cardiac or respiratory arrest, hypoxia via strangulation, carbon monoxide inhalation), showers of small emboli or hypotensive episodes. Patients' speech is characterized by echolalia; they involuntarily and compulsively repeat whatever they hear including long complex sentences. They are unable to carry a conversation, follow commands, or name objects.

Kaufman DM. *Clinical Neurology for Psychiatrists*. 5th ed. Philadelphia: WB Saunders; 2001: 176–177.

163. **Answer: D.** Aggression is a common and severe problem in patients with dementia. Some of the factors that have been associated with the presence of aggression in patients with dementia include: a premorbid history of conduct disorder, delusional thinking, and symptoms of depression. Aggressive acts also tend to occur more frequently during intimate care (bathing, getting dressed). During these situations patients can easily feel threatened or disrespected and they can react in an aggressive manner. The premorbid abuse of substances has not been associated with an increased risk of aggression in patients with dementia.

Pulsford D, Duxbuty J. Aggressive behaviour by people with dementia in residential care settings: a review. *J Psychiatr Ment Health Nurs*. 2006;13:611–618.

164. **Answer: A.** The superego is a concept of the structural, not topographical, model of the psyche. It is mostly unconscious. The superego maintains the moral conscience of an individual, and it includes parental values that have been internalized by a child by around age 5 years. Ego not superego functions primarily under the reality principle and is used in defense mechanisms.

Sadock BJ, Kaplan H. *Synopsis of Psychiatry*. 9th ed. Philadelphia: Lippincott Williams & Wilkins; 2003:204–205.

165. **Answer: E.** The hollow core of the embryonic neural tube develops into the continuous ventricular system. The large, paired lateral ventricles are found within the cerebral hemispheres to communicate through the interventricular foramina with the third ventricle of the diencephalon. The third ventricle communicates through the cerebral aqueduct with the fourth ventricle of the pons/medulla, and end in the rarely patent cerebral canal. The ventricles contain CSF, which protects the brain by allowing it to partially float, and is also a component of the system that regulates the composition of the extracellular fluid. The lateral and third ventricles only connect to the rest of the ventricular system, but the fourth provides flow of CSF to the subarachnoid space through the median and lateral apertures (not the rarely patent cerebral canal). The ventricles typically only contain about 20% of the total CSF with the majority found in the subarachnoid space. Disruption of CSF circulation causes hydrocephalus, almost always by some form of obstruction. Hydrocephalus is clinically divided into communicating and noncommunicating types, which do not differentiate causes, but provide partial location of the blockage. Blockage within the ventricular system is noncommunicating (both lateral ventricles have no access to the subarachnoid space) and outside is communicating.

Notle J. *The Human Brain: An Introduction to Its Functional Anatomy*. 4th ed. St Louis: Mosby; 1999:96–115.

166. **Answer: C.** Hallucinations are perceptions that occur in the absence of corresponding sensory stimuli, and phenomenologically are ordinarily subjectively indistinguishable from normal perceptions. They can affect any sensory system and can occur concurrently. Sometimes many normal people experience hallucinations, and hypnogogic and hypnopompic hallucinations are noted to be particularly common and occur during the moments of transition from wakefulness to sleep, or vice versa, and are of much less serious significance than are other types of hallucinations. Simple auditory hallucinations are more commonly associated with organic psychoses (i.e., delirium, seizures, encephalopathies) and are classically associated with schizophrenia or psychotic mood disorders. Visual hallucinations are generally assumed to reflect organic disorders, yet are seen in many Schizophrenic patients and occur in a wide variety of neurological and psychiatric disorders, including toxic disturbances, withdrawal syndromes from drugs, CNS lesions, and psychotic mood disorders. Olfactory and gustatory hallucinations have most often been associated with organic brain disease, particularly with complex partial seizures. Olfactory hallucinations may also be seen in psychotic depression, typically as odors of decay, rotting, or death. Haptic hallucinations involve touch, and simple haptic hallucinations are common in Alcohol Withdrawal or Cocaine Intoxication (i.e., formication), but some tactile ones (i.e., having intercourse with God) are highly suggestive of Schizophrenia, but can also occur in tertiary syphilis.

1. Kaplan HI, Sadock BJ. *Kaplan & Sadock's Synopsis of Psychiatry*. 8th ed. Philadelphia: Lippincott Williams & Wilkins; 1998:251.
2. Sadock BJ, Sadock VA. *Kaplan and Sadock's Comprehensive Textbook of Psychiatry*. 8th ed. Philadelphia: Lippincott Williams & Wilkins; 2005:987–989.

167. **Answer: A.** All of the symptoms listed are typically seen in opiate intoxication. Alcohol and lorazepam (both CNS depressants) are associated with sedation, impaired motor skills, and respiratory depression at higher concentrations. Cocaine, a stimulant, typically causes hypertension and papillary dilatation. Cannabis intoxication, associated with sedation and

euphoria, is rarely accompanied by physical exam findings.

Ebert M, Loosen P, Nurcombe B. *Current Diagnosis and Treatment in Psychiatry.* New York: McGraw-Hill; 2000. www.accessmedicine.com/content.aspx?aID=27152. Accessed October 24, 2007.

168. Answer: B. DSM-IV-TR defines a substance-induced persisting amnestic disorder as the development of impairment in the ability to learn new information or the inability to recall previously learned information. The memory disturbance causes impairment in social or occupational functioning and does not occur exclusively during the course of a delirium or dementia. There should be evidence from the history, physical, or laboratory findings that suggests an etiological link between the memory disturbance and the substance. As opposed to alcohol-induced persisting dementia, the cognitive deficit in alcohol-induced persisting amnestic disorder (or *Korsakoff's psychosis*) is much more discrete and limited to the realm of memory (though detailed neuropsychological testing may reveal deficits in additional cognitive domains). Wernicke's encephalopathy is an acute thiamine deficiency state characterized by confusion, lateral gaze palsy, nystagmus, and ataxia. The etiology of alcohol-induced persisting amnestic disorder is thought to be multiple episodes of Wernicke's encephalopathy, caused by thiamine deficiency. However, direct neurotoxic effects of alcohol and its metabolite acetaldehyde have also been implicated. Both delirium and dementia of the Alzheimer's type would typically present with deficits in memory as well as other cognitive domains (attention, language, praxis). This patient's presentation of a discrete, short-term memory impairment without additionally affected cognitive domains and an unremarkable neurological exam is most consistent with alcohol-induced persisting amnestic disorder.

1. American Psychiatric Association. *Desk Reference to the Diagnostic Criteria from DSM-IV-TR.* Washington: American Psychiatric Association; 2000:96–97.
2. Blazer DG, Steffens DC, Busse EW. *Textbook of Geriatric Psychiatry.* Washington: American Psychiatric Publishing; 2004:223–224.

169. Answer: D. The most frequently observed behavioral symptom in Alzheimer's disease is change in personality, of which apathy is most commonly seen, with a prevalence rate of 90% to 100% in patients. It has early onset and stays more or less constant. It is characterized by: (a) lack of interest, (b) reduced affection in personal relationships, (c) loss of enthusiasm, (d) reduction of initiative, and (e) social withdrawal.

Delusions are seen in approximately 16% to 70% of patients, and hallucinations are observed in 4% to 76% of patients. Depression is seen in about 40% to 50% of patients, whereas disinhibition is around 30% to 40% of patients.

1. Bassiony MM, Lyketsos CG. Delusions and hallucinations in Alzheimer's disease: review of the brain decade. *Psychosomatics.* 2003;44:388–401.
2. Cummings JL, Back C. The cholinergic hypothesis of neuropsychiatric symptoms in Alzheimer's disease. *Am J Geriatr Psychiatry.* 1998;6 (suppl 1):S64–S78.

170. Answer: C. Both familial-genetic studies (i.e., monozygotic versus dizygotic twin studies) and prospective follow-up studies show that genetic propensity to developing mood disorders (Major Depressive Disorder [MDD], Bipolar Affective Disorder [BPAD], Cyclothymia, Dysthymia) underlies milder versions of affective dysregulation as well and affects people in the community who never developed severe enough symptoms to look for treatment. Constitutional predisposition for affective dysregulation occurs in up to 30% of the general population. The proportion of 30% appears to be consistant across a variety of mood disorder models—including about one third of people who develop a major depressive episode after bereavement, one third of dogs who develop learned helplessness after inescapable shock, and one third of rhesus monkeys who develop depressive-like symptoms after a separation paradigm. Because rates of clinical mood disorders are lower than 30%, there appear to be multiple protective and other factors that determine whether one develops a full-blown mood disorder.

Sadock BJ, Sadock VA. *Kaplan and Sadock's Comprehensive Textbook of Psychiatry.* 8th ed. Philadelphia: Lippincott Williams & Wilkins; 2005:1612.

171. Answer: B. The most common anomalies associated with in utero valproic acid exposure are neural tube defects (NTD). NTD's are estimated to occur in 1% to 2% of fetuses exposed to valproic acid in utero. Other teratogenic effects of valproic acid include facial dysmorphism, congenital cardiac defects, limb reduction defects, and other skeletal anomalies. All pregnant women exposed to valproic acid should have a maternal serum alpha-fetoprotein screening and targeted ultrasonography. Periconceptual prophylaxis with high doses of folic acid is recommended for all women on valproic acid and counseling should also emphasize planning pregnancy to optimize folic acid supplementation.

Kennedy D, Koreng S. Valproic acid use in psychiatry: issues in treating women of reproductive age. *J Psychiatry Neurosci.* 1998;23:223–228.

172. **Answer: C.** Few controlled studies have evaluated the efficacy of antipsychotic medications in PTSD. Two recent controlled studies with risperdone showed an improvement in re-experiencing, sleep disturbances, impairment in social functioning, and global severity of PTSD symptoms in patients treated with risperidone in addition to standard treatment (e.g., SSRIs, benzodiazepines) when compared with patients on placebo. Although antipsychotic medications are not considered the first-line treatment for PTSD, they can be helpful adjuvants to target symptoms that are refractory to standard therapies.

Gao K, Muzina D, Gajwani P, et al. Efficacy of typical and atypical antipsychotics for primary and comorbid anxiety symptoms or disorders: a review. *J Clin Psychiatry*. 2006; 67:1327–1340.

173. **Answer: E.** In general, the nicotine based pharmacologic agents are equally effective, doubling the quit rate. A nicotine inhaler is also available. Bupropion is another option. Second line agents include clonidine and nortriptyline.

Sadock BJ, Sadock VA. *Kaplan and Sadock's Comprehensive Textbook of Psychiatry*. 8th ed. Philadelphia: Lippincott Williams & Wilkins; 2005:1262.

174. **Answer: B.** Respite care provides around-the-clock room and board to homeless patients discharged from a hospital, and encourages complying with posthospital rehabilitation. Many respite care centers also offer on-site medical care, social services, and transportation assistance to encourage continuity of care. In contrast, most shelters require homeless people to leave the shelter during the day and come back at night. It has been shown that the use of respite care centers reduces homeless patients' utilization of inpatient services and their use of future hospitalizations after being discharged from the hospital.

Buchanan D, Doblin B, Sai T, et al. The effects of respite care for homeless patients: a cohort study. *Am J Public Health*. 2006;96:1278–1281.

175. **Answer: C.** This patient has neuroleptic-induced Parkinsonism. All of the medications except bromocriptine are appropriate to use in the treatment of this disorder. Bromocriptine (as well as levodopa and pergolide) are contraindicated for patients with a history of psychosis.

1. Kaplan HI, Sadock BJ. *Kaplan & Sadock's Synopsis of Psychiatry*. 8th ed. Philadelphia: Lippincott Williams & Wilkins; 1998:1031–1032.
2. Katzung BG, Trevor AJ. *Examination and Board Review: Pharmacology*. 5th ed. Stamford: Appleton & Lange; 1998:214.

176. **Answer: B.** The major microscopic abnormalities of Alzheimer's disease are neurofibrillary tangles, senile (neuritic plaques), and amyloid angiopathy. Neurofibrillary tangles are composed of paired helical filaments of hyperphosphorylated forms of the protein tau, which is an axonal microtubule-associated protein that enhances microtubule assembly. They are not specific to the disease and are also found in progressive supranuclear palsy and postencephalitic Parkinson's disease. The dominant component of the neuritic plaque core is $A\beta$, a peptide of 40 to 43 amino acid residues derived from amyloid precursor protein. The $A\beta$ peptides aggregate and form the amyloid that is found in the brain parenchyma and around vessels. Lewy bodies are associated with Parkinson's disease and are demonstrable by immunohistochemistry for ubiquitin and $\acute{\alpha}$-synuclein. Hirano bodies are found in Alzheimer's disease in hippocampal cells. They are composed of paracrystalline arrays of beaded filaments with actin as the major component. Metachromatic leukodystrophy is an autosomal recessive disorder. It results from a deficiency of arylsulfatase A, resulting in the accumulation of sulfatides. This leads to myelin breakdown.

Cotran RS, Kumar V, Collins T. *Robbins Pathologic Basis of Disease*. 6th ed. Philadelphia: WB Saunders; 1999:1329–1340.

177. **Answer: E.** Epilepsy, mental retardation, autism, dyslexia, stuttering, and general clumsiness are all over represented in left-handed individuals. Left-handed individuals are also over represented among musicians, artists, and mathematicians. However, ADHD is not more common among left-handed children.

Kaufman DM. *Clinical Neurology for Psychiatrists*. 5th ed. Philadelphia: WB Saunders; 2001:176.

178. **Answer: D.** Opioid analgesics are the most potent pain-relieving drugs and have the broadest range of efficacy among analgesics. Some of their side effects include sedation, respiratory depression, pruritus, and constipation. Meperidine produces a metabolite, normeperidine, which causes hyperexcitability and seizures that are not reversible with naloxone.

http://www.wisc.edu/trc/projects/pop/DrugSpecific. html#mep. Accessed February 17, 2007.

179. **Answer: A.** Cocaine use is associated with all of the symptoms listed except decreased testosterone synthesis, which is usually seen in hypogonadism associated with alcohol use. Other common complications with cocaine use are sleep problems, sexual

disinterest, seizure, dystonia, arrhythmia, and cardiac ischemia.

Ebert M, Loosen P, Nurcombe B. *Current Diagnosis and Treatment in Psychiatry*. New York: McGraw-Hill; 2000. www.accessmedicine.com/content.aspx?aID=27152. Accessed October 24, 2007.

180. Answer: D. The EEG may have utility in assessment of certain patients with cognitive impairment (e.g., those with dementia accompanied by seizures), but is not generally considered part of the routine workup of dementia. Assessment of the patient with cognitive impairment in late life begins with a thorough history, including history from a collateral informant such as a relative or close friend. This is followed by mental status examination, including a formal cognitive rating scale, such as the Mini-Mental State Examination and physical examination with close attention to the neurological examination. An inventory of medications, both prescription and over-the-counter, is essential. Laboratory testing to rule out reversible causes of cognitive impairment should include complete blood count, electrolytes, blood urea nitrogen (BUN), creatinine, urinalysis, liver function tests, thyroid-stimulating hormone (TSH), B12, folate, and rapid-plasma regain (RPR) or Venereal Disease Research Laboratory test (VDRL). The routine use of neuroimaging in the workup of dementia has been debated, but the American Academy of Neurology has concluded that structural neuroimaging with either CT or MRI in the routine evaluation of patients with dementia is appropriate. Such imaging studies can help rule out the presence of potentially treatable intracranial abnormalities such as tumors, subdural hematomas, or NPH.

1. Blazer DG, Steffens DC, Busse EW. *Textbook of Geriatric Psychiatry*. Washington: American Psychiatric Publishing; 2004:208–210.
2. Knopman DS, DeKosky ST, Cummings JL, et al. Practice parameter: diagnosis of dementia (an evidence-based review). *Neurology*. 2001;56:1143–1153.

181. Answer: D. Intermittent Explosive Disorder (IED) includes discrete episodes of inability ro resist aggressive impulses, expressed out of proportion to precipitating stressors, and are not better accounted for by other physical, mental, or substance use disorders. IED is a diagnosis of exclusion, and thus a rare disorder. The other listed disorders may each have overlapping features of explosive aggression, but there is not enough criteria included in the vignette to diagnose any of them.

1. American Psychiatric Association. *Quick Reference to the Diagnostic Criteria from DSM-IV-TR*. Washington: American Psychiatric Association; 2000:281.

2. Hales RE, Yudofsky SC. *Textbook of Clinical Psychiatry*. 4th ed. Washington: American Psychiatric Publishing; 2003:781–785.

182. Answer: A. Criterion A 3 of DSM-IV-TR for MDD states that a person should have a change of more than 5% of body weight in a month or decrease or increase in appetite nearly every day. In children, consider failure to make expected weight gains. A 5% weight loss would be 8 lb (3.6 kg) for a 160 lb (73 kg) female and 9.5 lb (4.3 kg) for a 190 lb (86 kg) male.

American Psychiatric Association. *Quick Reference to the Diagnostic Criteria from DSM-IV-TR*. Washington: American Psychiatric Association; 2000:168–169.

183. Answer: E. Answers A-D are all possible side effects of valproic acid. The FDA has issued black box warnings for hepatic failure (occurs in 1 per 10,000 patients treated per year), hemorrhagic pancreatitis (occurs in 1 per 40,000 patients treated per year), and fetal neural tube defects (occurs in 1 to 2 per 100 pregnant patients). Thrombocytopenia, although not a black box warning, is significant and can result in platelet dysfunction and bleeding. Common side effects of valproic acid include gastrointestinal (nausea, vomiting, anorexia, diarrhea), neurological (sedation, tremor, ataxia), alopecia, and weight gain. Less common side effects include hyperammonemia, incoordination, asterixis, stupor, and coma. Hypothyroidism is not an adverse effect of valproic acid.

1. Prescribing information. *Physicians' Desk Reference®*. 59th ed. Montvale: Medical Economics; 2005.
2. Rosenbaum JF, Arana GW, Hyman SE, et al. *Handbook of Psychiatric Drug Therapy*. 5th ed. Philadelphia: Lippincott Williams & Wilkins; 2005:149–154.

184. Answer: B. Buspirone belongs to the azapirones and works as a partial 5-HT1a agonist. It does not have an immediate anxiolytic effect, because it has a slower onset of action (1 to 2 weeks). It does not produce the typical sedation or dependency seen with benzodiazepines. Some authors consider buspirone the drug of choice for patients with generalized anxiety disorder. Benzodiazepines bind to GABA-A receptors to exert their anxiolytic effect. Many antidepressants down regulate the 5HT-2 receptor, which is thought to be involved in the development of depression. 5HT-2 receptors mediate excitatory effects, whereas 5-HT1a receptors are involved in inhibitory effects in the brain.

1. Janicak PG, Davis JM, Preskorn SH, et al. *Principles and Practices of Psychopharmacotherapy*. 4th ed. Philadelphia: Lippincott Williams & Wilkins; 2006:465–475.
2. Sadock BJ, Sadock VA. *Kaplan and Sadock's Comprehensive Textbook of Psychiatry*. 8th ed. Philadelphia: Lippincott Williams & Wilkins; 2005:2958–2967.

185. Answer: D. MS is not an indication for ECT, all the others are. Additional indications include Mania, Schizophrenia (especially Catatonic subtype), and Schizoaffective disorder.

Sadock BJ, Sadock VA. *Kaplan and Sadock's Comprehensive Textbook of Psychiatry*. 8th ed. Philadelphia: Lippincott Williams & Wilkins; 2005:2972.

186. Answer: B. IDDT focuses on patients with both mental health and substance abuse problems. It believes that both mental health and substance abuse treatments should be integrated and delivered by a multidisciplinary team. Treatment is comprehensive and includes different therapeutic modalities. Treatment is offered in a long-term format and is provided in a stage-wise, flexible manner. Although most mental illnesses are chronic and have different levels of severity over time, treatment needs to be individualized for each patient's unique needs.

Brunette MF, Mueser KT. Psychosocial interventions for the long-term management of patients with severe mental illness and co-occurring substance use disorder. *J Clin Psychiatry*. 2006;67 (suppl 7):10–17.

187. Answer: A. Benztropine is an anticholinergic drug which blocks muscarinic receptors. Drugs such as bromocriptine and pergolide are partial agonists at D2 receptors. It may be that amantadine works by increasing the synthesis of dopamine or inhibiting its reuptake. The last choice (E) describes the mechanism of action of SSRIs such as fluoxetine.

Katzung BG, Trevor AJ. *Examination and Board Review: Pharmacology*. 5th ed. Stamford: Appleton & Lange; 1998:212–216.

188. Answer: E. A small minority of Alzheimer's disease is familial. Investigations have suggested a role for amyloid precursor protein (APP) and its processing to Aβ peptides in the pathogenesis of these cases. The gene which encodes APP is located on chromosome 21. Several forms of FAD (familial Alzheimer's disease) have been linked to mutations in the APP gene. The mutations lead to increased Aβ production and early-onset FAD. The development of Alzheimer's disease in trisomy 21 has been related to a gene dosage effect with increased production of APP and consequently Aβ. Two other genetic loci have been identified. They are on chromosome 14 (Presenilin-1) and chromosome 1 (Presenilin-2). They may actually account for the majority of early onset FAD. Mutations of these genes also lead to increased Aβ production. Last, one allele (ε4) of the apolipoprotein E gene located on chromosome 19, rather than causing Alzheimer's disease through mutation, can increase the risk of Alzheimer's disease and lower the age of onset of the disease.

Cotran RS, Kumar V, Collins T. *Robbins Pathologic Basis of Disease*. 6th ed. Philadelphia: WB Saunders; 1999:1329–1333.

189. Answer: E. Gerstmann's syndrome is accompanied by agraphia, acalculia, finger agnosia, and left-right confusion. Although the four abnormalities do not always occur simultaneously, making the syndrome somewhat controversial, clinically it is useful to check for the other deficits when one or more is present when evaluating patients after strokes and children with learning disabilities.

Kaufman DM. *Clinical Neurology for Psychiatrists*. 5th ed. Philadelphia: WB Saunders; 2001:185.

190. Answer: B. The effect of opioid analgesics is dose-dependent and there is great variability in regards to the doses that relieve pain for different patients. One of the most common mistakes in pain management is not prescribing an adequate dose of analgesics. One should repeat a patient's initial dose at the expected onset of peak effect to achieve an adequate control of the pain, as long as there are no signs of sedation.

Kasper DL, Braunwald E, Fauci AS, et al. *Harrison's Principles of Internal Medicine*. 16th ed. New York: McGraw-Hill; 2005:71–76.

191. Answer: D. Eugen Bleuler identified several primary, or fundamental, symptoms of schizophrenia including associational disturbances (particularly loose associations), autism, ambivalence, and affective disturbances. These are commonly summarized as the "4 A's:" associations, autism, ambivalence, and affect. "Audible thoughts" is one of the Schneiderian first-rank symptoms of Schizophrenia, but was not included in Bleuler's list.

Sadock BJ, Sadock VA. *Kaplan and Sadock's Synopsis of Psychiatry*. 9th ed. Philadelphia: Lippincott Williams & Wilkins; 2003:471–473.

192. Answer: C. The woman is suffering from Creutzfeldt-Jakob disease (CJD), the most common human transmissible spongiform encephalopathy. CJD is caused by a nonnucleic acid protein called a prion body. Iatrogenic cases have been reported in patients who received CNS tissue (e.g., corneal grafts, dura mater) from persons with CJD. CJD primarily affects people between the ages of 55 and 70 years; it is rare in the elderly population. The disease manifests as a rapidly progressing dementia accompanied by extrapyramidal signs, cerebellar signs, myoclonus, and seizures. Detection of 14-3-3 protein in the CSF has a sensitivity and specificity of 90% for sporadic

CJD. EEG reveals characteristic changes (1- to 2-per-second triphasic waves) in 80% of cases. CJD is uniformly fatal, with death typically occurring within 2 years from symptoms onset. There is no proven remedy for the disorder.

Levenson JL. *Textbook of Psychosomatic Medicine*. Washington: American Psychiatric Publishing; 2005:712–713.

193. Answer: C. Kleptomania involves the inability to resist stealing unneeded objects, which produces feelings of relief of tension or gratification, is not driven by anger/vengeance or psychosis, and is not better accounted for by other disorders which may have an overlapping symptom pattern. Chronic dysphoria is common in Kleptomania, but does not explain the behavior, nor does it necessarily mean she has a mood disorder. A pattern of disturbed sexual relationships is also common in kleptomania. An individual with Antisocial Personality Disorder would not be remorseful. OCD is often comorbid in Kleptomania, and may involve the relief of tension by certain acts, but is generally not limited to theft, and does not best explain this vignette.

1. American Psychiatric Association. *Quick Reference to the Diagnostic Criteria from DSM-IV-TR*. Washington: American Psychiatric Association; 2000:282.
2. Hales RE, Yudofsky SC. *Textbook of Clinical Psychiatry*. 4th ed. Washington: American Psychiatric Publishing; 2003:785–787.

194. Answer: A. In general, there is a linear relationship between the effectiveness of the TCAs and blood level: the higher the blood level, the more effective. However, an American Psychiatric Association task force after reviewing several studies concluded that a definitive relationship between plasma level and response has been documented for imipramine, desipramine, and nortriptyline; the therapeutic level for the latter being 50 to 150 ng/mL. The secondary amines are metabolites of the tertiary amines and have better side profiles; nortriptyline, for example, causes less orthostatic hypotension than amitriptyline owing to lesser a-adrenergic blocking activity.

Kaplan HI, Sadock BJ. *Comprehensive Textbook of Psychiatry*. 7th ed. Baltimore: Lippincot Williams & Wilkins; 2000:2494.

195. Answer: A. The brain is a highly aerobic tissue. It requires a constant supply of glucose and oxygen. In fact, its needs account for 15% of the resting cardiac output and 20% of the total body oxygen consumption. The brain may be deprived of oxygen either by functional hypoxia or by ischemia. Functional hypoxia occurs in the setting of low inspired partial pressure of oxygen; impaired oxygen-carrying capacity, or inhibition of oxygen use by tissue. Ischemia can be either transient or permanent. It occurs after interruption of normal blood flow. Cessation of blood flow can result from hypotension or blood vessel obstruction. Two types of ischemic injuries which occur are global cerebral ischemia and focal cerebral ischemia. Global cerebral ischemia results from cardiac arrest, shock, or server hypotension, while focal cerebral ischemia results from large vessel disease, such as embolic or thrombotic arterial occlusion, or small vessel disease, such as vasculitis. In global cerebral ischemia, there is a hierarchy of CNS cells that show selective vulnerability to the inadequate supply of oxygen. Neurons are the most sensitive cells, although glial cells, for example oligodendrocytes and astrocytes, are also susceptible. Of note, glial cells comprise the supporting system of neurons and their dendritic and axonal processes. The most susceptible structures to irreversible injury, in order, are pyramidal cells of the CA1 sector of the hippocampus; Purkinje cells of the cerebellum; and pyramidal neurons of the neocortex.

Cotran RS, Kumar V, Collins T. *Robbins Pathologic Basis of Disease*. 6th ed. Philadelphia: WB Saunders; 1999:1307–1308.

196. Answer: C. Patients with nonfluent aphasias are sometimes nonverbal or have a paucity of speech. The words that they use are usually nouns or verbs without modifiers. Their speech is slow and "telegraphic" and they are unable to name and repeat but can comprehend verbal and written language. The deficit is caused by a structural lesion on an infarction to Broca's area which is supplied by the left middle cerebral artery. Nonfluent aphasias are often accompanied by motor deficits in the right arm and lower face resulting in dysarthia because of the proximity of Broca's area to the motor cortex. With deeper lesions, patients can also develop a right homonymous hemianopsia and hemisensory loss.

Kaufman DM. *Clinical Neurology for Psychiatrists*. 5th ed. Philadelphia: WB Saunders; 2001:179–181.

197. Answer: C. Tricyclic antidepressants have been shown to be very helpful in the treatment of chronic pain. The mechanism of action of analgesia of tricyclic antidepressants is unknown. The analgesic effect of antidepressants has a shorter onset of action and occurs at a lower dose than the one needed for antidepressant effects. The following painful conditions have been shown to respond to tricyclic antidepressants: diabetic neuropathy, tension headache, migraine headache, rheumatoid arthritis, chronic low back pain, and cancer. Tricyclic antidepressants have not shown to be of help in the treatment of acute pain.

Kasper DL, Braunwald E, Fauci AS, et al. *Harrison's Principles of Internal Medicine*. 16th ed. New York: McGraw-Hill; 2005:71–76.

198. Answer: E. Trigeminal neuralgia consists of paroxysms of intense stabbing pain in the areas of the mandibular and maxillary divisions of the trigeminal nerve. The pain can be triggered by specific movements (such as chewing or brushing teeth), or it can come spontaneously. The treatment of this condition usually consists of anticonvulsant medications, such as carbamazepine, phenytoin, or valproic acid, which have shown to shorten the duration and the severity of the attacks. Baclofen is used as an adjunctive with anticonvulsants. When these treatments fail, patients recur to surgical procedures to destroy the trigeminal ganglion or nerve, such as the radiofrequency thermal rhizotomy, where a heat lesion is created in the ganglion or nerve. The pain of trigeminal neuralgia is so severe and intense that NSAIDs are usually ineffective in controlling the pain.

Rowland LP. *Merritt's Neurology*. 11th ed. Philadelphia: Lippincott Williams & Wilkins; 2005:528–529.

199. Answer: D. Opioid analgesics provide the most potent effect on pain. They have also been shown to reduce pain and disability in the long-term management of chronic pain. Patients with constant and severe chronic pain respond better to long-acting medications, such as the fentanyl patch, methadone, or sustained-release morphine, than to short acting medications, such as codeine, which produce a stronger and more frequent rebound effect. Although alternative therapies are commonly used to treat chronic pain, a patient with such severe and chronic pain will most likely need strong analgesic medications to control his pain.

South-Paul JE, Matheny SC, Lewis EL. *Current Diagnosis and Treatment in Family Medicine 2004*. Access Medicine: McGraw-Hill. http://www.accessmedicine.com/content.aspx?aID=8749711. Accessed February 17, 2007.

200. Answer: E. Individuals with intractable bilateral frontal seizures or infants with atonic seizures occasionally benefit from commissurotomy or corpus callostomy. In this procedure, the anterior two thirds or the entire corpus callosum is split longitudinally. This interrupts the spread of discharges between the cerebral hemispheres. Despite the extent of the surgery, postoperative deficits are subtle and specific tests are required to detect the major consequence of the surgery, split-brain syndrome. In this condition, each hemisphere can be tested individually by showing requests, objects, and pictures in the contralateral visual field. However, because the right hemisphere is unable to transmit information across the corpus callosum to the dominant left hemisphere, which controls language function, patients cannot read the requests or describe the objects. Conversely, written requests and objects shown in the right visual field are perceived by the left hemisphere. Patients can read and obey written requests and copy the objects with their right hand. However, because the language areas cannot send information through the corpus callosum to the right hemisphere, the left hand cannot do the same. Additionally, when patients describe emotions portrayed by the picture, their language lacks affect, because affect is derived from the nondominant hemisphere. The other choices (i.e., cognitive impairment, lethargy, confusion, stupor, coma, liver function abnormalities, bone marrow suppression, and rarely Stevens-Johnson syndrome) are all potential complications of therapy with antiepileptic drugs. Intoxication with phenytoin causes dysarthria, ataxia, and nystagmus.

Kaufman DM. *Clinical Neurology for Psychiatrists*. 5th ed. Philadelphia: WB Saunders; 2001:191–192, 247.

Questions

1. Elizabeth Kübler-Ross' five stages of reactions to impending death include all of the following EXCEPT:
   A. Denial
   B. Anger
   C. Bargaining
   D. Compensatory mania
   E. Acceptance

2. A 65-year-old, human immunodeficiency virus (HIV)-positive man presents with a gradual onset of "unintentional, forceful flinging movements of his right arm and leg." A rim-enhancing lesion is noted on a contrast-enhanced coronal magnetic resonance imaging (MRI). Which area of the brain would you expect to see a lesion causing this patient's condition?
   A. In the left subthalamic nucleus
   B. In the right caudate nucleus
   C. In the right substantia nigra
   D. In the left globus pallidus
   E. In the left primary motor cortex

3. Which one of the following terms was not described by Jean Piaget?
   A. *Schemas*
   B. *Accommodation*
   C. *Assimilation*
   D. *Adaptation*
   E. *Archetype*

4. In a recent study by Schneider, et al., evidence for increased mortality from atypical antipsychotic drug treatment for people with dementia was evaluated from various sources. Published and unpublished randomized placebo-controlled, parallel-group clinical trials of atypical antipsychotic drugs marketed in the United States to treat patients with Alzheimer's disease or dementia were selected by consensus of the authors. A total of 3,353 patients were randomized to the study drug and 1,757 were randomized to the placebo. Outcomes were assessed using standard methods (with random- or fixed-effects models) to calculate odds ratios (ORs) and risk differences based on patients randomized and relative risks based on total exposure to treatment. There were no differences in dropouts. Death occurred more often among patients randomized to drugs (118 [3.5%] versus 40 [2.3%]). The OR by meta-analysis was 1.54; 95% confidence interval [CI], 1.06 to 2.23; $p = 0.02$; and risk difference was 0.01; 95% CI, 0.004 to 0.02; $p = 0.01$). Sensitivity analyses did not show evidence for differential risks for individual drugs, severity, sample selection, or diagnosis. Based on this information, what would be the calculated number needed to harm (NNH) for atypical antipsychotic drugs compared to placebo in this population.
   A. 84
   B. 29
   C. 44
   D. 30
   E. 50

5. A manic patient is being evaluated by a psychiatrist for her recent behavior of leaving her husband of 30 years and traveling across the country to spend a large amount of money purchasing a new specialty store in the context of discontinuing her medications 1 month ago. During the psychiatric evaluation, the patient continues to demand for examples from the psychiatrist of manic behavior, refutes the examples given, and provides alternative explanations stating she had God-inspired feelings to change her life for the better. Which of the following areas of the mental status examination best describes the patient's problem?
   A. Insight
   B. Judgment
   C. Thought processes
   D. Thought content
   E. Perception

6. Which of the following is NOT TRUE of Antisocial Personality Disorder?
   A. It is more common in first-degree biological relatives of those with the disorder.
   B. The risk to biological relatives of women with the disorder tends to be higher than the risk to biological relatives of men with the disorder.
   C. Biological relatives of patients with this disorder are at an increased risk for Somatization Disorder.
   D. Only biological children of parents with Antisocial Personality Disorder have an increased risk of developing this disorder.
   E. All of the above.

7. To diagnose a Feeding Disorder of Infancy and Early Childhood according to DSM-IV-TR, the age of onset must be before which age?

A. 2 years
B. 4 years
C. 6 years
D. 8 years
E. 10 years

8. Neuroimaging studies in children and adults with Tourette's syndrome show which one of the following findings?

A. Smaller caudate volumes
B. Larger caudate volumes
C. Smaller dorsal prefrontal cortex
D. Smaller parieto-occipital cortex
E. Increased lateral ventricles

9. Which one of the following statements regarding cognitive deficits in Schizophrenia is TRUE?

A. The level of impairment worsens over time.
B. Impairment severity corresponds with symptom severity.
C. Evidence indicates cognitive deficits greatly improve with antipsychotics.
D. Early cognitive deficits are a risk factor for later emergence of psychosis.
E. Memory is most commonly impaired in Schizophrenia.

10. Which is the most common side effect of benzodiazepines?

A. Fatigue or drowsiness
B. Memory impairment
C. Impaired motor coordination
D. Depression
E. Behavioral disinhibition

11. Each one of the following statements regarding Alcoholics Anonymous (AA) is true EXCEPT:

A. In the mid-1930s, two recovering alcoholics initiated the self-help movement now known as AA.
B. Membership in AA is open to anyone who wants help with a drinking problem, regardless of age.
C. AA is a religious organization whose members are primarily Christian.
D. Patients with comorbid psychiatric illness can join AA, but may need education on how to cope if AA members suggest they stop taking medications.
E. AA is multiracial, apolitical, nonprofessional, and available almost anywhere.

12. A 13-year-old girl is brought by her mother to see you for an evaluation. Over the past year and a half the daughter has been increasingly bothered by involuntary, stereotyped movements of her face and hands. Recently, she has begun to periodically grunt several times a day. She is unable to suppress this grunt, and it is disruptive at school. Which of the following antipsychotic medications is most commonly used in the treatment of Tourette's syndrome?

A. Pimozide
B. Chlorpromazine
C. Thioridazine
D. Perphenazine
E. Quetiapine

13. Which of the following statements regarding Neuroleptic Malignant Syndrome is INCORRECT?

A. The association of the syndrome with neuroleptic agents is dose dependant.
B. The association of the syndrome with neuroleptic agents is idiosyncratic.
C. The onset of the syndrome is often associated with a recent switch from one agent to another.
D. Parenteral administration is considered a risk factor.
E. Mortality for the syndrome is currently estimated to be between 10% and 20%.

14. Which of the following drugs does NOT elevate the lithium level?

A. Nonsteroidal antiinflammatory drugs (NSAIDS)
B. Metronidazole
C. Hydrochlorothiazide
D. Acetazolamide
E. Captopril

15. Which one of the following is NOT a protective factor in preventing suicide?

A. Children at home
B. Sense of responsibility to family
C. White race
D. Pregnancy
E. Religiosity

16. Which artery provides the blood supply to the language center of the brain called the perisylvian arc?

A. Anterior cerebral artery
B. Middle cerebral artery
C. Posterior cerebral artery
D. Posterior inferior cerebellar artery
E. Posterior communicating artery

17. Which of the following is TRUE about a patient who is confabulating?

A. Amnesia is an important feature.
B. It occurs during an alert, unclouded state of consciousness.

C. It can occur in Korsakoff's syndrome.
D. Suggestibility is often a prominent feature.
E. All of the above.

18. Which one of the following is NOT TRUE of the genetics of mitochondrial disorders?

   A. Mutations can arise sporadically where there is no family history of the disease.
   B. They can be transmitted via maternal inheritance.
   C. Usually 50% of the mitochondria need to be abnormal before symptoms or signs manifest.
   D. Homoplasmy is the state of having uniformly normal or abnormal mitochondria in a tissue.
   E. Heteroplasmy is the mixture of normal and abnormal mitochondria in a single tissue.

19. Which one of the following is TRUE of the Minnesota Multiphasic Personality Inventory (MMPI)?

   A. The current version of the inventory for adults, 18 years or older, is the MMPI-4.
   B. The current version of the inventory has 500 items or questions.
   C. The current version of the inventory has 12 clinical scales.
   D. The current version of the inventory has three validity scales.
   E. Many items in the current version of the inventory are often seen in patients with neurological disorders.

20. Cardinal features of Parkinson's disease include all of the following EXCEPT:

   A. Postural instability
   B. Bradykinesia
   C. Rigidity
   D. Resting tremor
   E. Receptive aphasia

21. A 59-year-old woman who is morbidly obese and has an hemoglobin A1c of 11.9% presents with new onset ptosis in her left eye. When the lid is passively elevated, the eye is deviated outward and slightly downward. Which one of the following statements is TRUE regarding this disorder?

   A. There is unlikely to be any pain.
   B. These symptoms occur almost exclusively in diabetics.
   C. The prognosis for recovery is generally good.
   D. The pupil is likely to be sluggishly reactive.
   E. There will likely be findings in the right eye as well.

22. An immigrant child from a developing country arrives for an evaluation. His right arm is markedly weak, and he is unable to flex or rotate his arm. The child is in no distress. His mother reports having had a complicated delivery. Which one of the following is the most likely explanation for his limb weakness?

   A. Physical abuse
   B. Intracranial hemorrhage in the neonatal period
   C. Brachial palsy
   D. Congenital syphilis
   E. Toxoplasmosis infection

23. An 8-year-old boy was well until he started vomiting. Subsequently, he developed bouts of uncontrollable seizures, progressive mental retardation, hypotonia, spasticity, blindness, and jaundice. Given this presentation, what is the most likely diagnosis for his condition?

   A. Alpers' disease
   B. Multiple sclerosis (MS)
   C. Inhalant dependence
   D. X-linked adrenoleukodystrophy
   E. Wilson's disease

24. Which one of the following is NOT TRUE of neurosyphilis?

   A. Cerebrospinal fluid (CSF) invasion is common in early stages of untreated syphilis.
   B. If CSF abnormalities persist for over 5 years in the untreated patient, it is highly predictive of the development of clinical neurosyphilis.
   C. Tabes dorsalis is the most common type of neurosyphilis.
   D. Acute syphilitic meningitis is the earliest clinical manifestation of neurosyphilis.
   E. General paresis occurs due to tertiary syphilis and is now a rare condition.

25. Which one of the following statements regarding Creutzfeldt-Jakob disease (CJD) is NOT TRUE?

   A. CJD may be sporadic, infectious, or genetically inherited.
   B. Approximately 80% to 90% of the cases of CJD are sporadic.
   C. Familial CJD with an autosomal dominant mode of inheritance accounts for about 5% to 10% of cases of CJD.
   D. Sporadic CJD can spread like an ordinary infection as the agent has high infectivity.
   E. Those with prior head and neck trauma are at higher risk of acquiring CJD.

26. Surgical treatment options for Parkinson's disease include which one of the following?

   A. Thymectomy
   B. Commissurotomy
   C. Pallidotomy
   D. Labyrinthectomy
   E. Corpus callosotomy

27. Which of the following is the least likely to be the cause of chronic impotence in middle-aged men?

    A. Psychological disorders
    B. Normal aging
    C. Antidepressants
    D. Low testosterone levels
    E. Alcoholism

28. Which one of the following statements about autoreceptors is NOT TRUE?

    A. These are receptors that are located on the same type of neuron that releases the neurotransmitter that activates it.
    B. They are concerned with autoregulation of neuronal firing and terminal neurotransmitter release.
    C. The autoregulation is normally excitatory.
    D. Somatodendritic autoreceptors regulate neuronal firing.
    E. Terminal autoreceptors regulate neurotransmitter release.

29. Which one of the following statements is NOT TRUE of violence and culture?

    A. Across cultures, it is seen that men are more violent than women.
    B. The greater the degree of polygyny, the greater is the male–female disparity for violence.
    C. It is true that inclinations toward violence are influenced by cultural expectations.
    D. Difference between male and female homicide rates vary across cultures.
    E. Homicide rates are approximately 10 times higher in the United States than in Canada.

30. Which of the following is NOT an element of a malpractice claim?

    A. Duty
    B. Negligence
    C. Confidentiality
    D. Harm
    E. Causation

31. A 75-year-old woman is brought in by her daughter to a psychiatric clinic for the assessment of behavioral changes. The patient has refused to see a doctor for years, but was convinced by her daughter to see one for her sleep problems. The patient has been generally healthy and has not suffered any major illnesses or trauma. The patient's daughter states that her mother has become more confused over the last 5 years, often misplacing items and accusing the daughter of moving items or stealing things, and often forgets to turn off the lights or the oven. The patient responds minimally to questions, denies having memory problems, and states her daughter is making

up stories. Which of the following is the most appropriate test to detect cognitive deficits in this patient?

    A. Facial Recognition Test
    B. Mini-Mental State Examination (MMSE)
    C. Sentence Completion Test
    D. Thematic Apperception Test
    E. Wechsler Adult Intelligence Scale (Revised) (WAIS-R)

32. Which one of the following is NOT a feature of atypical depression?

    A. Laden paralysis
    B. Mood reactivity
    C. Weight gain or increase in appetite
    D. Loss of pleasure in all or almost all activities
    E. Hypersomnia

33. Which one of the following matches the DSM-IV-TR criteria for Tourette's syndrome?

    A. Onset before 18 years of age; both multiple motor and one or more vocal tics present at some time during the illness, occurring concurrently; duration of more than 1 year; no tic-free periods greater than 3 months.
    B. Onset before 18 years of age; both multiple motor and one or more vocal tics present at some time during the illness, not necessarily occurring concurrently; duration of more than 1 year; no tic-free period greater than 3 months.
    C. Onset before 18 years of age; both multiple motor and one or more vocal tics present at some time during the illness, occurring concurrently; duration of more than 1 year; no tic-free periods greater than 2 weeks.
    D. Onset before 18 years of age; both multiple motor and one or more vocal tics present at some time during the illness, occurring concurrently; duration of more than 6 months; no tic-free periods greater than 3 months.
    E. Onset before 21 years of age; both multiple motor and one or more vocal tics present during the illness, occurring concurrently; duration of more than 1 year; no tic-free periods greater than 3 months.

34. An 8-year-old boy with Tourette's syndrome and Obsessive-Compulsive Disorders (OCD) presents to his pediatrician complaining of sore throat. The throat pain resolves in a few days, but 3 weeks later, the child displays an exacerbation of tics and the obsessive-compulsive symptoms. Which one of the following infectious agents is the most likely cause for the worsening behaviors?

    A. Adenovirus
    B. Ebstein-Barr virus

C. Group A beta-hemolytic streptococci (GABHS)
D. Haemophilus influenza type b
E. Mycoplasma pneumoniae

35. A 36-year-old married, white woman with no prior psychiatric history presents for an outpatient psychiatric evaluation. She reports feeling depressed for the past year because she believes her husband is having an affair. For that past year, she confronts him daily about this alleged affair, which he denies. She recently lost her job as an editor because she was leaving work to follow him. She also reads his emails and calls his office many times each day. She does not report any hallucinations. There is no history of significant mood disorder, anxiety disorder, substance use disorder, or cognitive dysfunction. Given her presentation, what is the most likely diagnosis for her condition?

A. Schizophrenia
B. Delusional Disorder
C. Major depressive Disorder
D. Schizophreniform Disorder
E. Dementia

36. Each one of the following medications increases the blood level of benzodiazepines EXCEPT:

A. Cimetidine
B. Estrogens
C. Selective serotonin reuptake inhibitors (SSRIs)
D. Carbamazepine
E. Disulfiram

37. Which one of these instruments or modalities is NOT used in biofeedback?

A. Electromyograph (EMG)
B. Electrocardiogram (EKG)
C. Electroencephalograph (EEG)
D. Electrodermal response (EDR)
E. Perineometer

38. You have been treating a 28-year-old woman with Schizophrenia for the past year in your outpatient clinic. Six months ago you had switched her from a typical antipsychotic medication to an atypical antipsychotic medication to lower the risk of extrapyramidal symptoms (EPS). She has tolerated this new medication well without any return of psychosis. Today, however, she complains to you that she has not had her menstrual period for the past 3 months. A urine Beta- human chorionic gonadotropin (hCG) test is negative. Given this history, which of the following atypical antipsychotic medication has she been taking in the last 6 months?

A. Risperidone
B. Olanzapine

C. Quetiapine
D. Ziprasidone
E. Aripiprazole

39. Which one of the following is NOT a risk factor for the development of neuroleptic malignant syndrome (NMS)?

A. Age of the patient
B. Agitation
C. Dehydration
D. Use of restraints
E. Use of high potency typical antipsychotics

40. A 39-year old woman with a history of depression who has been taking fluoxetine 60 mg per day is admitted to the hospital after 10 days of working 24-hours a day on a new invention. Her husband tells you that this is atypical behavior for her, and that she has spent thousands of dollars in the last 10 days investing in this project. The patient reports that she has never felt better and endorses a decreased need for sleep as well as a plan to build three time machines in her backyard. Concerned that she is having a manic episode, you lower her dose of fluoxetine and begin treatment with lithium. She has no medical problems. Before starting the lithium, you should check all of the following in this patient EXCEPT:

A. Thyrotropin (TSH)
B. Triiodothyronine (T_3)
C. Serum urea nitrogen (BUN)/creatinine (Cr)
D. Beta-hCG
E. Sodium levels

41. Which one of the following statements regarding suicide and age is TRUE?

A. Thoughts of death are more common in younger than in older adults.
B. As people age, they are more likely to endorse suicidal ideation.
C. Suicidal elders give fewer warnings to others of their suicidal plans.
D. The ratio of attempted suicides to suicides in the elderly is as high as 200 : 1.
E. Self-destructive acts that occur in older people are less lethal.

42. Repeating or echoing of words said by others is termed *echolalia*, which is seen in a variety of disorders. In which of the following disorders is echolalia NOT commonly seen?

A. Isolation aphasia
B. Autism
C. Tourette's syndrome

D. Dementia

E. Epilepsy

43. Perceptual disturbances that occur during delirium tremens can be characterized by which of the following?

A. The patient has visual hallucinations of small animals or tiny men.

B. These hallucinations can change rapidly.

C. There is a strong affective response during the hallucinations.

D. It is usually associated with clouding of consciousness.

E. All of the above.

44. Which of the following disorders is caused by a trinucleotide repeat expansion mutation?

A. Huntington's disease

B. Myotonic dystrophy

C. Fragile X syndrome

D. Friedreich's ataxia

E. All of the above

45. The weight of the human brain increases by how much from birth to adulthood?

A. Twofold

B. Fourfold

C. Sixfold

D. Eightfold

E. Tenfold

46. All of the following statements are true of dopaminergic pathways EXCEPT?

A. Nigrostriatal pathway is involved with the initiation of motor plans and motor coordination.

B. Antipsychotic drugs produce motor disturbances by blocking the D2 receptors in the caudate-putamen.

C. Axons of the mesolimbic and mesocortical pathways arise from the dorsal tegmental area.

D. Axons of the mesolimbic and mesocortical pathways project to the nucleus accumbens, amygdale, and prefrontal cortex.

E. Mesolimbic and mesocortical pathways are associated with motivation and reward.

47. Which one of the following is the fundamental or basic rule of Freudian psychoanalysis?

A. Abreaction

B. Catharsis through hypnosis

C. Dreamwork

D. Free association

E. Uncovering childhood sexual seductions

48. Which of the following statements is TRUE of abandonment in a therapeutic relationship?

A. It is the unilateral termination of physician-patient relationship with reasonable justification.

B. A vacationing physician who provides coverage during her absence has a responsibility to ensure that such coverage is available and competent and could be liable for damages incurred during her absence.

C. Once made, claims of abandonment are almost always proven, as there are no mitigating factors against such claims.

D. A damage resulting from failure to provide adequate coverage during a physician's vacation is no grounds for abandonment claim since the therapeutic relationship is not severed during such absence.

E. There are absolutely no justifications for abandonment.

49. Which one of the following is a characteristic of the disorder-centered interviewing style?

A. It is based on an introspective model.

B. It focuses on the intra-psychic battle of conflicts.

C. It emphasizes the individuality of a patient.

D. It is sensitive to the patient's educational level.

E. It is based on a descriptive, atheoretical model.

50. Which one of the following is NOT a characteristic of melancholic depression?

A. Depression regularly worse in the morning

B. Early morning awakening

C. Psychomotor agitation

D. Mood reactivity

E. None of the above

51. The initial symptoms of Tourette's syndrome most frequently appear between which of the following age ranges?

A. 3 to 5 years

B. 5 to 8 years

C. 8 to 11 years

D. 11 to 14 years

E. 14 to 17 years

52. Which one of the following choices matches the DSM-IV-TR criteria for frequency and duration in enuresis?

A. A minimum frequency of once a month for 3 consecutive months.

B. A minimum frequency of three times a week for 1 month.

C. A minimum frequency of once a week for 3 consecutive months.

D. A minimum frequency of three times a week for 3 consecutive months.

E. No minimum frequency or duration.

53. Which one of the following is NOT a predictor of good outcome in first-episode Schizophrenia?

A. Negative symptoms

B. Acute onset

C. Late onset

D. Good premorbid functioning

E. Short time between the onset of psychotic phase and antipsychotic treatment

54. Which one of the following statements regarding the use of beta-blockers for anxiety is NOT TRUE?

A. Beta-blockers are competitive antagonists of norepinephrine (NA) and epinephrine at beta-adrenergic receptors.

B. Beta-blockers can be clinically useful in the treatment of performance anxiety.

C. Beta-blockers do not appear to induce tolerance nor do they have abuse potential.

D. The more lipophilic beta-blockers include propranolol and metoprolol.

E. Beta-blockers have a negative effect on memory and learning.

55. Which one of the following statements about zolpidem is NOT TRUE?

A. It is a nonbenzodiazepine hypnotic of the imidazopyridine class.

B. It has no muscle relaxant, anxiolytic, or anticonvulsant effects.

C. Its duration of action is 6 to 8 hours.

D. Its risk of abuse or dependence is low.

E. It has active metabolites.

56. Clozapine is an effective and unique antipsychotic medication which has affinity for multiple receptors, but its mechanism for efficacy remains unknown. Which of the following receptors does clozapine not have affinity for?

A. Muscarinic receptors

B. Serotonin receptors

C. N-methyl D-aspartate (NMDA) receptors

D. α-adrenergic receptors

E. Histamine receptors

57. While treating a 23-year-old agitated male with intramuscular (IM) haloperidol, he develops rigidity, hypertension, hyperthermia, and somnolence. What is the most appropriate first intervention for this patient?

A. Order a Creatinine kinase (CK) level.

B. Place the patient in a cooling blanket to lower his temperature.

C. Place an IV to begin aggressive hydration.

D. Make sure no further haloperidol is administered.

E. Administer dantrolene.

58. Which one of these medications is most likely to cause interdose rebound symptoms of anxiety?

A. Alprazolam

B. Clonazepam

C. Venlafaxine

D. Diazepam

E. Buspirone

59. Which one of the following statements about suicide and gender is NOT TRUE?

A. Suicide risk increases with age for both sexes, but the rates in older men are generally higher than those for women.

B. In the United States, men commit suicide four times more commonly than women, but women attempt suicide three times as often as men.

C. Men tend to use more lethal suicide methods than women.

D. Factors that contribute to these gender differences include the presence of depression and co-morbid alcohol and/or substance abuse.

E. In women, pregnancy is a time of significantly increased suicide risk.

60. There are a variety of apraxias that occur in various neurological disorders. Which type of apraxia is most commonly seen in normal pressure hydrocephalus (NPH)?

A. Conceptual

B. Ideational

C. Constructional

D. Gait

E. Buccofacial

61. Which of the following is NOT a dystonic reaction due to an antipsychotic medication?

A. Oculogyric crisis

B. Grimacing

C. Torticollis

D. Opisthotonus

E. Akathisia

62. Which one of the following is TRUE of temporal arteritis?

A. It occurs predominantly in men.

B. Blindness occurs in less than 10% of patients even if untreated.

C. Weight loss is the most common presentation.

D. Marked scalp tenderness is often present.

E. A normal erythrocyte sedimentation rate (ESR) excludes temporal arteritis.

63. Which one of the following is NOT TRUE of the Folstein Mini Mental State (MMSE)?

   A. It evaluates six areas of cognitive function.
   B. It correlates well with the Wechsler Adult Intelligence Scale Revised (WAIS-R).
   C. It should only be administered and scored by a qualified health care professional.
   D. A median score of 29 is normal for a person 18 to 24 years of age.
   E. A median score of 22 is normal for a person 80 years or older.

64. A 35-year-old African American woman presents to the emergency room (ER) complaining of an "explosive" headache and vomiting. Upon examination, she exhibits waxing and waning levels of consciousness. Her vitals are stable at this time. She is also pregnant and is currently in the third trimester of her pregnancy. She has a history of hypertension as well as current tobacco use. Given the high level of suspicion for subarachnoid hemorrhage, a computed tomography (CT) scan is performed and it does not reveal any clear signs of bleeding. What is the most reasonable next step in the evaluation and management of this patient?

   A. Prescribe analgesic medication and see if the headache resolves.
   B. Schedule a transthoracic echocardiogram to assess the presence of anatomic shunt, which could explain embolism to the brain.
   C. Perform a lumbar puncture to see if there is any blood in the CSF.
   D. Get a MRI to better assess possible anatomical contribution to the presentation.
   E. Schedule emergent surgery to repair the likely bleed.

65. A 26-year-old-man presents to your office. You note that his right arm and wrist are flexed and that he walks on his right toes, and he reports that he has had these deformities since childhood. Which one of the following disorders is he most likely to have?

   A. Hemiplegic cerebral palsy (CP)
   B. Diplegic CP
   C. Quadriplegic CP
   D. Extrapyramidal CP
   E. Dyskinetic CP

66. A 10-year-old girl presents to your office for an evaluation of Attention Deficit/Hyperactivity Disorder (ADHD). You note that she has microcephaly, short palpebral fissures, a hypoplastic philtrum with thin upper lip, and flattening of the maxillary area. Given this information, what do you think is the most likely diagnosis for her presentation?

   A. Down syndrome
   B. Williams syndrome
   C. Fragile X syndrome
   D. Fetal alcohol syndrome (FAS)
   E. Lead toxicity

67. An 80-year-old man from a skilled nursing facility presents to the ER with a 2-day history of high fever (102.0°F to 104.0°F), headache, vomiting, back and neck pain, and photophobia. Upon examination, he has neck stiffness with positive Kernig and Brudzinski signs. A lumbar puncture shows Gram-positive diplococci and a positive quellung reaction. He also has a history of chronic sinusitis and asplenism. Given this history, which of the following organisms is the most likely cause of his symptoms?

   A. *Hemophilus influenzae*
   B. *Streptococcus pneumoniae*
   C. *Neisseria meningitides*
   D. Group B *streptococcus*
   E. *Listeria monocytogenes*

68. Which of the following is NOT TRUE of tabes dorsalis?

   A. Tabes dorsalis affects the posterior columns of the spinal cord and of the dorsal roots.
   B. It manifests about 18 to 25 years after initial untreated infection.
   C. Occasionally patients may present with sensory loss or a positive Romberg sign.
   D. Argyll Robertson pupils (ARP) is seen in advanced cases, and it is pathognomonic of tertiary syphilis.
   E. Abnormal CSF findings are less common than in other types of neurosyphilis.

69. You are asked to evaluate a 35-year-old man with known acquired immunodeficiency syndrome (AIDS). He presented to the hospital with subacute monoparesis and diplopia. It is suspected that he has progressive multifocal leukoencephalopathy (PML). Which of the following is the gold standard for the diagnosis of this condition?

   A. PML is a clinical diagnosis, which is made on the basis of clinical presentation, history, and examination findings.
   B. Brain MRI
   C. Brain computed axial tomography (CAT) scan
   D. Brain biopsy
   E. Blood–JC virus (a human polyoma virus) assay

70. Corpus Callostomy is a treatment option for which of the following conditions?

   A. Myasthenia gravis
   B. Parkinson's disease

C. Bilateral frontal seizures
D. Ménière's disease
E. All of the above

71. The increase in size of the human brain from infancy to adulthood is most directly related to which one of the following?
   A. An increase in the number and density of neuronal cell bodies
   B. An increase in the number of layers of the cerebral cortex
   C. An increase in the number and density of gyri
   D. An increase in the fluid volume of the ventricles and cistern
   E. An increase in the number and branching of dendrites

72. Which one of the following statements regarding dopamine receptors is NOT TRUE?
   A. They consist of two families of receptors.
   B. D1-like receptors are positively coupled with cyclic adenosine monophosphate (cAMP).
   C. D2-like receptors inhibit cAMP or increase inositol 1,4,5-triphosphate (IP_3).
   D. D3 and D4 receptors are widely distributed in striatal, mesocortical, and hypothalamic areas.
   E. The D2 family of dopamine receptors is the most important group of dopamine receptors.

73. According to George Vaillant's classifications, which of the following defenses would be most likely to be seen in a child or psychotic patient?
   A. Asceticism
   B. Projection
   C. Rationalization
   D. Reaction formation
   E. Sublimation

74. Which one of the following statements regarding Medicare is NOT TRUE?
   A. It usually provides health insurance coverage for people who are 65 years of age and over.
   B. It also provides health insurance coverage for people who are under 65 years of age and are disabled or have end-stage renal disease (ESRD)
   C. It is partially financed by payroll taxes.
   D. Medicare Part A covers medical insurance.
   E. Medicare Part D provides prescription drug coverage.

75. Which of the following is thought to be the psychological process behind the defense mechanism of sublimation?
   A. Re-channeling of impulses into socially acceptable expressions

B. Changing anxiety into comedy
C. Replacing aggression by support
D. Intentional blocking of recall
E. Transferring a feeling from its actual object to a substitute

76. Who described schizophrenia symptoms using the term *dementia praecox*?
   A. Emil Kraepelin
   B. Thomas Szasz
   C. Eugen Bleuler
   D. Ewald Hecker
   E. Haslam Morel

77. What percentage of patients with Tourette's syndrome also meets the criteria for OCD by adulthood?
   A. 10%
   B. 20%
   C. 40%
   D. 60%
   E. 75%

78. A 6-year-old child who frequently urinates in his bed is brought in for evaluation. Which one of the following, if present, is least likely to preclude a diagnosis of enuresis?
   A. Functionally small bladder
   B. Diuretic treatment
   C. Diabetes
   D. Seizure disorder
   E. Mental retardation

79. Which one of the following is NOT associated with an early onset of Schizophrenia?
   A. Male gender
   B. Family history of Schizophrenia
   C. Birth complications
   D. Premorbid cognitive deficits
   E. Maladaptive parenting

80. Which one of the following antidepressants has NOT shown efficacy in the treatment of Posttraumatic Stress Disorder (PTSD)?
   A. Trazodone
   B. Mirtazapine
   C. Sertraline
   D. Venlafaxine
   E. Paroxetine

81. Which one of the following statements about zaleplon (Sonata) is NOT TRUE?
   A. It is a nonbenzodiazepine hypnotic.
   B. It is a pyrazolopyrimidine derivative.
   C. It has a half-life ($t_{1/2}$) of about 1 hour.

D. At the recommended dose of 10 mg, it is free of residual hypnotic or sedative effects.

E. In patients taking cimetidine, the dose of zaleplon used should be double the normal dose.

82. A 50-year-old African American woman with treatment-refractory Schizophrenia comes to the emergency department from her residential center complaining of a 1-week history of fever, chills, and productive cough. Several other residents have been sick with similar symptoms at her care facility. The patient is on metoprolol, lovastatin, albuterol, and clozapine (started 3 months ago) and has been medication compliant as the medications are administered by residential staff. She is fully oriented, pleasant, answers questions appropriately, and has no acute psychotic or mood symptoms. Her temperature is 101°F, blood pressure is 126/78 mm Hg, pulse is 100 beats/minute, and respirations are 20/minute. A chest x-ray is consistent with right lower lobe pneumonia. Which of the following is the most appropriate next step in the management of this patient's pneumonia?

A. Discharge the patient on oral antibiotics and have patient follow-up with her primary doctor.

B. Obtain a complete blood count with differential.

C. Obtain a serum chemistry including electrolytes and renal function.

D. Obtain sputum cultures and then start IV antibiotics.

E. Start antiseizure medication for prophylaxis in setting of clozapine treatment and fever.

83. An 81-year-old man is brought in for an evaluation by his daughter for "forgetfulness." The patient denies that there is any problem, but the daughter, who lives with the patient, notes a clear decline in memory over the past 6 months. Physical examination and laboratory testing are unremarkable. The patient scores a 21/30 on the MMSE, and the evaluation is not consistent with a depressive illness. You believe that the patient has Alzheimer's disease (AD). Which of the following statements regarding the pharmacological treatment for this disorder is TRUE?

A. Currently available treatments can alter the natural course of disease.

B. Rivastigmine typically has the least gastrointestinal side effects.

C. All of the available treatments are acetylcholinesterase inhibitors.

D. Donepezil is not contraindicated in patients with hepatic disease.

E. All of the available treatments can be given in once daily dosing.

84. Which one of the SSRIs is most effective in the treatment of Generalized Anxiety Disorder?

A. Paroxetine

B. Escitalopram

C. Citalopram

D. Sertraline

E. All SSRIs are equally effective

85. Which one of the following is NOT TRUE of Conversion Disorder?

A. There may be a biological component to the disorder.

B. Part of the treatment involves gently confronting the patient about the fact that symptoms do not reflect a genuine medical illness.

C. People with Conversion Disorder often are identifying with a family member with a medical illness.

D. Patients are not faking illness.

E. Some patients who have significant symptoms seem to be strangely indifferent to them.

86. A 73-year-old-man with a history of poorly controlled hypertension and diabetes presents with sudden onset of speech problems. His speech has normal volume, rate, and tone, and he is able to repeat phases but has difficulty following commands and naming objects. When asked to name a pen, he responds by saying "it's what you write with" and mimics writing with his right hand. When asked to name a wrist watch, he says "clock." Given this information, how would you classify his condition?

A. As fluent aphasia

B. As global aphasia

C. As nonfluent aphasia

D. As anomia

E. As agnosia

87. Which one of the following is NOT a part of Kurt Schneider's first-rank symptom of Schizophrenia?

A. Visual hallucinations

B. Voices commenting on the patient

C. Thought withdrawal

D. Delusions of being controlled

E. Somatic passivity

88. A 35-year-old man with a recent diagnosis of Huntington's disease asks you about the neuropsychiatric manifestations of this disorder. When giving an answer to his question, which one of the following statements will you make about this condition?

A. In Huntington's disease, long-term memory is usually worse than executive functions.

B. In Huntington's disease, speech deteriorates faster than comprehension.

C. In Huntington's disease, psychiatric and behavioral symptoms show a stepwise progression with disease severity.

D. In Huntington's disease, although depression occurs commonly, suicides are uncommon.

E. In Huntington's disease, mania and psychosis are uncommon.

89. A 65-year-old patient presents to the ER in an ambulance. Her husband found her collapsed in their living room. Her past medical history is notable for poorly controlled diabetes, hypertension, and stroke. She is unable to be aroused, and her respiratory pattern demonstrates rhythmic waxing and waning of respiratory amplitude. Dysfunction of which one of the brain areas would produce this respiratory pattern?

A. Dominant frontal lobe
B. Unilateral brain stem
C. Bilateral hemispheric dysfunction
D. Dominant occipital lobe
E. Spinal cord dissection

90. Which one of the deficits listed below is most characteristic of anterior spinal cord syndrome?

A. Bilateral loss of position sense below the level of the lesion
B. Autonomic instability
C. Contralateral loss of light touch below the level of the lesion
D. Ipsilateral loss of light touch below the level of the lesion
E. Flaccid paraplegia of tetraplegia below the level of the lesion

91. A child presents to your office for a psychiatric evaluation. You also learn he has a history of incontinence and gait disturbance. Given his history, which one of the following disorders is he most likely to have?

A. Spina bifida occulta
B. Frontal lobe tumor
C. Bell's palsy
D. CP
E. Hydrocephalus

92. A 7-year-old boy presents with gait disturbance and intellectual decline. Ataxia and upper motor neuron signs (weakness, hyperreflexia, and increased tone) are prominent on his physical examination. An MRI reveals symmetric white matter lesions and a blood test reveals that the activity of enzyme arylsulfatase-A is decreased. Given this information, what do you think is the most likely diagnosis?

A. Metachromatic leukodystrophy
B. Rett syndrome
C. Neurofibromatosis
D. Tuberous sclerosis
E. X-linked adrenoleukodystrophy

93. Which of the following is the commonest cause of acute bacterial meningitis in the United States?

A. *Hemophilus influenzae*
B. *Streptococcus pneumoniae*
C. *Neisseria meningitides*
D. Group B *streptococcus*
E. *Listeria monocytogenes*

94. Which one of the following statements is NOT TRUE of HIV-1-associated minor cognitive/motor disorder (MCMD)?

A. Patients with MCMD present with a clear consciousness.
B. Patients with MCMD do not have serious impairment in daily functioning.
C. The symptoms of MCMD are subtle and often missed.
D. MCMD is an early manifestation of HIV-associated dementia (HAD).
E. There are no controlled trials for the treatment of MCMD.

95. Which one of the following is the most common muscle group to be affected early in Guillain-Barré syndrome?

A. Proximal leg muscles
B. Facial muscles
C. Muscles of respiration
D. Fine muscles of the hand
E. Muscles lining the gastrointestinal tract

96. At what frequency of tension type headache occurrence would one consider starting a patient on prophylactic therapy?

A. Headache episodes less than 1 day per year
B. Headache episodes less than 1 day per 6 months
C. Headache episodes less than 1 day per month
D. Headache episodes 1 to 14 days per month
E. Headache episodes 15 or more days per month

97. Compared to healthy controls, volumetric analyses of MRIs of children with Schizophrenia demonstrate which one of the following findings?

A. ↑ total cerebral volume, ↓ ventricular volume, ↓ area of the thalamus
B. ↓ total cerebral volume, ↓ ventricular volume, ↓ area of the thalamus
C. ↓ total cerebral volume, ↑ ventricular volume, ↑ area of the thalamus
D. ↑ total cerebral volume, ↑ ventricular volume, ↑ area of the thalamus
E. ↓ total cerebral volume, ↑ ventricular volume, ↓ area of the thalamus

98. Which one of the following statements regarding noradrenergic (NA) neurotransmission is NOT TRUE?

   A. The principal noradrenaline containing neurons is the locus coeruleus.
   B. Axons project to the hypothalamus, cortex, and subcortical limbic areas.
   C. The main central nervous system (CNS) metabolite of noradrenaline is vanillylmandelic acid (VMA).
   D. Alpha1-receptors are excitatory and use inositol phosphate as the second messenger.
   E. Beta-adrenoceptors are stimulatory and increase cAMP.

99. According to George Vaillant's classifications, which of the following is considered to be a neurotic defense that is often encountered in an obsessive-compulsive patient?

   A. Distortion
   B. Introjection
   C. Isolation
   D. Regression
   E. Suppression

100. Which one of the following statements regarding hospice care in the United States is NOT TRUE?

   A. The contemporary hospice offers a comprehensive program of care to patients and families facing a life threatening illness.
   B. Hospice emphasizes palliative rather than curative treatment.
   C. Hospice affirms life and regards dying as a normal process and it neither hastens nor postpones death.
   D. Hospice coverage is provided by Medicaid in all the states.
   E. Most hospice patients are cancer patients, but hospices accept anyone regardless of age or type of illness, if they have limited life expectancy.

101. A 10-year-old boy goes to school after witnessing a violent fight between his parents. In school that day, he refuses to follow the teacher's instructions and pushes a schoolmate in the classroom. Which of the following defense mechanisms is this boy using to cope with his feelings?

   A. Passive aggression
   B. Projective identification
   C. Acting out
   D. Omnipotence
   E. Reaction formation

102. Which one of the following is a common characteristic of patients with Schizophrenia?

   A. Younger age of disease onset in females
   B. Low suicide rate

   C. Inhabitance in an urban area
   D. Low rates of substance abuse
   E. Low rates of assaultive behavior

103. In community surveys, up to what percentage of boys have been reported by their parents to have tics?

   A. 1%
   B. 6%
   C. 12%
   D. 18%
   E. 24%

104. Which one of the following treatments is most successful in the long-term remission of nocturnal enuresis?

   A. Imipramine
   B. Desmopressin (DDAVP)
   C. Alarm system
   D. Fluid restriction at night
   E. Reward system for delayed micturition

105. Which of the following is NOT a characteristic of a major Depressive Episode with Atypical Features according to the DSM-IV-TR?

   A. Leaden paralysis
   B. Hypersomnia
   C. Hyperphagia
   D. Decreased reactivity to positive events
   E. Increased rejection sensitivity

106. Which one of the following statements regarding alcohol detoxification is TRUE?

   A. Outpatient detoxification is a safe alternative to inpatient detoxification for healthy, motivated individuals.
   B. Patients at risk of complicated withdrawal include those with comorbidities, such as cardiac/pulmonary disease, infection, and recent surgery.
   C. It is safe to wait until symptoms of alcohol withdrawal develop before instituting pharmacologic treatment with benzodiazepines.
   D. Use of a standard rating scale such as the Clinical Institute Withdrawal Assessment (Revised) is preferable.
   E. All of the above.

107. Which of the following is NOT TRUE regarding eszopiclone (Lunesta)?

   A. It is a nonbenzodiazepine hypnotic that is structurally unrelated to zolpidem, zaleplon, benzodiazepines, or barbiturates.
   B. It is an S (+) enantiomer of racemic zopiclone.
   C. Its effect is believed to result from its interaction with γ-aminobutyric acid (GABA) receptor

complexes at binding domains located close to or allosterically coupled to benzodiazepine receptors.
D. Peak plasma concentrations are achieved within 1 hour after oral administration of this drug.
E. Its mean elimination half-life is approximately 2 hours.

108. A 40-year-old man with HIV is brought to the emergency department from his primary doctor's office, because he has lost a significant amount of weight by not eating and is endorsing new onset paranoid delusions that his food is being poisoned at his residential home. The patient is not agitated, denies any mood symptoms, and is not suicidal or homicidal. Review of records indicates this is the first time the patient is experiencing such delusions. Physical examination and a CT scan of the brain are unremarkable. The toxicology screen is negative, and the basic laboratory values are unremarkable from his baseline. The patient is admitted to psychiatry with a diagnosis of psychosis secondary to HIV infection. Given his history, which one of the following medications is the most appropriate treatment regimen for this patient's psychosis?

A. Clozapine 12.5 mg qhs
B. Haloperidol 10 mg BID
C. Lorazepam 1 mg BID
D. Olanzapine 10 mg qhs
E. Quetiapine 50 mg qhs

109. A 17-year-old man is brought in by his friends at 3AM after he "passed out" at a rave party. The patient is initially comatose, but on an intubation attempt, he becomes acutely agitated to the point of needing restraints. His friends are initially reticent about what drugs their friend may have taken, but eventually state that he used γ-hydroxybutyrate. Given this information, which one of the following statements is TRUE?

A. This patient should be given intravenous naloxone immediately.
B. A clinically significant withdrawal syndrome is quite rare.
C. Antipsychotics are recommended to treat the patient's agitation.
D. Physostigmine is a first line treatment for overdose.
E. Barbiturates are often useful in treating withdrawal.

110. Which one of the following is NOT a pharmacological property of the benzodiazepine receptor?

A. Hypnotic
B. Anxiolytic

C. Stimulant
D. Muscle relaxant
E. Anticonvulsant

111. You are called to evaluate a 55-year-old man for depression who was admitted to the hospital for pyelonephritis. The patient admits to you that for the last 7 months he has not been himself. His wife confirms that he has always had a zest for life, with many interests, and, in the past, has enjoyed his family and career and has had many hobbies. For the last year or so, he has become increasingly withdrawn and not interested in his usual activities. The patient himself endorses passive suicidal ideation (which is new for him), a 15-pound weight loss in the last few months, and a lack of desire or energy to do the things he used to enjoy. You notice that, when the patient was admitted to the medical ER, because the etiology of his symptoms was unclear, several labs were drawn, and, among other results, showed a normal blood urea nitrogen (BUN) and creatinine, and significantly elevated amylase level. You suspect the patient's symptoms of depression are likely secondary to which one of the following conditions?

A. The pyelonephritis
B. An undiagnosed pancreatitis
C. An occult stroke
D. A carcinoma
E. A silent myocardial infarction (MI)

112. All of the following descriptions are correctly matched EXCEPT:

A. Lipofuscin granules: cytoplasmic inclusions that are seen with aging
B. Lewy bodies: neuronal inclusions that are seen in Parkinson's disease
C. Hirano bodies: eosinophilic inclusions found in hippocampal neurons normally
D. Neurofibrillary tangles: degenerated cytoplasmic inclusions in AD
E. Melanin: a pigment in the substantia nigra that disappears in Parkinson's disease

113. All of the following are abnormal findings consistent with Bulimia Nervosa EXCEPT:

A. High estrogen level
B. Hypokalemia
C. Skin lesions on the dorsum of the hand
D. Hypochloremic alkalosis
E. Esophageal dysmotility

114. Which of the following is TRUE of patients with Huntington's disease (HD)?

A. Psychiatric symptoms may precede the onset of the movement disorder.

B. Unipolar major depression and bipolar disorder are extremely common.

C. Suicide rate has been found to be significantly higher than that found in the general population.

D. Hallucinations and delusions occur more frequently than in the general population.

E. All of the above.

115. A 55-year-old man with multiple vascular risk factors, as well as a family history of stroke, presents emergently with headache and aphasia. His speech is fluent with verbal output at approximately 120 words per minute. His expressive and sensory comprehension are poor. Assuming that his symptoms are the result of a cerebrovascular event, which one of the following regions is most likely to be affected?

A. Posterosuperior temporal region

B. Posteroinferior frontal region

C. Occipital region

D. Brain stem

E. Optic cortex

116. A 24-year-old man comes in for an evaluation of mid back pain that has been present for the past 2 years. An MRI of the mid back reveals a herniated disk at the level of T4. Given this finding, what anatomic region would you expect to have a sensory deficit in this patient?

A. Radial side of forearm

B. Ulnar side of forearm

C. Axilla

D. Nipple

E. Rib margin

117. A 31-week-old infant has a hematocrit drop of 25%. The CSF has many red blood cells and a protein content of 750 mg/dL. The child is lethargic, apneic, and bradycardic. These signs strongly suggest which one of the following disorders?

A. Periventricular intraventricular hemorrhage

B. Periventricular leukomalacia

C. Hypoxic-ischemic encephalopathy (HIE)

D. Neonatal herpes encephalitis

E. Descending aortic dissection

118. A 9-year-old boy presents to your office complaining of burning pain in his fingertips, legs, and feet, which is made worse by heat or exercise. On physical exam the child has a reddish-purple rash about his umbilicus and scrotum. Laboratory findings show a deficiency of α–galactosidase-A. Given this information, what do you think is the most likely diagnosis for his condition?

A. Fabry disease

B. Gaucher disease

C. Krabbe disease

D. Niemann-Pick disease

E. Metachromatic leukodystrophy

119. Which one of the following organisms is the most common cause of fatal sporadic encephalitis in the United States?

A. Varicella Zoster

B. Herpes Simplex virus (HSV)

C. Cytomegalovirus

D. Epstein Barr virus

E. Adenovirus

120. Which of the following statements is NOT TRUE of HIV-associated dementia (HAD)?

A. Since the introduction the advent of highly active antiretroviral therapy (HAART), the incidence of HAD has decreased.

B. There is growing evidence that HAART does not prevent neuropsychological impairment in HAD.

C. HIV disseminates to the CNS soon after primary infection via infected astrocytes.

D. Autopsy studies of HAD patients show characteristic white matter changes, demyelination, microglial nodules, multinucleated giant cells, and perivascular infiltrates.

E. It is also noted that basal ganglia and nigrostriatal structures are affected early in the course of the dementia.

121. A patient presents to the emergency department with progressive, symmetric muscle weakness as well as absent lower extremity deep tendon reflexes. Approximately 1 week ago, she had a mild gastrointestinal virus. A CT scan of the brain does not reveal any clear vascular events or anatomic causes for the presenting symptoms. In order to diagnose the patient with Guillain-Barré syndrome, a lumbar tap should reveal which of the following?

A. Normal CSF protein and normal CSF white count

B. Elevated CSF protein and normal CSF white count

C. Normal CSF protein and elevated CSF white count

D. Decreased CSF protein and decreased CSF white count

E. Decreased CSF protein and normal CSF white count

122. A 34-year-old man presents with cluster headaches. He describes them as three attacks of left-sided, throbbing, periorbital pain, occurring daily for the last 3 weeks. He states he had a similar episode approximately 6 months ago. What would be an appropriate abortive therapy for this patient?

A. Oxygen

B. Verapamil

C. Prednisone
D. Lithium
E. Indomethacin

123. What is meant by the term *lissencephaly*?
  A. A disorder of neuronal migration
  B. A disorder of neuronal differentiation
  C. A disorder of excessive synaptic elimination (pruning)
  D. A failure of synaptogenesis
  E. A disorder of brain size

124. Which of the statements regarding serotoninergic neurotransmission is NOT TRUE?
  A. The neurons containing serotonin are located in the midbrain and brainstem raphe nuclei.
  B. Ascending pathways innervate the hippocampus, striatum, amygdale, and hypothalamus.
  C. Descending pathways terminate in the dorsal and ventral horns of the spinal cord.
  D. Serotonin is formed by the sequential oxidation and hydrolysis of tryptophan.
  E. All the serotonin receptors are G protein coupled except 5-HT3.

125. Which of the following is NOT a mature defense mechanism?
  A. Humor
  B. Suppression
  C. Intellectualization
  D. Denial
  E. Undoing

126. According to Eugen Bleuler, which one of the following is not a fundamental symptom of schizophrenia?
  A. Disturbances of associations
  B. Hallucinations
  C. Autism
  D. Ambivalence in emotions
  E. Change or lack of emotional reactions

127. The progression of tics in Tourette's syndrome can best be described as which one of the following?
  A. Caudal-rostral
  B. Rostral-caudal
  C. Axial
  D. Variable
  E. Bimodal

128. Which one of the following theories has been proposed as an etiology for Enuresis?
  A. Delayed maturation of CNS regulatory functions
  B. Increased body mass index
  C. Aberrant nocturnal pituitary function

D. Decreased sodium re-absorption in the proximal renal tubule
E. Increased parathyroid hormone secretion

129. Which of the following statements is NOT TRUE?
  A. A person with systematized delusions can often go about his life unperturbed.
  B. A person with nonsystematized delusions often has hallucinations or affective instability, or mental confusion.
  C. A person with partial delusions never entertains doubts about the delusional beliefs.
  D. The distorted body images of body dysmorphic disorder serve as an example of overvalued ideas.
  E. Delusional atmosphere is accompanied by an uncanny feeling.

130. A 35-year-old man presents to his physician requesting help with smoking cessation. He currently smokes one pack of cigarettes daily (20 cigarettes). He and his physician decide to use nicotine replacement therapy in the form of the nicotine patch. Which dose of the nicotine patch should he begin using?
  A. 5 mg
  B. 7 mg
  C. 14 mg
  D. 21 mg
  E. 28 mg

131. Which one of the following drugs increases the risk of nephrolithiasis?
  A. Lithium
  B. Divalproex sodium
  C. Carbamazepine
  D. Lamotrigine
  E. Topiramate

132. A 45-year-old woman with treatment refractory schizophrenia has been almost free of psychotic symptoms since she was placed on clozapine 1 year ago, and the dose was titrated to 700 mg a day. Since that time, she has had two witnessed tonic-clonic seizures. Of the following, which one of the medications would be most appropriate for the treatment of this patient's seizure?
  A. Carbamazepine
  B. Lorazepam
  C. Phenobarbital
  D. Phenytoin
  E. Valproate

133. A 37-year-old man who was recently started on lithium develops nausea and anorexia. Given this information, which of the following statements is NOT TRUE about his condition?

A. The nausea and the anorexia are likely related to the dosing of lithium.

B. Suggesting that the patient take the lithium at meals may help with the nausea.

C. Giving a slow release preparation may help with the nausea, but may precipitate diarrhea.

D. If the nausea and anorexia had occurred later in the treatment, one would have to worry less about toxicity.

E. Use of an H_2-blocker might help ameliorate the nausea.

134. What is the mechanism of action of benzodiazepines?

A. Benzodiazepines enhance chloride channel opening when GABA simultaneously binds to the $GABA_A$ target receptor.

B. Benzodiazepines prevent chloride channel opening on the GABA neuron.

C. Benzodiazepines enhance chloride channel opening when GABA simultaneously binds to the $GABA_B$ receptor.

D. Benzodiazepines enhance calcium channel opening by binding at the $GABA_B$ receptor alone.

E. Benzodiazepines open chloride channels by binding at the $GABA_A$ receptor alone.

135. Which one of the following can cause paralysis of the abducent nerve (cranial nerve VI)?

A. Meningitis
B. Subarachnoid hemorrhage
C. Advanced syphilis
D. Trauma
E. All of the above

136. Which one of the following statements is TRUE of the QT interval on an EKG and the use of psychotropic medications?

A. A significantly decreased QT interval can lead to *torsades de pointes*.

B. Tricyclic antidepressants do not affect the QT interval.

C. The dose of haloperidol is not a factor in effecting QT interval length.

D. A QT interval of 550 is a cause of concern in a patient on haloperidol.

E. Gender is not a factor effecting QT interval length.

137. A 55-year-old woman presents to a neurology clinic with a chief complaint of left-sided facial numbness for several months. She has a history of breast cancer with chemotherapy and radiation treatment. Neurological examination is most notable for mild left-sided facial sensation around the eye and an absent left-sided corneal reflex. Her symptoms are most likely to be due to a lesion of which one of the following cranial nerves?

A. Left trigeminal V1
B. Right trigeminal V1
C. Left trigeminal V2
D. Right trigeminal V2
E. Right facial

138. An 18-year-old woman is brought into a neurology clinic on a referral from her primary care doctor. She has not menstruated for the last 4 months and has been found to have abnormal levels of luteinizing and follicle stimulating hormone. A plain film obtained revealed an enlarged sella turcica, and a follow-up MRI revealed a likely craniopharyngioma. Upon a neurologic examination, what visual field deficit would you expect to find in this patient?

A. No light perception in the left eye
B. Bilateral hemianopsia
C. Left homonymous hemianopia
D. No visual defects
E. Right homonymous upper quadrant defect

139. A full-term infant has seizure activity. Which of the following etiologies offers the best long-term prognosis for this infant?

A. Periventricular hemorrhage
B. Subarachnoid hemorrhage
C. Early-onset hypocalcemia
D. Infection
E. Hypoglycemia

140. A young child presents to your office with the following history: he had early normal development and then developed weakness, low energy, and poor tolerance for physical activity. He also had episodes of vomiting and headache, and lost some of his hearing. He eventually developed seizures and sudden onset hemiparesis. This presentation is most consistent with which of the following conditions?

A. Mitochondrial myopathy, encephalopathy, lactacidosis, and stroke (MELAS)

B. Myoclonic epilepsy and ragged-red fibers (MERRF)

C. Leigh syndrome

D. Neuropathy, ataxia, and retinitis pigmentosa (NARP)

E. Kearns-Sayre syndrome

141. Which of the following statements about the serology of syphilis is TRUE?

A. Isolation of *Treponema pallidum* is the most practical way of making a diagnosis of syphilis.

B. The Venereal Disease Research Laboratory (VDRL) test and the rapid plasma reagin (RPR) test are examples of tests based on the treponemal antibodies reaction with regain.

C. The RPR test remains the most suitable test for the CSF.

D. The CSF VDRL test is highly specific and false-positive reactions are uncommon.

E. For making the diagnosis of neurosyphilis an appropriate blood serology and a reactive CSF VDRL test is required.

142. Which one of the following is NOT seen in the brain of a patient with CJD?

A. Cerebral atrophy
B. Cytoplasmic vacuoles
C. Lewy bodies
D. Astrocytosis
E. Amyloid plaques

143. Who among the following is most likely to be affected by MS given their demographic and historical risk factors?

A. A 75-year-old man with hypertension and a history of heart disease
B. A 13-year-old girl with lupus
C. A 45-year-old man with inflammatory bowel syndrome
D. A 30-year-old woman with autoimmune thyroid disease
E. A 55-year-old woman with multiple cerebral infarcts

144. A 52-year-old woman with a history of recurring migraines reports that she continues to miss work at least 1 day per week due to her headaches. This interference with her daily routine persists despite abortive therapy. What would be the next step in managing her headaches?

A. Changing the triptan the patient is currently prescribed
B. IV metoclopramide
C. IV prochlorperazine
D. Topiramate
E. Rectal ergotamine

145. Synaptic density, through competitive synaptic elimination, reaches adult levels by which phase of development?

A. School age
B. Pre-puberty
C. Early adolescence
D. Late adolescence
E. Early adulthood

146. Which of the following statements about cholinergic transmission is NOT TRUE?

A. The most important cholinergic pathway originates from the nucleus basalis of Meynert with axons innervating the hippocampus.
B. The synthesis of acetylcholine is catalyzed by choline acetyltransferase.
C. Acetylcholine is hydrolyzed by acetylcholine esterase into choline and ethanol.
D. Nicotinic receptors are involved in fast excitatory synaptic transmission.
E. Muscarinic receptors either activate formation of inositol phosphate or inhibit cAMP.

147. What is the function of the Global Assessment of Functioning (GAF) scale in the DSM-IV-TR?

A. It rates the prognosis of various psychiatric disorders.
B. It rates the severity of symptoms and level of psychosocial functioning.
C. It rates the level of the patient's psychosis.
D. It rates a patient's level of safety.
E. It rates a patient's level of disability.

148. Two days after giving birth, a 27-year-old woman tells her family that the newborn is possessed by the devil. She refuses to eat because she believes the child is poisoning her food. What information from this woman's history would put her at greatest risk for postpartum psychosis?

A. Marital discord
B. Fetal distress
C. A family history of mood disorder
D. A history of postpartum psychosis
E. No previous pregnancies

149. The pattern of inheritance for Tourette's syndrome corresponds most closely to which one of the following?

A. Autosomal dominant
B. Autosomal recessive
C. X-linked recessive
D. X-linked dominant
E. Telomeric mutation

150. Which one of the following choices matches the frequency and duration criteria for Encopresis in DSM-IV-TR?

A. Once a week for 1 month
B. Once a week for 3 months
C. Twice a week for 1 month
D. Twice a week for 3 months
E. Once a month for 3 months

151. What is an autochthonous delusion?

A. A delusion that strikes like a bolt from the blue.
B. A delusion shared between a couple.

C. A delusion that a person close to you has been replaced by a double.

D. A delusion of misidentification in which strangers are identified as familiar persons.

E. A delusion that someone else has changed into oneself.

152. Which one of the following statements regarding the cognitive enhancer memantine is NOT TRUE?

   A. Memantine, an NMDA receptor antagonist, that may attenuate neurotoxicity caused by glutaminergic overstimulation.

   B. Memantine is excreted by the kidneys and doses may need to be reduced in patients with renal disease.

   C. The recommended daily dose of memantine is 20 mg twice a day.

   D. Clinical trials have shown that memantine slows cognitive and functional decline in patients with moderate to severe AD.

   E. Higher doses of memantine may cause confusion.

153. You are on call overnight in an urban ER. A 55-year-old disheveled, homeless man is brought in by the police after he was found climbing up a water tower so that he could receive transmission from Korea through the radio transmitter implanted in his brain by aliens. In the ER the patient is refusing medication, is agitated, hostile, and combative. After punching the security guard, he is placed in restraints. In considering your options for IM medications, which of the following is NOT among your available choices?

   A. Chlorpromazine

   B. Ziprasidone

   C. Haloperidol

   D. Olanzapine

   E. Aripiprazole

154. A 35-year-old man with paranoid schizophrenia has been hospitalized 8 times in the past 4 months for worsening psychosis due to medication noncompliance. During this hospitalization, he agrees to switch from his oral form of risperidone to the long-acting injectable form, Risperdal Consta. Of the following choices, which is the most appropriate treatment regimen for this patient?

   A. Give an injection every week for 1 month, then every 2 weeks.

   B. Give an injection every 2 weeks, and do not give any additional oral medication.

   C. Give an injection every 2 weeks, and provide oral medication until the second injection.

   D. Give an injection every 2 weeks, and provide oral medication for 3 weeks.

   E. Give an injection every 4 weeks, and provide oral medication for 2 weeks.

155. A 23-year-old woman is started on oral lithium at 300 mg three times a day. Assuming the patient is compliant with her medication, when would it be ideal to draw a lithium level?

   A. In 2 days

   B. In 5 days

   C. After 8 hours

   D. After 12 hours

   E. After 16 hours

156. Which of the following factors is NOT associated with severity of benzodiazepine withdrawal?

   A. Diagnosis of panic disorder

   B. Short half-life drugs

   C. Long duration of use

   D. Slow tapering

   E. High doses

157. Bell's palsy refers to which one of the following choices?

   A. A disorder causing bilateral facial weakness

   B. A disorder causing upper and lower facial weakness on one side

   C. A lower motor neuron lesion of cranial nerve V

   D. An upper motor neuron lesion of cranial nerve VII

   E. None of the above

158. SSRI antidepressant medications can help which of the following symptoms in Borderline Personality Disorder?

   A. Depressed mood

   B. Irritability

   C. Impulsive aggression

   D. Self mutilation

   E. All of the above

159. In examining an elderly man in a nursing home, you note that he has wasting of the muscles of the right shoulder. He is unable to shrug his shoulders against resistance, and there appears to be winging of his right scapula. His symptoms are most likely to be due to a lesion of which one of the following cranial nerves?

   A. Cranial nerve VIII

   B. Cranial nerve IX

   C. Cranial nerve X

   D. Cranial nerve XI

   E. Cranial nerve XII

160. What would be the appropriate strength level assigned to a muscle group that is able to perform active movement only with gravity eliminated?

   A. 1/5

   B. 2/5

C. 3/5

D. 4/5

E. 5/5

161. Which one of the following is NOT a factor influencing the decision to start symptomatic medical therapy of idiopathic Parkinson's disease?

A. Presence of significant akathisia

B. Effect of disease on dominant hand

C. Presence of significant gait disturbance

D. Degree to which the disease interferes with activities of daily living

E. The patient's attitude toward use of drugs

162. Myelination in the brain continues into which decade of life?

A. First decade

B. Second decade

C. Third decade

D. Fourth decade

E. Fifth decade

163. Which one of the following statements regarding glutamate neurotransmission is TRUE?

A. Glutamate is the major slow acting excitatory neurotransmitter in the brain.

B. Kainate, NMDA, and amino-3-hydroxy-5-methyl-4-isoxazole propionate (AMPA) receptors are metabotropic receptors.

C. There is a link between AMPA receptor activation and long-term potentiation in the hippocampus as the physiological substrate of memory.

D. Glutamate neurotransmission is implicated in anxiety but not schizophrenia.

E. Glutamate is the neurotransmitter implicated in neurodegeneration.

164. Which one of the following is NOT a useful intervention in a patient with Somatization Disorder?

A. Schedule frequent, short medical consultations

B. Establish a collaborative relationship with the patient's primary care provider

C. Include aspects of the patient's well being in general, including medical and psychological factors

D. Encourage urgent medical visits

E. Suggest nonstandard approaches when necessary, such as yoga or meditation

165. Which one of the following is not a diagnostic category in DSM-IV-TR?

A. Rumination Disorder

B. Pica

C. Failure to thrive

D. Feeding Disorder of Infancy or Early Childhood

E. Disorder of Infancy, Childhood, or Adolescence Not Otherwise Specified (NOS)

166. Which one of the following disorders is most frequently comorbid with Tourette's syndrome?

A. Bipolar disorder

B. ADHD

C. Major Depressive Disorder

D. Social Anxiety Disorder

E. Alcohol Abuse

167. What percent of 5-year-olds are supposed to have achieved bowel control in western culture?

A. 75%

B. 80%

C. 85%

D. 90%

E. 99%

168. Which of the following statements is NOT TRUE regarding Veraguth's fold?

A. It is due to changes in the tone of the corrugator and zygomatic facial muscles.

B. It is triangle shaped.

C. It is in the nasal corner of the upper eyelid.

D. It is exclusively seen in patients who suffer from clinical depression.

E. It was described by the Swiss neuropsychiatrist Otto Veraguth.

169. Which of the following is the most common side effect of cholinesterase inhibitors?

A. Fatigue

B. Gastrointestinal distress

C. Insomnia

D. Dizziness

E. Agitation

170. Typical antipsychotic medications have similar efficacy, but differ in their potency and side effect profile. The low-potency typical antipsychotic medications have all of the following side effects EXCEPT:

A. Constipation

B. Sedation

C. Hypotension

D. Cogwheel rigidity

E. Dry mouth

171. A 32-year-old man with paranoid schizophrenia has been noncompliant with oral medications because he "forgets" to take his medications. He is now agreeable to receiving a long-acting injectable form. When deciding between Risperdal Consta and haloperidol decanoate, which of the following statements is TRUE?

A. Unlike Risperdal Consta, haloperidol decanoate does not need an overlap of oral medications.

B. Unlike Risperdal Consta, haloperidol decanoate escapes first-pass metabolism by the liver.

C. Unlike Risperdal Consta, haloperidol decanoate is given every 4 weeks.

D. Unlike Risperdal Consta, haloperidol decanoate is not viscous and causes little, if any, swelling at the injection site.

E. Unlike Risperdal Consta, haloperidol decanoate requires patients to be exposed to the oral form first before an injection.

172. You decide to start a 33-year-old man with Bipolar Disorder with severe depressive episodes on lamotrigine. The patient currently takes valproic acid. Given this information, what dose of lamotrigine should you start this patient?

A. Prescribe 25 mg or less daily for 1 week and increase by 25 mg or less for the first 4 weeks.

B. Prescribe 50 mg daily for 1 week and increase by 50 mg for the first 4 weeks.

C. Prescribe 50 mg daily for 1 week and increase by 25 mg for the first 4 weeks.

D. Prescribe 75 mg daily for 1 week and increase by 50 mg for the first 4 weeks.

E. Given that the patient is on valproic acid, do not prescribe lamotrigine and find an alternative.

173. A 30-year-old graduate student experiences dry mouth, heart-pounding, tremor, and difficulty breathing only when he must speak in public. He has no prior psychiatric history and his medical workup is negative for any on ongoing illness. Given this information, what would be the most appropriate therapy for this patient?

A. Atenolol
B. Propranolol
C. Clonazepam
D. Methylphenidate
E. Lorazepam

174. A lesion of the vagal nerve (cranial nerve X) can result in which one of the following?

A. Dyspnea
B. Dysphagia
C. Dysarthria
D. Loss of the gag reflex
E. All of the above

175. Which of the following descriptions of psychodynamic interventions in patients with borderline personality disorder is NOT ACCURATE?

A. Interpretation is more of an exploratory, rather than supportive, intervention.

B. Confrontation involves addressing issues that the patient wishes to avoid.

C. In clarification, the patient's behavior is linked to its unconscious meaning.

D. Affirmation is a supportive intervention.

E. Praise helps to reinforce behaviors that are beneficial to the patient.

176. Which of the following is NOT an adverse effect of levodopa?

A. Nausea
B. Somnolence
C. Seizure
D. Dyskinesia
E. Headache

177. What is the minimum time period stipulated in the DSM-IV-TR to meet the diagnostic criteria for Pica?

A. 1 week
B. 1 month
C. 3 months
D. 6 months
E. 12 months

178. Which one of the following choices best matches the criteria for transient tic disorder in DSM-IV-TR?

A. Motor and/or vocal tics many times a day, nearly every day for at least 4 weeks, but no longer than 12 consecutive months.

B. Motor and/or vocal tics many times a day, nearly every day for at least 3 months, but no longer than 12 consecutive months.

C. Motor and/or vocal tics many times a day, nearly every day for at least 4 weeks, but no longer than 9 consecutive months.

D. Motor and/or vocal tics many times a day, nearly every day for at least 6 months but no longer than 12 consecutive months.

E. Motor and vocal tics many times a day, nearly every day for at least 4 weeks, but no longer than 12 consecutive months.

179. Which one of the following treatments is NOT used in a child with Encopresis?

A. Diet modification
B. Laxatives
C. Mineral oil
D. Timed intervals on the toilet
E. Alarm system

180. The prevalence of most Somatoform Disorders has been found to be higher in women than in men. In which of the following disorders is this NOT true?

A. Somatization Disorder
B. Conversion Disorder
C. Hypochondriasis

D. Pain Disorder
E. Body Dysmorphic Disorder

181. Which of the following statements regarding counseling for patients with Alcohol Dependence is NOT TRUE?
   A. In the first several months, counseling should focus on day-to-day life issues to help patients maintain motivation for sobriety and to enhance functioning.
   B. There is limited data to indicate that either individual or group therapy approaches are superior to the other.
   C. Psychotherapy techniques which require deep insights are useful toward maintaining abstinence.
   D. To optimize motivation, sessions should explore the consequences of drinking and the marked improvement that can be expected with abstinence.
   E. Counseling is usually offered for a minimum of 3 times per week for the first 2 to 4 weeks, followed by once a week for the following 3 to 6 months.

182. A 32-year-old woman with a diagnosis of Schizophrenia is referred to you by a colleague. She has a worrisome history of overdosing on prescribed medications with the intent to end her life. When considering antipsychotic options, you choose a medication that if taken in overdose is less likely to cause a seizure. Which of the following medications would you avoid using in this patient?
   A. Chlorpromazine
   B. Haloperidol
   C. Thioridazine
   D. Fluphenazine
   E. Olanzapine

183. A 30-year-old woman with Chronic Paranoid Schizophrenia has been maintained on one psychiatric medication for the past year. She now presents for a follow-up visit complaining of missing her last three menstrual periods. She has not had any sexual encounters in the past year and has never had a problem in the past with missing menstrual cycles. Which of the following medications is most likely the cause of her missing her menstrual periods?
   A. Clozapine
   B. Olanzapine
   C. Quetiapine
   D. Risperidone
   E. Ziprasidone

184. A 35-year-old woman with bipolar disorder and no past medical history has been on valproic acid for 6 months. Upon laboratory testing, you notice that the patient's platelets have dropped to 95,000/cmm. She is otherwise asymptomatic. Given this information, which one of the following statements is TRUE?
   A. Given that patients on valproic acid have a significant risk of developing a bleeding disorder, regardless of their other medical problems, should there be any evidence of thrombocytopenia, the medication should be stopped.
   B. Given that patients on valproic acid have a significant risk of developing a bleeding disorder, if the platelets drop 10,000 or more than at baseline, the medication should be stopped.
   C. This drop in platelet count is more likely to occur at doses of 250 mg/day.
   D. The patient should have her bleeding time and platelet count checked before having surgery.
   E. The drop in platelets is unlikely to be secondary to valproic acid.

185. What pharmacological action is shared by benzodiazepines and buspirone?
   A. Sedative
   B. Muscle relaxant
   C. Anticonvulsant
   D. Respiratory depression
   E. Anxiolytic

186. Which of the following is NOT TRUE of papilledema?
   A. It is caused by increased intracranial pressure.
   B. Brain tumors, subdural hematomas, and hydrocephalus are possible causes.
   C. It usually leads to blurred vision.
   D. It can cause increased blind spots in the visual fields.
   E. The optic disk is affected.

187. Klüver Bucy syndrome occurs when there is a lesion to which one of the following structures?
   A. Bilateral occipital lobe
   B. Bilateral frontal lobes
   C. Bilateral temporal lobes
   D. Bilateral parietal lobes
   E. Bilateral basal ganglia

188. A 60-year-old man with early Parkinson's disease is treated with the selective monoamine oxidase inhibitor, selegiline. Which of the following statements is NOT TRUE of this medication for the treatment of this condition?
   A. Modest effectiveness in monotherapy as symptomatic treatment
   B. There is risk of hypertensive crisis following ingestion of tyramine-containing foods
   C. It can cause insomnia due to its amphetamine metabolites

D. Risk of hypertensive crisis at higher doses due to nonselective inhibition

E. Headache and nausea are common adverse effects

189. An 8-month-old child is brought in for evaluation by his parents because of concerns about his feeding. The parents say the child eats and swallows but then brings the food back into his mouth; although he strains to bring the food up, he does not appear distressed. Which of the following diagnoses is most appropriate in this case?

A. Feeding Disorder of Infancy and Early Childhood

B. Infantile Anorexia

C. Feeding Disorder of Infant-Caregiver Reciprocity

D. Rumination Disorder

E. Sensory Food Aversions

190. A 20-year-old man presents to your office complaining of sudden, rapid facial movements, including blinking and grimacing. He also reports frequent sniffing behaviors that have been occurring many times a day nearly every day for more than a year and are worsening. You find no underlying medical condition for his presentation. Given his presentation, what is the most likely diagnosis?

A. Tourette's syndrome

B. Chronic Motor Tic Disorder

C. Transient Tic Disorder

D. Chronic Vocal Tic Disorder

E. Tic disorder NOS

191. All of the following are considered poor prognoses for encopresis EXCEPT?

A. Soiling at night

B. Nonchalant attitude

C. Conduct problems

D. Soiling as an expression of aggression

E. Elevated body mass index

192. A 19-year-old girl is brought to the emergency department by her distressed mother. In an anxious voice, the mother explains to the triage nurse that her daughter has suddenly become blind. Apart from the patient's subjective complaint of vision loss, a full physical examination is within normal limits and an extensive medical workup reveals no abnormalities. Psychiatric consultation is requested and a detailed history reveals that the family has been under considerable stress within the past week, as the patient's younger brother was involved in a serious farming accident. The patient was a witness to this event. When speaking with the patient, the psychiatrist is struck by her seemingly cavalier attitude toward the sudden blindness. Although the patient superficially endorses the serious nature of her acute symptoms,

she generally presents as quite unconcerned. Which of the following terms most accurately describes this aspect of the patient's presentation?

A. Astasia-abasia

B. Cataplexy

C. Pseudocyesis

D. La Belle indifference

E. Alexithymia

193. All of the following descriptions regarding memory are correctly matched EXCEPT:

A. Registration is the ability to remember data over a long period of time.

B. Retention is the ability to store knowledge.

C. Recall is the return of a memory into consciousness.

D. Semantic memory is the storage of information without regards to an emotional context.

E. Episodic memory refers to events based on an individual's personal experience.

194. Which of the following is NOT TRUE of the resting potential of a neuron?

A. The inside of the neuron is negative relative to the outside of the neuron.

B. Sodium-potassium pumps play a role in maintaining the resting potential across the membrane.

C. The concentration of potassium is higher outside of the cell than inside of the cell.

D. The resting cell membrane of a neuron is more permeable to potassium ions than to sodium ions.

E. In the refractory period, a neuron is capable of transmitting an action potential.

195. Which of the following is an indication to start antiepileptic therapy?

A. A grand mal seizure as the first seizure

B. A brain lesion on CT or MRI

C. A seizure due to a drug reaction

D. No history of serious brain injury

E. Absence of focal abnormalities on exam

196. A patient is recently diagnosed with generalized tonic-clonic seizures. Which of the following is an appropriate initial monotherapy for this patient's condition?

A. Levetiracetam

B. Tiagabine

C. Pregabalin

D. Vigabatrin

E. Gabapentin

197. A 20-year-old woman with partial onset seizures is referred for initiation of antiepileptic therapy.

Which of the following medications does NOT increase the risk of oral contraceptive failure in this patient?

A. Phenytoin
B. Carbamazepine
C. Valproate
D. Phenobarbital
E. Topiramate

198. A 28-year-old woman with a history of Major Depressive Disorder, currently treated with citalopram, was brought to the emergency department by her family for evaluation of fever, vomiting, and weakness. In the emergency department, her temperature was 39.5°C, her heart rate was 138 beats/minute, she was agitated and restless, and she was found to have hyperactive reflexes. Her symptoms started several hours after she used a new medication prescribed to her by her primary care physician. Which of the following is most likely to be the new medication?

A. Naproxen sodium
B. Topiramate
C. Acetaminophen with codeine
D. Sumatriptan
E. Propanolol

199. A 7-year-old girl is referred for evaluation of poor school performance. Her parents report that she frequently seems to "zone out" during the day, even when doing something she enjoys, such as watching a cartoon. Her teacher has noticed the same behavior at school. She frequently loses her homework, has difficulty completing assignments, and has very sloppy handwriting; school testing did not reveal any cognitive deficits or learning disabilities. Her neurologic exam was unremarkable until she was asked to keep blowing to keep a pinwheel rotating for as long as she could. After 30 seconds of hyperventilation, she stopped blowing on the pinwheel, developed a blank stare, and began blinking rapidly for the next minute. An EEG was done, which confirmed the diagnosis. Which of the following medications would be the best first-line therapy for this child's condition?

A. Phenytoin
B. Carbamazepine
C. Topiramate
D. Ethosuximide
E. Phenobarbital

200. The M'Naghten rule is associated with which of the following?

A. Guidelines for expert testimony
B. Maintaining confidentiality
C. Protocols for civil commitment
D. The insanity defense
E. The right to psychiatric treatment

Test 5

Answers

1. **Answer: D.** All are stages of the Kübler-Ross model except for D. Depression is the stage that is not listed in the answers. Although mood may improve and even seem euphoric during the acceptance stage, compensatory mania is not listed as a separate stage in this model.

Sadock BJ, Kaplan H. *Synopsis of Psychiatry*. 9th ed. Philadelphia: Lippincott Williams & Wilkins; 2003:60.

2. **Answer: A.** The lesion is in the contralateral (left) subthalamic nucleus and the condition is hemiballismus. The patient probably has toxoplasmosis. It is one of the more dramatic disorders caused by lesions to the basal ganglia and, as described previously, is characterized by wild flailing of one arm and leg. The subthalamic nucleus is connected by way of the globus pallidus and the substantia nigra to the ipsilateral motor cortex, which controls the motor function of the other side of the body. Lesions to the caudate nucleus would cause chorea (i.e., nearly continuous movements of the face, tongue, or limbs, as is found in Huntington's disease). Lesions to the substantia nigra would cause Parkinson's disease (i.e., resting tremor, bradykinesia, and rigidity). The globus pallidus regulates the output of the basal ganglia.

1. Notle J. *The Human Brain: An Introduction to Its Functional Anatomy*. 4th ed. St. Louis, MO: Mosby; 1999:450–467.
2. Provenzale JM, Scharzchild MA. Hemiballismus. *Am J Neuroradiol*. 1994;15:1377.

3. **Answer: E.** Jean Piaget was a Swiss philosopher, natural scientist, and developmental psychologist, who was well known for his work in studying children and for developing theories of cognitive development. Piaget noticed that even infants have certain skills by which they react to objects in their environment. These rudimentary skills were sensorimotor in nature, but were used by the infant to explore his or her environment and gain more knowledge of the world, and develop more sophisticated exploratory skills. Piaget termed these skills as schemas. Addition of new information to the preexisting schema was termed assimilation. Changing the preexisting schema based on the new information was called accommodation. According to Piaget, assimilation and accommodation are the two sides of adaptation, or

learning. Piaget saw adaptation as a broader learning experience than the kind of learning that behaviorists in the United States were describing. He envisaged it as a biological process that directs a balance between the structure of the mind and the environment. When there is congruency between the two, it would indicate that you have a good enough model of the universe and he called this ideal state "equilibrium." Carl Jung described archetypes as unlearned tendencies to experience things in a certain way. An archetype has no form of its own, but it acts as an "organizing principle" on the things we see or do. It works the same way that instincts work in Freud's theory.

1. Boeree CG. *Personality Theories. Carl Jung: 1875–1961*. http://www.ship.edu/~cgboeree/jung.html. Accessed December 12, 2006.
2. Boeree CG. *Personality Theories. Jean Piaget: 1896–1980*. http://www.ship.edu/~cgboeree/piaget.html. Accessed December 10, 2006.

4. **Answer: A.** NNH represents the number of patients who would need to be treated with a drug to produce one more adverse event than would have occurred with control treatment. The NNH is simply a reciprocal of the absolute risk increase (ARI). ARI is calculated as the difference between the experimental event rate (EER) and control event rate (CER). In this case, the ARI is 3.5% (EER) − 2.3% (CER) = 1.2% (or 0.012). The NNH then would be 1/0.012 = 84. An NNH of 84 means that 84 patients with dementia would have to be treated with an atypical antipsychotic drug before one more patient would have an adverse event (i.e., death).

1. Gray GE. *Evidence-Based Psychiatry*. Washington: American Psychiatric Publishing; 2004:155–156.
2. Schneider LS, Dagerman KS, Insel P. Risk of death with atypical antipsychotic drug treatment for dementia: meta-analysis of randomized placebo-controlled trials. *JAMA*. 2005;294:1934–1943.

5. **Answer: A.** Insight is defined as the patient's degree of awareness and understanding about being ill. This person clearly is in denial of her illness and places the blame for her behavior on external factors rather than the illness, showing lack of insight. Thought process refers to the way in which a person puts together ideas and associations and includes examples

275

like flight of ideas, tangentiality, circumstantiality, and thought blocking. Similarly, thought content refers to what a person is actually thinking about and includes examples like delusions, preoccupations, obsessions, phobias, and suicidal thoughts. Perception refers to experiencing sensory phenomenon as in hallucinations or illusions. Although this patient's judgment is shown to be poor, it has been markedly influenced by her lack of insight.

Kaplan HI, Sadock BJ. *Kaplan & Sadock's Synopsis of Psychiatry*. 8th ed. Philadelphia: Lippincott Williams & Wilkins; 1998:251–252, 254.

6. **Answer: D.** Antisocial Personality Disorder is more common in first-degree biological relatives of those with the disorder. The risk to biological relatives of women with the disorder tends to be higher than the risk to biological relatives of men with the disorder. Biological relatives of patients with this disorder are also at increased risk for somatization disorder and substance-related disorders. Within a family that has a member with Antisocial Personality Disorder, men often have Antisocial Personality Disorder and Substance-Related Disorders, whereas women more often have Somatization Disorder. But in such families, there is an increase in the prevalence of all of these disorders in both men and women compared to the general population. Both adopted and biological children of parents with Antisocial Personality Disorder have an increased risk of developing this disorder. Adopted-away children resemble their biological parents more than their adoptive parents, but the adoptive family environment influences the risk of developing a personality disorder and related psychopathology.

American Psychiatric Publishing. *Diagnostic and Statistical Manual of Mental Disorders (DSM-IV-TR) Personality Disorders- 301.7 Antisocial Personality Disorder*. http://www.psychiatryonline.com/content.aspx?aID=3928. Accessed April 16, 2007.

7. **Answer: C.** To diagnose a Feeding Disorder of Infancy and Early Childhood according to DSM-IV-TR, the age of onset must be before the age of 6 years. The feeding disturbance is manifested as a failure to eat adequately with significant failure to gain weight or significant loss of weight over at least 1 month. It is not attributable to a gastrointestinal or other medical condition or to lack of food.

American Psychiatric Association. *Diagnostic and Statistical Manual of Mental Disorders: DSM-IV-TR*. 4th ed. Washington: American Psychiatric Association; 2000:107–108.

8. **Answer: A.** A variety of basal ganglia abnormalities have been considered in Tourette's syndrome, including loss of normal right-left symmetry, increased dopamine receptor availability in more severely affected co-twins, changes in neuronal activity, and—more consistently—smaller caudate volumes.

1. Peterson BS, Thomas P, Kane MJ, et al. Basal ganglia volumes in patients with Gilles de la Tourette syndrome. *Arch Gen Psychiatry*. 2003;60:415–424.
2. Wiener JM, Dulcan MK. *Textbook of Child and Adolescent Psychiatry*. 3rd ed. Washington: American Psychiatric Publishing; 2004:715.

9. **Answer: D.** Studies have suggested cognitive compromises in patients with schizophrenia begin in early childhood, long before symptoms of psychosis. Cognitive deficits are largely independent of symptom severity in schizophrenia. Little evidence exists to suggest cognition improves with antipsychotic treatment. The level of cognitive impairment remains relatively stable from the time of a first psychotic break through late-middle age. Executive dysfunction is the most commonly impaired cognitive function in these patients.

Gold JM. Cognitive deficits as treatment targets in schizophrenia. *Schizophrenia Research*. 2004;72:21–28.

10. **Answer: A.** Fatigue and drowsiness are the most common side effects of benzodiazepines. Patients who are started on benzodiazepines should be cautioned to avoid driving or operating heavy machinery until they are certain the drug will not affect their performance. Impaired memory or other cognitive functions are also seen. Transient anterograde amnesia (inability to learn new information) may occur after an acute dose of benzodiazepines is given; this effect is worsened when benzodiazepines are combined with alcohol use. Impaired motor coordination is another, less common side effect of benzodiazepines. Depression is a potential side effect of all benzodiazepines, although a direct causative link has not been established. Patients who develop depressed mood on benzodiazepines may benefit from the addition of an antidepressant or switching to an antidepressant. Behavioral disinhibition (e.g., agitation, rage attacks) may occur as a paradoxical response to benzodiazepines, most notably among patients with personality disorders and a history of behavioral dyscontrol. When this occurs, antipsychotic medications are often effective in reversing the disturbances.

Rosenbaum JF, Arana GW, Hyman SE, et al. *Handbook of Psychiatric Drug Therapy*. Philadelphia: Lippincott Williams & Wilkins; 2005:178–182.

11. **Answer: C.** AA is a self-help group comprised of individuals who share one thing in common: a desire for

help with an alcohol-related problem. AA is multiracial, apolitical, nonprofessional, and available worldwide. There are no age or education requirements for membership. AA is not a religious organization and does not charge dues or fees. Members of AA often have help available 24 hours a day. AA is not a medical organization and does not provide medications or psychiatric advice. Patients with psychiatric comorbidities are welcome to join AA, but they may need education from physicians on how to cope should group members inappropriately suggest they stop taking medications. Similar organizations are available to family members and loved ones of alcoholics (Al-Anon and Alateen).

1. Alcoholics Anonymous. *Main Website*. http://www. alcoholics-anonymous.org. Accessed January 4, 2007.
2. Sadock BJ, Sadock VA. *Kaplan and Sadock's Comprehensive Textbook of Psychiatry*. 7th ed. Philadelphia: Lippincott Williams & Wilkins; 2000:970.

12. **Answer: A.** Pimozide and haloperidol are used in the treatment of Tourette's syndrome. The dose of pimozide is limited to 20 mg per day due to increased risk of prolonged QT interval (and risk of *torsades de pointe* and ventricular tachycardia) with higher doses.

Rosenbaum JR, Arana GW, Hyman SE, et al. *Handbook of Psychiatric Drug Therapy*. 5th ed. Philadelphia: Lippincott Williams & Wilkins; 2005:24.

13. **Answer: A.** While higher doses of neuroleptics are a risk factor for neuroleptic malignant syndrome, it is not a dose dependant phenomenon (i.e., the effects change when the dose of the drug changes). All of the other statements are true regarding neuroleptic malignant syndrome.

1. Keck PE, Pope HG, Cohen BM, et al. Risk factors for neuroleptic malignant syndrome. A case-control study. *Arch Gen Psychiatry*. 1989;46:914–918.
2. Wijdicks E. *Neuroleptic Malignant Syndrome*. http://www. uptodateonline.com/utd/content/topic.do?topicKey= medneuro/5946&type=A&selectedTitle=1~17. Accessed January 23, 2007.

14. **Answer: D.** NSAIDS, metronidazole, hydrochlorothiazide, and captopril (any Angiotensin-Converting Enzyme [ACE] inhibitor) increase lithium levels. Acetazolamide decreases the lithium levels.

Rosenbaum JF, Arana GW, Hyman SE, et al. *Handbook of Psychiatric Drug Therapy*. 5th ed. Philadelphia: Lippincott Williams & Wilkins; 2005:148.

15. **Answer: C.** Except "White race," all of the following are protective factors in preventing suicides. Other protective factors include life satisfaction, reality testing ability, positive coping skills, positive problem solving skills, positive social supports, and positive therapeutic relationships. White race is a risk factor for suicide.

American Psychiatric Association. *American Psychiatric Association's Practice Guideline for the Assessment and Treatment of Patients with Suicidal Behaviors. II. Assessment of Patients with Suicidal Behaviors*. http://www. psychiatryonline.com/content.aspx?aID=56135. Accessed January 14, 2007.

16. **Answer: B.** The middle cerebral artery supplies blood to the perisylvian arc, which includes Wernicke's area, the arcuate fasciculus, and Broca's area.

McCaffrey P. *SPPA 636, Neuropathologies of Language and Cognition. Unit 4. Medical Aspects: Blood Supply to the Brain*. http://www.csuchico.edu/~pmccaff/syllabi/ SPPA336/336unit4.html. Accessed December 13, 2006.

17. **Answer: E.** Confabulation is when a patient falsifies memories in a state of clear sensorium. It can occur during chronic alcohol abuse, which may lead to Korsakoff's syndrome, but also can occur in other causes of organic brain damage, embarrassment, and Schizophrenia.

Sims A. *Symptoms in the Mind*. 3rd ed. London: Elsevier Science; 2003:67–68.

18. **Answer C.** Mutations of mitochondrial deoxyribonucleic acid (DNA) causes a wide variety of clinical neuromuscular syndromes that can affect any part of the nervous systems, muscles, and other organs. Such mutations may arise sporadically where there is no family history of disease, or may be transmitted via maternal inheritance with up to 100% of a mother's offspring receiving the genetic defect. This is because all mitochondria are inherited from the ovum. Mitochondrial inheritance also arises from a mixture of normal and abnormal mitochondria within a single cell, but also in different tissues. Homoplasmy is the state of having uniformly normal or abnormal mitochondria in a tissue and heteroplasmy is the mixture of normal and abnormal mitochondria in a single tissue. Normally, 90% of the mitochondria need to be abnormal before abnormal symptoms and signs can manifest.

Goetz CG. *Textbook of Clinical Neurology*. 2nd ed. http:// home.mdconsult.com/das/book/67380190-2/view/1158. Accessed February 28, 2007.

19. **Answer: E.** The MMPI is one of the most frequently used personality tests. The original MMPI was developed at the University of Minnesota Hospital and was first published in 1942. The current standardized version for adults 18 years or older is the MMPI-2 which was first released in 1989. The MMPI-2

has 567 items, or questions (all true or false format), and takes approximately 60 to 90 minutes to complete. The short form of the test is comprised of the first 370 items on the long-form of the MMPI-2. It has ten clinical scales which are as follows: hypochondriasis, depression, hysteria, psychopathic deviate, masculinity-femininity, paranoia, psychasthenia, schizophrenia, mania, and social introversion. It also has four validity scales (i.e., if the test-taker was truthful, answered cooperatively, and not randomly) and assesses the test-taker's response style (i.e., cooperative). The four validity scales are the "cannot say" scale, the L (lie) scale, the F (deviant or rare response) scale, and the K (clinically defensive response) scale. Although its standardization sample was limited in racial diversity, this test has acceptable norms. When using the MMPI-2, care needs to be exercised in the interpretation especially when applied to patients with brain damage as many of the symptoms elicited by MMPI-2 questions are common to patients with neurological disorders.

Goetz CG. *Textbook of Clinical Neurology*. 2nd ed. Philadelphia: WB Saunders; 2003.

20. **Answer: E.** While it is possible for patients with Parkinson's disease to develop a concomitant aphasia, aphasia is not normally part of the presentation of Parkinson's disease. The other symptoms listed are commonly seen in patients with this movement disorder.

Goetz CG. *Textbook of Clinical Neurology*. 2nd ed. http://home.mdconsult.com/das/book/67380190-2/view/1158. Accessed February 28, 2007.

21. **Answer: C.** This patient is presenting with third nerve palsy, likely secondary to diabetic infarction of the third nerve. Damage to the nerve causes ptosis—drooping of the upper eyelid (because the levator palpebrae is supplied mainly by the third nerve)—and an inability to rotate the eye upward, downward, or inward. When the lid is passively elevated, the eye is found to be deviated outward and slightly downward because of the unopposed actions of the intact lateral rectus and superior oblique muscles. Common causes of this condition are neoplastic diseases, aneurysms and diabetic infarction. The palsy is usually chronic, progressive, and painless. Enlargement of the pupil is a sign of extramedullary third nerve compression because of the peripheral location in the nerve of the pupilloconstrictor fibers.

Infarction of the nerve in diabetics, however, usually spares the pupil. Because the damage is situated in the central portion of the nerve. It usually develops over a few hours and is accompanied by pain, usually severe, in the forehead and around the eye. The prognosis for recovery (as in other nonprogressive lesions of the oculomotor nerves) is usually good because of the potential of the nerve to regenerate. Usually the other eye is spared, but infarction may occur in the other optic nerve at a later date.

Ropper AH, Brown RH. *Adams and Victor's Principles of Neurology*. 8th ed. New York: McGraw-Hill; 2005:230–234.

22. **Answer: C.** A brachial plexus injury occurs when the plexus is stretched when the head is turned away from the shoulder. It is most likely to occur in a large infant with a cephalic presentation. Milder injuries involve cervical roots 5 and 6; more serious injuries involved the entire plexus. In milder cases, full recovery is expected. However, in more severe cases, consultation with a neurologist and surgeon is indicated to evaluate the need for intervention. Physical abuse always warrants exploration, but does not explain the finding nor would intracranial hemorrhage explain such a localized finding. Signs of congenital syphilis in a young child include notched teeth, clouded cornea, decreased hearing, bone pain, and bone problems of the lower legs, among others. In utero toxoplasmosis infection may lead to a range of outcomes, from mild to severe. At birth, severely infected newborns often have eye infections and an enlarged liver and spleen. If they recuperate, eventual problems may include mental retardation, seizures, CP, and severely impaired eyesight.

1. Center for the Evaluation of Risks to Human Reproduction. *Toxoplasmosis*. http://cerhr.niehs.nih.gov/common/toxoplasmosis.html. Accessed December 18, 2006.
2. Menkes JH, Sarnat HB, Maria BL. *Child Neurology*. 7th ed. Philadelphia: Lippincott Williams & Wilkins; 2006:417–418.
3. US Library of Medicine & National Institutes of Health. *Brachial Palsy in Newborns*. http://www.nlm.nih.gov/medlineplus/ency/article/001395.htm. Accessed December 17, 2006.

23. **Answer: A.** This patient has Alpers' disease which has an underlying metabolic defect. Death usually occurs within the first decade of life by unrelenting seizures, liver failure, or cardiorespiratory failure. Optic atrophy can lead to blindness. Dementia is also a common finding. Alpers' disease, however, is a rare condition.

National Institute of Neurological Disorders and Stoke. *NINDS Alpers' Disease Information Page*. http://www.ninds.nih.gov/disorders/alpersdisease/alpersdisease.htm. Accessed December 18, 2006.

24. **Answer: C.** Neurosyphilis occurs in many different forms and can manifest any time from a year

after the initial infection to 25 years later. Many different forms may overlap and coexist to confuse the making a diagnosis. CSF invasion is common in early stages of untreated syphilis. If CSF abnormalities persist for over 5 years in the untreated patient, it is highly predictive of the development of clinical neurosyphilis. Asymptomatic neurosyphilis can only be diagnosed via the examination of the CSF. Acute syphilitic meningitis is the earliest clinical manifestation of neurosyphilis and occurs within the first year of infection in most patients. It may occur later on in the course of the illness, if untreated. Meningovascular syphilis is more common than meningitis and can cause syphilitic endarteritis and resultant vascular occlusion and infarction. General paresis occurs due to tertiary syphilis, but is a rare condition. It presents with neuropsychiatric manifestations about 15 to 20 years after the initial infection due to the infection of the meninges and cerebral cortex. It results in changes in personality, delusions, mood lability, and dementia. Tabes dorsalis used to be the most common type of neurosyphilis, but is now rare. It affects the posterior columns of the spinal cord and the dorsal roots. It usually occurs 18 to 25 years after initial untreated infection and manifests with paresthesias, abnormal gait, and lightning pains of the extremities or trunk.

1. Rowland LP. *Merritt's Neurology*. 11th ed. Philadelphia: Lippincott Williams & Wilkins; 2005:236–242.
2. Sparling FP, Hicks CB. *Clinical Manifestations of Neurosyphilis*. http://www.uptodateonline.com/utd/content/topic.do?topicKey=stds/8400&type=A&selectedTitle=1 ~11. Accessed January 22, 2007.

25. Answer: D. The human prion diseases may be sporadic, infectious, or genetically inherited. Most of the cases of CJD (80% to 90%) are sporadic. Iatrogenic CJD and familial CJD (autosomal dominant inheritance) each account for about 5% to 10% of CJD cases. Sporadic CJD does not spread like an ordinary infection as the agent has low infectivity. Those with prior head and neck trauma or medical personnel are at higher risk because of increased exposure to the agent. CJD can be transmitted by implanting electrodes or during corneal transplants from infected patients. Iatrogenic disease may also occur due to dura mater grafts and administration of growth hormone extract prepared from pooled human pituitary glands. Mutations in the PrP gene causes the disease that are heritable and transmissible.

Rowland LP. *Merritt's Neurology*. 11th ed. Philadelphia: Lippincott Williams & Wilkins; 2005:265.

26. Answer: C. Surgical treatments of Parkinson's disease are thalamotomy or pallidotomy. They are helpful when patients become unresponsive to pharmacological treatment or develop intolerable adverse reactions to antiparkinsonian medications. Surgery is also sometimes more effective in young patients with mainly unilateral disease who have failed to respond to medications. Thalamotomy is more helpful for tremor, while pallidotomy is more helpful for hypokinesia. Contraindications include dementia or diffuse vascular disease. The rate of significant complications is less than 5% after unilateral surgery, but is about 20% or greater after bilateral procedures. Regarding the other choices, thymectomy is a treatment option in patients with uncomplicated myasthenia gravis who are between puberty and age 55 years. The remission rate is 35% and another 50% show some improvement. Response is usually evident after several months to 3 years. Individuals with intractable bilateral frontal seizures or infants with atonic seizures occasionally benefit from commissurotomy or corpus callosotomy. In this procedure, the anterior two thirds or the entire corpus callosum is split longitudinally. This interrupts the spread of discharges between the cerebral hemispheres. A complication of the surgery may be split-brain syndrome.

1. Greenberg DA, Aminoff MJ, Simon RP. *Clinical Neurology*. 5th ed. New York: McGraw-Hill; 2002:109–110, 183–186, 239–247.
2. Kaufman DM. *Clinical Neurology for Psychiatrists*. 5th ed. Philadelphia: WB Saunders; 2001:191–192, 247.

27. Answer: B. Psychological causes, rather than organic disorders, are more often the reason for chronic sexual impotence in middle-aged men. Alcohol, certain antidepressants, stress, and hormonal problems can cause impotence. Although sexual functioning may decline with age, chronic impotence is not a feature of normal mid-life aging.

Sadock BJ, Kaplan H. *Synopsis of Psychiatry*. 9th ed. Philadelphia: Lippincott Williams & Wilkins; 2003:47.

28. Answer: C. The autoregulation is normally inhibitory. The dopamine autoreceptor at both sites is the D2 receptor; similarly, the noradrenaline autoreceptor is the alpha2 receptor. With the serotonin neurons, the 5-HT1a receptor acts as the main somatodendritic autoreceptor, but the 5-HT1b/1D receptor is the terminal autoreceptor.

Anderson IM, Reid IC. *Fundamentals of Clinical Psychopharmacology*. London: Taylor & Francis Group; 2004:10.

29. Answer: D. It is seen across cultures that men are more violent than women. This observation is related to the biology of male/female differences and polygyny (where one male associates with multiple females). In all polygynous species, males are more prone to violence than are females, and the greater the degree of polygyny is, the greater the male/female disparity becomes for proneness to violence. This observation is probably related to adaptive need for males to succeed in competition with other males for a mate. Violence is also influenced by cultural expectations of male and female stereotypes. In most cultures, men are taught that aggression and violence are signs of "manliness," whereas it is "unfeminine" for women to be violent. It is the interaction between cultural expectation and the biological tendency for violence in men that ultimately results in higher rates of violence in men than in women. Although homicide rates vary substantially among different cultures, with rates being 10 times higher in the United States than in Canada, the difference in rates of homicide between male and female have remained remarkably constant regardless of the society and over time. Homicide rates are higher in poorer and less educated societies.

1. Peters J, Shackelford TK, Buss DM. Understanding domestic violence against women: using evolutionary psychology to extend the feminist functional analysis. *Violence Vict.* 2002;17:255–264.
2. Sadock BJ, Sadock VA. *Kaplan and Sadock's Comprehensive Textbook of Psychiatry.* 8th ed. Philadelphia: Lippincott Williams & Wilkins; 2005:635–637.

30. Answer: C. To prevail in a malpractice claim, the plaintiff must establish four elements: (i) physician is derelict in his duties, (ii) the defendant (physician) has a specific duty or obligation to the plaintiff (patient)—the existence of physician-patient relationship, (iii) the dereliction of duty is a direct cause of an injury, and (iv) economic, physical, emotional pain, and other types of damages must be proven. Although breach of confidentiality could result in emotional damages and may be grounds for a malpractice suit, it falls under the rubric of damages and by itself is not one of the four required elements of a malpractice suit.

Gutheil TG, Applebaum PS. *Clinical Handbook of Psychiatry and The Law.* 3rd ed. Philadelphia: Lippincott Williams & Wilkins; 2000:143–143.

31. Answer: B. The most widely used test of current cognitive functioning is the MMSE, which is used to detect cognitive impairments, follow the course of an illness, and monitor the patient's treatment responses. In this case, it would be the first appropriate test to use. The Facial Recognition Test is a test which requires the identifying a photograph of a face origi-

nally presented in a front view when it is included in various displays (i.e., side view, front view with shadows) and produces a high frequency of failure in patients with posterior right-hemisphere lesions. The WAIS-R is an assessment of intellectual abilities and gives intelligence quotient (IQ) scores. Some of the component tests hold up as aging progresses, while others do not, but this would not be the first test to use for detecting cognitive deficits in dementia. The Thematic Apperception Test and Sentence Completion Test are types of Projective Personality Assessments that are designed to tap into patient's emotions, motivations, and core personality conflicts, and are not helpful for detecting cognitive deficits in dementia.

Kaplan HI, Sadock BJ. *Kaplan & Sadock's Synopsis of Psychiatry.* 8th ed. Philadelphia: Lippincott Williams & Wilkins; 1998:197–203, 318–319, 1291.

32. Answer: D. Major Depressive Episode (MDE) with Atypical Features is defined by predominance of specific symptoms during the most recent 2 weeks of a current MDE in Major Depressive Disorder or Bipolar Disorder and is characterized by mood reactivity and two or more of the following: significant weight gain or increase in appetite, hypersomnia, laden paralysis, and long standing pattern of rejection sensitivity. In addition, criteria are not met for MDE with melancholic or with catatonic features. Loss of pleasure in all or almost all activities is a feature of Melancholic Depression.

American Psychiatric Association. *Quick Reference to the Diagnostic Criteria from DSM-IV-TR.* Washington: American Psychiatric Association; 2000:168–208.

33. Answer: B. DSM-IV-TR stipulates that both multiple motor and one or more vocal tics be present at some time during the illness but not necessarily concurrently (criterion A). The symptoms must last more than 1 year, and tic-free periods cannot last more than 3 months (criterion B). Criterion C refers to age of onset before 18 years and criterion D refers to exclusionary conditions.

American Psychiatric Association. *Diagnostic and Statistical Manual of Mental Disorders: DSM-IV-TR.* 4th ed. Washington: American Psychiatric Association; 2000:114.

34. Answer: C. GABHS can trigger a variety of immune mediated diseases in susceptible individuals. Pediatric autoimmune neuropsychiatric disorders associated with streptococcal infections (PANDAS) describes the exacerbation of tics or obsessive-compulsive symptoms triggered by GABHS autoimmune effects. The use of plasmapheresis or intravenous immunoglobulin infusion for PANDAS has been successful in limited trials but is not considered a standard of care.

1. Lewis M. *Child and Adolescent Psychiatry: A Comprehensive Textbook.* 3rd ed. Philadelphia: Lippincott Williams & Wilkins; 2002:739.
2. Swedo SE, Leonard HL, Mittleman BB, et al. Identification of children with pediatric autoimmune neuropsychiatric disorders associated with streptococcal infections by a marker associated with rheumatic fever. *Am J Psychiatry.* 1997;154:110–112.

35. **Answer: B.** A diagnosis of Delusional Disorder, Jealous type is the most likely diagnosis. Given this history, she does not have two or more characteristic symptoms needed for a diagnosis of Schizophrenia or Schizophreniform Disorder. Her delusions persist at times when there has been no mood disturbance, making Major Depressive Disorder an unlikely diagnosis. Given her age and the lack of cognitive dysfunction, a dementing illness is also unlikely.

Sadock BJ, Sadock VA. *Kaplan and Sadock's Comprehensive Textbook of Psychiatry.* 8th ed. Philadelphia: Lippincott Williams & Wilkins; 2005:1526.

36. **Answer: D.** Serious drug-drug interactions with benzodiazepines are rare, but may occur. Due to competition for microsomal enzymes, certain drugs (including cimetidine, estrogens, SSRIs, disulfiram, and erythromycin) increase blood levels of benzodiazepines. Carbamazepine, an inducer of liver enzymes, decreases blood levels of benzodiazepines. Antacids, as well as meals, tend to decrease benzodiazepine absorption; hence, patients taking these medications should be instructed to take them on an empty stomach and in the absence of antacids. Other interactions of concern with benzodiazepines include those drugs which may potentiate CNS depression, such as barbiturates, cyclic antidepressants, antihistamines, and alcohol. When taken together in overdose, alcohol and benzodiazepines may result in death.

Rosenbaum JF, Arana GW, Hyman SE, et al. *Handbook of Psychiatric Drug Therapy.* 5th ed. Philadelphia: Lippincott Williams & Wilkins; 2005:178–182.

37. **Answer: B.** EKG is not used in biofeedback. The EMG gives feedback of striate muscle tension. The EEG gives feedback of brain waves. The EDR involves feedback of sweat gland activity, measured from the fingers. The perineometer gives feedback of anal, sphincter, and pelvic floor muscles. Thermal feedback, which gives feedback of peripheral blood flow as monitored by skin temperature, is also used.

Jonas WB, Levin JS. *Essentials of Complementary and Alternative Medicine.* Philadelphia: Lippincott Williams & Wilkins; 1999:410.

38. **Answer: A.** Risperidone is most likely to elevate plasma prolactin levels resulting in prolactinemia. Prolactinemia in premenopausal women can result in hypogonadism, manifested by infertility, oligomenorrhea, or amenorrhea and, less often, galactorrhea. Prolactinemia also causes hypogonadotropic hypogonadism in men, which is manifest by decreased libido, impotence, infertility, gynecomastia, or rarely galactorrhea. In both men and women, there is an approximate correlation between serum prolactin levels and the presence of any of these symptoms. Other medications that can result in prolactinemia include metoclopramide, cimetidine, methyldopa, reserpine, and verapamil.

Rosenbaum JR, Arana GW, Hyman SE, et al. *Handbook of Psychiatric Drug Therapy.* 5th ed. Philadelphia: Lippincott Williams & Wilkins; 2005:35–36.

39. **Answer: A.** Available information indicates that age, sex, and time of year are not significantly correlated with risk of developing NMS. NMS is not specific to any neuropsychiatric diagnosis, but catatonic patients may be at risk of progressing to NMS after receiving antipsychotics. Agitation, dehydration, restraint, preexisting abnormalities of central nervous system dopamine activity or receptor function, and iron deficiency are all risk factors for NMS. Use of high-potency typical antipsychotics are associated with a greater risk compared to low-potency agents or atypical antipsychotics. Parenteral routes, higher titration rates, and total dose of drug administration have been associated with an increased risk of NMS.

Strawn JR, Keck PE Jr., Caroff SN. Neuroleptic malignant syndrome. *Am J Psychiatry.* 2007 Jun; 164(6):870–876.

40. **Answer: E.** Given the side effects of lithium, it is recommended that baseline levels of BUN, T_3, T4, T_3 resin uptake, and TSH be obtained prior to starting lithium. Women who could potentially bear children should have a beta-hCG checked. Patients who are over 50 years of age or have cardiac histories should receive an EKG. Although low sodium levels can lead to lithium toxicity, checking sodium levels is not one of the tests recommended as necessary before starting lithium.

Rosenbaum JF, Arana GW, Hyman SE, et al. *Handbook of Psychiatric Drug Therapy.* 5th ed. Philadelphia: Lippincott Williams & Wilkins; 2005:134, 148.

41. **Answer: C.** Although thoughts of death are more common in older than in younger adults, the elderly are less likely to endorse suicidal ideation than their younger counterparts. Suicide attempts are also less

frequent among the elderly than among the younger age group. The ratio of attempted suicides to suicides in adolescents is often as high as 200:1. In the elderly, the ratio is as low as one to four attempts for each suicide. Self-destructive acts that occur in the elderly are more lethal. This lethality is due to greater burden of illness, greater social isolation, and a greater determination to die. Elders give fewer warnings about their suicidal intent, use more violent and potentially deadly methods, and apply those methods with greater planning and resolve. Hence, suicide attempt in an older person confers a higher level risk for future suicides.

American Psychiatric Association. *American Psychiatric Association's Practice Guideline for the Assessment and Treatment of Patients with Suicidal Behaviors. II. Assessment of Patients with Suicidal Behaviors.* http://www.psychiatryonline.com/content.aspx?aID=56135. Accessed January 14, 2007.

42. Answer: E. Echolalia occurs in isolation aphasia and is in fact one of the key features of the syndrome. Echolalia is also seen in patients with autism, Tourette's syndrome, dementia, and Schizophrenia.

Kaufman DM. *Clinical Neurology for Psychiatrists.* 5th ed. Philadelphia: WB Saunders; 2001:182–183.

43. Answer: E. Delirium tremens is a serious form of alcohol withdrawal. Visual hallucinations of small animals or tiny men, known as Lilliputian hallucinations, can occur during delirium tremens. These hallucinations are usually characterized by all of the above noted features.

1. Sims A. *Symptoms in the Mind.* 3rd ed. London: Elsevier Science; 2003:105.
2. Wikipedia. *Delirium Tremans.* http://en.wikipedia.org/wiki/Delirium_tremens. Published January 5, 2007.

44. Answer: E. An important category of mutations is the trinucleotide repeat expansion mutations, characterized by an elongation of a gene region with repeats of a trinucleotide sequence. When the trinucleotides lie outside of the coding region, the expansions can reach a very large size. Some important disorders caused by the trinucleotide repeat expansion include Huntington's disease, Myotonic dystrophy, Fragile X syndrome, Friedreich, ataxia, and X-linked spinal and bulbar atrophy.

Goetz CG. *Textbook of Clinical Neurology.* 2nd ed. http://home.mdconsult.com/das/book/67380190-2/view/1158. Accessed March 1, 2007.

45. Answer: B. The human brain weighs approximately 350 grams at birth and approximately 1,450 grams by adulthood. This increase is mainly in the neocortex.

Sadock BJ, Sadock VA. *Kaplan and Sadock's Synopsis of Psychiatry.* 9th ed. Philadelphia: Lippincott Williams & Wilkins; 2003:23.

46. Answer: C. Axons of mesolimbic and mesocortical pathways arise from the ventral tegmental area. These pathways are an important site of action of antipsychotics (D2 and D4 antagonists). The tuberoinfundibular pathway arises from dopaminergic neuronal cell bodies in the median eminence that project to the pituitary. Release of dopamine inhibits prolactin release via activation of D2 receptors. Drugs that antagonize D2 receptors increase prolactin secretion causing amenorrhoea, lactation, and sexual dysfunction.

Anderson IM, Reid IC. *Fundamentals of Clinical Psychopharmacology.* London: Taylor & Francis; 2004:1.

47. Answer: D. The cornerstone of psychoanalytic theory is free association, in which patients say whatever comes to mind. It does more than provide content for the analysis; it induces the necessary regression and dependency connected with establishing and working through transference. Freud originally used the cathartic method in conjunction with hypnosis to attempt to remove hysterical symptoms through a process of recovering and verbalizing suppressed feelings with which the symptoms were associated, known as abreaction, but due to the forces of repression and resistance, he abandoned this cathartic method and switched to free association. He was originally convinced that childhood sexual seduction played a major role in causing the neuroses, but later shifted his thinking and placed much greater emphasis on childhood sexual fantasies as the core of neuroses. Freud believed that the interpretation of dreams was the road to understanding the unconscious. Dreamwork is defined as the unconscious mental operations by which latent dream content is transferred into manifest content.

Kaplan HI, Sadock BJ. *Kaplan & Sadock's Synopsis of Psychiatry.* 8th ed. Philadelphia: Lippincott Williams & Wilkins; 1998:206–211, 222, 887.

48. Answer: B. Claims of abandonment may be made if harm results from the unilateral termination of a therapeutic relation by the physician without consent or justification. Persistent no shows, violent behaviors, and noncompliance are likely justifications that could mitigate the claim of abandonment. Should termination of a therapeutic relationship become necessary, claims of abandonment may be ameliorated by making the following available to the patient: access to emergency care, referral to another clinician, medications in the period between termination, and appointment with another provider. A physican may be held liable for abandonment for failure to provide adequate and competent coverage in his/her absence. The very nature of a therapeutic relationship makes such a claim more likely to succeed regardless of whether the physician is physically present or not.

Gutheil TG, Applebaum PS. *Clinical Handbook of Psychiatry and The Law*. 3rd ed. Philadelphia: Lippincott Williams & Wilkins; 2000.

49. Answer: E. The disorder-centered interviewing style follows a descriptive and theoretical model of psychiatric disorders. It sees psychiatric disorders in a similar way to medical disorders, using specific diagnostic criteria. The patient-centered interviewing style is based on an introspective model, and it focuses on the intra-psychic battle of conflicts that each patient presents with. It is sensitive to a patient's educational, social, and emotional background, and it gives a lot of importance to the individuality of each patient.

Sadock BJ, Sadock VA. *Kaplan and Sadock's Comprehensive Textbook of Psychiatry*. 8th ed. Philadelphia: Lippincott Williams & Wilkins; 2005:794–800.

50. Answer: D. The specifier "with Melancholic Features" can be applied to depressive episodes occurring in Major Depressive Disorder, Bipolar I Disorder, or Bipolar II Disorder. It is characterized by either the loss of pleasure in all—or almost all—pleasurable activities or the lack of reactivity to usually pleasurable stimuli, in addition to the following: (i) distinct quality of depressed mood, (ii) depression worse in the morning, (iii) early morning awakening, (iv) marked psychomotor retardation or agitation, and (v) anorexia or weight loss and excessive or inappropriate guilt. Characteristics of an MDE with Atypical Features include mood reactivity and two or more of the following: (i) significant weight gain or increase in appetite, (ii) hypersomnia, (iii) laden paralysis, and/or (iv) long standing pattern of rejection sensitivity.

American Psychiatric Association. *Quick Reference to the Diagnostic Criteria from DSM-IV-TR*. Washington: American Psychiatric Association; 2000:168–208.

51. Answer: B. Initial symptoms of Tourette's syndrome generally appear in prepuberty between the ages of 5 and 8 years. Motor tics appear before vocal tics by age 1 or 2 years and are often simple tics initially such as eye blinking or grimacing.

Wiener JM, Dulcan MK. *Textbook of Child and Adolescent Psychiatry*. 3rd ed. Washington: American Psychiatric Publishing; 2004:711.

52. Answer: E. Voiding of urine into bed or clothes must occur twice a week for 3 consecutive months for the condition to meet the DSM-IV-TR criteria for Enuresis. However, in the presence of significant impairment or distress, the criteria for frequency and duration are not required. An age of at least 5 years or equivalent developmental level is required. The types to be specified are Nocturnal Only, Diurnal Only, or Nocturnal and Diurnal.

American Psychiatric Association. *Diagnostic and Statistical Manual of Mental Disorders: DSM-IV-TR*. 4th ed. Washington: American Psychiatric Association; 2000:121.

53. Answer: A. Presence of negative symptoms is associated with poor outcome in Schizophrenia. Acute onset, late onset, good premorbid functioning, and a short time between psychotic symptoms and medication initiation are predictors of good outcomes.

Sadock BJ, Sadock VA. *Kaplan and Sadock's Comprehensive Textbook of Psychiatry*. 8th ed. Philadelphia: Lippincott Williams & Wilkins; 2005:1551.

54. Answer: E. It has been hypothesized that NA systems are an integral component of fear and anxiety. As such, beta-blockers are competitive antagonists of norepinephrine and epinephrine at beta-adrenergic receptors. They may be clinically useful in the treatment of heightened anxiety states. Beta-blockers have not been convincingly shown to be useful for generalized social anxiety disorder, but may be more useful for anxiety limited to a specific situation (i.e., performance anxiety). When used for performance anxiety, a single dose of 10 to 40 mg of propranolol may be beneficial in reducing the peripheral effects of anxiety (i.e., dry mouth, palpitations, and tremors). Unlike benzodiazepines, which may also be helpful for heightened anxiety states, beta-blockers do not have an effect on memory or learning. They may, in fact, improve performance on tasks involving memory and learning by reducing anxiety levels, as such tasks are very sensitive to anxiety. In addition, beta-blockers do not induce tolerance nor do they have abuse potential like benzodiazepines. Lipophilic beta-blockers, including propranolol and metoprolol, cross the blood-brain barrier and have central, as well as peripheral, effects. Metoprolol and atenolol are considered selective beta-blockers, with greater activity at B1 then B2 receptors, thereby reducing the risk of bronchospasm with these medications. However, this selectivity is relative, and physicians must still exercise caution when using any beta-blocker in certain patient populations (i.e., those with asthma and those with diabetes, as beta-blockers may also mask the symptoms of hypoglycemia).

Rosenbaum JF, Arana GW, Hyman SE, et al. *Handbook of Psychiatric Drug Therapy*. 5th ed. Philadelphia: Lippincott Williams & Wilkins; 2005:188–191.

55. **Answer: E.** Zolpidem is a non-benzodiazepine hypnotic of the imidazopyridine class. It is primarily beneficial for sleep-onset-related insomnia but has no muscle relaxant, anxiolytic, or anticonvulsant effects. Zolpidem is rapidly absorbed after oral administration and reaches peak blood levels in about 2.2 hours. It is also highly protein bound. Its elimination half-life is 2 to 3 hours, and its duration of action is 6 to 8 hours. It does not have any active metabolites. Zolpidem has sleep-enhancing properties, but is less likely to affect sleep architecture. Zolpidem appears to be well tolerated in adults and in the elderly when administered appropriately. The available data indicates that when zolpidem is administered according to instructions the risk of abuse or dependence is low. Zolpidem has minimal rebound effects and less abuse potential than benzodiazepines. Its starting dose in adults is 10 mg orally immediately before bedtime, and its maximal dose is 20 mg. In the elderly, the starting dose is 5 mg immediately before bedtime.

1. Albers LJ, Hahn RK, Reist C. *Handbook of Psychiatric Drugs*. Laguna Hills: Current Clinical Strategies Publishing; 2005:66.
2. Rosenbaum JF, Arana GW, Hyman SE, et al. *Handbook of Psychiatric Drug Therapy*. 5th ed. Philadelphia: Lippincott Williams & Wilkins; 2005:260–261.

56. **Answer: C.** Clozapine has affinity for five types of receptors: dopamine, muscarinic, serotonin, alpha-adrenergic, and histamine receptors.

Rosenbaum JR, Arana GW, Hyman SE, et al. *Handbook of Psychiatric Drug Therapy*. 5th ed. Philadelphia: Lippincott Williams & Wilkins; 2005:34–35.

57. **Answer: D.** Although all of the above choices are treatment considerations in dealing with patients with neuroleptic malignant syndrome, the single most important intervention is discontinuation of the neuroleptic agent.

Wijdicks E. *Neuroleptic Malignant Syndrome*. http://www.uptodateonline.com/utd/content/topic.do?topicKey=medneuro/5946&type=A&selectedTitle=1~17. Accessed January 23, 2007.

58. **Answer: A.** A high potency, short-acting benzodiazepine, such as immediate release alprazolam, has an increased risk of interdose rebound symptoms. Clonazepam and diazepam are low-potency, longer-acting benzodiazepines. Venlafaxine and buspirone do not cause interdose rebound anxiety.

Rosenbaum JR, Arana GW, Hyman SE, et al. *Handbook of Psychiatric Drug Therapy*. 5th ed. Philadelphia: Lippincott Williams & Wilkins; 2005:178.

59. **Answer: E.** Suicide risk increases with age for both sexes, but the rates in older men are generally higher than those for women. In the United States, men commit suicide 4 times more commonly than women, but women attempt suicide 3 times as often as men. However, this female predominance among suicide attempters varies with age and the ratio of women to men approaches 1:1 in the elderly. Men also tend to use more lethal suicide methods than women (e.g., firearms or hanging, as compared to cutting or overdoses). Factors that contribute to these gender differences include the presence of depression and co-morbid alcohol and/or substance abuse. Men are also less likely to seek and accept help or treatment. Women tend to have lower rates of alcohol and substance abuse, are less impulsive, are more socially embedded, and are more willing to seek help. In women, pregnancy is a time of significantly reduced suicide risk. Women with young children in the home are less likely to kill themselves. But those women with a history of depression or suicide attempts are at greater risk during the postpartum period, as compared to women who don't have such a history. Suicide is most likely to occur in the first month after delivery, but the risk continues throughout the postpartum period. Teenagers, women of lower socioeconomic status, and women hospitalized with postpartum psychiatric disorders are particularly at increased risk in the postpartum period.

American Psychiatric Association. *American Psychiatric Association's Practice Guideline for the Assessment and Treatment of Patients with Suicidal Behaviors. II. Assessment of Patients with Suicidal Behaviors*. http://www.psychiatryonline.com/content.aspx?aID=56135. Accessed January 14, 2007.

60. **Answer: D.** Gait apraxia is seen in normal pressure hydrocephalus. Apraxia is characterized by the inability to perform learned or familiar movements on command, even though the command is understood and both sensory and motor functions are in tact. There are several different forms of apraxia. Ideomotor apraxia is the inability to carry out a command from the brain to mimic limb or head movements

performed or suggested by others. Conceptual apraxia is much like ideomotor ataxia but infers a more profound malfunctioning, in which the function of tools is no longer understood. Ideational apraxia is the inability to create a plan for a specific movement. Constructional apraxia affects the person's ability to draw or copy simple diagrams or to construct simple figures. Buccofacial apraxia (sometimes called facial-oral apraxia) is the inability to coordinate and carry out facial and lip movements such as whistling, winking, or coughing on command. This form includes verbal or speech developmental apraxia, perhaps the most common form of the disorder.

Kaufman DM. *Clinical Neurology for Psychiatrists*. 5th ed. Philadelphia: WB Saunders; 2001:186.

61. Answer: E. All of the choices from A to D are possible manifestations of an acute dystonic reaction. Dystonia can be a result of antidopaminergic medications and is manifested by muscular contractions, repetitive or abnormal movements, or abnormal postures. Akathisia is not classified as a dystonic reaction.

Sims A. *Symptoms in the Mind*. 3rd ed. London: Elsevier Science; 2003:36.

62. Answer: D. Temporal arteritis has an annual incidence of about 25 per 100,000 in people older than 50 years. It occurs predominantly in women (65%). The average age of onset is 70 years. Blindness occurs in about 50% of the patients, if untreated. Patients may also develop thrombosis of any predural artery or aortic aneurysm with rupture, if left untreated. The most common initial symptom is headache. It commonly occurs with malaise and myalgia. It may be unilateral or bilateral and is located to the temporal area in only about 50% of the patients. Headache, polymyalgia rheumatica, jaw or tongue claudication, fever, and weight loss can also occur. The pain usually develops slowly and is described as a dull ache with occasional sharp pains. Patients may have allodynia with marked scalp tenderness. Headaches are often worse at night and are worsened by exposure to cold. The ESR is often elevated, but a normal ESR does not exclude temporal arteritis. Serum viscosity and C-reactive protein levels are often elevated and may be helpful in the diagnosis or to follow-up the effect of treatment, in those with normal ESR. Plasma interleukin-6 (IL-6) is thought to be the most sensitive marker of disease activity. After temporal artery biopsy is done, prednisone therapy should be promptly initiated at 80 mg daily for 4 to 6 weeks.

1. Rowland LP. *Merritt's Neurology*. 11th ed. Philadelphia: Lippincott Williams & Wilkins; 2005:988–989.

2. Unwin B, Williams CM, Gilliland W. Polymyalgia rheumatica and giant cell arteritis. *Am Fam Physician*. 2006;74:1547–1554.

63. Answer: E. The Folstein MMSE is a brief examination consisting of 11 questions that evaluates an adult's level of cognitive functioning. Introduced in 1975, it is designed to evaluate cognitive functioning in elderly patients who are able to cooperate at an optimum level with an examiner for only a brief period of time. It is used most often to evaluate older adults for delirium or dementia. The MMSE can also be used to detect a decline in cognitive function, to follow the course of the patient's illness, and to monitor responses to treatment. It was recently approved as a measurement of the patient's ability to complete an advance directive (living will). The test has also been used in research studies. The MMSE evaluates six areas of cognitive function: orientation, attention, immediate recall, short-term recall, language, and the ability to follow simple verbal and written commands. It also provides a total score allowing the examiner to place the patient on a scale of cognitive function. It correlates well with a standard measure of cognition in adults like the WAIS-R. The results of the MMSE should be interpreted in the context of the patient's history, a full mental status examination, a physical examination, and laboratory findings. A score on the MMSE must be interpreted according to the patient's age and educational level. A median score of 29 is normal for a person 18 to 24 years of age, whereas a score of 25 is normal for someone 80 years or older. The median score is 22 for persons with a fourth-grade education or less, 26 for those who completed the eighth grade, and 29 for those who completed high school or college. The MMSE should only be administered and scored by a qualified health care professional.

1. Goetz CG. *Textbook of Clinical Neurology*. 2nd ed. http://home.mdconsult.com/das/book/67380190-2/view/1158. Accessed January 29, 2007.

2. Encyclopedia of Mental Disorders. *Mini-mental State Examination*. http://www.minddisorders.com/Kau-Nu/Mini-mental-state-examination.html. Accessed January 29, 2007.

64. Answer: C. When the index of suspicion is high for subarachnoid hemorrhage, but the CT scan does not reveal any bleeding, a lumbar puncture must be performed to rule out this high mortality condition (Note: 5% of cases can have normal CT scans). The patient's vascular risk factors (hypertension and tobacco use), as well as late stage pregnancy, increase the likelihood that subarachnoid hemorrhage is present. A CT scan is preferable to MRI when assessing intracerebral bleeding, and the utility of emergent surgery in subarachnoid bleeds has not been well established in research trials.

Goetz CG. *Textbook of Clinical Neurology*. 2nd ed. Philadelphia: WB Saunders; 2003:1009–1010.

65. Answer: A. The patient has hemiplegic CP. CP is a nonprogressive disorder, or static encephalopathy, consisting of abnormal movement or posture and is the result of an injury to the developing brain, usually before the age of 5. The three main types of CP are spastic, extrapyramidal, and mixed. Spastic CP is the most common. Spastic CP types are, in order of frequency, quadriplegia, hemiplegia, or diplegia. Extrapyramidal CP may consist of movement disorders such as chorea, athetosis, or dystonia. Extrapyramidal CP is also known as dyskinetic CP. Normal intelligence is found in 50% of patients with CP. Epilepsy is common.

Roberts KB. *Manual of Clinical Problems in Pediatrics*. 5th ed. Philadelphia: Lippincott Williams & Wilkins; 2001:384–385.

66. Answer: D. The Research Society on Alcoholism Fetal Alcohol Study group recommends the following criteria for FAS: (a) the presence of prenatal or postnatal growth retardation, (b) CNS dysfunction including developmental delay or intellectual compromise, and (c) at least two of the following: microcephaly, microphthalmia, short palpebral fissures, hypoplastic philtrum with thin upper lip and flattening of the maxillary area. In FAS, IQ is in the mild mental retardation to low average range. FAS occurs in 1 to 2 of 1,000 live births, while partial expression of the syndrome, fetal alcohol effects, occurs in 3 to 5 of 1,000 live births. ADHD is common in children with FAS. Down (Trisomy 21) syndrome includes microcephaly, upslanting palpebral fissures, open mouth with protruding tongue, and midface hypoplasia. Williams's syndrome consists of a microdeletion on chromosome 7. Craniofacial characteristics include "elfin-like" facies, medial eyebrow flare, stellate irises, mild microcephaly, and a long, flat philtrum. Lead toxicity may lead to symptoms of hyperactivity and other neuropsychiatric problems, but does not lead to characteristic craniofacial abnormalities.

Menkes JH, Sarnat HB, Maria BL. *Child Neurology*. 7th ed. Philadelphia: Lippincott Williams & Wilkins; 2006: 709–710.

67. Answer: B. This patient has acute meningitis from *S. pneumoniae*. The clinical symptoms, physical signs, and laboratory findings in pneumococcal meningitis are the same as those in other forms of acute purulent meningitis and the diagnosis is usually made by identifying Gram-positive diplococci in smears of the CSF or its sediment and a positive quellung reaction that serves to identify both the pneumococcus and its type. Particle agglutination of CSF and serum may be helpful in demonstrating pneumococcal antigen. *S. pneumoniae* is almost equal in frequency to meningococcus as a cause of meningitis, but it is seen more frequently in the elderly patients. It is usually a complication of otitis media, mastoiditis, sinusitis, fractures of the skull, upper respiratory infections, and infections of the lung. Alcoholism, asplenism, and sickle cell disease predispose patients to developing pneumococcal meningitis. More than 50% of the patients are younger than 1 year of age or older than 50 years of age.

Mortality rate is approximately 20% to 30%, with 30% of the survivors having permanent sequelae. Third-generation cephalosporin is the initial treatment for *S. pneumoniae*, until sensitivities are established, but vancomycin is often used as initial treatment. The treatment should be continued for 12 to 15 days. Chloramphenicol remains as an alternative drug for adults who are sensitive to the penicillins or cephalosporins.

Rowland LP. *Merritt's Neurology*. 11th ed. Philadelphia: Lippincott Williams & Wilkins; 2005:143.

68. Answer: D. Tabes dorsalis, formerly the most common type of neurosyphilis, is now rare. It affects the posterior columns of the spinal cord and of the dorsal roots. It manifests about 18 to 25 years after initial untreated infection and presents with paresthesias, abnormal gait, and lightning (sudden severe) pains of the extremities or the trunk. Upon physical examination, there is presence of reduced peripheral reflexes, loss of position and vibration senses, and occasionally a positive Romberg sign. Patients may also present with sensory losses. Vision can be poor due to optic atrophy. Patients may present with ARP in advanced cases, but are not pathognomonic of tertiary syphilis as it can occur in other conditions including diabetes. Abnormal CSF findings are less common than in other types of neurosyphilis, and the CSF VDRL can be normal in as many as one third of the cases.

1. Rowland LP. *Merritt's Neurology*. 11th ed. Philadelphia: Lippincott Williams & Wilkins; 2005:236–242.
2. Sparling FP, Hicks CB. *Clinical manifestations of neurosyphilis*. http://www.uptodateonline.com/utd/content/topic.do?topicKey=stds/8400&type=A&selectedTitle=1~11. Accessed January 22, 2007.

69. Answer: D. Clinical presentation and history are extremely useful in the diagnosis of PML. Typically, patients manifest with subacute neurologic deficits. If HIV positive, the CD4 count is frequently less than 200 per cubic mm. The typical appearance on neuroimaging is that of symmetric or asymmetric areas of white matter demyelination that are not consistent with a vascular territory. However, definitive diagnosis can only be made by brain biopsy, which should reveal JC virus infected oligodendrocytes, reactive gliosis, and macrophages with myelin and cellular debris. A JC virus polymerase chain reaction assay is useful in the diagnosis, but a CNS fluid sample should be used.

Koralnik I. *Progressive Multifocal Leukoencephalopathy.* http://www.uptodateonline.com/utd/content/topic.do? topicKey=demyelin/6861&type=A&selectedTitle=2~12. Accessed January 22, 2007.

70. Answer: C. Thymectomy is a treatment option in patients with uncomplicated myasthenia gravis who are between puberty and age 55 years. The remission rate is 35% and another 50% show some improvement. Response is usually evident after several months to 3 years. Individuals with intractable bilateral frontal seizures or infants with atonic seizures occasionally benefit from commissurotomy or corpus callostomy. A complication of the surgery may be split-brain syndrome. Surgical treatments for Parkinson's disease are thalamotomy and pallidotomy. In persistent, disabling, and drug-resistant Ménière disease cases, surgical procedures such as endolymphatic shunting, labyrinthectomy, or vestibular nerve section may be helpful.

1. Greenberg DA, Aminoff MJ, Simon RP. *Clinical Neurology.* 5th ed. New York: McGraw-Hill; 2002:109–110, 183–186, 239–247.
2. Kaufman DM. *Clinical Neurology for Psychiatrists.* 5th ed. Philadelphia: WB Saunders; 2001:191–192, 247.

71. Answer: E. All neurons are thought to be generated during gestation; thereafter, their differentiation continues, including the formation of synapses, and reaches a peak during the second year of life. The cell layers are established before birth. Fluid volume increases but is not the main reason for increased size and weight; the gyri represent underlying neuronal architecture, including dendritic branching.

1. Sadock BJ, Sadock VA. *Kaplan and Sadock's Synopsis of Psychiatry.* 9th ed. Philadelphia: Lippincott Williams & Wilkins; 2003:23.
2. Lewis M. *Child and Adolescent Psychiatry: A Comprehensive Textbook.* 3rd ed. Philadelphia: Lippincott Williams & Wilkins; 2002:40.

72. Answer: D. D3 and D4 receptors are localized in distribution, seen in mesolimbic, cortical, and hippocampal areas. There are two families of dopamine receptors: (a) D1-like receptors which include the D1 and D5 receptors, and (b) D2-like receptors which include D2, D3, and D4 receptors. The D1 and D2 receptors are widely distributed in the mesocortical, striatal, and hypothalamic areas.

Anderson IM, Reid IC. *Fundamentals of Clinical Psychopharmacology.* London: Taylor & Francis; 2004:12.

73. Answer: B. Narcissistic defenses are the most primitive and appear in children and people who are psychotically disturbed. These defenses include: denial, distortion, and projection. Projection is the perceiving and reacting to unacceptable inner impulses as though they were outside the self. On a psychotic level, this takes the form of frank delusions about external reality (usually persecutory) and includes both perception of one's own feelings in another and subsequent acting on the perception (psychotic paranoid delusions). Asceticism and sublimation are mature defenses. The former refers to the elimination of a pleasurable experience due to an assigned moral element to that experience. The latter refers to achieving impulse gratification and retention of goals, but by altering a socially objectionable aim to a socially acceptable one. Rationalization is a neurotic defense in which one offers rational explanations in an attempt to justify unacceptable attitudes or behaviors. Reaction formation is a neurotic defense involving transforming an unacceptable impulse into its opposite, and is characteristic of obsessional neurosis.

Kaplan HI, Sadock BJ. *Kaplan & Sadock's Synopsis of Psychiatry.* 8th ed. Philadelphia: Lippincott Williams & Wilkins; 1998:218–222.

74. Answer: D. Medicare is a health insurance program that is administered by the United States government and covers people who 65 years and above, or who are under 65 years but are disabled or have ESRD. It is administered by the Centers for Medicare and Medicaid Services, a component of the Department of Health and Human Services, which also administers Medicaid and other programs. Medicare is partially financed by payroll taxes imposed by the Federal Insurance Contributions Act and the Self-Employment Contributions Act of 1954. Individuals aged 65 years or older are eligible for Medicare if they (or their spouse) have worked for at least 10 years in Medicare-covered employment and are a citizen or permanent resident of the United States of America. Individuals who are under 65 years may also be eligible if they are disabled or have ESRD. These individuals must be receiving disability benefits from either Social Security or the Railroad Retirement Board for at least 24 months before automatic enrollment occurs.

There are four parts to Medicare. Part A of Medicare covers hospital stays. It will pay for nursing home stays as well, if certain criteria are met. The maximum length of stay that Medicare Part A will cover in a skilled nursing facility per ailment is 100 days. The first 20 of those days would be paid for in full by Medicare with the remaining 80 days requiring a copayment. Part B medical insurance helps pay for some services and products not covered by Part A, generally on an outpatient basis. Part B is optional and may be deferred if the beneficiary or their spouse is still actively working. Part B coverage includes physician and nursing services, x-rays, laboratory and diagnostic tests, influenza and pneumonia vaccinations, blood transfusions, renal dialysis, outpatient hospital procedures, and limited ambulance transportation. Part B also helps cover the cost of canes, walkers, wheelchairs, and mobility scooters for those with mobility impairments. In Part C of the plan, the Medicare beneficiaries are provided their benefits through private health insurance plans, instead of through the original Medicare plan (Parts A and B). These plans are now known as Medicare Advantage plans. They offer coverage comparable to Part A and Part B, and may also offer Part D coverage. Medicare Part D provides prescription drug plan. Anyone receiving Medicare Part A and B was eligible to enroll in Part D plan. The individual must enroll in a stand-alone Prescription Drug Plan or Medicare Advantage Prescription Drug Plan with prescription drug coverage. These plans are approved and regulated by the Medicare program, but administered by private health insurance companies.

Blazer DG, Steffens DC, Busse EW. *The American Psychiatric Association Textbook of Geriatric Psychiatry*. Washington: American Psychiatric Publishing; 2004:515–516.

75. Answer: A. Sublimation is a mature defense mechanism, where a patient rechannels unacceptable impulses into socially acceptable expressions. When using humor as a defense mechanism, a person changes his feelings of anxiety into comedy or irony. Altruism refers to replacing aggression and competition by support. When using suppression, there is an intentional blocking of a specific memory. In displacement, a patient transfers a feeling from its actual object to another object that is acting as a substitute.

Sadock BJ, Sadock VA. *Kaplan and Sadock's Comprehensive Textbook of Psychiatry*. 8th ed. Philadelphia: Lippincott Williams & Wilkins; 2005:800–810.

76. Answer: A. Positive and negative symptoms of schizophrenia were first described by Emil Kraepelin in an attempt to differentiate dementia praecox, also known as dementia of the young, from manic-depressive disorder. Eugen Bleuler introduced the term Schizophrenia and described the four primary symptoms of Schizophrenia. Thomas Szasz proposed Schizophrenia is a myth that enables society to manage deviant behavior. Ewald Hecker described hebephrenia, disorganized psychosis with early onset and poor prognosis. Haslam Morel described psychotic symptoms in patients at the end of the 18th century.

Sadock BJ, Sadock VA. *Kaplan and Sadock's Comprehensive Textbook of Psychiatry*. 8th ed. Philadelphia: Lippincott Williams & Wilkins; 2005:1329, 1418.

77. Answer: C. Tic-related OCD is thought to have an earlier age of onset and greater male preponderance. Obsessions tend to be concerned with religion, sex, and aggression. Tic-related compulsions are often driven by the desire to perform a task "just right" rather than by anxiety.

1. Leckman JF, Cohen DJ. *Tourette's Syndrome–Tics, Obsessions, Compulsions: Developmental Psychopathology and Clinical Care*. New York: Wiley;1999:43–62.
2. Wiener JM, Dulcan MK. *Textbook of Child and Adolescent Psychiatry*. 3rd ed. Washington: American Psychiatric Publishing; 2004:712.

78. Answer: A. A diagnosis of enuresis is excluded if voiding is the direct result of a medication effect or a medical condition and/or the child has mental retardation that puts the child below the equivalent developmental level of 5 years. Some children with enuresis have been found to have a functionally small bladder. Although the other options do not automatically exclude the diagnosis of enuresis, a functionally small bladder is least likely to do so.

1. American Psychiatric Association. *Diagnostic and Statistical Manual of Mental Disorders: DSM-IV-TR*. 4th ed. Washington: American Psychiatric Association; 2000: 121.
2. Lewis M. *Child and Adolescent Psychiatry: A Comprehensive Textbook*. 3rd ed. Philadelphia: Lippincott Williams & Wilkins; 2002:701.

79. Answer: E. Maladaptive parenting, including the concept of the "schizophrenogenic mother", was a once widely held and now debunked theory for the cause of Schizophrenia.

Sadock BJ, Sadock VA. *Kaplan and Sadock's Comprehensive Textbook of Psychiatry*. 8th ed. Philadelphia: Lippincott Williams & Wilkins; 2005:1390.

80. Answer: A. Only two SSRIs (paroxetine and sertraline) are approved by the Food and Drug

Administration (FDA) for the treatment of PTSD, although the other SSRIs are often used off-label. Fluoxetine has shown positive benefit in placebo-controlled studies. Dosing of SSRIs for the treatment of PTSD is similar to that for treatment of depression (e.g., equivalent of 50 to 200 mg of sertraline daily). There have been promising open trials of the serotonin-norepinephrine reuptake inhibitor (SNRI) venlafaxine, which has prompted the off-label use of this medication and fellow SNRI, duloxetine, for PTSD. Again, dosing is similar to that for depression (e.g., 75 to 225 mg of venlafaxine daily). Mirtazapine 15 to 45 mg daily has shown evidence of efficacy for the treatment of PTSD in a small placebo-controlled trial. There are no studies showing efficacy of trazodone or bupropion for the treatment of PTSD. Other antidepressant classes such as tricyclics and MAOIs have been used off-label for PTSD, generally only if all other classes of antidepressants have failed, given their side effect profile, drug-drug interactions, and lethality in overdose.

Rosenbaum JF, Arana GW, Hyman SE, et al. *Handbook of Psychiatric Drug Therapy*. 5th ed. Philadelphia: Lippincott Williams & Wilkins; 2005:199.

81. **Answer: E.** In patients taking cimetidine, the dose of zaleplon used should be half the regular dose as cimetidine increases its serum concentration by up to 80%. Zaleplon is a non-benzodiazepine hypnotic and is a pyrazolopyrimidine derivative. It has full agonist activity at central benzodiazepine (BZD2) receptors. As it has a very short half-life of almost 1 hour, it is useful in patients who have trouble falling asleep or for those who wake up at night and who have trouble falling back to sleep. It is rapidly absorbed after oral administration, and is metabolized in the liver by aldehyde oxidase and to a lesser extent by cytochrome P450 (CYP) 3A4. In recommended doses, it decreases the sleep latency with minimal effect on sleep stages. Zaleplon at the recommended dose of 10 mg is free of residual hypnotic or sedative effects even when administered 2 hours before waking in normal subjects. In the recommended dose of 10 mg, zaleplon does not significantly impair cognitive or psychomotor skills.

1. Janicak PG, Davis JM, Preskorn SH. *Principles and Practice of Psychopharmacotherapy*. 3rd ed. Philadelphia: Lippincott Williams & Wilkins; 2001:485.
2. Rosenbaum JR, Arana GW, Hyman SE, et al. *Handbook of Psychiatric Drug Therapy*. 5th ed. Philadelphia: Lippincott Williams & Wilkins; 2005:260–261.

82. **Answer: B.** Although this patient may have a community-acquired pneumonia that can be treated with a course of antibiotics, the fact that she was recently put on clozapine makes it imperative to obtain a complete blood count to rule out agranulocytosis (with a possible opportunistic infection). The incidence rate of agranulocytosis with clozapine is approximately 1% to 3%, and more than 95% of cases of agranulocytosis occur within the first 6 months of treatment, with the period of highest risk between weeks 4 and 18. Risk appears to increase in age and be higher in women. It is imperative to monitor white blood cell counts weekly for the first 6 months, then biweekly. Seizures can be an adverse side effect of clozapine and the risk of seizures increases significantly with dosages of 600 mg and above, from 1% to 2% to 3% to 5%. There is no clinical data, however, to support seizure prophylaxis in patients taking clozapine in the setting of a fever.

Rosenbaum JF, Arana GW, Hyman SE, et al. *Handbook of Psychiatric Drug Therapy*. 5th ed. Philadelphia: Lippincott Williams & Wilkins; 2005:50, 134–135.

83. **Answer: D.** The cholinergic system is important in cognitive processes, and most currently available treatments for AD are acetylcholinesterase inhibitors. Memantine, a low affinity NMDA receptor antagonist, is also approved, and can be used in conjunction with the acetylcholinesterase inhibitors (donepezil, rivastigmine, and galantamine). Despite their modest clinical effect, they are in wide spread use. Donepezil and memantine are given once a day, but the others have to be given twice because of their short half-life. Donepezil lacks hepatotoxicity, and has the least gastrointestinal side effects of the acetylcholinesterase inhibitors.

Rosenbaum JF, Arana GW, Hyman SE, et al. *Handbook of Psychiatric Drug Therapy*. 5th ed. Philadelphia: Lippincott Williams & Wilkins; 2005:269–274.

84. **Answer: E.** Although paroxetine and escitalopram are the only SSRIs approved by the FDA for use in treatment of Generalized Anxiety Disorder, no data suggests superior efficacy of one SSRI over another.

Rosenbaum JR, Arana GW, Hyman SE, et al. *Handbook of Psychiatric Drug Therapy*. 5th ed. Philadelphia: Lippincott Williams & Wilkins; 2005:177.

85. **Answer: B.** Confronting patients with Conversion Disorder about the unreal nature of their symptoms can make their condition worse. One of the distinguishing criteria of Conversion Disorders is that they contain one or more neurological symptoms that suggest a medical condition but cannot be explained by a medical or culturally sanctioned etiology (moreover, the symptoms cannot be faked). Some patients

who have severe symptoms exhibit what is called *la belle indifference*, an odd indifference to their symptoms. Patients sometimes model their symptoms on the real symptoms of a person (e.g., a loved, deceased person) with whom they identify. Studies are now finding that biological factors may be involved in conversion disorders.

Sadock BJ, Sadock VA. *Kaplan and Sadock's Comprehensive Textbook of Psychiatry*. 8th ed. Philadelphia: Lippincott Williams & Wilkins; 2005:1814–1818.

86. **Answer: A.** Patients with fluent aphasias have difficulty comprehending but have a normal quality of speech with paraphasic errors. Paraphasic errors can include circumlocution and related word substitutions as described above. They can also include unrelated words, generic substitutions, word altering, neologisms, clang associations, and tangential speech. The patient has normal prosody and tone consistent with their emotions, which indicates that the right cerebral hemisphere is intact. Fluent aphasias are usually caused by small strokes in the temporoparietal area or by diffuse disease as seen as AD.

Kaufman DM. *Clinical Neurology for Psychiatrists*. 5th ed. Philadelphia: WB Saunders; 2001:181–182.

87. **Answer: A.** Auditory, not visual, hallucinations are part of Schneider's first-rank symptoms of Schizophrenia. Primary delusions, as well as delusions of being controlled (including passivity over one's thoughts, feelings, or body), and thought withdrawal, insertion, or broadcasting are all included in Schneider's first-rank symptoms.

Sims A. *Symptoms in the Mind*. 3rd ed. London: Elsevier Science; 2003:414.

88. **Answer: B.** Patients with Huntington's disease often present with cognitive dysfunction. In these patients, long-term memory is spared, but executive functions (such as organizing, planning, checking, or adapting alternatives) and the acquisition of new motor skills are delayed. These functions worsen over time and it is noted that speech deteriorates faster than comprehension. In these patients, psychiatric and behavioral symptoms are often seen, but do not show stepwise progression with disease severity. Depression is common and suicide rates are 5 to 10 times that of the general population (5% to 10%). Manic and psychotic symptoms also commonly occur in these patients.

Walker FO. Huntington's disease. *Lancet*. 2007;369:218–228.

89. **Answer: C.** The respiratory pattern described is Cheyne-Stokes respirations. They are produced as a result of bilateral hemispheric dysfunction, and can frequently be seen with strokes, head injuries, brain tumors, and in patients with congestive heart failure.

Goetz CG. *Textbook of Clinical Neurology*. 2nd ed. Philadelphia: WB Saunders; 2003:9.

90. **Answer: E.** Due to the fact that the corticospinal tract is supplied by the anterior spinal artery, compromise of this artery causes motor deficits as listed in Choice E. Thermoanesthesia is also commonly seen due to the involvement of the spinothalamic tracts. As the dorsal columns are not supplied by the anterior spinal artery, light touch and position sense are not affected. Autonomic function is more associated with upper motor lesions.

Goetz CG. *Textbook of Clinical Neurology*. 2nd ed. Philadelphia: WB Saunders; 2003:416–417.

91. **Answer: A.** In spina bifida occulta, the posterior vertebral arches fail to fuse. It occurs in 5% of the population and is usually asymptomatic (often discovered incidentally on x-ray), but a small number of individuals have abnormalities that affect the spinal cord and these can lead to incontinence and gait disturbances. Other conditions involving problems of neural tube closure include: (i) meningocele, which involves protrusion of the meninges alone and does not lead to neurologic deficits, and (ii) myelomeningocele, which involves protrusion of the meninges and other elements of the spinal cord. Myelomeningocele is usually accompanied by major neurologic deficits; two common problems are paralysis of the lower extremities and bladder and bowel incontinence. An elevated maternal alpha-fetoprotein screen in the second trimester prompts an amniocentesis which confirms elevated alpha-fetoprotein in the amniotic sac. An ultrasound can then be used to visualize the myelomeningocele (or other causes of an elevated alpha-fetoprotein).

Roberts KB. *Manual of Clinical Problems in Pediatrics*. 5th ed. Philadelphia: Lippincott Williams & Wilkins; 2001: 384–385.

92. **Answer: A.** Leukodystrophies are inherited, progressive, neurodegenerative disorders of myelin formation. Metachromatic leukodystrophy is an autosomal recessive disorder and results from a deficiency in sulfatide sulfatase (arylsulfatase A). This leads to widespread loss of myelin in the brain and segmental demyelination of the peripheral nerves. The three forms are infantile, juvenile, and adult; the latter two often initially present with behavioral changes and a decline in school or work performance. Motor dysfunction is inevitable. Death ensues within 6 years

in the infantile and juvenile forms. The adult form progresses more slowly. Adrenoleukodystrophy has three forms, including X-linked adrenoleukodystrophy. Each form is characterized by excessive very long chain fatty acids and their elevation makes the diagnosis. It, too, may present with behavioral changes or decline in school performance and motor deficits. Seizures occur in 20% and can be the disease's first manifestation. The mean age of onset is 8 years. Progression of the disease results in psychomotor retardation, spasticity, and extensor posturing; death occurs within 10 years. Adrenal insufficiency (fatigue, anorexia, nausea/vomiting, and abdominal pain) is present in 40% of children.

McMillan JA, Feigin RD, DeAngelis C, Jones MD. *Oski's Pediatrics*. 4th ed. Philadelphia: Lippincott Williams & Wilkins; 2006:2350–2351.

93. Answer: B. Acute bacterial meningitis can be caused by an infection from almost any pathogenic bacteria, but in the United States, *S. pneumoniae* now accounts for about one half of cases with *N. meningitidis* accounting for about one fourth of the cases. In the neonatal period, group B *streptococci* and *Escherichia coli* are the most common causative agents and about 60% of all postneonatal bacterial meningitis of children used to be caused by *H. influenzae*.

Rowland LP. *Merritt's Neurology*. 11th ed. Philadelphia: Lippincott Williams & Wilkins; 2005:139.

94. Answer: D. HIV-1-associated MCMD is used to describe patients who demonstrate mild cognitive, motor, or behavioral problems associated with HIV but do not have serious impairment in daily functioning. MCMD is clinically diagnosed if the patient presents with at least two of the following symptoms: impaired attention or coordination, mental slowing, impaired memory, slowed movements, or incoordination. These patients with MCMD usually present with a clear consciousness. These symptoms are subtle and often missed. It is unclear as to if MCMD is a risk factor for or an early manifestation of HAD. To date there are no controlled trials for the treatment of MCMD.

Thompson AW, Pieper AA, Treisman GJ. *Dementia and Delirium in HIV-infected Patients*. http://www. uptodateonline.com/utd/content/topic.do?topicKey= hiv_infe/20631. Accessed January 23, 2007.

95. Answer: A. Guillain-Barré syndrome most commonly presents with proximal leg weakness. In approximately 10% of patients, it can begin with the muscles of the arms or face. In 30% of cases, severe respiratory muscle weakness can develop later in the disease course, necessitating mechanical ventilation. The involuntary muscles of the gut are not typically affected.

Vriesendorp F. *Clinical Features and Diagnosis of Guillain-Barré Syndrome in Adults*. http://www. uptodateonline.com/utd/content/topic.do?topicKey= muscle/14568&type=A&selectedTitle=1~57. Accessed January 22, 2007.

96. Answer: E. Prophylactic therapy is indicated for patients with chronic tension type headaches requiring daily or near-daily analgesics.

Bajwa ZH, Sabahat A. Approach to the Patient with Headache Syndromes Other Than Mirgaine. http:// www.uptodateonline.com/utd/content/topic.do?topic Key=headache/5253&type=A&selectedTitle=4~142. Accessed February 19, 2007.

97. Answer: E. Decreased total cerebral volume, increased ventricular volume and decrease in the area of thalamus are findings that are especially consistent with adult findings.

1. Hendren RL, De Backer I, Pandina GJ. Review of neuroimaging studies of child and adolescent psychiatric disorders from the past 10 years. *J Am Acad Child Adolesc Psychiatry*. 2000;39:815–828.
2. Kumra S, Shaw M, Merka P, et al. Childhood-onset schizophrenia: research update. *Can J Psychiatry*. 2001;46:923–930.
3. Lewis M. *Child and Adolescent Psychiatry: A Comprehensive Textbook*. 3rd ed. Philadelphia: Lippincott Williams & Wilkins; 2002:749.

98. Answer: C. The CNS of noradrenaline is 3-methoxy-4-hydroxyphenylglycol (MHPG). The cortical projections are involved with arousal and maintaining the cortex in an alert state. The limbic projections are concerned with drive, motivation, mood, and response to stress. The metabolite of noradrenaline in the periphery is VMA. NA release is under inhibitory autoreceptor (alpha2) feedback regulation. There are two types of NA receptors; alpha (alpha1 and alpha2) and beta (beta1, beta2, and beta3). Alpha2 receptors are inhibitory and inhibit cAMP.

Anderson IM, Reid IC. *Fundamentals of Clinical Psychopharmacology*. London: Taylor & Francis; 2004:16.

99. Answer: C. Neurotic defenses are encountered in obsessive-compulsive and hysterical patients, or adults under stress. These include: controlling, displacement, externalization, inhibition, intellectualization, isolation, rationalization, dissociation, reaction formation, repression, and sexualization. Isolation is splitting or separating an idea from the affect that accompanies it but is repressed. Distortion is a narcissistic defense and involves grossly reshaping external reality to suit inner needs and using entitlement. Introjection is an immature defense that involves internalizing the qualities of an object to obliterate the distinction between the subject and object (e.g., identification with the aggressor). Regression is an immature defense, an attempt to return to an earlier libidinal phase to avoid tension evoked at the present level of development. Suppression is a mature defense in which one consciously or semiconsciously postpones attention to a conscious impulse/conflict.

Kaplan HI, Sadock BJ. *Kaplan & Sadock's Synopsis of Psychiatry*. 8th ed. Philadelphia: Lippincott Williams & Wilkins; 1998:218–222.

100. **Answer: D.** Contemporary hospice offers a comprehensive program of care to patients and families facing a life threatening illness. Hospice is primarily a concept of care, and not a specific place of care. Hospice emphasizes palliative rather than curative treatment. The dying are comforted, professional medical care is given, and sophisticated symptom relief is provided. The patient and family are both included in the care plan and emotional, and spiritual and practical support is given based on the patient's wishes and family's needs. Hospice affirms life and regards dying as a normal process. It neither hastens nor postpones death. Hospice provides personalized services and a caring community so that patients and families can attain the necessary preparation for a death that is satisfactory to them. Hospice care is provided to patients who have a limited life expectancy and although most hospice patients are cancer patients, hospices accept anyone regardless of age or type of illness. These patients have also made a decision to spend their last months at home or in a homelike setting. Hospice is covered by Medicare nationwide and by Medicaid in 39 states, and by most private insurance providers. Medicare covers all services and supplies for the hospice patient related to the terminal illness.

Hospice Net. *The Hospice website*. http://www.hospicenet.org/. Accessed December 27, 2006.

101. **Answer: C.** This boy is using acting out as a defense mechanism to deal with the anxiety produced by his parent's fight. When a person is acting out, he is fulfilling a wish in a non-reflective and uncontrolled matter. Because this boy cannot confront, or show his anger directly to his parents, he fulfills his wish by showing off his anger in school. Passive aggression refers to the expression of hostility or resentment through inactivity. When using reaction formation, a person substitutes negative feelings (e.g., anger, hostility) by the opposite feelings (e.g., love, devotion).

Omnipotence refers to the substitution of feelings of low self-worth and failure by feelings of superiority and grandiosity. In projective identification, one converts one's own hostile impulses into acceptable reactions to other people's aggression.

Sadock BJ, Sadock VA. *Kaplan and Sadock's Comprehensive Textbook of Psychiatry*. 8th ed. Philadelphia: Lippincott Williams & Wilkins; 2005:802–804.

102. **Answer: C.** The incidence of Schizophrenia is greater in urban areas. Relative risk for Schizophrenia appears to be related to the degree of urbanization. The age of disease onset is lower in men than women. Patients with Schizophrenia are at increased risk for substance abuse, suicide, and assaultive behavior.

Sadock BJ, Sadock VA. *Kaplan and Sadock's Comprehensive Textbook of Psychiatry*. 8th ed. Philadelphia: Lippincott Williams & Wilkins; 2005:1331.

103. **Answer: D.** Prevalence estimates vary significantly depending on methods and wording used. However, as many as 18% of boys and 11% of girls are reported by their parents to have tics.

1. Leckman JF, Cohen DJ. *Tourette's Syndrome–Tics, Obsessions, Compulsions: Developmental Psychopathology and Clinical Care*. New York: Wiley;1999:177–193.
2. Wiener JM, Dulcan MK. *Textbook of Child and Adolescent Psychiatry*. 3rd ed. Washington: American Psychiatric Publishing; 2004:713.

104. **Answer: C.** The bell and pad alarm system has been found to work best for long-term remission. An alarm clock set to ring after 2 to 3 hours of sleep is also useful.

Lewis M. *Child and Adolescent Psychiatry: A Comprehensive Textbook*. 3rd ed. Philadelphia: Lippincott Williams & Wilkins; 2002:700–711.

105. **Answer: D.** The specifier "with Atypical Features" is used to describe a mood episode where the following features predominate during the most recent 2 weeks of a current MDE: (i) mood reactivity (the brightening of mood in response to actual or potential positive events), (ii) two or more of the following: significant weight gain/appetite increase, hypersomnia, leaden paralysis (or "heavy, leaden feelings in arms or legs"), or long-standing pattern of interpersonal rejection sensitivity (not limited to episodes of mood disturbance) resulting in significant social or occupational impairment, and (iii) criteria are not met for Mood Disorder with Melancholic Features or with Catatonic Features during the same mood episode.

Atypical Features of depression are reverse vegetative signs with rejection sensitivity, and are phenomenologically and pharmacologically at the other end of the spectrum from melancholia. They are a Major Depressive Disorder qualifier in up to a third of Major Depressive Disorders.

1. American Psychiatric Association. *Quick Reference to the Diagnostic Criteria from DSM-IV-TR*. Washington: American Psychiatric Association; 2000:203–204.
2. Sadock BJ, Sadock VA. *Kaplan and Sadock's Comprehensive Textbook of Psychiatry*. 8th ed. Philadelphia: Lippincott Williams & Wilkins; 2005:1618, 1628.

106. Answer: E. The pharmacologic treatment of alcohol withdrawal serves many purposes, namely to allow patients a comfortable detoxification and to prevent serious complications such as seizures and cardiac arrest. Healthy, motivated patients under the age of 45 are candidates for outpatient detoxification. In patients with a history of delirium tremens, alcohol-withdrawal seizures, or medical comorbidities, inpatient detoxification is necessary. Inpatients should be monitored every few hours to assess progression of alcohol withdrawal. Withdrawal symptoms for which to remain vigilant include autonomic arousal (elevated blood pressure and heart rate), diaphoresis, tremor, sleep-wake cycle disruption, nausea/vomiting, and cognitive changes. Use of a standard rating scale such as the Clinical Institute Withdrawal Assessment (Revised) for the evaluation of withdrawal progression is preferable. Benzodiazepines (e.g., lorazepam and chlordiazepoxide) are the mainstay of pharmacologic treatment for alcohol withdrawal, as they are agonists at GABA-A receptors and have cross-tolerance with alcohol. Clinicians may elect to start treatment with benzodiazepines immediately, or wait for withdrawal symptoms to develop. The latter may result in the use of lower total doses of benzodiazepines. Individual requirements of benzodiazepines to control symptoms are variable, and the dose may be titrated as needed to treat withdrawal symptoms and avoid excessive sedation.

Rosenbaum JF, Arana GW, Hyman SE, et al. *Handbook of Psychiatric Drug Therapy*. 5th ed. Philadelphia: Lippincott Williams & Wilkins; 2005:218–219.

107. Answer: E. Eszopiclone is an S (+) isomer of Zopiclone, which has been available as a hypnotic in Europe since 1992. It is indicated for the treatment of insomnia in patients ≥18 years of age and there is no restriction on its duration of use. It is a nonbenzodiazepine hypnotic that is structurally unrelated to pyrazolopyrimidines, imidazopyridines, benzodiazepines, or barbiturates. The precise mechanism of action of eszopiclone as a hypnotic is not known, but its effect possibly occurs from its interaction with GABA receptor complexes at the binding domains located close to or allosterically coupled to benzodiazepine receptors. Eszopiclone is rapidly absorbed following oral administration and achieves its peak plasma concentrations within 1 hour after oral administration. It is bound to plasma proteins about 52% to 59%. Eszopiclone is extensively metabolized in the liver by oxidation and demethylation by CYP3A4 and CYP2E1 enzymes. The mean elimination half-life of eszopiclone is approximately 6 hours and less than 10% of an oral dose is excreted in the urine as the parent drug. The two most frequent adverse side effects were headache and unpleasant taste. Dyspepsia, pain, diarrhea, somnolence, dry mouth, and nausea were also common in patients treated with eszopiclone. There are no known contraindications to eszopiclone, but this drug should be administered with caution in patients exhibiting signs and symptoms of depression as they can exhibit suicidal tendencies. There is no evidence for the development of tolerance in patients taking eszopiclone over a period of 6 months in clinical trials. The recommended starting dose for elderly patients is 1 mg immediately before bedtime with an increase to 2 mg, if clinically indicated. It has been assigned a category C for pregnancy, as there are no adequate, well-controlled studies of eszopiclone in pregnant women. It is not known whether eszopiclone is excreted in human milk and hence caution should be exercised when eszopiclone is administered to a nursing mother.

Brielmaier BD. Eszopiclone (Lunesta): a new nonbenzodiazepine hypnotic agent. *Proc (Bayl Univ Med Cent)*. 2006;19:54–59.

108. Answer: D. HIV infection, even in the absence of AIDS, can develop new onset psychotic symptoms. Patients with HIV are reportedly very sensitive to the EPS of neuroleptic medications so American Psychiatric Association guidelines recommend treating psychotic symptoms in HIV patients with an atypical antipsychotic at the lowest effective dose. Of the medications listed, Olanzapine is the treatment of choice as it is less prone to cause EPS when compared to haloperidol, a typical antipsychotic, and the dose is low yet in the therapeutic range for treating psychosis. Quetiapine is an atypical antipsychotic but the low dose of 50 mg would be ineffective at targeting the patient's psychotic symptoms. Although clozapine is also known to have decreased risk of EPS, it is not recommended in this patient already prone to neutropenia from his HIV given the risk of agranulocytosis associated with clozapine. The use of lorazepam, a benzodiazepine, is not indicated as the patient does not show any agitation or need for sedation.

American Psychiatric Association. *Practice Guideline for the Treatment of Patients with HIV/AIDS. VI. Data Regarding Psychiatric Treatments for Individuals with HIV Infection.* http://www.psychiatryonline.com/content.aspx?aID=44781. Accessed January 21, 2007.

109. Answer: E. γ-hydroxybutyrate is a sedative that acutely causes intoxication, sedation, euphoria, and sexual disinhibition. Overdose is characterized by stupor and respiratory depression. A rapid shift from unconscious apneic state to markedly agitated and combative is also often seen. Withdrawal is somewhat similar to alcohol. The major treatment in overdose is supportive care. Naloxone, flumazenil, and physostigmine have not been shown to have any benefits. Mild withdrawal can be treated with benzodiazepines, and barbiturates have also been useful. Antipsychotics can be used, but are not first-line because of the risk of seizures and neuroleptic malignant syndrome (NMS).

1. Kranzler HR, Ciraulo DA. *Clinical Manual of Addiction Psychopharmacology.* Arlington: American Psychiatric Publishing; 2005:244–255.
2. Li J, Stokes SA, Woeckener A. A tale of novel intoxication: a review of the effects of gamma-hydroxybutyric acid with recommendations for management. *Ann Emerg Med.*1998;31:729–736.

110. Answer: C. Two benzodiazepine receptor subtypes in the brain mediate hypnotic, anxiolytic, stimulant, and muscle relaxant pharmacological effects. Clinically, benzodiazepine receptor binding does not cause a stimulant effect.

Nishino S, Mishima K, Mignot E, et al. Sedative-hypnotics: benzodiazepines. In: Schatzberg AF, Nemeroff CB, eds. *Essentials of Clinical Psychopharmacology.* 2nd ed. http://www.psychiatryonline.com/content.aspx?aID=210307. Accessed February 2, 2007.

111. Answer: D. This patient's depressive symptoms are most likely secondary to pancreatic cancer, which should always be considered in depressed middle-aged patients. Although strokes and myocardial infarctions (MI) are also associated with depression, the elevated amylase and lack of symptoms suggesting these other etiologies favors pancreatic cancer. The elevated amylase admittedly could be related to kidney failure and, in this way, related to the pyelonephritis. However, a normal BUN and creatinine suggest that the pyelonephritis has not led to renal failure.

Kaplan HI, Sadock BJ. *Kaplan & Sadock's Synopsis of Psychiatry.* 8th ed. Philadelphia: Lippincott Williams & Wilkins; 1998:820.

112. Answer: C. All of the above are correctly matched except Choice C. Hirano bodies are eosinophilic inclusions in hippocampal neurons of patients who have AD.

Fix JD. *High-Yield Neuroanatomy.* Baltimore: Lippincott Williams & Wilkins;1995:24.

113. Answer: A. Patients with Bulimia Nervosa can have low estrogen levels and infrequent menstruation. They can also have esophagitis, esophageal dysmotility, dental caries, dehydration, hypokalemia, and hypochloremic alkalosis from vomiting. Laxative abuse can result in colonic dysmotility, hypomagnesemia, and hypophosphatemia. Russell's sign is scarring on the dorsum of the hand caused by self-induced vomiting. Other complications of bulimia nervosa include cardiomyopathy, peripheral myopathy, and enlarged parotid glands.

American Psychiatric Association. *Practice Guideline for the Treatment of Patients With Eating Disorders.* 3rd ed. http://www.psychiatryonline.com/content.aspx?aID=139788. Accessed January 9, 2007.

114. Answer: E. Huntington's disease is a neurodegenerative disorder with a prominent that follows an autosomal-dominant pattern of inheritance with 100% penetrance. The gene responsible for the disease has been located on the short arm of chromosome 4 and the manifestations are due to expanded trinucleotide repeats. In some patients with HD, psychiatric symptoms may precede the onset of the movement disorder. Both unipolar major depression and bipolar disorder are extremely common in these patients. Suicide rate has been found to be significantly higher than that found in the general population. Hallucinations and delusions also occur in frequencies above the rates found in the baseline population. Patients may also develop aggression, hypersexuality, and paraphilias sometime during the course of their illness.

1. Blass DM, Steinberg M, Leroi I, Lyketsos CG. Successful multimodality treatment of severe behavioral disturbance in a patient with advanced Huntington's disease. *Am J Psychiatry.* 2001 Dec;158(12):1966–1972.
2. Rosenblatt A, Leroi I. Neuropsychiatry of Huntington's disease and other basal ganglia disorders. *Psychosomatics.* 2000 Jan-Feb;41(1):24–30.

115. Answer: A. The aphasia described is a Wernicke's or a receptive type of aphasia. It is produced with damage to the auditory association cortex of the posterosuperior gyrus of the temporal lobe. Broca's aphasia, or expressive aphasia, results when there is damage to the posteroinferior frontal lobe.

Goetz CG. *Textbook of Clinical Neurology.* 2nd ed. Philadelphia: WB Saunders; 2003:88–90.

116. Answer: D. T4 supplies sensory input to the dermatome including the nipple region. The radial side of the forearm is innervated by levels C5 to C6. The ulnar side of the forearm is innervated by C8 to T1. The axilla is innervated by T3. The rib margin is innervated by T8.

Goetz CG. *Textbook of Clinical Neurology.* 2nd ed. Philadelphia: WB Saunders; 2003:339.

117. Answer: A. The incidence of intracranial hemorrhage in the pre-term newborn has decreased from 40% to 20% over the last two decades, but remains a common occurrence. It is also a common cause of CP. Parenchymal cerebral hemorrhage, originating in the periventricular area, periventricular intraventricular hemorrhage, is a common site of intracranial hemorrhage in infants of less than 32 weeks gestation. It is suggested by a fall in hematocrit of 20% or more and a CSF protein content of 250 mg/dL to 1250 mg/dL. Cribside sonography helps delineate the bleed. Severity is graded I through IV, with 50% mortality for Grade IV. Periventricular leukomalacia occurs in 50% of those with birth weights 500 g to 1000 g. MRI shows ventricular enlargement due to loss of white matter volume. Clinical manifestations include spastic diplegia. HIE is caused by abruptio placenta, uterine rupture, and umbilical cord or placental dysfunction. Low APGAR (Appearance, Pulse, Grimace, Activity, and Respiration) scores are present at birth (0 to 3 at 5 minutes). Microcephaly, developmental delay, and mental retardation are long-term consequences. Neonatal herpes encephalitis is manifested by fever, irritability, and seizures. It is diagnosed using polymerase chain reaction for herpes simplex virus (HSV)-type 2 (the most common herpes virus).

Rowland LP. *Merritt's Neurology.* 11th ed. Philadelphia: Lippincott Williams & Wilkins; 2005:563–573.

118. Answer: A. The options are all sphingolipidoses. These along with the mucolipidoses, polysaccharidoses, and gangliosidoses are inherited lysosomal storage diseases. The neurologic complications of Fabry disease arise from cerebral vascular accidents. The deficient enzyme in each disease is as follows: (i) Gaucher → glucocerebrosidase, (ii) Krabbe → galactocerebrosidase, (iii) Niemann-Pick → sphingomyelinase, and (iv) Metachromatic leukodystrophy → arylsulfatase A. Tay-Sachs is a gangliosidosis with hexaminidase A deficiency, and Hurler is a mucopolysaccharidosis with an a-L-iduronidase deficiency. Gaucher disease is the most common of the lipid storage diseases. Gaucher type 2 with onset in infancy has CNS involvement, causing developmental regression, seizures, eye muscle paralysis, and abnormal tone.

Becker KL. *Principles and Practice of Endocrinology & Metabolism.* 3rd ed. Philadelphia: Lippincott Williams & Wilkins; 2001:1720.

119. Answer: B. HSV is the single most important cause of fatal sporadic encephalitis in the United States. Early diagnosis is crucial because there is effective antiviral treatment. Of the two antigenic types, type 1 strains (HSV-1) is responsible for almost all cases of HSV encephalitis in adults. It also causes oral herpes. Type 2 strains (HSV-2) cause genital disease, but in the neonatal period, HSV-2 encephalitis can occur as part of a disseminated infection or as localized disease acquired during delivery. The route of HSV-2 spread in adults is by venereal transmission and it can cause aseptic meningitis. Varicella Zoster causes shingles, an inflammatory lesion of the posterior root ganglia, that causes pain and skin eruptions in the distribution of the affected ganglia. The CNS involvement is rare in the case of Varicella Zoster, but rarely, acute cerebellar ataxia, encephalitis, myelitis, and meningitis may occur. Cytomegaloviral infection of the CNS occurs in utero by transplacental transmission and can cause a granulomatous encephalitis, hydrocephalus, hydranencephaly, microcephaly, or cerebellar hypoplasia. Seizures or mental retardation occur commonly in infants who survive the infection. Epstein-Barr virus causes infectious mononucleosis or glandular fever. Rarely, it involves the CNS in children and young adults. Adenoviruses usually cause coryza, pharyngitis, pharyngoconjunctival fever, epidemic keratoconjunctivitis, pertussis-like syndrome, hemorrhagic, and pneumonia. CNS involvement is rare and when it occurs, it manifests as encephalitis or meningoencephalitis.

Rowland LP. *Merritt's Neurology.* 11th ed. Philadelphia: Lippincott Williams & Wilkins; 2005:191–198.

120. Answer: C. HIV disseminates to the CNS soon after primary infection via infected monocytes that traverses the blood brain barrier to replenish perivascular macrophages and not astrocytes. Since the advent of HAART, the incidence of HAD has declined from 20% to 30% to 10% to 15% in patients with advanced HIV infection. It is now noted that the proportion of new HAD cases occurring in patients with higher ranges of CD4 counts (200 to 350 cells) is increasing. There is growing evidence that HAART does not prevent neuropsychological impairment, but it may alter the type of impairment and delay the onset of dementia. Brain macrophages and microglia cells are usually infected with HIV and likely to be involved in the pathogenesis of HAD. There is little evidence that HIV infects other types of brain cells including astrocytes, neurons, or oligodendrocytes. Autopsy studies of HAD patients show characteristic white matter changes, demyelination, microglial nodules, multinucleated giant cells, and perivascular infiltrates. It is also noted that basal ganglia and nigrostriatal structures are affected early in the course of HAD. Later on in the illness, there is up to a 40% reduction in the number of neurons in the frontal and temporal lobes.

Thompson AW, Pieper AA, Treisman GJ. *Dementia and Delirium in HIV-infected Patients*. http://www.uptodateonline.com/utd/content/topic.do?topicKey= hiv_infe/20631. Accessed January 23, 2007.

121. **Answer: B.** Guillain-Barré syndrome is normally associated with albuminocytologic dissociation, or elevated CSF protein and normal white count (80% to 90% of cases 1 week after onset of symptoms). Normal CSF protein can be seen in up to one third of patients if tested earlier than 1 week following onset of symptoms.

Ropper AH, Wijdicks EFM, Truax BT. *Guillain-Barré Syndrome. Contemporary Neurology Series*. Philadelphia: FA Davis; 1991:57.

122. **Answer: A.** Inhalation of 100% oxygen is an effective abortive therapy for acute cluster headaches in the majority of patients. Verapamil, prednisone, lithium, and indomethacin are used as prophylactic therapy. Prophylactic therapy should be initiated at the onset of a cluster headache episode.

Bajwa ZH, Sabahat A. *Approach to the Patient with Headache Syndromes Other Than Migraine*. http://www.uptodateonline.com/utd/content/topic.do?topicKey= headache/5253&type=A&selectedTitle=4~142. Accessed February 19, 2007.

123. **Answer: A.** The term lissencephalies consist of several syndromes that involve disruption of normal neuronal migration during gestation, leading to four cortical layers, instead of the normal six, and a smooth cortical surface that lacks the normal pattern of gyri and sulci.

Lewis M. *Child and Adolescent Psychiatry: A Comprehensive Textbook*. 3rd ed. Philadelphia: Lippincott Williams & Wilkins; 2002:16.

124. **Answer: D.** Serotonin is formed by the sequential hydroxylation and decarboxylation of tryptophan. The ascending pathways are involved in a modulatory role in mood and behavior, sleep/wakefulness and regulation of circadian functions, control of behaviors (such as feeding and sex), body temperature, perceptions (hallucinations), and vomiting. The de-

scending pathways are involved in inhibition of pain transmission in the dorsal horn and in regulating motor neuron output in the ventral horn. The 5-HT3 receptor is a ligand gated cation channel. The 5-HT receptors are inhibitory and are negatively coupled to cAMP. The 5-HT2 receptors are excitatory and act through the phospholipase C/inositol phosphate pathways. The 5-HT4, 5-HT5, 5-HT6, and 5-HT7 receptors are positively coupled with cAMP and are excitatory.

The major mechanism for removal of 5-HT from the synaptic cleft is reuptake by the 5-HT transporter which is inhibited by SSRIs and tricyclic antidepressants. 5-HT is also metabolized by monoamine oxidase (MAO) to form 5-hydroxy-indole acetic acid (5-HIAA). The release of 5-HT at the terminals is subject to inhibitory regulation involving the 5-HT1B/1D receptor.

Anderson IM, Reid IC. *Fundamentals of Clinical Psychopharmacology*. London: Taylor & Francis Group; 2004:18.

125. **Answer: D.** Denial, in which a patient refuses to accept the awareness of a real fact, is considered an immature defense mechanism. Humor is a mature defense mechanism, in which a patient changes his feelings of anxiety into comedy or irony. Suppression is another mature defense mechanism, where a person intentionally blocks a memory that is either anxiety-provoking or unacceptable. When using intellectualization, a person removes the emotional component to an event to reduce the anxiety that it provokes. Undoing refers to a compulsive behavior to symbolically negate an unacceptable impulse, and it is commonly encountered in patients with OCD. Although intellectualization and undoing are not considered to be mature defense mechanisms, they are not considered to be as immature as denial.

Sadock BJ, Sadock VA. *Kaplan and Sadock's Comprehensive Textbook of Psychiatry*. 8th ed. Philadelphia: Lippincott Williams & Wilkins; 2005:802–804.

126. **Answer: B.** Bleuler described the "four As" as the primary symptoms of Schizophrenia: abnormal associations, autism, ambivalence, and inappropriate affect. Bleuler considered hallucinations, delusions, catatonia, and other behavioral abnormalities accessory symptoms.

Sadock BJ, Sadock VA. *Kaplan and Sadock's Comprehensive Textbook of Psychiatry*. 8th ed. Philadelphia: Lippincott Williams & Wilkins; 2005:1418.

127. **Answer: B.** Tics have been described as having a rostral-caudal progression. Initially, tics usually involve the head or upper extremities. Over time, they

tend to increase in diversity and distribution, often progressing to involve the trunk and legs.

Wiener JM, Dulcan MK. *Textbook of Child and Adolescent Psychiatry*. 3rd ed. Washington: American Psychiatric Publishing; 2004:711.

128. **Answer: A.** In a study comparing children with Enuresis to a control group, bone age was found to lag behind chronological age in children with enuresis, which has lead some to propose delayed maturation of the CNS as an etiology.

Lewis M. *Child and Adolescent Psychiatry: A Comprehensive Textbook*. 3rd ed. Philadelphia: Lippincott Williams & Wilkins; 2002:701.

129. **Answer: C.** Complete delusions are those which the person believes with certainty that their thoughts are absolutely true. Partial delusions are those in which the patient entertains doubts about the delusional beliefs. These doubts may represent the evolution of the delusion, the giving up of the delusion, or they may spring up intermittently in the course of the delusion. Systematized delusions are usually well circumscribed and are not associated with hallucinations or altered sensorium. Nonsystematized delusions are constantly evolving, and are being updated using more contemporary data from the world, to support their presence. A person with systematized delusions often goes about his life unperturbed by his delusional beliefs. A person with nonsystematized delusions usually displays some mental confusion, hallucinations, or affective instability. An overvalued idea is an unreasonable and sustained irrational belief. The ideas are, however, not bizarre or as obviously unbelievable as delusional content. The distorted body image of body dysmorphic disorder is the prototype of an overvalued idea. Delusional atmosphere, also known as delusional mood, is accompanied by an uncanny feeling. The person interprets ordinary events in a self-referential way, and even if the delusional interpretations are transient, the "odd feeling" stays.

Sadock BJ, Sadock VA. *Kaplan and Sadock's Comprehensive Textbook of Psychiatry*. 8th ed. Philadelphia: Lippincott Williams & Wilkins; 2005:977–978.

130. **Answer: D.** The nicotine transdermal patch is available in 7-mg, 14-mg, and 21-mg strengths. Patients who smoke greater than 10 cigarettes daily should begin treatment with the 21-mg patch. Those who smoke less than 10 cigarettes daily should begin with the 14-mg patch. The patch should be placed firmly on a region of the body with limited hair (e.g., upper arm or abdomen), and should be replaced every 24 hours. Patients should be warned that there is an initial lag time of 1 to 2 hours before nicotine is absorbed into the bloodstream, with peak concentration occurring around 6 to 12 hours after placement of the patch. The patch is generally well tolerated, with rare incidents of skin irritation at the site of the patch. After 6 weeks on the 21-mg patch, the patient may taper to the 14-mg patch for several more weeks before transitioning to the 7-mg patch for a few more weeks until discontinuation.

Rosenbaum JF, Arana GW, Hyman SE, et al. *Handbook of Psychiatric Drug Therapy*. 5th ed. Philadelphia: Lippincott Williams & Wilkins; 2005:218–240.

131. **Answer: E.** Among the following drugs, topiramate (Topamax) has the highest risk of nephrolithiasis. The incidence of renal stones in patients receiving topiramate is 2 to 4 times that is expected in the general population. However, the overall risk of developing renal stones with topiramate is only about 1%. Concomitant use of acetazolamide increases the risk of renal stones, while good hydration prevents it. More common side effects with topiramate include fatigue, somnolence, dizziness, nausea, anorexia, decreased concentration, ataxia, anxiety, parasthesias, weight loss, and hyperchloremic non-anion gap metabolic acidosis.

1. Albers LJ, Hahn RK, Reist C. *Handbook of Psychiatric Drugs*. Laguna Hills: Current Clinical Strategies Publishing; 2005:81–82.
2. Lamb EJ, Stevens PE, Nashef L. Topiramate increases biochemical risk of nephrolithiasis. *Ann Clin Biochem*. 2004;41:166–169.

132. **Answer: E.** Seizures can be an adverse side effect of clozapine therapy and the risk of seizures increases significantly with dosages of 600 mg and above, from 1% to 2% to 3% to 5%. Valproate is considered the safest and the best tolerated anticonvulsant for patients taking clozapine who experience seizures. Carbamazepine is contraindicated because the bone marrow suppression risk of this medication can increase clozapine's risk for agranulocytosis. There have been some reports of respiratory arrest in patients taking both clozapine and a high-potency benzodiazepine, so giving lorazepam in this patient would not be appropriate. Lorazepam is usually only used in acute settings of status epilepticus and not ideal for prophylaxis given its shorter half-life. Phenobarbital and phenytoin decrease serum clozapine levels, so these medications would not be the best choice for this patient who needed her clozapine titrated to that specific dose for resolution of symptoms.

Albers LJ, Hahn RK, Reist C. *Handbook of Psychiatric Drugs*. Laguna Hills: Current Clinical Strategies Publishing; 2005: 81–82.

133. **Answer: D.** Gastrointestinal side effects such as nausea, anorexia, vomiting, diarrhea, and abdominal pain are common with lithium use and are dose related. Nausea may be helped with dosing at meals, with the use of H_2 blockers, as well as with the use of slow-release preparations. However, the latter is more highly associated with diarrhea than is standard lithium. When gastrointestinal symptoms appear later in the course of treatment, that development should raise one's concern about toxicity.

Rosenbaum JF, Arana GW, Hyman SE, et al. *Handbook of Psychiatric Drug Therapy.* 5th ed. Philadelphia: Lippincott Williams & Wilkins, 2005:140.

134. **Answer: A.** Benzodiazepine binding at its receptor site on the $GABA_A$ receptor, with simultaneous binding of GABA at the $GABA_A$ receptor, allosterically modulates the receptor to exert a greater effect on the neuron's chloride channel opening. The effect on the neuron is inhibitory. Benzodiazepines have no effect on the $GABA_B$ receptor. Benzodiazepine binding without GABA binding cannot affect the calcium channel.

Nishino S, Mishima K, Mignot E, et al. Sedative-hypnotics: benzodiazepines. In: Schatzberg AF, Nemeroff CB, eds. *Essentials of Clinical Psychopharmacology.* 2nd ed. http://www.psychiatryonline.com/content.aspx?aID=210307. Published February 2, 2007.

135. **Answer: E.** Paralysis of the abducent nerve causes inability to abduct the eye and horizontal diplopia. It can be caused by all of the conditions that are listed as choices.

Fix JD. *High-Yield Neuroanatomy.* Baltimore: Lippincott Williams & Wilkins; 1995:56–57.

136. **Answer: D.** Tricyclic antidepressants and antipsychotic medications can increase the QT interval. Significant prolongation of the QT interval is associated with the *torsades de pointes* arrhythmia. Although *torsades de pointes* has been associated with uses of high doses of haloperidol, it also can occur at lower doses. A QTc interval (the QT corrected for heart rate) of 450 milliseconds or higher warrants caution with use of medications that can prolong this interval, and a cardiology consultation may be advised in cases of significantly prolonged QT (or QTc) intervals. Women tend to have a higher QT interval on average as compared to men.

1. Glassman AH, Bigger JT Jr. Antipsychotic drugs: prolonged QTc interval, torsade de pointes, and sudden death. *Am J Psychiatry.* 2001;158:1774–1782.
2. Reilly JG, Ayis SA, Ferrier IN, et al. QTc-interval abnormalities and psychotropic drug therapy in psychiatric patients. *Lancet.* 2000;355:1048–1052.

137. **Answer: A.** The symptoms described are most consistent with a lesion in the left trigeminal V1 (ophthalmic branch). The corneal reflex is formed with afferent fibers of the unilateral V1 and efferent fibers of the unilateral facial nerve (VII).

Goetz CG. *Textbook of Clinical Neurology.* 2nd ed. Philadelphia: WB Saunders; 2003:9.

138. **Answer: B.** Due to their location in the sella, craniopharyngiomas frequently impinge on the optic chiasm, which should cause a bilateral hemianopsia. Choice A would be caused by a left optic nerve lesion. Choice C would be caused by a lesion in the right occipital lobe. Choice E would be caused by a lesion in the left temporal lobe.

Goetz CG. *Textbook of Clinical Neurology.* 2nd ed. Philadelphia: WB Saunders; 2003:1033–1034.

139. **Answer: B.** Seizure activity as the result of a subarachnoid hemorrhage offers the best long-term prognosis, with 90% of infants having a normal outcome. The percentage of infants with a normal outcome is 10% for periventricular hemorrhage, 50% for early onset hypocalcemia (100% for late onset hypocalcemia), 50% for infection, and 50% for hypoglycemia. HIE, another cause of seizures, leads to a normal outcome in 50% of cases.

In descending order of frequency, the most common causes of seizures in the neonate are: HIE, intracranial hemorrhage (intraventricular > subarachnoid), hypoglycemia, infection, cerebral dysgenesis, and hypocalcemia.

MacDonald MG, Seshia MMK, Mullett MD. *Avery's Neonatology Pathophysiology and Management of the Newborn.* 6th ed. Philadelphia: Lippincott Williams & Wilkins; 2005:1386.

140. **Answer: A.** MELAS is probably the most common of the maternally inherited mitochondrial disorders. The other options are also diseases caused by mutations in maternally derived mitochondrial DNA. MERRF consists of progressive myoclonic epilepsy. Leigh syndrome presents variably but includes developmental regression, nystagmus, vomiting, dystonia, and abnormal respirations. NARP is an acronym for neuropathy, ataxia, and retinitis pigmentosa. Kearns-Sayre syndrome consists of pigmentary degeneration of the retina, ophthalmoplegia, and clinical onset before age 20. Leber hereditary optic neuropathy is another mitochondrial disease. In the mitochondrial diseases, think myopathy and degeneration suggestive of an inborn error.

McMillan JA, Feigin RD, DeAngelis C, Jones MD. *Oski's Pediatrics.* 4th ed. Philadelphia: Lippincott Williams & Wilkins; 2006:2336–2337.

141. Answer: E. Isolation of *T. pallidum* is impractical for clinical diagnosis and hence the diagnosis is made by detecting two categories of antibodies that are used as serologic tests for syphilis. The nontreponemal antibodies react with reagin, a complex of cardiolipin, lecithin, and cholesterol. The examples of tests based on the nontreponemal antibodies reaction with regain are the VDRL test and its variation called the RPR test. The RPR test remains unsuitable for testing of the CSF.

The CSF VDRL test is highly specific, but false-positive reactions may result from contamination of CSF by blood, high CSF-protein content, or the presence of paraproteinemia or autoimmune disease. The CSF VDRL test is not as reliable in following treatment (as the titers may not change), hence CSF pleocytosis is a more useful guide for monitoring treatment effects. The more specific test for syphilis is the fluorescent treponemal antibody (FTA-ABS) test. A positive FTA-ABS test in plasma has high specificity for making a diagnosis of syphilis. For making a diagnosis of syphilis a high titer in the blood on the VDRL test, ascertained by a positive FTA-ABS, is needed. For making a diagnosis of neurosyphilis, appropriate blood serology and a reactive CSF VDRL test is required. A reactive FTA-ABS in the blood indicates that the CSF VDRL result is not a false-positive response.

Rowland LP. *Merritt's Neurology.* 11th ed. Philadelphia: Lippincott Williams & Wilkins; 2005:237–238.

142. Answer: C. Lewy bodies are mainly seen in Parkinson's disease, but may also be present in the neurons of patients with Dementia of Lewy Body Type, the Lewy body variant of AD and Hallervorden-Spatz syndrome. They are spherical structures that displace other cell components. They are morphological of two types: classical (brain stem) Lewy bodies and cortical Lewy bodies. A classical Lewy body is a well defined eosinophilic cytoplasmic inclusion that is made of alpha-synuclein. A Lewy body may also contain other proteins like neurofilament protein and alpha-B crystallin. The cortical Lewy body in contrast is less well defined, but made of alpha-synuclein fibrils. The brain of patients present with atrophy and the microscopic findings include neuronal loss, astrocytosis, and the development of cytoplasmic vacuoles in neurons and astrocytes (status spongiosis). Amyloid plaques that contain the abnormal PrP are also found in the areas of brain affected with the disease. Usually there is inflammation of the affected tissues. The cortex and basal ganglia are commonly affected, but any part of the brain can be affected. Usually, gray matter is affected early and the lesions are more severe.

Rowland LP. *Merritt's Neurology.* 11th ed. Philadelphia: Lippincott Williams & Wilkins; 2005:266.

143. Answer: D. The mean age of onset for MS is 30 years. It is more frequently seen in women than in men, although 35% of cases are seen in males. Multiple studies have demonstrated that MS is frequently seen in patients with autoimmune disease, furthering the possible autoimmune basis for this disease.

Olek M. *Epidemiology, Risk Factors and Clinical Features of Multiple Sclerosis.* http://www.uptodateonline.com/utd/content/topic.do?topicKey=demyelin/4981&type=A&selectedTitle=2~54. Accessed January 22, 2007.

144. Answer: D. Prophylactic therapy is indicated in patients with recurring migraines that significantly impair daily function despite acute treatment. Topiramate is an approved medication for migraine prophylaxis. Triptans are not indicated in prophylactic treatment. Furthermore, no data suggests efficacy of one triptan over another. IV metoclopramide and prochlorperazine are indicated for treatment of patients who present to the emergency department with severe migraine. Ergotamine benefits few patients with migraines.

1. Bajwa ZH, Sabahat A. *Acute Treatment of Migraine in Adults.* http://www.uptodateonline.com/utd/content/topic.do?topicKey=headache/4364&type=A&selectedTitle=3~142. Accessed February 19, 2007.
2. Bajwa ZH, Sabahat A. *Preventive Treatment of Migraine in Adults.* http://www.uptodateonline.com/utd/content/topic.do?topicKey=headache/2543&type=A&selectedTitle=3~57. Accessed February 19, 2007.

145. Answer: C. Synaptogenesis starts in the second trimester and proceeds at a significant rate until the age of 10 or so, peaking in the first two postnatal years. By early adolescence synaptic density is at adult levels or 60% of the maximum.

Sadock BJ, Sadock VA. *Kaplan and Sadock's Synopsis of Psychiatry.* 9th ed. Philadelphia: Lippincott Williams & Wilkins; 2003:86, 478.

146. Answer: C. Acetylcholine is hydrolyzed to choline and acetic acid. There are two types of cholinergic receptors: nicotinic and muscarinic. Nicotinic receptors are of two types: muscle ganglionic and CNS types. Nicotinic receptors are coupled to cation channels. There are five muscarinic receptors. These are G protein coupled. They either activate the formation IP_3 (via M1, M3, and M5) or inhibit cAMP (M2, M4). The disruption of the pathway from the nucleus basalis to hippocampus is disrupted in AD and is probably associated with memory impairment.

Anderson IM, Reid IC. *Fundamentals of Clinical Psychopharmacology*. London: Taylor & Francis Group; 2004:20–23.

147. Answer: B. The GAF is a scale included in the DSM-IV-TR multiaxial diagnosis that provides an estimate of the severity of symptoms and level of psychosocial functioning of each patient. The scale (of 1 to 100) ranges from persistent danger to self and others with inability to maintain minimal personal hygiene to a superior level of functioning with no symptomatology.

American Psychiatric Association. *Desk Reference to the Diagnostic Criteria from DSM-IV-TR*. Washington: American Psychiatric Association; 2000:45–48.

148. Answer: D. A history of postpartum psychosis is the greatest risk factor for recurrence. The risk of relapse is as high as 70%. Other risk factors include a family history of postpartum psychosis, psychosocial stressors, and fetal distress or abnormalities. Primiparity may also be a risk factor.

Sadock BJ, Sadock VA. *Kaplan and Sadock's Comprehensive Textbook of Psychiatry*. 8th ed. Philadelphia: Lippincott Williams & Wilkins; 2005:1537.

149. Answer: A. In the late 19th century, Gilles de la Tourette first observed the strong familial nature of Tourette's syndrome. Several studies have concluded that the most likely mode of inheritance is autosomal dominant with sex specific penetrances.

Lewis M. *Child and Adolescent Psychiatry: A Comprehensive Textbook*. 3rd ed. Philadelphia: Lippincott Williams & Wilkins; 2002:423, 424.

150. Answer: E. Encopresis is the passage of feces in inappropriate places once a month for 3 months. Chronological age is at least 4 years or the equivalent developmental level. The subtypes are: (i) Encopresis With Constipation and Overflow Incontinence, and (ii) Encopresis Without Constipation and Overflow Incontinence.

American Psychiatric Association. *Diagnostic and Statistical Manual of Mental Disorders: DSM-IV-TR*. 4th ed. Washington: American Psychiatric Association; 2000:118.

151. Answer: A. An autochthonous delusion is a delusion that emerges fully formed, without any preceding event that could explain it, like "a bolt from the blue." A delusion shared between a couple/someone close is called *folie a deux*, whereas a delusion shared between family members is called *folie a famille*. The delusions of misidentification are: (i) Capgras syndrome, in which the person feels as though a person

he is close to has been replaced by a double (delusion of replacement of significant others), (ii) Fregoli syndrome, in which unfamiliar persons seem familiar (delusions of disguise), and (iii) subjective doubles, in which a person believes that another person has been physically changed into themselves (dopelganger).

Sadock BJ, Sadock VA. *Kaplan and Sadock's Comprehensive Textbook of Psychiatry*. 8th ed. Philadelphia: Lippincott Williams & Wilkins; 2005:978–979.

152. Answer: C. Memantine, the first NMDA receptor antagonist, is FDA-approved for the treatment of moderate to severe AD. Glutaminergic overstimulation may result in neurotoxicity; memantine may work by attenuating this neurotoxicity without disruption of glutamate's normal physiologic activity. Memantine is titrated from 5 mg daily to a total dose of 10 mg twice a day, over the course of 4 weeks. It is excreted renally and hence may require dosage adjustments in patients with renal disease. Memantine is generally well tolerated but may cause dizziness, fatigue, and confusion in higher doses. Clinical trials have shown that memantine has beneficial effects on cognition and functioning in donepezil-treated patients with moderate to severe AD.

Blazer DG, Steffens DC, Busse EW. *The American Psychiatric Association Textbook of Geriatric Psychiatry*. Washington: American Psychiatric Publishing; 2004:401.

153. Answer: E. Chlorpromazine, ziprasidone, haloperidol, and olanzapine are all available as IM preparations for the treatment of acute agitation. Aripiprazole is only available in the capsule form at present.

Rosenbaum JR, Arana GW, Hyman SE, et al. *Handbook of Psychiatric Drug Therapy*. 5th ed. Philadelphia: Lippincott Williams & Wilkins; 2005:12–14.

154. Answer: D. Risperdal Consta is a water-based suspension of the risperidone encapsulated in a carbohydrate polymer, and rather than the oil-based decanoate preparations, allows for gradual absorption that escapes first pass metabolism by the liver. Risperidal Consta is not viscous and causes little if any swelling or pain at the injection site. Absorption is gradual, taking over 3 weeks to reach peak concentration, thus requires an overlap of oral medications for at least 3 weeks after the first injection, and shots are given every 2 weeks, unlike Haldol decanoate which can be given every 4 weeks.

Rosenbaum JF, Arana GW, Hyman SE, et al. *Handbook of Psychiatric Drug Therapy*. 5th ed. Philadelphia: Lippincott Williams & Wilkins; 2005:32–33.

155. Answer: B. The half-life of lithium is about 25 hours. So, the blood sample should be drawn four to five half-lives later, when the drug is at its steady-state level. One will have to wait about 5 days before drawing a level.

Rosenbaum JF, Arana GW, Hyman SE, et al. *Handbook of Psychiatric Drug Therapy*. 5th ed. Philadelphia: Lippincott Williams & Wilkins; 2005:136.

156. Answer: D. A slow benzodiazepine taper reduces the risk of withdrawal symptoms, seizures, and rebound reactivation of the underlying anxiety disorder. Rapid tapering, diagnosis of panic disorder, short-half-life drugs, long duration of use, and high doses are thought to influence the severity of withdrawal.

Nishino S, Mishima K, Mignot E, et al. Sedative-hypnotics: benzodiazepines. In: Schatzberg AF, Nemeroff CB, eds. *Essentials of Clinical Psychopharmacology*. 2nd ed. http://www.psychiatryonline.com/content.aspx?aID=210307. Accessed February 2, 2007.

157. Answer: B. Bell's palsy is a lower motor neuron lesion of cranial nerve VII (the facial nerve), which results in ipsilateral weakness of the face. The upper and lower parts of the face are affected on the same side. By contrast, an upper motor neuron lesion of the corticobulbar tract would cause contralateral weakness of the lower face but would not affect the upper face. This is because the upper face is also innervated by the ipsilateral corticobulbar tract while the lower face only receives innervation from the contralateral corticobulbar tract.

Fix JD. *High-Yield Neuroanatomy*. Baltimore: Lippincott Williams & Wilkins; 1995:58.

158. Answer: E. SSRI antidepressants have been found to help depressed mood, irritability, impulsive aggression, self mutilation, and hostility in patients with borderline personality disorder in placebo-controlled, double-blind trials. Affective dysregulation and impulsivity are often prominent features of borderline personality disorder.

American Psychiatric Association. *Practice Guideline for the Treatment of Patients With Borderline Personality Disorder. VI. Review and Synthesis of Available Evidence*. http://www.psychiatryonline.com/content.aspx?aID=55433. Accessed January 9, 2007.

159. Answer: D. The spinal portion of cranial nerve XI (the spinal accessory nerve) innervates the sternocleidomastoid muscle and the trapezius muscle. The symptoms described are most likely the effect deficits in innervation of the trapezius.

Goetz CG. *Textbook of Clinical Neurology*. 2nd ed. Philadelphia: WB Saunders, 2003: 224–226.

160. Answer: B. A 1/5 strength level refers to a muscle group with only trace contractions and inability to perform active movement. A 2/5 strength level refers to a muscle group that can perform active movement only with gravity eliminated (i.e., along the top of a table). A 3/5 strength level refers to a muscle group that can perform active movement against gravity. A 4/5 strength level refers to a muscle group that can perform active movement against moderate resistance. A 5/5 strength level refers to normal muscle strength.

Goetz CG. *Textbook of Clinical Neurology*. 2nd ed. Philadelphia: WB Saunders; 2003:1033–1034.

161. Answer: A. The presence of significant bradykinesia is a factor in deciding to start symptomatic medical therapy for idiopathic Parkinson's disease. Other factors include the presence of significant gait disturbance, the effect of the disease on the patient's dominant hand, and the degree to which the disease interferes with work, activities of daily living, and leisure activities. Also, the patient's philosophy regarding the use of medications should be considered.

Tarsy D. *Pharmacological Treatment of Parkinson's Disease*. http://www.uptodateonline.com/utd/content/topic.do?topicKey=move_dis/4953&type=A&selectedTitle=2~33. Accessed February 19, 2007.

162. Answer: C. Myelination of axons starts in utero and is generally completed by early childhood in most brain regions. Myelination of the intracortical association areas continues into the third decade.

1. Lewis M. *Child and Adolescent Psychiatry: A Comprehensive Textbook*. 3rd ed. Philadelphia: Lippincott Williams & Wilkins; 2002:61.
2. Sadock BJ, Sadock VA. *Kaplan and Sadock's Synopsis of Psychiatry*. 9th ed. Philadelphia: Lippincott Williams & Wilkins; 2003:86.

163. Answer: E. Glutamate is derived from glutamine catalyzed by glutaminase. It is the major fast acting excitatory neurotransmitter in the brain. There are four main types of glutamate receptors: NMDA, AMPA, kainate receptors (which are all ionotropic receptors), and metabotropic receptors. Growing interest in brain glutamate was triggered by the possible link between excessive glutamate receptor activation and neurodegeneration caused by the loss of intracellular Ca^{2+} homeostasis. The physiological substrate of memory is putatively related to the activation of the NMDA receptors and long term potentiation in the hippocampus.

Glutamate neurotransmission is implicated in psychosis and anxiety. Activation of the metabotropic receptors causes the formation of IP_3, and the release of calcium ions, which may have a role in glutamate excitotoxicity and synaptic plasticity.

Anderson IM, Reid IC. *Fundamentals of Clinical Psychopharmacology*. London: Taylor & Francis Group; 2004:24–26.

164. **Answer: D.** Patients with Somatization Disorders are frequently difficult patients to interview and to establish an alliance with. They usually have seen many doctors before and continue to feel that their problem has not been solved. They feel that their symptoms are not being taken seriously. It is important for physicians to not undermine the patient's fears and anxiety, and to make sure that the patient does not feel that his/her symptoms are being dismissed. On the other hand, it is also important to reduce the harm from exposing a patient to potentially harmful and unwarranted medical interventions. It is important to establish a collaborative relationship with the patient's medical providers and to be aware of the extent of the patient's medical workup. When interviewing a patient, one should not only focus on the patient's medical complaint, but also explore other aspects of the patient's well being, such as social and psychological factors. One should try to encourage anything that can help the patient without causing harm, which sometimes includes using nonstandard approaches, such as yoga or meditation. Patients with Somatization Disorders usually respond better to frequent scheduled medical consultations instead of urgent medical visits, which can cause higher levels of anxiety and a recurrence of crises.

Sadock BJ, Sadock VA. *Kaplan and Sadock's Comprehensive Textbook of Psychiatry*. 8th ed. Philadelphia: Lippincott Williams & Wilkins; 2005:827–831.

165. **Answer: C.** Failure to thrive is not a DSM-IV-TR diagnostic category. It is a descriptive term that has a variety of definitions, each describing significantly lower than expected height and/or weight. Disorder of Infancy, Childhood, or Adolescence NOS is a residual category for disorders that do not meet the criteria for any specific disorder. The other options refer to the three diagnostic categories under Feeding Disorders of Infancy and Early childhood in DSM-IV-TR.

1. American Psychiatric Association. *Diagnostic and Statistical Manual of Mental Disorders: DSM-IV-TR*. 4th ed. Washington: American Psychiatric Association; 2000:103–108, 134.
2. Wiener JM, Dulcan MK. *Textbook of Child and Adolescent Psychiatry*. 3rd ed. Washington: American Psychiatric Publishing; 2004:639–657.

166. **Answer: B.** OCD and ADHD are especially common in children with Tourette's syndrome. ADHD symptoms often develop before the onset of tics. Some re-

searchers have attributed the frequent comorbidity of OCD, ADHD, and TD to common neurochemical or neuropathological problems in the basal ganglia.

Freeman RD, Fast DK, Burd L, et al. An international perspective on Tourette syndrome: selected findings from 3,500 individuals in 22 countries. *Dev Med Child Neurol.* 2000;42:436–447.

167. **Answer: E.** Ninety-five percent of children have achieved bowel control by 4 years of age and 99% by 5 years of age. This continues to decrease to a virtual absence by adolescence. Encopresis is more common in boys.

1. Sadock BJ, Sadock VA. *Kaplan and Sadock's Synopsis of Psychiatry*. 9th ed. Philadelphia: Lippincott Williams & Wilkins; 2003:1254.
2. Sheppard DM, Bradshaw JL, Purcell R, et al. Tourette's and comorbid syndromes: obsessive compulsive and attention deficit hyperactivity disorder. A common etiology? *Clin Psychol Rev.* 1999;19:531–552.

168. **Answer: D.** The fold of Veraguth is a psychomotor change of depression, manifesting as a perturbation of facial features. It was originally described by the Swiss neuropsychiatrist Otto Veraguth. It is a triangular-shaped fold seen in the nasal corner of the upper eyelid. It is not exclusively seen in clinical depression, and may also be observed in patients with a mild depressive affect. An EMG shows changes in the tone of the corrugator and zygomatic facial muscles.

Sadock BJ, Sadock VA. *Kaplan and Sadock's Comprehensive Textbook of Psychiatry*. 8th ed. Philadelphia: Lippincott Williams & Wilkins; 2005:1616.

169. **Answer: B.** Cholinesterase inhibitors, including donepezil, rivastigmine, and galantamine, are FDA-approved for the treatment of mild to moderate AD. Donepezil has recently been approved by the FDA for the treatment of severe AD. A fourth cholinesterase inhibitor, tacrine, is also available but is rarely used due to its risk of hepatotoxicity. The most common side effect of these medications is gastrointestinal distress, including nausea, vomiting, diarrhea, and anorexia. Other side effects include insomnia, dizziness, and agitation. Side effects occur as a result of the peripheral cholinergic effects of the medications, and are dose-dependent. Hence, slow titration of these medications is recommended.

Blazer DG, Steffens DC, Busse EW. *The American Psychiatric Association Textbook of Geriatric Psychiatry*. Washington: American Psychiatric Publishing; 2004:401.

170. **Answer: D.** All typical antipsychotic medications can achieve similar therapeutic benefits (efficacy) in patients with Schizophrenia. These medications however, differ in their potency and side effect profile.

Potency refers to the amount of drug needed to achieve a therapeutic effect. High potency drugs cause more EPS compared to the low potency drugs, which cause more sedation, hypotension, and anticholinergic side effects.

Rosenbaum JR, Arana GW, Hyman SE, et al. *Handbook of Psychiatric Drug Therapy*. 5th ed. Philadelphia: Lippincott Williams & Wilkins; 2005:8.

171. **Answer: C.** Risperdal Consta and haloperidol decanoate are two options for long-acting injectable forms of neuroleptics that are available to patients with chronic mental illness who relapse because of noncompliance. Because they are long-acting preparations, patients should be exposed to the oral form of the drug (regardless of which one) prior to their first injection to safeguard against the possibility of an idiosyncratic reaction that could last long if exposed the first time to the injection. Risperdal Consta is a water-based suspension of the risperidone encapsulated in a carbohydrate polymer, and rather than the oil-based decanoate preparations, allows for gradual absorption that escapes first pass metabolism by the liver. Unlike the decanoate preparations, the Risperdal Consta is not viscous and causes little if any swelling or pain at the injection site. Absorption is gradual, taking over 3 weeks to reach peak concentration, thus requires an overlap of oral medications for at least 3 weeks after the first injection, and shots are given every 2 weeks. Haloperidol decanoate injections, however, can be given every 4 weeks, but still require an overlap of oral medications.

Rosenbaum JF, Arana GW, Hyman SE, et al. *Handbook of Psychiatric Drug Therapy*. 5th ed. Philadelphia: Lippincott Williams & Wilkins; 2005:32–33.

172. **Answer: A.** Because of the risk of rash and the concomitant development of Stevens-Johnson syndrome or toxic epidermal necrolysis, lamotrigine should be started at a low dose and titrated slowly. The usual recommendation is to start at 25 mg per day and increase 25 mg per week for 4 weeks (and then at 100 mg per day usually to increase by 50 mg per week). Importantly, valproic acid raises the lamotrigine level, and so, if a patient is on valproic acid, one may want to consider lowering the lamotrigine dose by as much as a half of the usual dose.

Rosenbaum JF, Arana GW, Hyman SE et al. *Handbook of Psychiatric Drug Therapy*. 5th ed. Philadelphia: Lippincott Williams & Wilkins; 2005:154, 165–166.

173. **Answer: B.** A single dose of propranolol given 30 minutes prior to an anxiogenic event is used for the treatment of performance anxiety. Atenolol is

a less lipophilic beta-blocker; it crosses the blood-brain barrier poorly and has less potent CNS effects. Benzodiazepines such as clonazepam and lorazepam may cause sedation and induce tolerance. Methylphenidate is a stimulant and not indicated in the treatment of performance anxiety.

Rosenbaum JF, Arana GW, Hyman SE, et al. *Handbook of Psychiatric Drug Therapy*. 5th ed. Philadelphia: Lippincott Williams & Wilkins; 2005:188–191.

174. **Answer: E.** The vagal nerve innervates multiple body systems, including the palate, pharynx, larynx, thorax, and abdominal viscera. It is also involved in the parasympathetic autonomic nervous system response.

Fix JD. *High-Yield Neuroanatomy*. Baltimore: Lippincott Williams & Wilkins; 1995:61–62.

175. **Answer: C.** All of the above are accurate except the definition of clarification. In clarification, the therapist reformulates what the patient has said and reflects it back to the patient in a more coherent way. In interpretation, the therapist verbalizes how a patient's behavior, feeling, or thought is linked to its unconscious meaning.

American Psychiatric Association. Practice Guideline for the Treatment of Patients With Borderline Personality Disorder. VI. Review and Synthesis of Available Evidence. http://www.psychiatryonline.com/content.aspx?aID=55433. Accessed January 9, 2007.

176. **Answer: C.** Seizure is not a common adverse effect of levodopa. Nausea, somnolence, and headache are among the common adverse effects. At least 50% of patients may develop motor fluctuations, including dyskinesia, after 5 to 10 years of treatment with levodopa.

Tarsy D. *Pharmacological Treatment of Parkinson's Disease*. http://www.uptodateonline.com/utd/content/topic.do?topicKey=move_dis/4953&type=A&selectedTitle=2 ~33. Accessed February 19, 2007.

177. **Answer: B.** One month. The eating of nonnutritive substances is also inappropriate to developmental level, and the eating behavior is not part of a culturally sanctioned practice. If Pica occurs exclusively during another mental disorder, it is sufficiently severe to warrant separate clinical attention.

American Psychiatric Association. *Diagnostic and Statistical Manual of Mental Disorders: DSM-IV-TR*. 4th ed. Washington: American Psychiatric Association; 2000:103–105.

178. **Answer: A.** Tics in Transient Tic Disorder consist of motor or vocal tics or both. They last at least 4 weeks but do not last more than 12 consecutive months.

If motor tics or vocal tics persist for more than 12 months, the diagnosis of a Chronic Tic Disorder may be warranted. The diagnostic criteria for Chronic Motor Tic Disorder or Chronic Vocal Tic Disorder are similar to those of Tourette's syndrome with the exception that motor and vocal tics cannot be present together. If both motor and vocal tics are present for more than 12 months, a diagnosis of Tourette's syndrome may be warranted.

American Psychiatric Association. *Diagnostic and Statistical Manual of Mental Disorders*: DSM-IV-TR. 4th ed. Washington: American Psychiatric Association; 2000: 108–116.

179. Answer: E. Sitting on the toilet for 5 to 10 minutes, or 20 to 30 minutes after meals, makes use of the gastrocolic reflex. Diet modification includes increased fiber and water intake. Laxatives and mineral oils may be used if constipation is present.

Wiener JM, Dulcan MK. *Textbook of Child and Adolescent Psychiatry*. 3rd ed. Washington: American Psychiatric Publishing; 2004:747.

180. Answer: C. Men and women are equally affected by hypochondriasis. The prevalence of Hypochondriasis in general medical populations has been measured at 4% to 6%, but may be as high as 15%. In contrast, women with somatization disorder are thought to outnumber men 5 to 20 times, although the highest estimates may reflect a tendency to underdiagnose somatization disorder in male patients. The ratio of women to men among adult patients with Conversion Disorder is at least 2:1 and may be as high as 10:1. Pain Disorder is twice as frequent in women, as compared to men. Although Body Dysmorphic Disorder is a poorly studied condition, it is thought that women are affected more often than men.

Sadock BJ, Sadock VA. *Kaplan and Sadock's Synopsis of Psychiatry*. 9th ed. Philadelphia: Lippincott Williams & Wilkins; 2003:643–655.

181. Answer: C. In the first several months of counseling for Alcohol Dependence, the focus should be on day-to-day life issues with the goal of helping patients maintain a high level of motivation for abstinence. Techniques which provoke anxiety and require deep insights have not been shown to be useful during the early stages of recovery, and may even impair efforts at maintaining abstinence. In order to help patients maintain motivation, sessions should explore the negative consequences of drinking, the anticipated course of problems should drinking continue, and expected improvement with abstinence.

Both individual and group therapy approaches are useful, although there is limited data to indicate that one modality is superior to the other. In the early stages of treatment, whether inpatient or outpatient, counseling is usually offered at least three times per week. Less intense efforts follow after the first month.

Sadock BJ, Sadock VA. *Kaplan and Sadock's Comprehensive Textbook of Psychiatry*. 7th ed. Philadelphia: Lippincott Williams & Wilkins; 2000:969.

182. Answer: A. Chlorpromazine carries the highest risk of seizures among these antipsychotics. Among the typical antipsychotic medications, haloperidol, thioridazine, and fluphenazine carry a very low risk of seizure. Among the atypical antipsychotics, risperdal, olanzapine, quetiapine, and clozapine (dose less than 300 mg per day) have an incidence of seizure of 1%. In clozapine, at doses above 600 mg day, the incidence of seizure is 4%.

Kaufman DM. *Clinical Neurology for Psychiatrists*. 5th ed. Philadelphia: WB Saunders; 2001:233.

183. Answer: D. The combination of risperidone's D2 antagonism and high 5-HT2A affinity likely explains the medication's propensity to cause prolactin elevation, which accounts for the occasional reports of galactorrhea and menstrual irregularities in women. In men, hyperprolactinemia may cause impotence. Because of their low affinity for D2 dopamine receptors, clozapine and quetiapine have little or no effect on prolactin levels. Similarly, despite being reasonably potent D2 blockers, ziprasidone and olanzapine have also shown to have little effect on prolactin levels.

Rosenbaum JF, Arana GW, Hyman SE, et al. *Handbook of Psychiatric Drug Therapy*. 5th ed. Philadelphia: Lippincott Williams & Wilkins; 2005:36, 49.

184. Answer: D. Patients on valproic acid can develop thrombocytopenia and should have bleeding times and platelet counts checked before surgery. However, rarely do patients have significant clinical sequelae from thrombocytopenia secondary to valproic acid. Even in cases of clinically significant sequelae, it is not necessarily clear that valproic acid must be stopped. Thrombocytopenia occurs most commonly at high dosages (250 mg TID is a standard dose and 250 mg a day is a low dose).

1. Kaplan HI, Sadock BJ. *Kaplan & Sadock's Synopsis of Psychiatry*. 8th ed. Philadelphia: Lippincott Williams & Wilkins; 1998:1113.
2. Lackmann GM. Valproic-acid-induced thrombocytopenia and hepatotoxicity: discontinuation of treatment? *Pharmacology*. 2004;70:57–58.

3. Rosenbaum JF, Arana GW, Hyman SE, et al. *Handbook of Psychiatric Drug Therapy*. 5th ed. Philadelphia: Lippincott Williams & Wilkins; 2005:151, 153.

185. Answer: E. Because buspirone does not effect the benzodiazepine-GABA complex, it lacks benzodiazepines sedative, muscle relaxant, and anticonvulsant actions. Buspirone also does not depress respiration, which is a known adverse effect of benzodiazepines. Both benzodiazepine and buspirone share anxiolytic properties.

Schatzberg AF, Nemeroff CB. *Essentials of Clinical Psychopharmacology*. 2nd ed. http://www.psychiatryonline.com/content.aspx?aID=204268. Accessed February 2, 2007.

186. Answer: C. All the statements about papilledema are true except Choice C. Papilledema does not usually affect visual acuity.

Fix JD. *High-Yield Neuroanatomy*. Baltimore: Lippincott Williams & Wilkins; 1995:78.

187. Answer: C. The syndrome named after Heinrich Klüver and Paul Bucy is caused by injury or destruction of the temporal lobe bilaterally. In rhesus monkeys it is characterized by visual agnosia (can see, but are unable to recognize previously familiar objects or their use), emotional changes, altered sexual behavior, hypermetamorphosis (desire to explore everything), and oral tendencies (examine everything with their mouths, instead of their eyes). They would indulge in overt sexual behaviors including masturbation and heterosexual or homosexual acts. They became emotionally dulled with reduced facial expressions and vocalizations. They lacked fear and would approach dangerous situations willingly and this personality change is termed called "placidity." Humans with temporal lobes show oral or tactile exploratory behavior (socially inappropriate licking or touching), hypersexuality, overeating, forgetfulness, emotional flattening, and an inability to recognize objects or faces. Although the full syndrome rarely occurs in humans, parts of it are often seen in subjects with bilateral temporal lesions caused by herpes simplex encephalitis, trauma, cerebrovascular events, or neurodegenerative disorders like frontotemporal dementias.

Kaufman DM. *Clinical Neurology for Psychiatrists*. 5th ed. Philadelphia: WB Saunders; 2001:299, 402–403.

188. Answer: B. Higher doses of selegiline are of no additional benefit in patients with Parkinson's disease. Doses greater than 10 mg daily place the patient at risk for hypertensive crisis due to nonselective MAO inhibition. However, selegiline does not cause a hypertensive crisis when used with concomitantly ingested tyramine-containing foods. Headache, nausea, and insomnia are common adverse effects. Thus far, studies have shown that selegiline is modestly effective as a monotherapy.

1. Horn S, Stern MB. The comparative effects of medical therapies for Parkinson's disease. *Neurology*. 2004; 63(suppl 2):S7–S12.
2. Tarsy D. *Pharmacological Treatment of Parkinson's Disease*. http://www.uptodateonline.com/utd/content/topic.do?topicKey=move_dis/4953&type=A&selectedTitle=2~33. Accessed February 19, 2007.

189. Answer: D. In rumination disorder, the repeated regurgitation and rechewing of food must last for a period of at least a month following a period of normal functioning. The behavior is not attributable to gastrointestinal problems or other medical conditions. Infantile Anorexia, Feeding Disorder of Infant-Caregiver Reciprocity, and Sensory Food Aversions are all research diagnostic criteria.

1. American Psychiatric Association. *Diagnostic and Statistical Manual of Mental Disorders: DSM-IV-TR*. 4th ed. Washington: American Psychiatric Association; 2000: 103–108.
2. Wiener JM, Dulcan MK. *Textbook of Child and Adolescent Psychiatry*. 3rd ed. Washington: American Psychiatric Publishing; 2004:639–657.

190. Answer: E. The patient meets criteria for Tourette's syndrome except for age of onset. As a result, Tic disorder NOS is the appropriate diagnosis.

American Psychiatric Association. *Diagnostic and Statistical Manual of Mental Disorders: DSM-IV-TR*. 4th ed. Washington: American Psychiatric Association; 2000: 108–116.

191. Answer: E. Body mass index is not known to be correlated with prognosis in encopresis.

Wiener JM, Dulcan MK. *Textbook of Child and Adolescent Psychiatry*. 3rd ed. Washington: American Psychiatric Publishing; 2004:748.

192. Answer: D. *La belle indifférence* is an inappropriate attitude of calm or lack of concern about one's disability. The patient presents as inappropriately cavalier toward serious symptoms. Although not diagnostic of Conversion Disorder, this phenomenon can be seen in patients with Conversion. Astasia-abasia is a wildly ataxic gait sometimes seen in patients with Conversion Disorder. The staggering gait is usually accompanied by gross, irregular truncal and waving arm movements. Cataplexy, often associated with narcolepsy, is a temporary loss of muscle tone and weakness precipitated by a variety of emotional states. Pseudocyesis is a false belief of being pregnant, associated with objective signs of pregnancy.

Alexithymia is a person's inability to, or difficulty in, describing or being aware of emotions or mood.

Sadock BJ, Sadock VA. *Kaplan and Sadock's Synopsis of Psychiatry*. 9th ed. Philadelphia: Lippincott Williams & Wilkins; 2003:280–281, 649.

193. Answer: A. All are accurate except for Choice A. Registration is the ability to add new materials to one's memory, rather than related to the duration of one's memory. An example of semantic memory would be a fact, such as "Boston is a city." An example of episodic memory would be an event, such as "my family goes camping every summer."

Sims A. *Symptoms in the Mind*. 3rd ed. London: Elsevier Science; 2003:64.

194. Answer: C. The intracellular concentration of potassium ions is much greater than its concentration outside of the cell. The sodium-potassium ATPase (Na^+-K^+ ATPase) pump actively pumps three Na^+ out of the cell in exchange for two K^+ into the cell, in an ATP-dependent manner. The cell membrane is much more permeable to K^+ ions due to the presence of potassium leak channels that remain open, allowing diffusion of K^+ out of the cell. This diffusion of K^+ leads to a net negative charge inside of the cell, with the potential difference across the cell membrane approximately –70 mV. The diffusion of Na^+ is prevented during the resting state by closed voltage-gated sodium channels, helping maintain the membrane potential. When an excitatory stimulus is received by the neuron, membrane depolarization will lead to opening of the voltage-gated sodium channels, allowing an influx of Na^+ until a membrane potential of +40 mV is reached, causing the sodium channels to close, and voltage-gated potassium channels to open. The period after the action potential and membrane depolarization is called the refractory period, and during this time, the neuron is not capable of conducting any impulses.

Siegal GJ, Albers RW, Brady S, Price DL. *Basic Neurochemistry, Molecular, Cellular, and Medical Aspects*. 6th ed. Philadelphia: Lippincott Williams & Wilkins; 1999:119–139.

195. Answer: B. Starting antiepileptic therapy is warranted in patients with factors that increase risk of recurrent seizures. A brain lesion places a patient at increased risk of recurrent seizures. A grand mal seizure, seizure due to a resolvable cause, a nonfocal examination, and the absence of serious brain injury do not increase risk of additional seizures.

Schachter, SC. *Overview of the Management of Epilepsy in Adults*. http://www.uptodateonline.com/utd/content/topic.do?topicKey=epil_eeg/4878&type=A&selectedTitle=2~248. Accessed February 19, 2007.

196. Answer: A. Of the antiepileptic medications listed above, only levetiracetam is useful as an initial monotherapy for generalized tonic-clonic seizures. Tiagabine, pregabalin, vigabatrin, and gabapentin are initial monotherapies for partial onset seizures with or without secondary generalization.

Schachter, SC. *Overview of the Management of Epilepsy in Adults*. http://www.uptodateonline.com/utd/content/topic.do?topicKey=epil_eeg/4878&type=A&selectedTitle=2~248. Accessed February 19, 2007.

197. Answer: C. Many antiepileptic medications induce hepatic enzymes. Induction of hepatic enzymes enhances metabolism of oral contraceptives. This enzyme induction increases the expected contraception failure rate from 0.7 per 100 woman-years using oral contraception to 3.1 per 100 woman-years in patients who concomitantly take enzyme-inducing antiepileptic drugs. Valproate does not induce hepatic enzymes and is thus safer for this patient to take for her condition.

1. Schachter, SC. *Overview of the Management of Epilepsy in Adults*. http://www.uptodateonline.com/utd/content/topic.do?topicKey=epil_eeg/4878&type=A&selectedTitle=2~248. Accessed February 19, 2007.
2. Zupanc ML. Antiepileptic drugs and hormonal contraceptives in adolescent women with epilepsy. *Neurology*. 2006;66(suppl 3):S37–S45.

198. Answer: D. Of the medications listed for the acute treatment or prophylaxis of migraine headaches, sumatriptan is the most likely to be associated with the patient's presentation. There are several case reports of serotonin syndrome resulting from concomitant administration of an SSRI or SNRI with a selective serotonin agonist such as sumatriptan. The FDA has an advisory statement regarding treatments using an SSRI/SNRI with a triptan. Although, there is no absolute contraindication for simultaneous administration of these two drug classes, it is important to be aware of the potential for serotonin syndrome in this situation, to discuss the possibility with the patient, to be aware of the clinical presentation of serotonin syndrome, and to educate patients on the importance of making sure that all of their health-care providers are aware of all of their medications. Treatment of serotonin syndrome is largely supportive.

1. Food and Drug Administration. *Selective Serotonin Reuptake Inhibitors (SSRIs)*. http://www.fda.gov/cder/drug/InfoSheets/HCP/citalopramHCP.pdf. Accessed February 20, 2006.
2. Gardner DM, Lynd LD. Sumatriptan contraindications and the serotonin syndrome. *Ann Pharmacother*. 1998;32:33–38.

199. Answer: D. Ethosuximide is considered the drug of choice for control of absence seizures, diagnosed in this child. The EEG would show the characteristic 3 per second spike and wave pattern seen in childhood absence epilepsy. An absence seizure may be able to be provoked by hyperventilation such as having the child make a pinwheel move by blowing on it. The practitioner must be prepared for the possibility of a prolonged seizure during any provocative maneuver and act accordingly. Lamotrigine and valproic acid are also recommended first-line agents, and more than one drug may be necessary for seizure control. Phenytoin at therapeutic doses can actually worsen absence seizure control.

Beghi E. Efficacy and tolerability of the new antiepileptic drugs: comparison of two recent guidelines. *Lancet Neurol.* 2004;3:618–621.

200. Answer: D. The M'Naghten rule derives from the famous case of 1843 when Daniel M'Naghten murdered Edward Drummond, the private secretary of the Prime Minister, Robert Peel. M'Naghten suffered from delusions and thought he could correct the situation by murdering Peel. Instead, he accidentally murdered the secretary, Drummond. The jury found him not guilty by reason of insanity. According to the rule, the question is not whether the accused knows the difference between right and wrong in general, but whether he understood the nature and the quality of the act and whether he knew the difference between right and wrong with respect to the act. The current American Law Institute recommends that a person is not responsible for criminal conduct if, at the time of such conduct and as a result of mental disease, a person lacked substantial capacity either to appreciate the wrongfulness of the act or to conform conduct to the requirement of the law.

Kaplan HI, Sadock BJ. *Kaplan & Sadock's Synopsis of Psychiatry*. 8th ed. Philadelphia: Lippincott Williams & Wilkins; 1998:1314–1315.

Questions

1. A mother brings her 4-year-old child for a developmental assessment. Which one of the following skills would you NOT expect to find in this child?

   A. Hop on one foot
   B. Throw ball overhand
   C. Copy a triangle from a model
   D. Copy a bridge from a model
   E. Copy a cross and square from a model

2. Which one of the following statements is NOT TRUE about γ-aminobutyric acid (GABA)?

   A. It is the principal inhibitory neurotransmitter in the brain.
   B. An increase in the brain GABA levels may lead to convulsions.
   C. It is formed by the decarboxylation of glutamate by glutamate decarboxylase.
   D. It is degraded by GABA transaminase.
   E. Highest density of GABA is seen in the basal ganglia, hypothalamus, amygdala, and other limbic areas.

3. According to George Vaillant's classifications, all of the following are considered to be immature defenses which can be seen in adolescents and some depressed patients, EXCEPT:

   A. Blocking
   B. Introjection
   C. Reaction formation
   D. Schizoid fantasy
   E. Somatization

4. The most frequent issue in lawsuits against psychiatrists concerns which one of the following?

   A. Attempted or completed suicide
   B. Breach of confidentiality
   C. Improper commitment
   D. Incorrect diagnosis
   E. Incorrect treatment

5. During your initial interview, a 17-year-old boy reports occasional visual hallucinations while falling asleep. The rest of the mental status examination is unremarkable. Given this information, you would classify his visual hallucination as which one of the following?

   A. A brief psychotic disorder
   B. Prodrome of schizophrenia

   C. A hypnagogic hallucination
   D. A hypnopompic hallucination
   E. A part of Charles Bonnet syndrome

6. According to the DSM-IV-TR criteria for Delusional Disorder, a patient must never have met criteria A for Schizophrenia. However, which of the following types of hallucinations may be present in Delusional Disorder, if they are related to the delusional theme?

   A. Visual and auditory
   B. Visual and olfactory
   C. Tactile and auditory
   D. Auditory and olfactory
   E. Tactile and olfactory

7. A man of Thai origin seems to be petrified of dying. He believes that his penis is going to recede into his body, thereby precipitating his death. He has asked several of his friends and relatives to help prevent this retraction. He has even tried to use a pair of clamps to prevent his genital retraction. He does not appear to possess any other bizarre beliefs. What is the term used to describe the condition that he is suffering from at this time?

   A. *Dhat*
   B. *Koro*
   C. *Qi-Gong psychotic reaction*
   D. *Shin-Byung*
   E. *Rootwork*

8. Who was the first person to describe "hebephrenic" schizophrenia?

   A. Emil Kraepelin
   B. Kurt Schneider
   C. Ewald Hecker
   D. Karl Kahlbaum
   E. Eugen Bleuler

9. Which one of the following is TRUE of Dementia with Lewy Bodies (DLB)?

   A. Fluctuating mental status occurs in 50%–70% of patients
   B. Daytime sleep is only about 2–3 hours
   C. Staring into space occurs for long periods of time
   D. Flow of ideas are disorganized, unclear and illogical
   E. All of the above

10. What is a first-line treatment for Panic Disorder?
    A. Buspirone
    B. Alprazolam
    C. Gabapentin
    D. Sertraline
    E. Imipramine

11. Which of the following antidepressants is most likely to contribute to a geriatric patient's presentation of hyponatremia?
    A. Mirtazapine
    B. Imipramine
    C. Citalopram
    D. Trazodone
    E. Lithium

12. An 80-year-old man with moderate Alzheimer's type dementia has just been placed in a nursing home. He appears irritable, anxious, confused, his sleep-wake pattern is disturbed, and he is wandering throughout the unit at various times of the day and night. He takes no psychotropic medications and has no previous psychiatric history. Which one of the following interventions has the greatest potential to harm the patient?
    A. Educating staff and family about behavioral interventions, and his adjustment to the new environment.
    B. Considering cognitive enhancing agents such as cholinesterase or memantine.
    C. Considering a newer generation antidepressant for the treatment of anxiety or depression.
    D. In concert with the primary physician, attempting to reduce unnecessary medications, especially those that are highly anticholinergic.
    E. Prescribing antipsychotics or benzodiazepines to control his behavior and to correct his sleep-wake cycle.

13. Which of the following statements is TRUE of patients with Down syndrome (DS) and Alzheimer's disease (AD)?
    A. The age of onset of AD is earlier in patients with DS than in the general population.
    B. By 40 years of age, all patients with DS exhibit AD pathology in their brains.
    C. These patients first develop visual memory loss and impaired learning capacity when they develop AD.
    D. Magnetic resonance imaging (MRI) findings in these patients include cerebellar atrophy, basal ganglia calcification and hippocampal atrophy.
    E. All of the above.

14. A 35-year-old man is admitted to the psychiatric unit with a 2-month history of third-person auditory hallucinations and paranoid delusions. He is started on trifluoperazine. A week later, he develops fever with muscular rigidity, sweating, and confusion. He has a rapid pulse with fluctuating blood pressure. All of the following are TRUE statements of his condition EXCEPT:
    A. The prevalence is estimated to be approximately 5% in patients exposed to dopamine receptor antagonists.
    B. Laboratory findings include leucocytosis, abnormal liver function tests, myoglobulinemia, and elevated creatine kinase level.
    C. It can occur at any stage of treatment with these drugs.
    D. Renal failure is a known complication.
    E. Mortality ranges between 10% and 20%.

15. You are called to evaluate a 70-year-old patient with severe pneumonia who wants to leave the hospital against medical advice. You use the MacArthur Competence Assessment Tool for Treatment (MacCAT-T). All of the following are listed as components of capacity for medical decision-making with this tool EXCEPT:
    A. Factual understanding of the illness and risks and benefits of treatment alternatives
    B. Absence of delirium
    C. Appreciation for the fact that his or her decision will have consequences for him or her
    D. To be able to reason logically and realistically
    E. To be able to express a choice

16. Which of the following enzymes is involved in the rate-limiting step of serotonin biosynthesis?
    A. Aromatic amino acid decarboxylase
    B. Tryptophan hydroxylase
    C. Tyrosine hydroxylase
    D. Glutamic acid decarboxylase
    E. Phenylalanine hydroxylase (PAH)

17. A 28-year-old woman with Schizophrenia has been successfully maintained on risperidone for the past year. At her last medication evaluation appointment, she reported amenorrhea and a history of breast discharge. Pregnancy was ruled out by a urine test. Given this history, what is the most likely mechanism leading to her symptoms?
    A. Anovulatory cycles due to polycystic ovarian syndrome
    B. Inhibition of D2 receptor binding on pituitary cell membranes
    C. Increased oxytocin production in paraventricular hypothalamic neurons
    D. Drug-induced hypothyroidism
    E. Premature ovarian failure

18. Which of the following is TRUE of the genetics of Huntington's disease?

A. The gene for Huntington's disease is located on the short arm of chromosome 6.
B. The gene for Huntington's disease is associated with an expanded TAC repeats.
C. The expansion of the trinucleotide repeats account for the phenomenon of "anticipation" in this disease.
D. Even in identical twins, the age of onset of this disease remains highly variable.
E. All of the above.

19. You are asked to assist in the evaluation of a 35-year-old patient on the neurology service presenting with seizure activity. History reveals that he experiences full body tonic clonic seizures on a daily basis. He loses consciousness during these episodes, and following them, he has left-sided hand weakness. Based on this history, which one of the following is the most likely to be TRUE in this patient?
    A. Due to his age, the seizure activity is likely psychogenic in nature.
    B. As he is not noted to be incontinent of stool or urine during the seizure activity, the seizure focus is likely in the non-dominant hemisphere.
    C. There is too little objective data to make any accurate statements regarding his case.
    D. The seizure focus is likely to be in the left hemisphere.
    E. The seizure focus is likely to be in the right hemisphere.

20. A patient reports problems remembering personal experiences that took place at a particular place and time. Which type of memory is this patient referring to when talking about her problem?
    A. Semantic memory
    B. Episodic memory
    C. Non-declarative memory
    D. Implicit memory
    E. Immediate memory

21. Which one of the following is not usually seen in patients with normal pressure hydrocephalus (NPH)?
    A. Gait apraxia
    B. Dementia
    C. Urinary incontinence
    D. Headaches
    E. Frontal release signs

22. A 50-year-old man with human immunodeficiency virus (HIV) is admitted to the neurology service for insidious onset of confusion. Upon examination, he is found to have paresthesia along the C4-5 distribution. It is suspected that he has neurosyphilis, and a lumbar puncture (LP) is performed. The cerebrospinal fluid (CSF) is yellow in color. Which one of the following characteristics of neurosyphilis explains the color of the CSF?
    A. High red blood cell (RBC) concentrations in the CSF
    B. Elevated opening pressure of CSF
    C. High white blood cell (WBC) concentration
    D. High protein concentration
    E. There is no relationship between the CSF color and neurosyphilis.

23. A 45-year-old African American man presents to your office for an evaluation of polyuria, sleep disturbance, heat intolerance, and vestibular dysfunction. The patient has a history pertinent only for carpal tunnel syndrome, which was corrected surgically at the age of 38 years. An MRI of the brain reveals parenchymal inflammation with disruption of the blood brain barrier. LP yields a protein level of 100 mg/dL, glucose level of 30 mg/dL, WBC count of 50 PMN/mm^3 and an elevated serum angiotensin converting enzyme (ACE) level. Which of the following diagnosis is most consistent with this presentation?
    A. Hepatic encephalopathy
    B. Infection
    C. Carcinomatous meningitis
    D. Neurologic sarcoidosis
    E. Chronic cocaine intoxication

24. Which of the following is implicated in the pathophysiology of Rett syndrome?
    A. Presence of intranuclear hyaline inclusion disease
    B. Mutations of the MeCP2 gene, most commonly of the paternal X chromosome
    C. Mutations of the MeCP2 gene, most commonly of the maternal X chromosome
    D. Focal axonal swelling
    E. White matter changes compatible with leukodystrophy

25. Which of the following is LEAST likely to be associated with Rapid Eye Movement Sleep Behavior Disorder (RBD)?
    A. Shy-Drager syndrome
    B. Parkinson's disease
    C. Lewy body dementia
    D. Olivopontocerebellar disease
    E. Alzheimer's dementia

26. A 7-year-old girl is referred for evaluation of poor school performance. Her parents report that she frequently seems to "zone out" during the day, even when doing something she enjoys, such as watching a cartoon. Her teacher has noticed the same behavior at school. She frequently loses her homework, has difficulty completing assignments, and has very

sloppy handwriting; school testing did not reveal any cognitive deficits or learning disabilities. Her neurologic exam was unremarkable until she was asked to keep blowing to keep a pinwheel rotating for as long as she could. After 30 seconds of hyperventilation, she stopped blowing on the pinwheel, developed a blank stare, and began blinking rapidly for the next minute. An electrocephalogram (EEG) was done, which confirmed the diagnosis. Which of the following medications would be the best first-line therapy for this condition?

A. Phenytoin
B. Carbamazepine
C. Topiramate
D. Ethosuximide
E. Phenobarbital

27. A child is brought to his pediatrician for a routine visit. The pediatrician notices that the child knows his full name, refers to himself by the pronoun "I," helps put things away, and engages in pretend play. Given these observations, what would be the approximate age of this child?

A. 15 months
B. 18 months
C. 22 months
D. 26 months
E. 30 months

28. Which one of the following statements is TRUE regarding rivastigmine?

A. It is primarily metabolized by the liver.
B. It inhibits the activity of butyrylcholinesterase (BChE) and acetylcholinesterase (AChE).
C. It stops the progression of cognitive decline in patients with dementia.
D. It has no gastrointestinal side effects.
E. It must be taken four times daily.

29. All of the following are true statements regarding Erik Erikson's term *initiative versus guilt* EXCEPT:

A. If this stage is not mastered successfully, the psychopathological outcomes associated include Generalized Anxiety Disorder, phobias, or impotence.
B. Parents should make an issue about childhood sexual impulses by using punishment during this stage in order to repress those impulses until adolescence.
C. The end of this stage is marked by the establishment of a child's conscience, which sets the tone for the moral sense of right and wrong.
D. This stage corresponds to Freud's phallic-oedipal stage, which is when children will often manifest

their sexual curiosity by touching their genitalia or those of a peer.
E. This stage refers to ages 3 to 5 years but is an approximation, as stages are not fixed in time and development is continuous.

30. Of the following choices, which is the least frequent issue in lawsuits against psychiatrists?

A. Failure to manage suicide attempts
B. Improper supervision
C. Incorrect diagnosis
D. Incorrect treatment
E. Sexual involvement with patient

31. What score is considered to be the threshold for clinically significant anxiety when the Hamilton Anxiety Scale is administered?

A. 5
B. 9
C. 14
D. 18
E. 20

32. A 15-year-old man is brought to the emergency department (ED) by friends. His friends are initially elusive about their activities that evening, but state the patient became suddenly confused and agitated at a party, eventually running into traffic and screaming. In the ED, the patient remains agitated, disoriented, and is noted to be tachycardic and perspiring. One particularly worried friend later confesses that the group was experimenting with "Adam and Eve" prior to the patient's deterioration. In accordance with DSM-IV-TR classification, which class of substances is responsible for the patient's current presentation?

A. Amphetamines
B. Opioids
C. Hallucinogens
D. Inhalants
E. Steroids

33. A 30-year-old woman presents for a psychiatric evaluation. She complains of depressive symptoms such as low mood, anxiety, anhedonia, and marked irritability. She reports her symptoms seem to have a pattern: they occur in the week prior to menses and almost always remit within a few days after the onset of menses. Symptoms are noted to interfere with her work as a high school teacher. Given this history, which one of the following DSM-IV-TR diagnosis would be most appropriate for her condition?

A. Depressive Disorder Not Otherwise Specified (NOS)
B. Major Depressive Disorder (MDD)

C. Depressive Disorder due to a General Medical Condition

D. Dysthymia

E. Adjustment Disorder

34. Which one of the following is NOT part of the diagnostic criteria for Catatonic Schizophrenia according to DSM-IV-TR?

A. Catalepsy/stupor

B. Echolalia/echopraxia

C. Extreme negativism/mutism

D. Posturing

E. Hypertonia

35. Which of the following statements is TRUE of Frontotemporal Lobar Degeneration (FTLD)?

A. It is the second most common cause of cortical dementia

B. Pick's bodies are the defining histopathologic feature of FTLD

C. FTLD encompasses two pathologic substrates and three prototypic neurobehavioral syndromes

D. Patients are often clinically amnesic

E. None of the above

36. A 29-year-old military combat veteran presents with symptoms of hyperarousal, recurrent reexperiencing of his combat experience, and avoidance of environments that remind him of his time in combat. Which one of the following medications would be an appropriate initial treatment of his condition?

A. Sertraline

B. Lorazepam

C. Gabapentin

D. Risperidone

E. Buspirone

37. Which one of the following is most likely to contribute to a clinical presentation of polydipsia with dilute urine?

A. Mirtazapine

B. Citalopram

C. Imipramine

D. Trazodone

E. Lithium

38. Which of the following statements is NOT TRUE of phototherapy for the treatment of Seasonal Affective Disorder (SAD)?

A. Phototherapy is the most widely studied treatment for SAD.

B. The dosage often found to be effective is 2,500 lux per day.

C. Similar to antidepressant therapy for depression, phototherapy carries some risk of precipitating mania.

D. Phototherapy is most effective when administered earlier in the day.

E. None of the above.

39. A 35-year-old woman with Bipolar Disorder is admitted to the hospital for an acute manic episode. She is disorganized and intrusive and requires haloperidol injections every 6 hours to control her threatening behavior. She is placed on lithium and benztropine, but continues to require PRN haloperidol for agitation. All of the following are currently potential risk factors for development of Tardive Dyskinesia (TD) in this patient EXCEPT:

A. Intermittent dosing of benztropine and haloperidol

B. Patient's age

C. Patient's gender

D. Patient having a mood disorder

E. Switching intramuscular haloperidol to oral haloperidol for long term use

40. A 70-year-old woman with moderate vascular dementia demonstrates behavioral disturbances secondary to paranoid delusions. Routine investigations including complete blood screen and mid-stream urine examination fails to determine any underlying cause for her psychotic symptoms. Her general practitioner commences her on haloperidol 2 mg a day; this is increased to 5 mg once a day after 5 days. Ten days later, she is brought to the emergency room (ER) in a state of dehydration and rigidity. Investigations reveal acute renal failure with elevated creatine kinase and myoglobinuria. Neuroleptic Malignant Syndrome (NMS) is diagnosed in this patient. All of the following conditions are known risk factors for NMS EXCEPT:

A. Rapid dose increase of antipsychotic drugs

B. Abrupt discontinuation of anticholinergic drugs

C. Hypothyroidism

D. Parkinson's disease

E. Mental retardation

41. Which one of the following is NOT TRUE regarding hallucinations in the hospital setting?

A. The most common cause is Schizophrenia.

B. Sensory isolation is a common etiology of hallucinations in intensive care units.

C. Delirium tremens often occurs 3 to 4 days after hospitalization.

D. Brain tumors can cause hallucinations.

E. Systemic lupus erythematosus (SLE) can cause hallucinations.

42. Which of the serotonin receptors exerts its second messenger effects via a ligand-gated ion channel?
    A. $5-HT_{1A}$
    B. $5-HT_{1B}$
    C. $5-HT_{2A}$
    D. $5-HT_{2B}$
    E. $5-HT_3$

43. Which of the following statements about nitric oxide is NOT TRUE?
    A. Nitric oxide functions as an important neurotransmitter.
    B. Nitric oxide inhibits platelet aggregation.
    C. Nitric oxide is used as an anesthetic gas.
    D. Nitric oxide facilitates penile erections.
    E. Nitric oxide dilates blood vessels.

44. Which one of the following is TRUE of Wilson's disease?
    A. It is inherited as an autosomal dominant disorder.
    B. In occurs in 1 in 5,000 people.
    C. The symptoms of this disorder usually appear in the first decade of life.
    D. There is excess accumulation of copper in the liver because of increased absorption.
    E. None of the above.

45. A 45-year-old woman with Schizophrenia presents with galactorrhea and amenorrhea. A prolactin level is drawn and is found to be elevated. Which of the following should be considered in a patient with hyperprolactinemia?
    A. Use of antipsychotic medications
    B. Chronic renal failure
    C. Hypothyroidism
    D. Pituitary stalk damage
    E. All of the above

46. A 20-year-old woman college student presents to the ER with headache, fever, and lethargy. An LP is performed, and analysis of the cloudy fluid shows the following values: (i) WBC/mm: 450, (ii) proteins: 150 mg/100 mL, and (iii) glucose: 12 mg/100 mL. This profile is most consistent with which of the following?
    A. Normal CSF
    B. Bacterial meningitis
    C. Viral meningitis
    D. Subarachnoid hemorrhage (SAH)
    E. Intracranial mass

47. Which one of the following is the diagnostic test of choice for routinely detecting NPH in adults?
    A. Skull transillumination
    B. Plain skull radiograph
    C. LP
    D. CSF pulse wave analysis
    E. MRI of the brain

48. A patient presents with subacute onset of facial nerve palsy, ipsilateral decreased lacrimation, and ipsilateral ear pain. She had a viral syndrome several weeks prior to the onset of her neurologic symptoms. The symptoms worsened for a week and then appear to be resolving for the past week. An LP performed on this patient would likely reveal which of the following findings?
    A. Increased opening pressure
    B. Increased RBC concentration
    C. Increased protein concentration
    D. Decreased WBC concentration
    E. No abnormalities

49. Which one of the following statements regarding the Mini-Mental State Examination (MMSE) is NOT TRUE?
    A. It can be useful in detecting and estimating severity of cognitive deficits.
    B. It can overestimate cognitive impairment in people who are older and less educated.
    C. It does not distinguish various etiologies of dementia (e.g., Alzheimer's from vascular dementia).
    D. It distinguishes dementia from depression-induced memory impairment.
    E. It is used so widely that it is considered the standard in screening tests for cognitive impairment.

50. A 16-month-old child is brought to your office because the mother has noticed that in the past few months the child seems to be unable to move as quickly as before. He seems to be having problems carrying things, and he has not been reaching his developmental milestones on time. Upon your physical examination, you notice muscular atrophy and generalized hyperreflexia. A brain MRI shows diffuse and prominent hyperintensity of the cerebellar cortex, dentate nucleus, and pyramidal tracts. Given this history, what is this patient's most likely diagnosis?
    A. Rett syndrome
    B. Megalencephalic leukodystrophy
    C. Seitelberger disease
    D. Cockayne syndrome
    E. Juvenile Huntington's disease

51. A 73-year-old woman with a history of hypertension and hypercholesterolemia presents to the outpatient clinic with her daughter after a fall at home. In recent months, the patient has developed unsteadiness and

impaired balance. Her greatest difficulty has been with ambulating on stairs and curbs. Her daughter notes that the patient has been forgetting to take her medications and appears more apathetic. Given this history, which of the following is the most likely diagnosis?

A. Alzheimer's disease
B. NPH
C. Parkinson's disease
D. Vascular dementia
E. Pelvic fracture

52. A 25-year-old man presents seeking treatment for headaches. He started having headaches 6 years ago, usually accompanied by photophobia and phonophobia. He has noticed lately that he will be irritable for several hours before a headache starts, "before I even know it's on the way." He has not noticed any aura symptoms associated with the headaches, has not had any loss of consciousness, and has not had any weakness associated with the headaches. Although he may wake up in the morning with a headache, the pain does not rouse him out of sleep. His mother and a maternal aunt have migraines with aura. He had previously been treating the headaches with ibuprofen, but had been having two to three headaches per week for the last 3 months that were not very responsive to non-steroidal anti-inflammatory drugs (NSAIDs). Based on his history, he is diagnosed with migraines, given a prescription for sumatriptan, and asked to keep a headache diary until his follow-up appointment in 1 month. At the next visit, he reports that the sumatriptan has been effective in treating a migraine headache once it has started, but that he is still having at least one headache weekly. The headaches last 10 to 12 hours and are interfering with his ability to work. Which of the following drugs would be indicated for the prophylaxis of migraine headaches?

A. Daily acetaminophen
B. Topiramate
C. Caffeine
D. Zinc supplements
E. The patient does not meet criteria for prophylactic migraine therapy.

53. By what age is a child able to repeat sentences of at least ten syllables?

A. 30 months
B. 36 months
C. 42 months
D. 48 months
E. 60 months

54. Which one of the following disorders exhibits an autosomal recessive pattern of inheritance?

A. Homocystinuria
B. Neurofibromatosis type 1
C. Tuberous sclerosis
D. Huntington's disease
E. Turner's syndrome

55. According to Erik Erikson, a patient suffering from Obsessive Compulsive Personality Disorder might likely have not successfully mastered which of the following stages?

A. Basic trust versus basic mistrust
B. Autonomy versus shame and doubt
C. Initiative versus guilt
D. Identity versus role diffusion
E. Integrity versus despair and isolation

56. All of the following are true principles regarding psychiatric patients that were decided by landmark legal cases EXCEPT:

A. A clinician must notify the intended victim when there is an imminent threat posed by the patient.
B. Harmless mental patients cannot be confined against their will without treatment if they can survive in the community.
C. Patients committed to mental institutions have a constitutional right to receive individualized treatment plans.
D. Patients do not have a constitutional right to be discharged if they are involuntary status, even if they are not receiving treatment.
E. Patients have an absolute right to refuse treatment and to use an appeal process.

57. A 23-year-old combat veteran having his first psychiatric evaluation complains of insomnia and increased irritability. Upon further interviewing, he also reports hypervigilance and nightmares. Which of the following rating scales would you use to further clarify his diagnosis?

A. Yale-Brown Obsessive-Compulsive Scale (YBOCS)
B. Clinician-Administered Posttraumatic Stress Disorder Scale (CAPS)
C. Alcohol Use Disorders Identification Test (AUDIT)
D. Addiction Severity Index (ASI)
E. CAGE Questionaitte

58. According to the DSM-IV-TR, which of the following is NOT defined as a type of Delusional Disorder?

A. Paranoid type
B. Erotomanic type
C. Somatic type
D. Persecutory type
E. Grandiose type

59. Each one of the following is considered a risk factor for the development of MDD EXCEPT:

A. Female gender
B. Family history of depression
C. Separated or divorced marital status
D. Race/ethnicity
E. Lower socioeconomic status

60. A family brings in their 6-year-old son for evaluation to a psychiatrist. They report that they have noted that their son is unable to do many of the things that other children his age can do and that he looks a little odd. As part of the evaluation you note that the patient is short for his age, has a long face and large ears, there is joint laxity, and he has macroorchidism. An IQ test reports a score of 50. You suspect a diagnosis of Fragile X syndrome. In order to complete your workup for this patient, you recommend genetic testing. Which of the following results of the genetic testing would confirm the diagnosis?

A. Trisomy 21
B. Deletion in 15q12 of paternal origin
C. Deletion of 17p11.2
D. Deletion in 15q12 of maternal origin
E. Inactivation of FMR-1 gene at Xq27.3 due to CGG base repeats

61. Which of the following is/are difference(s) between FTLD and AD?

A. A predominantly "senile" onset
B. Absence of severe amnesia, visuospatial impairment, and myoclonus
C. The preponderance of neurofibrillary tangles (NFTs) over amyloid plaques
D. The presence of "bradyphrenia"
E. All of the above

62. A 22-year-old man was recently hospitalized following his first psychotic break. In this patient with Schizophrenia, what would be an important treatment modality to facilitate the reduction of stress at home?

A. Psychoanalysis
B. Cognitive behavioral therapy
C. Dialectal behavioral therapy
D. Family therapy
E. Motivational enhancement therapy

63. Which one of the following is the site most likely to be involved in the rare clinical presentation of Syndrome of Irreversible Lithium-Effectuated Neurotoxicity (SILENT)?

A. Cerebellum
B. Peripheral nerves
C. Orbitofrontal cortex

D. Dorsal columns (spinal cord)
E. None of the above

64. Which one of the following statements about clozapine is TRUE?

A. Phenytoin should be added to clozapine at doses above 600 mg per day.
B. The risk of seizure due to clozapine at doses 600 mg to 900 mg a day is 15%.
C. Valproic acid should be added to clozapine at doses above 600 mg per day.
D. The risk of seizure due to clozapine at doses 600 mg to 900 mg a day is 25%.
E. Carbamazepine should be added to clozapine at doses above 600 mg per day.

65. Regarding antipsychotic drugs in pregnancy and nursing, all of the following statements are true EXCEPT:

A. A breast-feeding infant of a mother treated with antipsychotics is at some risk for the development of extrapyramidal symptoms (EPS).
B. Chlorpromazine has been associated with an increased risk of neonatal jaundice in late pregnancy.
C. It is best if possible to avoid antipsychotic agents in pregnancy, especially in the first trimester.
D. There are no clear patterns of teratogenicity that have emerged with the use of antipsychotics in pregnancy.
E. To avoid EPS in the newborn, it has been recommended that an antipsychotic be discontinued 1 week before the due date.

66. The management of NMS includes all of the following EXCEPT:

A. Withdrawing the antipsychotic medication
B. Supportive management with monitoring of vital signs
C. Using dantrolene and bromocriptine
D. Avoiding benzodiazepines
E. Maintaining hydration

67. Each of the following statements about gender is true EXCEPT:

A. Gender refers to the phenotypic sex of an individual.
B. Gender is determined in part by expectations and behavioral patterns learned in early childhood.
C. Gender is determined in part by exposure to sex steroids.
D. Gender identity begins at age 3 to 4 years.
E. Gender identity generally occurs earlier in girls than in boys.

68. Occlusion of the vertebral artery produces ipsilateral Horner's syndrome along with ipsilateral loss of pain and temperature sensations of the face, cerebellar ataxia, weakness of the palate, pharynx, and vocal cords. It is also associated with contralateral loss of pain and temperature sensation to the body. This constellation of findings is found in which of the following syndromes?
   A. Anterior inferior cerebellar artery syndrome
   B. Wallenberg's syndrome
   C. Parinaud's syndrome
   D. Anterior spinal artery syndrome
   E. Weber's syndrome

69. Which of the following statements regarding mitochondria is NOT TRUE?
   A. Mitochondrial DNA is derived equally from both parents.
   B. Mitochondria produce approximately 90% of the body's energy requirement.
   C. Free radicals are highly toxic by-products of mitochondrial metabolism.
   D. Mitochondria produce the majority of their energy in the form of adenosine-triphosphate (ATP).
   E. Energy-producing enzymes of mitochondria are easily poisoned.

70. Which one of the following is TRUE of mood disorders in multiple sclerosis (MS)?
   A. Studies indicate that 10% of patients with MS will sometime during the course of their illness meet the formal diagnostic criteria for a major mood disorder.
   B. The rate of completed suicide is approximately twice that of the general population.
   C. Available data indicate that symptoms of affective disturbances correlate with severity of neurological disability.
   D. It has been noted that the severity of depression is negatively correlated with the disease duration.
   E. Patients with MS show 10 times the lifetime prevalence of bipolar affective disorder than the general population.

71. What is the Finger Tapping Test used for?
   A. To identify difficulties in adaptation
   B. To identify problems in sustained attention
   C. To identify subtle lateralizing motor damage
   D. To identify problems in visual shifting
   E. To identify problems in concept formation

72. A 20-year-old woman presents to the ED complaining of sudden onset of blurry vision with diplopia, nausea, malaise, and dry mouth. She had been healthy with no medical problems. She had a flu vaccine 1 week ago and just came home for the weekend to visit her family in Connecticut. When asked what she did the day prior to coming to the hospital, she stated she helped make pies with her parents while eating some home-canned foods, and went for a hike with her brother in the woods behind their house. Physical exam is notable for dysconjugate gaze, dilated pupils that react slowly, and decreased deep tendon reflexes. A chem-7 is unremarkable. Which of the following is the most appropriate diagnostic procedure at this time?
   A. A computed tomography (CT) scan of head to rule out stroke
   B. An LP to rule out bacterial meningitis
   C. An MRI of the brain to rule out Guillain-Barré syndrome
   D. Screen with an enzyme-linked immunosorbent assay for Lyme disease
   E. Serum detection of *Clostridium botulism* toxin

73. Which one of the following statements is NOT TRUE of idiopathic intracranial hypertension (IIH)?
   A. It is characterized by increased intracranial pressure (ICP) without any know cause.
   B. Spontaneous recovery is characteristic.
   C. It can sometimes cause serious threat to vision.
   D. Patients usually present with headaches which are usually worse in the evenings.
   E. These headaches are usually worse with coughing or straining.

74. You are asked to evaluate a 70-year-old woman admitted to the medical service for evaluation of confusion. She has poor short-term memory and her recall at 5 minutes is one out of three objects. She has also been incontinent of urine. Her gait is slow and wide based. Upon examination, the patient is found to be bradykinetic and has increased deep tendon reflexes diffusely. A CT scan of the brain reveals a hydrocephalus. An LP is performed to confirm the diagnosis of NPH. Given this history, what is the most likely opening pressure for this patient?
   A. 0 cm H_2O
   B. 5 cm H_2O
   C. 15 cm H_2O
   D. 30 cm H_2O
   E. 50 cm H_2O

75. An 80-year-old retired attorney presents with his wife to a psychiatrist for an evaluation of his cognitive impairment. His wife brings in records from his previous physician appointments. He was diagnosed with "Alzheimer's disease" 3 years prior by his primary care physician. He has never seen a psychiatrist. He has had complete laboratory and imaging workup,

with no apparent abnormalities. His records indicate that yearly MMSEs were obtained, with the patient scoring 25 or 26 out of 30 each year. Upon examination by the psychiatrist, the patient is noted to be psychomotorically slowed with a flat affect. He scores 25 out of 30 on the MMSE. Which of the following statements is TRUE about this patient's condition?

A. The diagnosis of AD should be reconsidered.
B. A depressive syndrome has been ruled out.
C. The patient's MMSE indicates severe dementia.
D. Neuropsychological testing would not be helpful in this case.
E. All of the above.

76. A 3-year-old boy is brought to your office for an initial consultation. You notice that the patient has unusually large ears and sunken eyes. The child is deaf, very thin, and has to be protected from the sun because his skin is extremely sensitive to sunlight. For the past year, the child has not been growing appropriately and he is not reaching his developmental milestones. Radiographic studies show kyphoscoliosis. The patient also has intracranial calcifications and an MRI of the brain reveals loss of white matter and white matter hyperintensities. Given this history, what is this child's most likely diagnosis?

A. Rett's disorder
B. Seitelberger disease
C. Cockayne syndrome
D. Krabbe disease
E. Juvenile Huntington's disease

77. A 23-year-old woman with a history of severe acne presents to the ER. She complains of a headache in the back of her head which has been present for the last 3 weeks. The headache is dull and constant. She has had occasional blurred vision and dizziness. She denies fever, neck stiffness, weight loss, recent falls, or other head trauma. A head CT is unremarkable, and on LP, the CSF pressure is elevated. Which of the following is the most likely cause of her condition?

A. Isotretinoin
B. Gliomatosis cerebri
C. Lead toxicity
D. Hyperparathyroidism
E. Systemic lupus erythematosus

78. Which one of the following statements is NOT TRUE of bladder care in a neurobehavioral rehabilitation program?

A. The first step in this process is the evaluation for non-neurologic causes of dysfunction.
B. These programs include the implementation of regular voiding programs for patients.

C. Avoid training families on the use of catheters as its use will cause major problems in the future.
D. Scheduled voiding every 2 hours may help with regaining bladder incontinence and preventing overflow incontinence.
E. For patients with a flaccid bladder, cholinergic drugs and intermittent catheterization may be helpful.

79. By what age is a child usually able to walk alone?

A. 9 months
B. 12 months
C. 15 months
D. 18 months
E. 24 months

80. A visual field cut can occur due to an injury in which one of the following areas?

A. Pons
B. Medulla
C. Midbrain
D. Cerebellum
E. Cerebrum

81. Erik Erikson used the term *generativity versus stagnation* to describe which conflict and stage of the life cycle?

A. Childhood
B. Adolescence
C. Young adulthood
D. Middle adulthood
E. Late adulthood

82. As a rule, a psychiatrist can share his patient's information without the patient's consent to which of the following people?

A. A consultant
B. An insurer
C. Patient's lawyer
D. Patient's parents
E. Patient's previous therapist

83. What is the Conner's Rating Scales most frequently used for?

A. Eating disorders
B. Personality disorders
C. Dementia
D. Anxiety disorders
E. Attention-Deficit/Hyperactivity Disorder (ADHD)

84. A psychiatric consultation-liaison service has asked you to see a 55-year-old woman who was brought to the hospital following an intentional polypharmacy overdose. The woman is a member of a tightly knit religious community and wishes to leave the hospital immediately, insisting that she must return home to

protect her husband. The childless couple lives alone, and the patient explains that they are constantly under attack by hateful neighbors. Prior to her hospitalization, the couple's fear had reached such a level that they decided that suicide was preferable to living under constant attack. The wife attempted suicide by overdose, but the husband changed his mind at the last minute. When the consultation team initially arrives on the medical floor, they are told by internal medicine staff that there is uncertainty regarding the reality of the couple's persecution by neighbors. Upon visiting his wife, the husband initially insists that the persecution is real, but other members of the couple's community disagree. Over the subsequent days of the patient's hospitalization, the husband's certainty regarding the persecution seems to lessen and he expresses doubt that the neighbors ever meant the couple any harm. Although the husband is not the patient under treatment, the consultation-liaison team may reasonably hypothesize that he may have been experiencing which of the following disorders?

A. Delusional Disorder
B. Shared Psychotic Disorder
C. Brief Psychotic Disorder
D. Schizophreniform Disorder
E. Schizophrenia

85. A 70-year-old widowed white man is seen by his primary care physician. When asked how he has been feeling, the patient begins to cry. Upon further questioning, he admits to 2 months of low mood, early morning awakening, anorexia with 20 lb. weight loss, and crying spells. He describes waking each morning feeling extremely depressed, a feeling which is described as being different than the sadness he experienced when his wife died. He notes that he is still able to enjoy some activities such as spending time with his grandchildren and going to church. When he speaks of his grandchildren, his affect brightens and he is proud to show off their pictures in his wallet. He denies suicidal ideation and states, "I could never do that to my family." Which of the following features of the man's depression is NOT consistent with melancholic depression?

A. Loss of appetite with twenty pound weight loss
B. Early morning awakening
C. Ability to enjoy and react to pleasurable activities
D. Lack of suicidal ideation
E. Depression regularly worse in the morning

86. Which one of the following is the most common chromosomal anomaly leading to mental retardation?

A. Trisomy 21
B. Deletion in 15q12 of paternal origin
C. Deletion of 17p11.2
D. Deletion in 15q12 of maternal origin
E. Inactivation of FMR-1 gene at Xq27.3 due to CGG base repeats

87. Which one of the following statements is TRUE of the genetics of AD?

A. Genetic factors have been linked to approximately 20% to 40% of patients with the far more frequent "sporadic" forms of AD, but most of these factors have not fully elucidated.
B. Multiple gene mutations involving amyloid precursor protein (APP), presenilin 1 and 2 on chromosome 14 and 1 are associated with familial early onset AD and accounts for all cases of autosomal dominant AD.
C. Multiple gene mutations involving APP, presenilin 1 and 2 on chromosome 14 and 1 account for 10% of AD in general.
D. Apolipoprotein E related to chromosome 19 is an essential risk factor in 40% of the frequent late onset form of AD.
E. The hereditary form of AD showing mutation in APP and presenilin genes is becoming increasingly common and has been found in over 1,000 families world wide.

88. Evidence suggests that family therapy in treatment of substance use disorders results in which of the following?

A. Worse outcomes overall compared to individual therapy
B. Greater motivation to remain in treatment
C. Worsened social functioning
D. No change in drug use
E. High treatment dropout rates

89. Which one of the following is known to cause clinically significant increases in warfarin levels?

A. Nefazodone
B. Haloperidol
C. Fluvoxamine
D. Escitalopram
E. None of the above

90. Which countertransference reaction is incorrectly paired with the personality structure?

A. Obsessive and compulsive character—annoyed impatience
B. Paranoid character—anxiety
C. Obsessive and compulsive character—obliteration
D. Paranoid character—hostility
E. Obsessive and compulsive character—boredom

91. An 80-year-old man with coronary artery disease, diabetes, and recurrent orthostatic hypotension is hospitalized for relapse of his major depression with psychotic features. Of the following choices, which one is the most appropriate antipsychotic medication for this patient?

    A. Chlorpromazine
    B. Clozapine
    C. Haloperidol
    D. Risperidone
    E. Thioridazine

92. A 35-year-old man, on risperidone for his Schizophrenic illness, develops NMS. You will consider the following principles in relation to restarting antipsychotic treatment EXCEPT:

    A. Allowing time for symptoms to resolve completely before rechallenge
    B. Consider using an antipsychotic structurally unrelated to that associated with the syndrome
    C. Begin with low doses and titrate upwards slowly
    D. Closely monitor vital signs and biochemical parameters
    E. Using depot preparation of antipsychotics as they are administered infrequently

93. What is the fastest growing segment of Internet users?

    A. Women age 14 to 24
    B. Women age 25 to 40
    C. Women age 41 to 54
    D. Women age 55 and older
    E. Men age 14 to 24

94. A 72-year-old man was brought to his primary care physician's office by his daughter. The daughter became concerned when she had gone to visit him at home after not seeing him for the past 2 weeks. He had weakness of his right hand and arm, and he spoke fluently with frequent word substitutions. During the physical examination, he was able to follow a three-step oral command as well as read and obey a written command. He was unable to repeat simple phrases. His physician determined that he had had a stroke, and ordered an MRI to confirm the location of the lesion. The pattern of language deficits exhibited by this patient is best described by which one of the following syndromes?

    A. Wernicke's aphasia
    B. Broca's aphasia
    C. Conduction aphasia
    D. Global aphasia
    E. None of the above

95. Expansion of trinucleotide (triplet repeat) sequences beyond their normal size have been associated with a number of neurodegenerative disorders. Which one of the following terms describes the further lengthening of trinucleotide sequences with successive generations, which results in earlier onset and more severe phenotypes?

    A. *Transcription*
    B. *Translation*
    C. *Substitution*
    D. *Anticipation*
    E. *Translocation*

96. When teaching a group of medical students about migraines, which one of the following statements would you NOT make regarding the epidemiology of this condition?

    A. Approximately 6% to 8% of men and 12% to 14% of women suffer from migraines.
    B. Before puberty, the prevalence of migraine is approximately 5% both in boys and girls.
    C. The highest incidence of migraine attacks is in the age between 15 and 25.
    D. The median duration of untreated migraine attacks is 6 hours.
    E. The median frequency of attacks is approximately once per month.

97. Which one of the following is NOT considered to be an executive functioning task?

    A. Problem solving
    B. Abstraction
    C. Ability to plan and organize
    D. Ability to maintain and terminate behaviors
    E. Construction and perception of spatial relations

98. A 15-year-old girl presents to the ED complaining of blurry vision and difficulty swallowing her food. She has also been feeling increasingly fatigued, especially toward the end of the day. Physical examination is notable for bilateral ptosis and normal deep tendon reflexes. Initial strength in her squeezing your fingers is normal, but repeated efforts reveal remarkable weakness. She is alert and oriented, and her parents note that she has not had any recent problems in memory or academic functioning. Of the following, which is the best diagnostic test for this condition?

    A. CSF analysis of leukocytes and glucose
    B. CSF analysis of oligoclonal bands
    C. Serum acetylcholine (ACh) receptor antibody level
    D. Serum botulism titer
    E. Serum creatinine phosphokinase

99. Which one of the following is NOT TRUE of Idiopathic Intracranial Hypertension (IIH)?

A. IIH remains a diagnosis of exclusion by ruling out the more common causes of increased ICP.

B. CT or MRI of the brain is the diagnostic imaging of choice for this condition.

C. Magnetic Resonance venography (MR venography) is mandatory to establish the diagnosis of IIH.

D. CSF fluid is otherwise normal except for protein content in the lower range of normal.

E. Lumboperitoneal shunts or optic-nerve decompressions are treatments of choice for progressive visual loss.

100. A 6-month-old infant is brought to a pediatrician's office for evaluation of recent onset seizure activity, vomiting, and fever. In the office, he appears to have a depressed level of consciousness, frequently closing his eyes despite verbal and tactile stimulation. At 4 months of age, he had a febrile illness with associated swelling of his parotid gland. His family recently immigrated to the United States from Asia, and his vaccination history is unclear. Given this history, what is the most likely finding on CSF analysis of this patient?

A. Positive bacterial culture

B. Positive bacterial gram stain

C. Elevated lactic acid

D. Decreased glucose

E. Lymphocytic pleocytosis

101. Which of the following tests would be LEAST useful in the workup of an adolescent or young adult with dementia?

A. Serum ceruloplasmin determination

B. Test for prion protein in the CSF

C. Urine toxicology screen

D. HIV test

E. Neuroimaging (CT or MRI)

102. Which one of the following is NOT a commonly found symptom in Friedreich's ataxia?

A. Truncal ataxia

B. Dysarthria

C. Atrophy of lower extremities

D. Scoliosis

E. Cataracts

103. Which one of the following is a potential complication of untreated pseudotumor cerebri?

A. Pontine hemorrhage

B. Hypoparathyroidism

C. Permanent visual loss

D. Glioblastoma multiforme

E. Astrocytoma

104. Which one of the following medications has not been found to be helpful for the treatment of neuropathic pain?

A. NSAIDs

B. Tramadol hydrochloride

C. Anticonvulsants

D. Tricyclic antidepressants (TCAs)

E. Selective serotonin reuptake inhibitors (SSRIs)

105. A mother brings her 4-year-old child to the pediatrician for a yearly follow-up appointment. She is concerned that her child has only gained 3 inches in height in the last year. When discussing her concerns, the pediatrician should make all of the following statements regarding growth in children between the ages of 3 and 5 years EXCEPT:

A. On average, a child gains approximately 7 cm (2 in) in height per year.

B. On average, a child gains approximately 2 kg (approximately 1 lb) in weight per year.

C. The head circumference increases by approximately 2 cm (1 in) each year.

D. Lordosis becomes more pronounced.

E. Legs usually grow faster than the trunk, head, and upper extremities.

106. You are asked to consult on a 70-year-old man who was admitted to the medical service from a skilled nursing home for recurrent urinary tract infections. Despite resolution of his urinary tract infection, the patient remains combative and psychotic. In addition, he has an unsteady gait, impaired sensations, and an abnormal pupil response to light. His MMSE score is 19 and he has a positive Romberg's sign. This patient is most likely suffering from which of the following diseases?

A. MS

B. Systemic lupus erythematosus

C. Neurosyphilis

D. Paranoid schizophrenia

E. NPH

107. A 68-year-old woman has had multiple plastic surgeries and never leaves the house without makeup or fashionable and young attire. When she hangs out with her daughter, she forbids being called "mom" and tells strangers that they are sisters. According to Erik Erikson, which conflict and stage of the life cycle is this woman having difficulty resolving?

A. Identity versus role diffusion

B. Industry versus inferiority

C. Initiative versus guilt

D. Integrity versus despair and isolation

E. Intimacy versus self-absorption or isolation

108. Which of the following statements regarding a psychiatrist's role in court is most accurate?

A. A psychiatrist qualifies as an expert witness when there is popular recognition in his or her clinical field outside of the court.

B. A witness of fact can express his or her own opinions or report others' statements.

C. A witness of fact may make the conclusion that a patient meets the criteria for a commitment or for an insanity defense.

D. An expert witness is often used to read portions of a medical record aloud in court to enter them into the legal record.

E. A psychiatrist at any level of training can fulfill the role of witness of fact, whereas one must qualify to be an expert witness.

109. Which of the following statements is TRUE of the use of interpreters in psychiatric interviews?

A. A professionally trained interpreter with mental health experience should be used whenever possible for evaluating patients with limited English proficiency.

B. In cooperative patients, over-the-phone language interpretation services can be used when other professionally trained interpreters are unavailable.

C. Family members or friends should not be used unless the patient refuses to use the professional interpreter or under emergency circumstances, in which case this should be noted in the patient record.

D. The interpreter should be instructed to translate the patient's own words and to avoid paraphrasing except as needed to translate the correct meaning of idioms and other culture-specific expressions.

E. All of the above.

110. According to the classification of schizophrenia proposed by T.J. Crow, which of the following is a characteristic of Type II Schizophrenia?

A. Delusions
B. Hallucinations
C. Normal brain structures on CT scans
D. Good treatment response
E. Poverty of speech

111. The National Comorbidity Survey (NCS) reported the lifetime prevalence of MDD to be which one of the following?

A. 1%
B. 5%
C. 10%

D. 17%
E. 25%

112. Which one of the following is the most preventable cause of mental retardation?

A. Lesh Nyhan's syndrome
B. Hurler's syndrome
C. Hunter's syndrome
D. Fetal alcohol syndrome
E. Phenylketonuria (PKU)

113. Which of the following statements is TRUE of the pathogenesis of AD?

A. Neuritic plaques and NFTs are pathognomonic of AD.

B. Neuritic plaques are intracellular lesions composed of a central core of aggregated amyloid-beta peptide surrounded by neurites, activated microglia, and reactive astrocytes.

C. NFTs are extracellular bundles of paired helical filaments and straight filaments.

D. Neuritic plaques and NFTs are at the root of the pathogenesis of AD and targeting the genesis of these proteinaceous lesions is believed to hold out hope for disease modifying therapeutic options.

E. Neuritic plaques and NFTs are peripheral to the pathogenesis of AD.

114. Which one of the following is the most effective treatment for adolescent delinquency and substance use disorders?

A. Medication management
B. Individual psychotherapy
C. Inpatient hospitalization
D. Day treatment programs
E. Family therapy

115. Which of the following causes the least pronounced orthostatic hypotension?

A. Nortriptyline
B. Desipramine
C. Amitriptyline
D. Clomipramine
E. None of the above

116. Which one of the following is NOT an effect of opioids mediated via the μ receptors?

A. Analgesia
B. Tachycardia
C. Sedation
D. Physical dependence
E. Respiratory depression

117. A 24-year-old homeless woman with a history of bipolar disorder with psychotic features presents to the ED in a manic state with auditory hallucinations. She is admitted to a medical floor with dehydration and a chest x-ray showing left lower lobe pneumonia. She is treated with lithium and haloperidol, and is also started on antibiotics. Over the next 2 days, the psychiatry consult service is called because, despite the use of increasing doses of lithium and haloperidol, the patient continues to present with confusion, agitation, and combative behavior, but she is now mute. When evaluated, the patient is verbally unresponsive, has bizarre and contorted posturing, marked diaphoresis, has a temperature of 103°F, a heart rate of 110 beats/minutes, blood pressure of 110/70 mm Hg, and a respiratory rate of 20 per minute. All of the following should be considered risk factors for this patient's presentation EXCEPT:

A. Coadministration of antibiotics with psychiatric medications
B. Coadministration of lithium with haloperidol
C. Dehydration
D. Poor nutrition
E. Repeated use of haloperidol

118. A 69-year-old woman with a history of psychotic depression is on long-term treatment with olanzapine and paroxetine. The neurologists recently diagnosed her with idiopathic Parkinson's disease and commence her on selegiline. Over the next 72 hours, she develops agitation, profuse sweating, myoclonus, and grand mal seizures. Upon admission to the medical unit, the selegiline is discontinued. The patient improves without sequelae 3 days later. All of the following would help differentiate serotonin syndrome from NMS EXCEPT:

A. The symptoms coincided with the introduction of selegiline.
B. Chorea or myoclonus is seen with NMS.
C. Lead pipe rigidity is seen with NMS.
D. Elevation in creatine kinase levels are more marked in NMS.
E. Hyperreflexia is seen more in serotonin syndrome.

119. Which one of the following statements is TRUE regarding healthcare issues in women?

A. Women have a lower incidence of diabetes mellitus.
B. Elderly women have decreased rates of orthostatic hypotension compared to elderly men.
C. Women die twice as often following their first myocardial infarction.
D. Women have larger heart vessels.
E. Women have an earlier onset of arteriosclerosis.

120. Bitemporal hemianopsia is associated with a lesion in which part of the visual pathway?

A. The optic chiasm
B. The left temporal lobe
C. The left occipital lobe
D. The left lateral geniculate nucleus
E. The right optic nerve

121. Involuntary movement disorders are characterized by Parkinsonism, athetosis, chorea, and hemiballismus. Which one of the following areas of the central nervous system (CNS) is affected when these signs are present?

A. Basal ganglia
B. Brainstem
C. Cerebellum
D. Spinal cord
E. Cerebral hemisphere

122. Which of the following is TRUE of apolipoprotein E (apo E) that is involved in the genetics of Alzheimer's disease (AD)?

A. It is synthesized and secreted by astrocytes and macrophages
B. It has four major isomeric forms
C. The isomeric forms arise from different alleles of a single gene on chromosome 1
D. The e2 allele is the most common of all alleles
E. All of the above

123. Which of the following tests is used to assess visuospatial functioning?

A. Clock Drawing Test
B. Trail Making Test
C. Wisconsin Card Sorting Test
D. Category Test
E. Wechsler Adult Intelligence Scale-Revised (WAIS-R)

124. A 75-year-old man is brought in by his family to the clinic due to concern that the patient has Alzheimer's dementia. The patient has had gradual memory loss, often wanders around the house confused, tends to get angry easily, and has fluctuating mood. The family does not know of any medical problems in the past given that he only recently came to live with them. After a complete physical including neurologic examination, and obtaining a complete blood count (CBC), chem-10, and urinalysis, which one of the following would be another initial diagnostic step in the workup of dementia for this patient?

A. Apolipoprotein E genotyping
B. CT scan of brain
C. HIV testing

D. Serum B_{12} and thyroid stimulating hormone (TSH) levels

E. Tau proteins in CSF

125. A 55-year-old woman presents to the clinic with a 9-month history of motor deficits, including left-hand weakness, right-foot drop, and a sixth cranial nerve palsy. She also develops optic neuritis during this time period. Preceding the onset of these symptoms, she had a prodrome of low-grade fever and myalgias. An MRI of the brain reveals multiple increased T2-weighted and decreased T1-weighted lesions. Her symptoms improve with a course on intravenous steroids, and she does not develop similar symptoms following this first episode. Given this history, which one of the following is the most likely diagnosis for her symptoms?

A. Acute disseminated encephalomyelitis

B. Relapsing-remitting MS

C. Secondary progressive MS

D. Schildler's myelinoclastic diffuse sclerosis

E. Cerebral vascular accident

126. A 45-year-old man comes to your office for evaluation of several symptoms that have developed gradually over the last several months. They include headaches, episodic seizure-like activity, nausea, vomiting, and intellectual decline. He has spent much of the last few years traveling in sub-Saharan Africa, and subsisted on a diet of mainly local meat products, such as pork. You have a high index of suspicion for neurocysticercosis and perform an LP to confirm this diagnosis. Which of the following immune cells is most characteristically found in the CSF of patients with this disorder?

A. Polymorphonuclear leukocytes (PMNs)

B. Eosinophils

C. Basophils

D. Mast cells

E. Dendritic cells

127. A 70-year-old man is being evaluated for cognitive impairment. On the mental status examination, he is noted to have impairment in memory, attention, and visuospatial abilities. His neurological examination is notable for the presence of masked facies, shuffling gait, and postural instability. Which of the following would help confirm the suspected diagnosis of DLB?

A. History of stroke

B. Detailed visual hallucinations

C. Severe auditory hallucinations

D. Lack of fluctuating cognitive impairment

E. All of the above

128. Which is the characteristic pathological finding of Charcot-Marie-Tooth disease?

A. Focal axonal swelling

B. Segmental demyelination and remyelination of peripheral nerves

C. Total loss of oligodendroglia

D. Diffuse cerebral atrophy with increased amounts of neuronal lipofuscin

E. Presence of neuroaxonal spheroids

129. Which one of the following is the most serious complication of lead poisoning in children?

A. Apathy

B. Ataxia

C. Encephalopathy

D. Irritability

E. Vomiting

130. Which one of the following factors has the highest correlation with disease relapse in MS?

A. Female sex

B. Younger age of onset

C. History of pregnancy

D. Psychosocial stress

E. Physical trauma

131. Which one of the following statements regarding pubertal development is NOT TRUE?

A. Breast bud development is usually the first pubertal change in girls.

B. Breast bud development in girls can be as late as 13 years.

C. In girls, menses usually begins sometime during breast Tanner stage IV.

D. In boys, the first sign of puberty is penile enlargement.

E. The onset of pubic hair growth occurs between the ages of 10 and 15 years.

132. Where is the primary auditory cortex located?

A. Parietal lobe

B. Frontal lobe

C. Temporal lobe

D. Occipital lobe

E. Insula

133. All of the following situations involve an obligation on the part of the treating physician to breach patient confidentiality and make a report to another authority EXCEPT:

A. A child who states that she is uncomfortable by the way a family member touches her "down there."

B. A patient who calls and states he is going to commit suicide by overdosing on pills and hangs up.

C. A patient who has fantasies about killing his step-father for years of abuse he endured as a child.

D. A patient who works as a school bus driver and presents to clinic intoxicated before his work shift.

E. A patient who states he has a plan to wait outside a person's home today and beat this person with a bat.

134. A 22-year-old woman with a history of anxiety, depression, and Borderline Personality Disorder is referred to you by her internist for a psychiatric evaluation. You learn that she is abusing lorazepam, which was prescribed by her internist for her symptoms of anxiety and may be contributing to her symptoms of depression. You request permission to share this assessment with the referring internist, but the patient refuses. What should you do in such a situation?

A. Abide by the patient's wish.

B. Tell the patient that you have to share the assessment anyway.

C. Agree with the patient, but share the assessment anyway.

D. Don't ask for the patient's permission and share the assessment with the internist.

E. None of the above.

135. According to the DSM-IV-TR, which of the following clinical descriptions would NOT be suggestive of a good prognosis in Schizophreniform Disorder?

A. The patient experiences acute onset of psychotic symptoms shortly after functional changes are noted by family.

B. In addition to psychosis, the patient displays broad-ranging and labile affect.

C. Prior to arrival at the ED, the patient assaults a family member who is attempting to soothe the patient.

D. Upon assessment in the ED, the patient appears confused and perplexed.

E. Prior to the acute presentation, the patient has been married, maintained numerous long-term friendships, and has been successful in a professional career.

136. Parents of a 10-year-old girl are concerned that their daughter is doing poorly in school. She only has a few friends and does not seem to be functioning at the same level as her peers. After a thorough evaluation, it is clarified that the patient meets the criteria for Mental Retardation. Her IQ is determined as being 45. Given this information, how would you code her condition on the DSM-IV-TR Multiaxial Diagnostic System?

A. Axis II: Mental Retardation, Severity Unspecified

B. Axis II: Mild Mental Retardation

C. Axis I: Severe Mental Retardation

D. Axis II: Moderate Mental Retardation

E. Axis I: Profound Mental Retardation

137. During a routine newborn screening test, it is noted that an infant has PKU. While explaining to the patient's parents about this disorder, how would you classify the mode of inheritance for this disorder?

A. Autosomal dominant

B. Autosomal recessive

C. X-linked recessive

D. Mitochondrial

E. Deletion of the short arm of chromosome

138. Which one of the following statements is TRUE of the physiology of glutamate and the N-methyl-D aspartate (NMDA) receptors?

A. Glutamate is the main inhibitory neurotransmitter in the CNS.

B. Glutamate excitotoxicity, mediated via excessive activation of NMDA receptors is believed to play a role in neuronal death observed in several degenerative diseases, including Parkinson's disease.

C. In AD, excessive activation of NMDA receptors has been reported to cause increase in extracellular calcium ions, leading to a cascade of events that ultimately cause neurodegeneration.

D. Memantine is a high affinity, competitive inhibitor of NMDA receptor.

E. None of the above.

139. Who developed Short-Term Anxiety Provoking Psychotherapy (STAPP)?

A. Habib Davanloo

B. Franz Alexander

C. Thomas French

D. Peter Sifneos

E. James Mann

140. A 50-year-old man develops high fever and severe sore throat. When you check a CBC with differential, you find that he has a granulocyte count of less than 500/cmm. Which of the following medications has most likely contributed to the patient's condition?

A. Ziprasidone

B. Mirtazapine

C. Diphenhydramine

D. Duloxetine

E. Haloperidol

141. According to the World Health Organization's (WHO) treatment guidelines for chronic pain, how should persistent moderate-to-severe pain be treated?

A. Nonopioid medication as needed
B. Opioids as needed
C. Opioids with nonanalgesic adjuvant medications as needed
D. Opioids on a fixed schedule
E. Nonopioids on a fixed schedule

142. Which of the following has the most evidence-based support for first-line use in the treatment of obsessive-compulsive disorder (OCD)?

A. Phenelzine
B. Trazodone
C. Mirtazapine
D. Desipramine
E. Clomipramine

143. A 74-year-old woman on long-term treatment with fluphenazine depot for Schizophrenia develops orobuccofacial dyskinetic movements. In the clinic, she complains that she is too embarrassed to go out because people stare at her which she finds distressing. To help this patient's plight, you will do all of the following EXCEPT:

A. Lower the dose of the depot
B. Consider stopping the depot altogether
C. Consider alternative antipsychotics
D. Consider other causes for her dyskinesia
E. Treat her with anticholinergics

144. Which one of the following neurotransmitters is involved in the neural pathway involving substantia nigra, amygdala, caudate and putamen, nucleus accumbens, olfactory tubercle, and arcuate nucleus?

A. ACh
B. Serotonin
C. Norepinephrine (NE)
D. Dopamine
E. GABA

145. You are completing a physical examination in the ED. While examining the cranial nerves of a patient you detect repetitive jerk-like eye movements when asking the patient to gaze to his far right and far left. Although the presence of nystagmus is nonspecific, your differential diagnosis would include all of the following EXCEPT:

A. Alcohol intoxication
B. Wernicke-Korsakoff syndrome
C. Viral labyrinthitis
D. Dilantin intoxication
E. Gerstmann's syndrome

146. What is the Token Test used for in neuropsychological testing?

A. It assesses problems in planning.
B. It assesses difficulties in problem solving.
C. It assesses problems in concept formation.
D. It assesses problems in verbal functioning.
E. It assesses problems in identifying similarities.

147. A 60-year-old man presents to the ED with signs and symptoms consistent with meningitis and has an LP performed. Based only on the CSF analysis of glucose showing a reduced level of less than 45 mg/dL, which of the following causes of meningitis is least likely?

A. Acute syphilitic
B. Bacterial
C. Fungal
D. Tuberculous
E. Tumor

148. Which one of the following is seen in the CSF examination of patients with MS?

A. Elevated immunoglobulin level
B. Elevated WBC count
C. Elevated protein level
D. Elevated opening pressure
E. Elevated RBC count

149. A 14-year-old girl comes to a pediatric clinic for evaluation of amenorrhea. Upon physical examination, the pediatrician finds that the girl has Tanner Stage IV development for both breast and pubic hair growth. Which one of the following is the most appropriate statement for the pediatrician to make at this time?

A. The patient is having normal development for her age.
B. The patient is lagging behind in her sexual development.
C. The patient has hormonal deficiency that is causing her amenorrhea.
D. The patient needs a thorough evaluation for her amenorrhea.
E. None of the above.

150. A 25-year-old man presents to the ED complaining of weakness of the shoulder and proximal muscles of the arm. He reports that a few days ago he developed sudden onset of severe right shoulder pain that radiated to the neck and the back. He had to keep his elbow flexed to be able to tolerate the pain. Given this history, what is the most likely diagnosis for this patient's complaints?

A. Parsonage-Turner syndrome
B. Amyotrophic lateral sclerosis (ALS)

C. Unilateral C1 lesion
D. Unilateral C2 lesion
E. Unilateral C3 lesion

151. Which one of the following is NOT an abnormality of thought content?

A. Obsession
B. Compulsion
C. Depersonalization
D. Preoccupation
E. Phobias

152. Which one of the following statements about OCD is NOT TRUE?

A. The occurrence of OCD shows a bimodal age distribution.
B. Treatment response in OCD is usually measured by a 30% to 35% reduction in symptoms on the YBOCS or a decline in symptoms below a threshold of 16.
C. Mirtazapine monotherapy has been shown to be lacking in efficacy.
D. Augmentation using antipsychotics is efficacious in patients refractory to SSRIs.
E. Ablative neurosurgery for OCD generally targets the cortico-striato-thalamo-cortical circuits.

153. A 12-year-old boy is brought to the child psychiatry clinic for an evaluation. From his medical records you gather that he has an IQ of 60. Given this history, what is his lifetime risk of developing a comorbid psychiatric disorder?

A. 33%
B. 25%
C. 67%
D. 75%
E. 50%

154. Velocardiofacial syndrome (VCFS) is caused by which one of the following genetic defects?

A. A defect in hypoxanthine guanine phosphoribosyltransferase (Xq26–q27.2)
B. Deficiency in α-L-iduronidase, located at 4p16.3
C. Deficiency of iduronate sulfatase, located at Xq28
D. A defect in PAH located at 12q.24.1
E. A deletion at 22q11.2

155. What is the prevalence of delirium superimposed on dementia in community dwelling elderly?

A. 5%
B. 8%
C. 10%
D. 13%
E. 20%

156. A 21-year-old undergraduate student was referred to a psychiatrist by her primary care physician. The patient reports having experienced moderate anxiety in social situations since she was in junior high school. She has noticed that she avoids going to parties or leaves early from most social events. At this time she is reluctant to initiate pharmacotherapy and would prefer to have a trial of psychotherapy. She informs you that she will be graduating from college shortly and is motivated to start treatment as soon as possible. After taking a detailed history and discussing various options with the patient, a trial of Short-Term Anxiety Provoking Psychotherapy was started. Which one of the following is NOT an inclusion criterion for this type of brief therapy?

A. A circumscribed chief complaint, which will be the focus of therapy.
B. Evidence to support the patient's involvement in at least one meaningful relationship during childhood.
C. Patient should have the ability to interact flexibly with the therapist.
D. Patient meets the criteria for alexithymia.
E. Patient must be motivated and willing for change.

157. Which of the following drugs is most likely to contribute to sudden-death in pediatric patients?

A. Mirtazapine
B. Sertraline
C. Desipramine
D. Atomoxetine
E. None of the above

158. Which of the following is not a component of an opioid contract?

A. Informed consent
B. Agreement by the patient to obtain prescriptions from the contracting physician only
C. Nonspecific, open-ended terms for contract violation
D. Agreement by the patient to take medication only as prescribed
E. Acknowledgement of patient responsibility for prescriptions and medications

159. Who was responsible for the development of Dialectical Behavior Therapy (DBT)?

A. Thomas French
B. Michael Balint
C. James Mann
D. Marsha Linehan
E. Habib Davanloo

160. A 34-year-old man is admitted to the psychiatric unit with hallucinations and grandiose delusions. He appears to be responding to auditory hallucinations and becomes severely agitated. He is administered haloperidol 5 mg intramuscularly when he fails to accept oral antipsychotic medication to alleviate his agitation. He soon becomes more settled. Two hours later the nurse informs you that he is now complaining of difficulty in closing his eyes and in swallowing. By the time you see him, he is complaining of breathlessness. All of the following are true of his condition EXCEPT:

A. Treatment with intramuscular anticholinergics will resolve the condition.
B. It can be painful and frightening.
C. It can affect future compliance with treatment.
D. It is commonest in older men.
E. It can occur on drug withdrawal.

161. A 61-year-old man with a longstanding history of alcohol dependence was found unconscious in a public park and brought to the ER by ambulance. Upon examination, the patient was not responsive to verbal stimuli and minimally responsive to noxious stimuli. Laboratory studies revealed macrocytic anemia with a hematocrit of 31%, a mean corpuscular volume of 104 fl, and thrombocytopenia with a platelet count of 80,000 per μL. Chemistry panel was significant for mild renal insufficiency (creatinine: 1.9 mg/dL; blood urea nitrogen [BUN]: 62) and hyperglycemia with blood glucose 286 mg/dL, and aspartate aminotransferase (AST) and alanine aminotransferase (ALT) within the normal range. Coagulation studies were abnormal with a prothrombin time of 21.0 seconds and an internationalized normalized ratio of 2.0. The initial ammonia level obtained was 123 μg/dL. The blood alcohol level was 299 mg/dL, and the remainder of the serum toxicology screen was negative. A CT scan of the head was obtained in the ER and it did not reveal any intracranial bleed, tumors, or skull fracture. There was also no radiographic evidence of spinal injury. Despite aggressive medical attention, the patient's condition continued to worsen and he died after 18 hours of treatment in the intensive care unit. Pathologic findings in the brain at autopsy would include which of the following?

A. Cellular swelling of astrocytes and brain edema
B. Demyelinated plaques
C. Lewy bodies
D. Perivascular hemorrhage
E. Brain mass

162. A 68-year-old man with diabetes mellitus and hypertension is brought to the ER. He states clearly that while having dinner with his wife he repeatedly

dropped his fork and also began to see double. Upon physical examination you find right hemiparesis and a left third cranial nerve palsy. Visual fields are full and visual acuity is 20/20 in both eyes with glasses. Where is his lesion located?

A. Pons
B. Midbrain
C. Medulla
D. Internal capsule
E. Spinal cord

163. Which one of the following drugs is NOT an AChE inhibitor?

A. Donepezil
B. Rivastigmine
C. Galantamine
D. Memantine
E. Tacrine

164. Which one the following choices regarding Tanner Staging of secondary sexual development is INCORRECT?

A. Tanner III: The pubic hair becomes more coarse and curly and begins to extend laterally.
B. Tanner III: The testicular volume is between 6 and 12 mL—the scrotum enlarges further and the penis begins to lengthen.
C. Tanner III: Breasts begin to become more elevated and extends beyond the borders of the areola, which continues to widen, but remains in contour with surrounding breast.
D. Tanner IV: The testicular volume is greater than 20 mL—there is an adult scrotum and penis.
E. Tanner V: Breast reaches final adult size—the areola returns to contour of the surrounding breast, with a projecting central papilla.

165. A 38-year-old man presents to your office complaining of gradual right arm weakness. Upon physical exam, you observe weakness of the wrist and finger flexion as well as weakness of the intrinsic hand muscles. Sensation is lost in the ulnar aspect of the hand. The rest of the neurological exam is unremarkable. The patient was recently diagnosed with lung cancer and is currently receiving chemotherapy. What is this patient's most likely diagnosis?

A. Upper brachial plexus paralysis
B. Middle brachial plexus paralysis
C. Lower brachial plexus paralysis
D. Lesion of the lateral cord of the brachial plexus
E. Lesion of the medial cord of the brachial plexus

166. Which one of the following tests is generally not required in healthy adult patients before starting treatment with lithium?

A. Thyroid function tests
B. Electrocardiogram (EKG)
C. EEG
D. BUN
E. Serum electrolytes

167. Amanda is a 4-year-old girl who, at the age of 15 months, began to exhibit retrogression from her previously acquired language skills. Her interest in her environment has also begun to diminish. She now displays abnormal truncal movements and difficulty in walking. Which one of the following is NOT TRUE regarding her condition?
A. Hand washing skills are lost early.
B. Abnormal head circumference is present at birth.
C. Apraxia develops later on in the illness.
D. Psychomotor retardation is usually present.
E. Impaired comprehension develops subsequently.

168. Which one of the following is NOT a group A criterion for the diagnosis of Schizophrenia using the DSM-IV-TR?
A. Hallucinations
B. Occupational and social impairment
C. Disorganized speech
D. Affective flattening/alogia/avolition
E. Delusions

169. Which one of the following disorders is NOT classified as a communication disorder in the DSM-IV-TR?
A. Expressive Language Disorder
B. Mixed Receptive-Expressive Language Disorder
C. Phonologic Disorder
D. Stuttering
E. Disorder of Written Expression

170. Which one of the statements regarding the prevalence of delirium is NOT TRUE?
A. The prevalence of delirium in the hospitalized medically ill ranges from 10% to 30%.
B. In hospitalized elderly, the prevalence of delirium ranges from 10% to 40%.
C. Approximately 25% of hospitalized cancer patients have delirium.
D. Between 30% and 40% of hospitalized acquired immunodeficiency syndrome (AIDS) patients develop delirium some time during the course of their illness.
E. As many as 30% of postoperative patients develop delirium.

171. Which one of the following is TRUE of the treatment of neuropathic pain?

A. Decompression or neurotomy should be considered in patients with pain in a single extremity and whose pain has a burning quality, made worse by cold, and is associated with swelling and/or sweating abnormalities.
B. Diagnostic sympathetic block should be considered in a patient that has pain associated with traumatic or compressive mononeuropathy.
C. Gabapentin is almost as effective as TCAs in the treatment of neuropathic pain with a more benign side effect profile.
D. Opioids are the first line of treatment for patients with chronic neuropathic pain.
E. The use of intraspinal opioids in chronic pain is supported by controlled clinical trials.

172. The mechanism of action for which of the following agents involves inhibiting both AChE and BChE?
A. Dihydroergotoxine
B. Galantamine
C. Donepezil
D. Rivastigmine
E. Memantine

173. Which of the following is TRUE of the treatment of chronic pain with TCAs?
A. Amitriptyline is the only TCA with an indication for chronic pain.
B. Doses of TCAs are typically lower than doses used in depression.
C. Analgesia typically occurs during the first days of treatment.
D. Nortriptyline is more likely to cause anticholinergic side effects than other TCAs.
E. TCAs are only effective in patients with comorbid chronic pain and depression.

174. There are four primary modes of treatment in DBT which include individual therapy, group skills training, telephone contact, and therapist consultation. All of the following are part of the modules in group skills training EXCEPT:
A. Core mindfulness skills
B. Interpersonal effectiveness skills
C. Emotion modulation skills
D. Distress tolerance skills
E. Therapy interfering behavior skills

175. Which of the following mechanisms of action of antipsychotic drugs is NOT correctly paired?
A. Acute Dystonia—due to dopaminergic hyperactivity in the basal ganglia that occurs when the CNS levels of the dopamine receptor antagonist drug begins to rise between doses.

B. Acute Akathisia—due to imbalance between the noradrenergic and dopaminergic system caused by the dopamine receptor antagonists.

C. Tardive Dysknesia—due to dopamine supersensitivity of the basal ganglia due to chronic dopamine blockade caused by the dopamine receptor antagonists.

D. NMS—due to rapid dopamine blockade in the basal ganglia and the hypothalamus.

E. Parkinsonism—due to blockade of dopaminergic transmission in the nigrostriatal pathway.

176. Degenerative changes found in the brain of a patient with Huntington's disease would include which of the following?

A. Loss of motor neurons in the anterior horn of the spinal cord

B. Atrophy of the caudate nucleus

C. Loss of dopaminergic neurons in the substantia nigra

D. NFTs in the cerebral cortex

E. Spongiform transformation of the cerebral cortex.

177. A homeless gentleman presents to the ED looking disheveled and gaunt. You notice that he has a broad-based, unsteady, and uncoordinated gait. His speech is poorly modulated with irregular cadence. You suspect damage to the cerebellum. All of the following toxins or deficiencies can lead to cerebellar dysfunction EXCEPT:

A. Vitamin E deficiency

B. Phenytoin intoxication

C. Alcohol intoxication

D. Thiamine deficiency

E. Vitamin C intoxication

178. A 72-year-old woman is seen in consultation at her skilled nursing facility for evaluation of increasing difficulty with her memory. Her score on the Folstein MMSE is 18 out of the possible 30 points. She is being treated with hydrochlorothiazide for hypertension and metformin for type 2 diabetes mellitus. She has a history of a femoral neck fracture secondary to osteoporosis. After she is started on donepezil, which side effect of the medication would be especially important to monitor?

A. Anorexia

B. Vertigo

C. Headache

D. Tachycardia

E. Decreased sweating

179. Which one of the following is the most common feature of caffeine withdrawal?

A. Drowsiness

B. Anxiety

C. Fatigue

D. Headache

E. Dysphoric mood

180. Which of the following is the hallmark of paranoid schizophrenia?

A. Preoccupation with one or more delusions or frequent auditory hallucinations

B. Presence of persecutory delusions

C. Presence of persecutory hallucinations

D. Preoccupation with delusions or hallucinations that is necessarily persecutory in nature

E. Disorganized speech and disorganized behavior

181. Which of the following statements is TRUE regarding DLB?

A. It is characterized by the presence of Lewy bodies restricted to the subcortical areas of the brain.

B. It is characterized by the presence of Lewy bodies restricted to the cortical areas of the brain.

C. NFTs are as common in the brain of patients with DLB as in Alzheimer's dementia.

D. DLB is characterized by the presence of Lewy bodies in the subcortical and cortical areas of the brain as well as amyloid plaques.

E. Specific risk factors for DLB have been described.

182. Which of the following is NOT characteristic of delirium?

A. Perceptual disturbances

B. Hypoactive psychomotor behavior

C. Sleep-wake disturbance

D. Gradual onset

E. Altered or labile affect

183. Which of the following is the most appropriate antidepressant augmentation strategy to treat depression?

A. Thyroxine (T_4)

B. Triiodothyronine (T_3)

C. Thyroid Stimulating Hormone (TSH)

D. Antithyroglobulin antibodies (Anti-Tg Ab)

E. None of the above

184. Which of the following is NOT considered an approved treatment for the cognitive and functional decline associated with dementia?

A. Rivastigmine

B. Donepezil

C. Quetiapine

D. Memantine

E. Galantamine

185. A 42-year-old man with chronic low back pain misses work several days per week due to complaints of pain. What psychologically-based treatment modality may help this patient decrease medication use and increase activity levels as a result of reinforcing positive behaviors and minimizing behaviors that maintain pain?

A. Cognitive Behavioral Therapy
B. Family Therapy
C. Hypnosis
D. Operant conditioning
E. Group Therapy

186. Who was responsible for developing the concept of Behavioral Psychology?

A. Joseph Wolpe
B. John B. Watson
C. Edmund Jacobson
D. Nathan Ackerman
E. Marsha Linehan

187. Which one of the following statement is TRUE?

A. The retinal pigmentation is reversible with thioridazine.
B. A condition dissimilar to retinitis pigmentosa occurs with thioridazine.
C. The retinal pigmentation associated with thioridazine can occur at any dose, if given on a long-term basis.
D. Chlorpromazine is associated with whitish brown granular deposits in the macula.
E. Retinal damage does not occur with chlorpromazine.

188. Which of the following statements is TRUE regarding circadian rhythms?

A. Melatonin blood levels peak at night.
B. Human body temperature displays a cyclic pattern, with a trough between 4 and 6 AM.
C. Daily oscillations in activity have been noted in many species.
D. Environmental factors called "*zeitgebers*" entrain free-running circadian rhythms up to a 24-hour period.
E. All of the above.

189. While performing a routine neurological examination, you notice that your patient is unable to maintain his balance while standing erect with his eyes closed. He also appears to have an abnormal steppage gait. Which of the following is NOT included in the differential diagnosis for a positive Romberg sign?

A. Tabes dorsalis

B. Friedreich's ataxia
C. Pernicious anemia
D. Malabsorption
E. ALS

190. A 26-year-old woman with partial epilepsy wished to change from treatment with valproate, which she felt had caused substantial weight gain, to monotherapy with lamotrigine. After a review of her records and seizure history, her neurologist saw no contraindication to making the transition in antiepileptic medication. Which of the following side effects would be most important to discuss with the patient before making the medication change?

A. Nausea
B. Headache
C. Rash
D. Somnolence
E. Dizziness

191. Which one of the following signs is NOT included in the DSM-IV-TR criteria for Hallucinogen Intoxication?

A. Sweating
B. Palpitations
C. Pupillary constriction
D. Incoordination
E. Tremors

192. Which one of the following symptoms precludes the diagnosis of Residual Schizophrenia using the DSM-IV-TR criteria?

A. Avolition
B. Alogia
C. Perceptual disturbances
D. Odd beliefs
E. Disorganized speech

193. Which of the following is NOT associated with DLB?

A. Fluctuating cognition
B. Visual hallucinations
C. Parkinsonism
D. RBD
E. Restless Leg Syndrome

194. Risk factors for delirium include all of the following EXCEPT:

A. Age
B. Preexisting cognitive impairment
C. Terminal illness
D. Hypoalbuminemia
E. Male gender

195. A 32-year-old woman presents to her primary care physician with complaints of extreme fatigue and lower extremity weakness for the last 2 months. She also reports a history of experiencing numbness and tingling in her hands 3 years ago. She attributed this to carpel tunnel symptoms from computer overuse, and had not sought medical attention. An MRI of the brain at this time revealed multiple periventricular T2 hyperintensities. Given this history, which one of the following statements are TRUE about her condition?

A. Cerebrospinal fluid examination would likely be normal.
B. Immunomodulators have been found to delay progression of disease or decrease severity of attacks.
C. Men and women are equally affected with this disorder.
D. Male offspring of the patient are likely to be affected.
E. The symptoms are most likely directly due to bacterial infection.

196. You are seeing a 45-year-old woman in your clinic for a medication follow-up visit. She started a new medication 1 week ago and currently denies any side effects except for blurred vision when she attempts to read the newspaper. Her visual acuity is otherwise normal and her extraocular muscles are not impaired. Which of the following medication is NOT likely causing this effect?

A. Clozapine
B. Paroxetine
C. Thioridazine
D. Imipramine
E. Haloperidol

197. A 15-year-old white man is brought to the ED by his friends, who stated that he started acting bizarrely, calling them names, and responding as if he were hearing voices. The patient admitted drinking alcohol earlier in the evening, but denied use of any illicit drugs. A urine toxicology screen was negative. His parents were contacted, who reported that he was being treated for depression with fluoxetine, but was otherwise healthy and on no medications. Upon reevaluation, the patient was drowsy, restless, and hyperthermic, and admitted to taking "some pills" he had obtained from another teen, but again denied use of any illicit drugs. Which of the following is the likely substance of abuse?

A. Diphenhydramine
B. Diazepam
C. Quetiapine
D. Methylphenidate
E. Dextromethorphan

198. Which of the following drugs is a dopamine receptor agonist?

A. Haloperidol
B. Pramipexole
C. Bupropion
D. Methylphenidate
E. Memantine

199. Which one of the following is NOT TRUE of the treatment of early stage Parkinson's disease?

A. Patients with early-stage Parkinson's disease include those who have had the disease for less than 5 years.
B. Most of these patients will not need treatment with levodopa or a dopamine agonist.
C. Levodopa is better than dopamine agonists to improve motor disability.
D. Dopamine agonists are initiated in patients with mild disease when the age of onset is at a younger age.
E. Levodopa is used when the age of onset is at an older age and the patient has more severe motor symptoms.

200. Which one of the following is NOT TRUE of the treatment of late stage Parkinson's disease?

A. This group includes all those patients who have been receiving treatment with carbidopa/levodopa and have developed motor complications.
B. Approximately 90% of all patients treated with levodopa develop motor fluctuations and dyskinesia.
C. Patients may experience a "wearing-off" effect from the levodopa.
D. Many of these patients may also experience an "on-off" effect from the levodopa.
E. These complications can be treated by adding a dopamine agonist, monoamine oxidase (MAO)-B inhibitor, catechol O-methyltransferase (COMT) inhibitor to the carbidopa levodopa combination.

Answers

1. Answer: C. A child of 4 years (48 months) should have acquired all of the following skills:

1. Motor skills: Throw a ball overhand, hop on one foot, climb well, and use scissors to cut.
2. Adaptive skills: Copy cross and square, copy a bridge from a model, imitate construction of "gate" of five cubes, draw a man with two to four parts besides his head, and name the longer of two lines.
3. Language skills: Tell a story and count four pennies accurately.
4. Social skills: Go to toilet alone and play with several children with beginning of social interaction and role-playing.

A child of 48 months would not be expected to copy a triangle from a model as this is acquired only by 60 months (5 years) of age.

Behrman RE, Kliegman RM, Jensen HB. *Nelson Textbook of Pediatrics*. 17th ed. Philadelphia: WB Saunders; 2004.

2. Answer: B. Decreased GABA levels may cause convulsions. GABA is chiefly confined to the brain and spinal cord. It acts as a postsynaptic inhibitory neurotransmitter in the cerebral and cerebellar cortices. In the spinal cord, it mediates the postsynaptic inhibition of the afferent pathways. Benzodiazepines, newer hypnotics such as zopiclone, and alcohol act on GABA-A receptors coupled to chloride ion channels, which on activation result in an influx of chloride ions and rapid depolarization causing inhibition. The GABA-B receptors in the brain increase K+ conductance and produce slow inhibitory potentials through inhibition of cyclic adenosine monophosphate (cAMP).

Sadock BJ, Sadock VA. *Kaplan and Sadock's Comprehensive Textbook of Psychiatry*. 8th ed. Philadelphia: Lippincott Williams & Wilkins; 2005:62–63.

3. Answer: C. Immature defenses are seen in adolescents and some non-psychotic patients, and include: acting out, blocking, hypochondriasis, introjection, passive-aggressive behavior, regression, schizoid fantasy, and somatization. Blocking is temporarily or transiently inhibiting thinking. Introjection is an immature defense that involves internalizing the qualities of an object to obliterate the distinction between the subject and object (e.g., identification with the aggressor). Schizoid fantasy is indulging in autistic retreat in order to resolve conflict and to obtain gratification (the person does not fully believe in the fantasies and does not insist on acting them out). Somatization is the conversion of psychic derivatives into bodily symptoms and reacting with somatic manifestations. Reaction formation is a neurotic defense involving transforming an unacceptable impulse into its opposite, and is characteristic of obsessional neurosis.

Kaplan HI, Sadock BJ. *Kaplan & Sadock's Synopsis of Psychiatry*. 8th ed. Philadelphia: Lippincott Williams & Wilkins; 1998:218–222.

4. Answer: E. Malpractice claims experienced by the Psychiatrist's Purchasing Group, the liability insurer of members of the American Psychiatric Association, reveal the following approximate frequencies of alleged claims by percentage: incorrect treatment (33%), attempted or completed suicide (20%), incorrect diagnosis (11%), improper supervision (7%), improper commitment (5%), breach of confidentiality (4%), undue familiarity (3%), libel or slander (2%), and other (i.e., abandonment, ECT, or third-party injury) (4%).

Sadock BJ, Sadock VA. *Kaplan and Sadock's Comprehensive Texbook of Psychiatry*. 8th ed. Philadelphia: Lippincott Williams & Wilkins; 2005:3969–3970.

5. Answer: C. This patient is most likely experiencing hypnagogic hallucinations. Hypnagogic and hypnopompic hallucinations are hallucinations that occur right before going to sleep and right after waking up, respectively. These can present in normal people and are also characteristic of narcolepsy. This patient does not meet criteria for brief psychotic disorder or schizophrenia. Charles Bonnet syndrome occurs in patients who become visually impaired and suffer from pseudo-hallucinations.

Sadock BJ, Sadock VA. *Kaplan and Sadock's Comprehensive Textbook of Psychiatry*. 8th ed. Philadelphia: Lippincott Williams & Wilkins; 2005:987–990.

6. Answer: E. The DSM-IV-TR states that tactile and olfactory hallucinations may be present in delusional disorder, if they are related to the delusional theme. Delusional disorder is characterized by nonbizarre delusions of a least 1 month's duration. Apart from the impact of the delusion(s) or its ramifications, the patient's functioning is not markedly impaired and behavior is not obviously odd or bizarre. The delusions cannot be due to a primary mood disorder, direct physiological effects of a substance, or a general medical condition.

American Psychiatric Association. *Quick Reference to the Diagnostic Criteria from DSM-IV-TR.* Washington, DC: American Psychiatric Association; 2000:159–160.

7. Answer: B. This man appears to be suffering from *Koro*. *Koro* is a term of Malaysian origin, and is the name given to the onset of sudden anxiety that the genitals will recede into the body, causing death. It has been reported in South and East Asia. It occasionally occurs in epidemic form in East Asian areas. This belief goes hand in hand with panic, fear, or anxiety. A proposed diagnostic criterion is that apart from the fear of death, the belief in genital retraction, and the efforts to prevent it, the individual should not have met criteria for any axis I disorder (other than somatoform disorder) and there are no organic explanations for this behavior. Dhat is an Indian culture-bound syndrome characterized by anxiety regarding the discharge of semen and feelings of weakness. Qi-Gong psychotic reaction is an episode characterized by dissociative/paranoid/psychotic/nonpsychotic symptoms associated with the Chinese health-enhancing practice of qi-gong. Rootwork is seen in the southern United States among African American, European American, and Caribbean societies. It is the attribution of illness to witchcraft, hexing, and sorcery. Shin-Byung is a Korean culture-bound syndrome characterized by a phase of anxiety, followed by dissociation and possession by ancestral spirits.

Sadock BJ, Sadock VA. *Kaplan and Sadock's Comprehensive Textbook of Psychiatry.* 8th ed. Philadelphia: Lippincott Williams & Wilkins; 2005:2286–2290.

8. Answer: C. Disorganized Schizophrenia was first described by Ewald Hecker, who called it *hebephrenia*. This term continues to be used in ICD-10. Karl Kahlbaum was his supervisor, and he coined the term *catatonia*. Kurt Schneider described the "first rank" symptoms of schizophrenia. Emil Kraepelin coined the term *dementia preacox* and distinguished Schizophrenia from affective psychosis. He provided detailed case presentations of Schizophrenia. Eugen Bleuler coined the term *Schizophrenia*.

Sadock BJ, Sadock VA. *Kaplan and Sadock's Comprehensive Textbook of Psychiatry.* 8th ed. Philadelphia: Lippincott Williams & Wilkins; 2005:1418–1419.

9. Answer: E. Fluctuating mental status occurs frequently in DLB, with some studies suggesting a prevalence of 50% to 70%. Fluctuations are often dramatic and mimic delirium. The delirium associated with DLB is characterized by daytime drowsiness and lethargy, daytime sleep of 2 or more hours, persistent motionless stare, and episodic flow of ideas which are disorganized, unclear, or not logical.

1. Ferman TJ, Smith GE, Boeve BF, et al. DLB fluctuations: specific features that reliably differentiate DLB from AD and normal aging. *Neurology.* 2004;62:181–187.
2. McKeith I, Mintzer J, Aarsland D, et al. Dementia with Lewy bodies. *Lancet Neurol.* 2004;3:19–28.

10. Answer: D. The safety and efficacy of the SSRIs, such as sertraline, make this class of medication the first-line treatment for Panic Disorder. Due to its risk for tolerance, dependence, and withdrawal, treatment with short-acting benzodiazepine monotherapy is not first-line. However, initial treatment with a longer-acting benzodiazepine in the short-term may be indicated while antidepressant treatment is titrated. No evidence exists for efficacy of gabapentin or buspirone in the treatment of Panic Disorder.

Hales RE, Yudofsky SC. *The American Psychiatric Publishing Textbook of Clinical Psychiatry.* 4th ed. http://www.psychiatryonline.com/content.aspx?aID=76499. Published February 2, 2007.

11. Answer: C. SSRI-induced syndrome of inappropriate secretion of antidiuretic hormone (SIADH) is not uncommon in elderly patients receiving SSRI therapy. In these patients, water excretion is impaired. Carbamazepine, oxcarbazepine, and neuroleptics are other possible offenders. Treatment of SIADH consists of fluid restriction, lithium or demeclocycline, and intravenous Sodium Chloride (NaCl). SIADH is contrasted with nephrogenic diabetes insipidus (NDI), which can occur with chronic lithium therapy. NDI consists of impaired renal conservation of water, and has a clinical presentation of polydipsia with dilute (not concentrated) urine.

1. Jacob S, Spinler S. Hyponatremia associated with selective serotonin-reuptake inhibitors in older adults. *Ann Pharmacother.* 2006;40:1618–1622.
2. Rai A, Whaley-Connell A, McFarlane S, et al. Hyponatremia, arginine vasopressin dysregulation, and vasopressin receptor antagonism. *Am J Nephrol.* 2006;26:579–589.
3. Romero S, Pintor L, Serra M, et al. Syndrome of inappropriate secretion of antidiuretic hormone due to citalopram and venlafaxine. *Gen Hosp Psychiatry.* 2007;29:81–84.

12. Answer: E. Although staff often would like patients to be sedated, this is a potentially harmful event. It may lead to aspiration, falls, and other complications. Benzodiazepines may disinhibit patients, interfere with cognition, and cause depression. Antipsychotics increase the risk for stroke, clotting, and cardiac complications. Reducing unnecessary medications, especially anticholinergic ones, is often beneficial to elderly patients. Cognitive enhancers and newer generation antidepressants (TCAs are often anticholinergic and are associated with cardiac arrhythmias) have some undesirable side effects, but are generally well tolerated, and often beneficial. Education of family and caregivers, as well as institution of appropriate behavioral interventions, should be used first-line and are among the least harmful of interventions when combined with judicious pharmacotherapy.

Sadavoy J, Jarvik LF, Grossberg GT, Meyers BS. *Comprehensive Textbook of Geriatric Psychiatry*. 3rd ed. New York: WW Norton; 2004:903–991.

13. Answer: E. All of the statements are true. Patients with DS start developing AD earlier than the general population. The incidence of AD in patients with DS is 75% by the age of 60 years, as compared to an incidence of less than 5% in the general population. By the age of 40 years, 100% of these patients show AD pathology in their brains. Visual memory loss and impaired learning capacity are the first symptoms of cognitive dysfunction in these patients. MRI findings in these patients include cerebellar atrophy, basal ganglia calcification, and hippocampal atrophy.

Menendez M. Down syndrome, Alzheimer's disease and seizures. *Brain Dev*. 2005;27:246–252.

14. Answer: A. The prevalence of NMS is estimated to be between 0.02% and 2.4% in patients exposed to dopamine receptor antagonists. It is an idiosyncratic rather than an allergic reaction. It is thought to be due to dopamine antagonism in the basal ganglia and the hypothalamus, leading to a resetting of the thermoregulatory systems and severe muscular spasm, which contributes to a considerable heat load that cannot be dissipated. The syndrome consists of generalized muscular rigidity, pyrexia, autonomic instability, lowered consciousness, akinesia, and mutism. It can occur at any stage of treatment with antipsychotic drugs. It can last for a few days up to 2 weeks. Renal failure can occur as a result of rhabdomyolysis triggering myoglobulinemia and myoglobinuria; this may be the main presentation without manifest rigidity. Respiratory failure may result from rigidity of the chest wall and requires ventilation. Other complications include infection such as pneumonia, hyperpyrexia, and cardiac failure. Mortality rates for NMS range from 10% to 20%.

1. Cookson J, Katona C, Taylor D. *Use of Drugs in Psychiatry: The Evidence From Psychopharmacology*. 5th ed. London: Gaskell Publications; 2002:88.
2. Kaplan BJ, Sadock HI. *Kaplan and Sadock's Synopsis of Psychiatry*. 9th ed. Philadelphia: Lippincott Williams & Wilkins; 2003:993–994,1060.
3. Taylor D, Paton C, Kerwin R. *The Maudsley 2005–2006 Prescribing Guidelines*. 8th ed. London: Taylor & Francis; 2005:9, 81–82.

15. Answer: B. The MacCAT-T contains the famous four criteria for capacity, or A, C, D, and E, as mentioned previously. Researchers have questioned whether or not these criteria genuinely provide a valid evaluation of capacity. Absence of delirium is not one of the four criteria; however, a delirious patient is unlikely to have the cognitive faculties necessary to fulfill the other four criteria.

1. Hudson SA, Raymont V. Mental incapacity and medical ethics. *Br J Psychiatry*. 2004;184:84–85.
2. Wyszynski AA, Wyszynski B. *Manual of Psychiatric Care for the Medically Ill*. Washington: American Psychiatric Publishing; 2005:222–223.

16. Answer: B. Serotonin is synthesized from tryptophan by tryptophan hydroxylase (the rate-limiting step), followed by aromatic amino acid decarboxylase, and is degraded by Monoamine oxidase (MOA) into 5-hydroxyindoleacetic acid (5-HIAA). Phenylalanine is converted to tyrosine by PAH, and tyrosine hydroxylase is the rate-limiting enzyme in the synthesis of DOPA, which is converted to dopamine by DOPA decarboxylase, followed by conversion to NE by dopamine B-hydroxylase. Glutamate is decarboxylated by glutamic acid decarboxylase to GABA.

Smith CUM. *Elements of Molecular Neurobiology*. 3rd ed. New York: John Wiley and Sons; 2002:366–400.

17. Answer: B. Although premature ovarian failure and polycystic ovarian syndrome can both lead to amenorrhea, galactorrhea is not present in either condition. Hypothyroidism is not an associated side effect of risperidone treatment. Prolactin secretion from the pituitary is under basal negative control by dopamine originating from the hypothalamus, and is stimulated by oxytocin release. Treatment with antipsychotics, particularly typical agents and risperidone, can lead to increased serum prolactin via inhibition of D2 receptors, removing the tonic inhibition of prolactin release, and leading to amenorrhea and galactorrhea. Discontinuation of the drug results in a return of the serum prolactin level to the normal range.

Larsen PR, Kronenberg HM, Melmed S, et al. *Williams Textbook of Endocrinology.* 10th ed. Philadelphia: WB Saunders; 2003:125–128.

18. Answer: C. The gene for Huntington's disease is located on the short arm of chromosome 4. This gene is associated with an expanded trinucleotide (CAG) repeats. Normal alleles at this site contain CAG repeats, but when these repeats reach 41 or more, the disease becomes fully penetrant. Incomplete penetrance occurs with 36 to 40 repeats and less than 35 repeats are not associated with the disorder. The number of CAG repeats accounts for as much as 60% of the variation in age of onset of the disease, with the remainder being caused by modifying genes and environment factors. Trinucleotide CAG, once it exceeds 28 repeats, start to show either expansion (73%) or contraction (23%). The expansion of the trinucleotide repeats account for the occurrence of anticipation, a phenomenon where the age of onset of Huntington's disease becomes earlier in successive generations, and the likelihood of paternal inheritance in children with juvenile onset symptoms. Also, new-onset cases of Huntington's disease with a negative family history usually occurs because of expansion of an allele in the borderline or normal range (28 to 35 CAG repeats), mostly from the paternal side. Identical twins with Huntington's disease typically have the age of onset of symptoms within a few years of each other, but may present with different clinical phenotypes. In homozygous cases of this disorder, there is no substantial difference in age of onset of the disease, but the rate of progress may be rapid.

Walker FO. Huntington's disease. *Lancet.* 2007;369:218–228.

19. Answer: E. The postictal extremity weakness described is referred to as Todd's paralysis, and is usually present on the contralateral side from the seizure focus. Seizure activity should not be suspected to be psychogenic in nature until a full workup is performed. The presence of bowel or bladder incontinence is not related to the origin of seizure activity.

Goetz CG. *Textbook of Clinical Neurology.* 2nd ed. Philadelphia: WB Saunders; 2003:1158.

20. Answer: B. Memory is the ability to record, retain, and retrieve knowledge. It is usually divided into declarative and non-declarative memory. Declarative memory is responsible for remembering everyday events and facts. It can be further subdivided into episodic memory, which refers to the ability to remember personal experiences that happened at a particular place and time, and semantic memory, which entails the remembrance of generic information. Non-declarative memory, which is also referred to as implicit memory, is not retrieved intentionally. It entails things such as remembering how to drive or run. Memory can also be divided in relation to time, such as immediate and long-term memory.

Goetz CG. *Textbook of Clinical Neurology.* 2nd ed. Philadelphia: WB Saunders; 2003:5.

21. Answer: D. NPH presents with an insidious onset and gradual development of symptoms over weeks to months. Patients usually present with the triad of dementia, gait apraxia, and urinary incontinence. Headache and signs of increased ICP do not occur in these patients. NPH may occur secondary to head trauma, infection, or SAH. In patients with more advanced disease, frontal release signs along with hyperactive tendon reflexes and Babinski signs may be elicited.

Rowland LP. *Merritt's Neurology.* 11th ed. Philadelphia: Lippincott Williams & Wilkins; 2005:354.

22. Answer: D. The normal color of CSF is clear, and xanthochromia refers to CSF that is not clear in color. Typical colors observed are yellow (due to a high protein concentration), pink (from hemoglobin in the CSF due to prior bleeding), and red (seen with high levels of oxyhemoglobin).

Goetz CG. *Textbook of Clinical Neurology.* 2nd ed. Philadelphia: WB Saunders, 2003:517, 930.

23. Answer: D. Neurologic sarcoidosis can occur in 5% of patients with sarcoidosis, and may follow an earlier diagnosis of sarcoidosis or manifest as the presenting symptoms in patients with this autoimmune disorder. It can affect any cranial nerve and commonly causes hypothalamic inflammation, which can lead to abnormal temperature sense, sleep patterns, and urinary habits. While the elevated ACE level is not specific for neurosarcoidosis (it can also be seen in infection or carcinomatous meningitis), it is supportive of this diagnosis when the symptoms constellation is consistent.

1. Goetz C. *Textbook of Clinical Neurology.* Philadelphia: WB Saunders; 2003:518.
2. Stern B. *Neurologic sarcoidosis.* UpToDate 2006. http://www.uptodateonline.com/utd/content/topic.do?topic Key=medneuro/7716&type=A&selectedTitle=1~6. Accessed January 27, 2007.

24. Answer: B. Rett syndrome is the second most common cause of mental retardation in women and it presents during childhood. The gene for Rett syndrome is located in the chromosome X, and mutations in the paternal chromosome account for the majority of these cases. The phenotypic expression of this entity is very variable. Patients, most frequently girls, develop normally until they reach 6 months to a year of age. At that point, there is a gradual deceleration in head growth, with the development of autistic-like behaviors and pyramidal signs. There is usually prolonged survival and patients tend to stabilize and sometimes improve by the second decade of life. In Alpers syndrome, which is characterized by gray matter degeneration, there are neuronal intranuclear hyaline inclusions. Neuroaxonal dystrophies, such as Seitelberger disease, cause focal axonal swelling in myelinated and nonmyelinated central and peripheral nervous system axons. Leukodystrophies are characterized by white matter changes.

Menkes JH, Sarnat HB, Maria BL. *Child Neurology*. 7th ed. Philadelphia: Lippincott Williams & Wilkins; 2006:210–215.

25. Answer: E. RBD is a parasomnia, commonly treated with clonazepam. RBD occurs frequently in synucleinopathies of which Parkinson's disease and Lewy body dementia are common synucleinopathies. Multiple-system atrophies are less commonly occurring synucleinopathies (including Striatonigral degeneration, Shy-Drager syndrome, and olivopontocerebellar atrophy). Alzheimer's dementia is not a synucleinopathy, because it is an amyloid and tauopathy. RBD is not frequently associated with Alzheimer's dementia.

1. Ferini-Strambi L, Fantini ML, Zucconi M, et al. REM sleep behaviour disorder. *Neurol Sci*. 2005;26(suppl 3):S186–S192.
2. Gagnon JF, Postuma RB, Mazza S, et al. Rapid-eye-movement sleep behaviour disorder and neurodegenerative diseases. *Lancet Neurol*. 2006;5:424–432.
3. Lauterbach EC. The neuropsychiatry of Parkinson's disease and related disorders. *Psychiatr Clin North Am*. 2004;27:801–825.

26. Answer: D. Ethosuximide is considered the drug of choice for control of absence seizures, diagnosed in this child. The EEG would show the characteristic 3 per second spike and wave pattern seen in childhood absence epilepsy. An absence seizure may be provoked by hyperventilation, such as having the child make a pinwheel move by blowing on it, although the practitioner must be prepared for the possibility of a prolonged seizure during any provocative maneuver and act accordingly. Lamotrigine and valproic acid are also recommended first-line agents, and more than one drug may be necessary for seizure control. Phenytoin at therapeutic doses can actually worsen absence seizure control.

Beghi E. Efficacy and tolerability of the new antiepileptic drugs: comparison of two recent guidelines. *Lancet Neurol*. 2004;3:618–621.

27. Answer: E. By the age of 30 months, children usually acquire the following skills:

1. Motor: Going up stairs with alternating feet.
2. Adaptive: Making a tower of nine cubes, making vertical and horizontal strokes, imitating circular strokes, and forming closed figures.
3. Language: Knowing his or her full name and referring to self with the pronoun "I."
4. Social: Engaging in pretend play and help put things away.

Behrman RE, Kliegman RM, Jensen HB. *Nelson Textbook of Pediatrics*. 17th ed. Philadelphia: WB Saunders; 2004.

28. Answer: B. Rivastigmine inhibits both BChE and AChE. It is metabolized at its site of action rather than in the liver. Patients often do experience gastrointestinal side effects such as nausea, vomiting, and diarrhea. Rivastigmine is prescribed twice daily. As with all the anticholinesterase medications, rivastigmine does not stop the progression of dementia but may slow the rate of cognitive decline.

Stern TA, Herman JB. *Massachusetts General Hospital Psychiatry Update and Board Preparation*. 2nd ed. New York: McGraw-Hill; 2004:55.

29. Answer: B. The *initiative versus guilt* term is Erikson's third stage in his theory of human development, refers to ages 3 to 5 years, but is not fixed in time as development is continuous. This stage corresponds to Freud's phallic-oedipal phase, where children's growing sense of sexual curiosity is manifested by engaging in group sex play or touching their own genitalia. If parents do no make an issue of these childhood impulses, the impulses are eventually repressed and reappear during adolescence as part of puberty. If parents make too much of the impulses, children may become sexually inhibited. By playing with peers, children learn how to interact with others and develop a sense of initiative and ambition. By the end of this stage, a child's conscience is established. If a child is made to feel excessively guilty, this may lead to a variety of conditions including generalized anxiety disorder, phobias, and if sexual fantasies are accepted as unrealizable, children may attempt to repress their wishes and deny them, and develop sexual inhibition, paralysis, or impotence.

Kaplan HI, Sadock BJ. *Kaplan & Sadock's Synopsis of Psychiatry*. 8th ed. Philadelphia: Lippincott Williams & Wilkins; 1998:234–239.

30. Answer: E. Malpractice claims experienced by the Psychiatrist's Purchasing Group, the liability insurer of members of the American Psychiatric Association, reveal the following approximate frequencies of alleged claims by percentage: incorrect treatment (33%), attempted or completed suicide (20%), incorrect diagnosis (11%), improper supervision (7%), improper commitment (5%), breach of confidentiality (4%), undue familiarity (3%), libel or slander (2%), and other (i.e., abandonment, ECT, or third party injury) (4%).

Sadock BJ, Sadock VA. *Kaplan and Sadock's Comprehensive Textbook of Psychiatry*. 8th ed. Philadelphia: Lippincott Williams & Wilkins; 2005:3969–3970.

31. Answer: C. The Hamilton-Anxiety Scale is used to evaluate somatic and cognitive anxiety symptomatology. It consists of 14 items, and each is rated from 0 to 4. This scale was designed to be administered by trained clinicians. The standard threshold for clinically significant anxiety is considered to be 14.

Sadock BJ, Sadock VA. *Kaplan and Sadock's Comprehensive Textbook of Psychiatry*. 8th ed. Philadelphia: Lippincott Williams & Wilkins; 2005:943–950.

32. Answer: A. This is a presentation of amphetamine intoxication. Substituted, or "designer," amphetamines include methylenedioxymethamphetamine (MDMA) (also referred to as ecstasy, XTC, and Adam), MDEA (also referred to as Eve), MMDA, and DOM (also referred to as STP). These substances have neurochemical effects on both the serotonergic and dopaminergic systems and have behavioral effects that reflect a combination of amphetamine-like and hallucinogen-like activities. Because they are so closely structurally related to the classic amphetamine drugs, they are classified with the amphetamines. Intoxication following the recent use of these substances includes maladaptive behavioral or psychological changes in addition to at least two of the following: (i) tachycardia or bradycardia, (ii) papillary dilation, (iii) elevated or lower blood pressure, (iv) perspiration or chills, (v) nausea or vomiting, (vi) evidence of weight loss, (vii) psychomotor agitation or retardation, (viii) muscular weakness, respiratory depression, chest pain, or cardiac arrhythmias, and (ix) confusion, seizures, dyskinesias, dystonias, or coma.

1. American Psychiatric Association. *Quick Reference to the Diagnostic Criteria from DSM-IV-TR*. Washington: American Psychiatric Association; 2000:122–125.
2. Sadock BJ, Sadock VA. *Kaplan and Sadock's Synopsis of Psychiatry*. 9th ed. Philadelphia: Lippincott Williams & Wilkins; 2003:413–419.

33. Answer: A. This woman has Premenstrual Dysphoric Disorder (PMDD), which is considered by the DSM-IV-TR, to be a depressive disorder NOS. PMDD includes symptoms of depression (markedly depressed mood, anxiety, mood lability, anhedonia) that occur during the last week of the luteal phase and that remit within a few days of the onset of menses. Symptoms

are entirely absent for at least 1 week after the completion of menses, and, when present, must be severe enough to interfere with work and school, for example. Other disorders classified as Depressive Disorder NOS include the following: Minor Depressive Disorder (2 weeks of depressive symptoms not meeting full criteria for MDD); recurrent Brief Depressive Disorder (depressive symptoms occurring from 2 days to 2 weeks at least once a month for 12 months); and Postpsychotic Depressive Disorder of Schizophrenia (a Major Depressive Episode occurring during the residual phase of Schizophrenia). Depressive Disorder NOS is also used to diagnose patients in whom the etiology of depression has not been fully elucidated (i.e., primary mood disorder versus mood disorder due to general medical condition or substance).

American Psychiatric Association. *Desk Reference to the Diagnostic Criteria from DSM-IV-TR*. Washington: American Psychiatric Association; 2000:178–179.

34. Answer: E. In order to diagnose Catatonic Schizophrenia based on the DSM-IV-TR, at least two of the following symptoms should be present:

1. Motoric immobility (catalepsy/stupor)
2. Excessive motor activity (purposeless, not influenced by external stimuli)
3. Extreme negativism/mutism
4. Peculiarities of voluntary movement, as evidenced by posturing, stereotyped movements, prominent grimacing, prominent mannerisms
5. Echolalia and echopraxia

American Psychiatric Association. *Desk Reference to the Diagnostic Criteria from DSM-IV-TR*. Washington, DC: American Psychiatric Association; 2000:153–158.

35. Answer: C. FTLD is the third most common cause of cortical dementia (after AD and DLB). It encompasses two major pathologic substrates affecting the frontal or temporal cortex, sometimes asymmetrically. Three clinical syndromes are produced by FTLD (Frontotemporal Dementia, Progressive Nonfluent Aphasia and Semantic Dementia). Although for a long time Pick's disease was used synonymously with FTLD, two histologic types have been described with the same underlying histopathologic features: prominent microvacuolar change devoid of specific histologic features and severe astrocytic gliosis with or without ballooned cells and inclusion bodies (Pick's disease).

1. Neary D, Snowden JS, Gustafson L, et al. Frontotemporal lobar degeneration: a consensus on clinical diagnostic criteria. *Neurology*. 1998;51:1546–1554.
2. The Lund and Manchester Groups. Clinical and

neuropathological criteria for frontotemporal dementia. *J Neurol Neurosurg Psychiatry.* 1994;57:416–418.

36. Answer: A. Antidepressants may be effective in the treatment of post-traumatic stress disorder (PTSD). Additionally, they also treat common comorbidities of PTSD. Atypical antipsychotics may be used as adjuncts when patients present with disorganized or explosive behavior. Benzodiazepines are not considered first-line therapy given the comorbidity of PTSD and substance abuse. The efficacy of anticonvulsants in PTSD has yet to be fully determined. Little evidence suggests efficacy of buspirone in treating PTSD.

Rosenbaum JR, Arana GW, Hyman SE, et al. *Handbook of Psychiatric Drug Therapy.* 5th ed. Philadelphia: Lippincott Williams & Wilkins; 2005:198–201.

37. Answer: E. Lithium is the most common cause of drug-induced NDI, with impaired renal conservation of water. Treatment approaches include lowering or discontinuing the lithium dose, adding amiloride/thiazide diuretics/carbamazepine, low salt diet, or Desmopressin acetate ((DDAVP). NDI is contrasted with SIADH, where patients present with impaired water excretion (not conservation) and concentrated (not dilute) urine output.

1. Khanna A. Acquired nephrogenic diabetes insipidus. *Semin Nephrol.* 2006;26:244–248.
2. Livingstone C, Rampes H. Lithium: a review of its metabolic adverse effects. *J Psychopharmacol.* 2006;20: 347–355.
3. Sadock BJ, Sadock VA. *Kaplan and Sadock's Comprehensive Textbook of Psychiatry.* 8th ed. Philadelphia: Lippincott Williams & Wilkins; 2005:1692.

38. Answer: B. Phototherapy is the most widely studied treatment for SAD. The dosage often found to be effective is 5,000 lux per day, given as 2,500 lux for 2 hours or 10,000 lux for 30 minutes. A recent meta-analysis of 23 studies of light therapy found that the odds ratio for remission was 2.9 (95% confidence interval, 1.6 to 5.4). Similar to antidepressant therapy for depression, phototherapy carries some risk of precipitating mania. Phototherapy is most effective when administered earlier in the day. Early morning light therapy regulates the circadian pattern of melatonin secretion, whereas the use of light in the evening delays the normal melatonin phase shift. To ensure adequate response, patients should be treated with phototherapy units that are specifically designed to treat SAD.

Lurie SJ, Gawinski B, Pierce D, et al. Seasonal affective disorder. *Am Fam Physician.* 2006;74:1521–1524.

39. Answer: B. TD is most commonly caused by the long-term use of typical antipsychotic medication. At least

20% of patients who are treated with first-generation antipsychotics long-term develop TD. TD rarely develops in patients who have had less than 3 to 6 months of antipsychotic drug exposure. The only firmly established risk factor for TD besides typical antipsychotic drug exposure is being older than age 50, although there is some evidence that women may be at greater risk than men (thus this patient's age of 35 years old is not a current risk factor for TD development). There is inconsistent evidence that patients with mood disorders may be at greater risk for developing TD and that intermittent dosing may increase the risk of TD. There is some suggestion that chronic use of anticholinergic compounds may increase the risk of TD.

Rosenbaum JF, Arana GW, Hyman SE, et al. *Handbook of Psychiatric Drug Therapy.* 5th ed. Philadelphia: Lippincott Williams & Wilkins; 2005:44–46.

40. Answer: C. Hyperthyroidism is one of the risk factors for NMS. Other risk factors include high-potency typical antipsychotic drugs, rapid or recent dose increase, organic brain disease, alcoholism, agitation, intercurrent infections, psychosis especially with catatonic features, dehydration, and abrupt withdrawal of dopamine precursor levodopa in patients with Parkinson's disease and mental retardation. Men are more commonly affected as are younger patients. Antipsychotic drugs with anticholinergic effects appear to be less likely to cause NMS. Mortality may be lower with atypicals but may be as high as 20% to 30% with depot dopamine receptor antagonists.

1. Cookson J, Katona C, Taylor D. *Use of Drugs in Psychiatry: The Evidence From Psychophamacology.* 5th ed. London: Gaskell Publications; 2002:88.
2. Kaplan BJ, Sadock HI. *Kaplan and Sadock's Synopsis of Psychiatry.* 9th ed. Philadelphia: Lippincott Williams & Wilkins; 2003:993–994, 1060.
3. Taylor D, Paton C, Kerwin R. *The Maudsley 2005–2006 Prescribing Guidelines.* 8th ed. London: Taylor & Francis; 2005:9, 81–82.

41. Answer: A. The most common etiology of hallucinations in the hospital setting is delirium tremens, which often occurs 3 to 4 days after hospitalization. Sensory isolation is a common cause of isolation in intensive care units (ICU's) and hallucination in this setting should encourage an evaluation of sensory isolation. Occipital lobe tumors as well as SLE are associated with hallucinations.

Kaplan HI, Sadock BJ. *Kaplan & Sadock's Synopsis of Psychiatry.* 8th ed. Philadelphia: Lippincott Williams & Wilkins; 1998:819–823.

42. Answer: E. 5-HT_3 is the only serotonin receptor that is not coupled to a G-protein receptor. The 5-HT_3

receptor is a ligand-gated Na^+, K^+ channel that leads to depolarization of the cell when serotonin binds to the 5-HT_3 receptor. The 5-HT_3 receptor is found in high concentrations in the brainstem and area postrema, and stimulates dopamine release when activated. Decreased release of dopamine in the area postrema is thought to be the anti-emetic mechanism of the 5-HT_3 antagonist, ondansetron. The remainder of the serotonin receptors are G-protein coupled receptors. The 5-HT_{1A} receptor is located with the highest concentrations in the hippocampus and the amygdala, though it is distributed throughout the brain. These receptors seem to be involved in reduction of anxiety when stimulated, and buspirone is an agonist at the 5-HT_{1A} receptor. The 5-HT_{1B} receptors are found mainly in the basal ganglia, striatum, frontal cortex, and raphe nuclei, and may play a role in circadian rhythms, and the response of migraines to sumatriptan. The 5-HT_{2A} receptor subtype is localized primarily in the cortex and basal ganglia, and interacts with the atypical antipsychotics, and may contribute to their therapeutic effects. Little is known about the 5-HT_{2B} receptor.

Webster RA. *Neurotransmitters, Drugs and Brain Function*. 1st ed. New York: John Wiley and Sons; 2001:187–209.

43. **Answer: C.** Nitric oxide is an important neurotransmitter which should not be confused with nitrous oxide (an anesthetic gas – "laughing gas"), which can become a drug of abuse. Nitric oxide inhibits platelet aggregation, dilates blood vessels, boosts host defenses against infections, and functions in a variety of CNS roles. From a neurological standpoint, its main functions are in regulating cerebral blood flow and facilitating penile erection.

Kaufman DM. *Clinical Neurology for Psychiatrists*. 5th ed. Philadelphia: WB Saunders; 2001:562.

44. **Answer: E.** None of the choices are true. Wilson's disease is a rare autosomal recessive genetic disorder of copper metabolism. The disease affects between one in 30,000 and one in 100,000 individuals. It is characterized by hepatic and neurological disease. The symptoms of this disorder usually appear in the second and third decades of life. In these individuals, there is accumulation of excess copper in the liver because of reduced excretion in the bile. Wilson's disease is a progressive disorder and if undiagnosed and treated can be fatal.

Ala A, Walker AP, Ashkan K, et al. Wilson's disease. *Lancet*. 2007;369:397–408.

45. **Answer: E.** Galactorrhea, or abnormal lactation, may be associated with various clinical conditions. Patients with galactorrhea usually have elevated serum prolactin levels; however, women who have breast-fed may experience mild galactorrhea for many years with a normal prolactin level. Hyperprolactinemia is often caused by medications, including antipsychotic medications, metoclopramide, and cimetidine. Apart from medications, the most common cause of hyperprolactinemia is a prolactin-secreting adenoma or a lesion in the pituitary or hypothalamus that interferes with dopamine secretion. (Prolactin secretion is inhibited by dopamine.) Other conditions associated with hyperprolactinemia include chronic renal failure, cirrhosis, hypothyroidism, stress, and, less commonly, medications such as opiates, SSRIs and TCAs.

Rosenburg RN, Pleasure DE. *Comprehensive Neurology*. 2nd ed. New York: John Wiley & Sons; 1998:554–555.

46. **Answer: B.** The previously mentioned CSF profile combined with the clinical presentation is most suggestive of a bacterial meningitis. Normal CSF is clear, with 0 to 4 WBC/mm, 30 to 45 mg protein/100 mL, and 60 to 100 mg glucose/100 mL. Bacterial meningitis is notable for very high WBC (100 to 500), above normal protein (75 to 200), and very low glucose (0 to 40). Viral meningitis, by contrast, shows more modest elevations in WBC (50 to 100) and protein (50 to 100), and little to no decrease in glucose (40 to 60). SAH is characterized by bloody fluid. LP would not be helpful in diagnosing an intracranial mass.

Kaufman DM. *Clinical Neurology for Psychiatrists*. 5th ed. Philadelphia: WB Saunders; 2001:532–533.

47. **Answer: E.** In infants, hydrocephalus can be distinguished from other forms of macrocephaly, such as subdural hematoma by skull transillumination or plain-skull radiograph. LP may be done to measure CSF pressure and to determine whether it contains blood, inflammatory material or infection. CSF-pulse-wave analysis may be more reliable than CSF pressure measurement alone in diagnosing hydrocephalus. Ultrasonography is useful in evaluating subependymal and intraventricular hemorrhages in infants. Cerebral angiography can be done to detect hydrocephalus due to intracranial mass lesions. However, CT scan or MRI of the brain remains the best diagnostic aids to detect all forms of hydrocephalus.

Rowland LP. *Merritt's Neurology*. 11th ed. Philadelphia: Lippincott Williams & Wilkins; 2005:355.

48. **Answer: E.** The syndrome described is most consistent with an idiopathic facial nerve palsy (Bell's palsy). The symptoms typically follow a viral prodrome,

resolve without treatment in ~3 weeks (in 85% of patients) and can include facial nerve weakness, ear numbness or pain, chorda tympani and reduction in tearing or salivary flow. In 70% of cases, full function is eventually regained with no treatment. Patients with Bell's palsy do not typically have abnormal CSF analyses.

Goetz CG. *Textbook of Clinical Neurology*. 2nd ed. Philadelphia: WB Saunders; 2003:192, 520–521.

49. Answer: D. The MMSE is a 30-point test whose purpose is to help clinicians screen for cognitive impairment. It includes tests of orientation, immediate and recent memory, language, attention, and visuospatial skills, among others. It was developed by Folstein and colleagues in 1975 and has since become the most widely used screening test for cognitive impairment. Screening tests such as the MMSE can be useful in detecting cognitive deficits and estimating their severity. Gender has no specific effect, though the MMSE may overestimate cognitive deficits in older people, members of ethnic minority groups, and those who are poorly educated (<8 years of school). However, there are corrections which can be applied for age/educational level. The MMSE does not distinguish between etiologies of dementia nor does it distinguish dementia from memory impairment due to depression ("pseudodementia").

1. Folstein M, Folstein S, McHugh P. Mini-Mental State. A practical method for grading the cognitive state of patients for the clinician. J Psych Res 1975;12:189–198.
2. Kaufman DM. *Clinical Neurology for Psychiatrists*. 5th ed. Philadelphia: WB Saunders; 2001:128–130.

50. Answer: C. Seitelberger syndrome is a neuroaxonal dystrophy which is rare and it is characterized by focal axonal swelling in myelinated and nonmyelinated central and peripheral nervous system. Patients usually develop symptoms between the first and second year of age, and the clinical picture is characterized by both upper and lower motor neuron disease. Patients present with weakness, muscular atrophy, urinary retention and optic atrophy. The most common neuroimaging finding is prominent and diffuse hyperintensity of the cerebellar cortex, dentate nucleus, and pyramidal tracts. Rett syndrome is usually seen in girls who develop normally until the first 6 to 12 months of life, when they develop deceleration of head growth and autistic-like symptoms. Cockayne syndrome is a disorder of DNA repair. Patients have a progeroid facies, progressive intellectual deterioration, lack of subcutaneous fat and hypersensitivity to sunlight. Juvenile Huntington's disease is characterized by mental deterioration, behavioral abnormalities, and gait disturbances.

Menkes JH, Sarnat HB, Maria BL. *Child Neurology*. 7th ed. Philadelphia: Lippincott Williams & Wilkins; 2006:165–225.

51. Answer: B. The patient has NPH. NPH is characterized by a triad of clinical findings including slowly progressive gait disorder, impaired mental function, and urinary incontinence. It may follow an SAH from either a ruptured aneurysm or head trauma; resolved acute meningitis or chronic meningitis. In most cases, a cause cannot be established. Gait disturbance, usually the earliest feature, often takes the form of unsteadiness and impaired balance. Weakness and tiredness of the legs are frequent complaints. Patients may take short steps and have stooped posture resembling Parkinson's disease. Unlike Parkinson's disease, there is no rigidity, slowness of alternating movements, or tremor. Mental changes are "frontal" in character. They include apathy, dullness in thinking and actions, inattention, and impaired memory. Urinary symptoms appear late in the disease. Initially, they consist of urgency and frequency. Later, urgency is associated with incontinence. Hydrocephalus can be treated with surgical shunting. Often a complete or nearly complete restoration of mental function and gait can be obtained. Memory disturbance in Alzheimer's dementia is usually insidious and the urinary incontinence with gait abnormality present at the onset of dementia can help to distinguish NPH from AD. Patients with vascular dementia often have a history of hypertension, a stepwise progression of deficits, abrupt onset of dementia, and focal neurological symptoms or signs. While this patient has several of these features, including abrupt onset of dementia and a history of hypertension, she does not have any focal neurological deficits or a history of stoke. Parkinson's disease is characterized by resting tremor, cogwheel rigidity, bradykinesia, and abnormal gait and posture. The patient has an abnormal gait but does not exhibit any other signs of Parkinson's disease. It should be noted that 10% to 15% of patients with Parkinson's disease develop dementia; the incidence of dementia increases with advancing age, and up to 65% above age 80 have it. The patient's fall may be complicated by a pelvic fracture. However, such a fracture would not explain her pre-existing impaired gait or memory disturbance.

1. Greenberg DA, Aminoff MJ, Simon RP. *Clinical Neurology*. 5th ed. New York: McGraw-Hill; 2002:62–63, 241–242.

2. Ropper AH, Brown RH. *Adams and Victor's Principles of Neurology.* 8th ed. New York: McGraw-Hill; 2005:529–545, 916–918.

52. Answer: B. Migraine without aura is more common than migraine with aura. It accounts for 80% of all migraines. An estimated 10% to 20% of the United States population has migraines, and there is a 3:1 female preponderance, although in childhood onset, men and women are equally affected. There is a family history in greater than 70% of migraine sufferers. Many patients can use only abortive therapies for treatment, such as ibuprofen or acetaminophen in less severe cases, and a serotonin receptor agonist (a triptan) for more severe migraines. Patients who are having disabling, frequent migraines may benefit from prophylactic therapy. Indications for prophylactic therapy are the presence of two or more headaches per month that cause at least 3 days of disability per month, use of abortive treatments more than twice a week, a contraindication to the use of abortive treatments, or unusual migraine conditions/variants, such as hemiplegic migraine or migrainous infarction. Medications that have been used for prophylaxis include beta blockers and valproate, but topiramate has recently shown efficacy in migraine prophylaxis and received United States Food and Drug Administration (FDA) approval. The doses of topiramate used for migraine prophylaxis are lower than those used for seizure control and thus more likely to be well tolerated by patients, and topiramate's lower risk of causing weight gain may make it more attractive in some patients, particularly those who are obese.

1. Linde M. Migraine: a review and future directions for treatment. *Acta Neurol Scand.* 2006;114:71–83.
2. Peres MF, Mercante JP, Tanuri FC, et al. Chronic migraine prevention with topiramate. *J Headache Pain.* 2006;7:185–187.
3. Snow V, Weiss K, Wall EM, et al. Pharmacologic management of acute attacks of migraine and prevention of migraine headache. *Ann Intern Med.* 2002;137:840–849.

53. Answer: E. By the age of 60 months, most children usually acquire the following skills:

1. Motor: Skipping
2. Adaptive: Copying triangles and naming heavier of two weights
3. Language: Repeating sentences of ten syllables, naming four colors, and counting up to ten pennies correctly
4. Social: Dressing and undressing, domestic role-playing, and asking the meaning of words

Behrman RE, Kliegman RM, Jensen HB. *Nelson Textbook of Pediatrics.* 17th ed. Philadelphia: WB Saunders; 2004.

54. Answer: A. Homocystinuria is an autosomal recessive condition. Neurofibromatosis type 1, tuberous sclerosis and Huntington's disease are inherited in an autosomal dominant fashion. Turner's syndrome is due to the complete or partial absence of one of the X chromosomes found in women.

Kaufman DM. *Clinical Neurology for Psychiatrists.* 5th ed. Philadelphia: WB Saunders; 2001:329–339.

55. Answer: B. Each stage of Erikson's life cycle has its own psychopathological outcome if it is not mastered successfully. If shame and doubt dominate over autonomy, compulsive doubting may occur and can produce an overly anal personality with people who are parsimonious, punctual, and perfectionistic. Too little autonomy can also lead to the development of paranoid personalities who feel that others are trying to control them. Prolonged separation during infancy can lead to anaclitic depression and in later life, this lack of trust can manifest as dysthymia, depression, or sense of hopelessness. Basic mistrust is also a major contribution to the development of Schizoid Personality Disorder, or more severely, schizophrenia, and can also lead to substance related disorders. Excessive guilt may lead to a variety of anxiety, phobias, or sexual inhibitions. Identity confusion can result in many disorders of adolescence, including Conduct Disorder, Disruptive Behavior Disorder, and Gender Identity Disorder, for example, and prolonged dependence may occur when there is an inability to separate from the parent. In older people who are not satisfied with their lives or feel they have not been generative, anxiety or depressive disorders often develop with increased suicide rates over the age of 65.

Kaplan HI, Sadock BJ. *Kaplan & Sadock's Synopsis of Psychiatry.* 8th ed. Philadelphia: Lippincott Williams & Wilkins; 1998:233–239.

56. Answer: D. In the 1966 *Rouse v. Cameron* case, the District of Columbia's Court of Appeals ruled that the purpose of involuntary hospitalization is treatment, and that a patient who is not receiving treatment has a constitutional right to be discharged from the hospital. In the 1976 case of *Tarasoff v. Regents of University of California*, physicians have the duty to warn and protect intended victims if there is reason to believe a patient may injure or kill someone. In the 1971 case of *Wyatt v. Stickney*, Judge Johnson ruled that people on civil commitment to a mental institution have a constitutional right to receive such individual treatment as will give them a reasonable opportunity to be cured or to have their mental condition improved. The result of this case was minimum requirements for staffing, specified physical facilities and nutritional standards, and required individualized treatment plans. In the 1976 *O'Conner v. Donaldson* case, the United States Supreme Court ruled that harmless mental patients cannot be confined against their will without treatment if they can survive in the community. As a result of the 1979 case of *Rennie v. Klein*, patients have the right to refuse treatment and to use an appeal process.

Kaplan HI, Sadock BJ. *Kaplan & Sadock's Synopsis of Psychiatry.* 8th ed. Philadelphia: Lippincott Williams & Wilkins; 1998:1308, 1310–1316.

57. **Answer: B**. The CAPS includes 17 items to make the diagnosis of PTSD according to DSM criteria. It is a helpful tool not only to make the diagnosis of PTSD, but also to assess the impact of the PTSD on social and occupational functioning and general severity of symptoms. The YBOCS measures the severity of obsessive-compulsive disorder symptoms. It includes ten items and it is administered in a semi-structured interview. The AUDIT was developed by the WHO as a brief screening tool for the detection of dangerous alcohol use. The threshold score for the diagnosis of alcoholism is considered to be between 8 and 10. The ASI provides a quantitative measure of symptoms and functional impairment due to alcohol or drug addictions. The CAGE Questionnaire is a brief screen for patients with significant alcohol problems that consists of four questions concerning the effect that drinking has on a person. Scores of 2 or more suggest significant alcohol problems.

Sadock BJ, Sadock VA. *Kaplan and Sadock's Comprehensive Textbook of Psychiatry.* 8th ed. Philadelphia: Lippincott Williams & Wilkins; 2005:943–950.

58. **Answer: A**. There are seven types of Delusional Disorder described by the DSM-IV-TR: erotomanic (delusions that another person, usually of higher status, is in love with the individual), Grandiose (delusions of inflated worth, power, knowledge, identity, or special relationship to a deity or famous person), Jealous (delusions that the individual's sexual partner is unfaithful), Persecutory (delusions that the person, or someone to whom the person is close, is being malevolently treated in some way), Somatic (delusions that the person has some physical defect or general medical condition), Mixed (delusions characteristic of more than one type, but no one theme predominates), and Unspecified Type. Paranoid Type is a subtype of Schizophrenia, but not Delusional Disorder.

1. American Psychiatric Association. *Quick Reference to the Diagnostic Criteria from DSM-IV-TR.* Washington: American Psychiatric Association; 2000:153–160.

2. Sadock BJ, Sadock VA. *Kaplan and Sadock's Synopsis of Psychiatry.* 9th ed. Philadelphia: Lippincott Williams & Wilkins; 2003:511–517.

59. **Answer: D**. Race or ethnicity has not been shown to be a significant risk factor for the development of MDD. Although some community studies have suggested a higher prevalence of depressive symptoms among African Americans, this racial disparity usually disappears when confounding factors such as age and socioeconomic status are controlled. With regards to other risk factors, women are at greater risk of developing MDD than men (in contrast to bipolar disorder, where gender is not a risk factor). People who are separated or divorced have a greater risk, as do people with a family history of depression. Those with lower socioeconomic status are at greater risk for the development of MDD as well. Other risk factors for the development of MDD include age (young at greater risk), childhood experiences (loss of parental figure and disruptive childhood environment), chronic stress, and residence (greater risk in urban areas than rural areas).

Sadock BJ, Sadock VA. *Kaplan and Sadock's Comprehensive Textbook of Psychiatry.* 7th ed. Philadelphia: Lippincott Williams & Wilkins; 2000:1303–1306.

60. **Answer: E**. Fragile X Syndrome is the second most common single cause of Mental Retardation. There is a high rate of ADHD, learning disorders, and Pervasive Developmental Disorders, such as Autism in children with Fragile X syndrome. The clinical features are as described in the question. Trisomy 21 is seen in Down syndrome, deletion of 15q12 of paternal origin is seen in Prader-Willi syndrome, deletion of 17p11.2 is seen in Smith-Magenis syndrome, and deletion of 15q12 of maternal origin is seen in Angelman's syndrome. They are all associated with mental retardation, but they have unique clinical features.

Sadock BJ, Sadock VA. *Kaplan and Sadock's Concise Textbook of Clinical Psychiatry.* 2nd ed. Philadelphia: Lippincott Williams & Wilkins; 1996:514, 517–518.

61. **Answer: B**. Patients with FTLD are occasionally misdiagnosed as Alzheimer's disease. Careful history taking and attention to certain aspects of presentation are likely to clarify diagnosis. FTLD has a predominantly "pre-senile" onset, whereas AD is more common in the elderly. Severe amnesia and visuospatial deficits and myoclonus characteristic of AD are often not described in the early stages of FTLD. Patients with FTLD are typically oriented and do not evidence significant deficits in negotiating their local environment. Profound alteration in personality in the early stages of a dementing illness suggests FTLD rather

than AD. Bradyphrenia is typical of subcortical vascular dementia.

1. Neary D, Snowden JS, Bowen DM, et al. Neuropsychological syndromes in presenile dementia due to cerebral atrophy. *J Neurol Neurosurg Psychiatry*. 1986;49:163–174.
2. Neary D, Snowden JS, Northern B, et al. Dementia of frontal lobe type. *J Neurol Neurosurg Psychiatry*. 1988;51:353–361.

62. Answer: D. Family therapy has been shown to be effective in teaching family members about Schizophrenia. In addition, family therapy can emphasize the reduction of expressed emotion and coping skill enhancement, which can improve the level of stress in the home. Family therapy has been shown to reduce post-hospitalization symptoms and recidivism.

Sadock BJ, Sadock VA. *Kaplan and Sadock's Comprehensive Textbook of Psychiatry*. 8th ed. Philadelphia: Lippincott Williams & Wilkins; 2005:2591.

63. Answer: A. The cerebellum is the site most commonly involved in Irreversible Lithium-Induced Neurotoxicity, although atypical effects have also been observed. Some less common presentations include extrapyramidal syndromes, brainstem dysfunction, and dementias of varying degrees. There is evidence that lithium can have both neuroprotective and toxic effects, possibly due to differential gene expression pathways.

1. Adityanjee, Munshi KR, Thampy A. The syndrome of irreversible lithium-effectuated neurotoxicity. *Clin Neuropharmacol*. 2005;28:38–49.
2. Janicak P, Davis J, Preskorn S, Ayd F, et al. *Principles and Practice of Psychopharmacotherapy*. 4th ed. Philadelphia: Lippincott Williams & Wilkins; 2006:433.
3. Sadock BJ, Sadock VA. *Kaplan and Sadock's Comprehensive Textbook of Psychiatry*. 8th ed. Philadelphia: Lippincott Williams & Wilkins; 2005:1692.

64. Answer: C. Clozapine is an atypical antipsychotic drug with minimal extrapyramidal toxicity and 30% efficacy for treatment-resistant Schizophrenic patients (approval by the FDA). The risk of seizure due to clozapine is in the range of 1% to 5%. In a chart review of 1,418 patients treated with clozapine in the United States between 1972 and 1988, 2.8% of patients had generalized tonic-clonic seizures during treatment with clozapine (1). Life-table analysis predicted a cumulative 10% risk of seizures after 3.8 years of treatment. Clozapine-related seizures appear to be dose-related. High-dose therapy (greater than or equal to 600 mg/day) was associated with a greater risk of seizures (4.4%) than medium (300 to 600 mg/day; 2.7%) or low doses (less than 300 mg/day; 1.0%). Also, rapid upward titration may increase seizure risk.

Good clinical practice includes anti-seizure prophylaxis with valproic acid at doses of clozapine above 600 mg a day. Phenytoin or carbamazepine should be avoided because they cause agranulocytosis and other hematologic abnormalities both independently and especially in combination with clozapine. In addition, phenytoin lowers clozapine levels.

1. Devinsky O, Honigfeld G, Patin J. Clozapine-related seizures. *Neurology*. 1991;41:369–371.
2. Sadock BJ, Sadock VA. *Kaplan and Sadock's Comprehensive Textbook of Psychiatry*. 8th ed. Philadelphia: Lippincott Williams & Wilkins; 2005:747–748.

65. Answer: E. Antipsychotic medications are all generally able to cross the maternal-placental barrier and be present in the fetus and amniotic fluid. Although some studies have investigated some agents with regard to teratogenicity, no clear pattern has emerged, yet given the relative lack of safety data it is best if possible to avoid agents during pregnancy, especially the first trimester. In late pregnancy, there are well-documented problems with chlorpromazine being associated with an increased risk of neonatal jaundice, and reports of women on antipsychotics giving birth to infants with EPS. Because the washout time for these drugs in the fetus is at least 7 to 10 days, the recommended time period to discontinue antipsychotics before a women's due date is 2 weeks (not 1 week). Antipsychotics have been shown to be secreted in breast milk; therefore, there is some risk for the development of EPS in breast-feeding infants of mothers treated with antipsychotics.

Rosenbaum JF, Arana GW, Hyman SE, et al. *Handbook of Psychiatric Drug Therapy*. 5th ed. Philadelphia: Lippincott Williams & Wilkins; 2005:39.

66. Answer: D. Because NMS is potentially fatal, it is imperative to seek the advice of the physicians. It may be possible to manage the patient on a psychiatric unit if the symptoms are relatively mild. However, more serious cases will require transfer to a medical unit or even the intensive care unit. Treatment is chiefly supportive with removal of the offending agent (i.e., discontinue the antipsychotic drug). Dopamine receptor agonists such as bromocriptine and amantadine are used to overcome the antipsychotic-induced dopamine receptor blockade. Avoid the use of anticholinergics as these may exacerbate the fever. Dantrolene is used as a muscle relaxant. Benzodiazepines may be used for sedation and muscle relaxation. Artificial ventilation may be required in the event of respiratory failure. ECT may be considered for psychosis.

1. Cookson J, Katona C, Taylor D. *Use of Drugs in Psychiatry: The Evidence From Psychopharmacology*. 5th ed. London: Gaskell Publications; 2002:88.
2. Kaplan BJ, Sadock HI. *Kaplan and Sadock's Synopsis of Psychiatry*. 9th ed. Philadelphia: Lippincott Williams & Wilkins; 2003:1060.
3. Taylor D, Paton C, Kerwin R. *The Maudsley 2005–2006 Prescribing Guidelines*. 8th ed. London: Taylor & Francis; 2005: 81–82.

67. Answer: A. Gender refers to one's sex-role identity, and is determined both by exposure and responsiveness to sex steroids as well as by expectations and behavioral patterns learned in early childhood. Gender identity begins at age 3 to 4 years, when a child perceives him- or herself as either male or female. The timing of gender identity varies widely among individuals, influenced in large part by sociocultural influences. Gender identity generally occurs earlier in girls than in boys and is very difficult to change after the age of four. *Gender roles* refer to behavior related to gender identity. The concept of certain behaviors as "masculine" or "feminine" is relatively fixed by age 4 or 5.

Sadock BJ, Sadock VA. *Kaplan and Sadock's Comprehensive Textbook of Psychiatry*. 7th ed. Philadelphia: Lippincott Williams & Wilkins; 2000:2546–2547.

68. Answer: B. Wallenberg's syndrome (lateral medullary syndrome) is a vertebrobasilar stroke syndrome caused by occlusion of the vertebral artery that leads to loss of pain and temperature sensation on the contralateral side of the body below the level of the lesion, accompanied by ipsilateral Horner's syndrome, motor and sensory loss in the face, and cerebellar ataxia. Anterior inferior cerebellar artery syndrome is associated with vertigo and nystagmus, ipsilateral deafness, ipsilateral Horner's syndrome, and contralateral loss of pain and temperature sensation in the body. Parinaud's syndrome is characterized by supranuclear paralysis of eye elevation and impaired gaze convergence. Anterior spinal artery syndrome is characterized by flaccid paralysis below the level of the lesion, with loss of pain and temperature sensation, though with preserved light touch, position sense, and vibration sense. Weber's syndrome results from infarction of the posterior cerebral artery (PCA) affecting the cerebral peduncle, which results in ipsilateral pupillary dilation, ipsilateral oculomotor paresis, and contralateral paralysis of the face, arm, and leg.

Goetz CG. *Textbook of Clinical Neurology*. 2nd ed. Philadelphia: WB Saunders; 2003:415–416.

69. Answer: A. In contrast to chromosomal DNA, mitochondrial DNA is derived entirely from the mother. Mitochondria produce about 90% of the body's energy requirement, mostly in the form of ATP. In generating energy, mitochondria must constantly remove free radicals, which are highly toxic byproducts of mitochondrial metabolism. The vital energy-producing enzymes of mitochondria are delicate and easily poisoned, as in cyanide poisoning.

Kaufman DM. *Clinical Neurology for Psychiatrists*. 5th ed. Philadelphia: WB Saunders; 2001:104.

70. Answer: D. Studies indicate that 50% of patients with MS will sometime during the course of their illness meet the formal diagnostic criteria for a major mood disorder. The rate of self harm in these patients is about 30% and the rate for completed suicide is about 7 times that of the general population. Available data indicate that symptoms of affective disturbances do not necessarily correlate with the severity of the neurological disability. Although patients with MS show higher rates of depression than the general population, it is often not possible to differentiate them successfully from individuals with other chronic illnesses. It has been noted that severity of depression is negatively correlated with the disease duration indicating that the reduction in depressive symptoms is due to improved coping skills with time. Patients with MS also show twice the lifetime prevalence of bipolar affective disorder than the general population.

Pinkston JB, Alekseeva N. Neuropsychiatric manifestations of multiple sclerosis. *Neurol Res*. 2006;28:284–290.

71. Answer: C. The Finger Tapping Test is included in the Halstead-Reitan Neuropsychological Test Battery. It tests fine motor speed and it is particularly useful in identifying subtle lateralizing motor damage. Normal young adults should be able to produce at least 50 taps per 10 seconds with their dominant hand. Tests, such as the Tactual Performance Test, are helpful in identifying difficulties in adaptation by brain-injured patients. Tests for executive functioning, such as the Trail Making Test (which evaluates visual shifting and sequencing), the Wisconsin Card Sorting Test, and the Category Test (which measures concept formations) are also very helpful tools in the neuropsychological assessment of a patient with suspected brain damage.

Ebert MH, Loosen PT, Nurcombe B. *Current Diagnosis & Treatment in Psychiatry*. New York: McGraw-Hill; 2006:12.

72. Answer: E. This patient presents with a history and classic signs and symptoms consistent with botulism. This disease is caused by *C. botulism* which is a common anaerobic gram-positive bacillus that produces several types of neurotoxins and can be foodborne (most cases caused by home-canned foods), with symptoms usually occurring within 18–36 hours after exposure. Dry mouth, blurred vision, and diplopia are usually the earliest neurologic signs, followed by dysphonia, dysphagia, and peripheral muscle weakness. A symmetric descending paralysis is characteristic of botulism (paralysis begins with cranial nerves, then upper extremities, then respiratory muscles), and is treated by antitoxin administration in severe cases. This patient is young with no medical problems, thus a stroke is of low suspicion and would be better evaluated by MRI. The patient does not present with other symptoms suggestive of meningitis: mental status changes, fever, headache, nuchal rigidity. Guillain-Barré syndrome is an ascending symmetric paralysis with proximal weakness that is usually diagnosed by history and with an LP in which the protein is elevated; it is not diagnosed with MRI. Lyme symptoms usually present weeks after infection and begin with a target appearing rash, and the disease is associated with Bell's palsy and does not present with the neurologic symptoms presented in this case.

Rowland LP. *Merritt's Neurology*. 11th ed. Philadelphia: Lippincott Williams & Wilkins; 2005:124, 245, 750, 886.

73. Answer: D. IIH is a heterogeneous group of disorders characterized by increased ICP without any known cause. It is also referred to by terms such as pseudotumor cerebri, "serous meningitis", and "otitic hydrocephalus." Although spontaneous recovery is characteristic, it can cause a serious threat to vision and hence accurate diagnosis and therapeutic interventions are needed. Differential diagnosis includes obstructive hydrocephalus, chronic meningitis (i.e., sarcoid, fungal, or neoplastic), hypertensive encephalopathy, pulmonary encephalopathy resulting from paralytic hypoventilation, obstructive pulmonary disease, or the Pickwickian syndrome (morbid obesity). Patients usually present with headache and impaired vision. These headaches are usually worse on awakening and aggravated by coughing and straining. Patients also present with blurred vision due to papilledema. Some patients may also complain of brief, dimming, or complete loss of vision, occurring many times during the day called amaurosis fugax. It can be worsened by coughing and straining. Once this happens, it is imperative to treat as vision is in jeopardy. Visual loss may often be minimal despite having severe chronic papilledema

or retinal hemorrhages, but blindness may develop rapidly. Visual fields usually present with enlargement of the blind spots, constriction of the peripheral fields, and central or paracentral scotoma. Diplopia caused by unilateral or bilateral sixth-nerve palsy may develop due to increased ICP. The neurological examination is otherwise normal. Patients with IIH usually look well except for the papilledema. This disorder may last for months to years without serious sequelae.

Rowland LP. *Merritt's Neurology*. 11th ed. Philadelphia: Lippincott Williams & Wilkins; 2005:360–364.

74. Answer: C. As would be expected from the name, the opening pressure of CSF in patients with NPH should be within the normal range. This range is between 10 cm H_2O and 20 cm H_2O in healthy adults.

Goetz CG. *Textbook of Clinical Neurology*. 2nd ed. Philadelphia: WB Saunders; 2003:515, 527.

75. Answer: A. The patient's MMSE score indicates mild, not severe, cognitive impairment. AD typically has a progressive course, and one would expect to see gradual decline over time on tests such as the MMSE. If MMSE scores remain stable over the course of two or more years, a diagnosis of AD should be reconsidered. If scores decline rapidly over a short period of time, a more rapidly progressing dementia such as Creutzfeldt-Jakob disease should be considered. In this case, the patient has some mental status findings suggestive of depression (flat affect, psychomotoric retardation), and this diagnosis should be explored. Dementias which may have a stable longitudinal course include alcohol-induced persisting dementia (if the patient ceases alcohol consumption) and dementia due to traumatic brain injury. Neuropsychological testing can be helpful in differentiating etiologies of dementia and in differentiating depression-induced memory impairment from dementia.

Kaufman DM. *Clinical Neurology for Psychiatrists*. 5th ed. Philadelphia: WB Saunders; 2001:128–131.

76. Answer: C. Cockayne syndrome is an autosomal recessive disorder caused by an abnormality of DNA repair. The most common features of the symptom are severe growth retardation that starts after the second year of life, microcephaly and mental retardation, The presence of other symptoms can vary between patients, and include a specific facies with enlarged ears and sunken eyes, cataracts, lack of subcutaneous fat, hypogonadism, deafness, and hypersensitivity to sunlight. Rett syndrome is usually seen in girls who develop normally until the first 6 to 12 months of life, when they develop deceleration of head growth and autistic-like symptoms. Patients with Seitelberger syndrome usually develop symptoms between the first and second year of age. The clinical picture is characterized by both upper and lower motor neuron disease. Juvenile Huntington's disease is characterized by mental deterioration, behavioral abnormalities, and gait disturbances. Krabbe disease is a leukodystrophy, which has three different clinical forms and usually has an abrupt onset at approximately 4 years of age. Children develop irritability, restlessness, and convulsions. Patients gradually develop flaccidity and bulbar signs.

1. Menkes JH, Sarnat HB, Maria BL. *Child Neurology.* 7th ed. Philadelphia: Lippincott Williams & Wilkins; 2006: 165–225.
2. Ozdirim E, Topcu M, Ozon A, et al. Cockayne syndrome: review of 25 cases. *Pediatr Neurol.* 1996;15:312–316.

77. Answer: A. Pseudotumor cerebri designates a syndrome consisting of headache, papilledema (unilateral or bilateral), minimal focal neurological signs, and elevated CSF pressure in the range of 250 to 450 mm H_2O. These findings all occur in the absence of enlarged ventricles or an intracranial mass. Headache is the cardinal symptom. It may be described as dull or a feeling of pressure. The headache can be occipital, generalized, or asymmetrical. Patients may also note blurred vision, vague dizziness, minimal horizontal diplopia, transient visual obscurations, or numbness of the face on one side. Rarely, a nasal CSF leak may be the presenting feature. Pseudotumor cerebri arises most commonly in obese adolescent girls and young women. It can be caused by covert occlusion of the dural venous sinuses, gliomatosis cerebri, occult arteriovenous malformation, and carcinomatous, infectious, or granulomatous meningitis. However, most commonly it results from idiopathic ("benign") IIH. Diseases associated with raised CSF protein can also give rise to a pseudotumor cerebri syndrome. The more frequent ones are Guillain-Barré syndrome, systemic lupus erythematosus, and spinal tumors. Lead toxicity in children may cause this condition, along with excessive doses of tetracycline and isotretinoin, which is an oral vitamin A derivative used in the treatment of severe acne. Ingestion of large quantities of animal (bear) liver is another source of vitamin A intoxication. Lastly, metabolic disturbances such as hyper- and hypoadrenalism, myxedema, corticosteroids, and hypoparathyroidism can be contributing factors.

Treatment for pseudotumor cerebri includes weight reduction, repeated therapeutic LP, lumbar-peritoneal shunting, corticosteroids, and fenestration of the optic nerve sheath.

Ropper AH, Brown RH. *Adams and Victor's Principles of Neurology.* 8th ed. New York: McGraw-Hill; 2005:529–545.

78. Answer: C. Neurorehabilitation program for bladder care is based on clinical observations about whether the patient has incontinence or retention. The first step in this process is to look for non-neurologic factors, like mechanical problems or infections that may cause the problem. These programs include the implementation of regular voiding programs, and training patients and their families in the use of urinary catheters. Scheduled voiding every 2 hours may also help with regaining bladder control and preventing overflow incontinence. For those patients retaining urine even after voiding, bladder antispasmodic drugs and intermittent catheterization may be helpful. For patients with a flaccid bladder, cholinergic drugs may improve emptying, but intermittent catheterization may be needed in some situations.

Rowland LP. *Merritt's Neurology.* 11th ed. Philadelphia: Lippincott Williams & Wilkins; 2005:1196–1197.

79. Answer: C. A child is usually able to walk alone by 15 months of age. By this age, the child is also able to crawl upstairs, make a tower of three cubes, draw lines, and insert pellets in a bottle. Other skills acquired by the child of this age include following simple commands, naming familiar objects, and making their needs known by pointing to objects. They may also be able to hug their parents on command.

Behrman RE, Kliegman RM, Jensen HB. *Nelson Textbook of Pediatrics.* 17th ed. Philadelphia: WB Saunders; 2004.

80. Answer: E. Only an injury to the cerebral hemisphere would result in a visual field loss. Injuries to the other areas may produce visual problems, but not a field cut.

Kaufman DM. *Clinical Neurology for Psychiatrists.* 5th ed. Philadelphia: WB Saunders; 2001:8–20.

81. Answer: D. The psychoanalyst Erik Erikson has theorized that ego development proceeds from birth through eight identifiable stages marked by specific psychosocial crises. Each stage represents a turning point where resolution of the crisis results either in psychological growth or regression. Generativity versus stagnation is the Eriksonian stage associated with middle adulthood, from the ages of 40 to 60 years, and represents the period of time when an individual starts to shift their goal of personal accomplishments to concern for the rest of society and future generations and develop a sense of altruism and creativity. This stage comes after the young adulthood stage of "intimacy vs. isolation," where the goal is to make and honor commitments to other people and to ideas by associating with an extended and diverse social group. The late adulthood stage of "integrity vs. despair" involves mastering integrity, which allows people to accept their place in the life cycle and to realize that life is each person's responsibility. The childhood stage is characterized by "industry vs. inferiority," which is equivalent to Freud's latency psychosexual stage, and involves learning to take pride in accomplishments with new skills. The adolescence stage is called "identity vs. role confusion," where the main task is to develop a solid sense of identity and role in society. The other three earlier stages include: (i) trust versus mistrust (birth to 18 months), coincides with Freud's oral stage, and if an infant's needs are promptly met, the infant sees the world as a nurturing place; (ii) autonomy versus shame (18 months to 3 years), corresponds to Freud's anal stage and Mahler's separation-individuation stage, where a child will acquire a healthy self-esteem if allowed to experiment with motility and curiosity about the environment; and (iii) initiative versus guilt (3 to 5 years), corresponds to Freud's phallic stage, when children expand their explorations and have omnipotent fantasies about their powers and can develop a capacity of self-reflection and establish a conscience, manifested by feeling guilty when rules are broken.

Kaplan HI, Sadock BJ. *Kaplan & Sadock's Synopsis of Psychiatry*. 8th ed. Philadelphia: Lippincott Williams & Wilkins; 1998:234–237.

82. **Answer: A.** Confidentiality is a professional obligation that binds physicians to hold secret all information given by patients. This applies to most populations, but the group that is within the circle of confidentiality that can share information without receiving specific consent from the patient includes: other staff members treating the patient, clinical supervisors, and consultants. Parties outside the circle include: patient's family, attorney, and previous therapist. Insurers cannot compel disclosure, but can withhold a benefit without it. Thus, patients must first authorize the psychiatrist to make any disclosures.

Kaplan HI, Sadock BJ. *Kaplan & Sadock's Synopsis of Psychiatry*. 8th ed. Philadelphia: Lippincott Williams & Wilkins; 1998:1307.

83. **Answer: E.** The Conner's Rating Scales are several tools designed to measure different childhood and adolescent disorders. However these scales are most commonly used for the diagnosis of ADHD. The scales include versions for patients, parents, and teachers. The validity of these scales is considered to be excellent in discriminating between patients with ADHD and normal subjects. However, the validity is not as good when it comes to discriminating between ADHD and other disruptive disorders.

Sadock BJ, Sadock VA. *Kaplan and Sadock's Comprehensive Textbook of Psychiatry*. 8th ed. Philadelphia: Lippincott Williams & Wilkins; 2005:948–950.

84. **Answer: B.** Shared Psychotic Disorder (also referred to as "*folie a deux*") is characterized by the transfer of delusions from one person to another. In its most common form, the individual who first has the delusion (the primary case) is often chronically ill and typically is the influential member of a close relationship with a more suggestible person (the secondary case) who also develops the delusion. If the pair is separated, the secondary case may abandon the delusion. The occurrence of the delusion is attributed to the strong influence of the more dominant member. The most common relationships in which this disorder occurs are sister-sister, husband-wife, and mother-child.

Sadock BJ, Sadock VA. *Kaplan and Sadock's Synopsis of Psychiatry*. 9th ed. Philadelphia: Lippincott Williams & Wilkins; 2003:517–520.

85. **Answer: C.** Melancholic features specifier can be applied to the current or most recent Major Depressive Episode in MDD or in Bipolar Disorder. Melancholic depression must include either: (i) loss of pleasure in all, or almost all, activities, or (ii) lack of reactivity to usually pleasurable stimuli (one does not feel better, even temporarily, when something good happens). The patient in this vignette described being able to enjoy time with his grandchildren and going to church; his affect brightened upon talking about his grandchildren. Although many of his other symptoms (early morning awakening, anorexia, excessive guilt, distinct quality of depressed mood, and depression worse in the morning) are consistent with melancholia, his lack of anhedonia and ability to react to pleasurable stimuli are not.

American Psychiatric Association. *Desk Reference to the Diagnostic Criteria from DSM-IV-TR*. Washington: American Psychiatric Association; 2000:202–203.

86. **Answer: A.** Nondisjunction of chromosome 21 results in DS, the most common chromosomal abnormality leading to mental retardation. Children with this syndrome have shown distinctive phenotypic, cognitive, and linguistic profiles. Deletion of 15q12 of paternal

origin is seen in Prader-Willi syndrome, deletion of 17p11.2 is seen in Smith-Magenis syndrome, and the deletion of 15q12 of maternal origin is seen in Angelman's syndrome. Inactivation of FMR-1 gene at Xq27.3 due to CGG base repeats results in Fragile X syndrome, the second most single cause of mental retardation. All these syndromes are associated with mental retardation, but they have unique clinical features.

1. Sadock BJ, Sadock VA. *Kaplan and Sadock's Concise Textbook of Clinical Psychiatry*. 2nd ed. Philadelphia: Lippincott Williams & Wilkins; 1996:514, 517–518.
2. Sadock BJ, Sadock VA. *Kaplan and Sadock's Comprehensive Textbook of Psychiatry*. 8th ed. Philadelphia: Lippincott Williams & Wilkins; 2005:3090–3094.

87. Answer: A. Major pathogenic factors in the development of AD are currently the subject of much discussion. One of the most important areas under consideration is the role of genetics. Apo E 4 allele is perhaps the most well known genetic risk factor. Related to chromosome 19, it is an essential risk factor in 20% of the more frequent late onset form of AD. More recently, the APP gene and presenilin 1 and 2 genes located on chromosomes 14 and 1 have been found to be associated with the rare familial, early onset AD, accounting for 30% to 50% of autosomal dominant AD cases (described in 400 families worldwide) and less than 1% of AD in general. In the larger proportion of patients with sporadic AD, genetic factors have been implicated in 20% to 40% of cases, however most of the specific elements of these factors are yet to be fully elucidated.

1. Goldgaber D. My story: the discovery and mapping to chromosome 21 of the Alzheimer amyloid gene. *J Alzheimers Dis*. 2006;9(suppl 3):349–360.
2. Schellenberg GD. Early Alzheimer's disease genetics. *J Alzheimers Dis*. 2006; 9(suppl 3):367–372.

88. Answer: B. Family involvement has been shown to motivate patients with substance use disorders to seek and remain in treatment. Studies favor family therapy over individual therapy for substance abuse treatment. Outcomes of family therapy include improved social functioning and decreased drug use.

Sadock BJ, Sadock VA. *Kaplan and Sadock's Comprehensive Textbook of Psychiatry*. 8th ed. Philadelphia: Lippincott Williams & Wilkins; 2005:2591.

89. Answer: C. Fluvoxamine increases warfarin levels via inhibition of the 2C family of CYP450 enzyme systems. Fluoxetine and sertraline are also inhibitors of the 2C system, but unlike fluvoxamine, they have not been demonstrated to cause clinically significant increase in warfarin levels.

Janicak P, Davis J, Preskorn S, Ayd F, et al. *Principles and Practice of Psychopharmacology*. 4th ed. Philadelphia: Lippincott Williams & Wilkins; 2006:433.

90. Answer: C. Countertransference with obsessional patients is an annoyed impatience, with wishes to get them to open up about ordinary feelings. Their combination of excessive conscious submission and powerful unconscious defiance can be maddening. Clinicians easily feel bored or distanced by the patient's unremitting intellectualization. However, feelings of insignificance and obliteration are not common during the treatment of obsessional patients (because they are with narcissistic patients who have obsessional defenses). There is something very object-related (as opposed to self-object) about their unconscious devaluation, and something touching about their efforts to be "good" in such childlike ways as cooperating and deferring. Countertransference to paranoid personality patients is usually either strongly anxious or hostile; in the less common instance of being regarded as a savior, it may be benevolently grandiose. Because of the combination of denial and projection that constitute paranoia, causing the repudiated parts of the self to be extruded, therapists of paranoid patients often find themselves consciously feeling the aspect of an emotional reaction that the patient has exiled from consciousness. For example, the patient may be full of hostility, while the therapist feels the fear against which hostility is a defense, or the patient may feel vulnerable and helpless, while the therapist feels sadistic and powerful.

McWilliams N. *Psychoanalytic Diagnosis: Understanding Personality Structure in the Clinical Process*. New York: Guilford Press; 1994.

91. Answer: C. Orthostatic hypotension is mediated by adrenergic blockade and is most common with low-potency dopamine receptor antagonists, particularly chlorpromazine, thioridazine, and clozapine. High-potency neuroleptics (haloperidol, fluphenazine) have lower anticholinergic side effects and adrenergic blockade than low-potency typicals, and are less likely to cause postural hypotension. Risperidone is an atypical neuroleptic that causes significant postural hypotension (more than haloperidol).

1. Kaplan HI, Sadock BJ. *Kaplan & Sadock's Synopsis of Psychiatry*. 8th ed. Philadelphia: Lippincott Williams & Wilkins; 1998:1029.
2. Rosenbaum JF, Arana GW, Hyman SE, et al. *Handbook of Psychiatric Drug Therapy*. 5th ed. Philadelphia: Lippincott Williams & Wilkins; 2005:9, 47.

92. Answer: E. NMS can occur with any antipsychotic including newer atypicals and clozapine. It is most commonly associated with haloperidol and the intramuscular depot fluphenazine. It has also been known to occur with lithium and antidepressants. Besides considering an antipsychotic structurally unrelated to that associated with the syndrome, antipsychotics with low dopamine affinity may be of benefit. Always start at low doses and increase very slowly, with close monitoring of vital signs. Avoid the use of depots due to their long duration of action, and high-potency typical antipsychotics. Close monitoring of vital signs and biochemical parameters is effective in reducing progression to full blown NMS. Successful rechallenge has been reported in two-thirds of the cases.

1. King DJ. *Seminars in Clinical Psychopharmacology*. 1st ed. London: Gaskell Publications; 1995:288.
2. Taylor D, Paton C, Kerwin R. *The Maudsley 2005–2006 Prescribing Guidelines*. 8th ed. London: Taylor & Francis; 2005:81–82.

93. Answer: D. The fastest growing segment of Internet users is women aged 55 years and over. Women are more likely to use the Web to send email, play games, obtain coupons, and get information on health, employment, and religion.

Sadock BJ, Sadock VA. *Kaplan and Sadock's Comprehensive Textbook of Psychiatry*. 8th ed. Philadelphia: Lippincott Williams & Wilkins; 2005:3822–3827.

94. Answer: C. Conduction aphasias are characterized by excess word production with paraphasic errors, as in Wernicke's aphasia, but comprehension is intact. Repetition is invariably impaired in conduction aphasias. The ability of the patient in the above scenario to follow oral and written commands suggests that comprehension is intact, a feature not found in Wernicke's aphasia, has grossly impaired comprehension as a hallmark feature. Broca's aphasia, by contrast, is characterized by sparse, telegraphic speech, produced with great effort, though comprehension is much better than expressive language. Global aphasia is a marked defect in all areas of expressive and receptive speech. Conduction aphasias result from infarction to the arcuate fasciculus in the dominant hemisphere (the left hemisphere in all right-handed people and approximately 70% or more of left-handed people).

Goetz CG. *Textbook of Clinical Neurology*. 2nd ed. Philadelphia: WB Saunders; 2003:87–92.

95. Answer: D. In many genes, short blocks of repeated sequences (e.g., CAGCAG... or CTGCTG) normally occur. Expansions of these trinucleotide or triplet repeat sequences beyond their normal size have been associated with a number of neurodegenerative disorders, including Fragile X syndrome (CGG), Friedrich's ataxia (GAA), Huntington's disease (CAG), myotonic dystrophy (CTG), and spinocerebellar atrophies (CAG). These expanded repeats are characteristically unstable and often lengthen with successive generations, producing the clinical phenomenon of anticipation. Anticipation results in an earlier age of onset and more severe phenotypes with successive generations. Transcription is the process by which RNA is synthesized from a DNA template. Translation is the process by which protein is synthesized from an RNA template. Substitution is the replacement of a single base pair (or longer sequence) with another. Translocation occurs when a portion of one chromosome is transferred to a different location on the same or another chromosome.

1. Kaufman DM. *Clinical Neurology for Psychiatrists*. 5th ed. Philadelphia: WB Saunders; 2001:610.
2. Rolak LA. *Neurology Secrets*. 2nd ed. Philadelphia: Hanley & Belfus; 1998:10–12.

96. Answer: D. Migraine is one of the most frequent headache disorders. It is characterized by moderate to severe, often unilateral, pulsating headaches which is aggravated by physical activity and is accompanied by nausea, vomiting, photophobia, and phonophobia. The duration of each attack lasts anywhere from 4 to 72 hours with at least five attacks needing to have occurred before the diagnosis can be established. Most of the patients suffer from migraine attacks without aura. However, many types of migraine syndromes with specific aura features and migraine syndromes with uncommon courses or complications are present. These syndromes have their own diagnostic criteria. About 6% to 8% of men and 12% to 14% of women suffer from migraines. Before puberty, the prevalence of migraine is about 5% both in boys and girls. The highest incidence of migraine attacks is in the age between 35 and 45 years with a female preponderance of 3:1. The median duration of untreated migraine attacks is 18 hours, with the median frequency of attacks being one per month. In children, migraine attacks can be as short as 1 to 2 hours.

1. Evers S, Afra J, Frese A, et al. EFNS guideline on the drug treatment of migraine-report of an EFNS task force. *Eur J Neurol*. 2006;13:560–572.
2. Lipton RB, Scher AI, Kolodner K, et al. Migraine in the United States: epidemiology and patterns of health care use. *Neurology*. 2002;58:885–894.
3. Rasmussen BK. Epidemiology of headache. *Cephalalgia*. 2001;21:774–777.

97. Answer: E. Executive functioning refers to the cognitive functions and areas of the personality that are served by the frontal lobes in interaction with other areas of the brain. These tasks include abstraction, problem solving, set generation and sequencing, ability to maintain or terminate behaviors, and ability to plan and organize. Visuospatial functioning refers to patient's ability to function within their environment with regard to recognition of objects and their construction and perception of spatial relations.

Ebert MH, Loosen PT, Nurcombe B. *Current Diagnosis & Treatment in Psychiatry*. New York: McGraw-Hill; 2006:12.

98. Answer: C. This patient has findings consistent with myasthenia gravis, which may typically occur during early adolescence. It is an autoimmune disorder with antibodies directed against ACh receptors in the neuromuscular junction. It classically presents with weakness and fatigability where weakness is worse with repetitive use and is relieved by rest, bilateral ptosis, facial weakness, and hypotonia. Because cranial muscles are involved early, other complaints may include difficulty chewing, dysarthria, and dysphagia. After a test dose of Tensilon or edrophonium, there is usually improvement in the eye muscles or increased strength in the extremities, as the drugs work by inhibiting the breakdown of ACh and increases the concentration of ACh at the neuromuscular junction. CSF analysis of leukocytes and glucose would be appropriate if meningitis was suspected, yet this patient does not present with classic signs of meningitis: change in mental status, fever, headache, and nuchal rigidity. CSF analysis of oligoclonal bands would be helpful in the diagnosis of MS, yet this is unlikely in this presentation given that MS tends to occur in women aged 20 to 40, tends to be associated with fatigue not associated with activity, and is diagnosed with a history of remitting symptoms over time. Botulism can give weakness and ptosis, but usually has other signs on physical exam, such as papillary changes and decreased deep tendon reflexes. Creatine phosphokinase (CPK) would be abnormal in muscle diseases, which often involves myalgias and proximal greater than distal muscle weakness.

Rowland LP. *Merritt's Neurology*. 11th ed. Philadelphia: Lippincott Williams & Wilkins; 2005:124, 877–881, 886, 894, 952.

99. Answer: C. LP and not MR venography is mandatory to establish the diagnosis of IIH. IIH remains a diagnosis of exclusion by ruling out the more common causes of increased ICP. CT scan or MRI of the brain are diagnostic imaging of choice for this condition. MR venography excludes venous occlusion, but is not mandatory of the diagnosis of IIH. LP is mandatory to establish the diagnosis of IIH. In IIH, CSF fluid is otherwise normal except for protein content in the lower range of normal at about 10 mg/dL to 20 mg/dL and an elevated CSF pressure, usually between 250 mmHg and 600 mmHg. A CSF protein content greater than 50 mg/dL, and decreased CSF glucose indicates other disease process. In the extremely obese patient, weight reduction is recommended. CSF-shunt procedure, such as a lumboperitoneal shunt, is useful in patients with intractable headache and progressive visual impairment. Dexamethasone has been used empirically to reduce cerebral edema after acetazolamide and furosemide fails to reduce the ICP. Acetazolamide has been used because this carbonic anhydrase inhibitor reduces CSF formation. Furosemide also reduces CSF formation. Lumboperitoneal shunts or optic-nerve decompressions are treatments of choice for progressive visual loss.

Rowland LP. *Merritt's Neurology*. 11th ed. Philadelphia: Lippincott Williams & Wilkins; 2005:360–364.

100. Answer: E. The patient described demonstrates the classic presentation of mumps meningitis. The prodrome as well as the presentation of symptoms are now rarely seen due to the great efficacy of the trivalent measle-mumps-rubella vaccine. As with other types of aseptic meningitis, bacterial culture and gram stain are negative by definition. It is also rare to see elevated lactic acid levels or decreased glucose concentrations with viral meningitis. However, aseptic meningitides are associated with an elevated lymphocyte count (300 to 600 cells/mm^3).

Goetz CG. *Textbook of Clinical Neurology*. 2nd ed. Philadelphia: WB Saunders; 2003:518, 900–901.

101. Answer: B. The common causes of dementia in adolescents and young adults differ from the common causes of dementia in older adults. The evaluation of dementia in young adults includes basic laboratory workup (CBC, electrolytes, BUN, creatinine, TSH, liver function tests) with special attention to other possible etiologies more likely to be seen in a younger population. Depending on the patient's clinical presentation and risk factors, evaluation may include an HIV test or tests for Wilson's disease (serum ceruloplasmin determination and slit-lamp examination). Urine toxicology screen can be very useful in this patient population, as drug and alcohol abuse and overdose are common causes of dementia in this age group. Neuroimaging can detect evidence of trauma or neoplasm. Testing CSF for traces of prion protein would not be useful in this age group. This test is useful in diagnosing Creutzfeldt-Jakob disease, a rare cause of rapidly-progressing dementia which primarily affects adults ages 60–65 years.

Kaufman DM. *Clinical Neurology for Psychiatrists*. 5th ed. Philadelphia: WB Saunders; 2001:131–149.

102. Answer: E. Friedreich's ataxia is characterized by a degenerative process where there is a dying back of neurons in certain systems from the periphery to the center with disappearance of the cell body. The clinical picture usually starts at approximately 10 years of age and includes progressive ataxia, spasticity, absent lower limb reflexes, scoliosis, cardiomyopathy, dysarthria, and progressive atrophy of lower extremities until affected children become wheelchair-bound. Other more infrequent symptoms include diabetes mellitus and hearing impairment. Cataracts are not usually associated with Friedreich's ataxia.

1. Corben LA, Georgiou-Karistianis N, Fahey MC, et al. Towards an understanding of cognitive function in Friedreich's ataxia. *Brain Res Bull*. 2006;70:197–202.
2. Menkes JH, Sarnat HB, Maria BL. *Child Neurology*. 7th ed. Philadelphia: Lippincott Williams & Wilkins; 2006:179–183, 190–215.

103. Answer: C. Disorders of CSF include hydrocephalus, pseudotumor cerebri, and syndromes produced by reduced pressure in the CSF compartment. Pseudotumor cerebri designates a syndrome consisting of headache, papilledema (unilateral or bilateral), minimal focal neurological signs, and elevated CSF pressure in the range of 250 to 450 mm H_2O, all occurring in the absence of enlarged ventricles or an intracranial mass. Headache is the cardinal symptom. Despite its name, there is no association between the syndrome and malignancy. If IIH and papilledema are left untreated, permanent visual loss from compressive damage to the optic nerve fibers and compression of the central retinal veins may result.

Ropper AH, Brown RH. *Adams and Victor's Principles of Neurology*. 8th ed. New York: McGraw-Hill; 2005:529–545.

104. Answer: A. Neuropathic pain is usually resistant to therapy with NSAIDs and acetaminophen. Narcotic analgesics are also less likely to provide pain relief in these patients. Tramadol hydrochloride has been found to be effective in the treatment of painful neuropathy. It acts by inhibiting NE and serotonin reuptake, and also has low affinity for the μ-opioid receptors. Anticonvulsants like carbamazepine, oxcarbazepine, and gabapentin may also be effective in treating neuropathic pain. Lamotrigine has proven efficacy in treating the pain of HIV neuropathy and in trigeminal neuralgia. TCAs like amitriptyline, desipramine, and nortriptyline are effective in treating neuropathic pain. Although the SSRIs have not been as extensively studied as the TCAs in the treatment of neuropathic pain, paroxetine and citalopram have been found to be more effective than placebo in treating these patients. Venlafaxine, a serotonin and NE reuptake inhibitor, has demonstrated efficacy in treating neuropathic pain. Lidocaine patch and capsaicin cream, which depletes substance P from the cutaneous-sensory nerves on topical use may be helpful in some patients.

Rowland LP. *Merritt's Neurology*. 11th ed. Philadelphia: Lippincott Williams & Wilkins; 2005:549–550.

105. Answer: D. Children grow at a much slower pace between the ages of 3 and 5 years, than they did in the first year of their life. The average child gains about 7 cm (2 inch) in height and 2 kg (approximately 1 lb) in weight per year. Boys gain slightly more than girls. Lordosis also becomes less pronounced, with the abdomen flattening and the body appears to be leaner. Head growth declines with head circumference increasing by only 2 cm (1 inch) each year. The face becomes elongated and by comparison, the legs grow faster than the trunk, head, or upper extremities.

Green-Hernandez C, Singleton JK, Aronzon D. *Primary Care Pediatrics*. 1st ed. Philadelphia: Lippincott Williams & Wilkins; 2001:131–132.

106. Answer: C. Tabes dorsalis, a form of neurosyphilis, degenerates the posterior columns of the spinal cord resulting in ataxia, paresthesias, decreased proprioception (positive Romberg's sign) and vibratory sense, Argyll Robertson pupil (pupil accommodates but does not react to light), neurogenic bladder, and painful sensations throughout the body. General paresis, another form of neurosyphilis, results in dementia, psychosis, depression, and changes in personality. It would be unlikely for MS, lupus, and schizophrenia to first present at age 70. NPH presents with dementia, incontinence, and ataxia but not with pupil abnormalities and impaired sensation.

Greenberg B, Tampi R. Cases that test your skills: beware the men with toupees. *Curr Psychiatry*. 2003;2:60–64.

107. Answer: D. Erik Erikson has theorized that ego development proceeds from birth through eight identifiable stages marked by specific psychosocial crises. Each stage represents a turning point where resolution of the crisis results either in psychological growth or regression. Integrity versus despair is the last of the Eriksonian stages and takes place after the age of 60. If this stage is mastered, the individual arrives at a peaceful acceptance of his or her mortality without losing interest in life. The woman in this case clearly has difficulties accepting the passage of time.

Kaplan HI, Sadock BJ. *Kaplan & Sadock's Synopsis of Psychiatry*. 8th ed. Philadelphia: Lippincott Williams & Wilkins; 1998:234–237.

108. **Answer: E.** Psychiatrists can act as two kinds of witnesses in the legal system: witnesses of fact and expert witnesses. Witnesses of fact have the same role as any other witness who is called to court to testify about facts. They may be asked to read aloud portions of a medical record to be entered legally in court, and a psychiatrist at any level of training could fulfill this role. A psychiatrist can qualify as an expert witness, however, when there is acceptance by the court and by advocates for both sides of the case that he or she is suitable to perform expert functions and is independent of actual expertise in a given area and is not based on popular recognition. The expertise is elucidated during direct and cross-examination, and when in the courtroom, an expert witness may draw conclusions from data and render an opinion. They play a role in determining the standard of care and reasonable practice of psychiatry.

Kaplan HI, Sadock BJ. *Kaplan & Sadock's Synopsis of Psychiatry*. 8th ed. Philadelphia: Lippincott Williams & Wilkins; 1998:1305.

109. **Answer: E.** A professionally trained interpreter with mental health experience should be used for evaluating patients with limited English proficiency and those who are deaf or have severely limited hearing and who prefer to communicate using sign language. The use of staff with bilingual and bicultural experience may also be helpful in such situations. When the patient is cooperative, over-the-phone language interpretation services can be used when other professionally trained interpreters are unavailable. However, establishing rapport with the patient is more difficult in such situations. Family members, community members, or friends of the patient should not be used unless the patient refuses to use the professional interpreter or under emergency circumstances, in which case this should be noted in the patient record. The interpreter should be instructed to translate the patient's own words and to avoid paraphrasing except as needed to translate the correct meaning of idioms and other culture-specific expressions.

American Psychiatric Association. *American Psychiatric Association Practice Guidelines for the Treatment of Psychi-

atric Disorders*. http://www.psychiatryonline.com/content.aspx?aID=137707. Accessed February 14, 2007.

110. **Answer: E.** TJ Crow proposed a classification of Schizophrenic Patients into Types I and II, on the basis of the presence or absence of positive ("productive") or negative ("deficit") symptoms. Positive symptoms include delusions and hallucinations. Negative symptoms include affective flattening or blunting, poverty of speech, poor grooming, lack of motivation, anhedonia, and social withdrawal. Type I patients tend to have mostly positive symptoms, normal brain structures on CT scans, and relatively good response to treatment. Type II patients tend to have mostly negative symptoms, structural brain abnormalities on CT scans, and poor response to treatment.

Sadock BJ, Sadock VA. *Kaplan and Sadock's Synopsis of Psychiatry*. 9th ed. Philadelphia: Lippincott Williams & Wilkins; 2003:490.

111. **Answer: D.** The NCS was the first national mental health survey to use a structured diagnostic interview to determine the prevalence and correlates of DSM-III disorders. Data from the NCS revealed that major depression and alcohol dependence are the two most common psychiatric disorders. The 1-year prevalence for MDD is reported to be 10.3%; the lifetime prevalence is 17.1%. The lifetime prevalence for MDD is higher in women (10% to 25%) compared to men (5% to 12%).

Stern TA, Herman JB. *Massachusetts General Hospital Psychiatry Update and Board Preparation*. 2nd ed. New York: McGraw Hill; 2002:484–485.

112. **Answer: D.** Fetal alcohol syndrome is the most preventable cause of mental retardation. It is seen in 1 in 3,000 live births in Western countries and is related to maternal alcohol consumption during pregnancy (third trimester > second trimester > first trimester). It is noted that as many as 1 in 300 children may have the effects of alcohol use. These children present with characteristic physical appearance or neurological dysfunction which may include all of the following:

1. Intrauterine growth retardation
2. Persistent postnatal poor growth in weight or height
3. Characteristic facial appearance including microcephaly, microphthalmia, short palpebral fissures, a thin upper lip, midface hypoplasia, and a smooth or long philtrum
4. Delayed development, hyperactivity, attention deficits, intellectual delays, learning disabilities, and occasionally seizures

Lesh Nyhan's syndrome is caused by a defect in hypoxanthine guanine phosphoribosyltransferase (Xq26-q27.2) and has a recessive inheritance and an estimated incidence of 1 in 38,000 live births. Hurler's syndrome is caused by an autosomal-recessive deficiency in α-L-iduronidase, located at 4p16.3 with an estimated prevalence of 1 in 144,000 live births. Hunter's syndrome is caused by the deficiency in iduronate sulfatase, which is located at Xq28, and has an estimated prevalence of about 1 in 111,000 births. PKU is caused by an autosomal-recessive defect in PAH located at 12q.24.1, or cofactor (biopterin synthetase, 11q22.3-q23.3), which results in an accumulation of phenylalanine. It has a prevalence of approximately 1 in 12,000.

1. Lewis M. *Child and Adolescent Psychiatry: A Comprehensive Textbook*. 3rd ed. Philadelphia: Lippincott Williams & Wilkins; 2003:449.
2. Sadock BJ, Sadock VA. *Kaplan and Sadock's Comprehensive Textbook of Psychiatry*. 8th ed. Philadelphia: Lippincott Williams & Wilkins; 2005:3090–3094.

113. Answer: D. Neuritic plaques and NFTs are characteristic hallmarks of AD and are considered central to its pathogenesis, making them targets of prospect and novel therapeutic interventions. However, they are by no means pathognomic of the disease as they are found in varying degrees in normal aging, minimal cognitive impairment, and several other dementias. Neuritic plaques are extracellular lesion, composed of a central core of aggregated amyloid-beta peptide, whereas NFTs are intracellular bundles of paired and straight filaments.

1. Iqbal K, Grundke-Iqbal I. Discoveries of tau, abnormally hyperphosphorylated tau and others of neurofibrillary degeneration: a personal historical perspective. *J Alzheimer Dis*. 2006;9(suppl 3):219–242.
2. Selkoe DJ. The genetics and molecular pathology of Alzheimer's disease: roles of amyloid and the presenilins. *Neurol Clin*. 2000;18:903–922.
3. Selkoe DJ. The molecular pathology of Alzheimer's disease. *Neuron*. 1991;6:487–498.

114. Answer: E. Family therapy has been shown to be more effective typically than medication, individual psychotherapy, inpatient, and day hospitalization for adolescent deliquency and substance use disorders. Family therapy yields positive changes in drug use, recidivism, and treatment compliance.

Sadock BJ, Sadock VA. *Kaplan and Sadock's Comprehensive Textbook of Psychiatry*. 8th ed. Philadelphia: Lippincott Williams & Wilkins; 2005:2592.

115. Answer: A. Orthostatic hypotension is among the most common reasons for discontinuation of tricyclic antidepressant treatment. It occurs with all of the tricyclics, but appears to be less pronounced with nortriptyline. The secondary tricyclics (i.e, nortriptyline and desipramine) are generally better tolerated than the tertiary tricyclics (i.e., amitriptyline, imipramine, and clomipramine), particularly in the elderly. Orthostasis is caused by α-1 blockade with these medications, and is more pronounced in patients with preexisting orthostatic hypotension or cardiac disease. Nortriptyline has a therapeutic window of 50 to 150 ng/mL. Desipramine has the most potent NE effect among the tricyclics. Clomipramine is the most potent serotonergic tricyclic, thus its common use in the management of OCD. Of note, there is a clinically significant interaction between clomipramine and fluvoxamine (both used to treat OCD), with fluvoxamine increasing clomipramine levels via CYP 1A2 inhibition, causing seizure and cardiac risks.

1. Janicak P, Davis J, Preskorn S, Ayd F, et al. *Principles and Practice of Psychopharmacotherapy*. 4th ed. Philadephia: Lippincott Williams & Wilkins; 2006:281.
2. Schatzberg A, Nemeroff C. *APPI Textbook of Psychopharmacology*. 3rd ed. Arlington: American Psychiatric Publishing; 2004:207–229.

116. Answer: B. Analgesia, bradycardia, sedation, physical dependence, and respiratory depression are effects mediated by the opioids via the μ receptors within the CNS. The receptors are found in large numbers in the midbrain periaquaductal gray and the substantial gelatinosa in the dorsal horn or the spinal cord.

Bajwa ZH, Warfield CA, Wootton RJ. Overview of the Treatment of Chronic Pain. http://www.uptodateonline.com/utd/content/topic.do?topicKey=genr_med/22160&type=A&selectedTitle=6~87. Accessed on February 19, 2007.

117. Answer: A. This patient's presentation is consistent with an NMS, which is a relatively rare but potentially fatal complication of neuroleptic treatment. Its main features are hyperthermia, severe muscular rigidity, autonomic instability, and changes in mental status. Although the cause of NMS is unknown, several risk factors for NMS have been implicated in various case reports, which include: dehydration, poor nutrition, repeated use of haloperidol, and co-administration of lithium with haloperidol. Co-administration of antibiotics with psychiatric medications has not been implicated as a potential risk factor.

1. Rosenbaum JF, Arana GW, Hyman SE, et al. *Handbook of Psychiatric Drug Therapy*. 5th ed. Philadelphia: Lippincott Williams & Wilkins; 2005:43.
2. Sadock BJ, Sadock VA. *Kaplan and Sadock's Comprehensive Textbook of Psychiatry*. 8th ed. Philadelphia: Lippincott Williams & Wilkins; 2005:2830.

118. Answer: B. Serotonin syndrome produces a clinical picture that is very similar to NMS. Both syndromes are associated with autonomic dysfunction, alteration of mental status, rigidity, and hyperthermia. Clinical differentiation between these syndromes is very important because management may differ. NMS develops in association with neuroleptics, whereas serotonin syndrome develops in association with serotonergic agents. NMS has a slow onset (days to weeks) and a slow progression of 24 to 72 hours, whereas serotonin syndrome has a more rapid onset and progression. NMS is associated with bradykinesia and lead pipe rigidity, whereas serotonin syndrome is associated with chorea, myoclonus, hyperkinesia, but less rigidity. NMS is an idiosyncratic reaction to therapeutic doses, whereas serotonin syndrome is a manifestation of toxicity, frequently generated from the combination of two drugs with serotonergic activity. However, they also share nonspecific symptoms such as hyperpyrexia, sweating, confusion, coma, and hypertension. In this case, the symptoms commenced soon after commencement of selegiline, a MAO inhibitor, which augmented the serotoninergic effects of paroxetine leading to serotonin excess. The resolution of the symptoms with the discontinuation of selegiline helps to strengthen this diagnosis. Most cases resolve without sequelae within 24 to 36 hours with adequate supportive measures.

1. Cookson J, Katona C, Taylor D. *Use of Drugs in Psychiatry: The Evidence From Psychophamacology*. 5th ed. London: Gaskell Publications; 2002:89.
2. Martin TG. Serotonin syndrome. *Ann Emerg Med*. 1996;28:520–526.
3. Sternbach H. The serotonin syndrome. *Am J Psychiatry*. 1991;148:705–713.

119. Answer: C. Women are older than men at the time of their first myocardial infarction. They are more likely to die following their first myocardial infarction. In addition, women have a higher incidence of diabetes mellitus and orthostatic hypotension. Women have smaller heart vessels than men as well as a later onset of arteriosclerosis.

Sadock BJ, Sadock VA. *Kaplan and Sadock's Comprehensive Textbook of Psychiatry*. 8th ed. Philadelphia: Lippincott Williams & Wilkins; 2005:3822–3827.

120. Answer: A. Bitemporal hemianopsia is associated with lesions of the optic chiasm, such as pituitary tumors or craniopharyngiomas. A lesion in the left temporal lobe portion of the visual pathway will result in a right homonymous upper quadrant defect. A lesion in the left occipital lobe will produce a right homonymous hemianopia, as can a lesion in the left lateral geniculate nucleus. Interruption in signals from the right optic nerve results in no perception of light from the right eye.

Goetz CG. *Textbook of Clinical Neurology*. 2nd ed. Philadelphia: WB Saunders; 2003:123–128.

121. Answer: A. The basal ganglia is composed of the globus pallidus, the putamen, the substantia nigra, and the subthalamic nucleus. Destruction of the basal ganglia gives rise to signs such as Parkinsonism, athetosis, chorea, and hemiballismus. Collectively this gives rise to the extrapyramidal tract which modulates the corticospinal tract. The corticospinal tract is directly responsible for the control of muscle tone and activity via the spinal cord and lower motor neurons. The extrapyramidal tract, however, does not directly act on the spinal cord or lower motor neurons. Therefore, in cases of Parkinsonism, athetosis, chorea, and hemiballismus, there will be no signs of corticospinal tract lesions (deep tendon reflexes [DTRs] abnormalities, paresis, or Babinski).

Kaufman DM. *Clinical Neurology for Psychiatrists*. 5th ed. Philadelphia: WB Saunders; 2001:14–15.

122. Answer: A. ApoE is a protein synthesized and secreted by astrocytes and macrophages in the nervous system. It is important in mobilizing lipids during the normal development of the nervous system and also for the regeneration of peripheral nerves after injury. Apo E has three major isomeric forms; the apoE2, apoE3, and apoE4. These isomeric forms arise from different alleles (e2, e3, and e4) of a single gene on chromosome 19q13.2. The e3 allele is the most common, accounting for about 75% of all alleles, while the e2 and e4 forms account for roughly 10% and 15%, respectively. The e4 allele is associated with increased risk for earlier onset of both familial and sporadic late-onset Alzheimer's disease, whereas the inheritance of e2 appears to be associated with decreased risk and later onset of the disease. As AD occurs in the absence of e4 and many people with e4 do not develop the disease, genotyping for apo E4 is currently not recommended as a genetic test for AD.

McPhee SJ, Ganong WF. *Pathophysiology of Disease*. 5th ed. Access Medicine: McGraw-Hill. 2006. http://www.accessmedicine.com/content.aspx?aID=2093796. Accessed October 29, 2007.

123. Answer: A. Visuospatial functioning refers to patients' ability to function within their environment with regard to recognition of objects and their construction and perception of spatial relations. Patients with AD or right strokes are especially sensitive to having deficits in these areas of functioning. Tests used to measure visuospatial functioning tasks include figure copying, clock drawing, visual organization of parts to whole, facial recognition, and map orientation. The Trail Making Tests, Wisconsin Card Sorting Tests, and Category Tests are all used to assess executive functioning. The WAIS-R is a commonly used test to measure intellectual functioning in adults.

Ebert MH, Loosen PT, Nurcombe B. *Current Diagnosis & Treatment in Psychiatry*. New York: McGraw-Hill; 2006:12.

124. **Answer: D.** The first thing to do is determine the reversibility of this condition. Checking B_{12} and TSH levels, as well as liver function tests (LFTs), are part of the initial workup for dementia to help determine if the symptoms are caused by any deficiencies or treatable conditions. CT scan is not the first diagnostic step; even though pathologic changes may be found, the better way to detect possible changes is by MRI, however, this increases the cost of the workup and is not routinely recommended. Performing an LP is not a first step in a dementia workup as noninvasive methods are preferred first. Furthermore, tau proteins are not routinely checked as the test is not reliable. Genotyping for apolipoproteins is a research tool that is helpful in determining the risk of AD in populations but it is of little value in making a clinical diagnosis and developing a management plan in individual patients. HIV testing is not a first step in dementia workup but should be done if everything else is excluded and there is significant suspicion that symptoms are related to HIV infection (patient has risk factors).

1. Kulgis RO. *Alzheimer Disease*. http://www.emedicine. com/NEURO/topic13.htm. Published February 23, 2007.
2. Rowland LP. *Merritt's Neurology*. 11th ed. Philadelphia: Lippincott Williams & Wilkins; 2005:779.
3. Santacruz KS, Swagerty D. *Early Diagnosis of Dementia*. http://www.aafp.org/afp/20010215/703.html. Accessed February 23, 2007.

125. **Answer: A.** The symptoms and neuroimaging findings described are consistent with a demyelinating process. Acute disseminated encephalomyelitis frequently presents with symptoms similar to MS, but generally occurs in an older population. Once symptoms have resolved, they usually do not recur. Given the lack of recurrent symptoms, MS (relapsing-remitting or secondary progressive) is unlikely. Schilder's myelinoclastic diffuse sclerosis can cause a similar symptom constellation, but it normally begins in childhood and is progressive. The symptoms are not likely due to a cerebral vascular accident due to their distribution and resolution with steroid treatment.

Goetz CG. *Textbook of Clinical Neurology*. 2nd ed. Philadelphia: WB Saunders; 2003:1061–1063.

126. **Answer: B.** Although some elevation of most immune cells would be expected in the CSF analysis of patients with neurocysticercosis, the most characteristic finding is elevated levels of eosinophils, which is typical with many parasitic infections.

1. Goetz C. *Textbook of Clinical Neurology*. Philadelphia: WB Saunders; 2003:518.
2. Leder K, Weller P. *Clinical Manifestation and Diagnosis of Cysticercosis*. http://www.uptodateonline.com/utd/content/topic.do?topicKey=parasite/13224&type=A&selectedTitle=1~9. Published January 27, 2007.

127. **Answer: B.** The diagnosis of DLB is primarily a clinical one. Patients must have evidence of dementia, with progressive cognitive decline and impairment in memory, attention, and visuospatial abilities. (Note: Unlike AD, memory impairment may not be the initial cognitive deficit and may occur later in the disease.) Core features of DLB include spontaneous Parkinsonism (masked face, postural instability), fluctuating level of cognitive function and/or alertness, and detailed visual hallucinations. Clinical features which further support the diagnosis of DLB include falls, syncope, systematic delusions, and neuroleptic sensitivity. Auditory hallucinations and a history of stroke are not typical features of DLB. Definitive diagnosis requires the extensive presence of Lewy bodies in the cerebral cortex; these intracytoplasmic neuronal inclusions are otherwise found only in the substantia nigra of patients with Parkinson's disease. Lewy bodies are confirmed histopathologically by an antiubiquitin antibody stain.

1. Kaufman DM. *Clinical Neurology for Psychiatrists*. 5th ed. Philadelphia: WB Saunders; 2001:131–149.
2. McKeith I, Mintzer J, Aarsland D, et al. Dementia with Lewy bodies. *Lancet Neurol*. 2004;3:19–28.

128. **Answer: B.** Charcot-Marie-Tooth disease is characterized by extensive segmental demyelination and remyelination, which causes a consequential thickening of peripheral nerves. On pathological examination, patients also have degeneration of the posterior columns, loss of anterior horn cells, and degeneration of the spinocerebellar tracts and the anterior posterior nerve roots. Patients usually show a delay in walking and progressive weakness and atrophy of upper extremities. They also present with pes cavus deformity, scoliosis, and contractures of the wrist and fingers. Neuroaxonal dystrophies, such as Seitelberger disease show focal axonal swelling in myelinated and nonmyelinated central and peripheral nervous system axons and neuroaxonal spheroids. Leukodystrophies, such as

Krabbe disease, develop almost total loss of oligo-dendroglia. Rett disorder is characterized by diffuse cerebral atrophy with increased amounts of lipofuscin and under-pigmentation of the substantia nigra.

Menkes JH, Sarnat HB, Maria BL. *Child Neurology*. 7th ed. Philadelphia: Lippincott Williams & Wilkins; 2006:170–215.

129. **Answer: C.** In the United States, lead poisoning is most often identified in 1- to 3-year-old children who live in old, deteriorated houses in urban slum areas; lead paint was used in many houses built before 1960. The chewing of lead paint is promoted by compulsive ingestion (pica) of paint from windowsills and plaster walls. Clinical symptoms develop over 3 to 6 weeks. Initially, the child becomes anorectic, less playful, less alert, and more irritable. Sometimes these signs are misinterpreted as mental retardation or a behavioral disturbance. If the child continues to ingest lead, manifestations of acute encephalopsy may develop. The development of acute encephalopathy is the most serious complication of lead toxicity. It results in death in 5% to 20% of cases and in permanent neurological impairment and mental deficits in >25% of survivors. With continued lead intake, vomiting also becomes more persistent; apathy progresses to drowsiness and stupor interspersed with periods of extreme irritability; and finally seizures and coma ensue. This syndrome can develop in the period of 1 week or less.

Ropper AH, Brown RH. *Adams and Victor's Principles of Neurology*. 8th ed. New York: McGraw-Hill; 2005:1034–1039.

130. **Answer: D.** Earlier data suggested that MS followed a more benign course in women than in men and that the onset of symptoms at an early age has a more favorable prognosis compared with onset at older age. However, subsequent data has showed that sex and age of onset are not independent prognostic factors. The relapsing form of MS is generally associated with a better prognosis than the progressive disease. Certain symptoms at disease onset were once thought to predict a favorable (sensory symptoms, optic neuritis) or unfavorable (pyramidal, brain stem, and cerebellar symptoms) prognosis, but recent data suggests that none of these symptoms are independent prognostic factors. There is no overall difference in prognosis between women who have been pregnant compared with those who have not been pregnant. Psychosocial stress has been found to have a significant correlation with MS exacerbations. There is no known association between physical trauma and disease induction or relapse.

1. Olek MJ. Diagnosis of Multiple Sclerosis in Adults. http://www.uptodateonline.com/utd/content/topic.do?topicKey=demyelin/4438&type=A&selectedTitle=1~60. Accessed February 24, 2007.
2. Rowland LP. *Merritt's Neurology*. 11th ed. Philadelphia: Lippincott Williams & Wilkins; 2005:124.

131. **Answer: D.** The first pubertal change in girls is the development of breast buds. It can appear as early as 7.5 years and as late as 13 years. Normally, pubic hair growth follows 6 months later. Menses usually begins sometime during breast Tanner stage IV. In boys, the first sign of puberty is testicular enlargement and scrotal skin thinning, which can appear as early as 9 years and as late as 13.5 years. The median age of occurrence is 11.5 years. The onset of pubic hair growth occurs between the ages of 10 and 15 years. Normally, pubic hair appears 6 months after testicular enlargement begins. Penile enlargement occurs between the ages of 10.5 years and 14.5 years, 1 year after testicular enlargement.

Green-Hernandez C, Singleton JK, Aronzon D. *Primary Care Pediatrics*. 1st ed. Philadelphia: Lippincott Williams & Wilkins; 2001:141–142.

132. **Answer: C.** The primary auditory cortex is located in the temporal lobe.

Burt AM. *Textbook of Neuroanatomy*. Philadelphia: WB Saunders; 1993:448.

133. **Answer: C.** There are some cases where a physician must breach patient confidentiality. By law, a physician must report any suspected child abuse to authorities. Other scenarios where confidentiality can be broken include: when the patient is suicidal, homicidal, or has potentially life-threatening responsibilities (i.e., driving a bus or plane with impaired judgment). The 1976 case of *Tarasoff v. Regents of University of California* recommend that physicians have the duty to warn and protect potential victims of patients, but that a clinician is not required to report a patient's fantasies.

Kaplan HI, Sadock BJ. *Kaplan & Sadock's Synopsis of Psychiatry*. 8th ed. Philadelphia: Lippincott Williams & Wilkins; 1998:1307–1308.

134. **Answer: A.** You should abide by the patient's wish, while advising the patient that lorazepam is contributing to her depressive symptoms and suggest that the patient reconsider her refusal to let you share your findings with her internist. Psychiatrists are bound by medical ethics not to divulge any information revealed to them unless the patient consents.

However, they must also protect patients and assume responsibility for seeing that no harm will come to patients by virtue of the patients' revealing information about themselves. In non-emergency situations like the one above, if the patient refuses to give permission to the psychiatrist to reveal information, even if it is to the referring provider, the psychiatrist must respect the patient's wishes. Only when patients are in danger of hurting themselves or others because of their mental state is the psychiatrist obliged to reveal such information in order to involuntarily hospitalize the patient.

Hales RE, Yudofsky SC. *American Psychiatric Publishing Textbook of Clinical Psychiatry*. 4th ed. http://www.psychiatryonline.com/content.aspx?aID=67867. Accessed February 14, 2007.

135. **Answer: C.** According to the DSM-IV-TR, Schizophreniform Disorder may be specified to have good prognostic features if at least two of the following are present: (i) onset of prominent psychotic symptoms within 4 weeks of the first noticeable change in usual behavior or functioning, (ii) confusion or perplexity at the height of the psychotic episode, (iii) good premorbid social and occupational functioning, and (iv) absence of blunted or flat affect. Aggressive or assaultive behavior is not considered a good prognostic feature in Schizophreniform Disorder.

1. American Psychiatric Association. *Quick Reference to the Diagnostic Criteria from DSM-IV-TR*. Washington: American Psychiatric Association; 2000:158.
2. Sadock BJ, Sadock VA. *Kaplan and Sadock's Synopsis of Psychiatry*. 9th ed. Philadelphia: Lippincott Williams & Wilkins; 2003:505–508.

136. **Answer: D.** Mental retardation is classified on axis II on the DSM-IV-TR Multiaxial Diagnostic System. An IQ of 45 falls in the range of Moderate Mental Retardation. The IQ range for Mild Mental Retardation is 50 to 55 to 70, Moderate Mental Retardation is 35 to 40 to 50 to 55, Severe Mental Retardation is 20 to 25 to 35 to 40, and Profound Mental Retardation is below 20 to 25. Mental Retardation severity is unspecified when the person's intelligence is untestable by standard tests for reasons like the individual is too impaired or uncooperative, or is an infant.

American Psychiatric Association. *Desk Reference to the Diagnostic Criteria from DSM-IV-TR*. Washington: American Psychiatric Association; 2000:52.

137. **Answer: B.** PKU is inherited as a simple recessive autosomal mendelian trait. It has a prevalence of approximately 1 in 12,000. Symptoms are usually absent neonatally, but untreated children with classic PKU fail to attain early developmental milestones,

develop microcephaly, hyperactivity, seizures (25% generalized), and have severe mental retardation. Patients also have "mousy" odor of skin, hair, and urine (due to phenylacetate accumulation) and a tendency to hypopigmentation and eczema. Early detection and treatment can reduce the likelihood of developing neurological problems, seizures and mental retardation. PKU is caused by a defective gene for the enzyme PAH; although a rare form of the disease can also occur when PAH is normal, but there is a defect in the biosynthesis or recycling of the cofactor tetrahydrobiopterin. In this disorder, there is no conversion of amino acid phenylalanine to tyrosine due to a faulty or missing enzyme and results in accumulation of phenylalanine with lower levels of tyrosine. PKU can be readily detectable within days of birth by the Guthrie heel prick test. Children can have normal brain development by eating a special diet low in phenylalanine for the rest of their life.

1. Sadock BJ, Sadock VA. *Kaplan and Sadock's Concise Textbook of Clinical Psychiatry*. 2nd ed. Philadelphia: Lippincott Williams & Wilkins; 1996:514.
2. Sadock BJ, Sadock VA. *Kaplan and Sadock's Comprehensive Textbook of Psychiatry*. 8th ed. Philadelphia: Lippincott Williams & Wilkins; 2005:3090–3094.

138. **Answer: B.** Glutamate is the main excitatory neurotransmitter in the CNS. Glutamate's physiologic and excitotoxic activities are mediated through stimulation of the NMDA receptor and result from the influx of calcium ions. Excitotoxicity is believed to play a role in the pathogenesis of several diseases, including Parkinson's disease and AD. Several NMDA receptor antagonists have been described. Phencyclidine (PCP) and MK-801 cause psychotomimetic side effects due to their activities on the NMDA receptors. Memantine, approved by the FDA for the treatment of moderate to severe AD is a noncompetitive NMDA receptor antagonist with moderate affinity which protects against excessive stimulation of the receptor while allowing normal physiologic activities unhindered.

1. Hynd MR, Scott HL, Dodd PR. Glutamate-mediated excitotoxicity and neurodegeneration in Alzheimer's disease. *Neurochem Int*. 2004;45:583–595.
2. Kornhuber J, Weller M. Psychotogenicity and N-methyl-D-aspartate receptor antagonism: implications for neuroprotective pharmacotherapy. *Biol Psychiatry*. 1997;41:135–144.
3. Sonkusare SK, Kaul CL, Ramarao P. Dementia of Alzheimer's disease and other neurodegenerative disorders-memantine, a new hope. *Pharmacol Res*. 2005;51:1–17.

139. **Answer: D.** During the 1950's Peter Sifneos developed STAPP at the Massachusetts General Hospital in

Boston. Habib Davenloo conducted Short Term Dynamic Psychotherapy. In the 1940s, Franz Alexander and Thomas French identified most of the basic characteristics of Brief Psychotherapy. During the 1970s, James Mann and his colleagues at Boston University developed Time-Limited Psychotherapy.

Sadock BJ, Sadock VA. *Kaplan & Sadock's Concise Textbook of Clinical Psychiatry*. 2nd ed. Philadelphia: Lippincott Williams & Wilkins; 2004:401–402.

140. Answer: B. Agranulocytosis is thought to be a rare idiosyncratic adverse effect of mirtazapine. Clozapine and carbamazepine are other medications that may cause such reactions. Mirtazapine's more common side effects include somnolence, increased appetite, and weight gain. The somnolence decreases with increasing dose, as NE effects begin to overtake histamine (H1) effects. Mirtazapine is not considered to have sexual side effects. Mirtazapine's mechanism of action includes antagonism at 5-HT_{2a}, 5-HT_{2c}, and 5-HT_3 receptors, as well as antagonism of presynaptic α-2 adrenergic autoreceptors. These actions result in an increase in 5-HT_{1a} transmission, and an increase in serotonin and NE release from their respective axon terminals.

1. Janicak P, Davis J, Preskorn S, et al. *Principles and Practice of Psychopharmacotherapy*. 4th ed. Philadelphia: Lippincott Williams & Wilkins; 2006:277.
2. Schatzberg A, Nemeroff C. *APPI Textbook of Psychopharmacology*. 3rd ed. Arlington: American Psychiatric Publishing; 2004:341–347.

141. Answer: D. The WHO recommends opioids for the treatment of moderate-to-severe pain that does not improve with nonopioids and adjuvant medications. In addition, a fixed dose schedule provides more consistent pain relief as the patient does not need to wait until the previous analgesic dose has largely worn off before receiving more analgesic. A fixed dosing schedule in moderate-to-severe pain enhances patient comfort and decreases the use of pain medication overall.

Bajwa ZH, Warfield CA, Wootton RJ. *Overview of the Treatment of Chronic Pain*. http://www.uptodateonline.com/utd/content/topic.do?topicKey=genr_med/22160&type=A&selectedTitle=6~87. Published February 19, 2007.

142. Answer: E. SSRIs are generally used as first-line treatment for OCD, but clomipramine is also an appropriate choice. Clomipramine is the most serotonergic tricyclic antidepressant, hence its utility in the treatment of OCD. Of note, there is a CYP 450 (2D6) interaction between the SSRI fluvoxamine (inhibitor) and clomipramine (substrate), which can lead to toxic clomipramine levels, potentially resulting in

cardiac arrhythmias, seizures, coma, and death. Desipramine is the most noradrenergic tricyclic. The other medications listed above do not have as much evidence for the treatment of OCD as in the case of clomipramine.

1. Denys D. Pharmacotherapy of obsessive-compulsive disorder and obsessive-compulsive spectrum disorders. *Psychiatr Clin North Am*. 2006;29:553–584.
2. Fineberg NA, Gale TM. Evidence-based pharmacotherapy of obsessive-compulsive disorder. *Int J Neuropsychopharmacol*. 2005;8:107–129.

143. Answer: E. Approximately 10% to 20% of people on treatment for more than 1 year with typical antipsychotics develop TD. Approximately 15% to 20% of long-term hospital patients have TD. TD is postulated to be due to dopamine supersensitivity of the basal ganglia due to chronic dopamine blockade. Risk factors include women, age >50 years, brain damage, children, and affective disorders. The aim is to prevent the development of TD by using medication only when indicated and at the lowest possible doses. Patients on dopamine receptor antagonists for TD should be regularly examined; consider a differential diagnosis when abnormal movements are detected. The psychiatrist may wish to reduce and perhaps stop the medication altogether. If this is not possible, alternative medications especially from the group of serotonin dopamine antagonists may be considered which may reduce the movements and have the lowest risk of exacerbating TD. Avoid the use of anticholinergics. Although TD was previously thought to be chronic and progressive, recent literature suggests that although TD develops rapidly and stabilizes, it often remits even when the patient continues on the same treatment. Eventually 5% to 40% of cases of TD remit. However, it is less likely to remit in older people than younger persons.

1. Kaplan BJ, Sadock HI. *Kaplan and Sadock's Synopsis of Psychiatry*. 9th ed. Philadelphia: Lippincott Williams & Wilkins; 2003:1060.
2. King DJ. *Seminars in Clinical Psychopharmacology*. 1st ed. London: Gaskell Publications; 1995:286–287.

144. Answer: D. Dopamine is the neurotransmitter involved in this pathway. The majority of dopaminergic cell bodies in the human brain are concentrated in the substantia nigra, and project via the nigrostriatal pathway to the caudate and putamen (striatum) and the amygdala. Another pathway projects inferiorly to the nucleus accumbens and the olfactory tubercle via the mesolimbic pathway. A separate dopamine pathway arises from the arcuate nucleus in the hypothalamus and regulates prolactin release from the pituitary gland.

Webster RA. *Neurotransmitters, Drugs and Brain Function*. 1st ed. New York: John Wiley and Sons; 2001:137–161.

145. Answer: E. Nystagmus occurs when there is injury to the vestibular nuclei located in the brainstem. This can result from intoxication with alcohol, Dilantin, or barbiturates intoxication. It can also occur when there is inflammation, as in viral labyrinthitis, or ischemia to the vestibular nuclei as a result of a compromised vertebrobasilar artery system. Damage to the medial longitudinal fasciculus in MS can result in nystagmus. Signs of Gerstmann's syndrome include, acalculia, agraphia, finger agnosia, and left right confusion, which are seen with lesions to the cerebral hemisphere, dominant not the brainstem.

Kaufman DM. *Clinical Neurology for Psychiatrists*. 5th ed. Philadelphia: WB Saunders; 2001:16.

146. Answer: D. The Token Test is a test commonly used to identify abnormalities in verbal functions. Patients are presented with tokens of different shapes, sizes, and colors and are then asked to perform different tasks with the tokens. This test is very sensitive in identifying problems with verbal functions, but further tests are usually required to identify the specific verbal problem. The category test is used to identify problems with concept formation. Tests for executive functions, such as the Wisconsin Card Sorting Test, are helpful for problem-solving difficulties and difficulties with planning. A subtest of the WAIS-III is specifically designed to test a patient's ability to identify common elements between two stimuli.

Goetz CG. *Textbook of Clinical Neurology*. 2nd ed. Philadelphia: WB Saunders; 2003:27.

147. Answer: E. In acute syphilitic meningitis, the CSF glucose is usually normal and rarely reduced. Normal values are around 45 to 80. In contrast, CSF glucose is characteristically low in acute purulent meningitis and is a usual finding in tuberculous and fungal meningitis. CSF glucose levels are usually normal in viral meningitis, although reduced in about 25% of mumps cases and in some cases of herpes simplex and zoster meningoencephalitis. Low CSF glucose concentrations can also be observed in CNS infections due to *M. pneumoniae* and noninfectious processes, including malignant processes infiltrating the meninges, SAH, and CNS sarcoidosis.

1. Johnson KS, Sexton DJ. *Cerebrospinal Fluid: Physiology and Utility of an Examination in Disease States*. http://www.utdol.com/utd/content/topic.do?topicKey=cns_infe/2328&type=A&selectedTitle=2~65. Accessed February 24, 2007.

2. Rowland LP. *Merritt's Neurology*. 11th ed. Philadelphia: Lippincott Williams & Wilkins; 2005:124–126.

148. Answer: A. A common finding in the CSF of patients with MS is an elevation of the immunoglobulin level relative to other protein components. The immunoglobulin that is present is of the predominantly IgG type although IgM and IgA levels are also increased. Among the IgG, the IgG lambda and kappa light chains predominate. An abnormality of CSF IgG production as measured by the IgG index or IgG synthesis rate is found in 90% of the patients with clinically definite MS. The CSF is grossly normal in MS. The CSF opening pressure is also normal in these patients. The total leukocyte count is normal in most patients with MS with the cell count rarely exceeding 50 cells/μL. Lymphocytes are the predominant cell type, with the majority being T cells. The CSF protein level is also usually normal. Elevated white cell count and protein level is usually seen in the CSF of patients with bacterial or tuberculous meningitis. Opening pressures are elevated in patients with hydrocephalus. RBCs are seen in traumatic tap and SAH.

Olek MJ. *Diagnosis of Multiple Sclerosis in Adults*. http://www.uptodateonline.com/utd/content/topic.do?topicKey=demyelin/4438&type=A&selectedTitle=1~60. Accessed February 24, 2007.

149. Answer: A. This 14-year-old has normal development of secondary sexual features like breast and pubic hair development. Given this normal development, it is highly unlikely that she has a hormonal deficiency and needs any evaluation at the present time. Menarche, or the beginning of menstruation, generally begins during Tanner stage IV to V and so this patient should have menarche any time in the near future. A thorough investigation is required only if she has Tanner stage V development for breast and pubic hair growth and still has not had any menstrual period. The Tanner stages first described by James Mourilyan Tanner are stages of physical development in children, adolescents, and adults. These stages define physical measurements of development based on external primary and secondary sex characteristics, such as the size of the breasts, genitalia, and development of pubic hair. Due to natural variation, individuals pass through the Tanner stages at different rates, depending in particular on the timing of puberty. Most of these changes take place in early adolescence and are completed by middle adolescence. The defining sequence in girls is related to the breasts and pubic hair. In boys, the sequence is based on changes in the genitals and pubic hair. The Tanner stages help to predict other physical changes important to adolescents, such as the growth spurt, menarche, and spermarche. Tanner stage I is child-like, and Tanner stage 5 is adult-like. In women, the physical change that marks progression from Tanner stage I to stage II is the development of the breast bud or thelarche, which occurs on average at age 11 years. The growth spurt, defined by peak height velocity, occurs in girls between Tanner stages II and III. Peak height velocity is recognized with the help of a growth chart. These stages can be divided into the following three categories:

1. **Pubic hair (both male and female)**

Tanner I: none (prepubertal state)

Tanner II: small amount of long, downy hair with slight pigmentation at the base of the penis and scrotum (men) or on the labia majora (women)

Tanner III: hair becomes more coarse and curly and begins to extend laterally

Tanner IV: adult-like hair quality, extending across pubis, but sparing medial thighs

Tanner V: hair extends to medial surface of the thighs

2. **Genitals (male)**

Tanner I: prepubertal (testicular volume less than 1.5 mL; small penis)

Tanner II: testicular volume between 1.6 and 6 mL; skin on scrotum thins, reddens, and enlarges; penis length unchanged

Tanner III: testicular volume between 6 and 12 mL; scrotum enlarges further; penis begins to lengthen

Tanner IV: testicular volume between 12 and 20 mL; scrotum enlarges further and darkens; penis increases in length and circumference

Tanner V: testicular volume greater than 20 mL; adult scrotum and penis

3. **Breasts (female)**

Tanner I: no glandular tissue; areola follows the skin contours of the chest (prepubertal)

Tanner II: breast bud forms with small area of surrounding glandular tissue; areola begins to widen

Tanner III: breasts begin to become more elevated and extend beyond the borders of the areola, which continues to widen, but remains in contour with surrounding breast

Tanner IV: increased breast size and elevation; areola and papilla form a secondary mound projecting from the contour of the surrounding breast

Tanner V: breasts reach final adult size; areola returns to contour of the surrounding breast with a projecting central papilla

Green-Hernandez C, Singleton JK, Aronzon, D. *Primary Care Pediatrics*. 1st ed. Philadelphia: Lippincott Williams & Wilkins; 2001:151–152.

150. Answer: A. Parsonage-Turner syndrome is characterized by acute and severe shoulder pain that radiates to the neck, arm, and back. It forces the patient to avoid using the affected arm and to adduct the shoulder and flex the elbow to tolerate the pain. After a few hours or days, the patient develops paresis of the affected shoulder and proximal muscles of the arm. Some patients may also develop unilateral or bilateral phrenic paralysis. Although the exact etiology is still unknown, it is thought to be due to a brachial plexitis or multiple mononeuritis, and it can occasionally present after viral illness, immunizations, or surgery. ALS is a motor neuron disease caused by degeneration of the anterior horn cells of the spinal cord, and it presents with signs and symptoms of both lower and upper motor neuron dysfunction. C1 lesions only produce motor deficits because there is no dorsal root from C1. C2 lesions produce alterations in head and neck movements and sensory perception. C3 lesions cause sensory deficits on the lower occiput, angle of the jaw, and upper neck. Motor abnormalities include muscles of the neck, trapezius, and sometimes phrenic paralysis.

1. Brazis PW, Masdeu JC, Billr J. *Localization in Clinical Neurology*. 5th ed. Philadelphia: Lippincott Williams & Wilkins; 2007:70–79.
2. Miller JD, Pruitt S, McDonald T. *Acute Brachial Plexus Neuritis: An Uncommon Cause of Shoulder Pain*. http://www.aafp.org/afp/20001101/2067.html. Published December 16, 2006.

151. Answer: C. All are abnormalities of thought content except depersonalization which is considered an abnormality of perception. Depersonalization describes the patient's feelings that they are not themselves, and that there is something different about themselves that they cannot account for. Derealization is the patient's expression of feeling that the environment is somehow different or strange but they cannot account for these changes. Delusions are false fixed beliefs that have no rational basis in reality and are deemed unacceptable by the patient's culture. Obsessions are marked by repetitive, unwelcome, and irrational thoughts that impose themselves on the patient's consciousness and over which he or she has no apparent control. Compulsions are repetitive, stereotyped behaviors that the patient feels impelled to perform ritualistically, even though he or she recognizes the irrationality and absurdity of the behaviors. *Preoccupation* is the term used to describe the patient's absorption with his or her own thoughts to such a degree that the patient loses contact with external reality.

Hales RE, Yudofsky SC. *American Psychiatric Publishing Textbook of Clinical Psychiatry*. 4th ed. Psychiatry

Online. American Psychiatric Association. 2003. http://www.psychiatryonline.com/content.aspx?aID=68501. Accessed October 29, 2007.

152. Answer: C. Mirtazapine monotherapy has been shown to have efficacy in relieving OCD symptoms. OCD occurrence shows a bimodal age distribution; pre-pubertal, which is associated with increased risk of tics and Tourette's syndrome, and during puberty/postpubertal, which does not tend to be associated with tics and Tourette's syndrome. SS-RIs constitute first-line therapy for OCD with augmentation using atypical and typical antipsychotics being useful in the treatment of SSRI-refractory patients. The Cortico-Striato-Thalamo-Cortical circuit has been implicated in OCD; hence, most ablative neurosurgery targets that circuit.

1. Coric V, Taskiran S, Pittenger C, et al. Riluzole augmentation in treatment-resistant obsessive-compulsive disorder: an open-label trial. *Biol Psychiatry.* 2005;58:424–428.
2. Pittenger C, Krystal JH, Coric V. Glutamate-modulating drugs as novel pharmacotherapeutic agents in the treatment of obsessive-compulsive disorder. *NeuroRx.* 2006; 3:69–81.

153. Answer: C Epidemiological surveys indicate that up to two-thirds of people with mental retardation have a comorbid mental disorder, and this rate is 2 to 5 times higher than that in non-mentally retarded community samples. There seems to be a correlation with the severity of mental retardation.

1. Sadock BJ, Sadock VA. *Kaplan and Sadock's Comprehensive Textbook of Psychiatry.* 8th ed. Philadelphia: Lippincott Williams & Wilkins; 2005: 3096–3097.
2. Sadock BJ, Sadock VA. *Kaplan and Sadock's Concise Textbook of Clinical Psychiatry.* 2nd ed. Philadelphia: Lippincott Williams & Wilkins; 1996:512.

154. Answer: E. Mutation causing VCFS is the deletion of genetic material on one of the two chromosome 22's. This deletion may arise spontaneously as a new mutation or may be inherited from an affected parent. When inherited from a parent, it has an autosomal dominant mode of inheritance. However, 90% of patients with the 22q11.2 deletion develop this mutation de novo. VCFS is commonly associated with cleft palate, cardiac malformations, severe speech problems, and learning disabilities. The high incidence of psychosis associated with VCFS may be related to the defect in the COMT which is also located at the 22q11.2 region. This enzyme is responsible for the catabolism of catecholamines neurotransmitters dopamine, epinephrine, and NE. Prevalence is 1 in 4,000 for deletion at 22q11.2 making it the second most common cause of congenital cardiac anomalies after DS. Because the signs and symp-

toms of 22q11.2 deletion syndrome are so varied, it is also referred to as the CATCH 22 syndrome and includes velocardiofacial syndrome, DiGeorge syndrome, hearing loss with craniofacial syndromes and conotruncal anomaly face syndrome, thymic hypoplasia, cleft palate, psychiatric disorders, and hypocalcemia. The 22q11.2 deletion syndrome is diagnosed by fluorescence in situ hybridization (FISH) using DNA probes from the DiGeorge chromosomal region. 95% of patients with 22q11.2 deletion syndrome have abnormal cytogenetic studies and positive FISH testing. Treatment is mainly symptomatic.

Sadock BJ, Sadock VA. *Kaplan and Sadock's Comprehensive Textbook of Psychiatry.* 8th ed. Philadelphia: Lippincott Williams & Wilkins; 2005:3090–3094.

155. Answer: D. Older studies had reported that delirium is present in 22% to 89% community dwelling elderly with dementia. However, a recent study showed that delirium was not that common in the demented elderly living in the community, with the rate being about 13%.

Fick DM, Kolanowski AM, Waller JL, et al. Delirium superimposed on dementia in a community-dwelling managed care population: a 3-year retrospective study of occurrence, costs, and utilization. *J Gerontol A Biol Sci Med Sci.* 2005;60:748–753.

156. Answer: D. According to Sifneos, patients must meet with all of the criteria except for choice D in order to participate in this type of therapy. Criterion four involves the therapist's assessment of the patient's intelligence and "psychological mindedness." Patients who are psychologically minded have the ability to associate fantasies and thoughts with their emotions. In contrast, patients who are alexithymic are affect deficient. Alexithymics are usually lonely, isolated, and suffer from substance abuse problems. They feel isolated from the world due to their affect deficits and are prone to develop psychosomatic illness. If a patient is alexithymic, then they are unfit for STAPP and require long-term psychotherapy.

Sadock BJ, Sadock VA. *Kaplan & Sadock's Concise Textbook of Clinical Psychiatry.* 2nd ed. Philadelphia: Lippincott Williams & Wilkins; 2004:401–402.

157. Answer: C. Tricyclics have been reported to contribute to pediatric sudden death. Risk may be related to increasing dose.

1. Ray WA, Meredith S, Thapa PB, et al. Cyclic antidepressants and the risk of sudden cardiac death. *Clin Pharmacol Ther.* 2004;75:234–241.
2. Varley CK. Sudden death related to selected tricyclic antidepressants in children: epidemiology, mechanisms

and clinical implications. *Pediatric Drugs*. 2001;3:613–627.

158. Answer: C. *Opioid contracts* include specified terms for contract violation. Often contracts clearly state that a lack of adherence may result in weaning and discontinuation of opioid therapy.

Bajwa ZH, Warfield CA, Wootton RJ. *Overview of the Treatment of Chronic Pain*. http://www.uptodateonline.com/utd/content/topic.do?topicKey=genr_med/22160&type=A&selectedTitle=6~87. Accessed February 19, 2007.

159. Answer: D. Marsha Linehan pioneered treatment with DBT, based on the idea that psychosocial treatment of those with Borderline Personality Disorder was as important in controlling the condition as traditional psycho- and pharmacotherapy were. Concomitant with this belief was a hierarchical structure of treatment goals. Paramount among these was reducing parasuicidal (self-injuring) and life-threatening behaviors. Next came reducing behaviors that interfered with the therapy/treatment process, and finally reducing behaviors that reduced the client's quality of life. In 1991, Linehan published results of a study that seems to do remarkably well at achieving these goals. Thomas French, Michael Balint, James Mann, and Habib Davenloo were all pioneers of Brief Therapy model.

1. Martinson D. *Dialectical Behavioral Therapy*. http://www.palace.net/~llama/psych/dbt.html. Accessed February 15, 2007.
2. Sadock BJ, Sadock VA. *Kaplan & Sadock's Concise Textbook of Clinical Psychiatry*. 2nd ed. Philadelphia: Lippincott Williams & Wilkins; 2004:412.

160. Answer: D. This patient is having neuroleptic-induced acute dystonia. It is commonest in men under 40 years of age. It can occur with any dopamine receptor antagonists but is commonest with intramuscular high-potency dopamine receptor antagonists. It is thought to be due to dopaminergic hyperactivity in the basal ganglia that occurs when the CNS levels of the dopamine receptor antagonist drug begins to fall between doses. Seen in 10% of the cases on dopamine receptor antagonists, it occurs in the first few hours or days of treatment. It can occur also on drug withdrawal. Differential diagnosis should include dissociation, malingering, seizures, and TD. It can lead to noncompliance if the patient fears recurrence of the condition in which case it would be advisable to use an alternative antipsychotic.

1. Kaplan BJ, Sadock HI. *Kaplan and Sadock's Synopsis of Psychiatry*. 9th ed. Philadelphia: Lippincott Williams & Wilkins; 2003:1058.

2. Taylor D, Paton C, Kerwin R. *The Maudsley 2005–2006 Prescribing Guidelines*. 8th ed. London: Taylor & Francis; 2005:7.

161. Answer: A. Cellular swelling of astrocytes secondary to failure of the cell's pump systems and brain edema. Hepatic encephalopathy produces nonspecific brain changes which are initially reversible, but fatal if untreated, leading to brainstem herniation because of pressure by the edematous brain. Other pathologic findings in the brain of a chronic alcoholic include atrophy and loss of granule cells in the anterior cerebellar vermis in alcoholic cerebellar degeneration. Wernicke-Korsakoff syndrome, characterized by psychosis, ophthalmoplegia, memory dysfunction, and confabulation, is caused by thiamine deficiency in the setting of chronic alcoholism. The initial stage of the two closely linked conditions, Wernicke encephalopathy, shows foci of hemorrhage and necrosis, particularly in the mamillary bodies. Subsequently, infiltration of macrophages occurs, and the presence of hemosiderin-laden macrophages and cystic spaces in the mamillary bodies and medial dorsal nucleus of the thalamus is characteristic of Korsakoff's syndrome.

Kumar V, Abbas AK, Fausto N. *Robbins and Cotran Pathologic Basis of Disease*. 7th ed. Philadelphia: WB Saunders; 2005:28, 904–907, 1399.

162. Answer: B. The combination of cranial nerve impairment and long tract signs are indicative of a brainstem lesion. Further support of a brainstem lesion would include the absence of visual field cuts and impaired visual acuity. In addition, the absence of cerebral hemisphere signs such as aphasia and pseudobulbar palsy further support brainstem lesions. Cranial nerves 3 and 4 are located in the midbrain; cranial nerves 5 through 7 are located in the pons; cranial nerves 8 through 12 are located in the medulla.

Kaufman DM. *Clinical Neurology for Psychiatrists*. 5th ed. Philadelphia: WB Saunders; 2001:16.

163. Answer: D. Alzheimer's disease is characterized by loss of cholinergic neurons in conjunction with NFTs and amyloid plaques, leading to decreased cholinergic neurotransmission in areas of the brain involved in learning and memory, and accelerated neuronal cell death. The majority of drug therapies currently available for treatment of AD inhibit the degradation of ACh in the synapse, increasing its availability for neurotransmission. The AChE inhibitors do not appear to be disease-modifying, and have significant gastrointestinal side effects, including anorexia, nausea and vomiting, and diarrhea, that may limit their use in some individuals. Memantine is an antagonist at the NMDA receptor that has been shown to modify the decline in cognitive ability and functioning in patients with moderate to severe AD. It binds near and blocks the magnesium channel of the NMDA receptor and prevents calcium influx through the channel in the resting state. During a transient rise in glutamate, memantine releases from the NMDA receptor and allows calcium influx, thus permitting normal neurotransmission and learning. In the presence of tonic high glutamate levels, as found in cell death, memantine becomes "trapped" in the channel, preventing calcium entry during pathologic activation. In animal studies, memantine was also found to be neuroprotective, reducing neuronal cell loss in response to injury.

1. Robinson DM, Keating GM. Memantine: a review of its use in Alzheimer's disease. *Drugs*. 2006;66:1515–1534.
2. Standridge JB. Pharmacotherapeutic approaches to the treatment of Alzheimer's disease. *Clin Ther*. 2004;26: 615–630.

164. Answer: D. Testicular volume greater than 20 mL and an adult scrotum and penis is Stage V on Tanner staging and not Stage IV. The Tanner Stages are stages of physical development in children, adolescents, and adults. These stages define physical measurements of development based on external primary and secondary sex characteristics, such as the size of the breasts, genitalia, and development of pubic hair. Due to natural variation, individuals pass through the Tanner stages at different rates, depending in particular on the timing of puberty. The Tanner stages help to predict other physical changes important to adolescents, such as the growth spurt, menarche, and spermarche. These stages can be divided into the following three categories:

1. **Pubic hair (both male and female)**

   Tanner I: none (prepubertal state)

   Tanner II: small amount of long, downy hair with slight pigmentation at the base of the penis and scrotum (men) or on the labia majora (women)

   Tanner III: hair becomes more coarse and curly and begins to extend laterally

   Tanner IV: adult-like hair quality, extending across pubis, but sparing medial thighs

   Tanner V: hair extends to medial surface of the thighs

2. **Genitals (male)**

   Tanner I: prepubertal (testicular volume less than 1.5 mL; small penis)

   Tanner II: testicular volume between 1.6 and 6 mL; skin on scrotum thins, reddens, and enlarges; penis length unchanged

   Tanner III: testicular volume between 6 and 12 mL; scrotum enlarges further; penis begins to lengthen

   Tanner IV: testicular volume between 12 and 20 mL; scrotum enlarges further and darkens; penis increases in length and circumference

   Tanner V: testicular volume greater than 20 mL; adult scrotum and penis

3. **Breasts (female)**

   Tanner I: no glandular tissue; areola follows the skin contours of the chest (prepubertal)

   Tanner II: breast bud forms with small area of surrounding glandular tissue; areola begins to widen

   Tanner III: breasts begin to become more elevated and extend beyond the borders of the areola, which continues to widen, but remains in contour with the surrounding breast

   Tanner IV: increased breast size and elevation; areola and papilla form a secondary mound projecting from the contour of the surrounding breast

   Tanner V: breasts reach final adult size; areola returns to contour of the surrounding breast with a projecting central papilla

Green-Hernandez C, Singleton JK, Aronzon, D. *Primary Care Pediatrics*. 1st ed. Philadelphia: Lippincott Williams & Wilkins; 2001:151–152.

165. Answer: C. This patient is presenting with the classical features of a lower brachial plexus paralysis. This lesion usually involves the C8 and T1 roots and it is characterized by weakness of wrist and finger flexion, as well as weakness of the intrinsic hand muscles. Sensation can be either intact or lost in the medial arm, medial forearm and ulnar part of the hand. The finger flexor reflex can be diminished or lost. If T1 is injured, patients also present with Horner syndrome. Upper brachial paralysis consists of lesion to C5 and C6 and it presents clinically with an internally rotated and adducted arm, while the forearm is extended and pronated. When there is a middle plexus paralysis (C7), patients present with weakness of the extensors of the forearm and fingers. Lesions of the lateral cord produce paresis of all muscles innervated by the median nerve with the exception of the intrinsic hand muscles. Lesions of the medial cord cause weakness of the muscles innervated by the ulnar nerve and the medial head of the median nerve.

1. Brazis PW, Masdeu JC, Billr J. *Localization in Clinical Neurology*. 5th ed. Philadelphia: Lippincott Williams & Wilkins; 2007:70–79.
2. Miller JD, Pruitt S, McDonald T. *Accute Brachial Plexus Neuritis: An Uncommon Cause of Shoulder*

Pain. http://www.aafp.org/afp/20001101/2067.html. Accessed December 16, 2006.

166. Answer: C. EEG is not a standard test done prior to starting a patient on lithium. Recommended pretreatment diagnostic evaluations include a CBC with differentials, serum electrolytes, BUN, serum creatinine, thyroid function tests, urinalysis, an EKG, and, sometimes, a 24-hour urine test for creatinine clearance. For women in childbearing age, a pregnancy test should be ordered to clarify the patient's childbearing status.

Hales RE, Yudofsky SC. *American Psychiatric Publishing Textbook of Clinical Psychiatry*. 4th ed. http://www.psychiatryonline.com/content.aspx?aID=69719. Accessed February 14, 2007.

167. Answer: B. Amanda suffers from Rett syndrome. In Rett syndrome, head circumference at birth is normal. There is no abnormality in prenatal and perinatal development, and no apparent psychomotor retardation until the age of 5 months. Typically, between the ages of 5 and 48 months, head growth decelerates. Hand skills that were acquired earlier are lost. Stereotypes including hand-wringing and handwashing may develop. The child stops engaging socially. Psychomotor retardation is present. Apraxia and ataxia develop subsequently. Although not included in the DSM criteria for diagnosis, the following features may also be present: seizures, breathholding spells, and periodic hyperventilation. There are severe problems, both in speaking and comprehending language. Rett syndrome is named after Andreas Rett, who originally described a case in 1966. If prenatal growth retardation or postnatal head trauma were present, these features go against the diagnosis of Rett syndrome.

1. Naidu SB. Rett syndrome. *Indian J Pediatr*. 1997;64:651–659.
2. Sadock BJ, Sadock VA. *Kaplan and Sadock's Comprehensive Textbook of Psychiatry*. 8th ed. Philadelphia: Lippincott Williams & Wilkins; 2005:3175, 3176.
3. Van Acker R. Rett syndrome: a review of current knowledge. *J Autism Dev Disord*. 1991;21:381–406.

168. Answer: B. According to DSM-IV-TR, for the diagnosis of Schizophrenia, the following group A criteria have to be met:

A. Two or more of the following symptoms present for a significant portion of a month (or less, if the symptoms are successfully treated):

  Delusions
  Hallucinations
  Disorganized speech

  Grossly disorganized or catatonic behavior
  Negative symptoms

  However, only 1 criterion A symptom is required if the delusions are bizarre, if the person hears two voices conversing with each other, or if the person hears a running commentary on his thoughts or actions.

B. Social or occupational dysfunction present since the onset of the disturbance

C. Continuous signs of the disturbance for at least 6 months, including 1 month of criterion A symptoms. In this period, allowance is made for residual or prodromal symptoms, which may either be only negative symptoms or attenuated forms of criterion A symptoms.

D. Schizoaffective and mood disorder have to be ruled out. No major depressive, manic, or mixed episode must occur concurrently with the active phase symptoms. If mood episodes occur, their duration must be brief compared to the duration of the active and residual periods.

E. Substance abuse and general medical conditions, which may cause the symptoms as direct effects, should be ruled out.

F. If a pervasive developmental disorder has already been diagnosed, the diagnosis of schizophrenia is made only if delusions or hallucinations are present for at least 1 month.

American Psychiatric Association. *Desk Reference to the Diagnostic Criteria from DSM-IV-TR*. Washington: American Psychiatric Association; 2000:153–158.

169. Answer: E. In the DSM-IV-TR, Expressive Language Disorder, Mixed Receptive-Expressive, Phonologic Disorder, Stuttering and Communication Disorder NOS are classified under Communication Disorders. Disorder of Written Expression, on the other hand, is categorized as a Learning Disorder.

American Psychiatric Association. *Desk Reference to the Diagnostic Criteria from DSM-IV-TR*. Washington: American Psychiatric Association; 2000:53–59.

170. Answer: E. The prevalence of delirium in postoperative patients is approximately 51% and not 30%. Delirium also develops in about 80% of patients with terminal illnesses closer to their time of death.

Trzepacz P., Breitbart W, Franklin J, et al. *Practice Guideline for the Treatment of Patients with Delirium*. http://www.psych.org/psych_pract/treatg/pg/DeliriumPG_05-15-06.pdf. Accessed December 17, 2006.

171. Answer: C. If there is evidence for sympathetic pain, the initial treatment step is a diagnostic sympathetic block. This should be considered in patients with pain in a single extremity and whose pain has a burning quality, is made worse by cold, and is associated with swelling and/or sweating abnormalities. If the patient has a good response, these blocks should be repeated when their pain reoccurs. If the patient has pain associated with a traumatic or compressive mononeuropathy and the pain is made worse by movement, such patients should have either a decompression or neurotomy and/or moving the nerve to reduce the traction on the nerve. Topical agents are considered in patients who experience cutaneous discomfort and are effective if the patients have allodynia or hyperalgesia to cutaneous stimulation. If the patient continues to have significant pain, then initiate therapy with gabapentin or a TCA. Gabapentin is almost as effective as the TCAs, and its side effect profile is more benign. If further relief is needed, a membrane-stabilizing drug like lidocaine infusion is used to evaluate the usefulness of this approach. If there is no relief with lidocaine, oral membrane-stabilizing drugs will not be effective. If there is pain relief with lidocaine infusion, oral mexiletine at high levels may be needed. Patients who do not respond to the above noted drugs either as monotherapy or in combination, opioids are indicated. For patients with lower extremity pain, more invasive approaches like an intraspinal opioid infusion pump is indicated, but its use in chronic pain is largely supported only by anecdotal data.

Schiffer RB, Rao SM, Fogel BS. *Neuropsychiatry.* 2nd ed. Philadelphia: Lippincott Williams & Wilkins; 2003:401–402.

172. **Answer: D.** As part of its mechanism of action, rivastigmine inhibits both the more centrally located AChE, and the more peripherally located BChE. Tacrine (not listed) also inhibits both. Donepezil and galantamine are more specific inhibitors of AChE. Memantine is an antagonist of the NMDA glycine receptor. Dihydroergotoxine (Hydergine) is an older drug, either an MAOI or weak vasodilator, which carried the vague FDA approval for "senile mental decline." It is unclear whether any of its benefits were specific to dementia pathology.

Sadavoy J, Jarvik LF, Grossberg GT, Meyers BS. *Comprehensive Textbook of Geriatric Psychiatry.* 3rd ed. New York: WW Norton; 2004:903–991.

173. **Answer: B.** Although amitriptyline has been widely studied for chronic pain, no TCA is indicated for use in chronic pain. TCAs appear to have an analgesic effect independent of antidepressant effects. The TCA doses used in pain management tend to be lower than to treat depression. Analgesia frequently takes

weeks to develop. Nortriptyline has less anticholinergic side effects than other TCAs such as amitriptyline.

Bajwa ZH, Warfield CA, Wootton RJ. *Overview of the Treatment of Chronic Pain.* http://www.uptodateonline.com/utd/content/topic.do?topicKey=genr_med/22160&type=A&selectedTitle=6~87. Published February 19, 2007.

174. **Answer: E.** One of the terms for a patient to participate in DBT is that they would not engage in therapy interfering behavior. The "core mindfulness skills" are techniques to enable one to become more clearly aware of the contents of experience and to develop the ability to stay with that experience in the present moment. The "interpersonal effectiveness skills," which are taught, focus on effective ways of achieving one's objectives with other people: to ask for what one wants effectively, to say no and have it taken seriously, to maintain relationships, and to maintain self-esteem in interactions with other people. "Emotion modulation skills" are ways of changing distressing emotional states and "distress tolerance skills" include techniques for putting up with these emotional states if they cannot be changed for the time being.

1. Kiehn B, Swales M. *An Overview of Dialectical Behaviour Therapy in the Treatment of Borderline Personality Disorder.* http://www.priory.com/dbt.htm. Accessed February 15, 2007.
2. Sadock BJ, Sadock VA. *Kaplan & Sadock's Concise Textbook of Clinical Psychiatry.* 2nd ed. Philadelphia: Lippincott Williams & Wilkins; 2004:412.

175. **Answer: A.** Acute dystonia is thought to be due to dopaminergic hyperactivity in the basal ganglia that occurs when the CNS levels of the dopamine receptor antagonist drug begins to fall between doses. This may explain why drug withdrawal may trigger a dystonic response.

1. Kaplan BJ, Sadock HI. *Kaplan and Sadock's Synopsis of Psychiatry.* 9th ed. Philadelphia: Lippincott Williams & Wilkins; 2003:1057–1060.
2. Taylor D, Paton C, Kerwin R. *The Maudsley 2005–2006 Prescribing Guidelines.* 8th ed. London: Taylor & Francis; 2005:7–9, 76–82.

176. **Answer: B.** Atrophy of the caudate nucleus is seen in patients with Huntington's disease. The brain is generally small in Huntington's disease, and may also show involvement in the putamen, the globus pallidus, and the frontal lobes. Huntington's disease is an autosomal dominant disease characterized by a jerky movement disorder and dementia, and death generally occurs within 15 years of onset. The mutation in Huntington's disease is mediated by trinucleotide repeat expansions in the Huntington's gene.

The function of the Huntington's gene product is unknown. Loss of motor neurons in the anterior horn of the spinal cord is found in ALS. Parkinson's disease is characterized by loss of dopaminergic neurons in the substantia nigra. The neuropathology of Alzheimer's dementia shows NFTs composed of hyperphosphorylated tau protein, neuritic plaques with amyloid cores, and cerebral amyloid angiopathy. Transmissible spongiform encephalopathies, the most well known of which is Creutzfeldt-Jakob disease, reveal spongiform changes in pathologic specimens, with multiple vacuoles within neurons.

Kumar V, Abbas AK, Fausto N. *Robbins and Cotran Pathologic Basis of Disease*. 7th ed. Philadelphia: WB Saunders; 2005:1385–1397.

177. **Answer: E.** Vitamin C is water soluble therefore would be excreted if excessive amounts were ingested. Deficiencies in vitamin E, a fat soluble vitamin, can result in cerebellar dysfunction as seen in a genetic disorder. Phenytoin is directly toxic to Purkinje cells, thus with chronic use can result in cerebellar signs and symptoms. Alcohol is directly toxic to the cerebellum in both acute and chronic use. Thiamine deficiency in any malnutritioned patient, in the setting of glucose ingestion, can result in Wernicke-Korsakoff syndrome and cerebellar dysfunction (ataxia).

Kaufman DM. *Clinical Neurology for Psychiatrists*. 5th ed. Philadelphia: WB Saunders; 2001:20.

178. **Answer: A.** Donepezil and other AChE inhibitors used in the treatment of mild to moderate Alzheimer's dementia have significant gastrointestinal side effects that may limit their use in some patients. Anorexia, nausea, vomiting, and diarrhea may significantly decrease dietary intake in some patients, leading to dehydration and weight loss. In the patient depicted in the example, anorexia coupled with treatment with metformin for diabetes mellitus could potentially lead to life-threatening hypoglycemia, so careful monitoring of oral intake would be very important. Additionally, depression in the elderly can present as pseudodementia, so careful attention to potential neurovegetative symptoms of depression, such as decreased appetite, would be important to assess prior to initiation of donepezil, to avoid the assumption that anorexia is a medication side effect.

Standridge JB. Pharmacotherapeutic approaches to the treatment of Alzheimer's disease. *Clin Ther*. 2004;26:615–630.

179. **Answer: D.** Headache is the most commonly observed feature of caffeine withdrawal. It is characteristically throbbing and generalized, responsive to caffeine consumption, and is worsened by exercise and Valsalva's maneuver. It usually begins from half a day to a day after the last consumption of caffeine. The other features include depression, sleepiness, fatigue, anxiety, nausea or vomiting, muscle aches and impaired cognitive performance, lack of motivation, irritability, and dysphoria. Low doses of caffeine can suppress caffeine withdrawal in individuals routinely exposed to moderate doses.

Sadock BJ, Sadock VA. *Kaplan and Sadock's Comprehensive Textbook of Psychiatry*. 8th ed. Philadelphia: Lippincott Williams & Wilkins; 2005:1207–1208.

180. **Answer: A.** Contrary to what the name suggests, delusions and hallucinations of paranoid schizophrenia do not have to be persecutory in nature. It suffices that there are one or more delusions, or frequent auditory hallucinations. This subtype has a relatively favorable prognosis, because the poor prognostic features, such as disorganized speech, disorganized behavior, and flat or inappropriate affect, are absent.

1. American Psychiatric Association. *Desk Reference to the Diagnostic Criteria from DSM-IV-TR*. Washington: American Psychiatric Association; 2000:153–158.
2. Sadock BJ, Sadock VA. *Kaplan and Sadock's Comprehensive Textbook of Psychiatry*. 8th ed. Philadelphia: Lippincott Williams & Wilkins; 2005:1420–1421.

181. **Answer: D.** Emerging consensus suggests that pathologically, DLB represents a distinct pathologic entity that lies somewhere between AD and Parkinson's disease. Whereas AD is associated with amyloid plaques and NFTs in the parietal, parieto-occipital and temporal cortex, Parkinson's disease is characterized by the presence of Lewy bodies in the subcortical regions of locus ceruleus and substantia nigra. On the other hand, DLB is associated with the presence of Lewy bodies in the subcortical and cortical areas, predominantly frontotemporal regions of the brain and amyloid plaques. NFTs are not common findings in DLB. No specific risk factors have been identified in DLB.

1. McKeith I, Mintzer J, Aarsland D, et al. Dementia with Lewy bodies. *Lancet Neurol*. 2004;3:19–28.
2. Nusshbaum RL, Ellis CE. Alzheimer's disease and Parkinson's disease. *N Engl J Med*. 2003;348:1356–1364.

182. **Answer: D.** DSM-IV-TR defines delirium as a disturbance of consciousness with reduced ability to focus, sustain, or shift attention. Delirium is characterized by a change in cognition (not better accounted for by an underlying dementia), which may include memory deficit (short- and long-term), language impairment (word-finding difficulty, dysgraphia, dysnomia), or disorientation (temporal or spatial).

Perceptual disturbances, including hallucinations and illusions, are not uncommon. Psychomotor behavior may be hyperactive or hypoactive; hypoactive delirium often goes undiagnosed or is misdiagnosed as depression. Mood may be labile, with periods of irritability and anger. Sleep-wake cycle may be disrupted or reversed. Although delirium and dementia may share several characteristics, a key distinguishing factor between the two is the abrupt onset of delirium, occurring over hours to days. This is in contrast to the usually gradual onset of dementia. Delirium typically has a fluctuating course with waxing and waning symptoms over a 24-hour period. Unlike most forms of dementia, delirium is reversible once the underlying condition is treated.

1. American Psychiatric Association. *Desk Reference to the Diagnostic Criteria from DSM-IV-TR*. Washington: American Psychiatric Association; 2000:83–84.
2. Levenson JL. *Textbook of Psychosomatic Medicine*. Washington: American Psychiatric Publishing; 2005: 91–92.

183. **Answer: B.** T$_3$ is used for antidepressant augmentation. T$_4$ is used to treat hypothyroidism, and is converted to T$_3$ peripherally. Anti-Tg Ab are involved in autoimmune thyroid disease. In the recent STAR*D project, T$_3$ augmentation was noted to be as effective as lithium augmentation, with less side effects reported. T$_3$ may be specifically effective with rapid cycling depressed patients.

1. Joffe RT, Sokolov ST, Levitt AJ. Lithium and triiodothyronine augmentation of antidepressants. *Can J Psychiatry*. 2006;51:791–813.
2. Lifschytz T, Segman R, Shalom G, et al. Basic mechanisms of augmentation of antidepressant effects with thyroid hormone. *Curr Drug Targets*. 2006;7:203–210.
3. Nierenberg AA, Fava M, Trivedi MH, et al. A comparison of lithium and T$_3$ augmentation following two failed medication treatments for depression: a STAR*D report. *Am J Psychiatry*. 2006;163:1519–1530.

184. **Answer: C.** Quetiapine is an atypical antipsychotic, which many use in the treatment of dementia, mostly focusing on psychotic symptoms, but it is not approved for use treating cognitive and functional decline. Rivastigmine, donepezil, and galantamine are cholinesterase inhibitors indicated in the treatment of cognitive and functional decline associated with dementia. Memantine is an NMDA receptor antagonist, which is indicated in certain dementia states for cognitive and functional decline.

1. Blazer DG, Steffens DC, Busse EW. *Textbook of Geriatric Psychiatry*. 3rd ed. Washington: American Psychiatric Publishing; 2004:387–411.

2. Sadavoy J, Jarvik LF, Grossberg GT, et al. *Comprehensive Textbook of Geriatric Psychiatry*. 3rd ed. New York: WW Norton; 2004:903–991.

185. **Answer: D.** Operant conditioning attempts to change learned behaviors in response to environmental cues. For example, medication or being excused from work may be the anticipated response to complaints of pain. Hypnosis is effective in relief of acute pain by teaching the patient to dissociate pain from the body. Cognitive Behavioral Therapy focuses on correcting a patient's distorted thinking. Group and Family Therapy may be used as adjuvant treatment for pain.

Hales RE, Yudofsky SC. *American Psychiatric Publishing Textbook of Clinical Psychiatry*. 4th ed. http://www. psychiatryonline.com/content.aspx?aID=87214. Accessed February 19, 2007.

186. **Answer: B.** Behavioral Psychology, also known as behaviorism, arose in the early 20th century in reaction to the method of introspection that was the psychology of that time. Joseph Wolpe developed the concept of Systematic Desensitization based on the behavioral principle of counter conditioning. Edmund Jacobson developed Progressive Relaxation Therapy. Nathan Ackerman defined goals of Couples Therapy and Marsha Linehan was the founder of DBT.

Sadock BJ, Sadock VA. *Kaplan & Sadock's Concise Textbook of Clinical Psychiatry*. 2nd ed. Philadelphia: Lippincott Williams & Wilkins; 2004:409–410.

187. **Answer: E.** The retinal pigmentation seen with thioridazine occurs with doses in excess of 800 mg a day; it is similar to that seen in retinitis pigmentosa and is irreversible. It can progress even after the discontinuation of thioridazine and can lead to blindness. Chlorpromazine is associated with a relatively benign pigmentation of the eyes, affecting commonly the lens and posterior cornea and, occasionally, the conjunctiva. Retinal damage does not occur with chlorpromazine and vision is only rarely impaired.

Kaplan BJ, Sadock HI. *Kaplan and Sadock's Synopsis of Psychiatry*. 9th ed. Philadelphia: Lippincott Williams & Wilkins; 2003:1057.

188. **Answer: E.** All of the statements are true. Circadian rhythms have been observed in species from *Drosophila* (fruit flies) to humans. In humans, the free-running circadian pattern is approximately 24.5 to 25 hours, with a peak blood melatonin concentration at night, and a body temperature variation of 1°C around 37°C, trough between 4 and 6 AM and peak between 4 and 6 PM. In the absence of *zeitgeibers* (time-givers), such as variation in light, temperature, and schedule regulation, sleep-wake

cycle periods can lengthen up to 30 to 50 hours, and become desynchronized from other body rhythms. Genes have been discovered in fruit flies, hamsters, and mice that have been shown to play a role in regulation of circadian periodicity. Abnormalities in circadian rhythms are thought to play a role in Major Depression, Bipolar Disorders, and SAD, and some antidepressants and lithium have been demonstrated to have an effect on circadian rhythms.

Refinetti R. *Circadian Physiology.* 2nd ed. CRC Press (Taylor & Francis Group) LLC, 2000:33–77.

189. Answer: E. A positive Romberg sign implies damage to the posterior columns (fasciculus gracilis and fasciculus cuneatus) and causes a loss of position sense. The loss of position sense becomes apparent in affected individuals when standing erect with their eyes closed. Tertiary syphilis causes damage to the posterior column. Friedreich's ataxia, an autosomal recessive disorder, also affects the posterior column as well as causes ataxia, cardiomyopathy, and pes cavus deformity. Pernicious anemia and malabsorption result in vitamin B12 deficiency which affects the posterior column. ALS results in the destruction of both upper and lower motor neurons but does not affect the posterior columns.

Kaufman DM. *Clinical Neurology for Psychiatrists.* 5th ed. Philadelphia: WB Saunders; 2001:24.

190. Answer: C. Although it is important to educate the patient about the possibility of all of the listed side effects, lamotrigine has been associated with a potentially fatal rash, Stevens-Johnson syndrome. The incidence of a rash associated with lamotrigine treatment ranges between 3.9% and 16.5% in clinical trials and post-marketing surveillance of lamotrigine treatment of epilepsy and bipolar disorders. Potentially serious rashes, such as in Stevens-Johnson syndrome, have a lower incidence, 0.1% in adults and 0.5% in children, and have been associated with concomitant valproate sodium treatment. A recent retrospective analysis found that a history of a rash associated with treatment with another antiepileptic drug was the greatest risk factor for development of a lamotrigine-associated rash. The utility of lamotrigine in treatment of seizure disorders and Bipolar Disorders, as well as its benign side effect profile and lower teratogenicity profile compared to other antiepileptic drugs, make rechallenge with the drug after an associated rash a consideration. Reintroduction of lamotrigine at a very slow titration rate may be possible, with titrations as slow as 5 mg every 2 weeks, retaining lamotrigine as a therapeutic option. Having patients avoid any new soaps, deter-

gents, cosmetic preparations, and skin lotions may help avoid the occurrence of a rash.

1. Goldsmith DR, Wagstaff AJ, Ibbotson T, et al. Lamotrigine: a review of its use in bipolar disorder. *Drugs.* 2003;63:2029–2050.
2. Hirsch LJ, Weintraub DB, Buchsbaum R, et al. Predictors of Lamotrigine-associated rash. *Epilepsia.* 2006;47:318–322.
3. P-Codrea Tigaran S, Sidenius P, Dam M. Lamotrigine-induced rash–worth a rechallenge. *Acta Neurol Scand.* 2005;111:191–194.

191. Answer: C. The DSM-IV-TR diagnostic criteria for Hallucinogen Intoxication are:

A. Recent use of a hallucinogen
B. Clinically significant maladaptive behavioral or psychological changes that develop during, or shortly after, hallucinogen use
C. Perceptual changes in a state of wakefulness or alertness occurring during or shortly after, hallucinogen use
D. Two or more of the following signs developing during or shortly after hallucinogen use:

  Pupillary dilatation
  Tachycardia
  Sweating
  Palpitations
  Blurring of vision
  Tremors
  Incoordination

E. The symptoms are not due to a general medical condition or better accounted for by another mental disorder

American Psychiatric Association. *Quick Reference to the Diagnostic Criteria from DSM-IV-TR.* Washington: American Psychiatric Association; 2000:134.

192. Answer: E. In residual schizophrenia, prominent delusions, hallucinations, disorganized speech, disorganized or catatonic behavior, must be absent. There should, however, be evidence of the ongoing illness, by means of negative symptoms, or attenuated criterion A symptoms.

American Psychiatric Association. *Desk Reference to the Diagnostic Criteria from DSM-IV-TR.* Washington: American Psychiatric Association; 2000:153–158.

193. Answer: E. Although the core symptoms of DLB are dementia, delirium, and visual hallucinations with Parkinsonism, a significant proportion of patients manifest extreme sensitivity to antipsychotic medications and rapid eye movement sleep behavior disorder that some authors have suggested these as defining features. An association between restless leg syndrome and DLB has not been described.

1. Knopman DS, Boeve BF, Petersen RC. Essentials of the proper diagnoses of mild cognitive impairment, dementia, and major subtypes of dementia. *Mayo Clin Proc.* 2003;78:1290–1308.
2. Stewart JT. Defining diffuse Lewy body disease. Tetrad of symptoms distinguishes illness from other dementias. *Postgrad Med.* 2003;113:71–75.

194. Answer: E. Many risk factors for delirium have been identified, though gender is not one of them. Particularly strong risk factors include age (with both children and the elderly at higher risk), preexisting cognitive impairment, severe comorbid illness, and medication exposure (implicated as a cause in 20% to 40% of cases). Polypharmacy and drug intoxication are probably the most common modifiable risk factors for delirium. In particular, benzodiazepines, opiates, and drugs with anticholinergic properties are associated with the development of delirium. Terminal illness is a risk factor for delirium, as is pain. Low serum albumin is an important risk factor at any age. It may represent poor nutrition, chronic disease, or renal or hepatic insufficiency. As many drugs are transported by albumin in the bloodstream, low serum albumin may result in greater bioavailability of these drugs with a subsequent increase in side effects, including delirium. Other risk factors for delirium include cardiac surgery, AIDS, and burn injuries.

1. Inouye SK, Bogardus ST, Charpentier PE, et al. A multicomponent intervention to prevent delirium in hospitalized older patients. *N Engl J Med.* 1999;340:669–676.
2. Levenson JL. *Textbook of Psychosomatic Medicine.* Washington: American Psychiatric Publishing; 2005:99–100.

195. Answer: B. MS is an autoimmune disorder of the CNS, affecting women more often than men in a 2:1 ratio. The prevalence throughout the world is highly variable, with more cases found further from the equator. The exact cause of MS is unknown, but genetic and environmental factors are thought to play a role in the pathogenesis of the disorder. The relative risk of developing MS is 20- to 40-fold higher in a relative of an affected patient, and an association between MS and the HLA-DR2 allele is well established. There is no clear transmission of the disorder to children of an affected person, decreasing the likelihood of single-gene inheritance. The lesions seen on MRI represent areas of demyelination, caused by antibody-mediated destruction of myelin by activated T cells and macrophages. CSF examination in the majority of patients with MS reveals oligoclonal

bands, IgG antibodies against myelin antigens. Treatment with immunomodulators, such as interferon or corticosteroids, can reduce severity of exacerbations and delay disease progression, but are not curative.

1. Frohman EM, Racke MK, Raine CS. Multiple sclerosis—the plaque and its pathogenesis. *N Engl J Med.* 2006;354:942–955.
2. Noseworthy JH, Lucchinetti C, Rodriguez M, Weinshenker BG. Multiple sclerosis. *N Engl J Med.* 2000;343:938–952.

196. Answer: E. The side effect that the patient is experiencing is drug-induced accommodation paresis secondary to anticholinergic actions of medications. Clozapine, paroxetine, thioridazine, and imipramine all have anticholinergic effects, which can cause paresis of accommodation. When looking closely at an object the accommodation reflex, which is parasympathetic mediated, constricts the ciliary bodies and allows the lens to focus the image on the retina. Haloperidol has minimal anticholinergic effects and thus drug-induced accommodation reflex is not a side effect of this medication.

Kaufman DM. *Clinical Neurology for Psychiatrists.* 5th ed. Philadelphia: WB Saunders; 2001:292.

197. Answer: E. The abuse of dextromethorphan is an important consideration in the evaluation of substance misuse, especially in adolescents. The misuse of dextromethorphan has been increasing due to its ready availability, low cost, and lack of stigma as a legal drug. The active metabolite, dextrorphan, binds to the NMDA receptor and causes dissociation, depersonalization, somnolence, "out-of-body" like experiences, and agitation when taken at supra-therapeutic doses. One particular formulation, Coricidin HBP Cold and Cough (called "triple Cs" or "C-C-C" on the street), is especially popular, as it comes in a pill form, reducing the need to drink the large volumes of cough syrup required for intoxication, which can cause nausea. This particular formulation, however, has been associated with many overdoses due to the presence of chlorpheniramine, an anticholinergic antihistamine that is one of the active ingredients. Dextromethorphan is metabolized in the liver by CYP 2D6. Genetic studies have determined that 5% to 10% of persons of Caucasian ancestry have a polymorphism in the gene for CYP 2D6 that causes them to be poor metabolizers of its substrates. One important consideration in this case is the information that the adolescent is taking fluoxetine for depression, as fluoxetine is an inhibitor of CYP 2D6. Taking fluoxetine alone can decrease metabolism enough to produce elevated drug levels, and when coupled with the poor metabolizer polymorphism, can lead to fatal overdose.

1. Miller SC. Coricidin HBP cough and cold addiction. *J Am Acad Child Adolesc Psychiatry*. 2005;44:509–510.
2. Schwartz RH. Adolescent abuse of dextromethorphan. *Clin Pediatr (Phila)*. 2005;44:565–568.
3. Wilkinson GR. Drug metabolism and variability among patients in drug response. *N Engl J Med*. 2005;352:2211–2221.

198. Answer: B. Pramipexole is a dopamine receptor agonist that binds the D2 and D3 receptors in the striatum and substantia nigra. It has a higher affinity for the D3 receptor, which may cause it to have a less pronounced effect on orthostatic blood pressure. Pramipexole has shown promise in the treatment of early Parkinson's disease, with decreased loss of dopaminergic neurons. Haloperidol is a D2 receptor antagonist. Bupropion works via increasing synaptic dopamine and NE concentrations, by inhibiting their reuptake. Methylphenidate and other stimulants induce release of dopamine from intracellular storage vesicles. Memantine is an NMDA receptor antagonist used in the treatment of AD.

Piercey MF, Hoffman WE, Smith MW, et al. Inhibition of dopamine neuron firing by pramipexole, a dopamine D3 receptor-preferring agonist: comparison to other dopamine receptor agonists. *Eur J Pharmacol*. 1996;312:35–44.

199. Answer: B. Patients with early-stage Parkinson's disease include those who have had the disease for less than five years or those who have not developed motor complications from the use of levodopa. In these patients, treatment with MAO-B inhibitor, amantadine(Symmetrel), or anticholinergics may modestly improve mild symptoms, but most patients will need treatment with levodopa or a dopamine agonist. The American Academy of Neurology recommends that levodopa or a dopamine agonist be used when dopaminergic agents are required. Levodopa is better to improve motor disability and dopamine agonists are used when motor complications need to be minimized. Dopamine agonists are initiated in patients with mild disease when the age of onset is at a younger age and with levodopa when the age of onset is at an older age and the patients have more severe motor symptoms.

Rao SS, Hofmann LA, Shakil A. Parkinson's disease: diagnosis and treatment. *Am Fam Physician*. 2006;74:2046–2054.

200. Answer: B. Patients with late-stage Parkinson's disease includes all of those who have already received carbidopa/levodopa treatment and have developed motor complications from these medications. About 40% of all patients treated with levodopa develop motor fluctuations and dyskinesia. Patients may experience a "wearing-off" effect, which is characterized by a shorter duration of benefit from each dose of levodopa. Many of these patients may also experience an "on-off" effect characterized by unpredictable, abrupt fluctuations in motor functioning when the medication is effective and symptoms are controlled ("on") to when parkinsonian symptoms worsen ("off"). These complications can be treated by adding a dopamine agonist, MAO-B inhibitor, or COMT inhibitor to the carbidopa levodopa combination.

Rao SS, Hofmann LA, Shakil A. Parkinson's disease: diagnosis and treatment. *Am Fam Physician*. 2006;74:2046–2054.

Questions

1. Which one of the following statements is NOT TRUE of fetal alcohol syndrome (FAS)?
   A. The prevalence in children of alcoholic mothers is 1 to 2 per 1,000 live births.
   B. They may present with intrauterine growth retardation.
   C. They may present with microcephaly and microphthalmia.
   D. Delayed development including learning and intellectual delays.
   E. Seizures may occur in a minority of children.

2. A 24-year-old woman comes to your office complaining of left shoulder pain. She spent the summer backpacking in Europe and has noticed this pain since her return home. She complains of weakness of the shoulder and finds it hard to raise her arm above the head when playing volleyball. When you ask the patient to hold her arms up in front of her body, the scapula becomes winged. Given this history and finding where would you localize the lesion?
   A. Suprascapular nerve
   B. Dorsal scapular nerve
   C. Thoracodorsal nerve
   D. Long thoracic nerve
   E. There is most likely no nerve lesion

3. Jean Piaget is best known for his theories on development of which of the following?
   A. Intelligence
   B. Interpersonal relationships
   C. Psychosexual functioning
   D. Psychosocial functioning
   E. Symbols and archetypes

4. Which one of the following terms refers to the doctrine that allows the state to intervene and to act as a surrogate parent for those who are unable to care for themselves or who may harm themselves?
   A. Actus reus
   B. Habeas corpus
   C. Mens rea
   D. Parens patriae
   E. Respondeat superior

5. Which one of the following statements is NOT TRUE of the blood level of lithium?
   A. Therapeutic blood levels for lithium in the treatment of acute mania is about 0.8 to 1.5 mEq/L.
   B. Stable, steady-state lithium levels are generally obtained about 7 to 10 days after either initiating lithium or adjusting the dose.
   C. Blood samples for lithium levels are generally drawn about 12 hours after the last dose of lithium.
   D. Maintenance therapy with lithium is at levels of 0.6 to 0.9 mEq/L.
   E. Lithium level can alter dramatically in patients who are taking thiazide diuretics.

6. Which one of the following statements regarding the use of electroencephalography (EEG) in delirious patients is TRUE?
   A. EEG is considered necessary to make a clinical diagnosis of delirium.
   B. The EEG in delirium tremens will show low-voltage fast activity.
   C. The EEG in children with delirium is notably different from that of adults.
   D. There is no correlation between the degree of EEG slowing and severity of delirium.
   E. The characteristic EEG in delirium has a 3-per-second spike and wave pattern.

7. In epidemiologic surveys, what is the past month prevalence for inhalant use in the United States?
   A. 1%
   B. 2%
   C. 4%
   D. 6%
   E. 8%

8. Which one of the following is the most common finding in depressed patients?
   A. Elevated levels of thyroid stimulating hormone (TSH)
   B. Elevated levels of antithyroid antibodies
   C. Decreased thyroid T3 hormone
   D. Decreased thyroid T4 hormone
   E. Blunted TSH response to thyrotropin releasing hormone (TRH) challenge

9. Which one of the following is NOT TRUE of the neuropsychiatric manifestations of multiple sclerosis?
   A. Impaired memory is the most common cognitive problem
   B. Patients commonly develop depression

C. Patients commonly develop a euphoric mood

D. Patients rarely develop personality changes

E. Patients rarely develop psychosis

10. A 29-year-old man is admitted with confusion and seizures after an overdose of 300 mg of haloperidol. He is treated symptomatically after gastric lavage. Each of the following is TRUE of overdose with dopamine receptor antagonists EXCEPT:

A. Extrapyramidal symptoms especially dystonia may occur.

B. Hypertension and hyperreflexia are other symptoms of such an overdose.

C. Haloperidol may be the safest of the dopamine receptor antagonists in overdose.

D. Death occurs from cardiovascular complications in the case of thioridazine.

E. The EEG shows diffuse slowing and low voltage.

11. Hyperprolactinaemia induced by antipsychotics can result in all of the following EXCEPT:

A. Unilateral gynaecomastia

B. Erectile failure

C. Hirsutism

D. Priapism

E. Reduced spermatogenesis

12. Which one of the following statements about the side effects of tricyclic antidepressant (TCA) is TRUE ?

A. Sexual dysfunction is most common early in treatment.

B. A rapid fine tremor is common and not dose responsive.

C. Orthostatic hypotension is only common with high plasma levels.

D. Tachycardia only occurs with highly anticholinergic agents.

E. There is no effect on chronic open angle glaucoma.

13. A 17-year-old woman is brought to your office by her mother who complains that her daughter is "unbearable" to live with for about 1 week each month. The other 3 weeks of the month, she is "an angel," pleasant to be around, and has a bright mood. She describes episodes of extreme mood lability and irritability as well as sleeping all day, overeating, and not involved in her usual activities that she normally enjoys. The daughter reluctantly agrees with her mother and adds that at these times she always has a headache, and feels bloated and "fat." Upon further questioning it appears that these symptoms are confined to the luteal phase of her menstrual cycle. Which one of the following medications has been most helpful for the treatment of premenstrual dysphoric disorder (PMDD)?

A. Selective Serotonin Reuptake Inhibitors (SSRIs)

B. Benzodiazepines

C. Nonsteroidal anti-inflammatory drugs (NSAIDs)

D. Antipsychotic medications

E. Monoamine oxidase inhibitors (MAOIs)

14. A female patient is angry with herself for not getting a promotion. She tells her psychiatrist "you are incompetent," and proceeds to belittle the psychiatrist's knowledge of medications. The next week, the psychiatrist discusses the side effects of a medication with this patient and incorrectly tells her that weight gain is not associated with this medication. He notices this mistake within a minute and corrects himself to her. Which one of the following best characterizes this process?

A. Projection

B. Denial

C. Acting out

D. Transference

E. Projective identification

15. Which one of the following statements is TRUE regarding the treatment of depression in pregnancy?

A. About 30% of pregnant women experience depressive episodes (major or minor).

B. The most extensive data on the prenatal use of antidepressants is for venlafaxine.

C. TCAs are contraindicated in the treatment of depression in pregnancy.

D. The MAOIs are commonly used to treat depression in pregnant women.

E. None of the above.

16. A 33-year-old man is brought to the emergency room (ER) by the police. At the ER, he is confused, agitated, and unable to provide any history. On physical examination, you find that he has abnormally large pupils. You suspect that he is intoxicated with a drug. Given this history, which one of the following drugs is he most likely to have ingested?

A. Phencyclidine

B. Heroin

C. Alcohol

D. Ecstasy

E. Atropine

17. Which one of the following is TRUE of reflex activity?

A. The basic unit of integrated reflex activity is the reflex arc.

B. Synapses are an integral part of the reflex arc.

C. Bell–Magendie law is the principle which states that in the spinal cord the dorsal roots are sensory and the ventral roots are motor.

D. A stimulus in the sensory receptor generates an all-or-none action potential in the afferent nerve.

E. All of the above.

18. A 50-year-old man was recently diagnosed with restless legs syndrome (RLS). He meets with you to discuss this diagnosis. When talking to him about his condition, which one of the following will you NOT be telling him?

A. It has a prevalence rate of about 7% to 10% of the general population in the United States and Northern Europe.

B. The prevalence and disease severity decreases with age.

C. The incidence in women is twice that of men.

D. It is more common in patients with iron deficiency anemia.

E. A strong family history is more closely correlated with an early age of onset (<45 years).

19. A 10-month-old girl is brought into the emergency department after she and her mother are involved in a motor vehicle accident. The child has had no previous health concerns and is on no medication. Which one of the following reflexes, if present, would still be considered normal for this child given her age?

A. Rooting reflex

B. Babinski reflex

C. Moro reflex

D. Tonic neck reflex

E. Palmar grasp reflex

20. A 73-year-old woman presents to the ER with right lower face and arm weakness of several hours duration. Her symptoms resolve while she is in the waiting room. Given this information, what is the most likely diagnosis for this patient's condition?

A. Transient ischemic attack (TIA)

B. Anterior cerebral stroke

C. Middle cerebral stroke

D. Posterior cerebral stroke

E. Wallenberg's syndrome

21. A 25-year-old woman has a history of recurrent attacks of severe abdominal pain that last for several days. The pain is generalized and comes and goes. During these attacks, she also develops constipation, muscle weakness, and depressed mood. Between attacks, she is pain free. She notes her father suffered from the same condition. Which one of the following drugs should this patient avoid taking?

A. Oral contraceptives

B. Methadone

C. Atropine

D. Metformin

E. Pyridoxine

22. All of the following are true of human immunodeficiency virus (HIV) associated dementia (HAD) EXCEPT:

A. It occurs in up to 50% of HIV infected persons.

B. It is almost always of sub-cortical origin.

C. It is important to consider other causes for the dementia in these patients.

D. It is a risk factor for suicide in HIV infected people.

E. Up to 75% of these patients with this illness die within 6 months.

23. A 27-year-old white woman is admitted with fever, olfactory, gustatory, and visual hallucinations, and marked memory impairment of 2 weeks duration. A diagnosis of herpes simplex encephalitis is being considered. All of the following investigations will be supportive or confirmatory of this diagnosis EXCEPT:

A. Magnetic resonance imaging (MRI) brain scan is sensitive in identifying early changes.

B. EEG shows early localization of spike and slow wave activity in one or both temporal lobes.

C. Rising titers of serum and cerebrospinal fluid (CSF) antibodies to the herpes simplex virus (HSV) antigen.

D. Demonstration of HSV DNA in CSF by polymerase chain reaction

E. Demonstration of HSV antigen or DNA in brain biopsy.

24. A 60-year-old truck driver comes to your clinic with his wife complaining of a 6-month history of poor concentration and impaired memory especially for recent events, affecting his ability to drive. His wife reports that he has been acting out of character for the past 12 months, being overly flirtatious with the women at the local store and making ribald jokes. You find him to be expansive in mood with what appears to be delusions of grandeur. On examination, you detect tremors, hyperreflexia, and Argyll-Robertson pupils. You suspect neurosyphilis and arrange a neurological consultation. All of the following are TRUE of neurosyphilis EXCEPT:

A. Neurosyphilis occurs at an average of 10 to 15 years from the time of initial infection.

B. It generally affects the frontal lobe of the brain.

C. Argyll-Robertson pupils are classically large, regular pupils which are nonreactive to accommodation.

D. Tabes dorsalis is associated with general paresis in 20% of cases.

E. Grandiose delusions are seen in 20% of cases.

25. Which one of the following is TRUE of Down syndrome and Alzheimer's disease (AD)?

    A. About 10% of the patients with Down syndrome above the age of 50 years develop AD.

    B. The presence of apolipoprotein E (ApoE) epsilon4 allele in Down syndrome patients is not a risk factor for developing AD.

    C. The presence of high levels of testosterone in Down syndrome patients is a risk factor for developing AD.

    D. Late-onset epilepsy in Down syndrome is associated with AD.

    E. In patients with Down syndrome, slowing of the dominant frontal rhythm is related to the development of AD.

26. Which one of the following is NOT a dopamine agonist used for treating Parkinson's disease?

    A. Bromocriptine (Parlodel)

    B. Pergolide (Permax)

    C. Selegiline (Eldepryl)

    D. Pramipexole (Mirapex)

    E. Ropinirole (Requip)

27. Which one of the following statements about child-parent relationship is NOT TRUE?

    A. *Goodness of fit* is a term used to describe the way in which infants and their parents achieve good adjustment to one another.

    B. *Poorness of fit* is a term used to describe the way in which infants and their parents have great difficulty adjusting to each other.

    C. Expert parents find it easy to care for all children.

    D. Some well behaved children may be disappointing to the caregivers because of their unconscious meaning.

    E. Problems in mutual adjustment interferes with parent–child relationship and result in deprivation and traumatic separation.

28. A 42-year-old man presents to your office complaining of recent onset of erectile impotence and occasional urinary incontinence. He reports that he decided to start biking several months ago to lose weight and now bikes several miles per day. Given his history, where would you expect to find a lesion that is causing his symptoms?

    A. Sciatic nerve proper

    B. Superior gluteal nerve

    C. Inferior gluteal nerve

    D. Tibial nerve

    E. Pudendal nerve

29. All of the following names are known for their relevant work on attachment theory EXCEPT:

    A. Harry Harlow

    B. Jean Piaget

    C. John Bowlby

    D. Mary Ainsworth

    E. Rene Spitz

30. A 35-year-old African American man is suing a covering psychiatrist for malpractice because he developed a painful case of priapism while hospitalized and given trazodone for insomnia. To successfully sue for malpractice, the patient must prove that there was deviation from standard of care which specifically caused damage to him, and which one of the following?

    A. Disrespect for autonomy

    B. Duty of care

    C. Failure at nonmaleficence

    D. Incompetence

    E. Mens rea

31. What is the only current Centers for Medicare & Medicaid Services (CMS) approved indication for a positron-emission tomography (PET) scan of the brain in routine clinical (nonresearch) patient care?

    A. To differentiate Lewy body dementia from Alzheimer's dementia

    B. To differentiate frontotemporal dementia from Alzheimer's dementia

    C. To differentiate vascular dementia from Alzheimer's dementia

    D. To differentiate Lewy body dementia from Parkinson's disease

    E. None of the above

32. A 70-year-old man is brought in to his physician's office by his daughter, who reports a recent change in her father's mental status. She notes him to be easily confused with irritability and depression. He has been complaining of weakness in his lower extremities and a tingling sensation in his feet. Notable findings on mental status examination include short-term memory impairment and disorientation to time. Neurological examination reveals weakness, hyperreflexia, and impairment in vibration and position sense in the lower extremities. What is the most likely diagnosis for this patient's condition?

    A. Dementia due to normal pressure hydrocephalus (NPH)

    B. Dementia due to hypothyroidism

    C. Dementia due to vitamin B_{12} deficiency

    D. Major depressive disorder (MDD)

    E. Dementia due to cerebrovascular event

33. Which alpha receptor subtype has been implicated in nicotine dependence?

    A. Alpha 2a

    B. Alpha 5

C. Alpha 7
D. Alpha 9
E. Alpha 2c

34. All of the following are TRUE EXCEPT:
    A. MDD is more heritable than bipolar disorder.
    B. An earlier age of onset of bipolar disorder is associated with great heritability.
    C. The depressed phase of bipolar disorder is often an atypical depression.
    D. Identical twins have greater heritability than fraternal twins in bipolar disorder.
    E. A mixed episode involves criteria met for both a manic and major depressive episode (MDE) (except for duration).

35. Which one of the following is NOT TRUE of post-stroke depressions?
    A. If a patient has post-stroke depression, it is most commonly associated with a lesion in the left-frontal lobe.
    B. Post-stroke depressions are associated with increased age.
    C. Medications used to prevent strokes can cause depression.
    D. Thirty to fifty percent of patients with cerebrovascular accidents develop symptoms of depression.
    E. Electroconvulsive therapy (ECT) is considered safe for patients with post-stroke depression.

36. Which one of the following antidepressant medications did the United States Food and Drug Administration (FDA) change from fetal risk classification class C to class D?
    A. Citalopram
    B. Fluoxetine
    C. Paroxetine
    D. Venlafaxine
    E. Sertraline

37. A 29-year-old man with treatment resistant Schizophrenia on clozapine 750 mg/day develops a generalized seizure. All of the following are TRUE of clozapine induced seizures EXCEPT:
    A. The risk of seizures in patients taking 600 mg or greater of clozapine is about 4%.
    B. Clozapine should be temporarily stopped if the patient has seizures.
    C. Treatment with an anticonvulsant must be initiated.
    D. Clozapine can be resumed at its previous dose.
    E. A previous history of head injury increases the risk of seizures during clozapine therapy.

38. Which one of the following medications is contraindicated prior to the administration of ECT?
    A. Amolidipine

B. Warfarin
C. Haloperidol
D. Lithium
E. Lisinopril

39. A 25-year-old woman has 1-month history of depressive symptoms characterized by an increase in appetite, sleeping up to 11 hours a night, being sensitive to rejection, and being tired all the time. Which of the following best describes her condition?
    A. Her mood episode can be characterized as a melancholic type of depression.
    B. An MAOI antidepressant is likely to be more effective than a TCA for her condition.
    C. Imipramine is likely to be more effective than phenelzine for her condition.
    D. SSRIs are first-line therapy for her condition.
    E. All of the above.

40. A male patient tells his psychiatrist of a humiliating incident in which his boss ridiculed him in front of his peers. This patient called in sick to work the next 2 days, though he did not have any physical symptoms other than a short-lived fatigue. He states that his boss' joke about him was pretty funny and that they are on good terms. The psychiatrist tells the patient that she noticed how the two sick days occurred soon after his boss made a joke about him in front of others. This is an example of the psychiatrist utilizing which of the following interventions?
    A. Interpretation
    B. Confrontation
    C. Clarification
    D. Empathic validation
    E. Affirmation

41. Which one of the following psychiatric disorders is most commonly associated with violence in the United States?
    A. Schizophrenia
    B. Bipolar disorder
    C. Major depression
    D. Anxiety disorders
    E. Antisocial personality disorder

42. A 45-year-old woman with a history of bipolar disorder is currently receiving ECT for her medication resistant depression. Following her third ECT treatment, her mental status begins to wax and wane with bouts of confusion and disorientation. Which of the following medications adds significant risk of delirium when combined with ECT?
    A. Lithium
    B. Divalproex
    C. Carbamazepine

D. Lamotrigine

E. Risperidone

43. Which one of the following pairings for nerve fibers is NOT CORRECT?

   A. Alfa: Proprioception

   B. B: Postganglionic autonomic function

   C. Beta: Touch, pressure, and motor function

   D. Gamma: Motor to muscle spindles

   E. Delta: Pain, cold, and touch sensations

44. Which of the following has an X-linked recessive mode of inheritance?

   A. Acute intermittent porphyria

   B. Lesch Nyhan syndrome

   C. Huntington's disease

   D. Spinocerebellar ataxias

   E. All of the above

45. A 50-year-old man with a 30-year history of alcohol dependence continues to drink daily. He now presents with complaints of unsteady gait, which has been slowly worsening over the last several months. He has a history, while detoxifying, of alcohol withdrawal delirium. On examination, he has an ataxic gait, ataxia on heel-knee-shin testing, sensory deficits in his feet, and absent ankle reflexes. Given this information, where would you most likely find the lesion for his symptoms?

   A. Corticospinal tract

   B. Superior vermis

   C. Nondominant parietal lobe

   D. Corticobulbar tract

   E. Subthalamic nucleus

46. A patient is being evaluated in a neurology clinic for a speech impediment. He is able to speak fluently, although he makes occasional errors in grammar. He is able to also follow verbal commands such as "close your eyes," but is unable to repeat the phrase "no ifs, ands, or buts." His examination is consistent with which one of the following aphasias?

   A. Broca's aphasia

   B. Wernicke's aphasia

   C. Conduction aphasia

   D. Transcortical motor aphasia

   E. Transcortical sensory aphasia

47. A 45-year-old woman has a two-year history of daily headaches that last from 2 to 45 minutes each. The headaches are unilateral, affect the temporo-orbital region, and are accompanied by tearing and conjunctival injection. They respond dramatically to indomethacin. Given this history, which one of the following is the most likely diagnosis?

   A. Tension headache

   B. Migraine without aura (common migraine)

   C. Tolosa-Hunt syndrome

   D. Chronic paroxysmal hemicrania

   E. Cluster headache

48. A 49-year-old HIV-positive white homosexual man in a monogamous relationship is brought to the ER by his partner, who describes a 2-week history of over-activity and confusion. The partner also informs that for the past 2 days the patient had been out late at night and that he had claimed that he had had sexual intercourse with two people whom he was unable to identify. The partner was worried that others may be at risk from his uncharacteristic promiscuity. This man has had HIV disease for 14 years and is on antiretroviral therapy and citalopram. A psychiatric consultation is requested as his mood appears to be elated. When he is seen by the psychiatrist, the patient claims to be the "god of love" and that he had to spread his love to all human beings by making love to them. The patient does not have any recollection of his alleged sexual encounters and is now threatening to leave the ER. In treating this patient, you should do all of the following EXCEPT:

   A. Arrange his involuntary hospitalization

   B. You suspect delirium and request a full medical workup

   C. Stop the citalopram

   D. Use antipsychotic medications at the usual adult doses

   E. Discuss his status with the hospital attorneys.

49. All of the following are TRUE of cerebral abscesses EXCEPT:

   A. The commonest organisms implicated in cerebral abscess are *staphylococci*.

   B. Hematogenous brain abscess are most commonly associated with pyogenic lung conditions.

   C. It occurs most commonly in the frontal lobe.

   D. MRI brain scans are more useful than computed tomography (CT) scans in the diagnosis and evaluation of the condition.

   E. Seizures are a recognized late complication in up to 70% of survivors.

50. Metastatic brain cancers occur commonly from all of the following primary cancers EXCEPT:

   A. Lung

   B. Pancreas

   C. Breast

   D. Melanoma

   E. Kidney

51. Which of the following statements is TRUE of patients with Down syndrome and Alzheimer's disease (AD)?

A. The age of onset of AD is earlier in patients with Down syndrome than in the general population.

B. By 40 years of age, all patients with Down syndrome show AD pathology in their brains.

C. These patients first develop visual memory loss and impaired learning capacity when they develop AD.

D. MRI findings in these patients include cerebellar atrophy, basal ganglia calcification, and hippocampal atrophy.

E. All of the above.

52. Which one of the following statements is NOT TRUE of catechol-O-methyl transferase (COMT) inhibitors used in the treatment of Parkinson's disease?

A. COMT inhibitors decrease the degradation of levodopa and extend its half-life.

B. They reduce the end-of-dose wearing-off effect and thereby reducing the *off* time.

C. Treatment with COMT inhibitors also modestly improves the motor symptoms and disability in patients with advanced Parkinson's disease.

D. Entocapone (Comtan) use requires close monitoring of liver function tests as they can rarely cause potentially fatal hepatotoxicity.

E. A combination of carbidopa/levodopa/entacapone (Stalevo) is currently available in the market.

53. Which one of the statements regarding lead poisoning in children is NOT TRUE?

A. It is the most common preventable pediatric health problem in the United States today.

B. People of any age, race, or economic level can get lead poisoning, but children are at the greatest risk.

C. Children also are more likely to absorb lead dust because they place hands and other objects in their mouths.

D. Lead poisoning has many obvious signs, and most children report severe headaches and abdominal pain.

E. All children 6 months through 6 years of age who are entering day care, preschool, or kindergarten must be assessed for lead poisoning.

54. A 56-year-old man was recently admitted to the intensive care unit for a cerebrovascular event. The patient presents with diminished facial sensation on the right side of the face, diminished sensation of the left trunk and leg, dysphagia and dysarthria, Horner syndrome, and right ataxia. Both propioception and

vibration are intact. The patient does not have any motor deficits. What is this patient's most likely diagnosis?

A. Wallenberg syndrome

B. Medial medullary syndrome (Dejerine syndrome)

C. Submedullary syndrome (Opalski's syndrome)

D. Lateral pontomedullary syndrome

E. Millard-Gubler syndrome

55. In Peanuts, the cartoon character Linus walks around with an old blanket wherever he goes and needs it to calm him when he is sad, upset, or wants to sleep. According to Psychologist Donald Winnicott, what is this blanket to this character?

A. A fetish

B. A transitional object

C. An archetype

D. An obsession

E. An imaginary friend

56. In a case-control study of the relationship between major depression and stressful life events, cases are more likely than controls to over-report stressful events. Which one of the following types of errors is most likely?

A. Selection bias

B. Ecological fallacy

C. Differential misclassification

D. Confounding

E. Random error

57. Which one of the following tests would best evaluate executive function?

A. Wisconsin Card Sort Test

B. Mini-Mental State Examination (MMSE)

C. Rorschach Test

D. Minnesota Multiphasic Personality Inventory

E. Vineland Adaptive Behavior Scale

58. A 35-year-old woman presents to her psychiatrist's office for an evaluation of mood symptoms. She reports "mood swings" of several years' duration, with alternating periods of depression and intense irritability. Her depressive episodes include 4 to 5 days of sad mood, crying spells, increased appetite, feelings of worthlessness, and impaired concentration. Her irritable episodes, which last for several days, include decreased need for sleep, hypersexuality, increased goal-directed activity, and racing thoughts. She denies any impairment in her ability to work as an advertising executive, though the symptoms do cause her distress and she has difficulty maintaining relationships. There is no history of psychiatric hospitalization, psychosis, or suicidal or homicidal ideation. She denies alcohol or drug use. Given her

history, this woman is suffering from which one of the following conditions?

A. Cyclothymia
B. Bipolar disorder type I
C. Bipolar disorder type II
D. Dysthymia
E. Borderline personality disorder

59. Which one of the following symptoms is NOT seen in opioid withdrawal?

A. Pupillary dilation
B. Diarrhea
C. Rhinorrhea
D. Fever
E. Hypersomnolence

60. What percentage of individuals who have one manic episode go on to have additional mood episodes?

A. 10%
B. 30%
C. 50%
D. 70%
E. 90%

61. A 70-year-old man presents with a few months history of worsening irritability, depressed mood, and waxing and waning consciousness. He has also complained of burning sensations in his feet. His family reports that he has been having four to seven watery bowel movements every day and that he is much more forgetful than before. They also report that he is a vegetarian. On examination, he is found to have red, thickened rashes with a bilateral distribution over several exposed areas of his body. Given his history and presentation, he is most likely suffering from which one of the following?

A. Thiamine deficiency
B. Niacin deficiency
C. Cobalamin (B$_{12}$) deficiency
D. Mercury poisoning
E. Manganese poisoning

62. You are asked to evaluate a 32-year-old woman with a history of MDD who is contemplating discontinuing her antidepressant medication prior to conceiving her first child. She has three prior episodes of major depression, which have resulted in profound impairment in functioning and inpatient hospitalizations. She is currently taking escitalopram and her mood has been euthymic for the past year and a half. After weighing the risks and benefits of continuing versus discontinuing her antidepressant medication she decides to continue to take her escitalopram throughout her pregnancy. The risks associated with in utero SSRI exposure include all of the following EXCEPT:

A. Low birth weight
B. Respiratory distress
C. Persistent pulmonary hypertension of the newborn
D. Neonatal abstinence syndrome
E. Left ventricular hypoplasia

63. Which one of the following is the longest acting orally administered antipsychotic?

A. Trifluoperazine
B. Olanzapine
C. Fluphenazine
D. Pimozide
E. Aripiprazole

64. Which one of the following drugs is NOT metabolized by the hepatic microsomal enzyme system (3A4 isoenzyme family)?

A. Triazolam
B. Temazepam
C. Flurazepam
D. Diazepam
E. Quazepam

65. Which one of the following statements is TRUE of bupropion?

A. It is primarily secreted unchanged in the urine.
B. It is not secreted in breast milk in measurable quantities.
C. There is a significant increased seizure rate at common dosages.
D. It is not associated with orthostatic hypotension.
E. Psychotic symptoms are commonly reported with its use.

66. Each of the following medications is correctly matched to its psychiatric side effect EXCEPT:

A. Interferon: Depressed mood
B. Acyclovir: Visual hallucinations
C. Sulfonamides: Psychosis
D. Zidovudine: Inability to dream
E. Corticosteroids: Mania

67. Compared with women in the general population, female murderers are more likely to present with which one of the following profiles?

A. Antisocial Personality Disorder
B. Alcohol/drug dependence and concomitant Personality Disorder
C. Alcohol/drug Dependence and concomitant Schizophrenia
D. After the first murder, 3% of these women studied committed another murder
E. All of the above

68. A 69-year-old woman with multiple medical problems including hypertension, diabetes mellitus, and hypercholesterolemia in the past year has suffered an ischemic brain stem stoke resulting in a bulbar palsy. She also has a history of bipolar disorder which has been well controlled with lithium. She was recently transferred from her nursing home to the hospital for what appeared to be another incidence of aspiration pneumonia. Considering that she is taking lithium, which one of the following antibiotic medication would you avoid to prevent renal failure?

A. Ciprofloxacin
B. Levaquin
C. Penicillin
D. Metronidazole
E. Clindamycin

69. Which one of the following statements about handedness in an individual is NOT CORRECT?

A. Right-handed individuals constitute 91% of the human population.
B. In 96% of the right-handed individuals, the left cerebral hemisphere is the dominant.
C. In 70% of left-handers, the right cerebral hemisphere is dominant.
D. Learning disabilities are more common in left-handed individuals.
E. Left-handers have slightly shorter lifespans than right-handers.

70. Which one of the following DOES NOT have an X-linked dominant mode of inheritance?

A. Incontinentia pigmenti
B. Fragile X syndrome
C. Rett syndrome
D. Aicardi syndrome
E. Subcortical band heterotopia

71. A 45-year-old man with a long history of alcohol dependence is diagnosed with Wernicke's encephalopathy. On examination, he is most likely to have ataxia, confusion, and which one of the following symptoms?

A. Dysarthria
B. Ophthalmoplegia
C. Nausea
D. Dysphagia
E. Vertigo

72. A 59-year-old man is brought to the ER by his wife. On examination, he repeatedly asks for the physician's name and why his wife has brought him to the hospital. He seems perplexed by his situation. He is unable to remember the events of the last several hours. His memory of personal information such as his address and telephone number remains intact. Given this information, what is the most likely diagnosis for this patient's condition?

A. Wernicke-Korsakoff syndrome
B. Transient global amnesia (TGA)
C. Dissociative amnesia
D. Dissociative fugue
E. Partial complex seizure

73. What is the mode of inheritance of acute intermittent porphyria?

A. Autosomal dominant
B. Autosomal recessive
C. X-linked recessive
D. X-linked dominant
E. Mitochondrial

74. All of the following are risk factors for completed suicide in acquired immunodeficiency syndrome (AIDS) patients EXCEPT:

A. Recent loss of friends who have died from the disease themselves
B. Recent notification of seropositivity
C. Relapse of illness
D. Older males
E. The presence of dementia or delirium

75. Which of these diseases is NOT inherited via an autosomal dominant transmission?

A. Creutzfeldt-Jakob disease (CJD)
B. Kuru
C. Familial fatal insomnia (FFI)
D. Gerstmann-Straussler-Scheinker (GSS) disease
E. Acute Intermittent Porphyria

76. Which one of the following is NOT TRUE of subdural hematomas?

A. The blood for subdural hematomas comes from the venous source.
B. Most subdural hematomas are located over the lateral cerebral convexities of the brain.
C. The risk of subdural hematomas is highest in young patients.
D. Patients with chronic subdural hematoma may present with altered mental status and are thought to have dementia.
E. Steroids do not have any role in the management of smaller, minimally symptomatic lesions.

77. A young man is admitted to a psychiatric hospital with a new onset psychotic disorder, and is immediately started on a neuroleptic medication. Within a couple of days, staff report that he is more agitated and constantly pacing the unit. The patient complains of anxiousness and feels like his legs cannot stop moving. Which of the following is TRUE of these symptoms?

A. Associated with typical antipsychotics, but not with atypical antipsychotics.

B. Due to worsening of the psychotic illness, warranting a higher potency antipsychotic.

C. Often noted in middle-aged women, who are at highest risk of developing them.

D. Persistent and typically do not remit even after medications are discontinued.

E. Temporary side effects to medication and will go away over time.

78. A 73-year-old man with Parkinsons disease presents for a follow-up appointment at the movement disorders clinic. He has been taking carbidopa/levodopa for the past 5 years, but now explains that his symptoms are worsening despite higher and more frequent doses. His physician wishes to prescribe a dopamine agonist. Which one of the following is NOT considered a dopamine agonist?

A. Bromocriptine
B. Pergolide
C. Pramipexole
D. Entacapone
E. Ropinirole

79. Which one of the following is NOT an effect of aging on pharmacokinetics and pharmacodynamics in the elderly?

A. Volume of distribution is increased due to an increase in lean muscle mass and a decrease in total body water.

B. Glomerular filtration rate (GFR) is reduced due to a decrease in renal mass and renal blood flow.

C. The elimination half-life of certain medications increases and may be affected by the relation between volume of distribution and clearance.

D. Age has no significant effect on drug absorption in the elderly.

E. The elderly are often more sensitive to medications, and drugs must often be started at lower doses.

80. A 45-year-old woman comes to your office complaining of gradual onset of bilateral upper limb tremors. The tremor is more evident while she is performing the finger-to-nose test. Given this history, what is this patient's most likely diagnosis?

A. Resting tremor due to a lesion in the basal ganglia

B. Resting tremor due to a lesion in the cerebellar pathways

C. Intention tremor due to a lesion in the basal ganglia

D. Intention tremor due to a lesion in the cerebellar pathways

E. Physiologic tremor

81. The example of big eyes in human infants evoking more caretaking behavior than do small eyes is best described by which of the following terms?

A. Displacement activities
B. Fitness
C. Imprinting
D. Innate releasing mechanisms
E. Temperament

82. You are reading about a new diagnostic measurement for depression in a leading psychiatric journal. The authors assert that their measurement is valid. What does it mean for the measurement to be described as having validity?

A. The extent to which multiple measurements of a characteristic are in agreement.

B. The ability to extrapolate study results to those not included in the study.

C. The ability to detect a true effect of a specified magnitude.

D. The extent to which measurements correctly reach a conclusion.

E. The probability of occurrence of a specific event.

83. A patient displays uncharacteristic impulsivity and disinhibition after a traumatic brain injury. Where is the lesion most likely to be seen on an MRI of the brain of this patient?

A. Orbitofrontal cortex
B. Mediofrontal cortex
C. Dorsolateral prefrontal cortex (DLPFC)
D. Occipital cortex
E. None of the above

84. Which one of the following statements regarding bipolar disorder type I is NOT TRUE?

A. Bipolar I disorder often starts with a depressive episode.

B. Ten to twenty percent of patients experience only manic episodes.

C. The male-to-female ratio of bipolar disorder is 2:1.

D. Patients with bipolar I have a poorer prognosis than patients with MDD.

E. The age of onset of bipolar I is earlier than that of MDD.

85. The action of phencyclidine (PCP) involves which neurotransmitter systems in the central nervous system (CNS)?

A. Dopamine
B. Norepinephrine
C. Serotonin

D. Acetylcholine

E. Glutamate

86. What is the lifetime prevalence for Bipolar Disorder in the United States?
    A. 1%
    B. 3%
    C. 5%
    D. 7%
    E. 9%

87. In the first phase of the Clinical Antipsychotic Trials of Intervention Effectiveness (CATIE), what percentage of patients with Schizophrenia who enrolled in the study discontinued the study antipsychotic before 18 months?
    A. 18%
    B. 25%
    C. 40%
    D. 66%
    E. 74%

88. A 27-year old woman, G2P1001, who is 33 weeks pregnant, goes into preterm labor. She has taken citalopram 60mg/day throughout her pregnancy with the plan to taper the medication prior to delivery. Given the abrupt and early onset of her preterm labor she was unable to taper her antidepressant prior to delivery. Which one of the following symptoms is NOT likely to occur in the infant after delivery?
    A. High-pitched cry
    B. Tremor
    C. Myoclonus
    D. Tachypnea
    E. Hypotension

89. Which one of the following is NOT a differential diagnosis for Tardive Dyskinesia (TD)?
    A. Hypoparathyroidism
    B. Hypothyroidism
    C. Wilson's disease
    D. Huntington's disease
    E. Sydenham's chorea

90. Which one of the following is NOT a risk factor for greater memory loss following ECT?
    A. Bilateral electrode placement
    B. Higher stimulus dosages
    C. Male sex
    D. Advancing age
    E. Lower premorbid intellectual function

91. Which of the following statements is TRUE of selective serotonin-norepinephrine reuptake inhibitors (SNRI)?
    A. Noradrenergic effects are most prominent at low therapeutic doses.

B. They are secreted primarily unchanged by the kidneys.

C. Risk of increased blood pressure is dose dependent in all SNRIs.

D. Sexual side effects are rare at therapeutic doses.

E. Nausea is more commonly seen in SNRIs than with SSRIs.

92. A 45-year-old white man with a 15-year history of alcohol dependence is now completing a 28-day inpatient program. He has been a model patient on the program and is very motivated to stay sober. He is physically healthy and has no acute medical problems. Prior to discharge, he asks you about naltrexone for the treatment of his alcohol dependence. Which one of the following statements would you NOT make to him regarding the use of naltrexone in the treatment of alcohol dependence?
    A. Naltrexone is an opioid-receptor antagonist.
    B. It is approved for use in the treatment of alcohol dependence in conjunction with psychosocial interventions.
    C. It is contraindicated in patients with hepatitis or liver failure.
    D. Nausea is the most commonly reported adverse effect.
    E. Evidence supporting long-term benefits with naltrexone therapy in alcohol dependant patients is good.

93. Which one of the following statements is NOT TRUE of mental illness and violence in the United States?
    A. Patients with serious mental illness are two to three times as likely as people without such an illness to be assaultive.
    B. The lifetime risk of schizophrenia was 5% among people convicted of homicide.
    C. The overall rate of violence in the general population attributable to mental illness is estimated to be 3% to 5%.
    D. The rates of violence in patients recently discharged to the community from a psychiatric hospital are higher than people without a psychiatric disorder.
    E. Homelessness is a risk factor for violence among psychiatric patients.

94. Which one of the following is TRUE of hormones?
    A. Hormones can be divided into two general classes by structure and by the location of their function.
    B. The proteins, polypeptides, and glycoproteins hormones are stored in vesicles and are lipid insoluble.
    C. The steroids and steroid-like compounds diffuse after synthesis and are lipid soluble.

D. Hormones can occasionally function independently as a neurotransmitter.
E. All of the above.

95. Which of the following statements about the neurobiology of learning is NOT TRUE?

A. Pre- and postsynaptic conduction can be increased or decreased on the basis of past experience.
B. Habituation occurs due to a decrease in intracellular calcium.
C. Sensitization occurs due to presynaptic facilitation.
D. Long-term potentiation (LTP) occurs due to a decrease in the intracellular calcium levels in the postsynaptic neuron.
E. LTP also involves protein synthesis and growth of the presynaptic and postsynaptic neurons and their connections.

96. Which one of the following is the second most common type of dementia in the United States?

A. AD
B. Vascular dementia
C. Lewy body dementia
D. Frontotemporal dementia
E. HIV associated dementia

97. Gerstmann's syndrome is characterized by all of the following findings EXCEPT:

A. Acalculia
B. Agraphia
C. Aphasia
D. Finger agnosia
E. Left-right confusion

98. To confirm a diagnosis of neurosyphilis, which one of the following tests should be ordered?

A. Venereal Disease Research Laboratory (VDRL) blood test
B. Fluorescent treponemal antibody absorption (FTA-ABS) blood test
C. CSF-VDRL
D. Rapid plasma reagin (RPR) blood test
E. CSF-FTA-ABS

99. A 34-year-old man was in a motor vehicle accident in which he struck his head against the steering wheel. Several days later he began to feel as if objects were spinning around him in circles. The sensation would often begin a few seconds after he lay down to sleep at night. He described sleeping on his left side. His symptoms were most likely accompanied by which of the following?

A. Dysarthria
B. Hyperreflexia

C. Nystagmus
D. Limb ataxia
E. Tinnitus

100. A 34-year-old lesbian woman is referred by her general practitioner who is concerned about her frequent requests for repeated serological tests despite several previous negative tests. You find her to be anxious about contracting the virus. All of the following are TRUE of this scenario EXCEPT:

A. She may not be suffering from any major psychiatric disorder at present.
B. She may be depressed or psychotic at present.
C. Her anxiety may progress to generalized anxiety disorder in the future.
D. Repeated reassurance is most likely to be helpful for her condition.
E. Cognitive behavioral strategy may be useful in treating her condition.

101. Which of the following is TRUE of the etiology and pathology of prion disease?

A. Prions are transmissible infectious viruses.
B. Prions contain nucleic acid.
C. The characteristic neuropathological changes are seen in the brainstem.
D. Amyloid plaques may or may not be present in the brain of these patients.
E. The human prion protein gene (PrP) is located on the short arm of chromosome 21.

102. Which one of the following is NOT a characteristic presentation of subarachnoid hemorrhage (SAH)?

A. Sudden severe headache
B. Early loss of consciousness
C. Early vomiting
D. Dense lateralizing neurological signs
E. Signs of meningeal irritation

103. A 25-year-old woman presents to the clinic with complaints of shaking of her hands, which she noted started a few years ago but has gotten worse over this period of time. The shaking is particularly bad when she is fatigued, hungry, or upset and makes writing and eating with utensils difficult. Her boyfriend notes that her shaking is not present when she is sleeping or when she is relaxed or has had a glass of wine. On physical examination, there is an action and postural tremor noted, as well as a mild head tremor. Otherwise, the examination is normal. Given this history, which of the following is the most likely diagnosis for this patient's condition?

A. Alcohol withdrawal tremor
B. Cerebellar tremor
C. Essential tremor

D. Physiologic tremor

E. Psychogenic tremor

104. Which one of the following medications used to treat Parkinson's disease works by its anticholinergic effect?

    A. Selegiline
    B. Trihexyphenidyl
    C. Bromocriptine
    D. Tolcapone
    E. Entacapone

105. A 60-year-old woman presents to her primary care physician complaining of sexual dysfunction. Further questioning reveals that the woman is in good physical health, does not smoke or drink alcohol, and has been happily married for 35 years. She is retired, but still enjoys volunteer work and time with her grandchildren. Her chief complaint is pain during intercourse. Which of the following is the most likely explanation for the patient's symptoms?

    A. Marital discord is causing a psychosomatic response of pain.
    B. Dyspareunia is likely a result of vaginal atrophy and reduced lubrication.
    C. Aging results in a significant decrease in sexual activity.
    D. Osteoporosis is contributing to pain during intercourse.
    E. Undiagnosed depression is the likely culprit.

106. A 64-year-old man is brought to the emergency department by his wife, due to a sudden change in his mental status. His wife reports that her husband became increasingly more somnolent during the day and forgot where he was or what his plan for the day was. He is usually a cheerful and outgoing man, but today he would not engage in conversations and seemed to be acting "strangely." During your interview the patient cannot recall what happened during the day. On your physical exam, you notice left hemiataxia and vertical gaze palsy. What is your most likely diagnosis?

    A. Infarct of the paramedian thalamic territory
    B. Infarct of the lateral thalamic territory
    C. Infarct of the anterolateral thalamic territory
    D. Infarct of the posterior choroidal arteries territory
    E. Wallenberg syndrome

107. Based on ethologist Konrad Lorenz's work, if an animal residing in the center of a marked territory were attacked, this animal is most likely to exhibit which of the following behaviors?

    A. Aggression and fight
    B. Displacement activities

C. Fear and flight

D. Imprinting behavior

E. Learned helplessness

108. What is the increased risk of developing Schizophrenia in a first-degree relative of a patient with the disorder, when compared to the general population?

    A. Five times greater
    B. Ten times greater
    C. Twenty times greater
    D. Fifty times greater
    E. None of the above

109. A patient displays amotivation, mutism, and akinesia after suffering from head trauma. Where is the lesion most likely to be seen on an MRI of the brain of this patient?

    A. Orbitofrontal cortex
    B. Mediofrontal cortex
    C. DLPFC
    D. Occipital cortex
    E. None of the above

110. What percent of individuals with Alcohol Dependence have Alcohol-Induced clinical syndromes that resemble an MDD, Panic Disorder, Generalized Anxiety Disorder, or other psychiatric conditions?

    A. 10%
    B. 20%
    C. 33%
    D. 50%
    E. 66%

111. What is the ratio of lethal to effective dose for benzodiazepines?

    A. 25:1
    B. 50:1
    C. 75:1
    D. 100:1
    E. 200:1

112. PMDD is classified under which one of the following categories in the DSM-IV-TR?

    A. Mood Disorder Not Otherwise Specified (NOS)
    B. MDD
    C. Depressive Disorder NOS
    D. Dysthymic Disorder
    E. Adjustment Disorder with Depressed Mood

113. A 15-year-old boy is brought in by his parents because they are concerned about two episodes of unusual behavior that he exhibited during the last 3 months. During each episode, lasting between 1 and 2 weeks, he wanted to sleep whenever possible and did not want to see his friends or spend time with

his family. Moreover, when awake, he would spend most of his time eating whatever he could get his hands on, which is also unlike his normal behavior. In between these periods, he excels at school, spends time with his many friends, and has a normal appetite and sleep schedule. Given his history, his most likely diagnosis is:

A. Normal adolescent development
B. Schizophreniform Disorder
C. Schizophrenia
D. Klein-Levin syndrome
E. Prader-Willi syndrome

114. A 36-year-old woman, on treatment with olanzapine 20 mg/day for Schizophrenia, gains 10 kg in weight in the following 3 months. She is unhappy about her weight gain and now wishes to change her medication. All of the following options to switch have a low risk for weight gain EXCEPT:

A. Haloperidol
B. Aripiprazole
C. Ziprasidone
D. Risperidone
E. Trifluoperazine

115. Which one of the following is NOT TRUE of barbiturates?

A. Barbiturates bind to their receptor sites that are part of the γ-aminobutyric acid (GABA) receptor complex.
B. Barbiturates inhibit the hepatic microsomal enzymes and increase the level of certain drugs.
C. In individuals using barbiturates, cross-tolerance may occur with alcohol.
D. Clonazepam may be used to reduce the severity of withdrawal symptoms from barbiturates.
E. Barbiturates should not be used in pregnancy.

116. Which one of the following is NOT a contraindication for prescribing a psychostimulant for Attention-Deficit/Hyperactive Disorder (ADHD)?

A. Presence of narrow-angle glaucoma
B. A personal history of drug abuse or dependence
C. Pregnancy
D. Co-administration with MAOIs
E. Hyperthyroidism

117. A 45-year-old woman is rushed to the ER in a semi-conscious state. Her 16-year-old daughter found her laying on the bed next to an empty bottle of pills. In her panic, the daughter forgot to bring the bottle, but remembers that it was an older antidepressant and that her mother has been depressed for many years. She knows that her mother has not been following

any special diets. Which one of the statements about the likely overdose is TRUE?

A. An overdose of two times the daily dose can be fatal.
B. Death most commonly occurs as a result of CNS depression.
C. Fatality is higher in patients with premature ventricular beats.
D. Acute hepatic failure is only seen in severe overdoses.
E. A low anticholinergic member of the family has the highest fatality rate.

118. A 50-year-old white man with a 25-year history of Alcohol Dependence is now completing an outpatient alcohol treatment program. He has been a model patient on the program and says that he is motivated to remain sober. He is physically healthy except for mild hepatic dysfunction. Prior to leaving the program, he enquires about the feasibility of taking disulfiram for the treatment of his Alcohol Dependence. Which one of the following statements would you NOT make to him regarding the use of disulfiram in the treatment of Alcohol Dependence?

A. Disulfiram was the first medication approved by the FDA for treatment of Alcohol Dependence.
B. Clinical studies clearly support the efficacy of disulfiram for the treatment of alcoholism in comparison to placebo.
C. Disulfiram alters normal metabolism of ingested alcohol to produce mildly toxic acetaldehyde, resulting in an aversive reaction.
D. Its use is contraindicated in patients with cardiovascular disease.
E. Definitive clinical trials evaluating disulfiram's use in dually diagnosed patients are still needed.

119. Which of the following statements is TRUE of criminal behaviors in the mentally ill?

A. Eight to ten percent of individuals with Schizophrenia manifested violent behavior within the last 12 months compared with 2% in the general population.
B. Drug abusers were at greater risk for presenting such behavior, regardless of whether or not they had a mental disorder.
C. Individuals with severe mental disorders are convicted of violent crimes more frequently than are other individuals.
D. The difference between those with mental disorders and those without in terms of the prevalence of committing a crime has been found to be greater for violent crimes than for nonviolent crimes.
E. All of the above.

120. Which of the following statements about leptin is NOT TRUE?

 A. It is a protein hormone.
 B. It is synthesized by the pituitary gland.
 C. The Ob(Lep) gene is located on chromosome 7 in humans.
 D. Binding of leptin to the ventral medial nucleus of hypothalamus results in satiety.
 E. Obesity is associated with leptin resistance.

121. Which one of the following statements about depression and thyroid dysfunction is TRUE?

 A. Depression and thyroid disease occur more often in men than in women.
 B. Peak incidence occurs in subjects aged 20 to 30 years.
 C. Most subjects with depression have biochemical evidence of thyroid dysfunction.
 D. Most subjects with depression have high thyroid hormone levels.
 E. Thyroid hormone levels are not correlated with severity of depression.

122. Which one of the following is NOT TRUE of dementia in Parkinson's disease?

 A. The prevalence of dementia in patients with Parkinson's disease can be as high as 40%.
 B. The risk of dementia is about four times higher in these patients compared to other people of the same age without Parkinson's disease.
 C. Development of visual hallucinations early in the disease is a risk factor for dementia.
 D. CT scan and MRI of the brain reliably distinguishes Parkinson's patients with from those without dementia.
 E. Dementia associated with Parkinson's disease is the third most common form of dementia.

123. A 72-year-old man is recovering from a recent stroke affecting the corticospinal tract. On physical examination, he is most likely to present with which of the following signs?

 A. Paresis
 B. Hypoactive deep tendon reflexes
 C. Negative Babinski reflex
 D. Muscle atrophy
 E. Muscle flaccidity

124. Which one of the following is the most reliable indicator of the body's thiamine status in a patient with Wernicke's encephalopathy?

 A. Urinary thiamine level
 B. Serum thiamine level
 C. Erythrocyte transketolase activity
 D. Urinary transketolase activity
 E. None of the above

125. All of the following are true of HIV transmission EXCEPT:

 A. Male-to-male transmission is the commonest route of sexual transmission in the western world.
 B. Male-to-female and female-to-male transmissions represent most of the sexual transmissions in the rest of the world.
 C. HIV can be transmitted through immune serum globulin.
 D. The presence of other sexually transmitted diseases increases the risk of transmission.
 E. Regular sexual partners of infected persons become infected themselves in 50% of the cases.

126. All the following are TRUE about herpes simplex encephalitis EXCEPT:

 A. It is the most commonly identified cause of acute sporadic viral encephalitis in the United States.
 B. HSV type 1 accounts for 95% of the cases.
 C. The clinical hallmark is acute onset of fever and focal neurological signs.
 D. It characteristically affects the parietal and occipital lobes.
 E. Mental retardation can arise as a long-term sequelae in children.

127. Variant CJD (vCJD) differs from CJD in all the following respects EXCEPT:

 A. It has a comparatively more protracted course.
 B. Psychiatric symptoms are often the presenting complaints that lead to referral.
 C. The EEG in vCJD is not dissimilar to that seen characteristically in CJD.
 D. Ataxia occurs early and myoclonus later than commonly seen in CJD.
 E. Amyloid plaques are a pathological feature of vCJD.

128. Which one of the following is NOT TRUE of epidural hematoma?

 A. Bleeding into the epidural space is most commonly due to a tear in one of the middle meningeal arteries.
 B. The majority of these bleeds are associated with a skull fracture.
 C. Most epidural hematomas are located in the middle cranial fossa.
 D. Epidural hematoma is primarily seen in the elderly.
 E. The dilation and fixity of the ipsilateral pupil is a sign of progression to brainstem compression.

129. A 60-year-old patient has trouble falling asleep because of unpleasant aching and drawing sensations in the calves and thighs. The patient also notes creeping or crawling feelings in the legs. The urge to move the legs can be suppressed voluntarily for a brief period, but is ultimately irresistible, and is relieved by movement. All of the following statements are true about this disorder EXCEPT:

A. It has a circadian rhythm and also occurs in children.
B. It has been associated with low serum ferritin.
C. Pramipexole is a usual first line of treatment, even in pregnant women.
D. The etiology remains unknown, although it appears to have a genetic component.
E. The prevalence is higher in women, and pregnancy appears to be a risk factor.

130. A 72-year-old man with Parkinson's disease presents with depressive symptoms. In this patient, which of the following medications when used with a SSRI increase the risk of serotonin syndrome?

A. Selegiline
B. Carbidopa/levodopa
C. Trihexyphenidyl
D. Bromocriptine
E. Entacapone

131. Which of the following medical conditions is associated with sexual dysfunction in late life?

A. Arthritis
B. Chronic obstructive pulmonary disease
C. Prostate disease and prostate surgery
D. Dementia
E. All of the above

132. A 82-year-old man died from dementia and coronary artery disease in the hospital and his family asks for an autopsy to be performed. His chart reveals that he had a progressive cognitive decline without any marked memory deficits. The pathologist reports round, eosinophilic, intracytoplasmic neuronal inclusions in the cerebral cortex and brainstem. What was the patient's most likely cognitive disorder?

A. AD
B. Dementia with Lewy bodies
C. Corticobasal ganglionic degeneration
D. AD with Lewy bodies
E. Progressive supranuclear palsy

133. Which of the following is TRUE of women and domestic violence in the United States?

A. Approximately one million women are assaulted by their partners annually.

B. Women are more likely to be assaulted by strangers.
C. Pregnant women are rarely victims of domestic violence.
D. Female victims of domestic violence and children of battered mothers are at risk to develop mainly just physical sequelae.
E. Women are often reluctant to reveal domestic violence.

134. A patient with a known intracranial tumor displays difficulty with planning and sequencing, loss of flexibility in dealing with novel situations, perseveration, and impaired foresight. Given this history, where is the tumor most likely to be seen on an MRI of the brain of this patient?

A. Orbitofrontal cortex
B. Mediofrontal cortex
C. DLPFC
D. Occipital cortex
E. None of the above

135. A mother reports that her 18-year-old son displays repetitive behaviors "that don't make sense." For example, he spent all evening rearranging items on the kitchen countertop and took apart the toaster oven to see what it was like. However, his father is most concerned about his paranoia. All these symptoms started suddenly about 3 months ago. As you gather more information, you should have a high index of suspicion for which of the following disorders?

A. Obsessive-Compulsive Disorder (OCD)
B. Amphetamine Abuse or Dependence
C. Schizophreniform Disorder
D. Schizotypal Personality Disorder
E. Wilson's disease

136. A 35-year-old postal worker who uses small doses of amphetamine for "more energy" finds herself written up for having failed to complete her route several times over the last 2 months because "the place I get is nowhere near my route, unfortunately." In the evening she has taken increasing amounts of oxycodone, prescribed for chronic back pain, "Because it helps with my lows after work." She also lets her husband put the kids to bed and read to them, which she says she used to enjoy, but "I just need time alone with a bath and a glass of wine." Given this history, which is the most appropriate diagnosis for her drug using the DSM-IV-TR criteria?

A. Amphetamine Abuse and Opioid Abuse
B. Amphetamine Abuse and Opioid Dependence
C. Polysubstance Abuse
D. Polysubstance Dependence

E. Amphetamine Abuse, Opioid Dependence, and Alcohol abuse

137. Which one of the following is the most important risk factor for the development of Postpartum Psychosis?

A. Being primigravida
B. Being unmarried
C. A history of postpartum psychosis
D. A history of psychiatric illness
E. A family history of psychiatric illness

138. A 55-year-old patient with a history of narcolepsy comes to his appointment with his wife. His wife tells you that he frequently kicks her at night, and now she has become frightened of him because he seemed to be trying to choke her the night before. He has never been violent towards her or others in any other circumstance and, prior to these episodes, has always been a loving partner. His behavior in general during the day is completely unremarkable. Having known this man for years, you are certain that he does not have a plot to kill his wife, but has one of the following disorders. Which one of the following disorders is he most likely to have?

A. Sleepwalking disorder
B. Rapid Eye Movement (REM) Sleep Behavior Disorder
C. Jactatio capitis nocturna
D. Sleep Terror Disorder
E. Psychotic Disorder (NOS)

139. Antipsychotics have long been associated with weight gain. All of the following are proposed mechanisms for weight inducing effects of these drugs EXCEPT:

A. 5 HT-2C antagonism
B. H1 antagonism
C. Hyperprolactinemia
D. Direct metabolic effect
E. Increased serum leptin

140. Desmethyl-diazepam is an active metabolite of which of the following drugs?

A. Diazepam
B. Chlordiazepoxide
C. Clorazepate
D. Halazepam
E. All of the above

141. Which one of the following is NOT TRUE of atomoxetine?

A. It is a presynaptic dopamine reuptake inhibitor.
B. It has shown efficacy in the treatment of ADHD in both children and adults.

C. Its pharmacokinetic half-life is 5 hours and hence it is generally dosed twice a day.
D. It should not be used concurrently with MAOIs.
E. It can be discontinued without a taper.

142. Which of the following is TRUE of the pharmacological treatments for Alcohol Dependence?

A. Naltrexone (Trexan) and acamprosate (Campral) are FDA-approved options for the treatment of Alcohol Dependence in conjunction with behavior therapy.
B. Disulfiram (Antabuse) does not increase abstinence rates or decrease relapse rates or cravings compared with placebo, and is not recommended for routine use in primary care.
C. Fluoxetine (Prozac) and other SSRIs are recommended for patients with comorbid depressive disorders in alcohol dependant patients.
D. Topiramate (Topamax) and ondansetron (Zofran) are recommended to reduce drinking frequency and increase abstinence in these patients.
E. All of the above.

143. A 40-year-old white man with a 25-year history of Alcohol Dependence is now completing a dual-diagnosis treatment program. He has been a model patient on the program and says that he is motivated to remain sober. He has severe hepatic dysfunction and is followed by a gastrologist for his liver disease. Prior to the completion of the program, he enquires about the use of acamprosate for the treatment of his Alcohol Dependence. Which one of the following statements would you NOT make to him regarding the use of acamprosate in the treatment of alcohol dependence?

A. It has been approved by the FDA for use in the treatment of Alcohol Dependence.
B. Although its exact mechanism remains unknown, it is thought to counteract alcohol use-related symptoms by modulating the glutamatergic and GABA-ergic systems.
C. It is metabolized by the liver.
D. Its use is contraindicated in renal disease.
E. If combined with alcohol, it does not induce unpleasant symptoms such as the aversive reactions secondary to disulfiram.

144. Which cell line is thought to be activated against self-antigens in the etiology of multiple sclerosis?

A. Macrophages
B. T cells
C. B cells
D. Oligodendrocytes
E. Schwann cells

145. Which one of the following is NOT TRUE of lithium-induced hypothyroidism?

   A. Lithium at therapeutic levels inhibits thyroid hormone release.
   B. At high levels it can also inhibit iodine uptake and organification.
   C. Symptoms of hypothyroidism develop in approximately 7% of patients taking lithium.
   D. The highest risk of developing this condition is in men.
   E. Rapid-cycling bipolar disorder is also a risk factor for developing this condition.

146. A 31-year-old man has had daily intense, nonthrobbing headaches for the last week. The headaches occur four to six times each night and last for about 25 minutes. They are localized to the left periorbital area and are accompanied by lacrimation and rhinorrhea. He notices that they are precipitated by drinking beer. He had a similar problem 3 years ago that lasted for 6 weeks. Given this information, what is his most likely diagnosis?

   A. Common migraine headache
   B. Tension headache
   C. Cluster headache
   D. Chronic paroxysmal hemicrania
   E. Tolosa-Hunt syndrome

147. An 18-year-old high school senior describes episodes of dizziness, "spacing out," and paresthesia around her mouth and fingertips. On occasions, her wrists bend and her fingers are pulled together. These episodes last for less than 5 minutes. You review an EEG performed during one of these episodes 2 years ago. It shows slowing of background activities and occasional bursts of high voltage. Which of the following is the most likely immediate cause of her symptoms?

   A. TIAs
   B. Petit mal seizures
   C. Panic attacks
   D. Post traumatic brain injury seizures
   E. None of the above

148. Which one of the following is part of the mechanism of action of triptans in the treatment of migraines?

   A. Enhancing the transmission in the trigeminal nucleus caudalis
   B. Inhibiting the release of vasoactive peptides
   C. Enhance afferent input to second order neurons
   D. Deactivating serotonin 1B/1D receptors in pain modulating pathways
   E. Promotion of vasodilation

149. Which one of the following statements about personality and aging is TRUE?

   A. Personality is strongly influenced by the sheer occurrence of positive or negative life events.
   B. Personality disorders "age out" and have little effect on older persons.
   C. Several longitudinal studies have shown that personality is stable across long periods of the lifespan.
   D. Personality has no influence on one's response to a stressful event.
   E. Personality is unaffected by increasing medical and neuropsychiatric comorbidity in late life.

150. Which one of the following statements is NOT TRUE of β-amyloid in AD?

   A. Its gene is located on chromosome 21.
   B. It is the principal constituent of neuritic plaques.
   C. It is formed due to an abnormal cleavage process.
   D. It accumulates extracellularly.
   E. Its gene is located on chromosome 19.

151. A 10-year-old girl presents to your office for an evaluation of mononeuritis myopathy, attentional deficits, and mood changes. She developed these symptoms after spending her vacation at her grandparents' home in Connecticut. You suspect that she has Lyme's disease. Which one of the following tests will confirm your suspicion of Lyme's disease?

   A. Positive fluorescent treponemal antibodies (FTAs)
   B. CSF 14-3-3 protein
   C. CSF borrelial DNA
   D. Positive anti-Hu antibody
   E. Abnormal niacin level

152. A 32-year-old patient with Chronic Schizophrenia reports daily consumption of eight cups of coffee. Use of which of the following agents would be of most concern given this information?

   A. Risperidone
   B. Olanzapine
   C. Quetiapine
   D. Clozapine
   E. Aripiprazole

153. A 26-year-old man is brought to an emergency department by the police. The police were called in by his wife after he punched her at home. He presents with irritability along with grandiose and paranoid delusions. His wife reports that he was diagnosed with Bipolar Disorder during a prior ER visit, but that he did not follow-up with his treatment. His wife also mentions that his symptoms seem confined mostly to the fall "when he tires himself out practicing for his rugby league." Given this history, you should consider obtaining a level for which of the following chemicals?

A. Testosterone
B. Luteinizing hormone (LH)
C. Prolactin
D. Ceruloplasmin
E. Adrenocorticotropin hormone

154. Which one of the following statements regarding Postpartum Psychosis is TRUE?

A. In the DSM-IV-TR, this disorder can be classified under a Brief Psychotic Disorder.
B. It has an incidence rate of about 1 to 2 per 10, 000 births.
C. Infanticide is common in this disorder.
D. Risk of puerperal relapse is close to 30%.
E. Natural labor is a risk factor for the development of this disorder.

155. Which one of the following is NOT considered a sleep hygiene technique?

A. An exercise program early in the day
B. Hot baths before bedtime
C. Getting up at that same time every day
D. Sleeping on a firm mattress
E. Progressive muscle relaxation

156. Many psychotropic drugs are associated with electrocardiogram (EKG) changes. Some are linked to prolongation of the cardiac QT interval, a risk factor for the development of ventricular arrhythmia 'Torsade de Pointes', which is occasionally fatal. All of the following antipsychotic drugs have either no effect or a low effect on the cardiac QT interval EXCEPT:

A. Fluphenazine
B. Risperidone
C. Aripiprazole
D. Ziprasidone
E. Clozapine

157. A 32-year-old single white woman presents with a depressed mood for 6 months and conflicts with her boyfriend. After discussing various options, you prepare to begin Interpersonal Therapy (IPT). Which one of the following statements about this therapy is TRUE?

A. It is not useful for patients with substance abuse disorders.
B. It is efficacious in major depression with psychotic features.
C. It is generally practiced as a time-unlimited psychotherapy.
D. Multiple interpersonal areas are covered during the course of treatment.
E. It is not useful in maintenance treatment of depression.

158. Although weight gain is a significant side effect of many atypical antipsychotic medications, this effect is even more severe among children and adolescents. Adjunctive metformin for children taking antipsychotic medications has been shown to keep weight stable or even decrease weight compared to those receiving antipsychotic medication alone. In addition to monitoring weight in children receiving antipsychotic medications, which one of the following is also important to monitor in patients receiving metformin?

A. Vitamin B_{12}
B. TSH
C. Prolactin
D. Vitamin B_6
E. Complete blood cell (CBC) count

159. Which of the following is an absolute contraindication for ECT?

A. Pregnancy
B. Seizure disorder
C. Myocardial infarction (MI) within past year
D. Hypertension
E. No absolute contraindications

160. A 50-year-old man with a 25-year history of Alcohol Dependence is finishing his detoxification at an inpatient psychiatric unit. His wife meets with you prior to his discharge to discuss his prognosis. When you discuss his prognosis with her, which one of the following would you NOT say to her about his condition?

A. Lower education and income is associated with less short- and long-term improvement.
B. As a man, his prognosis is better than a woman his age and ethnicity.
C. The relationship between age and long-term outcomes has not been established.
D. Long-term change typically does not occur with a single treatment episode and readmissions are important in promoting long-term recovery.
E. Improvements made in the short-term are often predictive of long-term outcomes.

161. Which one of the following statements about the neurotransmitter storage and release is NOT TRUE?

A. The presynaptic terminal releases the neurotransmitters into the synaptic cleft.
B. Most neurotransmitters are produced locally within the presynaptic terminal.
C. These neurotransmitters are stored in small presynaptic vesicles.
D. Neurotransmitters in the vesicles are released into the synaptic cleft via a process of exocytosis.
E. The release of neurotransmitters from vesicles is triggered by the entry of sodium ion into the presynaptic terminal.

162. Which one of the following is NOT a risk factor for lithium-induced hypothyroidsm?
    A. Female sex
    B. Patients with positive antithyroid antibodies
    C. Starting lithium at the ages of 20 to 30 years
    D. First 2 years of treatment in women
    E. Rapid cycling bipolar disorder

163. A 51-year-old woman with cervical dystonia is treated with botulinum toxin. Which one of the following is NOT a potential mechanism of this drug for pain relief?
    A. Enhancing alpha- and gamma-motor neurons
    B. Suppressing of neurogenic inflammation
    C. Releasing acetylcholine
    D. Changing regional blood flow
    E. Hindering muscle nociceptors

164. Which one of the following sleep changes is considered normal in the elderly?
    A. Decreased REM latency
    B. Decreased sleep latency
    C. Increased sleep efficiency
    D. Increased total REM time
    E. Increased NREM (slow-wave sleep) stages 3 and 4

165. Which is the most common human prion disease?
    A. Kuru
    B. Sporadic CJD
    C. Gerstmann-Straussler syndrome
    D. Fatal familial insomnia
    E. Familial CJD

166. A 43-year-old man presents for evaluation of recent onset seizures, cerebellar ataxia, extrapyramidal symptoms, and mild psychiatric disturbance. He owns a thriving company, and frequently travels back and forth to South America on business trips. You suspect neurocysticercosis. What test result would best support your diagnostic hypothesis accounting for his symptoms?
    A. Low serum B12 level
    B. Low serum TSH level
    C. MRI of the brain revealing mesial temporal sclerosis
    D. CT scan of the brain revealing "kissing" calcified cysts
    E. MRI of the brain with dilation of the third ventricle, lateral ventricles, and temporal horns, without cerebral atrophy

167. Which one of the following statements is NOT TRUE?
    A. Recreational doses of cannabis impair driving performance similar to blood alcohol concentrations of 0.08%.
    B. Cannabis can be detected in the urine for up to 11 weeks.
    C. An amotivational syndrome has not been demonstrated with its use in controlled studies.
    D. Blood levels of tetrahydrocannabinol (THC) peaks in 1 hour.
    E. Lifetime use of 12th-grade high school students is approximately 50%.

168. When considering the neurobiology of mood disorders, chronic stress has been shown to affect the gene coding for neurokinin brain-derived neurotrophic factor (BDNF) and neurogenesis in what ways?
    A. Increased BDNF and increased neurogenesis
    B. Decreased BDNF and decreased neurogenesis
    C. Increased BDNF and decreased neurogenesis
    D. Decreased BDNF and increased neurogenesis
    E. Decreased BDNF and no changes in neurogenesis

169. Which one of the following symptoms is NOT HELPFUL in differentiating an MDE from a "normal" grief according to the DSM-IV-TR?
    A. Guilt about things other than actions taken or not taken by the survivor at the time of death
    B. Thoughts of death other than the survivor feeling that he or she would be better off dead or should have died with the deceased person
    C. Insomnia
    D. Morbid preoccupations with worthlessness
    E. Marked psychomotor retardation

170. A 70-year-old man reports continued discomfort in his legs that is so persistent it keeps him awake at night. He describes the quality of the discomfort as a feeling of something is creeping in his calves, especially when he is sitting or lying down. Given his history all of the following are reasonable approaches to treatment for his condition EXCEPT:
    A. Clonazepam
    B. Pramipexole
    C. Fluoxetine
    D. Gabapentin
    E. Ropinirole

171. Physiological risk factors for QTc prolongation and arrhythmias include all of the following EXCEPT:
    A. Ischemic heart disease
    B. Hypokalemia
    C. Female gender
    D. Hypercalcemia
    E. Extreme physical exertion

172. Which of the following is an absolute contraindication for ECT?
    A. There are no absolute contraindications
    B. Brain tumor

C. Recent neurosurgical procedure
D. Recent MI
E. Recent stroke

173. Which one of the following medications has been shown to be most effective for the treatment of premature ejaculation?

A. Venlafaxine
B. Mirtazapine
C. Paroxetine
D. Imipramine
E. Buproprion

174. Which one of the following is NOT considered an important task to accomplish within the first few sessions of Interpersonal Psychotherapy (IPT), as developed by Gerald Klerman and Myrna Weissman?

A. Review of depressive symptoms and diagnosis
B. Evaluation of the need for medication
C. Gathering of an interpersonal inventory
D. Extensive exploration of the patient's childhood
E. Assignment of the "sick role" to the patient

175. All of the following are clearly associated with increased risk of violent behaviors EXCEPT:

A. Previous history of violence
B. Substance abuse
C. Psychiatric diagnosis
D. Neurologic impairment
E. None of the above

176. Which one of the following is NOT TRUE of postsynaptic receptors in the cell?

A. Postsynaptic receptors are either linked to ion channels or are linked to guanosine triphosphate binding proteins (G proteins).
B. The ion channels open to initiate the cell's response whereas the guanosine triphosphate binding proteins activate second messenger systems within the postsynaptic cell.
C. There are numerous types of receptors located at a single synapse.
D. The ion channel receptors are made of single protein subunits.
E. G-protein-linked receptors do not form channels, but function by altering the interaction of the intracellular portion of the receptors with G proteins.

177. Which one of the following is NOT TRUE of cholinergic projection within the CNS?

A. There are six major types of acetylcholine neurons within the CNS.
B. Motor neurons of the ventral horn of the spinal cord and the motor nuclei of the brainstem are the most numerous of these neurons.

C. The two major cholinergic projections in the brain are the one arising in the pedunculopontine nuclei and projections provided by the medial septal nucleus, the diagonal band of Broca, and the basal nucleus of Meynert.
D. The projections provided by the medial septal nucleus, the diagonal band of Broca, and the basal nucleus of Meynert connections are vital for regulating the sleep/wake cycles.
E. Neurons within the neocortex that function as local circuit neurons are important in the biology of movement disorders.

178. What class of medications is used as a levodopa extender in the treatment of Parkinson's disease?

A. Decarboxylase inhibitor
B. Anticholinergics
C. Dopamine agonists
D. COMT inhibitors
E. Monoamine oxidase (MAO)-B inhibitors

179. The potential medical complications of cocaine use include all of the following EXCEPT:

A. Seizures
B. Hyperpyrexia
C. Delayed rupture of the membranes during delivery
D. MI
E. Rhabdomyolysis

180. From a psychodynamic perspective, which one of the following descriptions best captures the presentation of depression?

A. Depression reflects poor self-esteem regulation and aggression turned inward, which exacerbates shame and guilt.
B. Depression is the projection of libidinal urges that cannot be met leading to aggression turned inward.
C. Depression reflects object loss, which creates shame and doubt and leads to aggression turned inward.
D. Depression reflects object loss which leads to projected hostility which then exacerbates feelings of inadequacy.
E. Depression reflects object loss, in reality or fantasy, leading to narcissistic injury and withdrawal.

181. According to the DSM-IV-TR, what is the usual time limit given for "normal" grief before a diagnosis of a MDE can be made in an individual who has suffered a loss?

A. 2 weeks
B. 4 weeks
C. 6 weeks

D. 2 months

E. 3 months

182. Which one of the following is the commonest substance of abuse among Schizophrenic patients?

A. Alcohol

B. Cannabis

C. Nicotine

D. Cocaine

E. Amphetamines

183. A 37-year-old man with Chronic Schizophrenia, who is currently asymptomatic on chlorpromazine, develops a moderate degree of hepatic impairment. A physician review advises discontinuation of chlorpromazine. You are anxious that he may suffer a relapse and would like to consider alternatives. All of the following antipsychotics are associated with a lower risk of hepatic impairment EXCEPT:

A. Olanzapine

B. Aripiprazole

C. Ziprasidone

D. Flupentixol

E. Phenothiazines

184. A 37-year-old woman presents with depressed mood. On interview, the patient reports a seasonal pattern of worsening symptoms in the winter. After discussing the various treatment options, the patient requests phototherapy. Which one of the following statements about this treatment is correct?

A. There are no reported cases of switches to mania.

B. It has no efficacy in bipolar depression.

C. Common side effect includes gastrointestinal distress.

D. The intensity of the light is unimportant.

E. Best response is generally with predawn exposure.

185. A 34-year-old woman with a history of Bipolar Disorder and Benzodiazepine Dependence is admitted to the psychiatric hospital in a manic state. In addition to her current mood stabilizer she is started on another medication, as well as her usual outpatient dose of clonazepam. Two days later she complains of increased anxiety and shaking. On physical examination, you note a tremor, tachycardia, and elevated blood pressure. Which one of the following medications was likely started on admission to the hospital and is likely precipitating benzodiazepine withdrawal?

A. Carbamazepine

B. Fluoxetine

C. Citalopram

D. Lithium

E. Lamotrigine

186. All of the following statements about the structural model of psychic structure are accurate EXCEPT:

A. It is divided into two components: The unconscious and conscious.

B. It is divided into three components: The ego, superego, and id.

C. It was introduced by Sigmund Freud.

D. This model was developed before the topographical model.

E. There can be conflict between different components of the psyche.

187. While observing a group session, it appears that the members of the group seem incapable of helping each other, but are idealizing the therapist. Given this scenario, which one of the following Bion's subgroups would best account for this behavior?

A. *Work* group

B. *Dependency* basic assumption group

C. *Fight or flight* basic assumption group

D. *Pairing* basic assumption group

E. None of the above

188. Which one of the following statements about the dexamethasone suppression test (DST) is TRUE?

A. DST is a routine diagnostic test in clinical psychiatry.

B. An abnormal DST is found in approximately 80% of patients with depression.

C. An abnormal DST is seen more frequently in patients with psychotic affective disorders and melancholia.

D. Abnormal DST is not seen in other psychiatric disorders.

E. The specificity of the test does not depend upon the population tested.

189. Which one of the following is NOT TRUE of the acetylcholine neurotransmitter system?

A. Acetylcholine is a major neurotransmitter of the peripheral motor system.

B. Acetylcholine interacts with postsynaptic receptors in a manner very similar to that of amino acids.

C. There is a high-affinity transport system for acetylcholine in the presynaptic neuron.

D. Drugs used to treat myasthenia gravis act by blocking the activity of acetylcholinesterase at the neuromuscular junction.

E. Centrally active inhibitors of acetylcholinesterase are now used in the treatment of AD.

190. A 42-year-old woman with a history of relapsing-remitting multiple sclerosis presents to the emergency department with a sudden impairment of vision. Her evaluation suggests this is an acute multiple sclerosis attack. Given this history, what is the most appropriate treatment for this patient's condition?

A. Glatiramer acetate

B. Corticosteroids
C. IFNB-1a
D. Natalizumab
E. IFNB-1b

191. Hallucinogens are thought to primarily involve which one of the following neurotransmitter systems in the CNS?
    A. Serotonin
    B. Dopamine
    C. Norepinephrine
    D. Epinephrine
    E. Acetylcholine

192. The following are part of the DSM-IV-TR criteria for the Atypical Features specifier of MDD EXCEPT:
    A. Leaden paralysis
    B. Hypersomnia
    C. Significant weight gain or increased appetite
    D. Mood unreactivity
    E. Interpersonal rejection sensitivity

193. Which one of the following conditions is most co-morbid with alcohol abuse?
    A. Antisocial Personality Disorder
    B. Bipolar I Disorder
    C. Schizophrenia
    D. Panic Disorder
    E. MDD

194. According to DSM-IV-TR, when should malingering be strongly suspected?
    A. When the person is referred by an attorney to the clinician for examination in a medicolegal context
    B. When there is marked discrepancy between the person's claimed stress or disability and objective findings
    C. When the subject fails to cooperate during the diagnostic evaluation and in complying with the prescribed treatment regimen
    D. When there is presence of antisocial personality disorder
    E. Any combination of the above

195. Which one of the following antiepileptic medications inhibits the metabolism of lamotrigine?
    A. Gabapentin
    B. Phenytoin
    C. Valproate
    D. Tiagabine
    E. Zonisamide

196. Which of the following drug classes is useful in re-ducing the prevalence of headaches?
    A. Thiazides
    B. Beta-blockers
    C. Angiotensin-converting enzyme (ACE) inhibitors

D. Angiotensin II receptor antagonists
E. All of the above

197. A 26-year-old woman with a 6-year history of mi-graines wants to start beta-blocker therapy for mi-graines. She is very healthy with no medical prob-lems. When you talk to her about the beta-blocker therapy, which one of the following drugs would you say is FDA approved for the prophylactic treatment of migraines?
    A. Timolol
    B. Metoprolol
    C. Nadolol
    D. Atenolol
    E. All of the above

198. A 30-year-old man with a 10-year history of mi-graines wants to start prophylactic therapy for migraines. He has a history of Bipolar Affective Dis-order and wants to know if any of the mood stabi-lizers are FDA approved for the prophylactic treat-ment of migraines. In answering his question, which one of the following mood-stabilizers would you say is FDA approved for the prophylactic treatment of migraines?
    A. Lithium
    B. Carbamazepine
    C. Lamotrigine
    D. Topiramate
    E. Oxcarbamazepine

199. EEG studies are useful as an adjunct in diagnosing certain neurological conditions. There are a few con-ditions however, that an EEG can be useful in mak-ing a specific diagnosis. In which condition would an EEG be most helpful in making a specific diagnosis?
    A. Subacute sclerosing panencephalitis (SSPE)
    B. Cerebral tumor
    C. Psychosis
    D. Multiple sclerosis
    E. Huntington's disease

200. Which one of the following statements about neuro-transmitter release is NOT TRUE?
    A. There are three kinds of synaptic vesicles that store the neurotransmitters in the presynaptic neurons.
    B. The clear synaptic vesicles contain acetylcholine, glycine, GABA, and /or glutamate.
    C. The small vesicles with a dense core contain cat-echolamines.
    D. Sodium triggers the exocytosis of neurotransmit-ters into the synaptic cleft.
    E. Usually, the synaptic vesicle discharges its con-tents through a small hole in the cell membrane, then the opening reseals rapidly and the main vesicle stays inside the cell.

Answers

1. Answer: A. Children with a history of in utero alcohol exposure are given a diagnosis of FAS if they have the characteristic physical appearance or neurological dysfunction, which may include all of the following:

1. Intrauterine growth retardation.
2. Persistent postnatal poor growth in weight or height.
3. Characteristic facial appearance including microcephaly, microphthalmia, short palpebral fissures, a thin upper lip, midface hypoplasia, and a smooth or long philtrum.
4. Delayed development, hyperactivity, attention deficits, intellectual delays, learning disabilities, and occasionally seizures.

In the general population, FAS occurs in about 1 per 3,000 live births. In alcoholic mothers the prevalence is much higher at about 2.5% to 10%. Even in the children who do not meet the full criteria for FAS, infants born to alcoholic mothers show an increased incidence of intellectual impairment, congenital anomalies, and decreased birth weight.

1. Lewis M. *Child and Adolescent Psychiatry: A Comprehensive Textbook*. 3rd ed. Philadelphia: Lippincott Williams & Wilkins; 2003:449.
2. Sadock BJ, Sadock VA. *Kaplan and Sadock's Comprehensive Textbook of Psychiatry*. 8th ed. Philadelphia: Lippincott Williams & Wilkins; 2005:3090–3094.

2. Answer: D. The long thoracic nerve is a motor nerve that arises from the C5–7 roots. It can be damaged due to pressure on the shoulder (sudden trauma or carrying heavy objects on the shoulder such as a backpack). Patients present with a winged scapula that is only apparent when the patient is asked to push the arm forward against resistance or hold the arms up in front of the body. Patients complain of shoulder weakness and get easily tired when they raise their arm above their head. When the suprascapular nerve is damaged or entrapped, patients may present with shoulder pain. Supraspinatus weakness causes weakness of arm abduction, whereas infraspinatus weakness causes impaired external rotation of the shoulder. Patients with dorsal scapular nerve injury are unable to press the elbow back against resistance. The thoracodorsal nerve

arises from C6–8 and it produces latissimus dorsi paresis.

Brazis PW, Masdeu JC, Billr J. *Localization in Clinical Neurology*. 5th ed. Philadelphia: Lippincott Williams & Wilkins; 2007:25–31.

3. Answer: A. Jean Piaget, a Swiss psychologist, emphasized the ways that children think and acquire knowledge, and described four major stages leading to the capacity for adult thought: (i) sensorimotor stage (up to 2 years of age), during which individuals acquire control of their motor functions and notion of object permanence, (ii) stage of preoperational thought (2 to 7 years), where symbols and language are used, notions of imminent justice and magical thinking exist, and children are egocentric, (iii) stage of concrete operations (7 to 11 years), where egocentric thought is replaced by operational thought, syllogistic reasoning occurs, conservation and reversibility are understood, and (iv) stage of formal operations (11 years through end of adolescence), which involves acquiring deductive reasoning skills and abstract thinking with use of complex language. Psychologists like Harry Stack Sullivan and Heinz Kohut emphasized the importance of interpersonal relationships. Freud's theories related to an individual's psychosexual development. Erik Erickson is best known for his theories of psychosocial development. Carl Jung defined archetypes as symbolic images that recur in dreams and are part of the collective unconscious.

Kaplan HI, Sadock BJ. *Kaplan & Sadock's Synopsis of Psychiatry*. 8th ed. Philadelphia: Lippincott Williams & Wilkins: 1998:140–143, 213, 227, 228, 232, 234.

4. Answer: D. The doctrine of *parens patriae* (father of his country) originally referred to a monarch's (King Edward I's) duty to protect the people. In United States common law, the doctrine has been transformed into a paternalism in which the state acts for people who are mentally ill and for minors and allows the state to intervene. *Actus rea* and *mens rea* are components in criminal law to determine if a crime has been committed: (i) *actus reus*, which means voluntary conduct, and (ii) *mens rea*, which refers to evil intent. There cannot be *mens rea* when an offender's mental status is so deficient, depriving him or her of the capacity of rational intent, which is the basis for the insanity defense. A writ of habeas corpus occurs when involuntary hospitalized patients who believe they have been illegally deprived of liberty ask for a legal proceeding in which a court decides if he or she has been hospitalized without due process of law. *Respondeat superior* is a Latin phrase that means *let the master answer for the deeds of the servant*, which refers to a person occupying a higher position in a hierarchy of responsibility being liable for the actions of people under his or her supervision (e.g., an attending psychiatrist being responsible for the clinical work of the resident that he or she is supervising).

Kaplan HI, Sadock BJ. *Kaplan & Sadock's Synopsis of Psychiatry.* 8th ed. Philadelphia: Lippincott Williams & Wilkins; 1998:1309, 1314, 1318.

5. **Answer: B.** Therapeutic blood levels for lithium in the treatment of acute mania is about 0.8 to 1.5 mEq/L. Patients who have serum lithium levels in the upper range should be alert for possible early signs of lithium toxicity. Stable, steady-state lithium levels are generally obtained about 4 to 5 days after either initiating lithium or adjusting the dose. Blood samples for lithium levels are generally drawn about 12 hours after the last dose of lithium. After resolution of an acute manic episode, maintenance therapy with lithium is at levels of 0.6 to 0.9 mEq/L. During maintenance therapy, lithium levels should be drawn every 1 to 3 months but more often if clinically indicated. The lithium level can alter dramatically in patients who are pregnant or immediately postpartum in patients who are taking thiazide diuretics or are dehydrated, and in patients with deteriorating renal function. In these situations, lithium levels should be drawn more frequently.

Hales RE, Yudofsky SC. *American Psychiatric Publishing Textbook of Clinical Psychiatry.* 4th ed. http://www.psychiatryonline.com/content.aspx?aID=69719. Accessed February 14, 2007.

6. **Answer: B.** The typical delirious patient will have an EEG pattern of diffuse theta or delta waves (i.e., diffuse slowing), poor organization of the background rhythm, and loss of reactivity to eye opening and closing. One exception to this pattern is the patient with delirium tremens, who will generally have a pattern of low-voltage fast activity. The pattern of 3-per-second spike and wave is typical of absence seizures, not delirium. Though the EEG is the only technological method to assist in the diagnosis of delirium, it is not necessary to make a clinical diagnosis in most cases. EEG is most useful when seizures are suspected or when the differential diagnosis is difficult. The EEG pattern in children with delirium is

similar to that of adults. The degree of EEG slowing correlates with the severity of delirium.

1. Jacobson SA, Jerrier S. EEG in delirium. *Semin Clin Neuropsychiatry.* 2000;5:86–93.
2. Levenson JL. *Textbook of Psychosomatic Medicine.* Washington: American Psychiatric Publishing; 2005:110–112.

7. **Answer: A.** The past month prevalence for inhalant use in the United States peaks at about 1.2% in 14- and 15-year-olds and declines thereafter, although prevalence of lifetime use increases with age.

Sadock BJ, Sadock VA. *Kaplan and Sadock's Comprehensive Textbook of Psychiatry.* 8th ed. Philadelphia: Lippincott Williams & Wilkins; 2005:1249.

8. **Answer: E.** Undetected thyroid dysfunction is found in 5% to 10% of depressed patients manifested by elevated basal TSH levels or increased TSH release in response to TRH. A larger number of patients, 20% to 30%, have a blunted TSH response when challenged by TRH. This type of response would suggest hyperthyroidism, but this is rare in depressed patients. Blunted TSH in a euthyroid person may result from downregulation at the pituitary level.

Sadock BJ, Sadock VA. *Kaplan and Sadock's Comprehensive Textbook of Psychiatry.* 8th ed. Philadelphia: Lippincott Williams & Wilkins; 2005:1600.

9. **Answer: D.** Many patients with multiple sclerosis suffer cognitive impairments, and difficulty with memory is the most common such impairment. Of the patients with multiple sclerosis, 40% to 60% complain of memory problems, which are thought to be associated with plaque formation in the temporal lobe and diencephalic areas. Moreover, approximately 25% of patients develop a type of euphoria that is not quite hypomanic and is often distinct from their mood before the onset of the disease; 25% to 50% develop depression associated with a higher rate of suicide; and 20% to 40% develop personality changes, which frequently include irritability and apathy. Psychosis can occur, but is considered rare.

Kaplan HI, Sadock BJ. *Kaplan & Sadock's Synopsis of Psychiatry.* 8th ed. Philadelphia: Lippincott Williams & Wilkins; 1998:347, 360.

10. **Answer: B.** Symptoms of overdose with dopamine receptor antagonists include extrapyramidal symptoms, mydriasis, tachycardia, hypotension, and diminished deep tendon reflexes. In severe cases, delirium, respiratory depression, seizures, and coma may occur. Overdose with dopamine receptor antagonists, especially haloperidol, generally has a favorable prognosis, unless complicated by ingestion of CNS depressants such as alcohol or benzodiazepines. Thioridazine and mesoridazine have the

worst prognosis owing to their cardiotoxicity in overdose.

Kaplan HI, Sadock BJ. *Kaplan and Sadock's Synopsis of Psychiatry*. 9th ed. Philadelphia: Lippincott Williams & Wilkins; 2003:1057.

11. Answer: D. Hyperprolactinemia associated with prolactinomata can result in loss of sexual desire, erectile failure, and reduced spermatogenesis in men. In women it can lead to altered ovarian cyclic function, amenorrhea, reduced sexual desire, and hirsutism. Conventional antipsychotic drugs can increase prolactin levels to a range associated with sexual dysfunction in nonpsychiatric patients, so hyperprolactinemia is a probable explanation of some of the sexual dysfunction seen during treatment with antipsychotics. Drug induced priapism results from alpha-adrenergic blockade and anticholinergic activity.

Haddad PM, Wieck A. Antipsychotic-induced hyperprolactinemia: mechanisms, clinical features and management. *Drugs*. 2004;64:2291–2314.

12. Answer: E. Tricyclics are effective antidepressants, but have a number of side effects that have caused them to fall out of favor as first-line agents. Anticholinergic side effects are common, including dry mouth, constipation, visual changes, urinary hesitancy, delirium, and an ocular crisis in patients with narrow-angle glaucoma. Tricyclic agents do not affect patients with chronic open-angle glaucoma. The central anticholinergic effects of the tricyclics can produce dose dependent delirium and seizures. A fine rapid tremor is fairly common and is also dose dependent. Tachycardia occurs with all the tricyclics, not just the more anticholinergic agents. Orthostatic hypotension is the most common reason for discontinuation, and often occurs at blood levels that are relatively low. Sexual dysfunction is a potential problem, and appears to be more frequent with clomipramine. It is often most bothersome to the patient in the second or third month of treatment, after the depression has improved.

Sadock BJ, Sadock VA. *Kaplan and Sadock's Comprehensive Textbook of Psychiatry*. 7th ed. Philadelphia: Lippincott Williams & Wilkins; 2000:2498–2499.

13. Answer: A. SSRIs are the treatment of choice for PMDD. The diagnosis of this disorder is done by prospectively charting mood and physical symptoms over the course of the menstrual cycle. According to the DSM-IV-TR, symptoms need to be present 5 days or less prior to menstruation and resolve by day 4 of menstruation. During this time patients need to endorse five out of eleven symptoms, one of which

needs to be related to mood (i.e., depressed mood, increased irritability, mood lability, anxiety, etc.). Somatic complaints only count as one of the five criteria for diagnosis, even if the person had multiple physical complaints. Other symptoms include changes in neurovegetative symptoms (i.e., changes in sleep, appetite, energy, and concentration). These symptoms should not be better accounted for by another axis I disorder.

1. American Psychiatric Association. *DSM-IV-TR, Diagnostic and Statistical Manual of Mental Disorders*. 4th ed. Text Revision. http://www.psychiatryonline.com/content.aspx?aID=5272#5272. Accessed March 4, 2007.
2. Kim DR, Gyulai L, Freeman EW, et al. Premenstrual dysphoric disorder and psychiatric comorbidity. *Arch Womens Ment Health*. 2004;7:37–47.

14. Answer: E. The patient is unable to tolerate an unpleasant internal object (i.e., viewing herself as incompetent) and projects this object onto the psychiatrist. This projection becomes projective identification because the psychiatrist begins to feel or react in a manner consistent with the patient's projection (i.e., the psychiatrist has identified with the internal object of the patient). There is no clear evidence that the patient is in denial of not getting the promotion or of being angry with herself. The patient may also have acting out behavior and a transference toward the psychiatrist, but these are not the most specific or key aspects of this example.

Gabbard GO. *Psychodynamic Psychiatry in Clinical Practice*. 3rd ed. Washington: American Psychiatric Press; 2000:40–43.

15. Answer: E. None of the statements are true. About 10% of pregnant women experience depressive episodes (major or minor). This rate is similar to that of nonpregnant women. Depressive episodes during pregnancy are usually associated with poor prenatal care, inadequate nutrition, a risk of postpartum depression, suicide, greater incidence of preterm deliveries, and small-for-gestational-age babies. Mild to moderate depressive episode can be treated by nonpharmacological treatment modalities such as psychotherapy and stress-reduction counseling. If patient's with severe symptoms fail to respond to nonpharmacological treatments, it mandates a trial of pharmacotherapy. Ideally, antidepressant medications should be withheld when possible during the first trimester, when major organogenesis occurs. Whenever possible, the dosage of drugs should be kept at the minimum necessary for symptom control. The most extensive data on the prenatal use of antidepressants is for fluoxetine. Prospective studies have not found an association between the use of fluoxetine during pregnancy and major congenital anomalies in the neonate. Studies have also evaluated the use of citalopram, sertraline, paroxetine, fluvoxamine, and venlafaxine during pregnancy and have found no link with congenital malformations. TCAs are not associated with congenital anomalies, although transient perinatal toxicity or withdrawal symptoms may be seen when they are used near the time of birth. If the decision is made to treat with a TCA, tertiary amines like nortriptyline or desipramine are preferable, given that they are less likely to cause anticholinergic and hypotensive side effects. Antidepressant dosages will need to be adjusted over the course of pregnancy as blood levels may fall, particularly after the patient begins the third trimester. There are no trial data for the use of bupropion, trazodone, venlafaxine, mirtazapine, or nefazodone in pregnancy. The MAOIs are contraindicated in pregnant women because of the risk of hypertensive crisis and interaction with tocolytic agents like terbutaline. There is no data as yet that children prenatally exposed to fluoxetine or TCAs have any difference in IQ, temperament, mood, behavior, or attention in children up to age 7 years compared to nonexposed children.

Hales RE, Yudofsky SC. *American Psychiatric Publishing Textbook of Clinical Psychiatry*. 4th ed. http://www.psychiatryonline.com/content.aspx?aID=98201. Accessed February 10, 2007.

16. Answer: E. Atropine is a sympathomimetic causing pupils to dilate. Heroin causes the pupils to constrict. Phencyclidine, alcohol, and ecstasy do not alter the size of the pupils.

Kaufman DM. *Clinical Neurology for Psychiatrists*. 5th ed. Philadelphia: WB Saunders; 2001:35–36.

17. Answer: E. The basic unit of integrated reflex activity is the reflex arc. It consists of a sense organ, an afferent neuron, one or more synapses that are generally in a central integrating station, an efferent neuron, and an effector. In humans, the connection between afferent and efferent somatic neurons occurs in the brain or the spinal cord. The afferent neurons enter via the dorsal roots or cranial nerves and have their cell bodies in the dorsal root ganglia or in the homologous ganglia on the cranial nerves. The efferent fibers leave via the ventral roots or corresponding motor cranial nerves. This principle in which the dorsal rods of the spinal cord are sensory and the ventral roots are motor is known as the Bell–Magendie law. When a stimulus arises in the sensory receptor, it generates an all-or-none action potential in the afferent nerve with the number of action potentials being proportional to the size of the generator potential.

All-or-none responses are also generated in the efferent nerve. When these reach the effector, they set up a graded response. The connection between the afferent and efferent neurons is usually in the CNS. The activity in the reflex arc is modified by the multiple inputs converging on the efferent neurons.

Ganong WF. *Review of Medical Physiology*. 22nd ed. http://www.accessmedicine.com/content.aspx?aID=707656. Accessed February 17, 2007.

18. Answer: B. RLS is a common and often disabling sensorimotor disorder with a prevalence rate of about 7% to 10% of the general population in the United States and Northern Europe. The prevalence and disease severity of this disorder increases with age. The incidence in women is twice that of men and higher-than-normal prevalence (from 25% to 30%) of RLS is found in patients with iron deficiency, pregnancy, and end-stage renal disease. Neurologic conditions linked with RLS include spinal cerebellar atrophy, Charcot-Marie-Tooth disease type 2, spinal stenosis, lumbar sacral radiculopathy, and Parkinson's disease. A strong family history of RLS is more closely correlated with an early age of onset (<45 years). RLS developing at an older age is more often associated with neuropathy and faster disease progression.

Gamaldo CE, Earley CJ. Restless legs syndrome: a clinical update. *Chest*. 2006;130:1596–1604.

19. Answer: B. Developmental reflexes present at birth include the following: the rooting reflex (puckering of lips in response to perioral stimulation), palmar grasp reflex, Babinski (extensor plantar response) reflex, startle (Moro) reflex, and the tonic neck reflex. In normal children, these reflexes disappear with development. The rooting reflex usually disappears by 3 months. The palmar grasp, Moro, and tonic neck reflexes usually disappear by 4 to 6 months. The Babinski reflex usually disappears by the twelfth month.

1. Rolak LA. *Neurology Secrets*. 2nd ed. Philadelphia: Hanley & Belfus; 1998:330.
2. Sadock BJ, Sadock VA. *Kaplan and Sadock's Synopsis of Psychiatry*. 9th ed. Philadelphia: Lippincott Williams & Wilkins; 2003:25–26.

20. Answer: A. TIAs are temporary interruptions in cerebral circulation. They give rise to constellations of deficits. They may occur in either the distribution of the carotid artery or of the basilar artery and typically last from 30 to 60 minutes but never more than 24 hours. TIAs can result from platelet emboli arising from extracranial arteries. They usually indicate underlying atherosclerotic cerebrovascular disease and signal an increased risk of sustaining a stroke; after a TIA, 4% of individuals develop a stroke within a month and 12% within a year. Strokes cause permanent physical and neuropsychiatric deficits. They can result from arterial thrombosis, embolus, or hemorrhage in the cerebral blood flow. Age, hypertension, and smoking are the greatest risk factors. Other risk factors are migraine headaches, diabetes mellitus, drug abuse, cardiac disease, vasculitis, and sickle-cell disease. In terms of distribution, anterior cerebral artery strokes are characterized by contralateral lower extremity paresis, mutism, apathy, and pseudobulbar palsy (with bilateral infarctions). Middle cerebral artery strokes are associated with contralateral hemiparesis, hemisensory loss, aphasia with dominant hemisphere lesions, and hemi-inattention with nondominant hemisphere lesions. These infarctions are the most common. Posterior cerebral artery strokes are connected with contralateral homonymous hemianopsia and alexia without agraphia. Wallenberg's syndrome results from lateral medullary infarction. It is caused by proximal vertebral artery occlusion. Clinical manifestations consist of vertigo, nausea, vomiting, dysphagia, hoarseness, nystagmus, ipsilateral Horner's syndrome, limb ataxia, impairment of all sensory modalities over the face, and loss of light touch and position sense in the limbs. There is also impairment of pinprick and temperature sensation in the contralateral extremities from involvement of the spinothalamic tract. Horner's syndrome results from involvement of the descending sympathetic tract. Hemiataxia stems from inclusion of the inferior cerebellar peduncle. Vertigo results from participation of the vestibular nuclei.

1. Kaufman DM. *Clinical Neurology for Psychiatrists*. 5th ed. Philadelphia: WB Saunders; 2001:268–290.
2. Ropper AH, Brown RH. *Adams and Victor's Principles of Neurology*. 8th ed. New York: McGraw-Hill; 2005:115–116.

21. **Answer: A.** This patient has acute intermittent porphyria, which is a disease inherited as an autosomal dominant trait. The metabolic defect is in the liver, and there is increased production and urinary excretion of porphobilinogen and its precursor d-aminolevulinic acid. The urine turns dark upon standing due to formation of porphobilin, which is an oxidation product of porphobilinogen. The initial and most prominent symptom is moderate to severe colicky abdominal pain. Pain may be generalized or localized. Constipation is frequent. Radiographs show intestinal distention or ileus. Attacks last for days to weeks, and repeated vomiting may occur. Neurological symptoms are those of an acute polyneuropathy involving the motor nerves more severely than the sensory ones. Often, the weakness predominates in the proximal muscles of the limbs and limb girdle. There may also be acute confusion, delirium, psychosis, depression, and/or convulsions. These attacks are usually recurrent. They are often precipitated by drugs, which induce the enzyme d-aminolevulinic acid synthetase such as sulfonamides, griseofulvin, estrogens, barbiturates, phenytoin, and the succinimide anticonvulsants (ethosuximide and methsuximide). Other precipitants include infection, fasting, pregnancy, or occasionally menses. The first attack rarely occurs before puberty or after late adulthood. The course of the disease is variable. Severe cases can lead to fatal respiratory or cardiac paralysis. Treatment is with intravenous glucose, which suppresses the heme biosynthetic pathway and intravenous hematin.

1. Greenberg DA, Aminoff MJ, Simon RP. *Clinical Neurology*. 5th ed. New York: McGraw-Hill; 2002:181–182.
2. Ropper AH, Brown RH. *Adams and Victor's Principles of Neurology*. 8th ed. New York: McGraw-Hill; 2005:1129.

22. **Answer: B.** The development of dementia is a poor prognostic sign with most patients dying within 6 months. The dementia may be cortical or subcortical in origin. The differential diagnoses include CNS infections, neoplasms, abnormalities caused by systemic disorders and endocrinopathies, and adverse reactions to pharmacotherapy.

Sadock BJ, Sadock VA. *Kaplan and Sadock's Synopsis of Psychiatry*. 9th ed. Philadelphia: Lippincott Williams & Wilkins; 2003: 374–376.

23. **Answer: B.** The EEG shows nonspecific slowing in the early stages with later localization of periodic spike and slow wave activity in one or both temporal lobes. CT scan of the brain may be normal initially. Later, the characteristic low density areas in one or both temporal lobes appear. MRI is more sensitive in the early stages when therapy is likely to be useful. Increased antibody titers are rarely present prior to 10 days into the illness; they are useful retrospectively but not usually useful in establishing the diagnosis early in the course of the illness. Brain biopsy provides the best means to diagnose and establish alternative causes of encephalitis.

1. Lishman WA. *Organic Psychiatry*. 3rd ed. Oxford: Blackwell Science; 1996:357.
2. Whitley RJ. Herpes simplex encephalitis: adolescents and adults. *Antiviral Res*. 2006;71:141–148.

24. **Answer: C.** Neurosyphilis may be meningeal, meningovascular, and parenchymatous. Parenchymatous type includes both general paresis and tabes dorsalis.

The interval from infection to symptoms range from a few months to 20 years for meningeal syphilis (usually in the first year) and meningovascular syphilis (average of 7 years), 20 years for general paresis and 20 to 25 years for tabes dorsalis. Meningeal syphilis may involve the brain or spinal cord; patients present with headache, nausea, vomiting, cranial nerve palsies, and changes in mental status. Meningovascular syphilis is associated with inflammation of the pia and arachnoid mater with focal or widespread involvement of small, medium, and large arteries. The commonest presentation is a stroke syndrome in a young person involving the middle cerebral artery. General paresis presents with symptoms relating to personality, affect, reflexes, eye, speech, intellect, and sensorium. Tabes dorsalis presents symptoms and signs of demyelination of the posterior columns, dorsal roots, and dorsal root ganglia. Symptoms include wide-based gait, paraesthesias, incontinence, areflexia, loss of position, vibration, deep pain, and temperature sensations. Atypical and attenuated presentations are common these days due to the partial suppression of the infection in earlier stages by antibiotics given for other purposes. Grandiose delusions are seen in 10% to 20% of affected persons with general paresis. The pupils are abnormal in two thirds of the patients. Argyll-Robertson pupils are small, irregular pupils, which are reactive to accommodation but not to light. Optic atrophy may develop in the absence of complaints about visual impairment. The classical Argyll-Robertson pupils are seen more commonly in the combined taboparetic type than with general paresis alone.

1. Lishman WA. *Organic Psychiatry*. 3rd ed. Oxford: Blackwell Science; 1996:343.
2. Rowland LP. *Merritt's Neurology*. 11th ed. Philadelphia: Lippincott Williams & Wilkins; 2005:236–242.
3. Sadock BJ, Sadock VA. *Kaplan and Sadock's Synopsis of Psychiatry*. 9th ed. Philadelphia: Lippincott Williams & Wilkins; 2003:363.

25. **Answer: D.** There are neuropathologic similarities between Down syndrome and AD. Neuropathologically, Alzheimer-type abnormalities are seen in demented and nondemented patients with Down syndrome and more than half of the patients with Down syndrome above the age of 50 years develop AD. The ApoE epsilon4 allele, oestrogen deficiency, high levels of Aβ1–42 peptide, elevated expression of BACE2, and valine polymorphism of PrP are associated with earlier onset of dementia in patients with Down syndrome. Up to 84% of demented individuals with Down syndrome develop seizures. Late-onset epilepsy in Down syndrome is associated with AD, while early-onset epilepsy is not. In patients with Down syndrome, slowing of the dominant occipital rhythm is related to AD and the frequency of the dominant occipital activity decreases at the onset of dementia.

Menendez M. Down syndrome, Alzheimer's disease and seizures. *Brain Dev*. 2005;27:246–252.

26. **Answer: C.** Dopamine agonists are those drugs that directly stimulate the dopamine receptors. The FDA approved dopamine agonists include bromocriptine (Parlodel), pergolide (Permax), pramipexole (Mirapex), and ropinirole (Requip). These drugs alone or combined with levodopa have been shown in studies to be effective in treating symptoms of early Parkinson's disease. Controlled studies comparing ropinirole or pramipexole to levodopa showed that levodopa was more effective in reducing the motor symptoms of Parkinson's disease, but the dopamine agonists had a lower incidence of motor complications. Selegiline (Eldepryl) is a MAO-B inhibitor that gives some mild symptomatic benefit to patients with early Parkinson's disease. Data indicates that in patients with Parkinson's disease, MAO-B inhibitors reduce disability, the incidence of motor fluctuations, and the need for levodopa without more adverse effects or increased mortality.

1. Kaufman DM. *Clinical Neurology for Psychiatrists*. 5th ed. Philadelphia: WB Saunders; 2001: 455–457.
2. Rao SS, Hofmann LA, Shakil A. Parkinson's disease: diagnosis and treatment. *Am Fam Physician*. 2006;74:2046–2054.

27. **Answer: C.** *Goodness of fit* and *poorness of fit* are terms used to describe the way in which children and parents adjust to one another. Even the most expert of parents may find it difficult to deal with some children. Difficult temperamental characteristics, unusual sensitivities, and developmental characteristics of activity and reactivity can make caregiving difficult. On the other hand, even some well behaved children may be disappointing to the caregivers because of their unconscious meaning. These problems of mutual adjustment interfere with parent-child relationship and may lead to various forms of deprivation and traumatic separation. Early recognition and intervention helps prevent such problems in reciprocity and mutual adjustment.

Lewis M. *Child and Adolescent Psychiatry: A Comprehensive Textbook*. 3rd ed. Philadelphia: Lippincott Williams & Wilkins; 2003:463.

28. **Answer: E.** The pudendal nerve arises from the first through fourth sacral segments. It may be damaged by buttock injections, pelvic fractures, surgery, and prolonged biking. It innervates areas of the anal sphincter, penis, clitoris, and scrotum. When damaged, patients present with sensory disturbances in

the innervated areas, as well as erectile impotence and difficulty with bladder and bowel control. The sciatic nerve proper is the largest of the body and it innervates areas starting around the gluteus and then divides into two different branches at the area of the apex of the popliteal fossa. When the superior gluteal nerve is damaged, patients tilt the pelvis toward the side of the unaffected raised leg. Patients with a lesion of the inferior gluteal nerve present with weakness when asked to extend the thigh against resistance. The tibial nerve is involved in innervating muscles in the feet.

1. Brazis PW, Masdeu JC, Biller J. *Localization in Clinical Neurology*. 5th ed. Philadelphia: Lippincott Williams & Wilkins; 2007:55–57.
2. Martinez JM. *Bicycle Seat Neuropathy*. http://www.emedicine.com/sports/TOPIC12.HTM. Accessed December 16, 2006.

29. **Answer: B.** Jean Piaget, a Swiss psychologist, emphasized the ways that children think and acquire knowledge, and described four major stages to accomplish that lead to the capacity for adult thought, including: (i) sensorimotor, (ii) preoperational thought, (iii) concrete operations, and (iv) formal operations. The other psychologists listed were all important contributors to work on attachment theory. John Bowlby formulated the theory that normal attachment in infancy is crucial to healthy development. Harry Harlow demonstrated the emotional and behavioral effects of isolating monkeys from birth and preventing formation of attachments. Mary Ainsworth expanded on Bowlby's work and is known for describing the "strange situation," the research protocol for assessing the quality and security of an infant's attachment. She observed that about 65% of infants are securely attached by the age of 24 months. Rene Spitz first described *anaclitic depression* after he studied the effects of emotional deprivation on normal attached infants when suddenly separated from their mothers and placed in institutions or hospitals.

Kaplan HI, Sadock BJ. *Kaplan & Sadock's Synopsis of Psychiatry*. 8th ed. Philadelphia: Lippincott Williams & Wilkins; 1998:140–147.

30. **Answer: B.** In a malpractice lawsuit, the plaintiff must show four elements of malpractice are present by a preponderance of evidence. There are the so-called four "Ds" of malpractice: (i) a doctor-patient relationship existed that created a duty of care; (ii) a deviation from standard of practice occurred; (iii) this deviation bore a direct causal relationship to the untoward outcome; and (iv) damage occurred as a result. Proof by a preponderance of the evidence as

required in a malpractice suit simply means more likely than not, or just enough evidence to tip the scale one way or the other.

Sadock BJ, Sadock VA. *Kaplan and Sadock's Comprehensive Textbook of Psychiatry*. 8th ed. Philadelphia: Lippincott Williams & Wilkins; 2005: 3969.

31. **Answer: B.** At this time, the only indication that CMS will reimburse the cost of a PET scan of the brain in routine clinical care is the differentiation of frontotemporal dementia from Alzheimer's dementia.

American College of Nuclear Physicians. *Summary of Coverage Criteria/Guidelines for AD and FTD PET Studies Effective September 15, 2004.* http://acnp.snm.org/index.cfm?PageID=3231&RPID=1951. Accessed December 31, 2006.

32. **Answer: C.** The patient's symptoms and exam findings are most consistent with dementia due to vitamin B_{12} deficiency. This is often considered a "reversible" form of dementia, as exogenous B_{12} replacement may result in improvement in neuropsychiatric symptoms if the condition is diagnosed early enough. The presence of subacute combined degeneration of the spinal cord (involvement of both posterior columns and pyramidal tracts) is indicated by weakness, hyperreflexia, and loss of position and vibration sense in the lower extremities. Though often associated with a macrocytic anemia, vitamin B_{12} deficiency can produce cognitive impairment in the absence of megaloblastic bone marrow changes. The pathophysiology of vitamin B_{12} deficiency may involve increased plasma homocysteine levels; elevated homocysteine may be associated with response to treatment of B_{12} deficiency in patients with dementia.

1. Blazer DG, Steffens DC, Busse EW. *The American Psychiatric Association Textbook of Geriatric Psychiatry*. Washington: American Psychiatric Publishing; 2004:221.
2. Nilsson K, Gustafson L, Hultberg B. Improvement of cognitive functions after cobalamin/folate supplementation in elderly patients with dementia and elevated plasma homocysteine. *Int J Geriatr Psychiatry*. 2001;16:609–614.
3. Wang HX, Wahlin A, Basun H, et al. Vitamin B_{12} and folate in relation to the development of Alzheimer's disease. *Neurology*. 2001;56:1188–1194.

33. **Answer: C.** The ion gated receptors alpha 7 and alpha 4/beta 2 are thought to be involved in nicotine dependence. They quickly desensitize and increase with nicotine use. The alpha 2 receptor is involved in norepinephrine regulation and is the site of action of clonidine and guanfacine (antihypertensives), also used in psychiatric treatment.

Sadock BJ, Sadock VA. *Kaplan and Sadock's Comprehensive Textbook of Psychiatry*. 8th ed. Philadelphia: Lippincott Williams & Wilkins; 2005:1258.

34. **Answer: A.** Bipolar disorder is more heritable than MDD. All the other options are correct.

   1. Benazzi F. Bipolar II disorder family history using the family history screen: findings and clinical implications. *Compr Psychiatry*. 2004;45:77–82.
   2. Sadock BJ, Sadock VA. *Kaplan and Sadock's Comprehensive Textbook of Psychiatry*. 8th ed. Philadelphia: Lippincott Williams & Wilkins; 2005:1595.

35. **Answer: A.** Patients displaying depressive symptoms after a stroke range from 30% to 50%. Though some strokes are associated with a lesion in the left frontal lobe, it is not necessarily the case that patients who display such symptoms must have lesions in the left frontal lobe. Such associations have been made with several other areas of the brain as well. Post-stroke depression is associated with increased age. ECT is considered safe for patients with such depression, though such patients may be more confused after receiving the treatment. Antihypertensive medications (e.g., reserpine) can induce depression as well.

   Kaufman DM. *Clinical Neurology for Psychiatrists*. 5th ed. Philadelphia: WB Saunders; 2001:278–279.

36. **Answer: C.** In 2005, the FDA warned of an increased risk in cardiac defects following in utero exposure to paroxetine and thus changed paroxetine's fetal risk classification from class C to class D. Two large unpublished studies showed a one and a half to two times increased risk of cardiac defects in newborns exposed to paroxetine in the first trimester. The most common cardiac defects included ventricular and atrial septal defects. Venlafaxine and mirtazapine have been examined in only one small study but to date has not been associated with any major malformations. The other SSRIs are classified as class C drugs in pregnancy.

   1. Grover S, Avasthi A, Sharma Y. Psychotropics in pregnancy: weighing the risks. *Indian J Med Res*. 2006;123:497–512.
   2. Thormahlen GM. Paroxetine use during pregnancy: is it safe? *Ann Pharmacother*. 2006;40:1834–1837.
   3. US Food and Drug Administration. *FDA Public Health Advisory: Paroxetine*. http://www.fda.gov/cder/drug/advisory/paroxetine200512.htm. Accessed February 27, 2007.

37. **Answer: C.** While the risk of seizures is about 1% for the other serotonin dopamine antagonists, the risk is higher for patients treated with clozapine. This effect is dose dependent with risk approaching 4% at or above 600 mg/day dosing. The clozapine should be stopped temporarily, but can be resumed at half the previous dose after commencing anticonvulsant treatment. Carbamazepine and phenytoin should not be used in these patients due to their risk of causing agranulocytosis. People with preex-

isting seizure disorders and with history of head injury are at greater risk of seizures during clozapine treatment.

Kaplan HI, Sadock BJ. *Kaplan and Sadock's Synopsis of Psychiatry*. 9th ed. Philadelphia: Lippincott Williams & Wilkins; 2003:1109.

38. **Answer: D.** The combination of ECT and lithium can result in confusional states and prolonged seizures. These adverse effects appear to be dose related. In an acute course of ECT, lithium should be discontinued. In continuation and maintenance ECT, lithium should be held for 24 hours prior to treatment. Maintenance antihypertensive medications should be administered prior to ECT. Anticoagulant medications also should be continued. Antipsychotic medications are safe to use in combination with ECT.

Sadock BJ, Sadock VA. *Kaplan and Sadock's Comprehensive Textbook of Psychiatry*. 8th ed. Philadelphia: Lippincott Williams & Wilkins; 2005:2979.

39. **Answer: B.** This patient has symptoms characteristic of an atypical depression, not a melancholic type of depression. For patients with atypical depression, MAOIs are thought to have the better efficacy than TCAs. SSRIs do not have proven efficacy for this condition.

   1. Frazer A. Antidepressants. *J Clin Psychiatry*. 1997;58 (Suppl 6):9–25.
   2. Stewart JW. Treating depression with atypical features. *J Clin Psychiatry*. 2007;68:25–29.

40. **Answer: B.** The psychiatrist is using confrontation, an intervention in which the subject that the patient does not want to accept or wants to avoid is presented to them. Unlike interpretation, confrontation does not necessarily pull something from the unconscious into consciousness. Confrontation introduces unspoken information or the psychiatrist's insight into the session, unlike clarification, which involves organizing and reflecting back information that the patient has already presented. Empathic validation and affirmation are more supportive interventions than confrontation.

Gabbard GO. *Psychodynamic Psychiatry in Clinical Practice*. 3rd ed. Washington: American Psychiatric Press; 2000:97–98.

41. **Answer: C.** The diagnoses related to the highest frequencies of violent behaviors are schizophrenia (14.8%), depression (28.5%), and bipolar disorder (22%). An important finding in these patients is that the strongest predictor of violent behavior was having a history of such behavior. Violent acts, including murder, are about eight times more common among the patients discharged from forensic hospitals than among those discharged from general

psychiatric hospitals. Mental disorders are significantly more common among homicidal individuals than among other criminals (35% versus 21%) with mental disorder being diagnosed prior to the murder. In summary, the association between severe mental disorders and violent or homicidal behavior has been demonstrated in all types of studies. As yet, no apparent association has been found between antisocial personality disorder (which generates behavior that is more violent than that generated by psychoses) and violent behavior. Some studies indicate that psychotic individuals are more likely to murder family members or close acquaintances, whereas the murder of strangers are more frequently perpetrated by abusers of alcohol or drugs.

Valenca AM, Moraes TM. Relationship between homicide and mental disorders. *Rev Bras Psiquiatr*. 2006;28:S62–68.

42. **Answer: A.** Although there are no absolute medication contraindications with ECT, concurrent use of lithium and ECT adds significant risk of post-ECT delirium. Risks associated with antiepileptic medications (i.e., valproate, carbamazepine, lamotrigine, gabapentin, and topiramate) are that they may inhibit seizure activity but do not cause post-ECT delirium. Carbamazepine may prolong the action of succinylcholine. The combination of antipsychotics and ECT as well as the combination of ECT with most antidepressants is well tolerated. Caution should be taken when combining ECT with MAOIs, especially the irreversible MAOIs, due to risk of catecholamine surge.

Naguib M, Koorn R. Interactions between psychotropics, anaesthetics and electroconvulsive therapy: implications for drug choice and patient management. *CNS Drugs*. 2002;16:229–247.

43. **Answer: B.** Of the following pairings, the only incorrect one is that of B fiber and postganglionic function. The B fiber is preganglionic autonomic in function. C fibers supply both postganglionic sympathetics and dorsal roots of spinal cord. In the dorsal root, they carry pain, temperature, some mechanoreception, and reflex responses. Erlanger and Gasser divided mammalian nerve fibers into A, B, and C groups, further subdividing the A group into α, β, γ, δ and fibers. The greater the diameter of a given nerve fiber, the greater its speed of conduction. The large axons are concerned primarily with proprioceptive sensation, somatic motor function, conscious touch, and pressure, while the smaller axons subserve pain and temperature sensations and autonomic function.

Ganong, WF. *Review of Medical Physiology*. 22nd ed. http://www.accessmedicine.com/content.aspx?aID=703497. Accessed February 18, 2007.

44. **Answer: B.** Among these disorders, Lesch Nyhan syndrome is the only one that has an X-linked recessive mode of inheritance. Acute intermittent porphyria, Huntington's disease, and spinocerebellar ataxias all have an autosomal mode of inheritance.

Rowland LP. *Merritt's Neurology*. 11th ed. Philadelphia: Lippincott Williams & Wilkins; 2005:686.

45. **Answer: B.** Ataxia is incoordination or clumsiness of movements. It is not the result of muscular weakness, but can be caused by vestibular, cerebellar, or sensory disorders. The clinical manifestations of cerebellar ataxia include irregularities in the rate, rhythm, amplitude, and force of voluntary movements. Alcoholic cerebellar degeneration is a syndrome which develops in chronic alcoholics. Affected patients often have a drinking history of 10 or more years which includes complications of alcoholism such as liver disease, delirium tremens, Wernicke's encephalopathy, and/or polyneuropathy. Alcoholic cerebellar degeneration is more common in men and has its onset between ages 40 and 60 years. The pathological finding is largely restricted to the superior vermis of the cerebellum. The disease is usually insidious in onset and is gradually progressive. Gait ataxia is a common feature. The gait is wide-based often with a staggering quality similar to drunkenness. Other commonly associated findings are distal sensory deficits in the feet and absent ankle reflexes, from polyneuropathy, and signs of malnutrition such as loss of subcutaneous tissue, generalized muscle atrophy, or glossitis. Less frequently ataxia of the arms, nystagmus, dysarthria, hypotonia, and truncal instability occurs. There is no specific treatment for this condition. Patients should receive thiamine because the syndrome is closely related to Wernicke's encephalopathy. Abstinence along with adequate nutrition leads to stabilization in most cases. The corticospinal tracts contain motor axons that originate in the cerebral cortex that pass through the internal capsule, the brainstem, and then cross over at the level of the medulla (lateral corticospinal tracts) and terminate by synapsing with the anterior horn cells of the spinal cord. The corticobulbar tract is an upper motor neuron (UMN) tract that innervates the brainstem motor nuclei and their nerves supplying the head and neck muscles. It is the cranial counterpart to the corticospinal tract. Bilateral cerebral hemisphere damage to the corticobulbar tract produces several disturbances including pseudobulbar palsy. This condition is characterized by emotional lability, dementia, and aphasia. Injury of the nondominant parietal lobe typically results in hemi-inattention. This is a constellation of disorders in which patients

neglect left-sided visual and tactile stimuli. The subthalamic nucleus is part of the basal ganglia which also includes the globus pallidus, the putamen, and the substantia nigra. The basal ganglia controls muscle tone, regulates motor activity, and generates the postural reflexes. The main feature of basal ganglia injury is often an involuntary movement disorder. Hemiballismus results from small infarctions of the contralateral subthalamic nucleus. It is associated with intermittent flinging of the arm and leg on one side of the body.

1. Greenberg DA, Aminoff MJ, Simon RP. *Clinical Neurology*. 5th ed. New York: McGraw-Hill; 2002:95–118.
2. Kaufman DM. *Clinical Neurology for Psychiatrists*. 5th ed. Philadelphia: WB Saunders; 2001:10, 13, 14–15, 51–52

46. Answer: C. Aphasia is a loss or impairment of the ability to produce or comprehend language due to an acquired lesion of the brain. It can be divided into two classes: fluent and nonfluent. There are three types of nonfluent aphasias: Broca's aphasia, transcortical motor aphasia, and global aphasia. Fluent aphasias include Wernicke's aphasia, conduction aphasia, and transcortical sensory aphasia. In terms of the nonfluent aphasias, Broca's aphasia is characterized by effortful but agrammatical speech. Comprehension is preserved, though repetition of language is impaired. Broca's is often associated with right arm and face weakness. It is localized to the frontal lobe. Global aphasia is another nonfluent aphasia where speech output is scant, comprehension is very impaired, and there is no repetition and there is often associated hemiplegia. This syndrome is due to destruction of the language zone, including both Broca's and Wernicke's areas and much of the territory between them. Lastly, transcortical motor aphasia is characterized by nonfluent speech, good comprehension, and intact repetition. The lesions are localized to either the anterior or superior to Broca's area. In terms of the fluent aphasias, in Wernicke's aphasia, speech is voluble and well articulated but lacking in meaning. Comprehension is greatly impaired and there is no repetition of words. It may be associated with hemi- or quadrantanopia, and there are usually no signs of paresis. The lesion is localized to the posterior temporal lobe. Conduction aphasia is another fluent aphasia where the patients are able to comprehend language, but unable to repeat phrases. There are no other associated signs. Localization is to the arcuate fasciculus. Finally, with transcortical sensory aphasia, patients have impaired comprehension similar to Wernicke's aphasia. Unlike Wernicke's aphasia, they are able to repeat phrases. The lesion is localized to the region surrounding Wernicke's area in the brain.

1. Greenberg DA, Aminoff MJ, Simon RP. *Clinical Neurology*. 5th ed. New York: McGraw-Hill; 2002:356.
2. Ropper AH, Brown RH. *Adams and Victor's Principles of Neurology*. 8th ed. New York: McGraw-Hill; 2005:417–423.

47. Answer: D. This patient has chronic paroxysmal hemicrania, a unilateral form of headache which resembles cluster headaches but with some distinctive features. These headaches are of short duration; they last from 2 to 45 minutes, usually affect the temporo-orbital region of the head, and are accompanied by tearing, conjunctival injection, rhinorrhea, and occasionally a partial Horner's syndrome. Unlike cluster headaches, attacks occur several times each day and recur daily over long periods of time. These headaches are more common in women than men by a ratio of 3:1; whereas cluster headaches occur predominantly in young men by a ratio of 5:1. Chronic paroxysmal hemicrania has a dramatic treatment response to indomethacin. Tension headaches are characterized by pressure, tightness, and aching. Their distribution is bilateral with occipitonuchal, temporal, or frontal predominance or diffuse extension over the top of the cranium. They occur mainly in adults and are more common in women. They occur with variable intensity and are provoked by fatigue or nervous strain. Tension headaches are associated with depression and anxiety, and can be treated with antianxiety and antidepressant drugs. Migraine without aura is also known as common migraine. These migraines are characterized by pulsatile, throbbing pain which is often worse behind one eye or ear. The headaches then become dull and generalized. Scalp sensitivity occurs, along with occasional nausea and vomiting. Common migraines occur in a frontotemporal, either unilateral or bilateral, distribution and are more common in women. They are seen in adolescents and young to middle-aged adults and last from 4 to 24 hours and occur either upon awakening or later in the day. Common migraines decrease in frequency during pregnancy and in middle age. Provoking factors include bright light, noise, tension, and alcohol. Headaches are relieved by darkness and sleep. Treatment includes ergotamine, sumatriptan, and/or NSAIDs. Propranolol and amitriptyline have been used for prevention. Tolosa-Hunt syndrome involves unilateral, mainly retro-orbital facial pain. The pain is intense, sharp, or aching. Ptosis and miosis are also observed. The syndrome is associated with granulomatous lesion of the cavernous sinus or superior orbital fissure. It is treated with corticosteroids.

Ropper AH, Brown RH. *Adams and Victor's Principles of Neurology*. 8th ed. New York: McGraw-Hill; 2005:144–167.

48. Answer: D. This patient appears manic. There are important confidentiality issues to consider when treating this patient so it is prudent to discuss his case with hospital attoneys. From the informant account, this patient may be putting others at risk of becoming infected and due to his lack of insight, has to be admitted involuntarily to prevent danger to others. He may be delirious and a full medical workup would be helpful in determining the onset of a new CNS related process. In the absence of any identifiable cause for his presentation, it is likely that he has progressed into the late stages of the disease. Manic symptoms most commonly arise in later stages of the disease complicated by neurocognitive impairment. As he is manic, the antidepressant would need to be discontinued. When antipsychotic medications are to be prescribed, they should be done so at lower doses as these patients are at higher risk of extrapyramidal side effects from these medications.

Sadock BJ, Sadock VA. *Kaplan and Sadock's Synopsis of Psychiatry*. 9th ed. Philadelphia: Lippincott Williams & Wilkins; 2003:374–377.

49. Answer: A. The commonest organisms implicated (in over 50% of cases) of cerebral abscess, are *streptococci*. *Staphylococci* are implicated in traumatic brain injury and neurosurgery. Brain abscesses occur in association with contiguous foci of infection (e.g., otitis or hematogenous) spread from distant sites (e.g., lung infections or from trauma). Hematogenous brain abscesses are likely to be multiple and are associated with higher mortality. Brain abscess occurs in the following regions of the brain in decreasing order of frequency: frontal > frontoparietal > parietal > cerebellar > occipital. Brainstem, basal ganglia, and thalamic abscesses are rare. MRI is more sensitive than CT scans in detecting early satellite lesions and extraparenchymal extension of an abscess, and is not hindered by bony artifacts whilst permitting mutiplanar imaging. Mortality rate is about 10%. Long term neurological sequelae occur in 30% to 50% of cases with up to 70% of survivors developing late seizures.

1. Carpenter J, Stapleton S, Holliman R. Retrospective analysis of 49 cases of brain abscess and review of the literature. *Eur J Clin Microbiol Infect Dis*. 2007; Jan;26:1–11.
2. Lishman WA. *Organic Psychiatry*. 3rd ed. Oxford: Blackwell Science; 1996:368.

50. Answer: B. Nonsmall-cell lung cancer is the most common primary lesion leading to a brain metastasis. Melanoma and small-cell lung cancer also have a great propensity to metastasize to the brain. Other primary cancers that commonly metastasize to the brain include breast, renal, and gastrointestinal (GI) cancers. Cancers of the prostate, pancreas, and uterus rarely metastasize to the brain. About 50% of all patients with brain metastases have a single lesions with an additional 20% having only two lesions.

Rowland LP. *Merritt's Neurology*. 11th ed. Philadelphia: Lippincott Williams & Wilkins; 2005:459–460.

51. Answer: E. All of the statements are true. Patients with Down syndrome start developing AD earlier than the general population. The incidence of AD in patients with Down syndrome is 75% by the age of 60 years compared with less than 5% in the general population. By the age of 40 years, 100% of these patients show AD pathology in their brains. Visual memory loss and impaired learning capacity are the first symptoms of cognitive dysfunction in these patients. MRI findings in these patients include cerebellar atrophy, basal ganglia calcification, and hippocampal atrophy.

Menendez M. Down syndrome, Alzheimer's disease and seizures. *Brain Dev*. 2005;27:246–252.

52. Answer: D. Entacapone (Comtan) and tolcapone (Tasmar) are COMT inhibitors that decrease the degradation of levodopa and extend its half-life. By doing so, they reduce the end-of-dose wearing-off effect and thereby reducing the "off" time. Compared to placebo, adjuvant COMT inhibitors treatment reduces the "off" time with levodopa dose and modestly improves the motor symptoms and disability in patients with advanced Parkinson's disease and motor complications. Tolcapone use requires close monitoring of liver function tests as they can rarely cause potentially fatal hepatotoxicity. A combination of carbidopa/levodopa/entacapone (Stalevo) is currently available in the market.

1. Kaufman DM. *Clinical Neurology for Psychiatrists*. 5th ed. Philadelphia: WB Saunders; 2001:455–457.
2. Rao SS, Hofmann LA, Shakil A. Parkinson's disease: diagnosis and treatment. *Am Fam Physician*. 2006; Dec 15;74(12):2046–2054.

53. Answer: D. Lead poisoning is the most common preventable pediatric health problem in the United States today. Lead is either eaten or breathed, in the form of dust. It accumulates in soft tissues and bones, where it can be stored for many years. It is currently estimated that more than 3 million children 6 years of age and younger have lead poisoning. Lead poisoning has no obvious signs, and most children do not report any abnormal symptoms. However, they may present with stomach aches, decreased appetite, hyperactivity, sleep problems, or irritability. Symptoms may mimic flu or common cold. In children elevated lead levels can cause learning disabilities, mental retardation, behavioral problems, lowered IQ, stunted growth, and hearing impairment. In serious cases, seizures, followed by coma and death can occur. Diagnosis of lead poisoning can be made by checking the blood level of lead. A level of 10 mcg/dL or greater is considered unsafe and all children between the ages of 6 months to 6 years of age who are entering day care, preschool, or kindergarten must be assessed for lead poisoning. Chelating drugs like ethylenediaminetetraacetic acid (EDTA) are used to treat children with very high blood lead levels. In cases of severe poisoning, repeated treatment with these drugs may be needed. Lead poisoning can be prevented by taking simple precautions around the house to remove or avoid lead contamination.

1. American Academy of Family Physicians. *Lead Poisoning in Children*. http://familydoctor.org/617.xml. Accessed December 5, 2006.
2. Illinois Dept of Pubic Health. *Childhood Lead Poisoning*. http://www.idph.state.il.us/public/hb/hblead.htm. Accessed December 5, 2006.

54. Answer: A. Lateral medullary syndrome (Wallenberg syndrome) is usually secondary to intracranial vertebral artery or posterior inferior cerebellar artery occlusion. Signs and symptoms arise from damage to an area of the lateral medulla and inferior cerebellum. The clinical picture varies widely and can include many different signs and symptoms, but the characteristic picture includes the following: (i) diminished ipsilateral facial pain and temperature perception, (ii) diminished contralateral trunk and extremity pain and temperature perception, ipsilateral palatal, pharyngeal, and vocal cord paralysis, and (iii) ipsilateral Horner syndrome, vertigo, and nausea and ipsilateral cerebellar signs and symptoms. Motor function, vibration and proprioception are spared. Medial medullary syndrome presents with ipsilateral paresis atrophy and fibrillation of the tongue, contralateral hemiplegia, and loss of position and vibratory sensation. Submedullary syndrome consists of signs and symptoms of Wallenberg syndrome in addition to ipsilateral hemiplegia. Lateral pontomedullary syndrome presents with ipsilateral facial weakness, tinnitus, and sometimes hearing disturbances. Millard-Gubler syndrome is caused by a unilateral lesion of the ventrocaudal pons and it presents with contralateral hemiplegia and ipsilateral lateral cranial nerves VI (CN VI) and VII (CN VII) paresis.

1. Brazis PW, Masdeu JC, Biller J. *Localization in Clinical Neurology*. 5th ed. Philadelphia: Lippincott Williams & Wilkins; 2007:351–357.
2. Montaner J, Alvarez-Sabín. *Opalski's Syndrome*. http://jnnp.bmj.com/cgi/reprint/67/5/688.pdf. Accessed December 16, 2006.
3. Vuillier F, Tatu L, Dietsch, et al. *Pontomedullary Sulcus Infarct: A Variant of Lateral Medullary Syndrome*. http://jnnp.bmj.com/cgi/reprint/77/11/1276. Accessed December 16, 2006.

55. Answer: B. Donald Winnicott, a British psychologist, was one of the central figures in the school of object relations theory instead of emphasizing instincts, and discussed the role of a transitional object. This is an object that a young child becomes attached to, provides a bridge between the child's inner and other worlds, and serves as a substitute for the mother during the infants' efforts to separate and become independent. Winnicott viewed the transitional object as an influence on the development of play, creativity, religion, and cultural life in general. Carl Jung was behind the term *archetype*, which he defined as symbolic images that recur in dreams and are part of the collective unconscious.

Kaplan HI, Sadock BJ. *Kaplan & Sadock's Synopsis of Psychiatry*. 8th ed. Philadelphia: Lippincott Williams & Wilkins; 1998:227, 233.

56. Answer: C. Bias is a systematic error in a study that leads to distortion of the results. Selection bias can occur when the selection process affects the type of patient that enrolls. In this study, the selection bias would be represented by patients with stressful events and depression being less likely to volunteer. Misclassification (or information) bias can occur when there is random or systematic inaccuracy in measurement. This bias comes in two types: differential (misclassification of one variable is dependent on the other variable) or nondifferential (misclassification is independent). This question is an example of differential misclassification bias, in which subjects are more likely to answer affirmatively about risk in an effort to explain their serious disease. Confounding is the mixing of the effect of an extraneous variable with the effects of the exposure and disease of interest such as if patients with a family history of depression being more likely to experience both stressful life events and depression. Confounding occurs when the effects of multiple factors on an event cannot be separated. Random error represents the variability seen during sampling a particular population.

Greenberg RS, Daniels SR, Flanders WD, et al. *Medical Epidemiology*. 3rd ed. New York: McGraw-Hill; 2001:144–150.

57. **Answer: A.** The Wisconsin Card Sort is a neuropsychological test commonly used to evaluate executive function. Others include the Stroop Test, Flanker Test, and the Tower Test. The MMSE does not thoroughly assess executive function, so additional ones are often performed in conjunction such as the Executive interview (EXIT) and Clock Drawing Test. Executive functions include planning, organizing, sequencing, problem solving, set-shifting, abstract thinking, judgement, and grasping similarities. Executive function is generally based in the frontal lobes of the cerebral cortex (although injury to other brain regions can produce similar impairments due to functional connections). The Rorschach is a projective test. The Vineland scale is used to evaluate functional ability of impaired (i.e., mentally retarded) individuals.

1. Goldberg E, Bougakov D. Neuropsychologic assessment of frontal lobe dysfunction. *Psychiatr Clin North Am*. 2005;28:567–580.
2. Mitchell AJ. *Neuropsychiatry and Behavioural Neurology Explained*. Philadelphia: WB Saunders; 2004:77–79.
3. Royall DR, Lauterbach EC, Cummings JL, et al. Executive control function: a review of its promise and challenges for clinical research. A report from the Committee on Research of the American Neuropsychiatric Association. *J Neuropsychiatry Clin Neurosci*. 2002;14:377–405.

58. **Answer: A.** The patient's symptoms are most consistent with cyclothymia. The lifetime prevalence of cyclothymic disorder is estimated to be about 1%. Patients with cyclothymic disorder may constitute 3% to 5% of all psychiatric outpatients, with a female to male ratio of 3:2. The DSM-IV-TR criteria for cyclothymia include at least 2 years of numerous periods with hypomanic symptoms and numerous periods with depressive symptoms that do not meet the criteria for MDEs. This is an important distinguishing factor between cyclothymia and bipolar disorder type II, which includes hypomanic episodes alternating with MDEs. For the diagnosis of cyclothymia to be made, there can be no episodes of mania or major depression in the 2-year period of mood disturbance. The patient's absence of psychiatric hospitalization and psychosis is important, as these symptoms, if occurring during a period of euphoric or irritable mood, would be more consistent with mania versus hypomania. Like dysthymic disorder, cyclothymic disorder frequently coexists with borderline personality disorder. Treatment of cyclothymia includes mood stabilizers and antimanic drugs as well as psychotherapy aimed at education to raise symptom awareness and increase coping skills.

Sadock BJ, Sadock VA. *Kaplan and Sadock's Synopsis of Psychiatry*. 9th ed. Philadelphia: Lippincott Williams & Wilkins; 2003:576–578.

59. **Answer: E.** Insomnia not hypersomnolence is common in opioid withdrawal. Piloerection, nausea, vomiting, lacrimation, muscle aches, and yawning are also common in withdrawal from opioid drugs.

Sadock BJ, Sadock VA. *Kaplan and Sadock's Comprehensive Textbook of Psychiatry*. 8th ed. Philadelphia: Lippincott Williams & Wilkins; 2005:1272.

60. **Answer: E.** Bipolar disorder is a recurrent disorder. An earlier onset increases the risk of recurrence. The time between episodes tends to decrease as the individual ages.

American Psychiatric Association. *Diagnostic and Statistical Manual of Mental Disorders: DSM-IV-TR*. 4th ed. Text Revision. http://www.med.yale.edu/library/. Published December 4, 2006.

61. **Answer: B.** The patient has pellagra, a disorder caused by niacin deficiency. It is associated with vegetarian diets, alcoholism, and extreme malnutrition, and the main results are commonly dermatitis, diarrhea, dementia, delirium, and death (the "five Ds"). The rashes are typically in a bilateral distribution in exposed areas, and patients often have peripheral neuropathies. Thiamine deficiency, vitamin B_{12} deficiency, mercury poisoning, and manganese poisoning can all cause neuropsychiatric symptoms of different constellations, some of which overlap with niacin deficiency. However, the rashes, the vegetarian diet, and diarrhea point to niacin deficiency. Mercury poisoning (associated with working in the lead industry and eating certain fish and grain) is classically associated with the Mad Hatter syndrome (depression, irritability, and psychosis) as well as, among other medical problems, visual field defects. A vitamin B_{12} deficiency arises from deficiency in intrinsic factor, which transports B_{12}, and, is therefore, necessary for absorption. This condition is classically associated with peripheral neuropathies, as well as dementia and other neuropsychiatric symptoms. Patients develop megaloblastic anemia, which can be seen on peripheral smear. Thiamine deficiency is associated with alcoholism and is classically associated with Wernicke-Korsakoff syndrome, as well as beriberi. Manganese poisoning in its early stages leads to "manganese madness," which includes joint pains, headaches, somnolence, and irritability.

It eventually leads to neuropsychiatric symptoms, among which the most prominent is the distinctive symptom of pathological laughter.

Kaplan HI, Sadock BJ. *Kaplan & Sadock's Synopsis of Psychiatry*. 8th ed. Philadelphia: Lippincott Williams & Wilkins; 1998:363.

62. Answer: E. A registry study of 119,547 births showed higher rates of respiratory distress and birth weight below the 10th percentile in SSRI exposed fetuses compared to nonexposed fetuses. In a case-control study, SSRI exposure during the second trimester was associated with persistent pulmonary hypertension (6 to 12 in 1,000 births) compared to nonexposure (1 to 2 per 1,000 births). Lastly, in a study of 120 term infants, 30% of the 60 infants with prolonged exposure to SSRIs (versus 0% of nonexposed infants) developed neonatal abstinence syndrome.

1. Oberlander TF, Warburton W, Misri S, et al. Neonatal outcomes after prenatal exposure to selective serotonin reuptake inhibitor antidepressants and maternal depression using population-based linked health data. *Arch Gen Psychiatry*. 2006;63:898–906.
2. Gentile S. The safety of newer antidepressants in pregnancy and breastfeeding. *Drug Saf*. 2005;28:137–152.

63. Answer: D. Pimozide has a half-life ranging between 29 to 150 hours. This may be of clinical importance in the treatment of patients who are irregularly compliant with their treatment.

Johnstone EC, Freeman CPL, Zealley AK. *Companion to Psychiatric Studies*. 6th ed. London: Churchill Livingstone; 1998:82–85.

64. Answer: B. Among the listed drugs, temazepam is the only one that is not metabolized by the hepatic microsomal enzyme system (3A4 isoenzyme family). The other benzodiazepines that are not metabolized by his system include lorazepam and oxazepam.

Albers LJ, Hahn RK, Reist C. *Handbook of Psychiatric Drugs*. Laguna Hills: Current Clinical Strategies Publishing; 2005:56–57.

65. Answer: D. Bupropion has dopaminergic and noradrenergic activity with no clinically significant effect on serotonin reuptake. It is rapidly absorbed from GI tract and is extensively metabolized by the liver with a pronounced first-pass effect. Only approximately 1% of bupropion is excreted unchanged in urine. Bupropion crosses the placental barrier, but fetal concentrations are lower than for maternal tissues. It is excreted in breast milk. The most commonly reported side effects are headache, nausea, dry mouth, and insomnia. Clinically, agitation, tremor, and insomnia are the most common side effects that limit treatment. Small increases in blood pressure are pos-

sible, but orthostatic hypotension has not been reported. Sexual dysfunction is uncommon, and sedation and weight gain are rare. Psychotic symptoms have been described in case reports but are rare and generally associated with complicating factors such as prior psychosis. The seizure rate at mild to moderate doses is 0.1%, which is comparable to other antidepressants. Increased rates of seizures are seen with higher doses of the intermediate release formulation, but the rates are not higher than the rates with higher doses of tricyclics.

Sadock BJ, Sadock VA. *Kaplan and Sadock's Comprehensive Textbook of Psychiatry*. 8th ed. Philadelphia: Lippincott Williams & Wilkins; 2005:2791–2796.

66. Answer: D. Zidovudine, which is used to treat HIV, can cause vivid dreams as a side effect, as well as insomnia, agitation, mania, auditory hallucinations, and confusion.

McDaniels SJ, Brown L, Cournos F, et al. *Quick Reference to the American Psychiatric Association Practice Guidelines for the Treatment of Psychiatric Disorders*. Arlington: American Psychiatric Association; 2004:53.

67. Answer: E. Female murderers are seventy times more likely than are women in the general population to present one of the following profiles: (i) Antisocial Personality Disorder, (ii) alcohol/drug dependence and concomitant Personality Disorder, and (iii) alcohol/drug dependence and concomitant schizophrenia. One study found that, after the first murder, 31 (23%) women studied committed subsequent crimes, 15% of which were violent crimes. Of the women presenting with criminal recidivism, 81% presented personality disorders and 10% presented psychosis. The remaining women presented no mental disorders. After the first murder, 3% of the women studied committed another murder. In a similar study involving males, 2% presented homicidal recidivism.

Valenca AM, Moraes TM. Relationship between homicide and mental disorders. *Rev Bras Psiquiatr*. 2006;28:S62–S68.

68. Answer: D. Antibiotic medications that should not be used concurrently with lithium include metronidazole and tetracycline. Metronidazole has been reported to cause serious renal toxicity when combined with lithium.

Rosenbaum JR, Arana GW, Hyman SE, et al. *Handbook of Psychiatric Drug Therapy*. 5th ed. Philadelphia: Lippincott Williams & Wilkins; 2005:148.

69. Answer: C. Hemispheric specialization of the brain is related to handedness of the individual. Handedness appears to be genetically determined. In 96% of the right-handed individuals, who constitute 91% of the human population, the left hemisphere is the dominant or categorical hemisphere. In the remaining 4%, the right hemisphere is dominant. In approximately 15% of left-handed individuals the right hemisphere is the categorical hemisphere, and in another 15% of left-handers there is no clear lateralization. However, in the remaining 70% of left-handers, the left hemisphere is the categorical hemisphere. Learning disabilities such as dyslexia are twelve times as common in left-handers than they are in right-handed individuals. The spatial talents of left-handers are above average as a disproportionately large number of artists, musicians, and mathematicians are left-handed, but for unknown reasons left-handers have slightly shorter lifespans than right-handers.

Ganong, WF. *Review of Medical Physiology*. 22nd ed. http://www.accessmedicine.com/content.aspx?aID=702666. Published February 19, 2007.

70. Answer: B. Of the following disorders, Fragile X syndrome does not have an autosomal dominant mode of inheritance. Fragile X syndrome is inherited as an X-linked recessive mode of inheritance.

Rowland LP. *Merritt's Neurology*. 11th ed. Philadelphia: Lippincott Williams & Wilkins; 2005:686.

71. Answer: B. Wernicke's encephalopathy is an acute disorder characterized by the clinical triad of ophthalmoplegia, ataxia, and confusion. It is caused by thiamine (vitamin B_1) deficiency and is most common in chronic alcoholics. Ataxia usually affects the gait and not the legs or arms. Dysarthria is rare, though an amnestic syndrome or global confusional state, horizontal or combined nystagmus, bilateral lateral rectus palsies, and absent ankle jerks may also be found. Diagnosis is established by response to administration of intravenous thiamine. Ocular palsies usually improve first and usually within hours. The remaining symptoms resolve within a few days. However, ataxia is fully reversible in only about 40% of patients.

Greenberg DA, Aminoff MJ, Simon RP. *Clinical Neurology*. 5th ed. New York: McGraw-Hill; 2002:114.

72. Answer: B. TGA is most likely caused by a basilar artery TIA. During a TGA attack, patients cannot memorize or encode new information (i.e., they have anterograde amnesia). They also cannot recall recently acquired information such as events of the last several hours or days, so they also have retrograde amnesia. They may lose track of their responses during an interview by a physician and ask several times for the same information to be repeated. However,

they retain their general knowledge and fundamental personal information. This helps to distinguish the condition from non-neurologic amnesia. Because the motor system is spared, patients walk and talk normally. TGA often occurs in middle-aged or older individuals in the midst of exertion. The onset is abrupt and usually the disorder resolves in several hours. The total duration, by definition, should not exceed 24 hours. Ten percent of patients have recurrent episodes. Wernicke-Korsakoff syndrome occurs with chronic, excessive alcohol consumption. The distinctive features of the disease are retrograde amnesia, anterograde amnesia, and confabulation. While it is often found in chronic alcoholics, it probably occurs from a profound nutritional deficiency of thiamine (vitamin B_1). Even with timely treatment with intravenous thiamine, only 25% of patients recover completely from the cognitive impairment associated with the illness. The pathologic changes are irreversible. In terms of differentiating TGA from Wernicke-Korsakoff syndrome, TGA patients do not confabulate. Partial complex seizures differ from TGA by producing dulling of the sensorium; simple repetitive actions, epileptiform EEG changes, and a high rate of recurrence. Dissociative amnesia consists of one or more episodes of amnesia for fundamental personal information. The amnesia may be highly selective for specific events and does not include an anterograde component. In dissociate fugue, individuals travel away from work or home. They may assume a new identity and are amnestic for personal information concerning their past life. Although they have retrograde amnesia, they do not have anterograde amnesia.

Kaufman DM. *Clinical Neurology for Psychiatrists*. 5th ed. Philadelphia: WB Saunders; 2001:143–144, 273–274.

73. Answer: A. Acute intermittent porphyria is inherited as an autosomal dominant trait. There is increased production and urinary excretion of porphobilinogen and its precursor δ-aminolevulinic acid. The urine turns dark upon standing due to formation of porphobilin, which is an oxidation product of porphobilinogen. Attacks are usually recurrent and are often precipitated by drugs, which induce the enzyme δ-aminolevulinic acid synthetase such as sulfonamides, griseofulvin, estrogens, barbiturates, phenytoin, and the succinimide anticonvulsants. Other precipitants include infection, fasting, pregnancy, or occasionally menses. Treatment is with intravenous glucose, which suppresses the heme biosynthetic pathway, and intravenous hematin.

Ropper AH, Brown RH. *Adams and Victor's Principles of Neurology*. 8th ed. New York: McGraw-Hill; 2005:1129.

74. Answer: D. Suicide attempts tend to cluster in the first 6 months after diagnosis. The risk factors for suicide also include previous psychiatric illness, alcohol and drug abuse, long term dependency, prospect of an inexorable terminal illness, social stigma and other difficult social issues relating to homosexuality, and inadequate social and financial support. Although males appear to be at increased risk of suicide, this appears not to be related to age.

1. Lishman WA. *Organic Psychiatry*. 3rd ed. Oxford: Blackwell Science; 1996:330–331.
2. Sadock BJ, Sadock VA. *Kaplan and Sadock's Synopsis of Psychiatry*. 9th ed. Philadelphia: Lippincott Williams & Wilkins; 2003:376–377.

75. Answer: B. GSS and FFI have autosomal dominant pattern of inheritance. Five to fifteen percent of CJD cases are familial with an autosomal dominant pattern of inheritance. Kuru was transmitted through of ingestion of infected brain material at cannibalistic rituals in Papua New Guinea with no new cases since the cessation of ritual cannibalism.

1. Lishman WA. *Organic Psychiatry*. 3rd ed. Oxford: Blackwell Science; 1996:473–479.
2. Rowland LP. *Merritt's Neurology*. 11th ed. Philadelphia: Lippincott Williams & Wilkins; 2005:264–268.

76. Answer: C. Subdural hematoma is caused by the filling of blood in the potential space between the dural and arachnoid membranes. In most cases, it comes from a venous source and from the tearing of veins that drain from the surface of the brain to the dural sinuses. Most subdural hematomas are located over the lateral cerebral convexities, but may also occur along the medial surface of the hemisphere, between the tentorium and occipital lobe, between the temporal lobe and the base of the skull, and in the posterior fossa. The risk of subdural hematomas is highest in the elderly and alcoholic patients who have cerebral atrophy. In these patients, hematomas may result from trivial injuries. In acute subdural hematomas, symptoms occur within 72 hours of injury. However, most patients have neurological symptoms from the moment of impact. Many patients (50%) with an acute subdural hematoma lose consciousness at the time of injury and about 25% will be in coma when they arrive at the hospital. Half of those patients who awaken will lose consciousness for a second time after a "lucid interval." Hemiparesis and pupillary abnormalities are the most common focal neurologic signs occurring in over 50% of all patients. Patients usually present with ipsilateral pupillary dilation and contralateral hemiparesis. Chronic subdural hematomas become symptomatic after about 3 weeks of the injury. They occur in older patients and in 50% of cases and there are no recognized head traumas. Many patients have histories of alcoholism, epilepsy, and previous traumas. Risk factors include overdrainage of ventriculoperitoneal shunts, bleeding disorders, and anticoagulant therapy. Most cases occur after mild trauma. CT scan of the brain typically shows an isodense or hypodense, crescent-shaped lesion that deforms the surface of the brain. Patients may present with altered mental status and this may be mistaken for dementia. Cerebral hygromas develop in some cases of chronic subdural hematoma. In both types, the main indication for surgery is the presence of symptomatic mass effect or seizures. The main treatment is the evacuation of the blood via craniotomy. The prognosis after surgical evacuation depends on the severity of the initial deficit and the interval from injury to surgery. Steroids do not have any role in the management of smaller, minimally symptomatic lesions.

Rowland LP. *Merritt's Neurology*. 11th ed. Lippincott Williams & Wilkins; 2005:487–488.

77. Answer: C. The patient described suffers from akathisia, which is characterized by a subjective feeling of restlessness and the need to move, especially in the legs. Patients often appear restless with symptoms of anxiety or agitation. Akathisia is a very common side effect of many conventional antipsychotic medications (dopamine receptor antagonists), with a greater likelihood from high-potency typical antipsychotics than with low-potency typical antipsychotics. It usually arises within the first few days of treatment, and although atypical antipsychotics have a lower prevalence than typicals, they still do occasionally have this side effect. Akathisia can be misdiagnosed for a worsening of the psychotic illness and will get worse if the antipsychotic is increased. Symptoms do not get better over time if the medication is left unchanged, but will tend to remit soon after medications are discontinued, unlike tardive extrapyramidal symptoms. Middle-aged women have been reported to be at the highest risk for developing akathisia.

1. Rosenbaum JF, Arana GW, Hyman SE, et al. *Handbook of Psychiatric Drug Therapy*. 5th ed. Philadelphia: Lippincott Williams & Wilkins; 2005:41–42.
2. Sadock BJ, Sadock VA. *Kaplan and Sadock's Comprehensive Textbook of Psychiatry*. 8th ed. Philadelphia: Lippincott Williams & Wilkins; 2005:2716, 2725, 2730, 2829.

78. Answer: D. There are currently four dopamine agonists available in the United States: bromocriptine, pergolide, pramipexole, and ropinirole. The older dopamine agonists, bromocriptine and pergolide, are ergot derivatives and carry the risk of complications such as vasoconstriction, exacerbation of peptic ulcer disease, and pulmonary/retroperitoneal fibrosis. Pramipexole and ropinirole are nonergoline agonists and carry a lower risk of such complications. Entacapone is a COMT inhibitor which works to preserve dopamine concentrations by retarding dopamine metabolism.

1. Kaufman DM. *Clinical Neurology for Psychiatrists*. 5th ed. Philadelphia: WB Saunders; 2001:455–457.
2. Rao SS, Hofmann LA, Shakil A. Parkinson's disease: diagnosis and treatment. *Am Fam Physician*. 2006;74:2046–2054.
3. Rolak LA. *Neurology Secrets*. 2nd ed. Philadelphia: Hanley & Belfus; 1998:147–148.

79. Answer: A. Pharmacokinetics and pharmacodynamics are significantly affected by changes in the body with aging. Volume of distribution is an important part of pharmacokinetics which is affected by aging. The elderly have a decrease in lean muscle mass and total body water, resulting in a decrease in volume of distribution. This is of particular importance when prescribing drugs, which are primarily distributed in water such as lithium. With a decrease in renal mass and renal blood flow with age, the elderly have a reduction in GFR, which can affect the rate at which some drugs are cleared from the body. In addition, hepatic blood flow declines with age, resulting in a decrease in hepatic drug clearance. Because of these changes in drug clearance and volume of distribution, the elimination half-life of some medications increases and doses should be adjusted accordingly. Certain changes with age result in an increase in drug absorption time (i.e., longer gastrointestinal transit time), while other changes result in a decrease in absorption time (i.e., reduction in acid secretion and gastrointestinal perfusion). The net result is no change in absorption with aging. With regard to pharmacodynamic effects of drugs, the elderly are often more sensitive to medications (e.g., those with anticholinergic properties) and often require lower starting doses.

Blazer DG, Steffens DC, Busse EW. *The American Psychiatric Association Textbook of Geriatric Psychiatry*. Washington: American Psychiatric Publishing; 2004:44–45.

80. Answer: D. This patient is presenting with intention (or kinetic) tremor, which is most likely secondary to a lesion in the cerebellar pathways. This tremor is most noticeable during goal-directed movements. Kinetic tremor can also occur with benign essential tremor, although the most characteristic tremor in this condition is postural tremor, which appears in extremities that are in an antigravity posture. Resting tremor appears in relaxed extremities and disappears, or becomes less noticeable, during movement of the extremity. It is secondary to diseases that affect the basal ganglia. Physiologic tremor can appear due to fatigue, anxiety, and alcohol or opiate withdrawal.

Brazis PW, Masdeu JC, Biller J. *Localization in Clinical Neurology*. 5th ed. Philadelphia: Lippincott Williams & Wilkins; 2007:440–447.

81. Answer: D. Ethologists Konrad Lorenz and Nikolaas Tinbergen described innate releasing mechanisms as animals' responses (i.e., sexual, aggressive, intimate, etc.), which are triggered and evoked by releasers or specific environmental stimuli (including shapes, colors, and sounds). Tinbergen described displacement activities as those that occur when a conflict arises and the need for fight and for flight are roughly equal strength, so the animal engages in behavior that appears to be irrelevant to the situation. *Fitness* is a term which sociobiologists postulate human behavior has evolved to achieve, and is defined as the highest measure of evolutionary success (i.e., the best genes are passed from one generation to the next). Temperament is mediated by genetics and plays a role in behavior (or personality).

Kaplan HI, Sadock BJ. *Kaplan & Sadock's Synopsis of Psychiatry*. 8th ed. Philadelphia: Lippincott Williams & Wilkins; 2005.

82. Answer: D. Validity is an important concept that concerns the degree to which a measurement or study reaches a correct conclusion. In general medicine, validity is often compared to the "gold standard" test, which is often nonexistent in psychiatry. Psychiatric validity is often based upon consistency of diagnosis over time and the ability of the test to predict long-term outcome. Choice A, B, C, and E describe reliability, generalizability, statistical power, and likelihood, respectively.

Greenberg RS, Daniels SR, Flanders WD, et al. *Medical Epidemiology*. 3rd ed. New York: McGraw-Hill; 2001:144.

83. Answer: A. There are three delineated frontal lobe behavioral syndromes: orbitofrontal, mediofrontal, and dorsolateral prefrontal. This patient displays behaviors typical with orbitofrontal lesions—disinhibition, impulsivity, and impaired judgment. Mediofrontal lesions, also known as anterior cingulated lesions, cause apathy and amotivation. DLPFC cause the classic "dysexecutive" syndrome with loss of cognitive flexibility, impaired planning, sequencing, and multitasking, difficulty with attention/distraction, and difficulty with foresight and monitoring of performance. Injuries to DLPFC also impair working memory, abstract thinking, and motor fluency.

1. Goldberg E, Bougakov D. Neuropsychologic assessment of frontal lobe dysfunction. *Psychiatr Clin North Am*. 2005;28:567–580.

2. Mitchell AJ. *Neuropsychiatry and Behavioral Neurology Explained*. Philadelphia: Saunders; 2004:77–79.
3. Royall DR, Lauterbach EC, Cummings JL, et al. Executive control function: a review of its promise and challenges for clinical research. A report from the Committee on Research of the American Neuropsychiatric Association. *J Neuropsychiatry Clin Neurosci*. 2002;14:377–405.

84. Answer: C. Unlike MDD, Bipolar disorder type I has an equal prevalence among men and women. The mean age of onset of Bipolar I is 30, generally earlier than that of MDD, which has a mean age of onset of 40. Bipolar I, a recurring mood disorder, most often starts with a depressive episode (75% of the time in women, 67% of the time in men). Approximately 10% to 20% of patients with Bipolar I experience only manic episodes, though the majority of patients experience both depressive and manic episodes. Patients with "rapid cycling" have four or more mood episodes per year, and constitute 5% to 15% of all patients with Bipolar I. Patients with Bipolar I have a poorer prognosis than those with MDD. Factors that contribute to a poorer prognosis include alcohol dependence, psychotic features, poor premorbid occupational status, interepisode depressive features, and male gender. Good prognostic indicators include advanced age at onset, few suicidal thoughts, few medical and psychiatric comorbidities, and short duration of manic episodes.

Sadock BJ, Sadock VA. *Kaplan and Sadock's Synopsis of Psychiatry*. 9th ed. Philadelphia: Lippincott Williams & Wilkins; 2003: 534–560.

85. Answer: E. PCP is thought to block the N-methyl-D-aspartate type receptor of the excitatory neurotransmitter glutamate.

Sadock BJ, Sadock VA. *Kaplan and Sadock's Comprehensive Textbook of Psychiatry*. 8th ed. Philadelphia: Lippincott Williams & Wilkins; 2005:1291.

86. Answer: A. The National Institutes of Mental Health (NIMH) Epidemiologic Catchment Area (ECA) study and the National Comorbidity Survey found a lifetime prevalence of 0.3% to 1.5%. The 6-month prevalence was not much lower, which suggests chronicity of the illness.

Gelder MG, Lopez Ibor JJ, Andreasen NC. *New Oxford Textbook of Psychiatry*. 1st ed. Oxford: Oxford University Press; 2000:696.

87. Answer: E. One of the important and disturbing findings of the first phase of the CATIE trial was that 74% of patients with Chronic Schizophrenia stopped taking their antipsychotic medications before the end of the 18-month trial. The lowest percentage of discontinuation occurred with patients who took olan-

zapine. However, even the percentage of patients who stopped taking olanzapine was 64%, suggests that, in terms of overall effectiveness, there is much room for improvement in the treatment of chronic schizophrenia.

Lieberman JL, Stroup TS, McEvoy JP, et al. Effectiveness of antipsychotic drugs in patients with chronic schizophrenia. *NEJM*. 2005;353:1209–1223.

88. Answer: E. Neonatal abstinence syndrome from SSRIs generally peak 48 hours after delivery and resolves in 4 days. Symptoms include high-pitched cry, sleep disturbance, tremor, hypertonicity or myoclonus, tachypnea, and gastrointestinal symptoms.

Sanz EJ, De-las-Cuevas C, Kiuru A, et al. Selective serotonin reuptake inhibitors in pregnant women and neonatal withdrawal syndrome: a database analysis. *Lancet*. 2005;365:482–487.

89. Answer: B. Hypothyroidism is the odd one out with thyroid overactivity being another differential diagnosis for Tardive Dyskinesia. Others include hepatic failure, postencephalitic, renal failure, SLE, brain tumors, torsion dystonia, chorea gravidarum of pregnancy, and drug-induced (antidepressants, levodopa, antimalarials, heavy metals, sympathomimetics, and antihistamines) Schizophrenic mannerisms and stereotypies.

Kaplan HI, Sadock BJ. *Kaplan and Sadock's Synopsis of Psychiatry*. 9th ed. Philadelphia: Lippincott Williams & Wilkins; 2003:1060.

90. Answer: C. A systematic review of patient views of ECT outcome found that significant persistent memory loss was reported by at least one third of patients. The incidence of memory loss with ECT is dependent upon treatment parameters including electrode placement, dose of stimulus, and type of stimulus used. Bilateral electrode placement, higher stimulus dosages, and sine wave form contribute to higher rates of cognitive and memory dysfunction. Other risk factors include advancing age, lower premorbid intellectual function, and female gender. Patients can develop either retrograde and/or anterograde amnesia. In retrograde amnesia, the memory of recent events is more impaired than that of remote events. Impersonal or public events are lost more frequently than autobiographical events. Retrograde memory loss recovers more slowly than anterograde loss and in some patients it may even be persistent. Degree of pretreatment global cognitive impairment and the length of postictal confusion are predictive of retrograde memory loss. Most patients do not suffer permanent anterograde memory loss and tend to improve within a few weeks to a few months.

1. Sackeim HA, Prudic J, Fuller R, et al. The cognitive effects of electroconvulsive therapy in community settings. *Neuropsychopharmacology*. 2007;32:244–254.
2. Tess A, Smetana GW. *Medical consultation for electroconvulsive therapy*. http://www.uptodateonline.com/utd/content/topic.do?topicKey=med_cons/7978&type=A&selectedTitle=1~13. Accessed March 6, 2007.

91. Answer: E. SNRIs are medications that have therapeutic effects that are presumably mediated by concomitant blockade of neuronal serotonin and norepinephrine uptake transporters. Two SNRIs are currently available in the United States: venlafaxine and duloxetine. Venlafaxine primarily blocks serotonin uptake at low therapeutic doses, with the noradrenergic effects more prominent in higher doses (above 150 mg approximately). There is minimal affinity for muscarinic, H_1histamine, and adrenergic receptors. After being metabolized by the liver, SNRIs are primarily eliminated by the kidneys. Clearance is reduced in patients with cirrhosis or severe renal disease, necessitating lower doses for such patients. Nausea is the most frequently reported adverse effect associated with SNRIs. An incidence of approximately 35% has been reported with venlafaxine (22% in duloxetine) in short-term placebo-controlled trials, which is higher than in trials with SSRIs. Therapy is associated with sexual side effects, predominantly decreased libido and a delay to orgasm or ejaculation. Higher-dose venlafaxine therapy is associated with an increased risk of sustained elevations of blood pressure. Duloxetine is also associated with increased blood pressure, but in contrast to venlafaxine, it does not appear to be a dose dependent phenomenon.

Sadock BJ, Sadock VA. *Kaplan and Sadock's Comprehensive Textbook of Psychiatry*. 8th ed. Philadelphia: Lippincott Williams & Wilkins; 2005:2881–2885.

92. Answer: E. Naltrexone is an opioid-receptor antagonist approved for use in the treatment of alcohol dependence in conjunction with psychosocial interventions. It is believed that naltrexone works through its blockage of μ-opioid receptors, which reduces the reinforcing effects of alcohol leading to decreased feelings of intoxication and fewer cravings. A systematic review found that naltrexone reduces short-term relapse rates in patients with alcohol dependence when combined with psychosocial treatments. Short-term outcomes that favor treatment with naltrexone included fewer patients relapsing to alcohol dependence (38% versus 60% with placebo), fewer patients returning to drinking (61% versus 69%), reduced cravings for alcohol, and fewer drinking days. The data showed one relapse was prevented for every five patients treated with naltrexone (i.e., number needed to treat [NNT] = 5). Another systematic review assessing medium-term outcomes (six to 12 months) indicated that there is no difference between naltrexone and placebo groups in the treatment of patients with alcohol dependence. In a recent trial comparing outcomes of three therapy groups (12 months of naltrexone therapy, 3 months of naltrexone followed by 9 months of placebo, and 12 months of placebo) found no significant differences among the groups in the number of days to relapse, number of drinking days, or number of drinks per drinking day. Hence the evidence supporting short-term benefit with naltrexone is good, but the evidence for long-term use is less compelling. Naltrexone has been shown to have dose-related hepatotoxicity, although it generally occurs at doses higher than those recommended for treatment of alcohol dependence. The drug also is contraindicated in patients with hepatitis or liver failure, and all patients should have hepatic transaminase levels checked monthly for the first 3 months and every 3 months thereafter. Nausea is the most common adverse effect (reported by 10% of patients), followed by headache, anxiety, and sedation. Naltrexone is FDA pregnancy category C.

1. Krystal JH, Cramer JA, Krol WF, et al. Naltrexone in the treatment of alcohol dependence. *N Engl J Med*. 2001;345:1734–1739.
2. Srisurapanont M, Jarusuraisin N. Opioid antagonists for alcohol dependence. *Cochrane Database Syst Rev*. 2005;1:CD001867.
3. Williams SH. Medications for treating alcohol dependence. *Am Fam Physician*. 2005;72:1775–1780.

93. Answer: D. The NIMH's ECA study, which examined the rates of various psychiatric disorders in a representative sample of 17,803 subjects in five United States communities showed that patients with serious mental illness (i.e., those with Schizophrenia, Major Depression, or Bipolar Disorder) were two to three times as likely as people without such an illness to be assaultive. Translated to absolute terms, the lifetime prevalence of violence among people with serious mental illness was 16%, as compared with 7% among people without mental illness. The lifetime risk of Schizophrenia was 5% among people convicted of homicide, a prevalence that is much higher than the rate of Schizophrenia in the general population. The presence of Schizophrenia, Major Depression, or Bipolar disorder is significantly associated with an increased risk of violence. The attributable risk of serious mental illness to violence has been estimated to be around 3% to 5%, much lower than that associated with Substance Abuse. Substance Abuse among the mentally ill compounds the increased risk of violence. Violence is independently correlated with several risk factors, including Substance Abuse, a history of having been a victim of violence, homelessness, and poor medical health. The 1-year rate of violent behavior for subjects with none or only one of these risk factors was 2%, a prevalence close to the ECA study's estimate for the general population. A study comparing the prevalence of violence in a group of psychiatric patients during the year after hospital discharge with the rate in the community in which the patients lived showed no difference in the risk of violence between treated patients and people without a psychiatric disorder. Thus, symptoms of psychiatric illness, rather than the diagnosis itself, appear to confer the risk of violent behavior.

Friedman RA. Violence and mental illness–how strong is the link? *N Engl J Med*. 2006;355:2064–2066.

94. **Answer: D.** Hormones can be divided into two general classes by structure and by the location of their function. On the basis of structure, they can be divided into (i) proteins, polypeptides, and glycoproteins; and (ii) steroids and steroid-like compounds. By location of function, they can be divided into three classes. The proteins, polypeptides, and glycoproteins hormones include, adrenocorticotropic hormone, beta-endorphin, thyrotropin-releasing hormone, LH, and follicle-stimulating hormone (FSH). They are stored in vesicles and are lipid insoluble. The steroids and steroid-like compounds include cortisol, estrogens, testosterone, progesterone, and dehydroepiandrosterone. They are not stored and diffuse after synthesis and are lipid soluble. The hormones can be divided into three classes by location of function into autocrine type which has self-regulatory effects, paracrine with local or adjacent cellular action and endocrine with distant target site activity. In addition to their action on a target tissue, they can also act as neuromodulators, regulating the effects of neurotransmitters or occasionally function independently as a neurotransmitter.

Sadock BJ, Sadock VA. *Kaplan and Sadock's Comprehensive Textbook of Psychiatry*. 8th ed. Philadelphia: Lippincott Williams & Wilkins; 2005:126.

95. **Answer: D.** Short- and long-term changes can occur in the synaptic function as a result of the history of discharge at a synapse. Pre- and postsynaptic conduction can be increased or decreased on the basis of past experience. Habituation occurs when a benign stimulus is repeated over and the response to the stimulus gradually weakens and disappears. Ha-

bituation is associated with decreased release of neurotransmitter from the presynaptic terminal because of decreased intracellular calcium. The decrease in intracellular calcium occurs due to a gradual inactivation of the calcium channels. This effect can occur for a short period or it can be prolonged if the exposure to the stimulus is repeated many times. Sensitization is the postsynaptic response to a habituated stimulus that is paired with a noxious stimulus. Sensitization occurs due to presynaptic facilitation. Sensitization can be a transient response, or prolonged if it is reinforced by additional pairings of the noxious stimulus and the initial stimulus. The prolongation of sensitization is due to a calcium mediated change in adenylyl cyclase activity that leads to a greater production of cyclic adenosine monophosphateAMP. LTP is the development of persistent enhancement of the postsynaptic potential responses to presynaptic stimulation after a brief period of rapidly repeated stimulation of the presynaptic neuron. It occurs by an increase in intracellular calcium levels in the postsynaptic neuron. LTP also involves protein synthesis and growth of the presynaptic and postsynaptic neurons and their connections.

Ganong, WF. *Review of Medical Physiology*. 22nd ed. http://www.accessmedicine.com/content.aspx?aID=707278. Accessed February 19, 2007.

96. **Answer: B.** Dementia associated with stroke (Vascular Dementia) is the second most frequent cause of dementia after AD, with as many as 15% to 20% of patients with acute ischemic stroke over age 60 years have dementia at the time of the stroke, and 5% per year become demented thereafter. Risk factors for development of Vascular Dementia include advancing age, diabetes, history of prior stroke, and the size and location of the stroke. The exact nature of complex interaction between stroke, vascular risk factors, and AD, remains unknown.

Rowland LP. *Merritt's Neurology*. 11th ed. Philadelphia: Lippincott Williams & Wilkins; 2005:771–780.

97. **Answer: C.** Gerstmann's syndrome occurs due to lesions in the angular gyrus of the dominant parietal lobe. It is accompanied by agraphia (inability to write), acalculia (impairment of arithmetic skills), finger agnosia (inability to identify fingers), and left-right confusion. Patients, however, rarely display all four of these components.

Kaufman DM. *Clinical Neurology for Psychiatrists*. 5th ed. Philadelphia: WB Saunders; 2001:9, 185–186.

98. **Answer: C.** Neurosyphilis is caused by persistent infection of the CNS by *Treponema pallidum*. Standard screening blood tests for syphilis include VDRL and RPR; neither is highly sensitive or specific. The newer

blood tests, FTA-ABS and the treponemal micro-hemagglutination assay, have improved sensitivity and specificity. If neurosyphilis is suspected, CSF testing should be done. The VDRL is the only currently available CSF test for neurosyphilis; however, it may have a false-negative rate of up to 40%. Additional findings in the CSF include elevated protein concentration (45 to 100 mg/dL) and a lymphocytic pleocytosis. The clinical presentation and CSF findings are usually adequate to make the diagnosis of neurosyphilis. Penicillin remains the gold-standard treatment for neurosyphilis.

Kaufman DM. *Clinical Neurology for Psychiatrists*. 5th ed. Philadelphia: WB Saunders; 2001:147–148.

99. **Answer: C.** The patient in the vignette has benign paroxysmal positional vertigo (BPPV). This is a peripheral vestibular disorder. BPPV is the most common cause of vertigo of peripheral origin and accounts for about 30% of cases. It is occasionally, though, due to central disease. BPPV occurs upon assuming a particular position, and is often caused by head trauma but may be idiopathic. It is characterized by brief episodes of severe vertigo that occur with any change in head position and may be accompanied by nausea and vomiting. Vertigo and nystagmus are often delayed in onset by several seconds after assumption of the precipitating head position. Usually, symptoms are most severe in the lateral decubitus position with the affected ear down. There is a tendency for the response to remit spontaneously (fatigue) and attenuate over time (habituation). BPPV continues for several weeks and often resolves spontaneously. Central BPPV has less severe vertigo, absent position nystagmus, and no latency, fatigue, or habituation. Treatment of BPPV is by the use of repositioning maneuvers. Vestibulosuppressant drugs (antihistamines, anticholinergics, benzodiazepines, and sympathomimetics) and vestibular rehabilitation may be helpful as well. Other peripheral vestibular disorders include Ménière disease, acute peripheral vestibulopathy, otosclerosis, cerebellopontine angle tumor, toxic vestibulopathy, and acoustic (cranial nerve VIII) neuropathy.

Greenberg DA, Aminoff MJ, Simon RP. *Clinical Neurology*. 5th ed. New York: McGraw-Hill; 2002:95–126.

100. **Answer: D.** This patient is one of those so called "worried well" who belong to the high risk groups but are seronegative, disease free, but anxious about contracting the virus. Some of these people may be reassured by repeated serum tests but others cannot be reassured. It is essential to rule out depression and psychosis in such patients. The worried well status may progress to Generalized Anxiety Disorder, Panic

Disorder, OCD, and Hypochondriasis, which may be delusional. Repeated reassurance is seen to be futile and merely serves to maintain the problem. A cognitive behavioral therapy-led approach based on cue exposure and response prevention with attempts at reinterpretation of symptoms in terms of their origin in anxiety, may prove more successful in managing her anxiety.

1. Lishman WA. *Organic Psychiatry*. 3rd ed. Oxford: Blackwell Science; 1996:331–332.
2. Sadock BJ, Sadock VA. *Kaplan and Sadock's Synopsis of Psychiatry*. 9th ed. Philadelphia: Lippincott Williams & Wilkins; 2003:376–377.

101. **Answer: D.** Prions are transmissible infectious proteins which do not contain nucleic acids, unlike viruses. The characteristic neuropathological changes include spongiform vacuolization, neuronal loss, and astrocyte proliferation in the cerebral cortex. Amyloid plaques may or may not be present; these are seen in vCJD, Kuru, and in the cerebellum in GSS disease. The PrP gene is located in the short arm of chromosome 20. PrP mutates into PrP-Super-C (PrP-Sc) that can replicate and is infectious. The characteristic neuropathological changes are thought to be due to the direct neurotoxic effects of PrP-Sc.

1. Rowland LP. *Merritt's Neurology*. 11th ed. Philadelphia: Lippincott Williams & Wilkins; 2005:264–268.
2. Sadock BJ, Sadock VA. *Kaplan and Sadock's Synopsis of Psychiatry*. 9th ed. Philadelphia: Lippincott Williams & Wilkins; 2003:364–365.

102. **Answer: D.** Sudden severe headache, an altered level of consciousness, early vomiting and loss of consciousness, signs of meningeal irritation and paucity of lateralizing neurologic signs are the characteristic features of SAH. Noncontrast CT scan of the brain with or without lumbar puncture remains the main diagnostic tool for SAH.

Singer RJ, Ogilvy CS, Rordof G. *Etiology, clinical manifestations, and diagnosis of aneurysmal subarachnoid hemorrhage*. http://www.uptodateonline.com/utd/content/topic.do?topicKey=cva_dise/7752&type=A&selectedTitle=1~62. Accessed on November 11, 2007.

103. **Answer: C.** This patient described in the vignette has an essential tremor, which is one of the most common movement disorders. This postural tremor may have its onset anywhere between the second and sixth decades of life, and its prevalence increases with age. The tremor typically affects the hands and also the head, voice, tongue, and legs and may be alleviated by alcohol. Women tend to have a head tremor more than men. An alcoholic withdrawal tremor affects only the hands, unlike the multiple sites of involvement of essential tremor and the

patient does not give a history of alcoholism. The cerebellar tremor is an intention or goal-directed tremor and increases in severity as the extremity approaches a target. A psychogenic tremor includes an abrupt onset, static course, spontaneous remission, and unclassified tremor that often increases with attention and decreases with distraction. The patient's response to alcohol and other symptoms make physiologic tremor unlikely, which can occur from medications or thyroid problems.

1. Kaufman DM. *Clinical Neurology for Psychiatrists*. 5th ed. WB Saunders; 2001:446–467, 474–476.
2. Tarsy D. *Overview of tremor*. http://www.utdol.com/utd/content/topic.do?topicKey=move_dis/4697&type=A&selectedTitle=1~5. Accessed February 23, 2007.

104. Answer: C. Trihexyphenidyl and benztropine are anticholinergic agents. Selegiline is a selective MAO-B. Bromocriptine is a synthetic dopamine agonist. Tolcapone and entacapone are COMT inhibitors, which are useful as a levodopa extender.

1. Kaufman DM. *Clinical Neurology for Psychiatrists*. 5th ed. Philadelphia: WB Saunders; 2001: 455–457.
2. Rao SS, Hofmann LA, Shakil A. Parkinson's disease: diagnosis and treatment. *Am Fam Physician*. 2006;74:2046–2054.

105. Answer: B. Menopause has several important consequences for older women. The number of ovarian follicles decreases with a resulting decrease in secretion of estrogen and androgens. The decline in estrogen levels results in atrophy of the uterus and vaginal endothelium, which, in combination with decreased lubrication during sexual intercourse, can result in dyspareunia. This is the most likely explanation for this patient's symptoms, as there is no evidence of marital discord or depression. The decline in estrogen does affect bone mass and places women at risk of osteoporosis, though this is less likely to be a contributing factor to dyspareunia than vaginal atrophy. With menopause, women lose the favorable effect of estrogen on lipids, resulting in an increase in low-density protein and subsequent increase in risk of cardiovascular disease. It is important to note that sexual activity continues throughout the life cycle, with the majority of individuals over the age of 60 remaining sexually active.

Blazer DG, Steffens DC, Busse EW. *The American Psychiatric Association Textbook of Geriatric Psychiatry*. Washington: American Psychiatric Publishing; 2004:42, 303.

106. Answer: A. Infarcts of the paramedian thalamic territory usually result in somnolent apathy, memory loss, and abnormal vertical gaze. Patients also present with behavioral changes, contralateral hemi-

ataxia, asterixis, or motor weakness, as well as delayed action tremor. Patients with an infarct to the lateral thalamic territory present with hemianesthesia, transient slight hemiparesis, hemiataxia, disequilibrium, and choreoathetoid movements and posture. An infarct to the anterolateral thalamic territory produces apathy and verbal perseveration, anterograde memory loss, the superimposition of temporally unrelated information, and hemineglect. Lesions to the posterior choroidal artery territory result in homonymous quadrantanopsia, decreased optokinetic nystagmus, mild hemiparesis, and transcortical aphasia. Wallenberg syndrome is a lateral medullary syndrome and consists of diminished ipsilateral facial pain and temperature perception, diminished contralateral trunk and extremity pain and temperature perception, ipsilateral palatal, pharyngeal, and vocal cord paralysis, as well as ipsilateral Horner syndrome, vertigo and nausea, and ipsilateral cerebellar signs and symptoms.

1. Brazis PW, Masdeu JC, Biller J. *Localization in Clinical Neurology*. 5th ed. Philadelphia: Lippincott Williams & Wilkins; 2007:423–425.
2. Perren F, Clarke S, Bogousslavsky J. The syndrome of combined polar and paramedian thalamic infarction. *Arch Neurol*. 2005;62:1212–1216.

107. Answer: A. Ethologist Konrad Lorenz studied aggression and wrote about the practical function of aggression. He showed that although aggression among members of the same species is common, under normal conditions it seldom leads to killing or serious injury. Rather, a certain balance appears between tendencies to fight and flight, with the tendency to fight being strongest in the center of the territory and the tendency to flight strongest at a distance from the center. Ethologist Nikolaas Tinbergen described displacement activities as those that occur when a conflict arises and the need for fight and for flight are of roughly equal strength, so the animal engages in behavior that appears to be irrelevant to the situation. The learned helplessness model of depression was developed by Martin Seligman, where he observed that dogs exposed to electric shocks from which they could not escape eventually gave up and made to more attempts to escape, and this behavior generalized no other situations. Imprinting was also studied by Lorenz and his work showed that during a certain short period of development, a young animal is highly sensitive to a certain stimulus that provokes a specific behavior pattern.

Kaplan HI, Sadock BJ. *Kaplan & Sadock's Synopsis of Psychiatry*. 8th ed. Philadelphia: Lippincott Williams & Wilkins; 1998:162–167.

108. Answer: B. Risk of developing Schizophrenia is ten times greater for individuals with one affected first-degree relative. Risk increases with greater number of affected family members, approaching nearly 50% if both parents are affected.

1. McGuffin P, Owen MJ, Farmer AE. Genetic basis of schizophrenia. *Lancet*. 1995;346:678–682.
2. Mueser KT, McGurk SR. Schizophrenia. *Lancet*. 2004; 363:2063–2072.

109. Answer: B. There are three delineated frontal lobe behavioral syndromes: orbitofrontal, mediofrontal, and dorsolateral prefrontal. This patient displays behaviors typical with mediofrontal (aka anterior cingulate) lesions—apathy and amotivation. Orbitofrontal lesions cause disinhibition, impulsivity, and impaired judgment. DLPFC lesions cause the classic "dysexecutive" syndrome, with loss of cognitive flexibility, impaired planning, sequencing, and multitasking, difficulty with attention/distraction, and difficulty with foresight and monitoring of performance. Injuries to DLPFC also impair working memory, abstract thinking, and motor fluency.

1. Goldberg E, Bougakov D. Neuropsychologic assessment of frontal lobe dysfunction. *Psychiatr Clin North Am*. 2005;28:567–580.
2. Mitchell AJ. *Neuropsychiatry and Behavioral Neurology Explained*. Philadephia: WB Saunders; 2004:77–79.
3. Royall DR, Lauterbach EC, Cummings JL, et al. Executive control function: a review of its promise and challenges for clinical research. A report from the Committee on Research of the American Neuropsychiatric Association. *J Neuropsychiatry Clin Neurosci*. 2002;14:377–405.

110. Answer: D. Approximately 40% to 50% of alcoholics develop symptoms suggestive of other disorders, which highlights the importance of obtaining a proper history and clarifying the diagnosis and etiology.

Sadock BJ, Sadock VA. *Kaplan and Sadock's Comprehensive Textbook of Psychiatry*. 8th ed. Philadelphia: Lippincott Williams & Wilkins; 2005:1160.

111. Answer: E. Respiratory depression is minimal with benzodiazepines. This contrasts with barbiturates which have a much lower margin of safety. Even in very high doses (e.g., 2 grams) respiratory suppression is rare. However, in the presence of other sedative hypnotics such as alcohol, smaller doses of benzodiazepines can cause death.

Sadock BJ, Sadock VA. *Kaplan and Sadock's Comprehensive Textbook of Psychiatry*. 8th ed. Philadelphia: Lippincott Williams & Wilkins; 2005:1311.

112. Answer: C. In the DSM-IV-TR, PMDD is classified under depressive disorder NOS. This category includes disorders with depressive features that do not meet the criteria for MDD, dysthymic disorder, adjustment disorder with depressed mood, or adjustment disorder with mixed anxiety and depressed mood. Other examples of depressive disorder NOS include:

1. Minor depressive disorder: Episodes of at least 2 weeks of depressive symptoms but with fewer than the five items required for MDD.

2. Recurrent brief depressive disorder: Depressive episodes lasting from 2 days up to 2 weeks, occurring at least once a month for 12 months (not associated with the menstrual cycle).

3. Postpsychotic depressive disorder of schizophrenia: A MDE that occurs during the residual phase of schizophrenia.

4. An MDE superimposed on delusional disorder, psychotic disorder NOS, or the active phase of schizophrenia.

5. Situations in which the clinician has concluded that a depressive disorder is present but is unable to determine whether it is primary, due to a general medical condition, or substance induced.

American Psychiatric Association. *Desk Reference to the Diagnostic Criteria from DSM-IV-TR*. Washington: American Psychiatric Association, 2000:178–179.

113. Answer: D. The patient has Klein-Levin syndrome, wherein patients have periods of prolonged sleep and hypersomnolence in between periods with normal sleep. The onset is usually between 10 and 21 years of age and, in early onset cases, typically remitting before the age 40. Patients may display a variety of neuropsychiatric symptoms (e.g., irritability, hallucinations, depression, etc.) and may eat voraciously or become sexually disinhibited. Patients with Schizophreniform Disorder and Schizophrenia do not classically exhibit such behaviors. Patients with Prader-Willi syndrome eat voraciously but such patients often have mental retardation and chronic oppositional behavior, as well as short statures, obesity, hypogonadism, and small hands and feet.

Kaplan HI, Sadock BJ. *Kaplan & Sadock's Synopsis of Psychiatry*. 8th ed. Philadelphia: Lippincott Williams & Wilkins; 1998:753, 1141.

114. Answer: D. Haloperidol, aripiprazole, trifluoperazine, and ziprasidone have low risk of weight gain. Chlorpromazine, risperidone, and quetiapine have moderate risk of weight gain. Thioridazine has a moderate to high risk while clozapine and olanzapine have high risk of weight gain.

Taylor D, Paton C, Kerwin R. *The Maudsley 2005–2006 Prescribing Guidelines: The South London and Maudsley NHS Trust & Oxleas NHS Trust*. 8th ed. London: Taylor & Francis; 2005:83.

115. Answer: B. Barbiturates induce hepatic microsomal enzymes and reduce the levels of medications like anticoagulants, TCAs, propanolol, carbamazepine, oral contraceptive pills, corticosteroids, quinidine, and theophylline. Use of barbiturates for over 4 weeks can result in the development of tolerance, dependence, and withdrawal symptoms. Cross-tolerance between barbiturates and alcohol and other sedative/hypnotic drugs can occur. Benzodiazepines with long half-life like clonazepam help reduce the severity of withdrawal symptoms. The rate of dose reduction determines the severity of withdrawal symptoms. Barbiturates should be avoided in pregnancy as they can cause severe respiratory depression or withdrawal symptoms in newborns.

Albers LJ, Hahn RK, Reist C. *Handbook of Psychiatric Drugs*. Laguna Hills: Current Clinical Strategies Publishing; 2005:68–69.

116. Answer: B. Stimulants should not be administered to patients with narrow-angle glaucoma as it can increase the intraocular pressure. Patients should not be on stimulants if they are pregnant or lactating, have a history of hyperthyroidism, or if they have a history of hypersensitivity to these agents. They should not be coadministered with MAOIs as it can precipitate hypertensive crisis or seizures. At least 14 days should elapse after the MAOI has been discontinued before initiating treatment with a stimulant. As these are controlled substances, they should be administered with caution in patients with a personal history of drug abuse or dependence. However, this is a caution and not a contraindication for psychostimulant use. Caution also should be maintained when using hypotensive agents such as guanethidine and clonidine with stimulants as adverse cardiovascular events and deaths reported with stimulants use (alone or combined with clonidine).

1. Albers LJ, Hahn RK, Reist C. *Handbook of Psychiatric Drugs*. Laguna Hills: Current Clinical Strategies Publishing; 2005:86–91.
2. Janicak PG, Davis JM, Preskorn SH. *Principles and Practice of Psychopharmacotherapy*. 3rd ed. Philadelphia: Lippincott Williams & Wilkins; 2001:588.

117. Answer: E. There are two older classes of antidepressants available, both of which can be fatal in overdose: MAOI and tricyclics. MAOIs require a tyramine-free diet, so this patient was taking a tricyclic. A tricyclic overdose of ten times the daily dose can be fatal. The tricyclics can cause a variety of anticholinergic side effects, but usually these are annoying but not serious. Use of nortriptyline or desipramine, which is less anticholinergic, can

help reduce the likelihood of these problems, but desipramine has the highest fatality rate (deaths per ingestions) among the tricyclics. Death most commonly occurs as a result of cardiac toxicity (type I antiarrhythmic effects), but seizures and CNS depression can occur. In patients without conduction delay, the tricyclics are well tolerated, and may be helpful in patients with premature ventricular beats. Acute hepatitis is not dose dependent. It develops idiosyncratically and quickly.

Sadock BJ, Sadock VA. *Kaplan and Sadock's Comprehensive Textbook of Psychiatry*. 7th ed. Philadelphia: Lippincott Williams & Wilkins; 2000: 2963–2965.

118. Answer: B. Although disulfiram was the first medication approved by the FDA for treatment of alcohol dependence, clinical studies to date, do not clearly support the efficacy of disulfiram for the treatment of alcoholism in comparison to placebo. The Veterans Affairs multisite cooperative study with more than 600 veterans showed that disulfiram and placebo-treated patients had similar outcomes with compliance with the study medication (disulfiram *and* placebo) being the best predictor of positive outcome. Disulfiram alters normal metabolism of ingested alcohol to produce mildly toxic acetaldehyde, resulting in an aversive reaction characterized by vomiting, flushing, headache, severe anxiety, and rarely even death. This reaction is severe enough that most individuals compliant to the medication completely stop drinking. This absolute prohibition of drinking is both the greatest strength and weakness of disulfiram. At doses of 250 to 500 mg, disulfiram is generally well tolerated. Its most common side effects include dermatitis, metallic taste, fatigue, headache, and sleepiness. It can also cause electrocardiogram changes, hypertension, and hypotension and hence it is contraindicated in patients with cardiovascular disease. Disulfiram has been associated with liver dysfunction, peripheral neuropathy with paresthesias, confusion, and optic neuritis. Adverse effects on the liver include elevated hepatic enzymes, hepatic failure, and hepatotoxicity. Disulfiram-induced hepatotoxicity generally occurs within 4 to 6 weeks after the beginning of disulfiram and may resolve within 2 weeks, although liver function may require up to 3 months to normalize. Some cases of hepatitis were irreversible and associated with liver transplantation or death. Consequently, caution is advised in patients with liver disease, and monitoring of liver function is recommended during treatment. Prompt discontinuation of the medication is associated with better clinical outcomes in cases of disulfiram-induced hepatitis. Nevertheless, definitive clinical trials evaluating disulfiram's use in dually diagnosed patients are still needed.

1. Buonopane A, Petrakis IL. Pharmacotherapy of alcohol use disorders. *Subst Use Misuse*. 2005;40:2001–20, 2043–2048.
2. Williams SH. Medications for treating alcohol dependence. *Am Fam Physician*. 2005;72:1775–1780.

119. Answer: E. All of the statements are true of criminal behaviors in the mentally ill. In addition, association between having a mental disorder and exhibiting criminal behavior (violent or nonviolent) has been shown to be stronger among women. Studies that compare criminal activity among individuals discharged from psychiatric hospitals with that observed among those without mental disorders residing in the same community indicate that the rate of criminality has been found to be higher among the individuals with severe mental disorders. Common diagnoses among these individuals were Depression (42%), Substance Abuse (21.8%), Schizophrenia (17%), Bipolar Disorder (14%), Personality Disorder (2%), and Psychotic Disorders (3%).

Valenca AM, Moraes TM. Relationship between homicide and mental disorders. *Rev Bras Psiquiatr*. 2006;28:S62–S68.

120. Answer: B. Leptin is a 16 kDa protein hormone that plays a role in regulating energy intake and energy expenditure, by regulating appetite and metabolism. It is synthesized by adipose tissue and is secreted in a pulsatile fashion. The Ob(Lep) gene (Ob for obese and Lep for leptin) is located on chromosome 7 in humans. Leptin interacts with six types of receptors (LepRa–LepRf). LepRb is the only receptor isoform that contains active intracellular signaling domains. This receptor is present in a number of hypothalamic nuclei, where it exerts its effects. Leptin binds to the ventral medial nucleus of the hypothalamus or the *satiety center*. Binding of leptin to this nucleus signals a sensation of satiety. Obesity is associated with leptin resistance. Leptin affects the hypothalamic-pituitary-gonadal axis, inhibits insulin-induced steroidogenesis and human chorionic gonadotropin–induced testosterone secretion. Substrates that mediate the action of leptin include orexigenic neuropeptides such as neuropeptide Y, galanin and galanin-like peptide, and melanin-concentrating hormone, and anorexigenic neuropeptides such as corticotropin-releasing hormone and alpha-melanocyte-stimulating hormone. Weight gain produced by some atypical antipsychotics may be mediated through increases in leptin.

Sadock BJ, Sadock VA. *Kaplan and Sadock's Comprehensive Textbook of Psychiatry*. 8th ed. Philadelphia: Lippincott Williams & Wilkins; 2005:129–130.

121. Answer: E. It appears that depression and thyroid disease occur more often in women than in men with the peak incidence occurring in women between the ages of 35 and 45 years. The prevalence of autoimmune thyroid disease is highest in women older than 40 years. Hypothyroidism shares many clinical features with depression. However, most subjects with depression do not have biochemical evidence of thyroid dysfunction. Several studies have found that many subjects with depression have high normal or borderline low thyroid hormone levels. In patients with unipolar depression rT3, the inactive analogue of T3, is increased. However, thyroid hormone levels are not correlated with severity of depression.

Schiffer RB, Rao SM, Fogel BS. *Neuropsychiatry*. 2nd ed. Philadelphia: Lippincott Williams & Wilkins; 2003:225–226.

122. Answer: D. The prevalence of dementia in patients with Parkinson's disease can be as high as 40%. The risk of dementia in these patients is about four times that of people of the same age without Parkinson's disease. The risk of dementia increases with age at diagnosis of Parkinson's disease, the presence of depression, visual hallucinations early in the disease, and advanced motor manifestations like bradykinesia or rigidity. Neither CT scan nor MRI of the brain can reliably distinguish patients with dementia from those without dementia. Dementia associated with Parkinson's disease is the third most common form of dementia.

Rowland LP. *Merritt's Neurology*. 11th ed. Philadelphia: Lippincott Williams & Wilkins; 2005:776–777.

123. Answer: A. Cerebral lesions that damage the corticospinal tract are characterized by signs of UMN injury. These signs include paresis with muscle spasticity, hyperactive deep tendon reflexes, and Babinski signs. Peripheral nerve lesions, including those of the anterior horn cells of the spinal cord or motor neuron disease, are distinguished by lower motor neuron injury. Signs of this include paresis with muscle flaccidity and atrophy, hypoactive deep tendon reflexes, and a negative Babinski reflex.

Kaufman DM. *Clinical Neurology for Psychiatrists*. 5th ed. Philadelphia: WB Saunders; 2001:8.

124. Answer: C. Urinary and serum thiamine levels do not reflect tissue concentrations accurately and hence are not reliable indicators of the body's thiamine status. The preferred test for the body's thiamine status is the erythrocyte transketolase activity. The other test to assess the body's thiamine stores is the assay or measurement of thiamine diphosphate in red blood cell hemolysates using high-performance liquid chromatography. As the erythrocyte transketolase activity normalizes quickly with treatment, blood samples should be drawn before initiation of treatment. Urinary transketolase activity is not a valid test.

Kumar N. Nutritional neuropathies. *Neurol Clin.* 2007;25: 209–255.

125. Answer: C. HIV is transmitted through whole blood, plasma, and clotting factors but not immune serum globulin or hepatitis B vaccine. In the West, those infected have mostly been homosexual men. In the rest of the world, the disease is mainly transmitted heterosexually. Sexually transmitted infections, such as herpes and syphilis, compromise the integrity of the skin and mucosa, thereby increasing the risk of transmission.

Sadock BJ, Sadock VA. *Kaplan and Sadock's Synopsis of Psychiatry.* 9th ed. Philadelphia: Lippincott Williams & Wilkins; 2003:371.

126. Answer: D. Herpes simplex encephalitis characteristically affects the temporal and frontal lobes. It affects all age groups but has a biphasic age distribution with peaks in the 5 to 30 years group and above 50 years. There is no seasonal variation. It may be a primary infection or a recrudescence of an established infection. The EEG shows nonspecific slowing in the early stages with later localization of periodic spike and slow wave activity in one or both temporal lobes. Similarly, CT of the brain may be normal initially, but later, characteristic low-density areas in one or both temporal lobes appear. MRI is more sensitive in the early stages when therapy is likely to be useful. Treatment is with intravenous antivirals such as acyclovir. Sequelae include mental retardation in children, dementia in adults, seizures, dysphasia, a Korsakoff-like syndrome, and personality changes. Neuropsychological testing may reveal the presence of cognitive impairment even among people who make apparently excellent recoveries after treatment with acyclovir.

1. Lishman WA. *Organic Psychiatry.* 3rd ed. Oxford: Blackwell Science; 1996:356–357.
2. Sadock BJ, Sadock VA. *Kaplan and Sadock's Synopsis of Psychiatry.* 9th ed. Philadelphia: Lippincott Williams & Wilkins; 2003:363.

127. Answer: C. vCJD's course is rather more protracted than CJD with a median of 12 months to death as opposed to 4 to 6 months in CJD. vCJD has mainly occurred in people younger than 30 years as opposed to middle-aged or older people in CJD. Behavioral and psychiatric symptoms are seen in young people with cerebellar signs such as ataxia and myoclonus, and should give rise to suspicion. Psychiatric symptoms are nonspecific and include de-

pression, anxiety, and sleep abnormalities. Neuropathological changes are similar to CJD with the addition of amyloid plaques. The EEG, although abnormal, lacks the characteristic features seen in CJD where a pattern of synchronous triphasic sharp wave complexes at 1 to 2 hz against a generalized slow background, occurs classically later in the disease. vCJD can be diagnosed by western blot immunostains to detect PrP-Sc in the tonsillar lymphoid tissue.

1. Rowland LP. *Merritt's Neurology.* 11th ed. Philadelphia: Lippincott Williams & Wilkins; 2005:264–268.
2. Sadock BJ, Sadock VA. *Kaplan and Sadock's Synopsis of Psychiatry.* 9th ed. Philadelphia: Lippincott Williams & Wilkins; 2003:364–365.

128. Answer: D. Epidural hematoma is a complication of head injury that occurs in 5% to 15% of autopsy series in patients with head injury. Bleeding into the epidural space is caused by a tear in the wall of one of the meningeal arteries most commonly the middle meningeal artery. However, in 15% of patients the bleeding can occur from one of the dural sinuses. In three fourths of these patients, it is associated with a skull fracture. Most epidural hematomas are located in the middle cranial fossa over the convexity of the hemisphere at the site of the impact. Epidural hematoma is primarily seen in young adults. It is rare in the elderly because the dura becomes increasingly adherent to the skull with advanced age. In one third of the patients, an immediate loss of consciousness is followed by a lucid interval, and then to a relapse into coma with hemiplegia. There is ipsilateral papillary dilation and fixity as the third cranial nerve is compressed by the hippocampal gyrus as it herniates over the free edge of the tentorium. The dilation and fixity of the pupil is a sign of impending brainstem compression. Progression to herniation and death occurs rapidly due to arterial bleeding. Mortality rates are close to 30% in treated patients with the rates approaching 100% in untreated patients. Early treatment is associated with better prognosis.

Rowland LP. *Merritt's Neurology.* 11th ed. Philadelphia: Lippincott Williams & Wilkins; 2005:488.

129. Answer: C. This patient suffers from RLS, which consists of random, irregular, spontaneous movements of the feet and legs associated with unpleasant paresthesias. These sensations occur only at rest, are relieved by movement, and tend to occur more during the evening and early portion of sleep. This circadian rhythm distinguishes it from akathisia. The prevalence of RLS has been noted to be almost twice as high for women compared to men, and pregnancy appears to be a risk factor for occurrence or worsening of RLS. RLS can also occur secondary to a number of disorders including iron deficiency (low serum ferritin), uremia, diabetes mellitus, rheumatic disease, and venous insufficiency. The cause of primary, idiopathic RLS is unknown, and a family history consistent with dominant inheritance has been implicated. Pramipexole is a usual first line of treatment, however, it is not recommended for pregnant women. Indeed, the treatment of RLS in pregnant women is complicated by the fact that nearly all of the drugs used for RLS are considered pregnancy risk factor C or D. If pharmacological treatment for RLS is necessary, opioids can be used in the second or third trimester.

1. Rosenbaum JF, Arana GW, Hyman SE, et al. *Handbook of Psychiatric Drug Therapy*. 5th ed. Philadelphia: Lippincott Williams & Wilkins; 2005:246–247.
2. Tarsy D, Sheon RP. *Restless Legs Syndrome*. http://www.utdol.com/utd/content/topic.do?topicKey=move_dis/2236&type=A&selectedTitle=1~2. Accessed February 23, 2007.

130. Answer: A. Selegiline's manufacturers have advised avoiding using this medication in combination with antidepressants due to the risk of serotonin syndrome. However, only a few cases of adverse effects of selegiline-antidepressant combinations have ever been published.

Tarsy D. *Comorbid Problems Associated with Parkinson's Disease*. http://www.uptodateonline.com/utd/content/topic.do?topicKey=move_dis/6536. Accessed March 4, 2007.

131. Answer: E. Medical and psychiatric disorders are the most common cause of sexual dysfunction in geriatric patients. In both men and women, medical conditions associated with sexual dysfunction include all those listed above, plus diabetes mellitus, cardiac disease, cancer, chronic renal or hepatic failure, multiple sclerosis, Parkinson's disease, and atherosclerosis (i.e., peripheral vascular disease and cerebrovascular disease). Psychiatric conditions associated with sexual dysfunction include MDD and other mood disorders, schizophrenia, and substance abuse. Medical and psychiatric conditions can result in primary and secondary effects on sexual functioning. Primary effects include the direct effects of the disease on sexual functioning (e.g., impaired vasocongestion due to peripheral vascular disease). The secondary effects of the condition can be just as impairing and include the indirect effects of the condition on sexual functioning (e.g., fatigue, pain, and low self-confidence). In addition, the effects of medications on sexual functioning are significant in the elderly population. Medications associated with sexual dysfunction are myriad and include, but are not limited to antidepressants, antihypertensives, antihis-

tamines, antipsychotics, corticosteroids, levodopa, and some cardiac medications.

Blazer DG, Steffens DC, Busse EW. *The American Psychiatric Association Textbook of Geriatric Psychiatry*. Washington: American Psychiatric Publishing; 2004:307.

132. Answer: B. This patient most likely suffered from dementia with Lewy bodies. Lewy bodies are round, eosinophilic, intracytoplasmic neuronal inclusions that are found in the cortex and brainstem. They contain α-syncline and tau-protein. This disorder is usually characterized by a progressive decline in cognitive function without such a marked memory loss as the one seen in AD. AD is the most common cause of dementia and it is pathologically characterized by the presence of β-amyloid and neurofibrillary tangles. A variant of AD can also present with Lewy bodies, but it behaves clinically in a similar way to AD. Corticobasal ganglionic degeneration is associated with parkinsonism, as well as with apraxias affecting the eye movements, speech, and limbs. Progressive supranuclear palsy mainly affects subcortical gray matter regions. Patients present with supranuclear ophthalmoplegia, pseudobulbar palsy, axial dystonia, and dementia.

1. Del Ser T, Hachinski V, Merskey H, et al. Clinical and pathologic features of two groups of patients with dementia with Lewy bodies: effect of coexisting Alzheimer-type lesion load. *Alzheimer Dis Assoc Disord*. 2001;15:31–44.
2. Greenberg DA, Aminoff MJ, Simon RP. *Clinical Neurology*. 6th ed. New York: McGraw-Hill; 2005:54–55.

133. Answer: E. Women are often reluctant to talk about abuse, so this should be routinely screened for with specific questions. Four million women or more (probably an underestimation) are assaulted by their partners each year in the United States. Present or former partners outnumber all other assailants combined. Women are more likely to be battered by someone they have a relationship with. At least 7% of pregnant women are victims of abuse. Pregnant women are more likely to be beaten in the abdomen, as opposed to the face. Beyond physical injury, both battered women and their children are at increased risk for mood, anxiety, eating, and substance abuse disorders. Children of abused women are at increased risk for substance abuse, behavior disorders, sleep problems, enuresis, and somatization.

Hales RE, Yudofsky SC. *Textbook of Clinical Psychiatry*. 4th ed. Washington: American Psychiatric Publishing; 2003:1511–1537.

134. Answer: C. There are three delineated frontal lobe behavioral syndromes: orbitofrontal, mediofrontal, and dorsolateral prefrontal. This patient displays behaviors typical with DLPFC lesions, the classic *dysexecutive syndrome*: loss of cognitive flexibility, impaired planning, sequencing, and multitasking, difficulty with attention/distraction, and difficulty with foresight and monitoring of performance. Injuries to DLPFC also impair working memory, abstract thinking, and motor fluency. Mediofrontal (also known as anterior cingulate) lesions cause apathy and amotivation. Orbitofrontal lesions cause disinhibition, impulsivity, and impaired judgement.

1. Goldberg E, Bougakov D. Neuropsychologic assessment of frontal lobe dysfunction. *Psychiatr Clin North Am.* 2005;28:567–580.
2. Mitchell AJ. *Neuropsychiatry and Behavioral Neurology Explained.* Philadelphia: WB Saunders; 2004:77–79.
3. Royall DR, Lauterbach EC, Cummings JL, et al. Executive control function: a review of its promise and challenges for clinical research. A report from the Committee on Research of the American Neuropsychiatric Association. *J Neuropsychiatry Clin Neurosci.* 2002;14:377–405.

135. **Answer: B.** Based on epidemiologic data, drug use should be suspected in an adolescent or young adult with new onset of psychiatric symptoms. Aside from repetitive behaviors, other symptoms of amphetamine use include elevated mood, talkativeness, irritability, decreased sleep and appetite, and paranoid thinking. Wilson's disease, a disorder of copper metabolism, which leads to psychosis and characteristic physical findings, is not suggested by the presentation. The other disorders could be considered in the evaluation, but are unlikely given the information as presented.

Sadock BJ, Sadock VA. *Kaplan and Sadock's Comprehensive Textbook of Psychiatry.* 8th ed. Philadelphia: Lippincott Williams & Wilkins; 2005:1195–1196.

136. **Answer: D.** Polysubstance Dependence involves the consumption of at least three groups of substances (excluding caffeine and nicotine) within the same 12 month period and requires meeting the criteria for Substance Dependence when considering the substances together. The use of each individual substance alone does not meet criteria. Here, the patient spends an inordinate amount of time to obtain amphetamine (criteria 5), she requires more heroin to achieve the desired effect (criteria 1), and she has given up a key social activity to drink wine (criteria 6). Polysubstance Abuse is not a disorder listed in the DSM-IV-TR.

American Psychiatric Association. *Desk Reference to the Diagnostic Criteria from DSM-IV-TR.* Washington: American Psychiatric Association; 2000:110–118, 148–149.

137. **Answer: C.** The most important risk factor for developing a postpartum psychosis is previous history.

The risk of puerperal relapse is about 70%. Other risk factors include being primigravida, being unmarried, having a cesarean section, having a female child, and a personal or family history of psychiatric illness.

Sadock BJ, Sadock VA. *Kaplan and Sadock's Comprehensive Textbook of Psychiatry.* 8th ed. Philadelphia: Lippincott Williams & Wilkins; 2005:1537.

138. **Answer: B.** This patient has REM Sleep Behavior Disorder, in which the regular inhibition of muscle tone is interrupted and, as a result, patients are able to act out dreams, which can be dangerous for their bed partners. This disorder occurs mainly in men and is chronic and progressive. This disorder has been reported in patients with narcolepsy who are treated with psychostimulants and TCAs, as well as in patients with depression and/or OCD on fluoxetine. Sleepwalking Disorder occurs during non-REM sleep and typically occurs in childhood. Sleep Terror Disorder also occurs during non-REM sleep, wherein patients usually scream or cry out and have intense anxiety and/or terror. Sleepwalking and Sleep Terror Disorder are particularly common in childhood. Jactatio capitis nocturna is sleep-related head banging or rocking. Given that the patient behaves normally during periods other than sleep, there is no indication that he has psychosis.

Kaplan HI, Sadock BJ. *Kaplan & Sadock's Synopsis of Psychiatry.* 8th ed. Philadelphia: Lippincott Williams & Wilkins; 1998:754–756.

139. **Answer: D.** There is no evidence that these drugs exert any direct metabolic effect to cause weight gain. The increase in weight appears to result from increased food consumption and reduced energy expenditure. Leptin is a protein hormone that plays a key role in regulating energy intake and energy expenditure, including the regulation of appetite and metabolism. Leptin binds to the ventromedial nucleus of the hypothalamus, known as the *satiety centre*. Binding of leptin to this nucleus signals to the brain that the body has had enough to eat (a sensation of satiety). Circulating leptin levels give the brain a reading of energy storage for the purposes of regulating appetite and metabolism. Although leptin is a circulating signal that reduces appetite, in general, obese people have an unusually high circulating concentration of leptin. These people are said to be resistant to the effects of leptin, in much the same way that people with type 2 diabetes are resistant to the effects of insulin. Thus, obesity develops when people take in more energy than they use over a prolonged period of time, and this excess food intake is not driven by hunger signals, occurring in spite of the antiappetite signals from circulating

leptin. The high sustained concentrations of leptin from the enlarged fat stores result in the cells that respond to leptin becoming desensitized. 5 HT-2C antagoniom, H1 antagonism & hyperprolactinemia are also proposed mechanisms for weight inducing effects of these drugs.

1. McIntyre RS, Mancini DA, Basile VS. Mechanisms of antipsychotic-induced weight gain. *J Clin Psychiatry*. 2001;62:23–29.
2. Taylor D, Paton C, Kerwin R. *The Maudsley 2005–2006 Prescribing Guidelines: The South London and Maudsley NHS Trust & Oxleas NHS Trust*. 8th ed. London: Taylor & Francis; 2005:83.

140. Answer: E. Diazepam, chlordiazepoxide, clorazepate, halazepam, and prazepam are all metabolized by the hepatic microsomal enzyme system (3A4 isoenzyme family) to produce an active metabolite desmethyl-diazepam. This active metabolite increases the half-life of these drugs to greater than 100 hours. These drugs can be given as once daily dosing, have less fluctuation in their serum levels, and have less severe withdrawal symptoms.

Albers LJ, Hahn RK, Reist C. *Handbook of Psychiatric Drugs*. Laguna Hills: Current Clinical Strategies Publishing; 2005: 56–57.

141. Answer: A. Atomoxetine is a presynaptic noradrenergic reuptake inhibitor that is superior to placebo in the treatment of ADHD in children, adolescents, and adults. It is metabolized by the cytochrome P 450 2D6 enzyme. As its pharmacokinetic half-life is 5 hours, it is generally dosed twice a day. Atomoxetine may also reduce tics and is thought to be effective in children with ADHD who have comorbid anxiety. The FDA has issued warnings regarding rare side effects of hepatotoxicity and suicidal ideation. It should not be used concurrently with MAOIs as it may precipitate a hypertensive crisis or seizures. It can be discontinued without a taper. It is not considered a psychostimulant and is not a controlled substance. Dosing in children (<70 kg) is about 1.2 mg/kg/day in two divided doses. In adults (>70 kg) the dose is 40 to 100 mg/day in two divided doses. Atomoxetine is category C in pregnancy.

1. Albers LJ, Hahn RK, Reist C. *Handbook of Psychiatric Drugs*. Laguna Hills: Current Clinical Strategies Publishing; 2005:91–92.
2. Pliszka SR. Pharmacologic treatment of attention-deficit/hyperactivity disorder: efficacy, safety and mechanisms of action. *Neuropsychol Rev*. 2007;17:61–72.

142. Answer: E. All of the statements are true. Till recently, counseling and twelve-step structured treatment programs have been the mainstays of the treatment of alcohol dependence, whereas pharmacologic treatments traditionally have played an adjunctive role. However, the FDA has recently approved three medications for the treatment of alcohol dependence: disulfiram (Antabuse), naltrexone (Trexan), and acamprosate (Campral). Despite their availability, only about 20% of the eligible patients receive them.

Williams SH. Medications for treating alcohol dependence. *Am Fam Physician*. 2005;72:1775–1780.

143. Answer: C. Acamprosate has been approved by the FDA for use in the treatment of Alcohol Dependence. Preclinical and clinical studies suggest that acamprosate reduces excessive drinking with favorable results with reductions in drinking days and increased length of abstinence. The exact mechanism of action of acamprosate remains unknown, but it counteracts alcohol-use-related symptoms by modulating the glutamatergic and GABA-ergic systems. It induces abstinence or improves relapse rates by possibly reducing "craving" and interfering with the processes of reward and conditioning in Alcohol Dependence. If combined with alcohol, acamprosate does not induce unpleasant symptoms as seen with disulfiram. Acamprosate is not metabolized by the liver and is excreted unchanged in the urine. It can be used in patients with liver disease but is contraindicated in renal disease. As only 10% of the oral dose is absorbed, 1 to 2 gram dosing per day is recommended. There are no interactions with concomitant use of alcohol, diazepam (Valium), disulfiram (Antabuse), or imipramine (Tofranil), so patients with alcohol dependence can continue to use acamprosate during a relapse. Acamprosate is FDA pregnancy category C (adverse effects on the fetus in animal studies, but no human trials).

1. Boothby LA, Doering PL. Acamprosate for the treatment of alcohol dependence. *Clin Ther*. 2005;27:695–714.
2. Buonopane A, Petrakis IL. Pharmacotherapy of alcohol use disorders. *Subst Use Misuse*. 2005;40:2001–2020, 2043–2048.
3. Williams SH. Medications for treating alcohol dependence. *Am Fam Physician*. 2005;72:1775–1780.

144. Answer: B. Of the immune cells listed (oligodendrocytes and Schwann cells are myelin producing supportive nerve cells), it is most likely that T cell activation against self-antigen is involved in the etiology of multiple sclerosis. Possible causes for this activation include molecular mimicry with viral antigen resembling self-antigen or compromise of the blood brain barrier exposing immune cells to CNS antigens.

Goetz CG. *Textbook of Clinical Neurology*. 2nd ed. Philadelphia: WB Saunders; 2003:1059–1062.

145. Answer: D. Lithium at therapeutic levels can inhibit thyroid hormone release by decreasing endocytosis of T3- and T4-laden thyroglobulin on the luminal side of the thyroid follicle. At higher levels, it can also inhibit iodine uptake and organification. Lithium is also thought to inhibit the peripheral conversion of T4 to T3. Symptoms of hypothyroidism develops in approximately 7% of patients taking lithium, over and above the rate expected for patients of the same age and sex not being treated with lithium. The highest risk is in women and patients with positive antithyroid antibodies. Other risk factors for developing this condition are starting lithium at the ages of 40 to 59 years, first 2 years of treatment in females, weight gain, iodine deficient diet, higher lithium levels, and rapid cycling bipolar disorder.

1. Livingstone C, Rampes H. Lithium: a review of its metabolic adverse effects. *J Psychopharmacol.* 2006;20: 347–355.
2. Schiffer RB, Rao SM, Fogel BS. *Neuropsychiatry.* 2nd ed. Philadelphia: Lippincott Williams & Wilkins; 2003:229–230.

146. Answer: C. This patient has a cluster headache. Cluster headaches commonly occur in young adult men from ages 20 to 50 years. The male to female ratio is 5:1. They are characterized by a consistent unilateral orbital localization. The pain is deep and felt around the eye. The headache is very intense but nonthrobbing. Pain may radiate into the forehead, temple, and cheek. Headaches can occur several times each day, more often at night, and may recur with regularity each day for periods extending from 6 to 12 weeks. Cluster headaches are also associated with vasomotor phenomena such as blocked nostrils, rhinorrhea, ptosis, miosis, injected conjunctiva, lacrimation, and flushing and edema of the cheek. Alcohol commonly precipitates these headaches. Treatment is with ergotamine before a suspected attack and abortive treatments include oxygen and sumatriptan.

Ropper AH, Brown RH. *Adams and Victor's Principles of Neurology.* 8th ed. New York: McGraw-Hill; 2005:144–167.

147. Answer: E. This patient is most likely experiencing carpopedal spasm and EEG slowing from hyperventilation. Although hyperventilation could result from panic attacks, there is insufficient information to reach that conclusion in this case. There is also insufficient information to suggest TIAs and posttraumatic brain injury. In addition, EEG slowing and carpopedal spasm are not features of these disorders. Although her complaints of spacing out and dizziness may indicate a petit mal seizure, absence of typical EEG findings (3 per second spike and wave) makes petit mal an unlikely diagnosis. Having the patient hyperventilate will most certainly recreate her symptoms, a useful bedside diagnostic test. Prolonged hyperventilation could result in altered consciousness, which is quickly aborted by breathing into a bag.

Eisendrath SJ. Factitious physical disorders. *West J Med.* 1994;160:177–179.

148. Answer: B. Triptans inhibit the release of vasoactive peptides and promote vasoconstriction. Triptans inhibit transmission in the trigeminal nucleus caudalis, which then blocks afferent input to second order neurons. Triptans may also activate serotonin 1B/1D receptors in the descending brainstem pain modulating pathway, inhibiting dural nociception.

Bajwa ZH, Sabahat A. *Acute Treatment of Migraines in Adults.* http://www.uptodateonline.com/utd/content/topic. do?topicKey=headache/4364&type=A&selectedTitle= 1~58. Accessed March 4, 2007.

149. Answer: C. Personality is defined as an individual's way of relating to others, interacting with the environment, and thinking about oneself. Although substantial changes in personality occur at ages 18 to 30, personality is relatively stable with only subtle changes during adulthood and later years. Increasing medical and neuropsychiatric comorbidity in late life, as well as normal psychosocial development, does affect the natural history of personality. Personality is largely resilient and uninfluenced by the sheer occurrence of positive or negative life events. It does, however, shape one's response to stressful life events. Personality disorders were previously thought to age out and have little effect on older persons, though recent study has shown the lifelong continuity of personality disorders in late life.

1. American Psychiatric Association. *Diagnostic and Statistical Manual of Mental Disorders: DSM-IV-TR.* 4th ed. (Text Revision). Washington: American Psychiatric Association; 2000.
2. Blazer DG, Steffens DC, Busse EW. *The American Psychiatric Association Textbook of Geriatric Psychiatry.* Washington: American Psychiatric Publishing; 2004:127–128, 369.

150. Answer: E. β-amyloid is the principal constituent of neuritic plaques. It is formed due to an abnormal cleavage of amyloid precursor protein in the brain. The abnormal β-amyloid accumulates in extracellular plaques and it is thought that this accumulation might result in neuronal death. The gene for the development of β-amyloid is located on chromosome 21 and not 19. The gene for the formation of ApoE is located on chromosome 19.

1. Edwardson J, Morris C. The genetics of Alzheimer's disease. The number of genetic risk factors associated with this disorder is increasing steadily. *BMJ.* 1998;317:361–362.

2. Greenberg DA, Aminoff MJ, Simon RP. *Clinical Neurology*. 6th ed. New York: McGraw-Hill Publishing; 2005: 46–50.

151. Answer: C. Lyme disease is caused by the spirochete *Borrelia burgdorferi* and is usually transmitted by tick bites. The infection becomes apparent 3 to 32 days after exposure with a characteristic acute rash (erythema migrans) surrounding the tick bite area. The rash is not always observed by the patient or family members. Approximately 10% to 15% of patients develop neurological symptoms such as chronic meningitis, progressive encephalomyelitis, encephalopathy, radiculopathy, mononeuritis multiplex, myopathy, cranial neuropathies (usually involving the seventh nerve), seizures, and occasionally mild cognitive impairment. The cognitive impairment of patients with Lyme disease is characterized by impaired executive function and reduced attention. Depression, emotional lability, irritability, and psychosis may also be present. As serological tests for B. burgdorferi are not sufficiently reliable, CSF examination may be required. The CSF often shows pleocytosis, elevated protein levels, oligoclonal bands, and borrelial DNA. In the presence of neurological symptoms, parenteral antibiotic treatment is recommended. FTA antibodies indicate spirochete infection, i.e., syphilis. 14–3-3 protein in CSF suggests CJD. Anti-Hu antibodies are associated with the paraneoplastic syndrome of limbic encephalitis. Niacin deficiency causes pellagra and the "5 Ds": dermatitis, diarrhea, dementia delirium and death. The rash in pellagra is symmetrical and occurs in sun-exposed areas. It begins with erythema and may become exudative. There is often a well-demarcated eruption on the front of the neck (Casal's necklace).

Almeida OP, Lautenschlager NT. Dementia associated with infectious diseases. *Int Psychogeriatr.* 2005;17:S65–S77.

152. Answer: D. Caffeine and clozapine are both metabolized by the CYP450 1A2 enzyme system. It has been detected that caffeine inhibits the metabolism of clozapine by CYP450 1A2 enzyme system and increasing its level by about 20%.

1. Raaska K, Raitasuo V, Laitila J, et al. Effect of caffeine-containing versus decaffeinated coffee on serum clozapine concentrations in hospitalised patients. *Basic Clin Pharmacol Toxicol.* 2004;94:13–18.
2. Sadock BJ, Sadock VA. *Kaplan and Sadock's Comprehensive Textbook of Psychiatry*. 8th ed. Philadelphia: Lippincott Williams & Wilkins; 2005:1203.

153. Answer: B. Anabolic steroid (AAS) use can cause symptoms of irritability, aggression, mania, and psychosis. LH and FSH are reduced in the presence of AASs. Testosterone levels vary according to the AAS used and the timing of the sample drawn. Liver function tests are often elevated, but certain liver functions can be elevated in weight-training athletes without the use of AASs.

Sadock BJ, Sadock VA. *Kaplan and Sadock's Comprehensive Textbook of Psychiatry*. 8th ed. Philadelphia: Lippincott Williams & Wilkins; 2005:1321.

154. Answer: A. In the DSM-IV-TR, the diagnostic specifier of Postpartum Psychosis can be applied to Mood Disorders, Brief Psychotic Disorder, and to Psychotic Disorder NOS, if the symptoms occur within 4 weeks of delivery. The incidence of Postpartum Psychsis is approximately 1 to 2 per 1,000 births, with psychotic symptoms usually appearing within the first week after childbirth. The most important risk factor for developing a postpartum psychosis is previous history. The risk of puerperal relapse is as high as 70%. Other risk factors include being primigravida, being unmarried, having a cesarean section, having a female child, and a personal or family history of psychiatric illness. Although more publicized, infanticide remains a rare complication of this illness.

1. American Psychiatric Association. *Desk Reference to the Diagnostic Criteria from DSM-IV-TR*. Washington: American Psychiatric Association; 2000:161, 165, 173–189.
2. Sadock BJ, Sadock VA. *Kaplan and Sadock's Comprehensive Textbook of Psychiatry*. 8th ed. Philadelphia: Lippincott Williams & Wilkins; 2005:1537–1538.

155. Answer: D. Sleep hygiene techniques or nonspecific measures to induce sleep in patients should consist of the following: (a) wake up at the same time every day, (b) stay in bed no more than they did before the onset of their sleeping difficulties, (c) stop their use of caffeine, nicotine, alcohol, and stimulants (with some exceptions), (d) avoid daytime naps, (e) exercise vigorously early in the day and develop a graded program for doing so, (f) avoid stimulation (e.g., television) at night, (g) take a very hot baths, (h) eat at regular meal times and avoid large meals before bed, (i) do relaxation routines in the evening, and (j) develop comfortable sleeping conditions, which do not necessarily include sleeping on a firm mattress.

Kaplan HI, Sadock BJ. *Kaplan & Sadock's Synopsis of Psychiatry*. 8th ed. Philadelphia: Lippincott Williams & Wilkins; 1998:747.

156. Answer: D. Ziprasidone, chlorpromazine, and quetiapine exert a moderate effect on the QTc interval. Sertindole, pimozide, and thioridazine exert a high effect on QTc interval. Amisulpride and aripiprazole have no reported effect on the QTc interval.

Clozapine, olanzapine, risperidone, fluphenazine, flupentixol, and sulpiride have a low effect on the QTc interval. No effect drugs are those in which QTc prolongation has not been reported at therapeutic doses or in overdose. Low effect drugs are those for which severe QTc prolongation has been reported ONLY following overdose or where only small increases (< 10 milliseconds) have been observed at therapeutic doses. Moderate effect drugs are those where the QTc interval is prolonged by an average of >10 milliseconds or where EKG monitoring is required in certain circumstances. High effect drugs are those for which the QTc is increased by an average of >20 milliseconds or where EKG monitoring is mandated by the manufacturer's data sheet.

1. Glassman AH, Bigger JT. Antipsychotic drugs: prolonged QTc interval, torsade de pointes, and sudden death. *Am J Psychiatry*. 2001;158:1774–1782.
2. Haddad PM, Anderson IM. Antipsychotic-related QTc prolongation, torsade de pointes and sudden death. *Drugs*. 2002;62:1649–1671.
3. Taylor DM. Antipsychotics and QT prolongation. *Acta Psychiatr Scand*. 2003;107:85–95.
4. Taylor D, Paton C, Kerwin R. *The Maudsley 2005–2006 Prescribing Guidelines: The South London and Maudsley NHS Trust & Oxleas NHS Trust*. 8th ed. London: Taylor & Francis; 2005:83.

157. Answer: D. Interpersonal Therapy is an evidence-based and time-limited therapy that is primarily used for acute and maintenance treatment of major depression, although studies have found some efficacy in bulimia. It is not useful in substance or psychotic disorders. There are three phases to the treatment, with the second phase focusing on the interpersonal area thought to be most relevant.

Sadock BJ, Sadock VA. *Kaplan and Sadock's Comprehensive Textbook of Psychiatry*. 7th ed. Philadelphia: Lippincott Williams & Wilkins; 2000:2178–2180.

158. Answer: A. In a 16-week double-blind, placebo-controlled trial, children and adolescents who were receiving at least one atypical antipsychotic medication for 1 year and had gained at least 10% of their pretreatment body weight, were randomly assigned to receive adjunctive metformin or placebo. In the children receiving adjunctive metformin, weight remained stable or decreased compared to those receiving antipsychotic medication alone. In another 16-week double-blind, placebo-controlled study, 390 patients with type II diabetes who were managed with insulin were randomly assigned to receive adjunctive metformin or placebo and were monitored for changes in homocysteine, folate, and Vitamin B$_{12}$. Metformin use was associated with a

significant decrease in folate and Vitamin B$_{12}$ levels secondary to an increase in homocysteine. Vitamin deficiencies are one of the few reversible causes of depression, and thus should be monitored in patients receiving metformin. TSH, prolactin, Vitamin B$_6$, and CBC count are not affected by metformin use.

1. Klein DJ, Cottingham EM, Sorter M, et al. A randomized, double-blind, placebo-controlled trial of metformin treatment of weight gain associated with initiation of atypical antipsychotic therapy in children and adolescents. *Am J Psychiatry*. 2006;163:2072–2079.
2. Wulffele MG, Kooy A, Lehert P, et al. Effects of short-term treatment with metformin on serum concentrations of homocysteine, folate and vitamin B$_{12}$ in type 2 diabetes mellitus: a randomized, placebo-controlled trial. *J Intern Med*. 2003 Nov;254(5):455–463.

159. Answer: E. There are no absolute contraindications to ECT, only situations in which patients are at increased risk and, therefore, require close monitoring. Pregnancy is not a contraindication to ECT, and fetal monitoring is generally not necessary unless the pregnancy is high risk or complicated. High-risk patients include those with space-occupying lesions, patients with increased intracerebral pressure or those at significant risk for intracerebral bleeding (e.g., patients with cerebrovascular diseases or aneurysms), and patients with recent MIs (though the risk is greatly diminished 2 weeks post-(MI) and even further reduced after 3 months). Patients with hypertension should be stabilized on antihypertensive medication before ECT is administered.

Sadock BJ, Sadock VA. *Kaplan and Sadock's Synopsis of Psychiatry*. 9th ed. Philadelphia: Lippincott Williams & Wilkins; 2003:1143.

160. Answer: B. Addiction is a chronic relapsing condition. It is still not clear from the literature as to how long interventions improve alcohol and drug problems and what kinds of interventions might extend these outcomes. We still do not know as to how individuals with poor short-term outcomes can most effectively be treated. Individual characteristics are the most consistent predictors of change in substance use. In general, socioeconomic status, particularly lower education and income, is associated with less short- and long-term improvement and stable employment contributes to better long-term outcomes. The relationship between gender and long-term outcomes is not well studied, but the few existing studies suggest that outcomes are similar or better for women than men. The role of ethnicity is also not well studied, because most studies have not had good distributions of ethnic groups. The relationship between age and long-term outcomes has not been established. Higher levels of alcohol and drug problems when entering treatment are consistently related to higher levels at later follow-ups, but the results appear to differ based on the diagnosis. Short-term studies have shown that retention, abstinence, and improvement rates are lower at follow-up for individuals who are drug dependent rather than alcohol-only dependent. The data also suggests that long-term change in drug problems typically does not occur with a single treatment episode and readmissions are important in promoting long-term recovery. The impact of short-term treatment success on long-term outcomes indicates that improvements made in the short-term are often predictive of longer-term outcomes. Data indicates that over the long-term a loss of treatment effect may occur if not reinforced by a social context supportive of abstinence.

Weisner C, Ray GT, Mertens JR, et al. Short-term alcohol and drug treatment outcomes predict long-term outcome. *Drug Alcohol Depend.* 2003;71:281–294.

161. Answer: E. In most cases, the release of neurotransmitters from the vesicles into the synaptic cleft follows the entry of calcium ion into the presynaptic terminal. Most of the neurotransmitters are produced locally by enzymes within the presynaptic terminal. After these neurotransmitters are synthesized, they are stored in small presynaptic vesicles. Neurotransmitters stored in presynaptic vesicles are released into the synaptic cleft through a process of exocytosis. This process requires that the membranes of the vesicles fuse with the membrane of the presynaptic terminal and release the vesicular contents into the synaptic cleft. This fusion and release occur along the presynaptic active zone. Calcium triggers a molecular cascade that results in the activation of molecular machinery that is responsible for the movement of presynaptic vesicles to the active zone and release of its contents.

Schiffer RB, Rao SM, Fogel BS. *Neuropsychiatry.* 2nd ed. Philadelphia: Lippincott Williams & Wilkins; 2003:188.

162. Answer: C. Symptoms of hypothyroidism develops in approximately 7% of patients taking lithium, over and above the rate expected for patients of the same age and sex not being treated with lithium. The highest risk is seen in women and patients with positive antithyroid antibodies. Other risk factors are starting lithium at the ages of 40 to 59 years, first 2 years of treatment in females, weight gain, iodine deficient diet, higher lithium levels, and rapid cycling bipolar disorder.

Lithium at therapeutic levels inhibits thyroid hormone release by decreasing endocytosis of T3- and

T4-laden thyroglobulin on the luminal side of the thyroid follicle. At higher levels, it can also inhibit iodine uptake and organification. It is also thought to inhibit the peripheral conversion of T4 to T3.

1. Livingstone C, Rampes H. Lithium: a review of its metabolic adverse effects. *J Psychopharmacol.* 2006;20: 347–355.
2. Schiffer RB, Rao SM, Fogel BS. *Neuropsychiatry.* 2nd ed. Philadelphia: Lippincott Williams & Wilkins; 2003:229–230.

163. Answer: A. Inhibition of alpha- and gamma-motor neurons by C is not a mechanism of action of botulinum toxin. Botulinum toxin prevents abnormal patterns of muscle contractions that activate muscle nociceptors. Other proposed mechanisms of action include acetylcholine release affecting emotional behavior and stress, suppression of neurogenic inflammation, and change of regional blood flow.

Malik AB, Bajwa ZH. Botulinum Toxins for Chronic Pain and Headache. *UpToDate.* http://www.uptodateonline.com/utd/content/topic.do?topicKey=headache/4364&type=A&selectedTitle=1~58. Accessed March 4, 2007.

164. Answer: A. Multiple normal changes occur in sleep patterns with age. These include less overall sleep and sleep that is fragmented. REM latency decreases and total REM sleep decreases. There is also an increase in sleep latency and a decrease in deep sleep.

Stern TA, Herman JB. *Massachusetts General Hospital Psychiatry Update and Board Preparation.* 2nd ed. New York: McGraw-Hill; 2004:174.

165. Answer: B. Although it is a rare illness, sporadic CJD is the most common form of the human prion disease. The neuropathological findings in sporadic CJD include neuronal loss, spongiform vacuolation, and reactive astrogliosis. The neuronal loss varies, and it is usually overshadowed by marked astrogliosis. Kuru is a prion disease first encountered in people of Papua New Guinea and was most likely transmitted by cannibalism. The disease starts insidiously and is usually fatal in 6 to 9 months. Gerstmann-Straussler syndrome has a longer duration than sporadic CJD, with a mean duration of 5 years. The pathological characteristics of Gerstmann-Straussler syndrome include amyloid plaques with a multicentric configuration within the cerebellum. Familial CJD is associated with a genetic point mutation. It is very similar to sporadic CJD, but it sometimes has an earlier onset of illness. Fatal familial insomnia is an autosomal dominant illness with incomplete penetrance. Patients develop nocturnal insomnia, excessive daytime sleepiness, and dysautonomia. The neuropathological findings are neuronal loss and astrocytic gliosis in the anterior ventral and dorsomedial nuclei of the thalamus.

Sadock BJ, Sadock VA. *Kaplan and Sadock's Comprehensive Textbook of Psychiatry*. 8th ed. Philadelphia: Lippincott Williams & Wilkins; 2005:462–480.

166. **Answer: D.** Cysticercosis cysts contain calcification and have little or no surrounding edema. These cysts have substantial cumulative mass effect and cause irritation to the cerebral cortex. Cysticercosis is caused by the parasite *Taenia solium*, and is the most common cerebral mass lesion in Central and South America. Toxoplasmosis is the most common cause of mass lesions in young and middle-aged adults in North America. Seizures are widely reported to be the most common symptom of neurocysticercosis, occurring in 70% to 90% of patients. There is no consistency in the reported distribution of seizure types. The clinical manifestations of neurocysticercosis are varied and probably depends on the number and location of cysts, as well as the host immune response to the parasite. Many syndromes have been described such as manifestations of brainstem dysfunction, cerebellar ataxia, sensory deficits, involuntary movements, stroke-like symptoms, extrapyramidal signs, and dementia. Other rare clinical manifestations, for instance, intrasellar cysticercosis and pseudotumor cerebri, have been reported. Low serum B12 or TSH alone would not account for this presentation. Mesial temporal sclerosis would account for seizures, but not all of the symptoms. Answer choice E describes NPH, which is clinically characterized by urinary incontinence, gait apraxia ("magnetized gait"), and dementia.

1. Carpio A. Neurocysticercosis: an update. *Lancet Infect Dis*. 2002;2:751–762.
2. Kaufman DM. *Clinical Neurology for Psychiatrists*. 5th ed. Philadelphia: WB Saunders, 2001:538–548.

167. **Answer: D.** THC levels peak in 10 minutes and declines to approximately 10% of their value in 1 hour. Performance impairments in laboratory tests and driving courses are similar to those found for blood alcohol levels of 0.07% to 1.0%. However, in normal driving conditions cannabis users drive more slowly and take fewer risks. Cannabis is usually detected from 4 days to 4 weeks but can be detected for up to 11 weeks. An amotivational syndrome has been described in case studies but has not been found in controlled studies.

Sadock BJ, Sadock VA. *Kaplan and Sadock's Comprehensive Textbook of Psychiatry*. 8th ed. Philadelphia: Lippincott Williams & Wilkins; 2005:1216–1218.

168. **Answer: B.** Chronic stress has been shown to decrease

BDNF and neurogenesis and thus affect the functional status of neurons and cause cell death.

Sadock BJ, Sadock VA. *Kaplan and Sadock's Comprehensive Textbook of Psychiatry*. 8th ed. Philadelphia: Lippincott Williams & Wilkins; 2005:1597.

169. **Answer: C.** Some grieving individuals as part of their reaction to loss may present with neurovegetative symptoms of an MDE. These may include feelings of sadness, insomnia, poor appetite, and weight loss. Sometimes, people may seek professional help during bereavement for symptoms like anorexia or insomnia. Although the duration and presentation of normal bereavement vary considerably among different cultural groups, a diagnosis of MDE is not usually made unless the symptoms persist for more than 2 months after the loss. Symptoms that may indicate an MDE and not normal grief include all of the following: (i) guilt about things other than actions taken or not taken by the survivor at the time of death, (ii) thoughts of death other than the survivor feeling that he or she would be better of dead or should have died with the deceased person, (iii) morbid preoccupations with worthlessness, (iv) marked psychomotor retardation, and (v) hallucinatory experiences other than thinking of hearing voices or transiently seeing images of the deceased person and prolonged and marked functional impairment.

American Psychiatric Association. *Desk Reference to the Diagnostic Criteria from DSM-IV-TR*. Washington: American Psychiatric Association; 2000:311–312.

170. **Answer: C.** The patient has RLS. In RLS, patients tend to have irrepressible desires to move their legs, particularly when sitting or lying down, and have associated paresthesias often described as creeping or crawling sensations in the legs. This disorder, which is disturbing enough to keep patients awake at night, is often underdiagnosed. First-line treatment consists of dopaminergic agonists, of which pramipexole and ropinirole are examples. Gabapentin (as well as opiates) is sometimes used as augmentation, and benzodiazepines can be used to help with sleep. Fluoxetine is not part of the treatment repertoire of RLS.

1. Kaplan HI, Sadock BJ. *Kaplan & Sadock's Synopsis of Psychiatry*. 8th ed. Philadelphia: Lippincott Williams & Wilkins; 1998:752.
2. Rosenbaum JR, Arana GW, Hyman SE, et al. *Handbook of Psychiatric Drug Therapy*. 5th ed. Philadelphia: Lippincott Williams & Wilkins; 2005:246–247.

171. **Answer: D.** Cardiac risk factors include history of ischemic heart disease, myocarditis, MI, long QT syndrome, cardiomyopathy, left ventricular hypertrophy,

bradycardia, and second- or third-degree heart block. Metabolic risk factors include hypokalemia, hypomagnesemia, hypocalcemia and severe renal or hepatic impairment. Stress or shock, extremes of age and female gender are other risk factors.

Taylor D, Paton C, Kerwin R. *The Maudsley 2005–2006 Prescribing Guidelines: The South London and Maudsley NHS Trust & Oxleas NHS Trust*. 8th ed. London: Taylor & Francis; 2005:83.

172. Answer: A. There is no absolute contraindication to ECT. Brain tumors used to be considered one, but there are numerous case reports of successful treatments. Patients with large lesions, midline shift, and increased intracranial pressure are at greater risk, and the decision to treat should be made in consultation with neurology. Neurosurgical procedures or skull fractures increase risk because bony defects offer a low resistance pathway for the electricity to enter the CNS. Electrodes should not be placed directly on the defects. Recent stroke or MI increases the risk of general anesthesia.

Sadock BJ, Sadock VA. *Kaplan and Sadock's Comprehensive Textbook of Psychiatry*. 7th ed. Philadelphia: Lippincott Williams & Wilkins; 2000:2512.

173. Answer: C. In a meta-analysis of 35 daily treatment studies with SSRIs and clomipramine, it was demonstrated that clomipramine had comparable efficacy with the SSRIs sertraline and fluoxetine in delaying ejaculation. It also demonstrated that the efficacy of SSRI paroxetine was greater than all other SSRIs and clomipramine in the treatment of premature ejaculation. It is also postulated that acute treatment with SSRIs, including those with short half-lives, will not produce an ejaculation delay equivalent to that induced by daily treatment of SSRIs.

Waldinger MD, Olivier B. Utility of selective serotonin reuptake inhibitors in premature ejaculation. *Curr Opin Investig Drugs*. 2004;5:743–747.

174. Answer: D. During the first few sessions of IPT, the therapist takes a clinical history which is focused on the patient's symptoms and current interpersonal situation. This allows the therapist to make a diagnosis and to select an interpersonal focus for treatment. During the first few sessions, an interpersonal therapist will: (i) review the depressive symptoms and make a diagnosis, (ii) explain depression and the various treatment options, (iii) evaluate the need for medication, (iv) take an *interpersonal inventory* in order to understand the context in which the depression has arisen, (v) present a formulation, linking the patient's illness to an interpersonal focus, (vi) make a treatment contract based on the formulation and explain what to expect in treatment, and (vii) give the patient the *sick role*. IPT generally deals with current, rather than past, interpersonal relationships and focuses on the patient's immediate social context.

1. Sadock BJ, Sadock VA. *Kaplan and Sadock's Synopsis of Psychiatry*. 9th ed. Philadelphia: Lippincott Williams & Wilkins; 2003:933–935
2. Weissman MM, Markowitz JC, Klerman, GL. *Clinician's Quick Guide to Interpersonal Psychotherapy*. New York: Oxford University Press; 2007:12.

175. Answer: C. Previous history, substance use, and certain neurologic impairments are clearly associated with increased risk of violence. Although a controversial issue, psychiatric diagnosis is not as clearly associated with risk of violence as the other choices listed.

1. Harris GT, Rice ME. Risk appraisal and management of violent behavior. *Psychiatr Serv*. 1997;48:1168–1176.
2. Norko M, Baranoski M. The state of contemporary risk assessment research. *Can J Psychiatry*. 2005;50:18–26.

176. Answer: D. Postsynaptic receptors are either linked to ion channels or are linked to guanosine triphosphate binding proteins (G proteins). The ion channels open to initiate the cell's response, whereas the guanosine triphosphate binding proteins activate second messenger systems within the postsynaptic cell. There are numerous types of receptors located at a single synapse. The effect of activation of the receptor on the postsynaptic neuron is dependent on the synapse's location on the postsynaptic neuron. The ion channel receptors, also called *ligand-gated ion channels*, are assembled from several protein subunits. Usually there are about four to five protein subunits that are coded by different genes. Each subunit has several membrane-spanning regions with the amino-terminal end of the protein being extracellular. The assembled subunits in turn form a pore through the membrane. When the receptor is activated, this pore allows the flux of ions driven by their concentration gradients. In most receptor families, the second membrane-spanning portion of each subunit forms the lining of this pore with specific amino acids in this region regulating which ions may permeate into the cell. G-protein-linked receptors usually have seven membrane-spanning regions. The amino-terminal end of the membrane-spanning region is extracellular. These receptors do not form channels but the binding of neurotransmitters to the extracellular part of the protein trigger conformational changes that alter the interaction of the intracellular portion of the receptors with G proteins.

Schiffer RB, Rao SM, Fogel BS. *Neuropsychiatry*. 2nd ed. Philadelphia: Lippincott Williams & Wilkins; 2003:189.

177. Answer: D. All are true except choice D. In the brain the two major cholinergic projections are the one arising in the pedunculopontine nuclei of the midbrain and projecting to the medulla, substantia nigra, thalamus, and globus pallidus and playing an important role in regulating the sleep/wake cycles. The other projection is provided by a complex set of nuclei, including the medial septal nucleus, the diagonal band of Broca, and the basal nucleus of Meynert. The neurons from these nuclei innervate the neocortex, the hippocampus, and the amygdala and are vital for learning and memory. These degenerate in AD. Some acetylcholine neurons within the neocortex also function as local circuit neurons. These are mainly seen in the caudate nucleus and putamen. These neurons participate in the cholinergic/dopaminergic balance that is important in the biology of movement disorders.

Schiffer RB, Rao SM, Fogel BS. *Neuropsychiatry*. 2nd ed. Philadelphia: Lippincott Williams & Wilkins; 2003:199–200.

178. Answer: D. COMT inhibitors may prolong and potentiate the effect of levodopa by reducing its methylation. COMT inhibitors are ineffective when given alone. A decarboxylase inhibitor blocks levodopa's conversion to dopamine in the systemic circulation and the liver before crossing the blood-brain barrier. Anticholinergic drugs improve symptoms by manipulating the dopamine acetylcholine electrochemical balance in the basal ganglia. Dopamine agonists are antioxidants and free-radical scavengers. MAO-B inhibitors block free radical formation and may inhibit apoptosis.

1. Kaufman DM. *Clinical Neurology for Psychiatrists*. 5th ed. Philadelphia: WB Saunders; 2001: 455–457.
2. Rao SS, Hofmann LA, Shakil A. Parkinson's disease: diagnosis and treatment. *Am Fam Physician*. 2006;74:2046–2054.

179. Answer: C. Obstetric complications of cocaine use include premature rupture of the membranes, spontaneous abortion, placenta previa, and placental abruption.

Sadock BJ, Sadock VA. *Kaplan and Sadock's Comprehensive Textbook of Psychiatry*. 8th ed. Philadelphia: Lippincott Williams & Wilkins; 2005:1229.

180. Answer: A. There are a number of dynamic theories to explain the development of depression. Two common themes among them are aggression turned inward and poor self-esteem. Object loss plays an important role in theories about depression, but none of the other answers capture this role adequately.

Sadock BJ, Sadock VA. *Kaplan and Sadock's Comprehensive Textbook of Psychiatry*. 8th ed. Philadelphia: Lippincott Williams & Wilkins; 2005:1606.

181. Answer: D. Although the duration and presentation of normal bereavement vary considerably among different cultural groups, a diagnosis of MDE is not usually made unless the symptoms persists for more than 2 months after the loss. Symptoms that may indicate an MDE and not normal grief include all of the following: (i) guilt about things other than actions taken or not taken by the survivor at the time of death, (ii) thoughts of death other than the survivor feeling that he or she would be better off dead or should have died with the deceased person, (iii) morbid preoccupations with worthlessness, (iv) marked psychomotor retardation, and (v) hallucinatory experiences other than thinking of hearing voices of or transiently seeing images of the deceased person, and prolonged and marked functional impairment.

American Psychiatric Association. *Desk Reference to the Diagnostic Criteria from DSM-IV-TR*. Washington: American Psychiatric Association; 2000:311–312.

182. Answer: C. Drug abuse is common in patients with Schizophrenia. The lifetime prevalence of any drug abuse (other than tobacco) is often greater than 50%. For all drugs of abuse (other than tobacco), abuse is associated with poorer function. The rate of Nicotine Dependence is especially high, with 80% to 90% of individuals with schizophrenia being regular cigarette smokers. These individuals tend to smoke heavily and tend to choose cigarettes with high nicotine content. Alcohol Abuse is also a serious problem in patients with Schizophrenia. The lifetime prevalence of Alcohol Abuse in patients with Schizophrenia is about 40%. Alcohol Abuse increases risk of psychotic symptoms and hospitalization. About 16% of subjects with Schizophrenia have a history of nonalcohol substance abuse with the use of amphetamine and cocaine being common. These drugs can worsen psychotic symptoms.

1. American Psychiatric Association. *DSM-IV-TR Diagnostic and Statistical Manual of Mental Disorders*. 4th ed. (Text Revision). http://www.psychiatryonline.com/content.aspx?aID=8939. Accessed January 10, 2007.
2. Sadock BJ, Sadock VA. *Kaplan and Sadock's Comprehensive Textbook of Psychiatry*. 8th ed. Philadelphia: Lippincott Williams & Wilkins; 2005:1433–1434.

183. Answer: E. No dose changes are necessary for aripiprazole in mild, moderate or severe hepatic impairment. No dosage adjustments are necessary for flupentixol, although caution is advised in significant hepatic impairment as it is metabolized hepatically. Similarly, for ziprasidone, no adjustments are necessary in mild to moderate impairment. Haloperidol and pimozide are other drugs that have a low risk of hepatic impairment, although dose adjustments may be necessary in severe impairment. Clozapine, loxapine, olanzapine, risperidone, quetiapine, phenothiazines, and sertindole have moderate risk of hepatic impairment. Clozapine and sertindole are contraindicated in severe hepatic impairment. Phenothiazines may cause hepatocanalicular cholestasis; there are suggestions of immunologically-mediated hepatic damage. Coma may be precipitated due to cerebral neuron sensitivity. Chlorpromazine is particularly hepatotoxic.

Bazire S. *Problem areas. Psychotropic Drug Directory 2005.* Wiltshire: Fivepin Limited; 2005:224–225.

184. Answer: E. Women represent at least 75% of all patients with seasonal depression, and the mean age of presentation is 40 years of age. Patients older than 55 years of age rarely present with seasonal affective disorder. Phototherapy (light therapy) is a treatment for seasonal affective disorder. The recommended treatment is 10,000 lux light for at least 30 minutes daily (can be as long as 2 hours) before dawn. A number of controlled studies suggest that phototherapy is as effective as monotherapy and as an adjunctive agent in the treatment of winter depressions. Studies have generally compared low-intensity light (<100 lux) with high-intensity light (>1,500 lux), and patients can usually differentiate low-intensity from high-intensity exposures. Bipolar depression with a seasonal component frequently appears responsive to phototherapy, and these patients also appear to be more susceptible to light-induced mania. Phototherapy tends to be well tolerated. Common side effects include irritability, headache, eyestrain, visual disturbances, nausea, sweating, and sedation. Ophthalmic damage is rare with currently used light sources. As with any effective antidepressant treatment, phototherapy has on the rare occasion been implicated in switching some depressed patients into hypomania or mania.

Sadock BJ, Sadock VA. *Kaplan and Sadock's Comprehensive Textbook of Psychiatry.* 7th ed. Philadelphia: Lippincott Williams & Wilkins; 2000:2522.

185. Answer: A. Carbamazepine induces cytochrome P450 enzymes and thus decreases plasma levels of benzodiazepines, and in this clinical case, precipitated withdrawal. Fluoxetine inhibits cytochrome P450 enzymes and thus would increase plasma levels of benzodiazepines. Citalopram also inhibits these enzymes but to a much lesser degree. Lithium does not inhibit or induce the cytochrome P450 system and is not metabolized by it. Lamotrigine is metabolized by the cytochrome P450 system but does not inhibit or induce it.

Rosenbaum JF, Arana GW, Hyman SE, et al. *Handbook of Psychiatric Drug Therapy.* 5th ed. Philadelphia:

Lippincott Williams & Wilkins; 2005:79–92, 122–149, 155–166.

186. Answer: A. All of the choices are accurate except choice A. The structural model was developed by Freud before he presented the topographical model. In the structural model, the psyche is envisioned as made of three parts: the ego, id, and superego. There can be conflict or tension among these components, thus producing anxiety.

Gabbard GO. *Psychodynamic Psychiatry in Clinical Practice.* 3rd ed. Washington: American Psychiatric Press; 2000:28–29.

187. Answer: B. Wilfred Bion worked to elucidate group dynamics at the Tavistock Institute in London, and described 2 main subgroups: the work group and the basic assumption group. The work group is involved in performing the actual task assigned to the group. The basic assumption group is divided into three categories: dependency, fight or flight, and pairing. These basic assumptions pertain to the unconscious fantasies of the group members, and they interfere with the accomplishment of the work group's task. The group members' behavior reveals which basic assumption predominates. In this vignette, the group members are dependent upon and idealizing the therapist, behavior which is a defense against depressive anxieties. Bion came from the school of Kleinian Object Relations, and he also developed the concept of psychiatrist as *container* for the patient in therapy.

1. Gabbard G. *Psychodynamic Psychiatry in Clinical Practice.* 4th ed. Washington: American Psychiatric Press; 2005:129–131.
2. Ganzarain RC. Psychotic-like anxieties and primitive defenses in group analytic psychotherapy. *Issues in Ego Psychology.*1980;3:42–48.
3. Sadock BJ, Sadock VA. *Kaplan and Sadock's Comprehensive Textbook of Psychiatry.* 8th ed. Philadelphia: Lippincott Williams & Wilkins; 2005:734–735.

188. Answer: C. The lack of inhibition of the hypothalamic-pituitary-adrenal axis by exogenous glucocorticoid in the presence of severe depression is found in children, adolescents, and adults. The DST is normal if there is suppression of the plasma cortisol level to less than 5 μg/dL 8 to 24 hours after an oral dose of 1 mg dexamethasone given at 11 PM. An abnormal DST is found in approximately 45% of patients with depression. The test has shown a specificity as high as 80% in some studies, but the specificity depends on the population tested. Abnormal DST are seen in other psychiatric disorders, including Anorexia Nervosa, Obsessive-Compulsive Disorder, Dementias, Mania, Schizophrenia, alcoholism, psychosexual dysfunction, and Schizoaffective disorder. They are also seen in Parkinson's disease and stroke. Other variables such as weight loss, acute hospitalization, and drug and alcohol withdrawal, can affect the test significantly, along with many commonly prescribed medications. Given this information, the DST is a more sensitive test for major depression in older persons and children and adolescents. It is abnormal more frequently in patients with psychotic affective disorders and melancholia (>50%) than in those with minor depression (23%) or grief reactions (10%). The exact reason for the nonsuppression is not known. The DST has not evolved into a routine diagnostic test in clinical psychiatry because of its lack of specificity.

Schiffer RB, Rao SM, Fogel BS. *Neuropsychiatry*. 2nd ed. Philadelphia: Lippincott Williams & Wilkins; 2003:221.

189. **Answer: C.** Acetylcholine is a major transmitter of the peripheral motor system, the presynaptic autonomic nervous system, the postsynaptic innervation of sweat glands, and the entire postsynaptic parasympathetic system. It also serves as a neurotransmitter in a number of CNS pathways. Acetylcholine released from presynaptic terminals interacts with postsynaptic receptors similar to that of amino acids. There is no high-affinity transport system for acetylcholine, instead it is broken down within the synaptic cleft by the enzyme, acetylcholinesterase to form choline and acetyl coenzyme A. The choline is taken back up into the presynaptic nerve terminal by a transporter and used for synthesis of new acetylcholine. Drugs useful in treating myasthenia gravis act by blocking the activity of acetylcholinesterase at the neuromuscular junction. Centrally active inhibitors of acetylcholinesterase are now used in the treatment of AD.

Schiffer RB, Rao SM, Fogel BS. *Neuropsychiatry*. 2nd ed. Philadelphia: Lippincott Williams & Wilkins; 2003:199.

190. **Answer: B.** Corticosteroids are the treatment of choice for acute multiple sclerosis attacks. The glatiramer acetate, IFNB-1a, IFNB-1b, and natalizumab are disease-modifying treatments.

Olek MJ. Treatment of Relapsing-Remitting Multiple Sclerosis. http://www.uptodateonline.com/utd/content/topic.do?topicKey=demyelin/2880&type=A&selectedTitle=2~6. Accessed March 4, 2007.

191. **Answer: A.** Hallucinogens bind to one or more of the serotonin receptor subtypes and act as agonists or partial agonists. Dopamine receptors may also play a role, but less so than the serotoninergic system.

Sadock BJ, Sadock VA. *Kaplan and Sadock's Comprehensive Textbook of Psychiatry*. 8th ed. Philadelphia: Lippincott Williams & Wilkins; 2005:1243.

192. **Answer: D.** Criterion A requires mood reactivity. Criterion B requires 2 of 4 of the other options (leaden paralysis, hypersomnia, weight gain or increased appetite, and longstanding interpersonal rejection sensitivity). Criterion C requires that the criteria for Melancholic or Catatonic features are not met.

American Psychiatric Association. *Desk Reference to the Diagnostic Criteria from DSM-IV-TR*. Washington: American Psychiatric Association; 2000:203–204.

193. **Answer: A.** Three diagnoses (Antisocial Personality Disorder, Schizophrenia, and Bipolar I Disorder) are most likely to run a course independent of Alcohol Abuse or Dependence and be true comorbid conditions. Helzer and Pryzbeck in their pivotal study used data from the ECA survey and found that every one of the psychiatric diagnoses examined was more likely to occur in alcoholics than in nonalcoholics. Associations were particularly strong with Antisocial Personality Disorder, other substance use and Mania. They found an odds ratio of 21.0 for a comorbid diagnosis of alcoholism and Antisocial Personality Disorder followed by drug dependence (11.2), Mania (6.2), Schizophrenia (4.0), Panic Disorder (2.4), and Major Depression (1.7). About 80% of people with Antisocial Personality Disorder are likely to develop severe alcohol problems in the course of their lives. A diagnosis of preexisting Antisocial Personality Disorder with subsequent Alcohol Abuse or Dependence indicates a poorer prognosis as they are more likely than the average Alcohol-Dependent person to have severe coexisting drug problems, to be violent, to discontinue treatment prematurely, and to have a less-than-optimistic prognosis.

1. Helzer JE, Pryzbeck TR. The co-occurrence of alcoholism with other psychiatric disorders in the general population and its impact on treatment. *J Stud Alcohol*. 1988;49:219–224.
2. Sadock BJ, Sadock VA. *Kaplan and Sadock's Comprehensive Textbook of Psychiatry*. 8th ed. Philadelphia: Lippincott Williams & Wilkins; 2005:1182–1183.

194. **Answer: E.** Malingering is the intentional production of false or grossly exaggerated physical or psychological symptoms, motivated by external incentives such as avoiding work, obtaining financial compensation, drugs, or evading criminal prosecution or military duty. According to the DSM-IV-TR, malingering should be strongly suspected when any combination of the above noted findings are present.

American Psychiatric Association. *DSM-IV-TR Diagnostic and Statistical Manual of Mental Disorders*. 4th ed. (Text Revision). http://www.psychiatryonline.com/content.aspx?aID=11409. Accessed January 14, 2007.

195. Answer: C. Valproate inhibits the metabolism of lamotrigine thereby increasing the plasma concentration of lamotrigine. Gabapentin, phenytoin, tiagabine, and zonisamide do not appear to effect lamotrigine's metabolism.

Schachter SC. Overview of the Management of Epilepsy in Adults. http://www.uptodateonline.com/utd/content/topic.do?topicKey=epil_eeg/4878&type=A&selectedTitle=2~268. Accessed March 4, 2007.

196. Answer: E. In a meta-analysis of 94 randomized placebo-controlled trials of four different classes of blood pressure-lowering drugs (thiazides, beta-blockers, ACE inhibitors, and angiotensin II receptor antagonists) in fixed doses treatment with any one of the drugs resulted in one third fewer patients on average reporting headache in the treated groups (8.0%) compared to placebo groups (12.4%) (odds ratio, 0.67; 95% CI, 0.61 to 0.74; $p <0.001$). Approximately 1 in 30 treated persons benefited by having the headache prevented. The prevalence of headache was reduced ($p <0.001$) in trials of each of the four classes of drugs. This effect seen with pharmacologically unrelated classes of drugs indicates that the headache reduction is most likely to be due to the reduction in blood pressure per se, the only recognized action that the drugs have in common.

Law M, Morris JK, Jordan R, Wald N. Headaches and the treatment of blood pressure: results from a meta-analysis of 94 randomized placebo-controlled trials with 24,000 participants. *Circulation*. 2005;112:2301–2306.

197. Answer: A. The only FDA approved beta-blockers for the prophylaxis of migraines are propranolol and timolol. Propranolol, nadolol, atenolol, metoprolol, and timolol have been shown to be effective although metoprolol, nadolol, and atenolol are commonly used. These drugs take several weeks for them to become effective and the dose should be titrated and maintained for at least 3 months before it is considered to be ineffective. These drugs should be used cautiously with erectile dysfunction, peripheral vascular disease, Raynaud's disease, and in patients with bradycardia and hypotension. They must also be used cautiously in patients with asthma, diabetes mellitus, and those with cardiac conduction disturbances or sinus node dysfunction.

Bigal ME, Lipton RB. The preventive treatment of migraine. *Neurologist*. 2006 Jul;12(4):204–13.

198. Answer: D. Although divalproex sodium, topiramate, and gabapentin have demonstrated efficacy in the prophylaxis of migraines, only divalproex sodium and topiramate are FDA approved for the prophylaxis of migraines. These drugs are especially useful when migraine occurs in patients with comorbid epilepsy, anxiety disorder, or manic-depressive illness. They can also be safely administered in patients with depression, Raynaud disease, asthma, and diabetes, when beta-blocker use is contraindicated. The efficacy of topiramate is supported by two large clinical trials which indicated that the target dose of topiramate for patients with migraines should be about 100 mg/day for most patients. These studies also indicated that the treatment effect of topiramate is seen within two weeks of initiation of therapy and its efficacy progressively increases over several months. Chronic use of topiramate has been associated with weight loss. Topiramate should be started at a dose of 15 to 25 mg/day at bedtime and increased weekly to 100 to 200 mg/day in divided doses. Side effects of this drug include weight loss, paresthesias, and cognitive dysfunction, which can often be prevented by slow gradual dose escalation. This drug should also be used with caution in patients who have a history of renal calculi.

1. Bigal ME, Lipton RB. The preventive treatment of migraine. *Neurologist*. 2006;12:204–213.
2. Bren L. *Managing Migraines*. http://www.fda.gov/fdac/features/2006/206_migraines.html. Published March 6, 2007.

199. Answer: A. The EEG is often used as an adjunctive tool to aid in the diagnosis of certain neurological conditions. However in SSPE, the EEG shows distinct periodic complexes that are diagnostic. There are four other conditions that EEG is also helpful in diagnosing. These include CJD, hepatic encephalopathy, psychogenic seizures, and pseudodementia.

Kaufman DM. *Clinical Neurology for Psychiatrists*. 5th ed. Philadelphia: WB Saunders; 2001:231.

200. Answer: D. Inside the presynaptic terminal there are many membrane-enclosed vesicles, which contain the neurotransmitters. There are three kinds of synaptic vesicles: (i) small, clear synaptic vesicles that contain acetylcholine, glycine, GABA, or glutamate, (ii) small vesicles with a dense core that contain catecholamines, and (iii) the large vesicles with a dense core that contains neuropeptides. The vesicles and the proteins contained in their walls are synthesized in the neuronal cell body and transported along the axon to the endings by fast axoplasmic transport. Usually, the synaptic vesicle discharges its contents through a small hole in the cell membrane, then the opening reseals rapidly and the main vesicle stays inside the cell. However, the small clear vesicles and the small dense-core vesicles are recycled.

The large dense-core vesicles are located throughout the presynaptic terminals and release their neuropeptide contents by exocytosis from all parts of the terminal. On the other hand, the small vesicles located near the synaptic cleft fuse to the membrane, discharging their contents very rapidly into the cleft in areas of membrane thickening called active zones. These active zones contain many proteins and rows of calcium channels. Voltage-gated Ca^{2+} channels are present very close to the release sites at the active zones as it is the Ca^{2+} that triggers exocytosis of neurotransmitters into the synaptic cleft.

Ganong, WF. *Review of Medical Physiology*. 22nd ed. http://www.accessmedicine.com/content.aspx?aID=707278. Accessed February 17, 2007.

Questions

1. Which one of the following is considered normal in an aging man?
   A. Impotence
   B. Retarded ejaculation
   C. Hypoactive sexual desire
   D. Increased time needed to achieve an erection
   E. Premature ejaculation

2. Which of the following pathological findings is more commonly seen in patients with Schizophrenia?
   A. Cortical gliosis
   B. Thalamic gliosis
   C. Decreased prefrontal gray matter
   D. Enlarged hippocampus
   E. Decreased thalamic density

3. Which of the following statements is best supported by Konrad Lorenz's work on aggression in animals?
   A. Aggression is not commonly seen among members of the same species, as it is between species.
   B. An animal that is consistently attacked will eventually give up and make no attempt to escape.
   C. Aggression between the members of the same species often leads to serious injury or death.
   D. In any conflict situations, animals will display displacement activities.
   E. There is a practical function of aggression, and a balance between tendencies to fight and flight.

4. Incidence of which of the following psychiatric disorders has the highest female to male ratio?
   A. Social Phobia
   B. Schizophrenia
   C. Bipolar Disorder
   D. Alcohol Dependence
   E. Major Depression

5. Positron emission tomography (PET) scan of a patient with obsessive compulsive disorder (OCD) symptoms would likely reveal increased activity in all of the following regions EXCEPT:
   A. Orbitofrontal (anterior cingulate) cortex
   B. Caudate nucleus
   C. Thalamus
   D. Midbrain
   E. Putamen

6. Which one of the following statements is TRUE?
   A. In Factitious Disorder, the motivation for symptom production is an external incentive.
   B. In Malingering, the motivation for symptom production is an intrapsychic conflict and the need to maintain the sick role.
   C. In Conversion Disorder, there is no intentional production of symptoms or obvious external incentives associated with it.
   D. In Malingering, symptom relief is often obtained by suggestion or hypnosis.
   E. All of the above.

7. A 65-year-old woman with hypertension and diabetes, both well controlled with antihypertensives and oral hypoglycemic agents, is brought by her daughter to a psychiatrist for an evaluation. The patient's husband of 40 years died 1 month ago, and the patient has been hearing the voice of her deceased husband. She admits to feeling sad, has difficulty concentrating on reading and is tearful when she thinks of her husband and sometimes hears his voice calling her. She states she is sleeping well, has a good appetite, and that she enjoys spending time with her grandchildren and wants to see them grow up. She scores a 25/30 on the Mini Mental Status Examination (MMSE). Which of the following is the most appropriate next step in the management of this patient's condition?
   A. Admit the patient for an in-patient hospitalization and obtain a brain CT scan
   B. Prescribe a low dose antipsychotic agent for auditory hallucinations
   C. Prescribe an acetylcholinesterase inhibitor for the beginning stages of dementia
   D. Prescribe a selective serotonin reuptake inhibitor (SSRI) for depression
   E. Reassure the patient and family that she is experiencing normal grieving

8. All of the following are TRUE of Postpsychotic Depressive Disorder of Schizophrenia EXCEPT:
   A. It is thought to occur in approximately 25% of patients with Schizophrenia.
   B. Symptoms experienced by patients with this disorder are the equivalent of negative symptoms of Schizophrenia.

437

C. There is evidence that there is a correlation between the disorder and extrapyramidal symptoms.

D. There is evidence that antidepressants can be useful as a treatment.

E. Depressive symptoms must occur during the residual phase of schizophrenia.

9. A 42-year-old man previously diagnosed years ago with Schizophrenia for bizarre delusions, now lives with his parents, and continues to report some unusual perceptions, expresses some mild odd beliefs, and eccentric behavior. He no longer has frank delusions or hallucinations. He appears emotionally blunted, and spends much of his time alone doing very little. Which is the most likely subtype diagnosis for his Schizophrenia?

A. Undifferentiated type
B. Disorganized type
C. Residual type
D. Catatonic type
E. Paranoid type

10. While observing a group session, there seems to be a theme that the group members have rallied around two individuals who are romantically involved and whose love will help save the group. Which of the following Bion subgroups would best account for this scenario?

A. *Work* group
B. *Dependency* basic assumption group
C. *Fight or Flight* basic assumption group
D. *Pairing* basic assumption group
E. None of the above

11. Which of the following is an important consideration in the referral of patients to specialized long-term alcohol rehabilitation program?

A. Living in an unstable environment
B. Polysubstance Dependence
C. Multiple treatment failures
D. Dual diagnoses: Comorbid severe mental illness and Alcohol Dependence
E. All of the above

12. Which psychodynamic characteristic of Passive-Aggressive subtype of Dependent Personality structure is incorrectly paired?

A. Central preoccupation: Tolerating mistreatment versus getting revenge
B. Central affects: Anger, resentment, and pleasure in hostile enactments
C. Pathogenic belief about self: I am entitled to hurt and humiliate others
D. Pathogenic belief about others: People all want me to conform to their rules

E. Central defenses: Projection, externalization, denial, and rationalization

13. Which of the following is TRUE of behavioral and relaxation approaches to treating chronic pain?

A. Available data indicates that cognitive behavioral therapy (CBT) is the most effective treatment for this condition.
B. The evidence is strong for the effectiveness of relaxation in reducing chronic pain in a variety of medical conditions.
C. The evidence supporting the effectiveness of hypnosis in alleviating chronic pain associated with cancer is weak.
D. The evidence is weak for the effectiveness of biofeedback (BF) in relieving chronic pain.
E. None of the above.

14. Which one of the following is NOT TRUE of venlafaxine?

A. Venlafaxine is a serotonin-norepinephrine reuptake inhibitor (SNRI).
B. It does not have an active metabolite.
C. Steady-state concentrations is attained in the blood within 3 days.
D. It should never be used in conjunction with a monoamine oxidase inhibitor (MAOI).
E. Caution should also be used in those patients with a seizure disorder.

15. Which individual diagnosis listed below carries the greatest risk of completed suicide?

A. Schizophrenia
B. Schizoaffective Disorder
C. Major Depressive Disorder (MDD)
D. Bipolar Disorder
E. Alcohol Abuse

16. During a neurological examination you notice that a patient does not have taste sensation in the anterior two thirds of the tongue. Which cranial nerve is most likely to be affected in this case?

A. CN IV
B. CN V
C. CN VI
D. CN VII
E. CN IX

17. A 25-year-old woman presents to a clinic with complaints of sudden onset of blindness in her right eye with right-sided paresis and right-sided sensory loss. Funduscopic exam is normal and extraocular movements are intact. Pupils are round and reactive to light and accommodation. She is unable to lift her right leg against resistance and drags her right leg behind her when she walks. A magnetic resonance

imaging (MRI) would most likely reveal which of the following:

A. A lesion in the cerebellum
B. A lesion in the cerebrum
C. A lesion in the midbrain
D. A lesion in the pons
E. No lesion

18. Which one of the following is NOT TRUE of Lambert-Eaton syndrome?

A. It is an autoimmune disorder where antibodies directed against voltage-gated calcium channels develop in the peripheral nerve terminals.
B. It develops in adults, and occurs in 60% of patients with small cell carcinoma of the lung.
C. In patients with small cell carcinoma of the lung, neurologic symptoms usually precede those of the tumor.
D. In those patients who have the syndrome without any tumors, they have the human leucocyte antigen (HLA)-B8 and DR-3 haplotype.
E. The diagnosis is confirmed by the characteristic reduction in response to repetitive nerve stimulation.

19. An 18-year-old high school senior describes episodes of dizziness, "spacing out," and paresthesia around her mouth and fingertips. On occasions, her wrists bend and her fingers are pulled together. These episodes last for less than 5 minutes. You review an electroencephalogram (EEG) performed during one of these episodes 2 years ago. This shows slowing of background activities and occasional bursts of high voltage. You can attempt to confirm your diagnosis by which of the following bedside maneuvers?

A. Valsalva maneuver
B. Asking her to stand up rapidly from a supine position
C. Have the patient hyperventilate
D. Simulating a populated room
E. Exposing her to sudden loud noise

20. Which of the following represents the rate-limiting step in the metabolic synthesis of norepinephrine?

A. Tyrosine hydroxylase
B. Dehydroxyphenyl alanine (DOPA) decarboxylase
C. Dopamine beta-hydroxylase (DβH)
D. Catechol-O-methyltransferase (COMT)
E. Norepinephrine transporter (NET)

21. A 35-year-old man presents to clinic with complaints of shaking of his hands. The shaking began a year ago and is particularly bad when writing or eating. He noticed that stress often makes the shaking worse, but having a glass of wine before meals allows him to eat without dropping food. He remembers his father had similar complaints before passing away from a tragic car accident. Given his history, which one of the following is the most likely diagnosis for his condition?

A. Essential tremor
B. Huntington's disease
C. Multiple sclerosis (MS)
D. Parkinson's disease (PD)
E. Wilson's disease

22. The presence or absence of all of the following clinical features is useful in distinguishing between cervical spondylotic myelopathy (CSM) and amyotrophic lateral sclerosis (ALS) EXCEPT:

A. Tongue fasciculations
B. Atrophy of arms
C. Atrophy of legs
D. Denervation
E. Sensory loss

23. A 30-year-old white woman is diagnosed with Guillain-Barré syndrome (GBS). While deciding on the appropriate treatment for this condition, which one of the following choices would you NOT take into account as the information is NOT CORRECT?

A. Plasma exchange or IV immunoglobulins (IVIG) hastens the recovery from GBS
B. The beneficial effects of plasma exchange and IVIG are equivalent
C. Combining plasma exchange and IVIG is much better that monotherapy with either drug alone
D. Plasma exchange should be given to non-ambulatory adult patients with GBS who start treatment within four weeks of the onset of neurologic symptoms
E. IVIG is recommended for non-ambulatory adult patients with GBS who start treatment within two or possibly four weeks of the onset of neurologic symptoms

24. All of the following are TRUE of the neuropathological features of Creutzfeldt-Jakob disease (CJD) EXCEPT:

A. Neuronal degeneration and astrocytic proliferation are commonly seen
B. The grey matter shows a characteristic spongy appearance
C. Circumscribed atrophy is often seen in the parietal and occipital lobes
D. Neurofibrillary tangles are commonly seen
E. Cortical status of spongiosus is not entirely pathognomonic of this disorder

25. Which of the following choices is NOT TRUE of akathisia?

A. Akathisia is an extremely unpleasant sensation that manifests itself as an inability to sit still.

B. In certain cases, the dysphoria can be so severe that patients may attempt suicide.

C. It may often be misdiagnosed as an anxiety disorder.

D. It may also be seen in Parkinson's disease.

E. Benztropine is the drug of choice to treat this condition.

26. A 70-year-old white woman presents with sudden onset of right unilateral temporal scalp pain and reduced vision in the right eye. Given this history, which one of the following should be the next best step in the management of this patient's condition?

A. Start treatment with intravenous methylprednisone

B. Get a temporal artery biopsy to confirm diagnosis

C. Order an erythrocyte sedimentation rate (ESR) to confirm diagnosis

D. Start treatment with acetaminophen

E. Start treatment with methotrexate

27. Which one of the following statements about suicide and gender is NOT TRUE?

A. Suicide risk increases with age for both sexes, but the rates in older men are generally higher than those for women.

B. In the United States men commit suicide four times more commonly than women, but women attempt suicide three times as often as men.

C. Men also tend to use more lethal suicide methods than women.

D. Factors that contribute to these gender differences include the presence of depression and comorbid alcohol and/or substance abuse.

E. In women, pregnancy is a time of significantly increased suicide risk.

28. Which one of the following is a characteristic of the tau-protein?

A. They normally maintain the cytoskeleton, axonal flow, and nerve cell circuitry.

B. They are neuropil threads.

C. They can be visualized with anti-A β antibodies.

D. They generate a glial response.

E. They are thought to be a degeneration of the neuronal cytoskeleton.

29. A 12-year-old Haitian girl is referred from school for an evaluation of potential psychosis after a teacher overheard the patient talking to spirits in an empty classroom. She is well groomed and engaging, has many friends at school, is doing well academically, and is an active participant in many school activities and sports. The patient is embarrassed to admit to feeling "spirits" of her deceased ancestors around her most of the time and states conversing with them helps her relax when nervous. The patient's parents and grandparents also believe in the presence of these spirits but are willing to follow any suggestions from the psychiatrist. The patient denies any history of drug use and denies any recent or current feelings of depression or suicidal ideation, intent, or plan. Which one of the following is the most appropriate intervention at this time for this patient?

A. Admit the patient to an in-patient unit for workup of psychosis.

B. Prescribe a low-dose antipsychotic agent and follow the patient as an outpatient.

C. Reassure the patient and family that there is no obvious psychiatric illness.

D. Recommend family counseling to treat delusional disorder among the family.

E. Separate the patient from her parents and look into foster care.

30. Which of the following is TRUE regarding the treatment of psychotic disorders during pregnancy?

A. Low potency antipsychotics are believed to have lower teratogenicity compared to higher potency antipsychotics.

B. First-trimester use of mood stabilizers (such as lithium, carbamazepine, or valproic acid) is considered safe.

C. Antidepressant use during pregnancy is recommended and completely safe.

D. There is no need to avoid routine benzodiazepine use during pregnancy.

E. Non-pharmacologic treatment methods are preferable during pregnancy.

31. A patient with chronic renal failure and on dialysis presents with recent history of personality changes, hallucinations, dysarthria, and dyspraxia associated with myoclonic jerks. Which of the following most likely contributed to this presentation?

A. Lead

B. Mercury

C. Selenium

D. Aluminum

E. None of the above

32. An 18-year-old college student is studying for the current semester's final exams. In order to stay awake studying into the wee hours of the morning, she consumes multiple cups of black coffee. Just as she is about to lie down for an hour or two of sleep, she begins to feel restless and nervous. Her stomach becomes upset and she finds it necessary to

make multiple trips to the bathroom. Despite believing that she should really take a nap, she is unable to fall asleep as thoughts race through her mind. She becomes fearful that in this state, she is likely to fail her exam in the morning. She is otherwise healthy, has no prior psychiatric history, and is not taking any medications. Given her symptoms, approximately how much caffeine is she likely to have consumed?

A. <25 mg
B. 50 to 100 mg
C. 250 to 500 mg
D. 1 to 5 g
E. >10 g

33. Based on the demographic data, which of the following individuals is most likely to be addicted to cocaine?

A. A 45-year-old woman who is a homemaker
B. A 25-year-old unemployed man living in an urban area
C. A 13-year-old high school student in a rural setting
D. A 75-year-old nursing home resident with dementia
E. A 35-year-old manual laborer living in the Pacific Northwest

34. According to the DSM-IV-TR all of the following disorders are classified as learning disorders EXCEPT:

A. Reading Disorder
B. Stuttering
C. Mathematics Disorder
D. Disorder of Written Communication
E. Learning Disorder, Not Otherwise Specified

35. Which of the following factors would favor a better long-term prognosis in an individual diagnosed with Schizophrenia?

A. Social isolation
B. A history of childhood behavioral problems
C. Prior history of psychiatric treatment
D. Being married
E. Longer duration of psychotic episode

36. Which of the following regarding naltrexone therapy for Alcohol Dependence is NOT TRUE?

A. It is given in a dose of 50 mg orally per day.
B. It can be administered concurrently with opioid analgesics in patients with severe pain.
C. It is contraindicated in patients with acute hepatitis or liver failure.
D. Effective response is usually evident in 10 days or less.
E. It should be discontinued in patients who have not responded in 10 days.

37. Which one of the following is TRUE of buprenorphine?

A. Buprenorphine is a full agonist at the mu-opioid receptor.
B. It has a low affinity for and a fast dissociation from mu-opioid receptors.
C. Buprenorphine displaces other opioids from the mu receptor, and can cause withdrawal symptoms in patients who have used opioids recently.
D. Its oral formulation has excellent bioavailability.
E. Its mean plasma elimination half-life is 10 hours.

38. Which psychodynamic characteristic of Schizoid Personality structure is incorrectly paired?

A. Central preoccupation: Fear of closeness versus longing for closeness
B. Central affects: Emotional pain when overstimulated
C. Central pathogenic belief about self: Dependency and love are dangerous
D. Central pathogenic belief about others: People who really get to know me will reject me
E. Central defenses: Withdrawal into fantasy and idiosyncratic preoccupations

39. Which one of the following is NOT TRUE of behavioral treatments for sleep?

A. Behavioral treatments are most helpful for sleep latency and time awake after sleep onset.
B. Relaxation and BF are both effective in alleviating insomnia.
C. Cognitive forms of relaxation such as meditation are slightly better than somatic forms of relaxation such as progressive muscle relaxation (PMR).
D. Sleep restriction is better than stimulus control and multimodal treatments for reducing insomnia.
E. Improvements seen at treatment completion are maintained at follow-ups averaging 6 months in duration.

40. Which one of the following is TRUE of bupropion?

A. It is an SNRI.
B. It is excreted unchanged by the kidneys.
C. It can be used concomitantly with MAOIs.
D. Its combination with nicotine replacement therapies can cause hypotension.
E. It is a category B in pregnancy.

41. Which of the following is the best predictor of future violent behavior in a patient?

A. Intense paranoia
B. Substance Intoxication or Abuse
C. Antisocial Personality

D. History of fire-setting, enuresis, and cruelty to animals

E. None of the above

42. Which of the following clinical findings is NOT associated with bulbar palsy?

A. Nasal intonation during speech

B. Dysphagia

C. Loss of gag reflex

D. Depressed jaw jerk reflex

E. Loss of taste in anterior two thirds of tongue

43. A 62-year-old man with hypertension and diabetes, but no past psychiatric history, presents to the emergency department (ED) because of a change in mental status over the past several days. His daughter states he is usually happy and enjoys spending time with his grandchildren and playing word puzzles, but over the past few days has been apathetic, refuses to go out or play, and has been tired and had difficulty concentrating. Physical examination is unremarkable. An MRI of the brain would likely reveal a lesion in which of the following structures?

A. A lesion in the frontal lobe

B. A lesion in the occipital lobe

C. A lesion in the parietal lobe

D. A lesion in the temporal lobe

E. No lesion, as this patient has a primary depressive disorder

44. Which one of the following statements about the concept of linkage analysis is correct?

A. It is essential to have a candidate gene in mind before beginning the study.

B. Polygenic traits are difficult to map with linkage analysis.

C. Classic linkage analysis is useful in tracking most psychiatric disorders.

D. Individual genes always independently assort.

E. It depends on the identification of a chromosomal abnormality.

45. Which of the following are prognostic indicators for traumatic brain injury (TBI)?

A. Duration of loss of consciousness (LOC)

B. Duration of post-traumatic amnesia (PTA)

C. Glasgow coma scale

D. All of the above

E. None of the above

46. Which is the major excitatory neurotransmitter in the central nervous system (CNS)?

A. Glutamate

B. γ-aminobutyric acid (GABA)

C. Glycine

D. Norepinephrine

E. Dopamine

47. Which of the following movement disorders carries the highest probability of genetic transmission for the child of an affected patient?

A. Parkinson's disease (PD)

B. Huntington's disease

C. Lesch-Nyhan syndrome

D. Sydenham's chorea

E. Wilson's disease

48. A 28-year-old man presents to the ED after a severe motor vehicle accident. He has stable vital signs, but has left-sided leg paresis with hyperactive deep tendon reflexes (DTRs) and a Babinski sign. He also has impairment of vibration and position sense of the left leg, and loss of temperature and pain sensation in the right leg. This patient's condition is most consistent with which of the following spinal cord injuries?

A. Anterior-cord syndrome

B. Brown-Sequard syndrome

C. Central cord transection

D. Complete cord transection

E. Posterior-cord syndrome

49. Which one of the following is the most common type of diabetic neuropathy?

A. Polyneuropathy

B. Autonomic neuropathy

C. Mononeuropathy affecting the oculomotor and median nerve

D. Thoracic and lumbar polyradiculopathies

E. Mononeuritis multiplex

50. You have a 49-year-old patient who was diagnosed with Huntington's disease 4 months ago. He has been managing his illness well, but recently his involuntary movements have begun to interfere with his activities of daily life. Which of the following medications would be helpful in treating his involuntary movements?

A. Pramipexole

B. Benztropine

C. Ropinirole

D. Haloperidol

E. Levodopa

51. A 55-year-old patient with PD is thinking of undergoing deep brain stimulation (DBS). When counseling this patient on DBS, which one of the following statements should you make to describe this procedure?

A. DBS of the globus pallidus (GPi) is the treatment of choice for patients with intractable PD.

B. DBS is destructive and can only be done as a unilateral procedure.

C. It can be modified over time to deal with changing or progressing symptoms.

D. It is most helpful for axial symptoms.

E. It does not slow the progression of the underlying neurodegenerative disease.

52. Each of the following medications induces the hepatic metabolism of other drugs EXCEPT:

A. Phenytoin
B. Phenobarbital
C. Carbamazepine
D. Primidone
E. Divalproex sodium

53. Guidance, care, productivity, and creativity are characteristics of which stage in Erik Erikson's Epigenetic Model of Development?

A. Identity versus role confusion
B. Intimacy versus isolation
C. Generativity versus stagnation
D. Ego integrity versus despair
E. Industry versus inferiority

54. Which one of the following diseases is NOT associated with the development of neurofibrillary tangles?

A. Alzheimer's disease
B. Dementia pugilistica
C. Subacute sclerosing panencephalitis
D. Normal aging
E. Huntington's disease

55. According to generally accepted current psychoanalytic theory, which of the following statements about therapist self-disclosure and countertransference is correct?

A. It is generally a good idea to discuss process rather than self disclose.

B. If a patient is making you angry, you should say so without hesitation.

C. If a patient demands to know the therapist's personal feelings, it is often more harmful not to disclose.

D. There are well-accepted psychoanalytic guidelines about policies of self-disclosure.

E. Self-disclosure by the therapist usually constitutes a boundary violation.

56. Which of the following conditions is NOT required to find a physician liable in a medical malpractice case?

A. A professional treatment relationship existed under which the physician owed the patient a duty.

B. The physician deviated from the standard of care in breaching a duty to the patient.

C. The physician deviated from published guidelines in the care of the patient.

D. Actual damages occurred, from which the patient suffered.

E. Any damages were directly caused by the deviation from standard practice.

57. You are evaluating a patient for cognitive decline with a movement disorder. Computed tomography (CT) scan of the head without contrast reveals atrophy of the caudate nuclei and enlarged, *bat–wing*, lateral ventricles. Given this information, what is the most likely diagnosis for this patient?

A. Huntington's disease
B. Alzheimer's disease
C. PD
D. Wilson's disease
E. None of the above

58. A patient diagnosed with Schizophrenia is most likely to meet criteria for comorbid dependence on which of the following substances?

A. Cocaine
B. Alcohol
C. Cannabis
D. Nicotine
E. Phencyclidine

59. Abrupt cessation of daily cocaine use can result in all of the following EXCEPT?

A. Depressed mood
B. Difficulty concentrating
C. Increased dreaming
D. Arrhythmias
E. Increased sleep

60. A 10-year-old boy is brought in for evaluation by his parents for school related problems. His parents report that the child's teachers have reported that he has been exhibiting disruptive behavior in class, with difficulties in concentration. His teachers have noted that he is also reluctant to read in class. After an extensive evaluation, it is determined that the child has a Reading Disorder. Given this information, what is the best intervention for this child's reading difficulties?

A. Initiate therapy with a stimulant medication
B. Initiate therapy with an antidepressant medication
C. Recommend the child be home schooled
D. Recommend remedial education therapy
E. No specific interventions required at this time

61. Which of the following statements regarding the epidemiology of Schizophrenia is NOT TRUE?

    A. Women generally develop schizophrenia at an earlier age than men.
    B. Prevalence rates for schizophrenia are relatively consistent worldwide.
    C. Diagnosis of schizophrenia has been associated with lower socioeconomic status.
    D. Schizophrenia is associated with increased rates of mortality.
    E. About one in three people with schizophrenia will attempt suicide, and about one in ten will complete suicide.

62. Which of the following correctly describes the behavioral changes related to Alcohol Dependence treatment?

    A. Drinker is in denial or has no desire to effect lifestyle changes: Pre-contemplation
    B. Drinker knows alcohol use is a problem but appears ambivalent towards lifestyle changes: Contemplation
    C. Drinker makes half-hearted changes: Preparation
    D. Drinker consolidates new behaviors: Maintenance
    E. All of the above

63. A 25-year-old African-American who is on 90 mg a day of methadone maintenance therapy for his opioid dependence enquires about treatment of his addiction with buprenorphine. When discussing this treatment option with him, you should inform him about all of the following EXCEPT:

    A. Methadone maintenance therapy is cheaper than buprenorphine maintenance therapy.
    B. Buprenorphine maintenance therapy is more effective in patients with higher tolerance to opioids.
    C. Buprenorphine maintenance therapy has lower treatment retention rates than methadone maintenance therapy.
    D. Buprenorphine has lower risk of toxicity at higher doses when compared to methadone.
    E. Buprenorphine has less severe withdrawal symptoms after discontinuation when compared to methadone.

64. Which transference reaction is incorrectly paired with its personality structure?

    A. Manic character: Patients need and deserve to be rescued
    B. Depressive character: Patients idealize and respect the clinician
    C. Masochistic character: Patients fear that the therapist is an uncaring authority who will abandon them

D. Manic character: Patients appear insightful and fascinating
E. Depressive character: Patients anticipate disapproval

65. Which one of the following is TRUE of varenicline?

    A. It is a partial agonist selective for the alfa$_4$ beta$_2$ nicotinic acetylcholine receptor subtype.
    B. It has a half-life of 8 hours.
    C. Dosage adjustments are required in patients with hepatic insufficiency.
    D. It is a known inhibitor of the hepatic cytochrome P450 enzyme system.
    E. It is a known teratogen.

66. A 37-year-old man is brought to the emergency room (ER) after attacking his wife because he believed that she was possessed by evil spirits. A urine toxicology screen is positive for cocaine. All of the following are true of cocaine intoxication EXCEPT:

    A. Most patients will have dilated pupils.
    B. Patients are at increased risk of developing strokes.
    C. Patients are at increased risk of developing seizures.
    D. Patients are at increased risk of developing hyperthermia.
    E. Given increased risk of morbidity and mortality, patients should be hospitalized if their cocaine-induced paranoia lasts for more than 8 hours.

67. According to the Epidemiological Catchment Area (ECA) survey, which of the following psychiatric diagnoses, is associated with the greatest base rate of violence?

    A. Bipolar Disorder
    B. Schizophrenia
    C. Major Depression
    D. Cannabis-related disorders
    E. No psychiatric diagnosis

68. A 55-year-old man has tongue deviation to the right, when he is asked to stick out his tongue during a neurological examination. The rest of the examination is unremarkable. Which cranial nerve is most likely to be affected in his case?

    A. Left CN IX
    B. Right CN IX
    C. Left CN XII
    D. Right CN XII
    E. Left CN X

69. A 60-year-old right-handed man presents to the ED after being in two car accidents in a day. However, he appears unconcerned with what happened. He reports that the first accident occurred because he lost vision in his left eye and was hit by a car on the left.

He got back into his car and then hit the passenger side mirror of another car to his left because he did not see it. He reports having some transient left arm numbness and a mild right-sided headache during the time of the accidents but feels fine currently. Physical examination is notable for a blood pressure of 160/90 mm Hg, and he is alert and oriented. He has normal visual acuity, and has full visual fields with left-sided visual extinction during double simultaneous stimulation. The rest of the physical exam is unremarkable. An MRI of the brain would most likely show a lesion in which one of the following structures?

A. Left parietal lobe
B. Right parietal lobe
C. Left temporal lobe
D. Right temporal lobe
E. Right pons

70. Cerebellar degeneration is associated with the abuse of which of the following drugs?

A. Alcohol
B. Opiates
C. Benzodiazepines
D. Cannabis
E. All of the above

71. Which one of the following is NOT an essential function of the cerebrospinal fluid (CSF)?

A. Protecting the brain and spinal cord from mechanical injury
B. Removing waste products from cerebral metabolism
C. Buffering and protecting the CNS from acute changes in venous pressure
D. Helping to provide a stable chemical environment for neurons, demyelinated fibers, and support cells
E. Actively participate in the metabolism of cells of the brain and spinal cord

72. Which of the following is the predominant inhibitory neurotransmitter in the brain?

A. Glutamate
B. GABA
C. Glycine
D. Serotonin
E. Acetylcholine

73. A type of vocal tic that involves the repetitions of one's own sounds is called:

A. Coprolalia
B. Copropraxia
C. Echolalia
D. Echopraxia
E. Palilalia

74. Which one of the following is the most common cause of autonomic neuropathy in the United States?

A. Diabetes mellitus
B. Amyloidosis
C. Thallium poisoning
D. Porphyria
E. GBS

75. Which one of the following drugs has been Food and Drug Administration (FDA) approved for the treatment of painful diabetic polyneuropathy?

A. Tricyclic antidepressants (TCAs)
B. Pregabalin
C. Gabapentin
D. Capsaicin cream
E. Mexiletine

76. An unconscious 16-year-old man is brought to the ER by ambulance. His mother states that her son was "fine" when she picked him up from football practice. He mentioned that he had a "hard hit" during practice and that he did not remember for a brief period of time, but then was "fine." When the son returned home, he had dinner and went to his room to finish his homework. When she checked in on him a few hours later, he was unconscious. This presentation is most characteristic of which of the following head traumas?

A. Epidural hemorrhage
B. Subarachnoid hemorrhage
C. Subdural hemorrhage
D. Intracranial hemorrhage
E. Petechial hemorrhage

77. A 55-year-old white man with Down syndrome dies due to pneumonia. His family donates his brain to the local brain bank for further studies. Which one of the following will NOT be seen on the evaluation of the brain of this patient?

A. The brain is small with fewer secondary sulci than normal.
B. The superior temporal lobes are hypoplastic with prominent sylvian fissure.
C. There is deposition of sodium in the hippocampus, basal ganglia, and cerebellum.
D. The pyramidal cells show reduced number of apical dendrites and synapses.
E. There is degeneration of the cells in the nucleus basalis of Meynert.

78. Lamotrigine requires a dose reduction and slower titration when co-administered with which of the following medications?

A. Fluoxetine
B. Divalproex sodium

C. Carbamazepine
D. Olanzapine
E. Lithium

79. What is the lifetime prevalence of Schizophrenia?
   A. 0.01%
   B. 0.1%
   C. 1.0%
   D. 2.0%
   E. 10.0%

80. Which one of the following statements about the medial temporal lobe is NOT TRUE?
   A. The neurons of the hippocampal region are arranged in one cellular layer.
   B. Most hippocampal pyramidal neurons are GABA-ergic.
   C. This region is important for the formation of declarative memory.
   D. The hippocampus may modulate emotion through its connections with the limbic system.
   E. This region contains the serial circuitry for long-term potentiation.

81. During a cognitive behavioral session, your patient states that he will never be able to do anything right. After you ask him what that means, he replies that he is inadequate. You astutely recognize this as a core belief. Which one of the following statements about core beliefs is correct?
   A. Most authors recognize three broad categories of core beliefs.
   B. Core beliefs are usually generated on a rational basis.
   C. They often only become activated during a depressed state.
   D. Core beliefs are usually unmodifiable in therapy.
   E. Cognitive theory never explores the childhood origins of the beliefs.

82. Which of the following criteria is required and sufficient for involuntary hospitalization?
   A. The patient is mentally ill.
   B. The patient is substance addicted.
   C. The patient is dangerous to self or others.
   D. The patient is unable to provide for his or her basic needs.
   E. The specific legal requirements vary by state.

83. Which one of the following statements is NOT TRUE of the plasma level of TCAs?
   A. Plasma levels are useful in determining patient compliance.
   B. Plasma levels are useful in patients with a poor response to a "typical" antidepressant dose.

C. Plasma levels are useful in patients who are potentially very sensitive to side effects.
D. Steady-state plasma levels are achieved in about 2 days after either initiating the medication or changing the medication dose.
E. These levels are generally obtained about 9 to 12 hours after the last dose.

84. A single man in his 20s is repeatedly admitted to the hospital with a diagnosis of "Schizophrenia." At the time of his presentations, he is malodorous and unkempt, often incoherent, and his actions seem lacking in purpose. On the inpatient unit he intermittently jumps up suddenly, grinning in an odd fashion. He then resumes his previous activity or state of rest. He has been unemployed for the past 5 years and is living on the street. Previous organic workups have been negative. His psychiatric treatment team is unable to elicit any specific delusional or hallucinatory experiences. With which one of the following subtypes of schizophrenia should this patient be diagnosed?
   A. Paranoid Type
   B. Disorganized Type
   C. Catatonic Type
   D. Undifferentiated Type
   E. Residual Type

85. While working in the psychiatric ER, you are asked to treat an acutely cocaine intoxicated patient. He is 25-years-old, and had been brought in by police when he became paranoid and agitated at a party. Which of the following initial therapeutic approaches would be most beneficial in the treatment of this patient?
   A. Medicate him with an antipsychotic agent to treat his substance induced psychosis.
   B. Provide assistance with immediate needs (pain relief, bathroom), reassure him that his thoughts are the result of his cocaine use, and attempt to provide reality orientation.
   C. Restrain the patient to prevent him from harming himself or ER staff.
   D. Initiate treatment with an antidepressant as he is likely using the cocaine to self-medicate a mood disturbance.
   E. Have him escorted out of the ER as his mental status will likely clear once he is no longer intoxicated.

86. All of the following factors in preschoolers increase the risk of developing a Reading Disorder EXCEPT:
   A. Difficulty learning the alphabet and failure to recognize letters by the start of kindergarten

B. Delayed or impaired speech and language
C. Difficulties with rhyming game
D. Failure to be completely potty trained by age 4
E. Family history of learning disability or difficulty with speech, language, spelling, or reading

87. Which of the following correctly depicts the manner in which having relatives suffering from Schizophrenia increases lifetime risk for an individual to develop Schizophrenia?

    A. Multiple family members with Schizophrenia > two family members with Schizophrenia > single family member with Schizophrenia
    B. Adopted with Schizophrenic biological mother > adopted with non-schizophrenic biological mother
    C. Monozygotic twin with Schizophrenia > dizygotic twin with Schizophrenia
    D. Both parents with Schizophrenia > one parent with Schizophrenia
    E. All of the above

88. Which of the following is NOT TRUE of Alcoholics Anonymous (AA)?

    A. It emphasizes the principle of "one day at a time."
    B. It stresses reliance on "one's higher power," and spirituality.
    C. It has been found to be exceptionally useful in patients with severe psychopathology.
    D. It affords immediate accessibility and connection to sponsors who are often sober supportive individuals in the community.
    E. It has free, unlimited 24/7 access.

89. Which one of the following is TRUE of debriefing after a traumatic event?

    A. Single session individual debriefing reduces psychological distress.
    B. Single session individual debriefing prevents the onset of Posttraumatic Stress Disorder (PTSD).
    C. Available evidence indicates that debriefing reduced general psychological morbidity.
    D. There was no evidence that debriefing reduces depression or anxiety.
    E. All of the above.

90. Which countertransference reaction is incorrectly paired with the personality structure?

    A. Masochistic character: Being excessively generous
    B. Depressive character: Benign affection
    C. Masochistic character: Sadistic
    D. Manic character: Overestimating the degree of suffering

    E. Depressive character: Fantasy of being God or the Good Mother

91. Which one of the following is NOT TRUE of sleep deprivation?

    A. Total sleep deprivation (TSD) for one whole night improves depressive symptoms in 40% to 60% of treatments.
    B. Response to sleep deprivation shows up in the sleep deprived night or the following day.
    C. After recovery sleep, 50% to 80% of day 1 responders suffer a complete or partial relapse.
    D. The best predictor of a therapeutic effect is a small variability of mood.
    E. The mechanism of action for sleep deprivation is still unknown.

92. Which one of the following is NOT TRUE of sexual education in post-menopausal women with sexual dysfunction?

    A. It should include basic information on genital anatomy and physiology following sexual stimulation.
    B. The role of hormones in maintaining genital structure and genital function should be discussed.
    C. It should be provided to all women being managed for their sexual health concerns.
    D. It should be only provided to the patient and not the partner due to confidentiality issues.
    E. It allows for patient preferences to be considered when deciding between the various types of treatments.

93. Which of the following is NOT TRUE of violent behavior?

    A. Men are three times more likely than women to engage in serious violence.
    B. In adults, younger age is associated with an increased risk of violence.
    C. Lower intelligence increases the risk of violence.
    D. Cluster B personality disorder diagnosis increases the risk of violent behavior.
    E. All of the above are true.

94. A 30-year-old woman comes for an initial visit to your office. During the neurological examination you notice that the patient has nystagmus of the abducting eye and failure of the adducting eye to cross the midline. Given this information, which structure is most likely to be damaged?

    A. CN I
    B. CN II
    C. Medial longitudinal fasciculus
    D. Pons
    E. Medulla

95. A 65-year-old man with poorly controlled hypertension and diabetes presents to the ED with complaints of acute right-sided weakness for the past 5 hours. He denies any sensory complaints, visual changes, or language impairments. On physical examination, his blood pressure is 160/100 mm Hg, and he is alert and speaks fluently. There is no visual field deficit and he has some mild drooping of his right lower face, clumsiness of his right hand, and drags his right leg. Sensory examination is normal. An MRI of the brain would most likely show a lesion occurring in which of the following structures?

A. Left internal capsule
B. Left thalamus
C. Right internal capsule
D. Right pons
E. Right thalamus

96. Typical findings of fetal-alcohol syndrome (FAS) include all of the following EXCEPT:

A. Microcephaly
B. Epicanthal eye fold
C. Absent philtrum
D. Small ears
E. Mental retardation

97. Which one of the following statements regarding the CSF is TRUE?

A. It is produced in the arachnoid granulations.
B. The blood brain barrier prevents rapid shifts in water and sodium to and from blood and CSF.
C. Diffusion gradients determine carbon dioxide exchange and the entry of proteins into CSF.
D. The CSF replenishes itself on average every 4 to 5 days.
E. Electrolytes and glucose equilibrate via exchange occurs at a very specialized location in the CSF pathway.

98. Which of the following is a major inhibitory neurotransmitter in the spinal cord?

A. Glutamate
B. Dopamine
C. Glycine
D. Serotonin
E. Acetylcholine

99. A 55-year-old man with a history of systemic lupus erythematosus presents to the ED with acute onset or sudden and severe back pain that started 1 hour ago. It is associated with bilateral lower extremity weakness, paresthesias, and sensory loss. While waiting in the ED, the patient develops loss of sphincter control and is unable to void. Which one of the following spinal cord disorders is the most likely cause of this patient's symptoms?

A. Acute transverse myelopathy
B. GBS
C. Mass lesion in spinal canal
D. Spinal cord stroke
E. Viral myelitis

100. Which one of the following is TRUE of autonomic neuropathy?

A. Patients with this condition can present with tachycardia.
B. Patients with this condition can present with sweating.
C. Patients with this condition can present with anhidrosis.
D. Autonomic neuropathy is commonly associated with symmetric distal polyneuropathy.
E. All of the above.

101. All of the following are neuropathological features seen in herpes simplex encephalitis EXCEPT:

A. Cowdry type A inclusion bodies are often seen
B. Perivascular inflammation of lymphocytes and histiocytes in the cortex
C. Proliferation of microglia
D. Glial nodules
E. The lesions are symmetrical

102. Which one of the following statements is NOT CORRECT?

A. Tremors are rhythmic oscillatory movements caused by the alternating contractions of opposing muscle groups.
B. Myoclonus is a rapid shocklike movement that arises from the contractions or inhibitions of muscle groups.
C. Chorea is a rapid, brief, irregular contraction that is not as fast as myoclonic jerks.
D. Ballism is a jerk of large amplitude that produces flinging movements of the affected limbs.
E. Athetosis is a simple or complex jerky movement that appears suddenly and intermittently.

103. Which one of the following is the most common disorder associated with the inborn error of metabolism of sulfur containing amino acids?

A. Homocystinuria and mild homocystinemia
B. Cystathioninuria
C. Homocystinuria with megaloblastic anemia
D. Homocystinuria
E. Sulfite oxidase deficiency

104. Which one of the following is the main mode of action of valproate?

A. Inhibition of voltage-dependent sodium channels

B. Agonist at the benzodiazepine-binding site of the GABA-A receptor

C. Inhibition of glutamate release

D. Antagonism of kainite at amino-methylphenyl-acetic acid (AMPA) receptors.

E. Increase brain levels of GABA

105. Which of the following physiologic changes is NOT typical in patients with advancing age?

A. Blood vessels stiffen, cardiac output and reserve decrease

B. Lungs lose elastic tissue, alveolar ducts and bronchioles enlarge

C. Small bowel transit slows, with increased vitamin and mineral absorption

D. Kidneys decrease in size, with cortical nephron loss and decreased creatinine clearance

E. Bone marrow mass decreases and is slower to respond, with decreased ability to respond to infections

106. Which one of the following statements is NOT TRUE?

A. The neurons of the hippocampal region are arranged in one cellular layer.

B. Most hippocampal pyramidal neurons are glutaminergic.

C. Medial temporal lobe is important for the formation of nondeclarative memory.

D. The hippocampus may modulate emotion through its connections with the limbic system.

E. Medial temporal lobe contains the serial circuitry for long-term potentiation.

107. Which one of the following statements is NOT TRUE of the neurobiology of aggression?

A. Increased CSF levels of 3-hydroxy, 4-methoxyphenylglycol (MHPG) are found in subjects with a history of aggressive behavior and personality disorders.

B. β-adrenergic antagonist propranolol has been effective in the treatment of episodic aggressive behavior in subjects with head injuries.

C. Personality disordered subjects have a CSF 5-HIAA level that is inversely correlated with clinician or self-reports of lifetime aggression.

D. Injuries involving the parietal cortex are associated with aggressive behaviors.

E. As men are more aggressive than women, there may be a role for the Y chromosome in the neurobiology of aggression.

108. Which of the following represents a potential exception to the requirement for obtaining informed consent before an intervention?

A. An emergency

B. The patient has been deemed incompetent

C. Therapeutic privilege

D. The patient has waived his or her right for informed consent

E. All of the above

109. Which one of the following is currently NOT part of the routine pretreatment workup for electroconvulsive therapy (ECT)?

A. A complete blood count (CBC) with differential

B. A chem-20 profile

C. A urinalysis

D. An electrocardiogram (EKG)

E. Spinal X rays

110. According to the DSM-IV-TR, which one of the following is NOT one of the criteria for Pain Disorder?

A. Pain in one or more anatomical sites is the predominant focus of the clinical presentation and is of sufficient severity to warrant clinical attention.

B. The pain causes clinically significant distress or impairment in social, occupational, or other important areas of functioning.

C. Psychological factors are judged to have an important role in the onset, severity, exacerbation, or maintenance of the pain.

D. The pain is intentionally produced or feigned.

E. The pain is not better accounted for by a mood, anxiety, or psychotic disorder and does not meet criteria for dyspareunia.

111. A 30-year-old man who has had a long history of heroin dependence with multiple failed attempts at abstinence is considering methadone maintenance. He is concerned that he will not be able to continue his employment as a construction worker as methadone will sedate him. What should you tell him about the use of methadone in response to his query?

A. Clients on a stable dose of methadone can safely operate machinery and drive without difficulty.

B. He may have to change his job to a position where he is not operating heavy machinery.

C. He needs to prioritize his health as continued heroine use will likely cause long term medical problems.

D. You are not able to advise him on deciding between his health and his employment.

E. He will be able to collect unemployment given his psychiatric condition, and so should not be concerned about losing his job.

112. All of the following are traditionally considered indicative features of Bipolar Depression (versus Unipolar Depression) EXCEPT:

    A. 1:1 sex ratio
    B. Hypersomnia > insomnia
    C. Psychomotor retardation > agitation
    D. Later age of onset
    E. Postpartum episode

113. Which of the following is the most consistent and best-replicated neuroanatomic finding in Schizophrenia?

    A. Enlarged temporal lobes
    B. Decreased frontal lobe size
    C. Cerebral ventricular enlargement
    D. Sulcal enlargement
    E. Increased thalamic size

114. A 23-year-old heroin-dependent woman presents to your ER in labor. Which of the following statements regarding opiate-dependent pregnant women is TRUE?

    A. Fifty percent of infants born to mothers addicted to opiate experience syndrome of opiate withdrawal.
    B. Providing methadone replacement therapy to opiate-dependent pregnant women is rarely if ever recommended.
    C. Should methadone be provided to opiate dependent pregnant women, the recommended dose is 40 mg/day orally.
    D. Opiate dependent pregnant women on methadone doses above 20 mg/day should be tapered slowly to lower doses during weeks 14 to 32 of pregnancy.
    E. There are no known pharmacologic remedies for infants withdrawing from opiate.

115. A 23-year-old man is brought in to the psychiatric ER by the police. They report that the family called the police because their son was increasingly agitated and was threatening to the family. The family states that for the past few days, the patient has been behaving oddly, has not been going to work, has remained isolative, and stays up most of the night. The family also reports that the patient does not have any medical problems and he does not take any medications. He also does not have any known drug allergies. While in the ER, the patient is noted to be pacing back and forth in his room and is refusing to answer questions. He then throws the chair to the ground, removing the sheets on the bed, and jumping up and down on the bed. You and the support staff are able to talk down the patient and for the moment he is calmly sitting on the chair in his room. Given this information, what is the next step in management of this patient's behavior?

    A. Discharge the patient to police custody
    B. Discharge the patient home to his family
    C. Order an antipsychotic and benzodiazepine immediately
    D. Refer the patient for outpatient detoxification
    E. Refer the family for family therapy

116. Which countertransference reaction is incorrectly paired?

    A. Narcissistic character: Being ignored
    B. Hysterical (histrionic) character: Distancing
    C. Narcissistic character: Grandiose expansion
    D. Hysterical character: Infantilization
    E. Narcissistic character: Being seduced

117. Which one of the following is NOT TRUE of AA?

    A. It is not a professionally delivered treatment program.
    B. It is a mutual-help group that offers peer support.
    C. It is always available and is free of charge.
    D. The philosophical foundation of AA is the Twelve Steps.
    E. It is opposed to the use of medication for alcohol-dependent individuals.

118. Which of the following psychosocial factors contributes to the failure of medical treatment in sexual dysfunction?

    A. Patient variables such as performance anxiety and depression
    B. Partner variables such as poor mental or physical health and partner disinterest
    C. Interpersonal nonsexual variables such as quality of the overall relationship
    D. Contextual variables such as current life stresses with money or children
    E. All of the above

119. Which of the following is the single strongest risk factor for future violent behavior?

    A. A combination of fire-setting, enuresis, and cruelty to animals
    B. Psychotic symptoms such as intense paranoia or command hallucinations
    C. Previous personal history of violent behavior
    D. A history of being physically abused as a child
    E. Poor social support

120. Which of the following structures carry light touch sensation?

    A. Anterior spinothalamic tracts
    B. Lateral spinothalamic tracts
    C. Posterior columns

D. Spinocerebellar tracts
E. Fasciculus gracilis

121. A 35-year-old patient presents with a one-month history of worsening headaches, episodic mood swings, and occasional hallucinations with visual, tactile, and auditory content. A CT scan of the head is most likely to reveal a tumor in which of the following areas?

A. Cerebellum
B. Frontal lobe
C. Occipital lobe
D. Parietal lobe
E. Temporal lobe

122. All of the following are TRUE of Wernicke's disease and Wernicke-Korsakoff syndrome EXCEPT:

A. It results from thiamine deficiency.
B. Wernicke's disease is characterized by the triad of mental disturbance, ataxia, and ophthalmoplegia.
C. Korsakoff's psychosis cannot be prevented by thiamine supplementation.
D. Intravenous glucose prior to thiamine administration can precipitate Wernicke's disease in alcoholics.
E. Ocular palsies in Wernicke's disease respond within hours of treatment.

123. Two weeks after a mild upper respiratory illness, a 61-year-old woman develops tingling and numbness in her toes, which then develops into weakness over the next several days. The weakness then ascends up to involve her trunk muscles. She is moved to the ICU as she starts to develop respiratory difficulties. A lumbar puncture is performed to clarify the diagnosis. Given this information, her cerebrospinal fluid (CSF) is most likely to show which of the following findings?

CSF	Color	WBC	Protein	Glucose
A.	Clear	Normal	High	Normal
B.	Clear	Normal	Normal	Normal
C.	Turbid	High	High	Low
D.	Turbid	High	High	Normal
E.	Clear	High	Elevated	Normal

124. In general, hyperactive DTRs suggest an injury at which location?

A. CNS and cortical spinal tracts
B. Neuromuscular junction
C. Peripheral nerve
D. Muscle
E. Anterior horn cells

125. A 58-year-old man presents to the ED complaining of sudden onset of bilateral lower extremity weakness, paresthesias, and sensory loss. Neurologic examination reveals symmetric weakness in the lower extremities, with inability to sense pain and temperature, but with preservation of light touch and position and vibratory sense. What is the most likely cause of this patient's symptoms?

A. ALS
B. Occlusion of ventral artery
C. Poliomyelitis
D. Tabes dorsalis
E. Vitamin B_{12} neuropathy

126. Which one of the following is NOT TRUE of GBS?

A. It is an acute inflammatory demyelinating neuropathy.
B. Its incidence gradually increases with age.
C. It affects men more than women.
D. The severity of neurologic abnormalities in this condition is not related to the degree of conduction slowing.
E. Early plasmapheresis or intravenous infusion of human gamma globulins can improve its long term prognosis.

127. The characteristic pathological features in general paresis include all of the following EXCEPT:

A. The brain is usually small and atrophied.
B. The neuronal loss is seen especially in temporal and occipital regions.
C. There is prominent neuroglial proliferation.
D. The pathognomonic histopathological feature is rod cells staining with Prussian blue to show iron containing pigments.
E. There is widespread dense perivascular collection of lymphocytes and plasma cells throughout the cortex.

128. Which one of the following is NOT TRUE of Friedreich ataxia?

A. It is the most common type of hereditary ataxia.
B. It has an autosomal dominant type of inheritance.
C. It is caused by the loss of function mutations in the frataxin gene (FXN gene).
D. Patients can manifest with hypertrophic cardiomyopathy.
E. Diabetes mellitus occurs in approximately one third of the patients.

129. A patient diagnosed with an acoustic neuroma presents with tinnitus and imbalance, in addition to unilateral hearing impairment and facial weakness. Given these symptoms, which of the following cranial nerves are most likely involved?

A. CN 7+8
B. CN 5+7
C. CN 5+8
D. CN 5,7+8
E. CN 8 only

130. Which one of the following statements regarding the use of antiepileptic drugs (AEDs) in pregnancy is NOT TRUE?
    A. Malformations associated with AEDs are probably induced during the first trimester.
    B. The rate of fetal malformations in mothers with epilepsy is 5% (twice that of nonepileptic mothers), exclusive of AED-induced malformations.
    C. Neural tube defects are several times more likely to occur as a result of maternal valproate use than maternal carbamazepine use.
    D. No one AED exclusively induces a particular fetal malformation.
    E. To reduce the risk of neural tube defects, women should take folic acid before conception and during the pregnancy.

131. In the absence of disease, which of the following nervous system changes is not part of normal aging?
    A. Cerebral blood flow decreases
    B. Brain weight declines
    C. Cortical myelin content decreases
    D. Brain size declines
    E. Neurotransmitter production uniformly declines

132. Which one of the following is the most heritable of all psychiatric disorders?
    A. Autism
    B. Schizophrenia
    C. Bipolar Disorder
    D. Attention-Deficit/Hyperactivity Disorder (ADHD)
    E. OCD

133. Which measure describes the number of persons in a given population who are initially free of a disorder and develop that disorder over a given period of time?
    A. Frequency
    B. Prevalence
    C. Odds ratio
    D. Incidence
    E. Relative risk

134. Which of the following is NOT usually included in the lithium baseline pretreatment and periodic follow-up tests?
    A. Blood urea nitrogen (BUN) and serum creatinine
    B. Thyroid stimulating hormone (TSH)
    C. Urine pregnancy test in women

D. White blood cell (WBC) count
E. Platelets

135. Withdrawal from which of the following substances does NOT carry a risk of seizures?
    A. Alcohol
    B. Lorazepam
    C. Chlordiazepoxide
    D. Secobarbital
    E. Cocaine

136. A 35-year-old woman is admitted to the general adult inpatient psychiatric unit for depression and suicidality in the setting of a recent divorce. She is currently being treated with sertraline and bupropion. She is also on methadone maintenance for her chronic heroine dependence. What would be the most appropriate decision regarding her methadone dose while she is in the hospital?
    A. Discontinue the methadone, as the CNS depressive effect can be contributing to her depression
    B. Taper her slowly from the methadone, as it has likely become another addiction for her
    C. After confirming the dose with the methadone maintenance program, continue it while she is hospitalized
    D. Switch her to a fentanyl patch of equivalent dose, as it requires less frequent dosing
    E. Begin treatment with naltrexone to assist with long term abstinence

137. All of the following are true statements regarding post-stroke depression EXCEPT?
    A. Severity of the stroke is predictive of depression
    B. Physical disability after the stroke is predictive of depression
    C. Cognitive impairment after the stroke is predictive of depression
    D. Early post-stroke onset of depression has worse prognosis than later onset
    E. None of the above

138. Which of the following is TRUE regarding Schizophrenia?
    A. Lower social class and inner cities breed Schizophrenia.
    B. Schizophrenia can be caused by emotionally cold and distant parenting.
    C. The stress of emigration causes Schizophrenia.
    D. Those suffering from Schizophrenia often drift into urban areas and lower socioeconomic class.
    E. Social isolation causes Schizophrenia.

139. A 23-year-old heroin-dependent woman presents to your ER in labor. She gives birth to a 7 lb baby girl. You consider neonatal opiate withdrawal as a

complication of this delivery. All of the following are common symptoms of this syndrome EXCEPT:

A. Hyperphagia
B. Hyperactivity
C. Diaphoresis
D. Tremors
E. Mottling

140. Which psychodynamic characteristic of dependent personality structure is incorrectly paired?

A. Central preoccupation: Keeping versus losing relationship
B. Central affects: Pleasure (with secure attachment), and sadness and fear (with being alone)
C. Pathogenic belief about self: I am impotent, inadequate, and needy
D. Pathogenic belief about others: Others are powerful and I need their care
E. Central defenses: Projection, rationalization, and denial

141. Which countertransference reaction is incorrectly paired with the personality structure?

A. Obsessive and compulsive character: Annoyed impatience
B. Paranoid character: Anxiety
C. Obsessive and compulsive character: Obliteration
D. Paranoid character: Hostility
E. Obsessive and compulsive character: Boredom

142. Which one of the following is TRUE of the treatment of Alcohol Dependence?

A. Pharmacotherapy should never be combined with psychosocial treatments.
B. Cognitive behavior therapy is the best psychosocial treatment for Alcohol Dependence.
C. Combination of pharmacotherapy and psychosocial treatments worsens the outcome for these patients.
D. Prescribing clinicians have no role in providing psychosocial treatments for these patients.
E. None of the above.

143. Which of the following is NOT TRUE of psychological treatments for Hypoactive Sexual Desire Disorder (HSDD) in women?

A. The outcomes for psychological treatments are worse when the female partner has lower desire than her male partner.
B. CBT has reported efficacy in the treatment of these patients.
C. CBT has been shown to produce significant improvements in the quality marital life of these patients.

D. CBT has been shown to reduce symptoms of depression and anxiety in these patients.
E. CBT has been shown to improve self esteem in these patients.

144. Which one of the following is NOT TRUE of Substance P?

A. It belongs to the tachykinin neuropeptide family.
B. It functions as a neurotransmitter and as a neuromodulator.
C. It is a neurotransmitter whose primary role is in pain transmission.
D. It can produce hypertension.
E. Capsaicin produces anesthesia by depleting the Substance P in the affected nerves.

145. Symptoms of unilateral hearing loss associated with vertigo, unsteadiness with falls and headaches, mild facial weakness, and ipsilateral limb ataxia is most commonly associated with tumors in which of the following locations?

A. Cavernous sinus
B. Cerebellopontine angle
C. Jugular foramen
D. Parasellar region
E. Superior orbital fissure

146. Noradrenergic neurons project diffusely from which one of the following brain regions?

A. Nucleus basalis of Meynert
B. Ventral tegmental area
C. Substantial nigra
D. Locus coeruleus
E. Dorsal raphe nuclei

147. Which of the following is a sign of an upper motor neuron (UMN) lesion?

A. Paresis with muscle flaccidity
B. Hypoactive DTRs
C. Babinski signs
D. Sensory loss
E. Atrophy

148. A 70-year-old man with rigidity, bradykinesia, and resting tremor has been prescribed trihexyphenidyl. This medication is LEAST likely to cause which of the following side effects?

A. Delirium
B. Urinary retention
C. Memory impairment
D. Diarrhea
E. Dry mouth

149. According to Erikson's stage-theory concept of epigenesis, which one of the following is a major developmental task of old age?

A. Industry versus inferiority
B. Ego integrity versus despair
C. Generativity versus stagnation
D. Identity versus role confusion
E. Trust versus mistrust

150. A 23-year-old white man with no previous psychiatric history is recently diagnosed with Schizophrenia, based on the DSM-IV-TR criteria. His parents ask you about the risk of this patient's only brother, who is 20 years old, of developing Schizophrenia. What would you tell them about the risk of this patient's brother developing Schizophrenia?
   A. 1%
   B. 5%
   C. 10%
   D. 15%
   E. 20%

151. Which of the following is NOT included in the valproate baseline pretreatment and periodic follow-up tests?
   A. BUN and serum creatinine
   B. Liver function tests
   C. Urine pregnancy test
   D. WBC count
   E. Platelets

152. All of the following can be co-morbid with Conversion Disorder EXCEPT:
   A. MDD
   B. Anxiety Disorders
   C. Schizophrenia
   D. Factitious Disorder
   E. Personality Disorder

153. A 14-year-old boy is brought in to the ED due to bizarre behaviors. On examination, he is disoriented, with facial flushing and dilated pupils, and appears to be hallucinating. His clothing has a strong chemical odor, and a piece of gauze with a similar odor is found in his pocket. Which treatment modality should be carefully avoided in the management of this patient?
   A. Intravenous fluids to prevent dehydration
   B. Mechanical restraints to manage behavioral problems
   C. Oxygen therapy to correct hypoxemia
   D. Catecholamines as a treatment for hypotension, should it occur
   E. Antibiotic therapy to treat concomitant infection

154. All of the following are personality traits commonly shared by patients with Anorexia Nervosa (AN) and Bulimia Nervosa (BN) EXCEPT?

A. Neuroticism
B. Perfectionism
C. Novelty seeking
D. Low cooperativeness
E. Obsessive-compulsiveness

155. You are asked to consult on a 61-year-old widowed housewife who is 5 months status post-left anterior cerebral artery stroke. She has been increasingly depressed, unmotivated, anhedonic, and psychomotorically slowed over the past 2 months. Her symptoms have begun to interfere with her participation in her rehabilitation program, which initially went well. She has no prior psychiatric history. Her sensorium is clear, and she correctly scores 25 out of 30 on her Folstein MMSE. CT scan shows changes consistent with an old left-anterior, cerebral artery stroke, and laboratories (including chemistries, CBC, urinalysis, vitamin B$_{12}$, folic acid, rapid plasma reagin (RPR), iron studies, and thyroid and parathyroid studies) are all unremarkable. Given this history, what is the most appropriate diagnosis for this patient according to the DSM-IV-TR?
   A. MDD, Single episode
   B. Dementia, Vascular Type with Depression
   C. Depressive Disorder due to Stroke
   D. Adjustment Disorder with Depressed Mood
   E. Delirium

156. A 23-year-old heroin-dependent woman presents to your ER in labor. She gives birth to a 7 lb baby girl. You consider neonatal opiate withdrawal as a complication of this delivery. Given this information, which of the following is TRUE of this condition?
   A. Mild symptoms of neonatal opiate withdrawal require no treatment.
   B. No treatment is necessary in neonatal opiate withdrawal.
   C. No treatment has proven efficacy or safety therefore, they are to be avoided.
   D. Paregoric is recommended for mild withdrawal symptoms.
   E. Phenobarbital is recommended for mild withdrawal symptoms.

157. Which psychodynamic characteristics of psychopathic personality structure are incorrectly paired?
   A. Central preoccupation: Manipulating versus being manipulated
   B. Central affects: Rage and envy
   C. Central pathogenic belief about self: I can make anything happen
   D. Central pathogenic belief about others: The world is full of potential attackers
   E. Central defenses: Omnipotent control

158. Which of the following pairs are not correctly matched?
    A. Narcissistic character: Self-object transference
    B. Hysterical (Histrionic) character: Object transference
    C. Narcissistic character: Guilt
    D. Hysterical character: Shame
    E. Hysterical character: Idealization and devaluation

159. When a court of law requests records on a patient from a psychiatrist, the psychiatrist has the right to do which of the following?
    A. Check with the court regarding the adequate need for disclosure
    B. Only disclose information that is relevant to the legal question in hand
    C. When in doubt, give the right of the patient to confidential and unimpaired treatment
    D. Refuse to send the records, if it is harmful to his patient's care
    E. All of the above

160. Which one of the following is TRUE of sex therapy for Erectile Dysfunction?
    A. It involves interventions like systematic desensitization and sensate focus.
    B. Systematic desensitization has the best evidence for efficacy.
    C. Men with acquired disorders tend to fare better than those with lifelong problems.
    D. Long-term follow-up indicates that relapse rates may be as high as 75%.
    E. Relapses may be prevented by periodic booster or maintenance sessions.

161. Gerstmann's syndrome, characterized by right-left disorientation, finger agnosia, acalculia (impaired calculation), and agraphia (impaired writing) is caused by a dysfunction of which one of the following structures?
    A. Dominant frontal lobe
    B. Dominant parietal lobe
    C. Dominant occipital lobe
    D. Non-dominant frontal lobe
    E. Non-dominant parietal lobe

162. Motor abnormalities seen in Huntington's disease, Tourette's disorder, and OCD are due to dysfunction of which one of the basal ganglia nuclei?
    A. Caudate nucleus
    B. Globus pallidus (GPi)
    C. Lenticular nucleus
    D. Substantia nigra
    E. Subthalamic nucleus (STN)

163. A 70-year-old white man with a 3-year history of PD is seen in a neurology clinic for worsening tremors. When educating him and his wife on the treatments for this condition, which one of the following statements would you NOT make to them?
    A. Anticholinergics like trihexyphenidyl are effective in the treatment of this condition.
    B. Anticholinergics are generally not recommended to patients with cognitive decline or elderly patients over 65 years of age.
    C. Dopaminergics are more effective than anticholinergic agents to treat parkinsonian tremor.
    D. Pramipexole and ropinirole, are probably the most effective antitremor drugs among all dopaminergic treatments.
    E. Dopamine agonists are also useful in advanced PD patients with tremor that are refractory to treatment with levodopa or anticholinergics drugs.

164. Each of the following statements regarding long-term care of the elderly is true EXCEPT:
    A. The majority of older patients with deficits in self-care live in the community.
    B. The emergence of assisted living facilities has added an alternative to nursing homes for those who require residential care.
    C. Some nursing homes now include sub-acute rehabilitative units and dementia care units, in addition to the traditional long-term care units.
    D. The majority of long-term care for older patients is provided in the nursing home setting.
    E. The growth of in-home health services has allowed many older patients to remain in the home longer.

165. Which one of the following is NOT TRUE of the synthesis of norepinephrine?
    A. Dopamine and epinephrine are synthesized from tyrosine.
    B. It is converted from dopamine by beta hydroxylase.
    C. Tyrosine hydroxylase is the enzyme in the rate-limiting step of its synthesis.
    D. It is produced in the raphe nuclei of the pons.
    E. It is produced in the lateral tegmentum.

166. Which of the following is NOT included in the routine TCA baseline pretreatment and periodic follow-up tests?
    A. EKG and vital signs
    B. Liver function tests
    C. Serum prolactin level
    D. CBC with differential
    E. Serum electrolytes

167. Which of the following Personality Disorders is thought to have significant comorbidity with and may predispose patients to PTSD?
    A. Schizoid Personality Disorder
    B. Narcissistic Personality Disorder
    C. Borderline Personality Disorder
    D. Obsessive-Compulsive Personality Disorder
    E. Schizotypal Personality Disorder

168. A 26-year-old man with Schizophrenia is thought to have a family with high expressed emotion. Which of the following is TRUE regarding families with high expressed emotion?
    A. It is correlated with higher relapse rates for psychiatric illness.
    B. Families with high expressed emotion tend to have several members who have experienced manic episodes secondary to Bipolar I.
    C. It is thought that Schizophrenia is frequently the result of a patient's being raised in a family with high expressed emotion.
    D. Intervention with families with high expressed emotion does not improve relapse rates.
    E. The development of expressed emotion and its relationship to Schizophrenia was developed by Gregory Bateson.

169. Who proposed the *kindling* hypothesis for mood disorders?
    A. Kraeplin
    B. Sullivan
    C. Meyer
    D. Pinel
    E. Post

170. You have been periodically following a 45-year-old man for the past 6 years for depression, and he has been stable on 40 mg/day of fluoxetine. He has no history of psychosis or substance abuse, nor any family history of psychiatric illness. Out of concern for his behavior, his family schedules him early for a visit. He has not been sleeping for several days, his mood is labile (ranging from irritable to euphoric), his speech is pressured, and his thoughts are tangential and distractible with mild paranoid ideation. He has been home from work for the past week because of a bronchitis for which he was prescribed azithromycin and prednisone. His laboratories (including chemistries, CBC, drug screen, and thyroid functions) show a mild leukocytosis and hyperglycemia, but are otherwise normal. His lungs are now clear and his chest X-ray is negative. You suspect his change in behavior is most likely due to which one of the following conditions?

A. Bipolar Disorder
B. Antidepressant-induced mania
C. Cocaine Intoxication
D. Infection
E. Mood changes due to corticosteroids

171. A 23-year-old heroin-dependent woman presents to your ER in labor. She gives birth to a 7 lb baby girl. The new mother is admitted to a methadone substitution program where 20 mg/day of methadone is administered. A week later, she is brought back to your ER by ambulance after she became unresponsive. On examination, she is lethargic and hypotonic. Her respiratory rate is 5 per minute and effort shallow. Her pupils are constricted bilaterally. What is the most likely explanation for her symptoms?
    A. Her methadone substitution is inadequate.
    B. Postpartum volume shift has rendered her current dose of methadone ineffective.
    C. Postpartum volume shift has led to toxic blood levels of opiate.
    D. She may have ingested additional opiate from an external source.
    E. All of the above.

172. Which psychodynamic characteristic of depressive personality structure is incorrectly paired?
    A. Central preoccupation: Good versus badness of self or aloneness versus relatedness of self
    B. Central affects: Sadness, guilt, and shame
    C. Pathogenic belief about self: I need to be perfect to feel okay
    D. Pathogenic belief about others: People who really get to know me will reject me
    E. Central defenses: Introjection, devaluation of self, and idealization of others

173. Which one of the following statements is NOT TRUE of narcissistic and psychopathic personality disorders?
    A. Both have subjectively empty internal world
    B. Both depend on external events to provide self-esteem
    C. Both have a sense of self-inflation
    D. Both depend on omnipotent control
    E. Narcissistic people rely on defenses of idealization and devaluation, while psychopathic people rely on defenses of projective identification and acting out

174. Which of the following is a risk factor for developing post-stroke depression (PSD)?
    A. Functional impairments
    B. Increasing age
    C. Past history of depression

D. Post-stroke social isolation

E. All of the above

175. Which one of the following is TRUE of hypnosis?

A. It is most commonly used as a stand alone therapy.

B. It is difficult to integrate hypnosis with other psychotherapeutic or behavioral treatments.

C. Hypnosis has the best evidence for treating PTSD.

D. The mechanism of action of hypnosis has been clearly understood.

E. None of the above.

176. Which one of the following hypothalamic nuclei is responsible for inhibiting the urge to eat?

A. Anterior nucleus

B. Posterior nucleus

C. Mamillary nucleus

D. Suprachiasmatic nucleus

E. Ventromedial nucleus

177. The syndrome that is characterized by psychic blindness (inability to identify friends and relatives), pathological overeating, hyperorality, placidity, heightened sexual activity, altered emotional responses, and constant shifting of attention is a result of damage to which of the following brain structures?

A. Arcuate fasciculus

B. Bilateral amygdale

C. Bilateral mamillary bodies

D. Reticular activating system

E. STN

178. Which of the following is TRUE of cognitive dysfunction seen in MS?

A. Cognitive dysfunction is seen in about 25% of patients with MS.

B. Cognitive dysfunction only occurs late in the course of the illness.

C. Cognitive difficulties lead to disability independent of the physical disability of the illness.

D. Drugs like beta-interferons and glatiramer have not been beneficial in slowing down the progression of the cognitive decline in this illness.

E. Cholinesterase inhibitors like donepezil, rivastigmine, or galantamine are not helpful in treating patients with cognitive impairment from MS.

179. All of the following are true of the epidemiology of Schizophrenia EXCEPT:

A. It is equally prevalent in men and women.

B. It is evenly distributed geographically.

C. A higher preponderance of patients who develop schizophrenia were born in the winter.

D. A higher preponderance of patients who develop schizophrenia were born in early spring.

E. Fifty percent of patients with schizophrenia attempt suicide.

180. Which of the following neurotransmitters have been implicated in the pathogenesis of schizophrenia?

A. Dopamine only

B. Dopamine and glutamate

C. Dopamine, glutamate, and GABA

D. Dopamine, glutamate, norepinephrine, and GABA

E. Dopamine, norepinephrine, and glutamate

181. A 19-year-old college student is brought in by friends for an evaluation. For the past 6 weeks she has been carrying a doll down to a nearby fountain. She believes that by baptizing it daily, she will keep it from becoming ill. Her friends report she has not been herself since starting college less than a year ago. She has not been concentrating well, misses classes, and does not care for herself as usual. On examination, she has a flat affect and reports hearing voices of angels. She does not use drugs or alcohol, and denies any mood disturbance. Given this history, what is her most likely diagnosis?

A. Brief psychotic disorder

B. Schizophreniform disorder

C. Schizoaffective disorder

D. Delusional disorder

E. Schizophrenia

182. A 27-year-old woman is brought to the ER in a frankly psychotic state. She has also been complaining of abdominal pain for the last 24 hours. On examination there is also evidence for muscle weakness and peripheral neuropathy. Initial routine laboratory data and imaging results are inconclusive. Further history reveals that she has had several such acute episodes in the past, and several close family members have experienced similar episodes throughout their lifetime. Which of the following tests should you order to confirm your suspicion?

A. Serum ceruloplasmin

B. Ophthalmologic examination

C. Urine porphobilinogen

D. Antineutrophil antibodies (ANA)

E. CSF examination for oligoclonal bands

183. A 23-year-old heroin-dependent woman presents to your ER in labor. She gives birth to a 7 lb baby girl. The new mother is admitted to a methadone substitution program where 20 mg/day of methadone is administered. A week later, she is brought back to your ER by ambulance after she became unresponsive. On examination, she is lethargic and hypotonic. Her respiratory rate is 5 per minute and effort shallow. Her pupils are constricted bilaterally. What is the most likely explanation for her symptoms? At this point interventional strategy should consist of the following EXCEPT:

A. Cardiopulmonary support

B. Hospitalization

C. Naloxone therapy given intramuscularly as a one-time bolus dose

D. Repeated doses of naloxone given intravenously

E. All of the above

184. Which psychodynamic characteristic of obsessive-compulsive personality structure is incorrectly paired?

A. Central preoccupation: Submission to versus rebellion against controlling authority

B. Central affects: Anger, fear, guilt, and shame

C. Central pathogenic belief about self: I am in constant danger from forces unknown

D. Central pathogenic belief about others: Others try to exert control, which I must resist

E. Central defenses: Isolation of affect, reaction formation, intellectualizing, and undoing

185. Which of the following is NOT TRUE of phototherapy for Seasonal Affective Disorder (SAD)?

A. Phototherapy has been the most widely studied treatment for SAD.

B. Phototherapy is most effective when administered later in the day.

C. Similar to drug therapy for depression, phototherapy carries some risk of precipitating mania.

D. The dosage most often found to be effective is 5,000 lux per day, given as 2,500 lux for 2 hours or 10,000 lux for 30 minutes.

E. All of the above.

186. Which one of the following is TRUE of duloxetine?

A. It blocks dopamine reuptake.

B. No dosage adjustment is needed in geriatric patients.

C. No discontinuation syndrome is seen even with abrupt cessation of treatment.

D. It is excreted unmetabolized by the kidneys.

E. It has a half-life of 100 hours.

187. A resident physician asks you about couples therapy. When giving him an answer, which one of the following would you NOT include as an indication for this mode of treatment?

A. The problem involves two or more family members.

B. A sexual problem or sexual dissatisfaction is present.

C. The couple's problems are ego syntonic.

D. A developmental transition or crisis causes disruption in the family structure.

E. The onset of symptoms is connected to relationship disharmony.

188. A patient diagnosed with central diabetes insipidus would have a lesion in which one of the following hypothalamic nuclei?

A. Suprachiasmatic nucleus

B. Lateral nucleus

C. Paraventricular nucleus

D. Arcuate nucleus

E. Medial preoptic nucleus

189. A 32-year-old woman with a 10-year history of MS is suffering from severe depression. She is unable to work secondary to her physical condition and has been sleeping more than 12 hours each day. Which of the following is most closely associated with severe depressive symptoms in patients with MS?

A. Cerebral involvement

B. Spinal involvement

C. Physical disability

D. Few social supports

E. Duration of illness

190. A 60-year-old white man with a 35-year history of alcohol dependence is being seen at the ER of a tertiary care hospital for a 1-week history of worsening confusion. On examination, he is very confused and scores 8/30 on the Folstein MMSE. Staff at the ER, who have known him for the last 10 years, indicate that he is much more confused than before and is also confabulating. He is also very unsteady on his feet and is exhibiting horizontal nystagmus on lateral gaze. The blood alcohol level is zero and the urine drug screen is negative for any illicit drugs. A CT scan of the head does not show any acute changes. His blood sugar is low at 50 mg/dl, but the rest of the laboratory data is normal including the liver function test. You discuss this information with the attending physician who indicates that the patient should be treated with thiamine. Which one of the following is NOT TRUE of the treatment of this man's condition?

A. He should receive parenteral thiamine before administration of glucose or parenteral nutrition.

B. He should receive intravenous thiamine followed by oral maintenance doses of thiamine.

C. Even if he is treated with parenteral thiamine, his mortality rate is between 10 to 20%.

D. Improvement in his gait and memory will happen within a day of treatment with parenteral thiamine.

E. Ocular signs improve in this patient in a few hours of treatment with parenteral thiamine.

191. Which of the following statements regarding delirium tremens (DTs) is TRUE?

A. It is the most severe on the spectrum of alcohol-withdrawal syndromes.

B. It is defined by a change in cognition that occurs over a short period of time and includes a fluctuating level of consciousness.

C. Compared to milder forms of withdrawal, which begin within hours of the last drink, DTs usually begin within 2 to 4 days after the last drink.

D. Although the average length of DTs is less than one week, there are reports of DTs lasting weeks to months.

E. All of the above.

192. A 67-year-old patient with Chronic Paranoid Schizophrenia is receiving social skills training. Social skills training in these patients target all of the following EXCEPT:

A. Verbal communication

B. Ability to read another person's emotions

C. Ability to understand oneself

D. Dating skills

E. Job interview skills

193. Which of the following symptom(s) of duration of 1 month is not clearly a potential symptom pattern of Schizophrenia?

A. Hearing voices of demons chattering with each other

B. The belief that ones neighbor is stealing from them

C. Speaking in a newly bizarre manner that is difficult to comprehend

D. Negativism, stupor and waxy flexibility

E. Social withdrawal, poverty of thought, and blunted affect

194. A 38-year-old woman presents to your office for an evaluation. She complains of gradually worsening anxiety, restlessness, and inability to sleep for over a month. She reports racing thoughts, palpitations, diarrhea, and weight loss. On examination her pulse is 115 beats/minute, and she has a mild tremor. She does not drink, smoke, or use drugs. She does not have regular medical care. Given this history, what should be the next step in the management of this patient's condition?

A. Prescribe alprazolam and follow her up next week

B. Teach her relaxation techniques using a cognitive behavioral approach

C. Prescribe paroxetine and educate her it may take four to six weeks on the appropriate dose for a response

D. Check laboratories, including chemistries and thyroid function tests, and encourage her to establish a primary care provider

E. Perform a dexamethasone suppression test to determine if this is physiological in origin

195. A 72-year-old man with history of coronary artery disease, hypertension, and diabetes presents to the ED with complaints of sudden onset of speech difficulty for the past few hours. When attempting to speak, he appears very frustrated and has difficulty getting words out. He appears to understand everything that is said to him and is able to follow commands correctly. A magnetic resonance angiography (MRA) of the brain would most likely show a problem in which of the following structures?

A. Basilar artery

B. Left middle cerebral artery

C. Left posterior cerebral artery

D. Right middle cerebral artery

E. Right posterior cerebral artery

196. Which of the following molecules is classified as an amino acid neurotransmitter?

A. GABA

B. Serotonin

C. Neurotensin

D. Cholecystokinin octapeptide

E. Acetylcholine

197. A 25-year-old woman has recently been diagnosed with migraine. She is 8 weeks pregnant and does not want to take any medications for her migraines, lest it affect the development of her baby. She asks you about non-pharmacological treatments for migraines. When giving her this information, which one of the following statements would you NOT make regarding non-pharmacological treatments for migraines?

A. Clinical trials support the notion that non-pharmacological therapies can be a first choice for patients with migraines.

B. The most common therapies include relaxation, cognitive-behavioural therapy, and BF.

C. Among these therapies, CBT is the most effective.

D. These therapies reduce the headache index by 50% or more in 30% to 60% of patients, identical to the effect of commonly used prophylactic drugs.

E. The initial effects from these therapies appear to be maintained for several years.

198. A 25-year-old man with a recent diagnosis of migraine asks you about pharmacological treatments for migraines. When giving him this information, which one of the following statements would you

NOT make regarding the pharmacological treatments for migraine?

A. For acute treatment of migraine attacks, oral nonsteroidal anti-inflammatory drugs (NSAIDs) and triptans are first line treatments.

B. In very severe attacks, intravenous acetylsalicylic acid or subcutaneous sumatriptan are drugs of first choice.

C. Status migrainous can probably be treated by steroids.

D. Amitriptyline and naproxen are drugs of first choice for prophylaxis.

E. Valproic acid and topiramate are also drugs of first choice for prophylaxis.

199. A 24-year-old man is seen status post motor vehicle related head trauma. He has been referred for post-TBI rehabilitation. You are told that his Rancho Los Amigos Level of Cognitive Scale is VI. Given this information, which of the following best describes his current status?

A. Unresponsive to sound, light, touch or pain

B. Purposeful appropriate: Alert and oriented. He is able to recall and integrate past and current events

and demonstrates carry-over of new learning and evidences independence with limitations

C. Confused and appropriate: Alert and inconsistently oriented to time and place. Follows simple directions and begins to show carry over of new learning

D. Generalized response: Reacts inconsistently in a nonspecific manner to stimulation. Unintelligible vocalization. Response to stimuli is frequently delayed

E. Automatic appropriate: Oriented to person, place, and time but shows a shallow awareness of mental condition. Performs basic activities of daily living (ADLs) with supervision and in robot-like manner

200. Which of the following is a highly significant risk factor for development of neuropsychiatric sequelae from TBI?

A. History of premorbid psychiatric illness

B. Poor premorbid social functioning

C. Older age at injury

D. History of alcoholism

E. All of the above

Answers

1. Answer: D. Impotence, retarded and premature ejaculation, and hypoactive sexual desire are all sexual disorders. Needing more time and more direct stimulation to achieve an erection is common in an aging man.

1. Sadock BJ, Sadock VA. *Kaplan and Sadock's Synopsis of Psychiatry*. 9th ed. Philadelphia: Lippincott Williams & Wilkins; 2003:701–708.
2. Stern TA, Herman JB. *Massachusetts General Hospital Psychiatry Update and Board Preparation*. 2nd ed. New York: McGraw Hill; 2004:155.

2. Answer: C. The prefrontal cortex of patients with Schizophrenia is thinner when compared to normal subjects. This thinning is thought to be mainly due to loss of neuropil; the area between neuronal and glial cell bodies. The absence of gliosis in brains of subjects with Schizophrenia most likely points to the absence of an inflammatory process in the pathogenesis of this illness. The hippocampus is smaller in size and functionally abnormal in patients with Schizophrenia. Studies of the thalamus have revealed controversial data. Some authors have found a reduced number of neurons in the medial dorsal nucleus of the thalamus, whereas others have found no differences.

Sadock BJ, Sadock VA. *Kaplan and Sadock's Comprehensive Textbook of Psychiatry*. 8th ed. Philadelphia: Lippincott Williams & Wilkins; 2005:1409–1415.

3. Answer: E. Ethologist Konrad Lorenz is well known for his study of aggression. He wrote about the practical function of aggression and showed that although aggression among members of the same species is common, it seldom leads to killing or serious injury under normal conditions. Rather, a certain balance appears between tendencies to fight and flight, with the tendency to fight being strongest in the center of the territory and the tendency to flight strongest at a distance from the center. The learned helplessness model of depression was developed by Martin Seligman, where he observed that dogs exposed to electric shocks from which they could not escape eventually gave up and made no more attempts to escape, and this behavior generalized to other situations. Ethologist Nikolaas Tinbergen described displacement activities as those that occur when a conflict arises and the need for fight and for flight are of roughly equal strength, so the animal engages in behavior that appears to be irrelevant to the situation.

Kaplan HI, Sadock BJ. *Kaplan & Sadock's Synopsis of Psychiatry*. 8th ed. Philadelphia: Lippincott Williams & Wilkins; 1998:162–167.

4. Answer: A. Incidence of Social Phobia is estimated at 4:1 ratio for female:male. Most other anxiety disorders (with the exception of OCD) have a female:male ratio close to that of Major Depression, which is 2:1. Schizophrenia and Bipolar Disorders have roughly equal female:male ratios overall for lifetime. For most substance abuse disorders (the main exception being cocaine and stimulant abuse), including alcoholism, the male:female ratio approaches 2:1. Although not listed, gender differences are greatest for eating disorders, with female:male ratios ≥10:1.

Hales RE, Yudofsky SC. *Textbook of Clinical Psychiatry*. 4th ed. Washington: American Psychiatric Publishing; 2003: 1511–1537.

5. Answer: D. PET scans show that OCD is associated with increased glucose metabolism in the orbitofrontal cortex (a.k.a., anterior cingulate cortex), caudate, thalamus, and putamen. This overactivity trends back toward normal with response to treatment. The brainstem (midbrain) is not thought to be significantly involved in OCD.

1. Friedlander L, Desrocher M. Neuroimaging studies of obsessive-compulsive disorder in adults and children. *Clin Psychol Rev*. 2006;26:32–49.
2. Sadock BJ, Sadock VA. *Kaplan and Sadock's Comprehensive Textbook of Psychiatry*. 8th ed. Philadelphia: Lippincott Williams & Wilkins; 2005:1755.

6. Answer: C. In Malingering, the motivation for symptom production is an external incentive, whereas in Factitious Disorder there are no external incentives. In Factitious Disorder, there is evidence of an intrapsychic conflict and the need to maintain the sick role. In Conversion Disorder, there is no intentional production of symptoms and no obvious external incentives associated with it. In Malingering, in contrast to Conversion Disorder, there is usually no symptom relief from suggestion or hypnosis.

American Psychiatric Association. *Diagnostic and Statistical Manual of Mental Disorders American Psychiatric Association*. 4th ed. (Text revision). http://www.psychiatryonline.

com/content.aspx?aID=11409. Accessed January 14, 2007

7. **Answer: E.** This patient does not show any signs of a pathologic bereavement, and a diagnosis of MDD is generally not given unless symptom criteria for depression are still present after 2 months. In acute bereavement, up to 50% of grieving spouses have reported hearing a recently deceased loved one's voice or feeling the presence of the deceased. The patient does not show evidence of a primary psychosis requiring treatment with an antipsychotic, and her current condition does not warrant hospitalization or head imaging at this time as she does not show any suicidality, homicidality, or psychotic symptoms. The patient scored within normal range for her age on MMSE, does not give evidence of a dementing illness with complaints of memory loss, and does not need medication for dementia at this time.

1. Kaplan HI, Sadock BJ. *Kaplan & Sadock's Synopsis of Psychiatry*. 8th ed. Philadelphia: Lippincott Williams & Wilkins; 1998:857.
2. Sadock BJ, Sadock VA. *Kaplan and Sadock's Comprehensive Textbook of Psychiatry*. 8th ed. Philadelphia: Lippincott Williams & Wilkins; 2005:988.

8. **Answer: B.** Postpsychotic Depressive Disorder of schizophrenia requires depressive symptoms, including depressed mood, that occur only during the residual phase of Schizophrenia. It is estimated that approximately 25% of patients with Schizophrenia develop the disorder. Although the depressive symptoms can be hard to distinguish from negative symptoms, the symptoms are not identical and refer to two distinct diagnostic entities. Antidepressants have been used as treatment and several studies have found a positive effect. There is a significant correlation between Postpsychotic Depressive Disorder and extrapyramidal symptoms secondary to antipsychotic medications.

Kaplan HI, Sadock BJ. *Kaplan & Sadock's Synopsis of Psychiatry*. 8th ed. Philadelphia: Lippincott Williams & Wilkins; 1998:494–495, 479–480.

9. **Answer: C.** Residual Schizophrenia is diagnosed via DSM-IV-TR criteria in patients who once met full criteria for Schizophrenia and no longer have prominent psychotic symptoms, but still have some evidence of ongoing illness, often in an attenuated form. They may have ongoing negative symptoms, as in this case, or also attenuated positive symptoms. The Paranoid subtype presents with prominent delusions or hallucinations, often with preserved cognition. The Disorganized subtype presents with prominent disorganization of speech or behavior, inappropriate

affect, with severe social impairment, and poor long-term functioning, and was once termed *hebephrenia*. Catatonic Schizophrenia presents with at least two catatonic symptoms, a prominent psychomotor disturbance, with early onset, and poor prognosis. The Undifferentiated subtype is the most commonly diagnosed subtype of schizophrenia, where criteria are met for the active phase but do not fully meet criteria for any of the other subtypes of the illness.

1. American Psychiatric Association. *Diagnostic and Statistical Manual of Mental Disorders American Psychiatric Association*. 4th ed. (Text Revision). http://www.psychiatryonline.com/content.aspx?aID=9070. Accessed February 17, 2007.
2. Hales RE, Yudofsky SC. *Textbook of Clinical Psychiatry*. 4th ed. Washington: American Psychiatric Publishing; 2003:379–439.

10. **Answer: D.** Wilfred Bion worked to elucidate group dynamics at the Tavistock Institute in London, and described two main subgroups: the work group and the basic assumption group. The work group is involved in performing the actual task assigned to the group. The basic assumption group is divided into three categories: dependency, fight or flight, and pairing. These basic assumptions pertain to the unconscious fantasies of the group members and they interfere with the accomplishment of the work group's task. The group members' behavior reveals which basic assumption predominates. In this vignette, the group members are focusing on one pair whose love is hoped will rescue/save the group; behavior that is a defense against negative emotions (hate and hostility) within the group. Bion came from the school of Kleinian object relations, and he also developed the concept of the psychiatrist as the *container* for the patient in therapy.

1. Gabbard G. *Psychodynamic Psychiatry in Clinical Practice*. 4th ed. Washington: American Psychiatric Press; 2005:129–131.
2. Ganzarin RC. Psychotic-like anxieties and primitive defenses in group analytic psychotherapy. *Issues Ego Psychol*.1980;3:42–48.
3. Sadock BJ, Sadock VA. *Kaplan and Sadock's Comprehensive Textbook of Psychiatry*. 8th ed. Philadelphia: Lippincott Williams & Wilkins; 2005:734–735.

11. **Answer: E.** Several factors have been shown to negatively affect successful nonspecialized short-term alcohol rehabilitation. These include unstable living environment (homelessness), additional substance related disorders, serial treatment failures, and the presence of concomitant serious mental illnesses. The presence of any of these factors is a red flag for possible poor outcome and an

indication for referral to specialized long-term treatment program.

Sadock BJ, Sadock VA. *Kaplan and Sadock's Comprehensive Textbook of Psychiatry*. 8th ed. Philadelphia: Lippincott Williams & Wilkins; 2005:1186.

12. Answer: C. Unlike the straightforward presentation of uncomplicated characterological dependency, individuals with Passive-Aggressive subtype of Dependent Personality Disorder resent being tied to another, yet cannot separate psychologically. Their dependency has a hostile edge and manifests itself via a tendency to punish others indirectly. Normal aggression is expressed obliquely in an effort to vent negative affect without threatening attachment. Dependent Passive-Aggressive individuals define themselves by reference to others, but with a negative valence (e.g., "I am the husband of that bitch"). Like paranoid patients, they attack to preempt expected attack by others, but they do so indirectly. Like masochistic patients, they expect mistreatment, but they fight back, albeit insidiously. They have core narcissistic concerns, but are more interpersonally engaged than characterologically narcissistic people. Because they locate themselves in opposition to others' agendas, it is hard for them to conceive of and to pursue their own goals. The Passive-Aggressive subtype of Dependent Personality disorder's pathogenic belief about self is that "The only route to dignity is to sabotage the achievements of others." In contrast, sadistic personality disorder's pathogenic belief about self is that "I am entitled to hurt and humiliate others."

1. McWilliams N. *Psychoanalytic Diagnosis: Understanding Personality Structure in the Clinical Process*. New York: The Guilford Press; 1994:257–277.
2. PDM Task Force. *Psychodynamic Diagnostic Manual*. Silver Spring: Alliance of Psychoanalytic Organizations; 2006:40–42, 50–53.

13. Answer: B. Evaluation of behavioral and relaxation interventions for chronic pain in adults found the following: (i) relaxation, (ii) hypnosis, (iii) CBT, (iv) BF, and (v) multimodal treatment were all helpful in pain reduction. The evidence is strong for the effectiveness of the *relaxation* class of techniques in reducing chronic pain in a variety of medical conditions. The evidence supporting the effectiveness of *hypnosis* in alleviating chronic pain associated with cancer seems strong. In addition, data suggests that it is effective in other chronic pain conditions, which include irritable bowel syndrome, oral mucositis, temporomandibular disorders, and tension headaches. The evidence is moderate for the usefulness of *CBT* in chronic pain. CBT has been found to be superior to placebo and to routine care for alleviating low back pain and both rheumatoid arthritis and osteoarthritis-associated pain, but inferior to hypnosis for oral mucositis and to electromyography (EMG) BF for tension headache. The evidence is moderate for the effectiveness of *BF* in relieving many types of chronic pain. Data shows that EMG BF to be more effective than psychological placebo for tension headache but equivalent in results to relaxation. For migraine headache, BF is better than relaxation therapy and better than no treatment, but superiority to psychological placebo is less clear. Several meta-analyses have examined the effectiveness of *multimodal treatments* in clinical settings. Although relatively good evidence exists for the efficacy of several behavioral and relaxation interventions in the treatment of chronic pain, the data are insufficient to conclude that one technique is usually more effective than another for a given condition. For any given individual patient, however, one approach may be more appropriate than another.

NIH Technology Assessment Panel on Integration of Behavioral and Relaxation Approaches into the Treatment of Chronic Pain and Insomnia. Integration of behavioral and relaxation approaches into the treatment of chronic pain and insomnia. *JAMA*. 1996;276:313–318.

14. Answer: B. Venlafaxine is an SNRI. It works by blocking the serotonin (5-hydroxytryptamine) and norepinephrine (noradrenaline) reuptake. Venlafaxine is well absorbed with at least 92% of an oral dose being absorbed into systemic circulation. It is extensively metabolized in the liver via the CYP2D6 isoenzyme to O-desmethylvenlafaxine, which is just as potent an SNRI as the parent compound. This means that the differences in metabolism between extensive and poor metabolizers are not clinically important. Steady-state concentrations of venlafaxine and its metabolite are attained in the blood within 3 days and therapeutic effects are usually achieved within 3 to 4 weeks. The half-life of venlafaxine is about 5 hours for venlafaxine and 10 hours for its active metabolite O-desmethylvenlafaxine. It can produce withdrawal symptoms even with missing a single dose.

Venlafaxine is not recommended in patients hypersensitive to venlafaxine. It should never be used in conjunction with an MAOI, due to the potential to develop serotonin syndrome. Caution should also be used in those with a seizure disorder as it has a seizure risk of about 0.3%. The clearance of venlafaxine is reduced in patients with hepatic and renal disease, and hence the dosage should be reduced by 50% in these patients. Venlafaxine should only be used during pregnancy if clearly needed. It is contraindicated in breast-feeding.

Albers LJ, Hahn RK, Reist C. *Handbook of Psychiatric Drugs.* Laguna Hills: Current Clinical Strategies Publishing; 2005:21–22.

15. Answer: D. Bipolar disorders are prevalent, disabling illnesses with elevated lethality largely due to completed suicide. Suicide rates average approximately 1% annually, sixty times higher than the international population rate of 0.015% annually. Suicidal acts typically occur early in the illness and usually associated with severe depressive or mixed states. The high lethality of suicidal acts in Bipolar Disorders is suggested by a much lower ratio of attempts:suicide (approximately 3:1) than in the general population (approximately 30:1).

1. Baldessarini RJ, Pompili M, Tondo L. Suicide in bipolar disorder. *CNS Spectrums.* 2006;11:465–471.
2. Valtonen HM, Suominen K, Mantere O, et al. Suicidal behaviour during different phases of bipolar disorder. *J Affect Disord.* 2007;97:101–107.

16. Answer: D. Taste sensation is provided by two different cranial nerves. The facial nerve (CN VII) provides sensation in the two anterior thirds of the tongue, whereas the glossopharyngeal nerve (CN IX) is responsible for taste sensation in the posterior third of the tongue. Cranial nerves IV, V, and VI are not involved in taste sensation.

Kaufman DM. *Clinical Neurology for Psychiatrists.* 5th ed. Philadelphia: WB Saunders; 2001:35–55.

17. Answer: E. The patient's symptoms cannot be explained by a single lesion, and a blatant psychogenic gait impairment occurs when patients drag a "weak" leg. In contrast, patients with a true hemiparetic gait end up swinging their leg outward with a circular motion. If she had a left cerebral lesion causing a right hemiparesis, then the patient's visual deficit should be a right homonymous hemianopia, and there should be the usual accompanying symptom of aphasia. There are no physical exam findings to indicate any cranial nerve deficits that would make one suspect a lesion in the brainstem, and a cerebellar lesion would be associated with ipsilateral limb ataxia. The patient's symptoms cannot be confirmed by objective signs, and her gait is suggestive of an absence of a true neurologic disease.

1. Kaufman DM. *Clinical Neurology for Psychiatrists.* 5th ed. WB Saunders; 2001:29.
2. Rowland LP. *Merritt's Neurology.* 11th ed. Lippincott Williams & Wilkins; 2005:295–296, 299–302.

18. Answer: E. The Lambert-Eaton syndrome is an autoimmune disorder where antibodies directed against voltage-gated calcium channels develop in the peripheral nerve terminals. It usually occurs in adults, and is seen in about 60% of patients with small cell carcinoma of the lung. In these patients, the neurologic symptoms mostly precede those of the tumor by almost 5 years in some cases. About 33% of cases of Lambert-Eaton syndrome are not associated with any tumors. These patients tend to have the HLA-B8, DR-3 haplotype. The diagnosis is made based on the clinical manifestations and is confirmed by the characteristic incremental response to repetitive nerve stimulation which is the opposite of the pattern in myasthenia gravis.

Rowland LP. *Merritt's Neurology.* 11th ed. Philadelphia: Lippincott Williams & Wilkins; 2005:887.

19. Answer: C. This patient is most likely experiencing carpopedal spasm and EEG slowing from hyperventilation. Having the patient hyperventilate will most certainly recreate her symptoms, a useful bedside diagnostic test. Prolonged hyperventilation could result in altered consciousness which is quickly aborted by breathing into a bag. All the other techniques mentioned are not useful in recreating a popedal spasm.

Eisendrath SJ. Factitious physical disorders. *West J Med.* 1994;160:177–179.

20. Answer: A. Tyrosine hydroxylase converts the amino acid tyrosine into DOPA, and is the rate-limiting step in the production of both dopamine and norepinephrine. DOPA is converted into dopamine by the action of DOPA decarboxylase (a.k.a., L-aromatic amino acid decarboxylase). DβH converts dopamine to norepinephrine, but is not the rate-limiting step. COMT degrades intrasynaptic norepinephrine after it is formed. NET removes norepinephrine to intracellular monoamine oxidases (MOAs) for degradation, not formation, and is the primary means of norepinephrine removal. Neither COMT nor NET is active in production or synthesis of norepinephrine.

Kaufman DM. *Clinical Neurology for Psychiatrists.* 5th ed. Philadelphia: WB Saunders; 2001:552–569.

21. Answer: A. The patient described has an essential tremor, which is one of the most common movement disorders. This postural tremor may have its onset anywhere between the second and sixth decades of life, and its prevalence increases with age. The positive family history and improvement with alcohol are typical features of essential tremor. Parkinson's disease typically has a characteristic resting tremor that appears like a "pill-rolling" motion and begins asymmetrically. The patient is young and does not present with other common signs of Parkinson's disease: rigidity, bradykinesia, and postural instability. The patient's history is not consistent with MS, which is a demyelinating illness. Huntington's disease is characterized by a choreiform movement disorder and a myriad of psychiatric manifestations, which this patient does not present with at this time. He is not presenting with symptoms of Wilson's disease (hepatolenticular degeneration), which is characterized by a Parkinson-like tremor and ataxia, or a characteristic wing-beating tremor where patients move their arms as if they were attempting to fly. It is an autosomal recessive genetic illness that is characterized by the development of dementia with involuntary movements from copper deposits in the brain and other organs, and symptoms tend to manifest by adolescence.

1. Kaufman DM. *Clinical Neurology for Psychiatrists*. 5th ed. WB Saunders; 2001:446–467, 474–476.
2. Rowland LP. *Merritt's Neurology*. 11th ed. Philadelphia: Lippincott Williams & Wilkins; 2005:48, 661, 804, 807, 827.

22. Answer: B. Atrophy of arms is present in both conditions, thus would not be a clinical feature useful in making a diagnosis between CSM and ALS. However, tongue fasciculations, atrophy of legs, and denervation are all present in ALS, but are absent in CSM. Likewise, sensory loss is present with CSM, but is absent in ALS.

1. Rowland LP. *Merritt's Neurology*. 11th ed. Philadelphia: Lippincott Williams & Wilkins; 2005:519, 866–867.
2. Young WF. Cervical spondylotic myelopathy: a common cause of spinal cord dysfunction in older persons. *Am Fam Physician*. 2000;62:1064–1070, 1073.

23. Answer: C. The American Academy of Neurology (AAN) practice parameter on immunotherapy for GBS states that plasma exchange or IVIG hastens the recovery from GBS. The beneficial effects of plasma exchange and IVIG are equivalent and that combining the two treatments has not been found to be beneficial. They also state that treatment with steroids alone is not beneficial in these patients. The AAN recommends plasma exchange for nonambulatory adult patients with GBS who start treatment within 4 weeks of the onset of neurologic symptoms. Plasma exchange is also recommended for ambulatory patients who start treatment within 2 weeks of the onset of neurologic symptoms. IVIG is recommended for non-ambulatory adult patients with GBS who start treatment within 2 or possibly 4 weeks of the onset of neurologic symptoms.

Vriesendrop FJ. *Treatment and Prognosis of Guillain-Barré Syndrome in Adults*. http://www.uptodateonline.com/utd/content/topic.do?topicKey=muscle/8595&type=A&selectedTitle=3~57. Accessed February 27, 2007.

24. Answer: C. The essential features of CJD are neuronal degeneration, astrocytic proliferation, and status spongiosus of the cortical grey matter. The cortex is almost always involved with relative sparing of the parietal and occipital lobes. The corticospinal and extrapyramidal pathways are often severely affected. Whilst being characteristic of CJD, status spongiosus is not entirely pathognomonic of this disorder, as it is sometimes seen in other degenerative conditions such as Alzheimer's disease and Wilson's disease. There are no neurofibrillary tangles as seen in Alzheimer's disease or massive circumscribed atrophy as in frontotemporal dementias such as Pick's disease. There is no evidence of an inflammatory reaction.

1. Lishman WA.*Organic Psychiatry*. 3rd ed. Oxford: Blackwell Science; 1996:478.
2. Rowland LP. *Merritt's Neurology*. 11th ed. Philadelphia: Lippincott Williams & Wilkins; 2005:266.

25. Answer: E. Akathisia is an extremely unpleasant subjective sensation of "inner" restlessness that manifests itself as an inability to sit still or remain motionless. It ranges from mild to a total inability to sit still with overwhelming anxiety and severe dysphoria. In severe cases, the dysphoria can be so severe that patients may attempt suicide. It may often be misdiagnosed as an anxiety disorder. It can be measured by using the Barnes Akathisia Scale. Akathisia is most often seen as a side effect of antipsychotic drug therapy, either as acute akathisia or tardive akathisia. It may also be seen in encephalopathies, in some dementias, and in Parkinson's disease. Paroxetine, tricyclics antidepressants, trazodone, promethazine, diphenhydramine, metoclopramide, and prochlorperazine may also cause akathisia. Drugs of abuse like gammahydroxybutyrate (GHB) and 3,4-methylenedioxymethamphetamine (MDMA, ecstasy) may cause akathisia in overdoses. Treatment includes the reduction or discontinuation of the offending agent. Propranolol is often considered as the drug of choice for the treatment of akathisia. Cyproheptadine or benztropine may be second-line agents for the treatment of this condition.

1. Pierre JM. Extrapyramidal symptoms with atypical antipsychotics: incidence, prevention, and management. *Drug Saf*. 2005;28:191–208.
2. Rathbone J, Soares-Weiser K. Anticholinergics for neuroleptic-induced acute akathisia. *Cochrane Database Syst Rev*. 2006;4:CD003727.

26. Answer: A. Blindness occurs in about 50% of the patients with temporal arteritis, if left untreated. In patients with visual symptoms, treatment should be initiated with intravenous formulations such as methylprednisolone (Medrol). Treatment should not be delayed while awaiting temporal artery biopsy. Corticosteroid therapy has no effect on biopsy results for up to 4 weeks after initiation of treatment. Hence, prompt treatment should be initiated on suspicion of this condition. Patients may also develop thrombosis of any peridural artery or an aortic aneurysm with rupture if left untreated. The ESR is often elevated in these patients, but a normal ESR does not temporal arteritis. Serum viscosity and C-reactive protein levels are often elevated and may be helpful in the diagnosis or to follow-up the effect of treatment, in those with normal ESR. Plasma interleukin-6 (IL-6) is thought to be the most sensitive marker of disease activity. Treatment with methotrexate is not routinely recommended, as studies using methotrexate in temporal arteritis are still inconclusive.

1. Rowland LP. *Merritt's Neurology*. 11th ed. Philadelphia: Lippincott Williams & Wilkins; 2005:988–989.
2. Unwin B, Williams CM, Gilliland W. Polymyalgia rheumatica and giant cell arteritis. *Am Fam Physician*. 2006; 74:1547–1554.

27. **Answer: E.** Suicide risk increases with age for both sexes, but the rates in older men are generally higher than in those for women. In the United States, men commit suicide four times more often than women, but women attempt suicide three times as often as men. However, this female predominance among suicide attempters varies with age and the ratio of women to men approaches 1:1 in the elderly. Men also tend to use more lethal suicide methods than women (e.g., firearms or hanging compared to cutting or overdoses). In the United States, women in middle ages are at highest risk of suicide than at any other time in their lives. Suicide attempts are also more common in women with borderline personality disorder, those with a history of domestic violence, and a history of physical and/or sexual abuse. In women, pregnancy is a time of significantly reduced suicide risk. Women with young children in the home are less likely to kill themselves. But those women with a history of depression or suicide attempts are at greater risk during the postpartum period compared to women who don't have such a history. Suicide is most likely to occur in the first month after delivery, but the risk continues throughout the postpartum period. Teenagers, women of lower socioeconomic status, and women hospitalized with postpartum psychiatric disorders are particularly at increased risk in the postpartum period.

American Psychiatric Association. *American Psychiatric Association Practice Guidelines for the Treatment of Psychiatric Disorders: Compendium 2006*. http://www.psychiatryonline.com/content.aspx?aID=56135. Accessed January 15, 2007.

28. **Answer: A.** Tau-protein normally binds to microtubules and stabilizes the neuronal skeleton, axonal flow, and cell circuitry. In Alzheimer's disease, tau-proteins become hyperphosphorylated and this weakens its affinity for the microtubules. Neurofibrillary tangles are filaments found in axonal processes throughout the neuropil in brains of patients with Alzheimer's disease.

Amyloid plaques are universally immunoreactive to anti-Aβ antibodies because the Aβ peptide is the most common protein in these lesions. Neuritic plaques are associated with a glial response, which is thought to produce a chronic state of proinflammatory activation. Hirano bodies are eosinophilic inclusions found most commonly in the hippocampus. They are thought to represent degeneration of the neuronal cytoskeleton.

1. Bugiani O. Neuropathology of the dementias other than Alzheimer's. *Neurol Sci*. 2006;27 (suppl 1):S44–S46.
2. Mott RT, Hulette CM. Neuropathology of Alzheimer's disease. *Neuroimaging Clin N Am*. 2005;15:755–765.

29. **Answer: C.** Delusions are disturbances in content of thought that are fixed, false beliefs out of keeping with the patients' cultural background. In this well related patient, belief in spirits is a part of the patient's cultural background and is supported by her family. The patient does not show any other signs concerning for psychiatric illness and is functioning optimally in academic and social settings. She does not require in-patient hospitalization, nor does her cultural belief require an antipsychotic prescription that would be helpful in patients with frank delusions. There is no indication that the patient is being neglected or abused by her parents; situations that would warrant separation and referral to foster care. It would be inappropriate to recommend family counseling for a cultural belief that is not a delusional disorder and would not be sensitive to cross-cultural beliefs.

Kaplan HI, Sadock BJ. *Kaplan & Sadock's Synopsis of Psychiatry*. 8th ed. Philadelphia: Lippincott Williams & Wilkins; 1998:252.

30. **Answer: E.** As our knowledge of the effects of most psychotropic medications on the developing fetuses is limited, nonpharmacologic treatments (e.g., psychotherapy, support groups, lifestyle modification, etc.) should be the preferred choice whenever possible. Higher potency antipsychotics are believed to confer lower risk of congenital malformation than low potency antipsychotics. Also, extrapyramidal symptoms and anticholinergic agents are associated with increased risk of congenital anomalies. First trimester lithium use has been

associated with increased risk of congenital mal-formations, notably cardiac anomalies (Ebstein's anomaly). Valproic acid and carbamazepine are as-sociated with increased incidence of fetal neural tube defects due to their anti-folate effect. Of note, bipo-lar women not treated with mood stabilizers during pregnancy are at increased risk for postpartum de-compensation. Antidepressants should also be ap-proached with the risk:benefit ratio in mind. Fluox-etine and TCA have been studied and were found to have increased risk for transient perinatal symp-toms in newborns. Studies suggest that antidepres-sants are not associated with an increased risk of major malformations, but most studies are limited or small, and none are definitive. Many antidepres-sants have not been adequately studied during preg-nancy, and MAOIs increase the risk of hypertensive crisis. Although some consider the judicious use of benzodiazepines during pregnancy safe, it is con-troversial, and some studies show an association with cleft palate (especially for alprazolam and di-azepam). Newborns may also be at risk for intoxica-tion or withdrawal.

Hales RE, Yudofsky SC. *Textbook of Clinical Psychia-try*. 4th ed. Washington: American Psychiatric Publishing; 2003:1511–1537.

31. Answer: D. Aluminum is the offending agent in *dialysis dementia*, being a contaminant of dialysis fluid or a component of phosphate-binding compounds.

Schofield P. Dementia associated with toxic causes and autoimmune disease. *Int Psychogeriatrics*. 2005;17:S129–S147.

32. Answer: C. The DSM-IV-TR specifies diagnostic cri-teria for caffeine intoxication, including the recent consumption of an amount of caffeine usually in ex-cess of 250 mg. Clinical signs and symptoms associ-ated with caffeine intoxication include restlessness, nervousness, excitement, insomnia, flushing, diure-sis, gastrointestinal disturbance, muscle twitching, rambling flow of thought and speech, tachycardia, periods of inexhaustibility, and psychomotor agita-tion. Consumption of more than 1 g of caffeine is likely to additionally cause confusion, cardiac ar-rhythmias, tinnitus, and visual hallucinations. Con-sumption of more than 10 g of caffeine can cause generalized tonic-clonic seizures, respiratory failure, and death. On the positive side, ingestion of 50 to 100 mg of caffeine can produce increased alertness, a mild sense of well-being, and a sense of improved verbal and motor performance.

1. American Psychiatric Association. *Quick Reference to the Diagnostic Criteria from DSM-IV-TR*. Washington: Amer-ican Psychiatric Association; 2000:105–151.

2. Sadock BJ, Kaplan VA. *Kaplan and Sadock's Synopsis of Psychiatry*. 9th ed. Philadelphia: Lippincott Williams & Wilkins; 2003:419–423.

33. Answer: B. While cocaine use occurs in all socioeco-nomic demographics, the highest prevalence is in males between the ages of 20 to 30 years, who are unemployed, live in urban areas, and have no more than a high school education.

Gorelick D. *Cocaine Abuse in Adults*. http://www.uptodate-online.com/utd/content/topic.do?topicKey=genr_med/15206&type=A&selectedTitle=1~59. Accessed January 22, 2007.

34. Answer: B. The DSM-IV-TR classifies all of the above disorders as learning disorders except Stuttering which is classified as a Communication Disorder.

American Psychiatric Association. *Desk Reference to the Di-agnostic Criteria from DSM-IV-TR*. Washington: American Psychiatric Association; 2000:53–55.

35. Answer: D. Being unmarried, along with social iso-lation, longer duration of psychotic episode, and a history of childhood behavioral problems and prior psychiatric treatment are the five most powerful indi-cators of poor outcome in Schizophrenia, according to the World Health Organization International Pilot Study on Schizophrenia. Other poor prognostic fac-tors in Schizophrenia include younger age at onset, male gender, low socioeconomic status, positive fam-ily history of Schizophrenia, a history of peri-natal complications, poor premorbid functioning, insidi-ous onset, chronic course, clear sensorium, negative symptoms, lack of mood disturbance, neurological soft signs, and structural brain abnormalities. Being married is a relatively protective factor in predict-ing long-term outcome in Schizophrenia. Even with modern treatment, less than one third to one half of patients will have a recovery of any kind.

Hales RE, Yudofsky SC. *Textbook of Clinical Psychiatry*. 4th ed. Washington: American Psychiatric Publishing; 2003: 379–439.

36. Answer: B. Naltrexone is an opiate receptor antago-nist that reduces craving in alcohol dependent pa-tients. Given at a dose of 50 mg/day orally, it is con-traindicated in patients receiving concurrent opioid analgesic (it inhibits and renders opioid analgesics ineffective) and liver impairments. Naltrexone is in-dicated in patients who crave alcohol but are moti-vated to quit drinking. Naltrexone leads to reduced craving or drinking in positive responders in 7 to 10 days, failure to respond in 10 days is suggestive of failed therapy and an indication for discontinuation.

O'Malley SS, Jaffe AJ, Chang G, et al. Naltrexone and coping skills therapy for alcohol dependence. A controlled study. *Arch Gen Psychiatry*. 1992 Nov;49(11):881–887.

37. Answer: C. Buprenorphine is a partial agonist of the mu-opioid receptor. It is different from a full opioid agonist, like methadone and heroin, in that the receptor activation increases as the dose increases until it reaches a plateau. For full opioid agonists, higher doses continues to create greater receptor activation. Because of this partial activation, chronic opioid users are less likely to abuse buprenorphine. It has high affinity for and a slow dissociation from mu-opioid receptors and can block other opioids temporarily. Due to its high affinity, buprenorphine displaces opioids from the mu receptor, causing withdrawal in patients who have used opioids recently. It is absorbed through gastrointestinal and mucosal membranes, but the oral formulation has poor bioavailability due to its extensive metabolism in the gastrointestinal tract. Sublingual buprenorphine has a bioavailability ranging from 30% to 50% of the intravenous dose. Maximal plasma concentration that is reached within 1 hour of oral dosing and it is metabolized primarily in the liver via the cytochrome P450. The majority of buprenorphine and its metabolites are excreted in the feces; less than 30% are eliminated in the urine. Its mean plasma elimination half-life is 37 hours.

1. Donaher PA, Welsh C. Managing opioid addiction with buprenorphine. *Am Fam Physician.* 2006;73:1573–1578.
2. Kuhlman JJ Jr, Lalani S, Magluilo J Jr, et al. Human pharmacokinetics of intravenous, sublingual, and buccal buprenorphine. *J Anal Toxicol.* 1996;20:369–378.
3. Mendelson J, Upton RA, Everhart ET, et al. Bioavailability of sublingual buprenorphine. *J Clin Pharmacol.* 1997;37:31–37.

38. Answer: D. Individuals with Schizoid Personality structure believe that the social world is dangerously engulfing. They are highly sensitive and reactive to interpersonal stimulation, which they tend to respond to with defensive withdrawal. They easily feel in danger of being engulfed, enmeshed, controlled, intruded upon, and traumatized; dangers that they associate with becoming involved with other people. In contrast, individuals with depressive personality structure believe that people who really get to know them will reject them because they believe that there is something essentially bad or incomplete about them. When mistreated, rejected, or abandoned, they tend to believe that they are somehow at fault. This belief may be a residue of the familiar tendency of children in difficult family situations to deny that their caregivers are negligent, abusive, or fragile—ideas that are too frightening. Instead, they attribute their suffering to their own badness—something they can try to change.

1. McWilliams N. *Psychoanalytic Diagnosis: Understanding Personality Structure in the Clinical Process.* New York: Guilford Press; 1994:189–204, 227–256.
2. PDM Task Force. *Psychodynamic Diagnostic Manual.* Silver Spring: Alliance of Psychoanalytic Organizations; 2006:33, 44–46.

39. Answer: D. Available evidence indicates that behavioral treatments produce improvements in sleep architecture, which are most pronounced for sleep latency and time awake after sleep onset. Relaxation and BF were both found to be effective in alleviating insomnia. Cognitive forms of relaxation, such as meditation, were slightly better than somatic forms of relaxation such as PMR. Sleep restriction, stimulus control, and multimodal treatment were the three most effective treatments in reducing insomnia. Improvements seen at treatment completion were maintained at follow-ups averaging 6 months in duration. Although these effects are statistically significant, it is questionable whether the magnitude of the improvements in sleep onset and total sleep time are clinically meaningful. Integration of behavioral and relaxation approaches into the treatment of chronic pain and insomnia can be synergestic.

NIH Technology Assessment Panel on Integration of Behavioral and Relaxation Approaches into the Treatment of Chronic Pain and Insomnia. Integration of behavioral and relaxation approaches into the treatment of chronic pain and insomnia. *JAMA.* 1996;276:313–318.

40. Answer: E. Bupropion is a dopamine and norepinephrine reuptake inhibitor. It is about twice as potent inhibitor of dopamine uptake than norepinephrine uptake. Bupropion is metabolized in the liver. It has at least three active metabolites: hydroxybupropion, threohydrobupropion and erythrohydrobupropion. These active metabolites are further metabolized to inactive metabolites and eliminated through excretion into the urine. The half-life of bupropion and hydroxybupropion is 20 hours. Threohydrobupropion's half-life is 37 hours and erythrohydrobupropion's is 33 hours. The therapeutic benefit of bupropion can be attributed to its active metabolites. It is contraindicated in epilepsy and other conditions that lower the seizure threshold (alcohol withdrawal, active brain tumors, etc.). It should not be use concomitantly with MAOIs. When switching medications, it is important that there be a short period of about 2 weeks between the medications in order to reduce risk of complications that might lead to things such as a decrease in seizure threshold. It should be used with caution in patients with AN and bulimia as they have decreased seizure thresholds. Bupropion is primarily metabolized to hydroxybupropion by the CYP2B6 isoenzyme. Combination of bupropion with nicotine replacement therapies can elevate blood pressure, so it is recommended that the patient's blood pressure is monitored. It is a category B in pregnancy.

Albers LJ, Hahn RK, Reist C. *Handbook of Psychiatric Drugs*. Laguna Hills: Current Clinical Strategies Publishing; 2005:16–17.

41. Answer: E. Psychiatrists are not able to accurately predict future behavior of patients, but are able to assess the risk of future violent behavior. Each of the other answers represents risk factors for an increased probability of future violence. Not listed, a prior history of violent behavior is perhaps the strongest risk factor for future violent behavior. Male gender is another strong risk factor for future violent behavior.

Cohen BJ. *Theory and Practice of Psychiatry*. New York: Oxford University Press; 2003:445–466.

42. Answer: E. Bulbar palsy is caused by cranial nerve injury within the brainstem or along the course of the nerves. Patients usually have a thick, nasal intonation while talking, dysphagia due to impaired palatal and pharyngeal movement, loss of the gag reflex, and, in some cases, a depressed jaw jerk reflex. If the bulbar damage is extensive, the medullary respiratory center might be affected and patients may present with respiratory depression. Taste sensation in the two thirds of the tongue is provided by the facial nerve (CNVII).

Kaufman DM. *Clinical Neurology for Psychiatrists*. 5th ed. Philadelphia: WB Saunders; 2001:35–55.

43. Answer: A. Given that this patient's depressive presentation is recent and sudden, it is likely due to a medical disorder rather than a primary psychiatric disorder. Lesions of the frontal lobe may present with a clinical syndrome indistinguishable from a depressive illness. The frontal lobes play a major role in personality, especially in acquired social behavior, and lesions here often result in a change in personality as an apathetic dementia results. Occipital lobe tumors are associated with hemianopia and unformed visual disturbances. Parietal lesions present with language and speech difficulties if in the dominant hemisphere, or with visuospatial integration problems and neglect syndromes. Temporal lobe lesions are also associated with language disturbance from the dominant hemisphere, olfac-

tory and partial-complex seizures, and visual field deficits.

1. Patten J. *Neurological Differential Diagnosis*. 2nd ed. New York: Springer; 2003:54, 61, 114.
2. Rowland LP. *Merritt's Neurology*. 11th ed. Philadelphia: Lippincott Williams & Wilkins; 2005:295, 374.
3. Sadock BJ, Sadock VA. *Kaplan and Sadock's Comprehensive Textbook of Psychiatry*. 8th ed. Philadelphia: Lippincott Williams & Wilkins; 2005:362, 367.

44. Answer: B. Linkage analysis is one of a number of techniques that molecular geneticists use to map the location of genes that contribute to psychiatric disorders. It depends on the law of independent assortment. Genes are typically inherited independently (because of recombination and segregation), unless they are located close together on a chromosome. When genes are relatively close together, the likelihood of recombination is proportional to the distance between the genes. It is an essentially hypothesis-free approach (i.e., it is not essential to have a candidate gene in mind before beginning). Classical linkage analysis is most useful in mapping traits caused by single genes, and has to be modified for use in polygenic disorders, which include most psychiatric disorders. Identification of a chromosomal abnormality is not necessary; this is important for cytogenetic studies.

1. Lachman HM. An overview of the genetics of substance use disorders. *Curr Psychiatry Rep*. 2006;8:133–143.
2. Stern TA, Herman JB. *Massachusetts General Hospital Psychiatry Update & Board Preparation*. 2nd ed. McGraw-Hill: Medical Publishing Division; 2004:493–494.

45. Answer: D. The severity of TBI is perhaps the most important determinant of outcome. Severity is estimated by one of the following three parameters: length of LOC, duration of PTA, and the Glasgow Coma Scale. The longer the length of LOC, the worse the prognosis of a given TBI, as this represents a more severe TBI. PTA is defined as the time interval between the attainment of full consciousness following TBI and the time at which new memories are formed. Longer periods of PTA portends worse prognosis. The Glasgow Coma Scale is a 15-item scale with scores ranging from 3 to 15. The lower the score the more severe the injury.

Ashman TA, Gordon WA, Cantor JB, et al. Neurobehavioral consequences of traumatic brain injury. *Mt Sinai J Med*. 2006;73:999–1005.

46. Answer: A. Glutamate (an amino acid) is the major excitatory neurotransmitter in the CNS. Glucose and glutamine are converted to, via the enzyme glucan mayonnaise, and to glutamate. It is widely distributed in the CNS, and receptors include N-methyl-D-aspartic acid (NMDA), AMPA, and kainate receptors (each inotropic), and some metabotropic receptors. Excess glutamatergic stimulation may result in seizures or neuronal damage (*kindling*). Decarboxylase of glutamate via glutamic acid decarboxylase (GAD) forms GABA, a major inhibitory neurotransmitter in the brain. Glycine is a major inhibitory neurotransmitter in the spinal cord. Norepinephrine and dopamine function vary depending on involved tracts.

Kaufman DM. *Clinical Neurology for Psychiatrists*. 5th ed. Philadelphia: WB Saunders; 2001:552–569.

47. Answer: B. Huntington's disease is a genetic disorder that is inherited as an autosomal dominant trait, thus each child of a parent who is carrying a defective gene has a 50% risk of inheriting the disease gene. There are several genes that are known to cause PD but they account for a very small minority of cases. Parkinson's mutations are the most common genetic cause of PD (causes young-onset PD) but still account for less than 1% of all cases, and is thought to be inherited in an autosomal recessive pattern. Sydenham's chorea is a neurologic movement disorder that frequently occurs in children or adolescents following acute rheumatic fever, and appears to result from an autoimmune or antibody-mediated inflammatory response involving certain regions of the basal ganglia and is not genetically transmitted. Wilson's disease is a genetic disorder that is inherited as an autosomal recessive trait and causes neurological and psychiatric symptoms and liver disease. Lesch-Nyhan syndrome is inherited as an x-linked recessive trait and involves an enzyme deficiency that results in hyperuricemia, with associated mental retardation, choreoathetosis, and self-destructive biting of the lips and fingers.

1. Rowland LP. *Merritt's Neurology*. 11th ed. Philadelphia: Lippincott Williams & Wilkins; 2005:620, 661, 804, 807–808, 832–833.
2. Worldwide Education and Awareness for Movement Disorders. *We Move Main Website*. http://www.wemove.org/. Published February 23, 2007.

48. Answer: B. This patient presents with signs consistent with Brown-Sequard syndrome, which refers to hemisection of the spinal cord. The following signs are found in this syndrome: ipsilateral paresis, ipsilateral corticospinal signs (hyperactive DTRs and Babinski), contralateral loss of pain and temperature sensation (from injury of the spinothalamic tract), and ipsilateral impairment of vibration and joint-position sense (from posterior column

injury). The loss of pain sensation contralateral to the paresis is the readily identifiable hallmark of this syndrome. Complete transection of the cord results in permanent bilateral motor, sensory, and autonomic paralysis below the level of the lesion. The central-cord syndrome is characterized by weakness that is more marked in the arms than the legs, with urinary retention and sensory loss below the level of the lesion. The arms or hands may be paralyzed or moderately weak. In the legs there may be severe paresis or only minimal weakness, overactive tendon reflexes, and Babinski signs. Micturition may be normal. While complete-cord transection may be diagnosed at first because there seems to be no cord function below the level of the lesion, careful testing may reveal sacral sparing, showing an incomplete lesion. In the anterior-cord syndrome, immediate complete paralysis is associated with mild-to-moderate impairment of pinprick response and light touch below the injury, with preservation of position and vibration sense (from dorsal columns). This syndrome may be caused by an acutely ruptured disc, fracture, or dislocation in the cervical region impinging on the anterior spinal artery and compromising blood flow to the anterior cervical spine. The posterior-cord syndrome is characterized by pain and paresthesia in the neck, upper arms, and trunk, which is usually symmetric and has a burning quality. The sensory manifestations may be combined with mild paresis of the arms and hands, but the long tracts are only slightly affected.

Rowland LP. *Merritt's Neurology*. 11th ed. Philadelphia: Lippincott Williams & Wilkins; 2005:505.

49. Answer: A. Diabetic polyneuropathy is the most common type of neuropathy in the Western world affecting up to half of all diabetic patients. Longer the duration of diabetes, greater is the chance of the patient developing neuropathy. Diabetic neuropathy can be classified into various distinct clinical syndromes which are characterized by a characteristic set of signs and symptoms. The common types of diabetic neuropathies are distal symmetric polyneuropathy, autonomic neuropathy, mononeuropathy mainly affecting the oculomotor and median nerves, thoracic and lumbar polyradiculopathies, and mononeuritis multiplex.

Feldman EL. *Classification of Diabetic Neuropathy*. http://www.uptodateonline.com/utd/content/topic.do?topicKey=neuropat/5373&type=A&selectedTitle=1~37. Accessed February 28, 2007.

50. Answer: D. Huntington's disease is a rare autosomal dominate neurodegenerative disease. There are no available disease-modifying treatments, only treatments to manage symptoms associated with the disease. Huntington's chorea is characterized by involuntary muscle movements usually of the limbs that can be somewhat reduced by the D2 blockade action of haloperidol. Pramipexole, ropinirole, and L-dopa all act to increase dopamine transmission and would likely worsen Huntington's chorea. Benztropine would likely have no effect on Huntington's chorea.

1. Kaufman DM. *Clinical Neurology for Psychiatrists*. 5th ed. Philadelphia: WB Saunders; 2001:461.
2. Rowland LP. *Merritt's Neurology*. 11th ed. Philadelphia: Lippincott Williams & Wilkins; 2005:806.

51. Answer: C. DBS of the STN is an effective therapeutic modality for well selected patients with medically intractable symptoms of PD. GPi DBS, although a safe treatment, is yet to be studied on its strength of effect to treat patients with PD. DBS is nondestructive and may be a bilateral procedure of low neurologic morbidity. It can be modified over time to deal with changing or progressing patient symptoms, but it is not helpful for axial symptoms (i.e., such as postural instability or speech problems) and it does not slow the progression of the underlying neurodegenerative disease. It is also expensive and can introduce infection into the brain. It may also have mechanical breakdowns and need reprogramming.

1. Horstink M, Tolosa E, Bonuccelli U, et al. Review of the therapeutic management of Parkinson's disease. Report of a joint task force of the European Federation of Neurological Societies (EFNS) and the Movement Disorder Society-European Section (MDS-ES). Part II: late (complicated) Parkinson's disease. *Eur J Neurol.* 2006;13:1186–1202.
2. Tarsy D. Kleiner-Fisman G. *Surgical Treatment of Parkinson's Disease*. http://www.uptodateonline.com/utd/content/topic.do?topicKey=move_dis/5608&type=A&selectedTitle=8~34. Accessed March 2, 2007.

52. Answer: E. Many drugs prescribed by neurologists and psychiatrists have significant drug–drug interactions of which clinicians must be aware. Common inducers of hepatic drug metabolism include phenytoin, phenobarbital, carbamazepine, primidone, and rifampin. Of the list above, only divalproex sodium (Depakote) is an *inhibitor* of drug metabolism. Other inhibitors of drug metabolism that psychiatrists in particular should be aware of include SSRIs (except citalopram and escitalopram), TCA, bupropion, methylphenidate, and disulfiram.

Stern TA, Herman JB. *Massachusetts General Hospital Psychiatry Update and Board Preparation*. 2nd ed. New York: McGraw Hill; 2002:377.

53. Answer: C. Erik Erikson described generativity as a process by which adults contribute to the next generation through guidance, care, productivity, creativity, and raising children.

Sadock BJ, Sadock VA. *Kaplan and Sadock's Synopsis of Psychiatry*. 9th ed. Philadelphia: Lippincott Williams & Wilkins; 2003:46, 214.

54. Answer: E. Neurofibrillary tangles are fibrillary intracellular deposits found in dendrites of neurons, especially pyramidal neurons. These pathological lesions are not unique to Alzheimer's disease, and have also been found in normal aging, some frontotemporal dementia subtypes, dementia pugilistica, and subacute sclerosing panencephalitis. Neurofibrillary tangles are not commonly associated with Huntington's disease.

Mott RT, Hulette CM. Neuropathology of Alzheimer's disease. *Neuroimaging Clin N Am*. 2005;15:755–765.

55. Answer: A. A psychiatrist cannot avoid some manner of self-disclosure, even if it is just their office decoration and style of dress. Most agree that some form of self-disclosure is not only unavoidable, but also often useful, but there are no generally accepted technical guidelines. Generally, if the therapist's feelings are obvious to the patient, such as if the therapist has become angry, it is disingenuous not to disclose. One should still disclose with caution, and it is generally a good idea to discuss process. While some have argued for select disclosure of countertransference love, most argue for extreme caution, as such feelings can be deeply disturbing to the patient, even without actualization in action.

Gabbard GO, ed. *Countertransference Issues in Psychiatric Treatment. Review of Psychiatry Series*. Vol. 18. Washington: American Psychiatric Press, 1999:14–17.

56. Answer: C. Although published clinical practice guidelines may be considered in malpractice cases, they are not comprehensive or without fault, and should never supersede professional judgment. It is not required that the physician deviated from guidelines for malpractice. Any carefully crafted guideline will have an opening disclaimer that it does not represent the standard of care. The four requirements for malpractice are summed up in the remaining answers. They may also be described in the four D's of malpractice: duty, deviation, damages, and direct causation.

Hales RE, Yudofsky SC. *Textbook of Clinical Psychiatry*. 4th ed. Washington: American Psychiatric Publishing; 2003:1585–1628.

57. Answer: A. This patient has Huntington's disease. It is inherited as an autosomal dominant allele on chromosome 4. Patients develop dementia and chorea, with deficient GABA activity. Huntington's disease is also an excessive trinucleotide repeat disorder. Radiological findings in these patients include the atrophy of caudate nuclei and the presence of *bat wing* lateral ventricles. Other excessive trinucleotide repeat disorders include myotonic dystrophy, Fragile-X syndrome, Friedrich's ataxia, and the spinocerebellar degenerations.

1. Kaufman DM. *Clinical Neurology for Psychiatrists*. 5th ed. Philadelphia: WB Saunders; 2001:459–461, 542.
2. Montoya A, Price BH, Menear M, et al. Brain imaging and cognitive dysfunctions in Huntington's disease. *J Psychiatry Neurosci*. 2006;31:21–29.
3. Rosenblatt A, Leroi I. Neuropsychiatry of Huntington's disease and other basal ganglia disorders. *Psychosomatics*. 2000;41:24–30.

58. Answer: D. Nicotine dependence amongst patients with schizophrenia is extremely common and has been found to range from 75% to 90%. Nicotine is by far the most common substance of dependence for patients with Schizophrenia. Comorbidity of Schizophrenia and other substance use disorders is also common. Thirty to fifty percent of patients with Schizophrenia have been found to meet the diagnostic criteria for Alcohol Abuse/Dependence. Other commonly used substances are cannabis (approximately 15% to 25%) and cocaine (approximately 5% to 10%).

Sadock BJ, Sadock VA. *Kaplan and Sadock's Synopsis of Psychiatry*. 9th ed. Philadelphia: Lippincott Williams & Wilkins; 2003:444, 476.

59. Answer: D. Unlike opiates and sedatives, cocaine withdrawal includes mainly psychological symptoms and is not usually medically serious. Depressed mood, problems concentrating, increased dreaming (due to increased rapid eye movement [REM] sleep), anhedonia, fatigue, and cocaine craving are often experienced. Occasionally, an initial period of severe symptoms occurs, during which the patient may become severely depressed and suicidal. However, typically symptoms are milder, and resolve within 2 weeks.

Gorelick D. *Cocaine Abuse in Adults*. http://www.uptodateonline.com/utd/content/topic.do?topicKey=genr_med/15206&type=A&selectedTitle=1~59. Published January 22, 2007.

60. Answer: D. The treatment of choice for Reading Disorder is first an accurate assessment of the child's specific deficits and weakness and matching them appropriately to an educational approach. A spe-

cific method developed by Samuel Orton suggests therapeutic attention to the mastery of simple phonetic units, followed by the blending of these units to words and sentences. An approach that systematically engages several senses is recommended. Children should be placed in a grade as close as possible to their social functional level and should receive special remedial work in reading. Coexisting emotional and behavioral problems should be treated by appropriate psychotherapeutic means. Parent counseling may also be helpful.

Kaplan HI, Sadock BJ. *Kaplan & Sadock's Synopsis of Psychiatry Behavioral Sciences/Clinical Psychiatry*. 8th ed. Philadelphia: Lippincott Williams & Wilkins; 1998:1159.

61. Answer: A. Although the sex ratio for rates of Schizophrenia is still debated, it does seem that men generally develop Schizophrenia at an earlier age than women. Despite some pockets of high and low rates of Schizophrenia, with clearly defined criteria the incidence and prevalence is relatively consistent worldwide. The association with lower socioeconomic class is thought to be explained by the *downward drift* hypothesis. Even with improved treatments, persons with Schizophrenia do suffer higher mortality rates, largely due to suicide and accidents, but also from poorer general medical health. Rates of attempted and completed suicide remain high in Schizophrenia.

Hales RE, Yudofsky SC. *Textbook of Clinical Psychiatry*. 4th ed. Washington: American Psychiatric Publishing; 2003:379–439.

62. Answer: E. Prochaska and DiClemente have provided a model for change in addictive behaviors. According to this paradigm, patients move through several distinct stages beginning with problematic drinking and ending with stable sobriety. Movement through these stages may be progressive but not necessarily chronologic. It is important for clinicians to recognize the specific stage a given patient has attained to be able to deploy the most effective motivational change strategy. In the *precontemplation stage*, patients are in denial of their drinking difficulties and have no desire to engage in meaningful lifestyle changes to address their drinking problem. Patients in contemplation stage are no longer in denial but evidence profound ambivalence towards the habit: they acknowledge all the ill effects of excessive alcohol consumption but are unable to take specific remedial actions. Patients who have made a decision to quit drinking and indeed able to make gestures (initiate small changes) are said to be in the *preparation stage*, whereas patients who go beyond making symbolic gestures and actually initiate specific changes, including accepting pharmacologic or psychological interventions are in the *action stage*. In the *maintenance stage*, new behavior pattern is applied consistently and consolidated. Because maintenance of sobriety is fraught with several remissions and relapses, the authors recognize that positive changes that have necessitated sobriety may be abandoned (i.e., the *relapse stage*).

Prochaska J, DiClemente C, Norcross J. In search of how people change. Applications to addictive behaviors. *Am Psychol*. 1992;47:1102–1114.

63. **Answer: B.** Studies comparing buprenorphine to methadone maintenance therapy for opioid dependence have shown that buprenorphine (less than 40 mg) is as effective as low-dose methadone (less than 40 mg). However, high-dose methadone (greater than 60 mg) may be more effective than buprenorphine. Hence, patients requiring higher methadone doses may not be good candidates for buprenorphine. A Cochrane meta-analysis reviewed the use of buprenorphine as maintenance treatment. This review demonstrated the superior efficacy of buprenorphine maintenance treatment when compared with placebo, as well as treatment retention and heroin suppression efficacy comparable with that of low-dose methadone maintenance. However, high-dose methadone demonstrated superior heroin suppression efficacy compared with buprenorphine. Advantages of buprenorphine over methadone include higher doses having lower risk of toxicity, potential effectiveness at less than recommended daily dosage, less severe withdrawal symptoms after discontinuation, less abuse potential, and more accessible for office-based treatment programs. Advantages of methadone maintenance over buprenorphine maintenance therapy include lower cost of treatment, more effective in patients with higher tolerances, and higher treatment retention rates.

1. Donaher PA, Welsh C. Managing opioid addiction with buprenorphine. *Am Fam Physician*. 2006;73:1573–1578.
2. Mattick RP, Kimber J, Breen C, et al. Buprenorphine maintenance versus placebo or methadone maintenance for opioid dependence. *Cochrane Database Syst Rev*. 2003;2:CD002207, DOI10, 1002/14651858, CD002207.
3. Sung S, Conry JM. Role of buprenorphine in the management of heroin addiction. *Ann Pharmacother*. 2006;40:501–505.

64. **Answer: A.** Masochistic patients tend to reenact with a therapist the drama of the child who needs care but can only get it if they are demonstrably suffering and helpless. The therapist may be seen as a parent who must be persuaded to save and comfort the patient,

who is too weak, threatened, and unprotected. The patient's subjective task is thus to persuade the therapist that they both need and deserve to be rescued. Coexisting with these aims is the fear that the therapist is an uncaring, critical, selfish, and abusive authority. They fear that the therapist will expose their worthlessness, blame the victim for being victimized, and abandon the relationship. To combat such fears, they try to make obvious both their helplessness and their efforts to be good. On the other hand, manic patients tend to be winsome, insightful, and fascinating. They also tend to be confusing and exhausting. Depressive patients attach quickly to the therapist, ascribe benevolence to their aims, work hard to be "good" in the patient role, and appreciate bits of insight as if they were morsels of life-sustaining food. They tend to idealize the clinician as morally good, in contrast to their subjective badness. Depressive patients try hard not to be burdensome. At the same time, they project onto the therapist their internal critics or harsh superego. Depressive patients are subject to the chronic belief that the therapist's concern and respect would vanish if they really knew the patient.

1. McWilliams N. *Psychoanalytic Diagnosis: Understanding Personality Structure in the Clinical Process*. New York: Guilford Press; 1994:239–241, 251, 268–271.
2. PDM Task Force. *Psychodynamic Diagnostic Manual*. Silver Spring: Alliance of Psychoanalytic Organizations; 2006:40–44, 44–46.

65. **Answer: A.** Varenicline acts as a partial agonist selective for the alfa$_4$ beta$_2$ nicotinic acetylcholine receptor subtype. Maximal plasma concentrations are reached within 3 to 4 hours and it reaches a steady-state concentration within 4 days. It has a half-life of 24 hours and its oral bioavailability is not affected by food or time of administration. It has linear pharmacokinetics and low plasma protein binding ($\leq$20%) regardless of a patient's age and renal function. Pharmacokinetic studies in the elderly have demonstrated activity similar to that observed in young adults. Dosage adjustments are not required in patients with hepatic insufficiency. It has no clinically significant drug–drug interactions. In vitro studies do not demonstrate a cytochrome P450 enzyme effect. The safety of coadministration of nicotine replacement products with varenicline has not been established. No significant differences in dosing have been established with regards to age, race, gender, tobacco use, or concurrent use of other drugs. Clinical trials indicate that varenicline was superior to sustained-release bupropion and placebo in two trials with regards to the incidence of abstinence,

adverse event rate, and tolerability. Varenicline has also been shown to increase long-term abstinence from cigarette smoking compared with placebo. Nausea was the most common adverse event associated with varenicline use. A dose reduction should be considered in patients with intolerable nausea. Varenicline has been designated as a pregnancy category C drug. Since there are no studies that have been conducted to investigate whether varenicline is excreted in human milk, it should be avoided in lactating women. Teratogenicity with varenicline is unknown.

Zierler-Brown SL, Kyle JA. Oral varenicline for smoking cessation. *Ann Pharmacother*. 2007;41:95–99.

66. Answer: E. During intoxication, patients will typically have dilated pupils and, at high doses, are at increased risk of developing autonomic instability and hyperthermia, strokes, and seizures. Patients experiencing cocaine toxicity, especially chronic users, may experience paranoia as this patient has done. If patients continue to exhibit paranoia after 12 hours, one should consider hospitalization and, if not, ensure that the patient is discharged to the care of someone reliable.

Bernstein C, Ishak WW, Weinder E, et al. *On Call Psychiatry*. 2nd ed. Philadelphia: WB Saunders; 2001:128–129.

67. Answer: D. Psychiatric diagnoses fall into the category of static risk factors. According to ECA data, the base rate of violent behavior amongst those without a psychiatric diagnosis is 2%. Amongst those with a DSM-III psychiatric diagnosis of OCD, Panic Disorder, Major Depression, Bipolar Disorder, or Schizophrenia, the base rate is about 12%. The base rate of violence jumps dramatically for any substance related disorder (with cannabis-related disorders at 19%, alcohol-related disorders at 25%, and other drug-related disorders at 35%). Do not be fooled that marijuana is calming and reduces rates of violence. Substance-related disorders react synergistically with other diagnoses to increase violence rates even further. Substance abuse of any kind is the most significant axis I risk factor for violent behavior. Chronic abuse and intoxication are the most important. Half to two thirds of violent offenders were drinking just before committing the violent act, and an additional 20% to 25% similarly used other drugs.

Cohen BJ. *Theory and Practice of Psychiatry*. New York: Oxford University Press; 2003:445–466.

68. Answer: D. The hypoglossal nerve (CN XII) innervates the tongue muscles. If one of the nerves is damaged it becomes weak and the tongue then deviates toward the weakened side, pointing towards the side of the lesion. The glossopharyngeal nerve (CN IX) provides taste sensation to the posterior third of the tongue, but it is not involved in tongue muscle movements. The vagus nerve (CN X) is not involved in tongue muscle movements.

Kaufman DM. *Clinical Neurology for Psychiatrists*. 5th ed. Philadelphia: WB Saunders; 2001:35–55.

69. Answer: B. This presentation is classic for a right parietal syndrome that includes neglect of the contralateral side of the world, and anosognosia (denial of illness). Left parietal lesions may present largely with language and speech difficulties, in addition to ideomotor apraxia, in which the patient may not perform learned motor acts on command but may describe the act. Temporal lobe lesions are also associated with language disturbance from the dominant hemisphere, olfactory and partial-complex seizures, and visual field deficits. Pontine lesions would be manifested by cranial nerve signs and multiple motor and sensory deficiencies.

Rowland LP. *Merritt's Neurology*. 11th ed. Philadelphia: Lippincott Williams & Wilkins; 2005:295, 297, 301.

70. Answer: A. Cerebellar degeneration is associated with the abuse of alcohol. It is characterized by unsteadiness of gait, problems with standing, and mild nystagmus. It is caused by the effects of alcohol and acetaldehyde, along with vitamin deficiencies. Treatment consists of complete abstinence and vitamin supplementation. Complete recovery is not common.

Sadock BJ, Sadock VA. *Kaplan and Sadock's Comprehensive Textbook of Psychiatry*. 7th ed. Philadelphia: Lippincott Williams & Wilkins; 2000:955.

71. Answer: E. The brain and spinal cord float in CSF, which provides buoyancy. They essentially weigh less than supporting structures while suspended in CSF, as it is 80% water. There is no CNS lymphatic system, so the CSF performs this function, and helps eliminate carbon dioxide, lactate, and hydrogen ions from the CNS. The CSF and the brain's intercellular fluid are chemically maintained within narrow limits to provide a stable environment for all the cells of the CNS. Despite being maintained within these limits, to date there is no reason to believe that CSF is active in brain and spinal cord metabolism.

Ropper AH, Brown RH. *Adams and Victor's Principles of Neurology*. 8th ed. New York: McGraw-Hill; 2005:529–545.

72. Answer: B. GABA is the major inhibitory neurotransmitter in the brain. It is formed from glutamate via the enzyme GAD. GABA$_A$ receptors have five types of subunits that form a chloride channel. Benzodiazepines bind to the alpha subunit of the GABA$_A$ receptors, and require GABA to bind to the beta subunit for their action to keep the chloride channel open. Barbiturates and ethanol bind to the chloride channel and increase its open time, but neither requires the presence of GABA. GABA$_B$ receptors act via potassium and calcium channels to prolonged inhibition of neurons. GABA is deactivated by sodium-dependent GABA uptake transporters, which remove GABA from the synapse. Gabapentin affects this step. Glycine is an inhibitory neurotransmitter predominant in the spinal cord. Glutamate is an excitatory neurotransmitter. Serotonin and acetylcholine function vary depending on which tracts and receptors are involved.

Kaufman DM. *Clinical Neurology for Psychiatrists*. 5th ed. Philadelphia: WB Saunders; 2001:552–569.

73. **Answer: E.** Tics may be simple jerks or complex sequences of coordinated movements that appear suddenly and intermittently. When simple, the movements resemble a myoclonic jerk. Complex tics often include head-shaking, eye-blinking, sniffing, shoulder-shrugging, facial distortions, arm-waving, touching parts of the body, jumping movements, making obscene gestures (copropraxia), or mimicking movements (echopraxia). In addition to motor tics, vocalizations may be a manifestation of tics. These vocalizations range from sounds (such as barking, throat-clearing, or squealing) to verbalizations, which can include the utterance of obscenities (coprolalia) and the repetitions of one's own sounds (palilalia) or the sounds of others (echolalia).

1. Kaufman DM. *Clinical Neurology for Psychiatrists*. 5th ed. Philadelphia: WB Saunders; 2001:476.
2. Rowland LP. *Merritt's Neurology*. 11th ed. Philadelphia: Lippincott Williams & Wilkins; 2005:49.

74. **Answer: A.** The most common cause of predominantly autonomic neuropathy in the United States is diabetes mellitus. Amyloidosis, thallium poisoning, porphyria, and GBS are other causes of autonomic neuropathy.

Rowland LP. *Merritt's Neurology*. 11th ed. Philadelphia: Lippincott Williams & Wilkins; 2005:735–736.

75. **Answer: B.** While smaller clinical trials have reported on the efficacy of TCA, gabapentin, capsaicin cream, mexiletine, and opiates for the treatment of painful diabetic polyneuropathy, none of these drugs are formally approved by the FDA for the treatment of this condition. Only duloxetine and pregabalin are approved by the FDA for the treatment of painful diabetic polyneuropathy. Both drugs appear to have equal efficacy in treating this condition.

Feldman EL, McCulloch DK. *Treatment of Diabetic Neuropathy*. http://www.uptodateonline.com/utd/content/topic. do?topicKey=neuropat/6605&type=A&selectedTitle= 9~37. Accessed November 18, 2007.

76. **Answer: A.** A head injury resulting in LOC followed by a lucid interval of a few hours and then rapidly progressing to a coma is most consistent with an epidural hemorrhage.

1. Kaufman DM. *Clinical Neurology for Psychiatrists*. 5th ed. Philadelphia: WB Saunders; 2001:582.
2. Rowland LP. *Merritt's Neurology*. 11th ed. Philadelphia: Lippincott Williams & Wilkins; 2005:483–489.

77. **Answer: C.** The brain of patients with Down syndrome is small with fewer secondary sulci than normal. The superior temporal lobes are usually hypoplastic with prominent sylvian fissure. There is also a reduction in neuronal density in many cortical areas. The pyramidal cells show reduced numbers of apical dendrites and synapses. There is also deposition of calcium in the hippocampus, basal ganglia, and cerebellum. The cerebellum is small with a higher number of undifferentiated fetal cells. There is degeneration of the cells in the nucleus basalis of Meynert with decreased choline acetyltransferase and pigmentary degeneration of neurons, along with accumulation of senile plaques and neurofibrillary tangles.

Rowland LP. *Merritt's Neurology*. 11th ed. Philadelphia: Lippincott Williams & Wilkins; 2005:608.

78. **Answer: B.** Because lamotrigine is metabolized by the liver, its clearance is potentially affected by medications which inhibit or induce hepatic drug metabolism. As an inhibitor of hepatic enzymes, divalproex sodium (Depakote) can dramatically increase lamotrigine blood levels. This is of significance due to the increased risk of rash and Stevens-Johnson syndrome with lamotrigine. When lamotrigine is initiated in a patient taking Depakote, the dose must be reduced and the titration slowed. On the other hand, carbamazepine is an inducer of hepatic enzymes, thereby decreasing lamotrigine blood levels. When lamotrigine is given to a patient taking carbamazepine, the dose of lamotrigine should generally be increased. Lithium is excreted by the kidney, not metabolized by the liver, and should not have a significant drug–drug interaction with lamotrigine. Neither fluoxetine (an inhibitor of the 2D6 isoenzyme of the cytochrome P450 enzymes) nor olanzapine (a substrate of the 1A2 isoenzyme) require

lamotrigine dose adjustment when the two medications are co-administered.

Stern TA, Herman JB. *Massachusetts General Hospital Psychiatry Update and Board Preparation*. 2nd ed. New York: McGraw Hill; 2002:378–380.

79. Answer: C. The lifetime prevalence of schizophrenia is estimated to be 1%.

Sadock BJ, Sadock VA. *Kaplan and Sadock's Synopsis of Psychiatry*. 9th ed. Philadelphia: Lippincott Williams & Wilkins; 2003:472.

80. Answer: B. The medial temporal lobe contains the amygdala, the hippocampal region, and the parahippocampal gyrus. The neurons of the hippocampal region are arranged in one cellular layer, the pyramidal layer. Most hippocampal pyramidal neurons are glutamatergic, and this region contains the serial circuitry for long-term potentiation through the NMDA receptor. Connections with the limbic system are important for the regulation of emotion, and connections with the frontal lobes are important for declarative memory.

Stern TA, Herman JB. *Massachusetts General Hospital Psychiatry Update & Board Preparation*. 2nd ed. New York: McGraw-Hill; 2004:267.

81. Answer: C. Beginning in childhood, people generate beliefs about themselves and the world. The most fundamental of these are the *core beliefs*. These are regarded as absolute truths, rigid, and are global, rigid, and overgeneralized. However, negative core beliefs are sometimes only activated in a depressed state. Two broad kinds of core beliefs are recognized, which can be categorized as "I'm helpless" or "I'm unlovable." These beliefs rarely stand up to a rational analysis when the patient is depressed. They are based on childhood experiences, and it is sometimes necessary to explore these origins in therapy. It is the goal of CBT to modify the core beliefs.

Beck J. *Cognitive Therapy: Basics and Beyond*. New York: Guilford Press; 1995:15–16, 166–168.

82. Answer: E. Laws for involuntary commitment vary by state. Typically no single criterion is sufficient for involuntary hospitalization. Requirements may have the basic components that the patient be mentally ill (which may be narrowly or broadly defined) and a danger to self (possibly unable to care for self) or others. Multiple caveats and variations exist, especially for special populations (mentally retarded, disabled, substance addicts, minors, etc.). Familiarize yourself with the specifics of the laws in the state in which you practice. Remember that, as a physician, you do not commit patients, a court or judge does. You should merely initiate proceedings in a good faith manner, and respect the rule and responsibility of the court.

Hales RE, Yudofsky SC. *Textbook of Clinical Psychiatry*. 4th ed. Washington: American Psychiatric Publishing; 2003:1585–1628.

83. Answer: D. The steady-state blood levels of the TCA are frequently not achieved until about 5 days after either initiating or changing the medication dose. The plasma-level measurements of imipramine, desipramine, and nortriptyline are useful in certain situations, which include all of the following: patients who have questionable compliance, patients with a poor response to a "typical" antidepressant dose, patients who experience side effects at a very low dose, patients who are potentially very sensitive to side effects, and patients for whom treatment is urgent and who require potentially therapeutic blood levels in as short a period as possible. These levels are generally obtained about 9 to 12 hours after the last dose (usually in the morning after a nighttime dose).

Hales RE, Yudofsky SC. *American Psychiatric Publishing Textbook of Clinical Psychiatry*. 4th ed. http://www.psychiatryonline.com/content.aspx?aID=69719. Accessed February 15, 2007.

84. Answer: B. The Disorganized Type is a type of Schizophrenia in which disorganized speech, disorganized behavior, and flat or inappropriate affects are all prominent. Furthermore, patients must not meet criteria for Catatonic Type. The disorganized type of Schizophrenia was formerly called *hebephrenic* and is characterized by primitive, disinhibited, and unorganized behavior. The onset of this subtype is generally early (usually before the age of 25). These patients show poor contact with reality and their personal appearance is often dilapidated. The Paranoid type of Schizophrenia is characterized by preoccupation with one or more delusions or frequent auditory hallucinations. The classic feature of Catatonic Schizophrenia is a marked disturbance in motor function and may involve immobility, excessive motor activity, extreme negativism, posturing, and/or echolalia/echopraxia. Patients who meet criteria for Schizophrenia, but not one of these three subtypes, are classified with Undifferentiated Type. The Residual Type of Schizophrenia is characterized by continuing evidence of the Schizophrenic disturbance in the absence of a complete set of active symptoms.

1. American Psychiatric Association. *Quick Reference to the Diagnostic Criteria from DSM-IV-TR*. Washington: American Psychiatric Association; 2000:153–165.

2. Sadock BJ, Sadock VA. *Kaplan and Sadock's Synopsis of Psychiatry*. 9th ed. Philadelphia: Lippincott Williams & Wilkins; 2003:485–488.

85. Answer: B. The San Francisco's Haight-Ashbury Free Clinic has developed the Acceptance, Reassurance, Talkdown (ART) approach to interact with acutely intoxicated patients. It involves acceptance of the patient's immediate needs, reassurance that the condition is due to intoxication and will resolve within a few hours, and talk down to provide reality orientation. Neuroleptics and restraints may be required, but should not be part of the initial treatment strategy.

Gorelick D. *Cocaine Abuse in Adults*. http://www.uptodateonline.com/utd/content/topic.do?topicKey=genr_med/15206&type=A&selectedTitle=1~59. Accessed January 22, 2007.

86. Answer: C. All of the answers, except a child's difficulty with rhyming game, are significant risk factors for developing reading disability. For those children who cannot read by the middle to end of their first-grade year, a thorough evaluation for the source of their reading difficulties is warranted. Children receiving intervention (e.g., speech and language therapy, Head Start programs) for identified risk factors remain at a higher risk of reading difficulties than other children.

Hamilton SS, Glascoe, FP. Evaluation of children with reading difficulties. *Am Fam Physician*. 2006;74:2079–2084.

87. Answer: E. Family, twin, and adoption studies have consistently provided ample evidence to confirm there is a biological component to Schizophrenia. The more family members with Schizophrenia, who are closely related genetically to an individual, the greater that individual's risk of developing Schizophrenia in their lifetime. However, even the numbers for monozygotic twins only approach 50%, not 100%. Therefore, studies also suggest that environmental factors also play a significant role in the development of the disorder.

Hales RE, Yudofsky SC. *Textbook of Clinical Psychiatry*. 4th ed. Washington: American Psychiatric Publishing; 2003:379–439.

88. Answer: C. To the plurality of patients with alcohol related disorders, AA is a major resource in their attempt to navigate the rehabilitation progress and in maintaining sobriety. Founded in 1933 by a surgeon and a stockbroker, it relies on group support, the assignment of a sponsor (an individual who has maintained sobriety for a prolonged period), emphasizes the here and now (one day at a time), and stresses reliance on a higher power and spirituality. Providers

of substance dependence rehabilitation have found AA very useful for several reasons including efficacy, accessibility, and reliability (it provides round the clock support to members). However AA is not universally effective. Nonreligious patients may find the premise of reliance on a "higher power" overbearing. In addition, patients with severe psychopathology may find the self group dynamic threatening and uncomfortable.

1. Chappel JN, DuPont RL. Twelve-step and mutual-help programs for addictive disorders. *Psychiatr Clin North Am*. 1999;22:425–446.
2. Ferri M, Amato L, Davoli M. Alcoholics Anonymous and other 12-step programmes for alcohol dependence. *Cochrane Database Syst Rev*. 2006;3:CD005032.

89. Answer: D. Over the last 2 decades, early psychological *debriefing* has been increasingly used to treat psychological trauma. Although these interventions have become popular and their use spread over several settings, their efficacy had largely not been tested empirically. A Cochrane review of the effectiveness of brief psychological debriefing for the management of psychological distress after trauma and the prevention of PTSD showed that most of the studies were generally of poor quality. It also showed that single session individual debriefing did not reduce psychological distress nor prevent the onset of PTSD. Those who received the intervention showed no significant short-term (3 to 5 months) increased risk of PTSD (odds ratio [OR]: 1.22; 95% confidence interval [CI]: 0.60 to 2.46). At 1 year, one trial reported that there was a significantly increased risk of PTSD in those receiving debriefing (OR: 2.88, 95% CI: 1.11 to 7.53). There was also no evidence that debriefing reduced general psychological morbidity, depression, or anxiety. The reviewers concluded that there is no current evidence that psychological debriefing is a useful treatment for the prevention of PTSD after traumatic incidents. Compulsory debriefing of victims of trauma should cease.

Rose S, Bisson J, Churchill R, et al. Psychological debriefing for preventing post traumatic stress disorder. *Cochrane Database Syst Rev*. 2002;2:CD000560.

90. Answer: D. Masochistic patients reenact with a therapist the drama of the child who needs care, but can only get it if they are demonstrably suffering. The most frequent pattern of practitioner response is first to be excessively (and masochistically) generous, and attempting to persuade the patient that one appreciates their suffering and can be trusted not to attack. When this approach only seems to make the patient more helpless and wretched, the therapist notices ego-alien feelings of irritation and fantasies of sadistic retaliation toward the "help-rejecting complainer."

Countertransference with depressive individuals runs the gamut from benign affection to omnipotent rescue fantasies. The therapeutic fantasy is that one can be God or the Good Mother, or be the sensitive, accepting parent that the patient never had. These longings can be understood as a response to the patient's unconscious belief that the cure for depressive dynamics is unconditional love and total understanding (dangerously incomplete approach). In therapists working with manic personality structured people, the most dangerous countertransference tendency is underestimation of the degree of suffering and potential disorganization that lie beneath their engaging presentation. What may appear to be a congenial observing ego and a reliable working alliance may be the operation of manic denial and defensive charm.

1. McWilliams N. *Psychoanalytic Diagnosis: Understanding Personality Structure in the Clinical Process*. New York: Guilford Press; 1994:239–241, 251, 268–271.
2. PDM Task Force. *Psychodynamic Diagnostic Manual*. Silver Spring: Alliance of Psychoanalytic Organizations; 2006:40–44, 44–46.

91. Answer: D. TSD for one whole night improves depressive symptoms in 40% to 60% of treatments. The degree of clinical change spans a continuum from complete remission to worsening (in 2% to 7%). Side effects of sleep deprivation are sleepiness and (hypo-) mania. Response to sleep deprivation shows up in the night of deprivation or the following day. About 10% to 15% of patients respond after recovery sleep. After recovery sleep, 50% to 80% of day-1 responders suffer a complete or partial relapse, but improvement may last for weeks. Sleep leads to relapse, although this is not necessarily the case. Treatment effects may be stabilized by antidepressant drugs, lithium, shifting of sleep time, or light therapy. The best predictor of a therapeutic effect is a large variability of mood. The present opinion is that partial sleep deprivation (PSD) in the second half of the night is equally effective as TSD. Early PSD (i.e., sleeping between 3:00 AM and 6:00 AM) has the same effect as late PSD given equal sleep duration. Newer data available has cast doubt on the time-honoured conviction that REM sleep deprivation is more effective than non-REM sleep deprivation. Both may work by reducing total sleep time. Sleep deprivation still remains an unspecific therapy with the main indication for the depressive syndrome. However, some studies show positive effects in PD also. The mechanism of action for sleep deprivation is still unknown.

Giedke H, Schwarzler F. Therapeutic use of sleep deprivation in depression. *Sleep Med Rev*. 2002;6:361–377.

92. Answer: D. Educational topics for menopausal women with sexual dysfunction include basic information on the genital anatomy and physiology following sexual stimulation, especially clitoral and vaginal engorgement, lubrication, and increases in vaginal vault width and length. The role of hormones in maintaining genital structure and genital function should also be discussed. Education provided to the menopausal woman and her partner is an essential component in the overall successful management of women's sexual dysfunction. While the educational style and content needs to be adapted to each clinical situation, educational opportunities should be provided to all women being managed for their sexual health concerns. Education can facilitate the patient and partner's comprehension of her sexual health concern. Education enables the results of her diagnostic assessment to be appreciated. Education also allows for patient preferences to be considered when deciding between the various type of treatments: psychologic or biologic treatments. Patient education is also critical in promoting a trusting patient–physician and patient–partner relationship.

Goldstein I. Current management strategies of the postmenopausal patient with sexual health problems. *J Sex Med*. 2007;4 (suppl 3):235–253.

93. Answer: E. Although women actually engage in as much or more aggressive behaviors than men, men are significantly more likely to engage in serious violent acts. This does not account for those with severe mental illness, where serious violence rates between men and women are similar but are expressed in different forms. Younger adults in general are at increased risk for violent behavior. However, there is another smaller peak after the age of 70 years due to dementia-related violent behavior. Lower intelligence does not just mean mental retardation, but those with learning disabilities and ADHD (which both predispose to conduct disorder) are also at an increased risk of violent behavior. Cluster B personality disorders increase the risk of violence via core symptoms of impulsivity. All of the answers are true. Of note, a history of childhood abuse or neglect also increases the risk of future violent behavior.

Cohen BJ. *Theory and Practice of Psychiatry*. New York: Oxford University Press; 2003:445–466.

94. Answer: C. The medial longitudinal fasciculus syndrome, also known as internuclear ophthalmoplegia, is characteristic of MS. It consists of nystagmus of the abducting eye and failure of the adducting eye to cross the midline. The medial longitudinal fasciculus is located in the brainstem and it is a common site of brainstem injury that affects the oculomotor nerves.

Kaufman DM. *Clinical Neurology for Psychiatrists*. 5th ed. Philadelphia: WB Saunders; 2001:35–55.

95. Answer: A. This patient is presenting with a pure motor hemiparesis, which is most likely secondary to a subcortical ischemic stroke. There are no other symptoms that would localize the patient's stroke to the cortex (i.e., aphasia, visual field deficit, and face and arm weakness, more than leg weakness). Pure motor hemiparesis was the first clinically recognized lacunar syndrome and typically localizes to the contralateral internal capsule or contralateral basis pontis. The thalamus, however, is associated with a different type of lacunar syndrome known as a pure sensory stroke, and involves numbness and sensory loss over one side of the body but does not affect motor strength.

1. Papamitsakis NIH. *Lacunar Syndromes*. http://www.emedicine.com/neuro/topic695.htm. Published February 24, 2007.
2. Rowland LP. *Merritt's Neurology*. 11th ed. Philadelphia: Lippincott Williams & Wilkins; 2005:301, 308.

96. Answer: D. Alcohol and acetaldehyde can both cross the placenta, and can cause fetal death and spontaneous abortion. The surviving infants of alcoholic mothers can evidence features of FAS that may include a small head, facial abnormalities (a flat bridge of nose, an epicanthal eye fold, and an absent philtrum), severe mental retardation, a diminished physical size, an atrial septal defect, and sundactyly. Small ears are not characteristic of the phenotypy of the FAS. These defects are irreversible. The exact amount of alcohol required or the most vulnerable period of pregnancy associated with FAS is unknown, therefore, any amount of alcohol at any stage of pregnancy is contraindicated.

Sadock BJ, Sadock VA. *Kaplan and Sadock's Comprehensive Textbook of Psychiatry*. 7th ed. Philadelphia: Lippincott Williams & Wilkins; 2000:958.

97. Answer: C. In general, diffusion gradients do seem to determine the entry of proteins into CSF and for carbon dioxide exchange. Most CSF is produced in the choroid plexuses (located on the floor of the lateral and third and fourth ventricles). However, if they are removed, the brain continues to produce some CSF. CSF production at these sites does require active transport and energy dependent secretion. The blood brain barrier does not prevent the flow of water and sodium between blood and CSF, which readily occurs, explaining why hypotonic/hypertonic solutions may have such a rapid effect. Electrolytes and glucose equilibrate at all points in the ventricular and subarachnoid spaces. With choroid plexuses intact, the CSF replenishes itself up to 4 to 5 times per day, making about 500 mL/day. The blood brain barrier is located at various specialized points to control access of large molecules (e.g., albumin and bound molecules) between blood and CSF. Metabolic products of the brain defused rapidly into CSF, which acts like a "sink," and are removed into the blood. CSF is removed through the arachnoid granulations to the dural venous sinuses.

Ropper AH, Brown RH. *Adams and Victor's Principles of Neurology*. 8th ed. New York: McGraw-Hill; 2005:529–545.

98. Answer: C. Glycine, an amino acid, is an inhibitory neurotransmitter in parts of the spinal cord system. GABA is another major inhibitory neurotransmitter, with some action in the spinal cord, but is not among the answers. Glutamate is an excitatory neurotransmitter. Dopamine, serotonin, and acetylcholine function varies depending on involved tracts and receptors.

1. Kaufman DM. *Clinical Neurology for Psychiatrists*. 5th ed. Philadelphia: WB Saunders; 2001:552–569.
2. Ropper AH, Brown RH. *Adams and Victor's Principles of Neurology*. 8th ed. New York: McGraw-Hill; 2005: 40–41.
3. Sadock BJ, Sadock VA. *Kaplan & Sadock's Comprehensive Textbook of Psychiatry*. 7th ed. Philadelphia: Lippincott Williams & Wilkins; 2000:50–59.

99. Answer: D. The spinal cord stroke, either ischemic or hemorrhagic, has an acute and often apoplectic onset evolving over minutes. This is drastically different from all other spinal cord disorders including acute transverse myelopathy, viral myelitis, GBS, and mass lesions in the spinal canal, which all develop over 24 to 72 hours with an acute but discernibly slower evolution than the vascular lesions. The first symptom of most spinal infarcts may be radicular back pain, either lancinating or burning in quality, and sensory symptoms are followed by the rapid onset of leg weakness.

1. Hogan E. *Spinal Cord Infarction*. http://www.emedicine.com/neuro/topic348.htm. Published February 24, 2007.
2. Rowland LP. *Merritt's Neurology*. 11th ed. Philadelphia: Lippincott Williams & Wilkins, 2005:343–344.

100. Answer: E. Common symptoms seen in patients with autonomic neuropathy are tachycardia, rapid alterations in blood pressure, flushing, sweating, and changes in gastrointestinal motility. Other symptoms include miosis (small pupil), anhidrosis (impaired sweating), orthostatic hypotension, sphincter symptoms, impotence, and vasomotor abnormalities. Autonomic neuropathy is also more commonly associated with symmetric distal polyneuropathy. In patients with autonomic neuropathy, these symptoms can occur without other symptoms of neuropathy like pain, paresthesias, or sensory loss.

Rowland LP. *Merritt's Neurology*. 11th ed. Philadelphia: Lippincott Williams & Wilkins; 2005:735–736.

101. Answer: E. Pathological lesion of herpes simplex encephalitis is seen in neurons, astrocytes, and oligodendrocytes. The inclusion bodies are seen as large eosinophilic intranuclear masses surrounded by a clear halo and displacing the nucleolus to the periphery. Perivascular inflammation of lymphocytes and histiocytes in the cortex and adjacent white matter, microglial proliferation, and glial nodule formation are changes characteristic of all forms of encephalitis. In areas of maximal involvement, there is necrosis with softening, hemorrhage, and loss of all neuronal and glial elements. These lesions are usually asymmetric and more often affect the medial temporal and orbital areas.

1. Lishman WA. *Organic Psychiatry*. 3rd ed. Oxford: Blackwell Science; 1996:346.
2. Rowland LP. *Merritt's Neurology*. 11th ed. Philadelphia: Lippincott Williams & Wilkins; 2005:192.

102. Answer: E. Tremors are rhythmic oscillatory movements that result from the alternating contractions of opposing muscle groups, whereas myoclonus is a brief shocklike movement that occurs due to the contraction or inhibition of muscle groups. On the other hand, chorea are brief, irregular contractions that are not as rapid as myoclonus. Ballism is a choreic jerky movement of large amplitude that produces flinging movements of the affected limbs. Tics are simple jerks or complex movements that occur suddenly and intermittently. Athetosis is a continuous and slow writhing movement of the limbs, trunk, head, face, or tongue.

Rowland LP. *Merritt's Neurology*. 11th ed. Philadelphia: Lippincott Williams & Wilkins; 2005:48–49.

103. Answer: D. The most common disorder associated with the inborn error of metabolism of sulfur containing amino acids is homocystinuria. It occurs in 1:45,000 newborns and has an autosomal-recessive mode of inheritance. It is second only to phenylke-

tonuria among inborn errors of metabolism responsible for brain damage. It is caused by the absence of activity of the enzyme cystathionine β-synthase that catalyzes the formation of cystathionine from homocysteine and serine. As the enzyme activity is absent, homocystine and its precursor methionine accumulate in the body and are seen in excessive amounts in the urine and plasma of these patients.

Rowland LP. *Merritt's Neurology*. 11th ed. Philadelphia: Lippincott Williams & Wilkins; 2005:614–615.

104. Answer: E. Valproate (valproic acid and divalproex sodium, also known as Depakene and Depakote, respectively) is an anticonvulsant that is FDA-approved for the treatment of acute mania, seizure disorders, and migraine headaches. Its mechanism of action is to increase brain levels of GABA, the principle inhibitory neurotransmitter. Carbamazepine (Tegretol) decreases the rapid firing of neurons by inhibiting voltage-dependent sodium channels. Clonazepam (Klonopin) is a high-potency benzodiazepine that acts as an agonist at the benzodiazepine-binding site of the GABA-A receptor. Lamotrigine, now approved for treatment of bipolar depression, is thought to act by inhibition of excitatory neurotransmitter glutamate as well as inhibition of sodium channels. Finally, topiramate (Topamax) has multiple mechanisms of action, including inhibition of sodium channels, enhancing the effect of GABA at the GABA$_A$ receptor, and antagonizing kainite at AMPA receptors. Other anticonvulsants of interest to psychiatrists include gabapentin (Neuronton), which interacts with the GABA transporter and increases GABA levels in the brain, and tiagabine (Gabitril), which blocks the reuptake of GABA and elevates extracellular levels of GABA.

Stern TA, Herman JB. *Massachusetts General Hospital Psychiatry Update and Board Preparation*. 2nd ed. New York: McGraw Hill; 2002:359–363.

105. Answer: C. Although transit time is usually unchanged for the small bowel, transit time through the large bowel is slower. In general there are fewer myenteric ganglion cells, so contractions are less coordinated and less forceful. Despite this, vitamin and mineral absorption often declines because of decreased perfusion and membrane transport. Increased transit time usually increases the absorption of medications. The other changes in cardiovascular, respiratory, renal, and hematological/immune systems generally are true for advancing age. Other physiological changes with age include slower drug metabolism through the liver due to decreased hepatic blood flow and slower oxidation in the cytochrome p450 system.

1. Blazer DG, Steffens DC, Busse EW. *The American Psychiatric Association Textbook of Geriatric Psychiatry.* Washington: American Psychiatric Publishing; 2004:37–51.
2. Sadavoy J, Jarvik LF, Grossberg GT, et al. *Comprehensive Textbook of Geriatric Psychiatry.* 3rd ed. New York: WW Norton & Company; 2004:105–130.

106. Answer: C. The medial temporal lobe contains the amygdala, the hippocampal region, and the parahippocampal gyrus. The neurons of the hippocampal region are arranged in one cellular layer: the pyramidal layer. Most hippocampal pyramidal neurons are glutamatergic, and this region contains the serial circuitry for long-term potentiation through the NMDA receptor. Connections with the limbic system are important for the regulation of emotion, and connections with the frontal lobes are important for declarative memory.

Stern TA, Herman JB. *Massachusetts General Hospital Psychiatry Update & Board Preparation.* 2nd ed. New York: McGraw-Hill; 2004:267.

107. Answer: D. Researchers have found increased CSF levels of MHPG in subjects with a history of aggressive behavior and in subjects with personality disorder. Reports indicate that the β-adrenergic antagonist propranolol may be effective in the treatment of episodic aggressive behavior in subjects with head injuries. Animal studies indicate that the stimulation of the amygdala produces sham rage and is associated with a fall in brainstem and brain levels of norepinephrine. Some animal models also indicate that shock-induced fighting, are induced more readily with lowered brain norepinephrine levels. The most consistent data indicating the role of the serotonergic system in human aggression comes from personality disordered subjects. Their CSF 5-HIAA level was inversely correlated with clinician or self-reports of lifetime aggression. Some investigators also reported negative correlations of CSF 5-HIAA with irritability, hostility, impulsive homicide, fire-setting, and maternal aggression, as well as self-rated behavioral difficulties during childhood. A correlation has also been found between the genotype for a polymorphism in the gene for tryptophan hydroxylase and levels of CSF 5-HIAA in impulsive, aggressive individuals. This suggests a link between a gene involved in the serotonergic system and impulsive aggression. Because the serotonergic system is under significant genetic control, there is a genetic contribution to aggressivity and part of genetic vulnerability to aggression may be explained by low CSF 5-HIAA as an inherited trait. Injuries involving the prefrontal cortex are associated with aggressive behavior. Seizures, especially those involving the temporal lobe, are also associated with episodic and impulsive aggression. These studies suggest that lesions to the prefrontal cortex and certain limbic areas interfere with mechanisms involved with inhibiting aggressive behaviors. Aggression also involves increased dopaminergic activity. Dopaminergic agents like amphetamine and the antiaggressive effects of dopamine antagonists support the hypothesis that increased dopaminergic activity may underlie some forms of aggression. Individuals with additional Y chromosomes are also overrepresented in violent, criminal populations. As men are more aggressive than women, there may be a role for the Y chromosome in the neurobiology of aggression.

1. Blake P, Grafman J. The neurobiology of aggression. *Lancet.* 2004;364 (suppl 1):S12–S13.
2. Kavoussi R, Armstead P, Coccaro E. The neurobiology of impulsive aggression. *Psychiatr Clin North Am.* 1997; 20:395–403.
3. Mann JJ. *Neurobiology of Suicide and Aggression.* http://www.acnp.org/g4/GN401000185/CH181.html. Published February 11, 2007.

108. Answer: E. Exceptions to the usual requirement for providing informed consent for a medical intervention exist. An exception exists in serious and imminent emergencies where interventions may be lifesaving, and either time does not permit consent, and/or someone is not available to authorize to consent for the patient. Incompetent patients may not legally provide informed consent, and a surrogate decision-maker should provide consent. Patients may knowingly and voluntarily waive their right to informed consent for treatment. Therapeutic privilege is more difficult to apply, but may be used when the clinician judges that disclosure of full informed consent (risks, alternatives, etc.) would be harmful to the patient.

Hales RE, Yudofsky SC. *Textbook of Clinical Psychiatry.* 4th ed. Washington: American Psychiatric Publishing; 2003: 1585–1628.

109. Answer: E. The routine pretreatment workup for ECT includes a CBC with differential, chem-20 profile, a urinalysis, a chest X ray, and an EKG. In addition, a CT scan and an EEG may be ordered if indicated by medical history or by the physical, neurological, or mental status examination. Spinal X rays are currently ordered less often than in the past because of the reportedly lower incidence of orthopedic complications associated with the administration of ECT. Routine pre-ECT screening does not include checking for abnormal pseudocholinesterase activity. It may be checked if there is a history of prolonged succinylcholine-induced apnea in the patient or in a blood relative.

Hales RE, Yudofsky SC. *American Psychiatric Publishing Textbook of Clinical Psychiatry.* 4th ed. http://www.psychiatryonline.com/content.aspx?aID=69719. Accessed February 15, 2007.

110. **Answer: D.** All are DSM-IV-TR criteria for pain disorder, except for D. In pain disorder, the symptom or deficit is NOT intentionally produced or feigned (as it is in factitious disorder or malingering).

American Psychiatric Association. *Quick Reference to the Diagnostic Criteria from DSM-IV-TR.* Washington: American Psychiatric Association; 2000:229–236.

111. **Answer: A.** Studies have shown that patients on a stable methadone dose can safely operate heavy machinery and drive. However, certain occupations, such as those in public safety, health care, and transportation of heavy machinery, do require that patients be drug free, precluding methadone maintenance.

Hauri-Bionda R, Bar W, Friedrich-Koch A. Driving fitness/riving capacity of patients treated with methadone. *Schweiz Med Wochenschr.* 1998;128:1538.

112. **Answer: D.** Bipolar Depression usually has an earlier onset than unipolar depression. Hypersomnia and psychomotor retardation are "atypical" depressive features, which are traditionally thought to be more common in Bipolar Depression. Postpartum Depression is more closely associated with Bipolar than Unipolar Depression. Individuals with Bipolar Disorder spend a majority of time in depressed states, compared to hypomanic or manic states. Clinically, it is thus imperative to distinguish Bipolar from Unipolar Depression, as treatment approaches (and consequences) are different. In an attempt to clarify the paradox of agitated Bipolar Depression, it has also been pointed out that, perhaps contrary to traditional thinking, the opposite of psychomotor retardation is actually acceleration (and not agitation).

American Psychiatric Association. *Diagnostic and Statistical Manual of Mental Disorders American Psychiatric Association.* 4th ed. (Text revision). http://www.psychiatryonline.com/content.aspx?aID=2444. Accessed February 6, 2007.

113. **Answer: C.** Cerebral ventricular enlargement has been found consistently in the studies of patients with Schizophrenia, and is perhaps one of the most consistent findings in psychiatry. The enlargement occurs early at onset, perhaps present from the beginning, and does not progress faster than age-matched controls. Ventricular enlargement is associated with poorer prognosis and treatment outcomes, and is not believed to be secondary to medication treatment. It is also associated with negative symptoms, cognitive impairment, and poor premorbid functioning. Ventricular enlargement is not specific to Schizophrenia. Sulcal enlargement, suggestive of atrophy, has been found, but not as consistently as ventricular enlargement. However, recent meta-analyses have reported a small but significant difference, with smaller brain volumes and intracranial size in schizophrenics compared with normals. Decrease in frontal lobe size, or *hypofrontality*, has been suggested. However, there are multiple negative studies, and dysfunction may be more related to circuitry than size. There may be a decrease (not an increase) in thalamic size, which has been more difficult to study with current techniques. Temporal lobes have also been difficult to study, but may involve decreased volumes. Midline and other neurodevelopmental abnormalities may be better understood with time.

Hales RE, Yudofsky SC. *Textbook of Clinical Psychiatry.* 4th ed. Washington: American Psychiatric Publishing; 2003:379–439.

114. **Answer: D.** Opiate-related disorders in pregnant women have far-reaching ramifications, including abortion, contracting and transmitting human immunodeficiency virus (HIV), and the development of specific neonatal opiate withdrawal syndrome. Studies indicate that more than 70% of neonates born to opiate-dependent mothers manifest symptoms of withdrawal at birth. Methadone substitution and maintenance therapy is becoming increasingly common. While the dosing schedules of such therapy are not universal, the consensus appears to favor a dose high enough to eliminate craving (and hence the possibility of resorting to external use) and low enough to decrease neonatal withdrawal symptoms at birth. A daily dose of 20 mg is generally recommended. If an expectant mother stable on daily methadone doses higher than 20 mg is admitted to a methadone maintenance program, the goal is to attempt to taper this by 1 to 2 mg weekly at gestation week 14 through week 32. A specific, opiate-withdrawal syndrome in infants born to opiate-dependent mothers has been described. Most infants manifest mild withdrawal symptoms (hyperactivity, exaggerated reflexes, diaphoresis, mottling, yawning, high-pitched cry, anorexia) that require no specific pharmacologic interventions. A few infants may experience more severe symptoms (vomiting, seizure, fever) and will require treatment with paregoric or phenobarbital.

1. Ebner N, Rohrmeister K, Winklbaur B, et. al. Management of neonatal abstinence syndrome in neonates born

to opioid maintained women. *Drug Alcohol Depend*. 2007; 87:131–138.

2. Galanter M, Kleber HD. *Textbook of Substance Abuse Treatment*. 2nd ed. Washington: American Psychiatric Press; 1999:271–279.

3. Osborn DA, Jeffery HE, Cole M. Opiate treatment for opiate withdrawal in newborn infants. *Cochrane Database Syst Rev*. 2005;3:CD002059.

115. Answer: C. Acute aggression is treated with the sedative properties of antipsychotics or benzodiazepines. In treating chronic aggression, it is essential to evaluate and diagnose and treat the underlying disorders and use, when possible, antiaggressive agents specific to those disorders. When there is partial response after a therapeutic trial with a specific medication, adjunctive treatment with a medication that has a different mechanism of action should be instituted.

Hales RE, Yudofsky SC. *American Psychiatric Publishing Textbook of Clinical Psychiatry*. 4th ed. http://www. psychiatryonline.com/content.aspx?aID=89808. Accessed March 2, 2007.

116. Answer: E. Countertransference with hysterical patients may include both defensive distancing and infantilization. The therapeutic dyad in which the potentials are most problematic is that of the male therapist and the female patient. It can be hard to respectfully attend to what feels like a pseudoaffect in histrionic patients. The self-dramatizing quality of these chronically anxious patients invites ridicule. Related to the condescending and hostile reaction to a histrionic woman is the temptation to treat her like a little girl. The problem with being too indulgent with a hysterical person is that the patient's diminished self-concept will be reinforced. Another problematic countertransference is the therapist's reaction to the hysteric's defensive seductiveness. Countertransference of having been obliterated and ignored as a real person as a result of either patients' idealization or devaluation is diagnostic of a narcissistic dynamic. Other countertransferences to narcissistic patients include boredom, extreme drowsiness, irritability, or a sense of grandiose expansion.

McWilliams N. *Psychoanalytic Diagnosis: Understanding Personality Structure in the Clinical Process*. New York: Guilford Press; 1994:178–181, 313–316.

117. Answer: E. AA is the best known and the most frequently recommended intervention for alcohol-dependent patients. It is not a professionally delivered treatment, and is a mutual-help group that offers peer support, role modeling, hope, practical problem-solving advice, a built-in social support network, sober activity, and structure. A great advan-

tage of AA is that it is always available and is free of charge. The philosophical foundation of AA is the twelve steps. Of these, only one (Step 1) actually mentions alcohol, while the other steps focus more on personal growth. When compared to those who do not attend AA meetings, individuals who participate in AA meetings typically have better drinking outcomes and fewer health-related expenditures. AA is not for everyone, as some people object to what they perceive to be religious overtones. Others do not like group approaches and some object because they believe that AA is opposed to the use of medication for alcohol-dependent individuals. The official position of AA is that the individuals should follow their physician's advice regarding the use of medication and that AA members should not tell others to stop their medications.

Weiss RD, Kueppenbender KD. Combining psychosocial treatment with pharmacotherapy for alcohol dependence. *J Clin Psychopharmacol*. 2006;26(suppl 1):S37–S42.

118. Answer: E. While medical therapies are generally efficacious (50% to 90%) for the treatment of sexual dysfunction, about 50% of individuals fail to continue treatment. Reasons include the failure to address all of the following: patient variables (such as performance anxiety and depression), partner variables (such as poor mental or physical health and partner disinterest), interpersonal nonsexual variables (such as quality of the overall relationship), interpersonal sexual variables (such as the interval of abstinence and sexual scripts), and contextual variables (such as current life stresses with money or children).

Althof SE, Leiblum SR, Chevret-Measson M, et al. Psychological and interpersonal dimensions of sexual function and dysfunction. *J Sex Med*. 2005;2:793–800.

119. Answer: C. Although psychiatrists cannot predict future behavior with certainty in any case, past behavior is the best predictor of future actions. A previous history of violent behavior is the single strongest risk factor for future violence, and the risk is greater with the increased number of incidents and greater intensity of prior acts. Although it is is not the single best predictor, the triad of fire-setting, enuresis, and cruelty to animals as a child has been associated with sociopathy. Intense paranoia and command hallucinations may be dynamic risk factors for violence, but their clinical presentation is variable, such that neither is the "single best" predictor of violence. Actually, the MacArthur Study of Mental Disorder and Violence has brought into question whether these psychotic symptoms are associated with a higher (in truth it may possibly be a lower rate) rate of violence. A prior history of abuse or neglect also predisposes to future violence, but not to the degree that a prior personal history of violence does.

Cohen BJ. *Theory and Practice of Psychiatry*. New York: Oxford University Press; 2003:445–466.

120. Answer: A. The anterior spinothalamic tracts carry light touch sensation to the thalamus. The lateral spinothalamic tracts carry temperature and pain sensation to the thalamus. The posterior columns, which include the fasciculus cuneatus and fasciculus gracilis, carry position and vibration sensation to the thalamus. The spinocerebellar tracts carry joint position and movement sensations to the cerebellum.

Kaufman DM. *Clinical Neurology for Psychiatrists*. 5th ed. Philadelphia: WB Saunders; 2001:21.

121. Answer: E. Tumors in different locations tend to create a typical constellation of symptoms. This patient presents with symptoms most consistent with a temporal lobe lesion, which is associated with behavioral changes, language disturbance from the dominant hemisphere, olfactory and partial-complex seizures, and visual field deficits. Patients who have temporal lobe seizures often have hallucinations that are tactile, auditory, or olfactory. Cerebellar tumors cause headache, ataxia, nystagmus, and occasionally neck pain. Tumors in the frontal lobe frequently cause seizures, behavioral changes, dementia, gait disorders, hemiparesis, and expressive aphasia from the dominant hemisphere. Occipital lobe tumors are associated with hemianopia and unformed visual disturbances. Parietal lesions present with language and speech difficulties if in the dominant hemisphere, or with visuospatial integration problems and neglect syndromes, when it involves the nondominant lobe.

1. Rowland LP. *Merritt's Neurology*. 11th ed. Philadelphia: Lippincott Williams & Wilkins; 2005:295, 374.
2. Sadock BJ, Sadock VA. *Kaplan and Sadock's Comprehensive Textbook of Psychiatry*. 8th ed. Philadelphia: Lippincott Williams & Wilkins; 2005:362, 364, 367.

122. Answer: C. Alcoholics are at higher risk for thiamine deficiency that can lead to Wernicke's disease and Wernicke-Korsakoff syndrome. Wernicke's disease presents with an acute onset, and is characterized by the triad of mental disturbance, ataxia, and paralysis of eye movements resulting from bilateral sixth cranial nerve palsy. Mental disturbances typically involve a global confusion, apathetic state, or a disorder of retentive memory. Wernicke's disease is a neurologic emergency that should be treated with immediate parenteral administration of thiamine, with a dose of 50 mg intravenously and 50 mg in-

tramuscularly. The risk of permanent memory loss increases with the delay in thiamine administration. Intravenous glucose prior to thiamine administration can precipitate Wernicke's disease by exhausting a patient's vitamin B reserve. Therefore, intravenous glucose must be accompanied by the administration of glucose in the alcoholic patient. Ocular palsy responds within hours, while the gait and cognitive problems of Wernicke's resolve slowly. Upon resolution of confusion and apathy, the patient may sometimes be left with a permanent defect in retentive memory and learning called *Korsakoff's psychosis*. To reduce the risk of Korsakoff's psychosis, all patients presenting with alcohol withdrawal should be administered parenteral thiamine on presentation, followed by oral supplementation for several weeks.

Graham AW, Schultz TK, Mayo-Smith MF, et al. *Principles of Addiction Medicine*. 3rd ed. Maryland: American Society of Addiction Medicine; 2003:629.

123. Answer: A. This patient has GBS. Just about any type of acute febrile illness (and even immunization) may come in the weeks before a GBS episode. Nondescript antecedent upper respiratory infections (URIs) are most common, although *Campylobacter jejuni* may be identified in cases when gastrointestinal illnesses precede the episode. GBS may occur in any season, over a broad age range (more common in the sixth and seventh decades), and females are slightly more susceptible. GBS presents with a characteristic ascending and progressive paralysis. GBS has a characteristic CSF profile on lumbar puncture with high protein concentration, with slight to no increase in cell count. Answer B is normal CSF. Answer C is characteristic of bacterial meningitis and Gram stain may reveal organisms. Answer D is characteristic of viral meningitis. Answer E is more characteristic of an infection such as neurosyphilis (WBCs will be mostly lymphocytes), and the distinguishing factor is that there are more WBCs and it may be Venereal Disease Research Laboratory (VDRL) positive.

1. Kaufman DM. *Clinical Neurology for Psychiatrists*. 5th ed. Philadelphia: WB Saunders; 2001:532–551.
2. Ropper AH, Brown RH. *Adams and Victor's Principles of Neurology*. 8th ed. New York: McGraw-Hill; 2005:1117–1128.

124. Answer: A. Hyperactive reflexes suggest CNS injury, specifically those involving cortical spinal tracts. Injuries to peripheral nerve, anterior horn cells, neuromuscular junction or the muscle, typically result in hypoactive reflexes.

Kaufman DM. *Clinical Neurology for Psychiatrists*. 5th ed. Philadelphia: WB Saunders; 2001:3–7.

125. Answer: B. This patient presents with sudden onset of symptoms that is consistent with a vascular etiology, rather than a slower, more progressive course of other spinal cord diseases (like ALS, tabes dorsalis, or Vitamin B_{12} neuropathy) and has a neurological exam consistent with occlusion of the ventral artery. Proprioception and vibratory sensations are spared because the posterior columns are supplied by the posterior arterial plexus. If proprioception and vibration sensation are impaired, the lesion is most likely not an anterior spinal artery infarction, but is rather a myelopathy of nonvascular origin. Spastic weakness in the legs results from lesions of the lateral corticospinal tract, and the loss of temperature and pain sensation is a result from lesions of the lateral spinothalamic tracks. ALS is a disease of unknown etiology in which there is degeneration of both upper and lower motor neurons, thus clinically there is both lower motor neuron signs (weakness, wasting, and fasciculation) and UMN signs (hyperactive DTRs, Babinski sign, clonus, Hoffmann signs) in the same limbs. Sensation, however, is not clinically affected, thus pain and paresthesia are impermissible with this diagnosis. Paralytic poliomyelitis is caused by the polio virus, and has thus become a clinical rarity because of the advent of vaccines. The symptoms at the onset are similar to those of any acute infection, and paralysis may develop between the 2nd and 5th day, or may be delayed longer when the virus invades the nervous system. The virus causes degenerative changes of the anterior horn (motor neuron) cells of the spinal cord and lower brainstem, and only causes lower motor neuron signs: paresis that is typically asymmetric, muscle fasciculations, and absent DTRs. Tabes dorsalis, also called *progressive locomotor ataxia*, results from tertiary syphilis and is manifested by lancinating or lightning-like pains, progressive ataxia, loss of tendon reflexes, loss of proprioception, dysfunction of sphincters, and impaired sexual function in men. The chief signs is loss of tendon reflexes at the knees and ankles, impaired vibratory and position sense in the legs, and abnormal pupils. Vitamin B_{12} neuropathy is characterized by predominantly sensory loss and sensory ataxia, as the dorsal columns, lateral corticospinal tracks (resulting in weakness), and spinocerebellar tracts (resulting in loss of joint position and movement sensation) are affected.

Rowland LP. *Merritt's Neurology*. 11th ed. Philadelphia: Lippincott Williams & Wilkins; 2005:178, 239, 343–344, 471, 865, 1096.

126. Answer: C. GBS is an acute inflammatory demyelinating neuropathy characterized by sudden onset of peripheral and cranial nerve dysfunction. It is the most frequent acquired demyelinating neuropathy, and its incidence gradually increases with age. It affects men and women equally and is often preceded by days to weeks by viral respiratory or gastrointestinal infection, immunization, or surgery. It consists of rapidly progressive symmetric muscle weakness, loss of tendon reflexes, impaired sensation in the hands and feet, and in severe cases oropharyngeal and respiratory paresis. The severity of neurologic abnormalities is not related to the degree of conduction slowing. The symptoms of the condition worsen for several weeks, followed by a period of stability and then gradual improvement to almost normal function. The long-term prognosis can be improved by early plasmapheresis or intravenous infusion of human gamma globulins.

Rowland LP. *Merritt's Neurology*. 11th ed. Philadelphia: Lippincott Williams & Wilkins; 2005:748–749.

127. Answer: B. General paresis is the only syphilitic disease where the spirochetes can be demonstrated in brain tissues. The dura mater is thickened and opaque, and the pia mater is firmly adherent to the underlying cortex. The brain is small and atrophied with widening of cerebral sulci and ventricular dilatation. Inflammatory lesions are seen throughout the cortex. Degenerative changes with neuronal loss are especially seen in the frontal and parietal regions. Enlarged microglial cells are characteristically arranged in rows (rod cells) and when stained with Prussian blue reveal iron-containing pigments in their cytoplasm, which is considered to be pathognomonic for general paresis.

1. Lishman WA. *Organic Psychiatry*. 3rd ed. Oxford: Blackwell Science; 1996:339.
2. Rowland LP. *Merritt's Neurology*. 11th ed. Philadelphia: Lippincott Williams & Wilkins; 2005:239–240.

128. Answer: B. Friedreich ataxia is the most common hereditary ataxia, which occurs with a frequency of 1 in 50,000 in the white population. It has an autosomal recessive type of inheritance and affects the CNS, the spinal cord, and peripheral nerves along with the heart and pancreas. Most cases of Friedreich ataxia are caused by the loss of function mutations in the FXN gene located on chromosome 9q13. Most patients have expanded trinucleotide (GAA) repeat in intron 1 of the FXN gene. Patients with Friedreich ataxia can manifest with hypertrophic cardiomyopathy. Patients with hypertrophic cardiomyopathy can present with serious arrhythmia or sudden cardiac death. Impaired glucose tolerance and diabetes mellitus occurs in about one-third of patients with Friedreich ataxia and it occurs with higher frequency in siblings of diabetics. Patients with onset of symptoms at a later age have a better prognosis, but most die between the ages of 30 and 40 years.

1. Opal P, Zoghbi HY, Cruse RB. *Friedreich Ataxia*. http://www.uptodateonline.com/utd/content/topic.do?topic-Key=ped_neur/6520&type=A&selectedTitle=3~97. Accessed March 1, 2007.
2. Rowland LP. *Merritt's Neurology*. 11th ed. Philadelphia: Lippincott Williams & Wilkins; 2005:783–786.

129. Answer: A. The covering of the acoustic (eighth cranial) nerve sometimes proliferates to form a relatively benign tumor called an acoustic neuroma. The tumor develops in the internal auditory canal and cerebellopontine angle where it may compress adjacent structures, particularly the fifth (trigeminal) and seventh (facial) cranial nerves. Acoustic neuromas generally cause unilateral hearing impairment, in addition to symptoms of tinnitus, imbalance, and vertigo, which result from eighth cranial nerve involvement. If the acoustic neuroma compresses the fifth cranial nerve, patients can develop facial sensory loss. If it compresses the seventh cranial nerve, patients can develop facial weakness.

Kaufman DM. *Clinical Neurology for Psychiatrists*. 5th ed. Philadelphia: WB Saunders; 2001:520.

130. Answer: C. Epilepsy itself carries a risk of fetal malformations (5%), independent of fetal exposure to AEDs. No one AED exclusively causes a particular fetal malformation, and no AED is risk-free. The majority of malformations are induced during the first trimester of pregnancy, a time when the CNS and vital organs are developing. Neural tube defects are associated nearly equally with valproate (1%) and carbamazepine (0.5%), but these malformations are not exclusively associated with these particular anticonvulsants. Fetal hydantoin syndrome, associated most commonly with phenytoin use, includes craniofacial and limb defects. Physicians caring for pregnant women taking AEDs should carefully inform the patient of the risks and benefits of using the AED during pregnancy. If it is deemed clinically appropriate, the AED should be tapered and discontinued prior to conception through at least the first trimester. If an AED is felt to be necessary, monotherapy is recommended and the lowest dose necessary should be used. To reduce the risk of neural tube defects, women who are trying to conceive should take folic acid and continue it through the pregnancy.

Kaufman DM. *Clinical Neurology for Psychiatrists*. 5th ed. Philadelphia: WB Saunders; 2001:246–247.

131. Answer: E. Changes in neurotransmitter function are variable with aging, and may vary throughout location in the brain. In general, cholinergic and dopaminergic function are thought to decline, but not uniformly. Cell loss occurs relatively at random with age, although there is also some clustered loss, particularly in the cerebellum, locus coeruleus, and substantia nigra. Loss of brain mass is reflected in both decreased size and weight. Myelin loss is noticeable in cortical white matter. Despite this, there is less neuronal loss with normal aging than was previously thought. Cerebral blood flow decreases significantly (perhaps by 20%) with age, even in the absence of disease.

1. Blazer DG, Steffens DC, Busse EW. *The American Psychiatric Association Textbook of Geriatric Psychiatry*. Washington: American Psychiatric Publishing; 2004:37–51.
2. Sadavoy J, Jarvik LF, Grossberg GT, et al. *Comprehensive Textbook of Geriatric Psychiatry*. 3rd ed. New York: WW Norton; 2004:105–130.

132. Answer: A. Among all psychiatric disorders, Autism has the highest heritability at about 90%. Schizophrenia and Bipolar Disorder have a heritability rate of 75% each followed by ADHD and OCD at 60%. The heritability rate for major depression, panic disorder, and alcoholism is about 40%.

Sadock BJ, Sadock VA. *Kaplan and Sadock's Comprehensive Textbook of Psychiatry*. 8th ed. Philadelphia: Lippincott Williams & Wilkins; 2005:239.

133. Answer: D. The question gives the definition for incidence, which measures new-onset of a diagnosis of a particular disorder in a specific period of time. Prevalence measures the proportion of individuals who have a particular disorder during a specific time period, not necessarily new onset cases. Both are measures of frequency, but incidence is a more specific answer. Odds ratio and relative risk are both measures of association between two variables.

Tohen M, Bromet E, Murphy JM, et al. Psychiatric epidemiology. *Harv Rev Psychiatry*. 2000;8:111–125.

134. Answer: E. Baseline pretreatment studies and periodic follow-up tests for lithium should include monitoring of renal and thyroid function. Renal function is monitored using BUN, serum creatinine, and a urinalysis. Because of the lithium's ability to impair the release of thyroid hormone from the thyroid gland, a baseline screening assessment of thyroid function is usually obtained. These tests are usually repeated every 6 months to every year. Clinicians also should obtain thyroid studies in patients taking lithium who experience fatigue or asthenia, cold intolerance, or changes in skin, voice, or weight (symptoms of impaired thyroid function). Before the administration of lithium in women of childbearing age, a screening urine pregnancy test generally should be obtained. Lithium is contraindicated during the first trimester of pregnancy owing to risk of congenital heart disease. Clinicians should advise women taking lithium to use adequate contraception. Because lithium can elevate the WBC count, a pretreatment WBC count also is usually obtained. Platelets are not routinely checked in patients taking lithium, unlike in patients who take valproic acid.

1. Albers LJ, Hahn RK, Reist C. *Handbook of Psychiatric Drugs*. Laguna Hills: Current Clinical Strategies Publishing; 2005:71–73.
2. Sadock BJ, Sadock VA. *Kaplan and Sadock's Comprehensive Textbook of Psychiatry*. 8th ed. Philadelphia: Lippincott Williams & Wilkins; 2005:923.

135. **Answer: E.** Although withdrawal from cocaine is experienced as being very unpleasant, it does not carry a risk of seizures. Cocaine withdrawal is generally associated with dysphoric mood, in addition to fatigue, vivid dreams, sleep disturbance, increased appetite, and/or psychomotor retardation/agitation. Both alcohol and those medications which are classified as "sedatives, hypnotics, or anxiolytics" carry the same DSM-IV-TR criteria for withdrawal, which include a risk of seizures. Seizures are a serious and well-known risk of withdrawal from alcohol, benzodiazepines (including lorazepam and chlordiazepoxide), and barbiturates (including secobarbital).

1. American Psychiatric Association. *Quick Reference to the Diagnostic Criteria from DSM-IV-TR*. Washington: American Psychiatric Association; 2000:105–151.
2. Sadock BJ, Sadock VA. *Kaplan and Sadock's Synopsis of Psychiatry*. 9th ed. Philadelphia: Lippincott Williams & Wilkins; 2003:380–470.

136. **Answer: C.** When a patient is hospitalized for non-substance abuse related issues, methadone should be continued at the current dose for patients on methadone maintenance. Dosages need to be confirmed with the maintenance program, and the treating team should communicate with the maintenance program at the time of discharge. Treatment with an antagonist, such as naltrexone, could cause abrupt onset of withdrawal, as it would displace methadone from the mu-receptor.

Weaver M, Hopper J. *Heroine and Other Opioids, Management of Chronic Abuse*. http://www.uptodateonline.com/utd/content/topic.do?topicKey=genr_med/32913&type=A&selectedTitle=1~4. Accessed January 22, 2007.

137. **Answer: D.** Depression occurring within a few days after a stroke is more likely to be associated with spontaneous remission than is onset of depression 7 weeks or later after a stroke. Left-sided lesions (especially in anterior and basal ganglia) are associated with depression. The association between lesion location and poststroke depression is stronger in the early poststroke period. Social isolation is an important risk factor 1 year after the stroke, but not immediately after the stroke. Severity of stroke, disability after stroke and cognitive impairment after stroke are all predictors for post stroke depression.

Newberg AR, Davydow DS, Lee HB. Cerebrovascular disease basis of depression: post-stroke depression and vascular depression. *Int Rev Psychiatry*. 2006;18:433–441.

138. **Answer: D.** The "drift hypothesis" likely best explains the on-average downward drift in socioeconomic status of those suffering from Schizophrenia. However, not all schizophrenics drift down in socioeconomic standing, especially those still living with family, which are more evenly spread across geographic areas and socioeconomic classes. Isolation, lower class, and inner city life have been thought to "breed" schizophrenia in the past, but newer studies indicate that those with Schizophrenia choose to live more isolated and urban lifestyles. The idea of an emotionally cold parent, such as a "schizophrenogenic mother," is no longer generally accepted as causative in schizophrenia. Immigrant populations are more likely to come from lower socioeconomic classes, and perhaps psychotic disorders are over-represented in such classes. Although stress may precipitate psychotic episodes, migration itself is not believed to be causative of psychotic disorders such as Schizophrenia.

Hales RE, Yudofsky SC. *Textbook of Clinical Psychiatry*. 4th ed. Washington: American Psychiatric Publishing; 2003:379–439.

139. **Answer: A.** There are studies indicating that more than 70% of neonates born to opiate-dependent mothers manifest symptoms of withdrawal at birth. Methadone substitution and maintenance therapy is becoming increasingly common. While the dosing schedules of such therapy are not universal, the consensus appears to favor a dose high enough to eliminate craving (and hence the possibility of resorting to external use) and low enough to decrease neonatal withdrawal symptoms at birth. A daily dose of 20 mg is generally recommended. If an expectant mother stable on daily methadone doses higher than 20 mg is admitted to a methadone maintenance program, the goal is to attempt to taper this by 1 to 2 mg weekly at gestation week 14 through week 32. A specific, opiate-withdrawal syndrome in infants born to opiate-dependent mothers has been described. Most infants manifest mild withdrawal symptoms (hyperactivity, exaggerated reflexes, diaphoresis, mottling, yawning, high-pitched

cry, anorexia) that require no specific pharmacologic interventions. A few infants may experience more severe symptoms (vomiting, seizure, fever) and will require treatment with paregoric or phenobarbital. Hyperphagia has not been described in neonatal opiate withdrawal.

1. Ebner N, Rohrmeister K, Winklbaur B, et al. Management of neonatal abstinence syndrome in neonates born to opioid maintained women. *Drug Alcohol Depend.* 2007;87:131–138.
2. Galanter M, Kleber HD. *Textbook of Substance Abuse Treatment.* 2nd ed. Washington: American Psychiatric Press; 1999:271–279.
3. Osborn DA, Jeffery HE, Cole M. Opiate treatment for opiate withdrawal in newborn infants. *Cochrane Database Syst Rev.* 2005;3:CD002059.

140. Answer: E. Individuals with dependent personality structure define themselves in relation to others and seek security and satisfaction predominantly in interpersonal contexts. They feel ineffectual when left to themselves and tend to regard others as powerful and effective. Psychological symptoms appear when something goes wrong in a primary relationship. Emotional preoccupations include performance anxiety and fears of criticism and abandonment. In therapy, they are compliant to a fault. They idealize the therapist, ask for advice, and seek reassurances that they are a "good patient." Countertransference is benign at first, then increasingly characterized by a sense of burden. The therapist needs to resist seduction into the role of omniscient authority, encourage the patient toward autonomous functioning, and contain anxieties that arise in the process. Dependent personality central ways of defending include avoidance, regression, and reversal. In contrast, individuals with passive-aggressive subtype of dependent personality disorder use projection, externalization, rationalization, and denial as part of hostile dependency.

1. McWilliams N. *Psychoanalytic Diagnosis: Understanding Personality Structure in the Clinical Process.* New York: Guilford Press; 1994:101–103, 107–112, 120–122, 124–125, 133–135.
2. PDM Task Force. *Psychodynamic Diagnostic Manual.* Silver Spring: Alliance of Psychoanalytic Organizations; 2006:50–52, 52–53.

141. Answer: C. Countertransference with obsessional patients is an annoyed impatience, with wishes to get them to open up about ordinary feelings. Their combination of excessive conscious submission and powerful unconscious defiance can be maddening. Clinicians easily feel bored or distanced by the patient's unremitting intellectualization. However,

feelings of insignificance and obliteration are not common during the treatment of obsessional patients, as they are with narcissistic patients. There is something very object-related (as opposed to self-object) about their unconscious devaluation. There is also something touching about their efforts to be "good" in childlike ways such as cooperating and deferring. Countertransference to paranoid personality patients is usually either strong anxiety or hostility. Furthermore, countertransference may be benevolently grandiose in the less common instance of being regarded as a savior. Because of the combination of denial and projection that constitute paranoia, causing the repudiated parts of the self to be extruded, therapists of paranoid patients often find that they consciously feel the aspect of an emotional reaction that the patient has exiled from consciousness. For example, the patient may be full of hostility, while the therapist feels fear (against which hostility is a defense), or the patient may feel vulnerable and helpless, while the therapist feels sadistic and powerful.

McWilliams N. *Psychoanalytic Diagnosis: Understanding Personality Structure in the Clinical Process.* New York: Guilford Press; 1994:216–217, 292–294.

142. Answer: E. The pharmacotherapy for Alcohol Dependence should never be delivered in a vacuum. General medical management should include maintaining an optimistic and helpful attitude, asking about drinking in a nonjudgmental manner, inquiring about adherence, and recommending participation in support groups such as AA. However, there is no evidence that any single form of psychosocial treatment is the treatment of choice for Alcohol-Dependent patients receiving pharmacotherapy. Psychosocial treatments may vary depending on the medication used. However, very few trials have compared different psychosocial approaches in conjunction with specific medications. One study found that adding medical management therapy and pills to a specialty psychosocial therapy improved the outcomes. It is important for the prescribing clinicians to realize the importance of their role in both providing psychosocial treatment themselves and referring their alcohol-dependent patients for adjunctive psychosocial treatment, as indicated.

1. Anton RF, O'Malley SS, Ciraulo DA, et al. Combined pharmacotherapies and behavioral interventions for alcohol dependence: the COMBINE study: a randomized controlled trial. *JAMA.* 2006;295:2003–2017.
2. Weiss RD, Kueppenbender KD. Combining psychosocial treatment with pharmacotherapy for alcohol dependence. *J Clin Psychopharmacol.* 2006;26(suppl 1):S37–S42.

143. Answer: A. HSDD is the most prevalent female sexual complaint. It has a prevalence of about 30% to 35%. Sexual desire problems may be alleviated largely or completely in 56% of the couples following treatment. However, a majority (75%) of the sample relapsed at 1- to 6-year follow-up. The outcome is poorer when the male partner has less desire than the partner. Efficacy of CBT for women with HSDD has been reported in two studies. A study by Mc-Cabe found that of the 43% of women complaining of HSDD who underwent ten sessions of CBT, 54% continued to complain of low desire following treatment. Overall, improvement was noted for only 44% of the women. The findings of this study are limited, given that many of these women had multiple sexual dysfunctions and there was no control group. In the study by Trudel et al., comparing cognitive-behavioral interventions specifically formulated to address desire disorders with a control group, 74% had improvement in function compared to 26% in the control group. Compared with the control group, CBT resulted in significant improvement in quality of sexual and marital life, sexual satisfaction, perception of sexual arousal, sexual self-esteem, and less depression and anxiety.

1. Althof SE, Leiblum SR, Chevret-Measson M, et al. Psychological and interpersonal dimensions of sexual function and dysfunction. *J Sex Med.* 2005;2:793–800.
2. McCabe MP. Evaluation of a cognitive behaviour therapy program for people with sexual dysfunction. *J Sex Marital Ther.* 2001;27:259–271.
3. Trudel G, Marchand A, Ravart M, et al. The effect of a cognitive behavioral group treatment program on hypoactive sexual desire in women. *Sex Rel Ther.* 2001;16:145–164.

144. Answer: D. Substance P is a short-chain polypeptide that belongs to the tachykinin neuropeptide family and functions as a neurotransmitter and a neuromodulator. Its primary role is in pain transmission. Stimulation of Substance P fibers produces burning pain. Capsaicin produces local anesthesia by depleting Substance P in the affected nerves. In the brain, Substance P neurons are concentrated in the nucleus of the tractus solitarius, around the cranial nerve nuclei, medullary tegmental nuclei, and in the parabrachial nucleus. They are also present in pontine nuclei, as well as in the caudal parts of the substantia nigra. They are also present in the cortex. Substance P can cause vasodilaton by the local release of nitric oxide from the endothelium, thus causing hypotension.

Schiffer RB, Rao SM, Fogel BS. *Neuropsychiatry.* 2nd ed. Philadelphia: Lippincott Williams & Wilkins; 2003:211.

145. Answer: B. The hallmark of a lesion in the region of the cerebellopontine angle is clinical evidence of damage to the seventh and eighth cranial nerves, so that a wide range of vestibular, auditory, and motor abnormalities occur. Common signs include: ipsilateral deafness, facial numbness, weakness, and ataxia. Tumors in the cavernous sinus may compromise third, fourth, or sixth cranial nerve functions, resulting in diplopia. Tumors affecting the jugular foramen affect cranial nerves IX, X, and XI, resulting in hoarseness, dysphagia, and pain in pharynx. The parasellar region is associated with cranial nerves II, IV, VI, and V_1, resulting in unilateral frontal headache, diplopia, and facial numbness. Superior orbital fissure location results in palsies of cranial nerves III, IV, and V, affecting the extraocular muscles.

1. Patten J. *Neurological Differential Diagnosis.* 2nd ed. New York: Springer; 2003:54, 61, 84.
2. Rowland LP. *Merritt's Neurology.* 11th ed. Philadelphia: Lippincott Williams & Wilkins; 2005:379, 422.

146. Answer: D. Noradrenergic neurons project diffusely from the locus coeruleus. Cholinergic neurons project diffusely from the nucleus basalis of Meynert and the basal forebrain/brainstem. Dopaminergic neurons project diffusely from the ventral tegmental area and substantia nigra. Serotoninergic neurons project diffusely from the dorsal raphe nuclei.

Kaufman DM. *Clinical Neurology for Psychiatrists.* 5th ed. Philadelphia: WB Saunders; 2001:552–569.

147. Answer: C. Typical signs of UMN injury include paresis with muscle spasticity (not flaccidity), hyperactive DTRs, and Babinski signs. Paresis with muscle flaccidity, atrophy, hypoactive DTRs, and lack of Babinski signs are all signs of lower motor neuron injury. Sensory loss by itself is not related to motor neuron injury.

Kaufman DM. *Clinical Neurology for Psychiatrists.* 5th ed. Philadelphia: WB Saunders; 2001:8–25.

148. Answer: D. Trihexyphenidyl (Artane) and benztropine (Cogentin) are anticholinergic medications that are sometimes used to treat parkinsonism. Common side effects of anticholinergic medications include dry mouth, urinary retention, and constipation (but not diarrhea). Anticholinergics can also cause memory impairment, and possibly precipitate a delirium in vulnerable patients such as those with underlying dementia.

Kaufman DM. *Clinical Neurology for Psychiatrists.* 5th ed. Philadelphia: WB Saunders; 2001:456.

149. Answer: B. According to Erikson, the major developmental task for old age is to look back across life (not forward as in other stages) and seek meaning, and maintain more integrity than despair in one's life. Conflicts of earlier life stages should be reconciled and integrated with this stage for resolution of earlier conflicts. Generativity versus stagnation is the directly preceding task in Erikson's stage theory, appropriate for mid-adulthood. Identity versus role confusion is appropriate for adolescence, industry versus inferiority for school-aged children, and trust versus mistrust for infancy. Developmental stages of Erikson's that are not mentioned in the answer set are autonomy versus shame for toddlerhood, and initiative versus guilt for preschool aged children.

1. Blazer DG, Steffens DC, Busse EW. *The American Psychiatric Association Textbook of Geriatric Psychiatry*. Washington: American Psychiatric Publishing; 2004:369–376.
2. Hales RE, Yudofsky SC. *Textbook of Clinical Psychiatry*. 4th ed. Washington: American Psychiatric Publishing; 2003:107–152.

150. Answer: C. The population prevalence for schizophrenia is about 1%. The risk of this illness developing in a first-degree relative (i.e., parents, siblings, and offspring) is about 10% (i.e., ten times more than the general population). When this is expressed as the recurrence risk ratio, the disease risk to first-degree relatives (i.e., parents, siblings, and offspring) divided by the population prevalence, the figure would be 10. The highest risk ratio among all psychiatric disorders is for Autism at about 50 to 100. For all other major psychiatric disorders like Bipolar Disorder, Major Depression, Alcoholism, and Panic Disorder, the risk ratio varies from 3 to 10.

Sadock BJ, Sadock VA. *Kaplan and Sadock's Comprehensive Textbook of Psychiatry*. 8th ed. Philadelphia: Lippincott Williams & Wilkins; 2005:239.

151. Answer: A. Pretreatment liver function tests are usually obtained because of the risk of hepatotoxicity, which range from mild dysfunction to hepatic necrosis. More commonly, valproate may cause a sustained, mild elevation in liver transaminase levels (as much as three times the upper limit of normal). Hepatic necrosis is rare and is more likely to occur in the young (younger than 2 years of age) and in those individuals taking multiple anticonvulsants. Valproate may also increase the risk of birth defects. A pretreatment urine pregnancy test is usually obtained in women of childbearing years. Women should be cautioned to use adequate contraception.

Hematological abnormalities are also possible and include leukopenia and thrombocytopenia. Hence, WBC and platelet counts are usually obtained. Acute pancreatitis may also occur, but amylase and lipase are not routinely followed. Renal function tests are routinely followed in patients taking lithium, not valproate.

1. Albers LJ, Hahn RK, Reist C. *Handbook of Psychiatric Drugs*. Laguna Hills: Current Clinical Strategies Publishing; 2005:82–85.
2. Sadock BJ, Sadock VA. *Kaplan and Sadock's Comprehensive Textbook of Psychiatry*. 8th ed. Philadelphia: Lippincott Williams & Wilkins; 2005:924.

152. Answer: D. Although conversion disorder is often comorbid with MDD, Anxiety Disorders, Schizophrenia, and Personality Disorders, it cannot be comorbid with Factitious Disorder because part of the diagnostic criteria, per the DSM-IV-TR, states that the "symptom or deficit is not intentionally produced or feigned (as in factitious disorder or malingering)."

Kaplan HI, Sadock BJ. *Kaplan & Sadock's Synopsis of Psychiatry*. 8th ed. Philadelphia: Lippincott Williams & Wilkins; 1998:634–636.

153. Answer: D. Many of the inhaled volatile gases of abuse (such as adhesives, nail polish removers, paint thinner, and gasoline) sensitize the myocardium to the effects of catecholamines, and can result in fatal arrhythmias. All of the other treatment modalities are not contraindicated in the management of the patient presenting with acute volatile gas intoxication.

Endom E. Inhalant Abuse in Children and Adolescents. http://www.uptodateonline.com/utd/content/topic.do? topicKey=ped_tox/6962&type=P&selectedTitle=3~5. Accessed January 22, 2007.

154. Answer: C. Personality traits have been implicated in the onset, expression, and maintenance of eating disorders. AN and BN are both consistently characterized by perfectionism, obsessive-compulsiveness, neuroticism, negative emotionality, harm avoidance, low self-directedness, low cooperativeness, and traits associated with avoidant personality disorder. Consistent differences that emerge between the eating disorder groups are high constraint and persistence and low novelty seeking in AN, as well as high impulsivity, sensation seeking, novelty seeking, and traits associated with Borderline PD in BN. A meta-analysis, which found PD rates of 0% to 58% among individuals with AN and BN, documented that self-report instruments greatly overestimate the prevalence of every PD.

Cassin S, von Ranson K. Personality and eating disorders: a decade in review. *Clin Psychol Rev*. 2005;25:895–916.

155. Answer: C. This patient meets most criteria for MDD, except for one important feature. MDD requires that potential medical causes be ruled out. Depression is common 6 months to a year after a stroke, and is usually more than just an adjustment to losses due to the illness. Formerly nonposterior, left hemisphere strokes were believed to be more likely than those in other locations to result in depression, but this is now being questioned. Despite some mild deficits on cognitive examination (MMSE: 25/30), there is not enough information to diagnose a vascular dementia. Such deficits may be due to her depression, as there are well known cognitive deficits that may appear somewhat like a dementia (e.g., *pseudodementia* or dementia of depression). The subtype of Vascular Dementia with Depression would first require that a dementia be diagnosed. Also, Delirium is less likely with a clear sensorium.

American Psychiatric Association. *Diagnostic and Statistical Manual of Mental Disorders American Psychiatric Association*. 4th ed. (Text revision). http://www.psychiatryonline.com/content.aspx?aID=2715. Accessed February 17, 2007.

156. Answers: A. Opiate-related disorders in pregnant women have far reaching ramifications, including abortion, contracting and transmitting HIV, as well as the development of specific neonatal opiate withdrawal syndrome. There are studies indicating that more than 70% of neonates born to opiate dependent mothers manifest symptoms of withdrawal at birth. Methadone substitution and maintenance therapy is becoming increasingly common. While the dosing schedules of such therapy are not universal, the consensus appears to favor a dose high enough to eliminate craving (and hence the possibility of resorting to external use) and low enough to decrease neonatal withdrawal symptoms at birth. A daily dose of 20 mg is generally recommended. If an expectant mother stable on daily methadone doses higher than 20 mg is admitted to a methadone maintenance program, the goal is to attempt to taper this by 1 to 2 mg weekly at gestation week 14 through week 32. A specific, opiate-withdrawal syndrome in infants born to opiate-dependent mothers has been described. Most infants manifest mild withdrawal symptoms (hyperactivity, exaggerated reflexes, diaphoresis, mottling, yawning, high-pitched cry, and anorexia) that require no specific pharmacologic interventions. A few infants may experience more severe symptoms (vomiting, seizure, and fever) and will require treatment with paregoric or phenobarbital.

1. Ebner N, Rohrmeister K, Winklbaur B, et al. Management of neonatal abstinence syndrome in neonates born to opioid maintained women. *Drug Alcohol Depend*. 2007;87:131–138.
2. Galanter M, Kleber HD. *Textbook of Substance Abuse Treatment*. 2nd ed. Washington: American Psychiatric Press; 1999:271–279.
3. Osborn DA, Jeffery HE, Cole M. Opiate treatment for opiate withdrawal in newborn infants. *Cochrane Database Syst Rev*. 2005;3:CD002059.

157. Answer: D. Individuals with psychopathic personality structure believe that everyone is selfish, manipulative, and dishonorable. They believe that love and kindness are illusory, and consequently devalue those who manifest these qualities. For instance, the therapist's empathy is seen as a weakness. Therefore, the most important features of treatment become incorruptibility of the therapist, the frame, and the conditions that make the therapy possible. In contrast, individuals with paranoid personality structure believe that the world is full of potential attackers. They tend to have histories marked by felt shame and humiliation. Hence, they expect to be humiliated by others and may attack first to spare themselves the agony of waiting for the inevitable attack from the outside. In addition, individuals with paranoid personality are capable of experiencing guilt, love, and empathy, unlike those with psychopathic personality structure.

1. McWilliams N. *Psychoanalytic Diagnosis: Understanding Personality Structure in the Clinical Process*. New York: Guilford Press; 1994:151–167, 205–226.
2. PDM Task Force. *Psychodynamic Diagnostic Manual*. Silver Spring: Alliance of Psychoanalytic Organizations; 2006:34–35, 36–37.

158. Answer: C. People whose personalities are organized around maintaining their self-esteem through affirmation from external sources are called *narcissistic* by psychoanalysts. Both narcissistic and hysterical individuals have basic self-esteem defects, deep shame, and the compensatory need for attention and reassurance (both idealize and devalue). But the sources of these similarities differ. For the hysterical person, self-esteem problems are related to gender identification or to particular conflicts, while with narcissistic people, they are diffuse. Self-psychologists have coined the term *self-objects* for the people in our lives who nourish our sense of identity and self-regard by their affirmation, admiration, and approval. The narcissistic person needs self-objects so greatly that other aspects of any relationship pale in comparison. Thus, the most grievous cost of a narcissistic orientation is a stunted capacity to love. Despite the importance of other people to the equilibrium of a narcissistic person, their need for reassurance about self-worth leaves no energy for others except in their function as self-objects and narcissistic extensions. On the other hand, hysterical people are warm and loving. They are capable of relating to others as objects, unlike narcissistic people who relate to others as self-objects. Hence, narcissistic patients require therapeutic attention to self-object phenomena, while hysterical patients thrive with an attention to object transferences. Guilt is the conviction that one is sinful or has committed wrongdoings. It is easily conceptualized in terms of an internal critical parent or superego. Shame is the sense of being seen as having an inherent defect, and therefore being bad or wrong (the audience is outside the self). Both narcissistic and hysterical self-assessment process leads to feeling inadequate, falling short of an ideal that one should be, and hence, ashamed. At the core of a narcissist's inner world is a secret wish to exhibit themselves in a grandiose manner, which leads to a deep sense of shame. Being confronted with deficiencies in one's abilities or the recognition of unsatisfied needs leads narcissistic people to feel humiliated and painfully exposed. As a result, their typical defenses (including defenses of idealization and devaluation) are designed to prevent awareness of such feelings. On the other hand, hysterical people idealize and devalue in specific, often gender-related, ways. In contrast, narcissistic people habitually rank all others in terms of better or worse, without the press of object-directed affects. Whereas guilty persons may feel they are not living up to a standard, they do not have the sense of being irreparably defective in the same way that narcissistic persons do. Guilt carries with it a sense of an active potential for evil, while shame has connotations of helplessness, ugliness, and impotence.

1. Gabbard GO. *Psychodynamic Psychiatry in Clinical Practice*. 3rd ed. Washington: American Psychiatric Press; 2000:468.
2. McWilliams N. *Psychoanalytic Diagnosis: Understanding Personality Structure in the Clinical Process*. New York: Guilford Press; 1994:168–188, 301–322.

159. **Answer: E.** When the psychiatrist is ordered by the court to reveal the confidences entrusted to them by patients, they may comply or they may ethically hold the right to dissent within the framework of the law. When the psychiatrist is in doubt, the right of the patient to confidentiality and, by extension, to unimpaired treatment should be given priority. The psychiatrist should reserve the right to raise the question of adequate need for disclosure. In the event that the necessity for legal disclosure is demonstrated by the court, the psychiatrist may request the right to disclosure of only that information which is relevant to the legal question at hand.

American Psychiatric Association. *The Principles of Medical Ethics*. http://www.psych.org/psych_pract/ethics/medical-ethics.cfm. Accessed March 29, 2007.

160. **Answer: C.** Sex therapy treatment of Erectile Dysfunction consists of a variety of interventions including: systematic desensitization, sensate focus, interpersonal therapy, behavioral assignments, sex education, communications and sexual skills training, and masturbation exercises. As of today, it has not been possible to statistically analyze the precise contribution of any of these single interventions to overall success. Men with lifelong and acquired erectile dysfunction typically achieve significant improvements early on and over the long term following participation in sex therapy. It has been found that men with acquired disorders tend to fare better than those with lifelong problems. Long-term follow-ups indicate that erectile dysfunction has a tendency to relapse and these rates may be up to 75%. Relapses may be prevented by periodic booster or maintenance sessions following termination of the initial therapy.

1. Althof SE, Leiblum SR, Chevret-Measson M, et al. Psychological and interpersonal dimensions of sexual function and dysfunction. *J Sex Med*. 2005;2:793–800.
2. Hawton K, Catalan J, Martin P, et al. Long-term outcome of sex therapy. *Behav Res Ther*. 1986;24:665–675.

161. **Answer: B.** Gerstmann's syndrome characterized by right–left disorientation, finger agnosia, acalculia (impaired calculation), and agraphia (impaired writing) occurs due to a dysfunction of the angular gyrus of the left hemisphere (parietal lobe). The treatment is mainly symptomatic supportive. Occupational and speech therapies may reduce dysgraphia and apraxia.

Waxman S. *Clinical Neuroanatomy*. 25th ed. http://www.accessmedicine.com/content.aspx?aID=152446. Accessed February 21, 2007.

162. **Answer: A.** The basal ganglia are essentially composed of five subcortical, macroscopic nuclei: the caudate nucleus and the putamen (which form the corpus striatum), the GPi, the STN, and the substantia nigra. When properly functioning, the caudate nucleus acts as a gatekeeper to allow the motor system to perform only those acts that are goal directed. When it fails, extraneous acts are performed, as in OCD or Tourette's. In Huntington's disease, the caudate shrinks dramatically and results in choreiform movements. The GPi may be severely damaged in Wilson's disease and in carbon monoxide poisoning, which are characterized by dystonic posturing and flapping movements of the extremities. GPi and the putamen form the lenticular nucleus, and pathology involving the lentiform nucleus occurs in neurodegeneration with brain iron accumulation, Wilson's disease, and infarction resulting in dystonia. Part of

the substantia nigra is what degenerates in Parkinson's. Lesions in the STN yield ballistic movements.

1. Kaplan HI, Sadock BJ. *Kaplan & Sadock's Synopsis of Psychiatry*. 8th ed. Philadelphia: Lippincott Williams & Wilkins; 1998:87.
2. Rowland LP. *Merritt's Neurology*. 11th ed. Philadelphia: Lippincott Williams & Wilkins; 2005:821.

163. Answer: C. Randomized controlled trials assessing the efficacy of medications for the treatment of tremors in early PD indicate that although anticholinergics like trihexylphenidyl are effective in the treatment of this condition, they are now rarely used because of their side effect profile. These drugs are generally not recommended for elderly patients over 65 years of age or for patients with cognitive decline. Both dopaminergic and anticholinergics agents are equally effective in treating parkinsonian tremors, but dopaminergic agents additionally treat other parkinsonian symptoms. Dopamine agonists like pramipexole and ropinirole are probably the most effective antitremor drugs among all the dopaminergic agents. They should be considered in the treatment of tremors in all newly diagnosed PD patients who have no cognitive impairment. Other dopamine agonists like pergolide and bromocriptine also treat tremors in PD patients. Dopamine agonists are also useful in advanced PD patients with tremor, who are refractory to treatment with L-dopa or anticholinergics drugs.

Bhidayasiri R. Differential diagnosis of common tremor syndromes. *Postgrad Med J*. 2005;81:756–762.

164. Answer: D. Most long-term care of older patients with disabilities is provided in the home. Family members provide much of this care informally. However, home health services comprise another important part of care for the elderly. In-home assistance has allowed many older adults to remain in the home longer. Additionally, the emergence of assisted living facilities has offered an alternative to the nursing home for many people who require some assistance with instrumental activities of daily living. However, nursing homes remain a vital residential care setting for the oldest and most disabled individuals. Perhaps in response to the trend of shortened length of hospital stays, nursing homes now often include subacute rehabilitation units. Dementia care units are available at some nursing homes and specialize in the care of patients with dementia, who may be prone to wandering and other behavioral disturbances.

Sadavoy J, Jarvik LF, Grossberg GT, et al. *Comprehensive Textbook of Geriatric Psychiatry*. New York: WW Norton & Company; 2004:1071–1073.

165. Answer: D. The catecholamines (including norepinephrine, epinephrine, and dopamine) are products of enzymatic reactions beginning with the substrate tyrosine. The rate-limiting step in the synthesis of catecholamines occurs when tyrosine is converted to DOPA via tyrosine hydroxylase. Dopamine is converted to norepinephrine by beta-hydroxylase. Norepinephrine is produced in the lateral brainstem tegmentum and the locus ceruleus of the pons, not the raphe nuclei – where serotonin is produced.

Kaplan HI, Sadock BJ. *Kaplan & Sadock's Synopsis of Psychiatry*. 8th ed. Philadelphia: Lippincott Williams & Wilkins; 1998:107, 113–115.

166. Answer: C. Routine laboratory tests before the initiation of TCAs or tricyclic antidepressants typically include a CBC, serum electrolytes, and liver function tests. Liver function tests allow monitoring for the TCA hepatotoxicity with hepatitis and potential hepatic failure. CBC allows monitoring for the rare TCA side effects of agranulocytosis, neutropenia, and anemia. Serum electrolytes allow monitoring for the syndrome of inappropriate antidiuretic hormone secretion with hyponatremia, which has been reported in patients receiving tricyclics and other antidepressants (including SSRIs). Because TCAs effect cardiac conduction, clinicians may obtain an EKG to rule out abnormal cardiac rhythms and prolonged PR interval, QRS complexes and QTc interval, before the initiation of these medications. When the QTc interval is longer than 0.440 seconds, a patient is at increased risk for potentially fatal cardiac arrhythmias such as torsade de pointes. Heart rate may also be increased from the anticholinergic effects of the medication. Pretreatment EKGs are commonly obtained in patients older than 40 years of age to exclude a QTc interval of longer than 0.440 seconds, a QRS interval of longer than 0.10 seconds, or bundle branch block. TCAs could affect prolactin secretion by disturbing the balance of catecholaminergic inhibition and serotonergic stimulation of prolactin release, although any change is less than with antipsychotic therapy. Clomipramine and nortriptyline had been reported to stimulate prolactin release whereas amitriptyline, desipramine, and imipramine had been reported to be without effect. Such stimulation may account for symptoms of galactorrhea or amenorrhoea reported with some tricyclics. However, prolactin level is not monitored routinely in TCA therapy.

1. Albers LJ, Hahn RK, Reist C. *Handbook of Psychiatric Drugs*. Laguna Hills: Current Clinical Strategies Publishing; 2005:23–27.

2. Sadock BJ, Sadock VA. *Kaplan and Sadock's Comprehensive Textbook of Psychiatry*. 8th ed. Philadelphia: Lippincott Williams & Wilkins; 2005:924.

167. **Answer: C.** There is a high comorbidity between PTSD and Borderline Personality Disorder and there may be a causal relationship. As many as 68% of patients with PTSD have Borderline Personality Disorder and there is a suggestion that patients with Borderline Personality Disorder are more predisposed to developing PTSD.

1. Classen CC, Pain C, Field NP, et al. Posttraumatic personality disorder: a reformulation of complex posttraumatic stress disorder and borderline personality disorder. *Psychiatr Clin North Am*. 2006;29:87–112, viii–ix.
2. Kaplan HI, Sadock BJ. *Kaplan & Sadock's Synopsis of Psychiatry*. 8th ed. Philadelphia: Lippincott Williams & Wilkins; 1998:621.

168. **Answer: A.** Psychiatric patients who come from families with what is called *high expressed emotion* do have increased relapse rates. Such families are overly involved and their overinvolvement can take the form of criticism, hostility, and/or infantilizing behavior. However, it is not known to be associated with mania or bipolar disorder in many family members. Intervention with such families is thought to help lower relapse rates of psychiatric illness. There is no clear evidence that high expressed emotion causes Schizophrenia. Gregory Bateson developed the concept of the *double bind*, another theory about families of patients with schizophrenia. The idea behind this theory is that patients with Schizophrenia come from families where they receive contradictory messages from their parents regarding, e.g., their behavior and feelings. (Studies have not borne out this theory as a causal explanation for Schizophrenia.)

1. Kaplan HI, Sadock BJ. *Kaplan & Sadock's Synopsis of Psychiatry*. 8th ed. Philadelphia: Lippincott Williams & Wilkins; 1998:466.
2. Sadock BJ, Sadock VA. *Pocket Handbook of Clinical Psychiatry*. 3rd ed. Philadelphia: Lippincott Williams & Wilkins; 2001:106–107.

169. **Answer: E.** Robert Post and colleagues put forth the idea that an oligoepisodic disorder initially triggered by environmental stressors could assume an autonomous and polyepisodic course. Kindling represents a process in which increasing behavioral and convulsive responses occur to repetition of the same stimulus over time.

1. Post RM. Neurobiology of seizures and behavioral abnormalities. *Epilepsia*. 2004;45(supp 2):5–14.
2. Post RM, Uhde TW, Putnam FW, et al. Kindling and carbamazepine in affective illness. *J Nerv Ment Dis*. 1982;170:717–731.

3. Sadock BJ, Sadock VA. *Kaplan and Sadock's Comprehensive Textbook of Psychiatry*. 8th ed. Philadelphia: Lippincott Williams & Wilkins; 2005:1571.

170. **Answer: E.** Mania can present for the first time at age 45, but other potential likely causes would need to be ruled out. Corticosteroids are a common cause of iatrogenic mania and/or psychosis. His behavior change occurred after treatment was begun for his infection, and leukocytosis and hyperglycemia can be explained by the steroids; otherwise, there are no signs of infection in this patient. Antidepressants may induce mania; however, this patient had been stable on fluoxetine for years, so this is less likely. Acute drug intoxication (with cocaine or others) could result in a similar presentation, but the drug screen is negative, he has no history of drug use, and there is another common explanation. Of note, certain antibiotics, especially quinolones, are often the cause of altered mentation and mood.

Brown ES, Suppes T, Khan DA, et al. Mood changes during prednisone bursts in outpatients with asthma. *J Clin Psychopharmacol*. 2002;22:55–61.

171. **Answer: D.** While the dosing schedules of methadone substitution and maintenance therapy in pregnancy are not universal, the consensus appears to favor a dose high enough to eliminate craving (and hence the possibility of resorting to external use) and low enough to decrease neonatal withdrawal symptoms at birth. A daily dose of 20 mg is generally recommended. If an expectant mother stable on daily methadone doses higher than 20 mg is admitted to a methadone maintenance program, the goal is to attempt to taper this by 1 to 2 mg weekly at gestation week 14 through week 32. Patients on methadone replacement and maintenance therapy require close monitoring, as some of these patients have been known to ingest additional amounts of opiate derived from "non-treatment" sources, potentially leading to opiate intoxication. Although postdelivery volume shifts may affect the bioavailability of pharmacologic agents, in a patient previously tolerant of a given dose of methadone, an external source of opiate is the most likely explanation for sudden onset of intoxication. Acute opioid intoxication accompanied by respiratory suppression or coma is a medical emergency and treatment is best accomplished in the hospital setting. Therapeutic strategies include cardiopulmonary resuscitation and the administration of intravenous naloxone at a dosage 0.4 mg to be repeated several times at an interval of 2 minutes until adequate spontaneous respiratory effort is achieved.

1. Galanter M, Kleber HD. *Textbook of Substance Abuse Treatment*. 2nd ed. Washington: American Psychiatric Press; 1999:271–279.

2. Wilbourne P, Wallerstedt C, Dorato V, et al. Clinical management of methadone dependence during pregnancy. *J Perinat Neonatal Nurs*. 2001;14:26–45.

172. Answer: C. Individuals with depressive personality structure believe that there is something essentially bad or incomplete about them. They look inward to find the explanation for painful experiences. When mistreated, rejected, or abandoned, they tend to believe they are somehow at fault. This belief may be a residue of the familiar tendency of children in difficult family situations to deny that their caregivers are negligent, abusive, or fragile (ideas that are too frightening). Instead, they attribute their suffering to their own badness (something they can try to change). Thus, depressive people work hard to be "good," but rarely succeed to their own satisfaction.

In contrast, individuals with narcissistic personality structure believe that they need to be perfect to feel okay. The characteristic subjective experience of narcissistic individuals is a sense of inner emptiness and meaninglessness that requires recurrent infusions of external confirmation of their importance and value.

1. McWilliams N. *Psychoanalytic Diagnosis: Understanding Personality Structure in the Clinical Process*. New York: Guilford Press; 1994:168–188, 227–256.
2. PDM Task Force. *Psychodynamic Diagnostic Manual*. Silver Spring: Alliance of Psychoanalytic Organizations; 2006:38–39, 44–46.

173. Answer: D. There is a very close connection between psychopathic and narcissistic conditions. Both character types reflect a subjectively empty internal world and a dependence on external events to provide self-esteem. Kernberg and Meloy put psychopathy and narcissism on one dimension, characterized overall as narcissistic; thus, the psychopath is considered to be on the pathological end of the narcissistic continuum. McWilliams argues that antisocial and narcissistic people are different enough to warrant a continuum for each. Most psychopathic people do not idealize repetitively and most narcissistic ones do not depend on omnipotent control. But many people have aspects of both character types, and self-inflation can characterize either one.

Omnipotent control is the fantasy that one is in control of all they come in contact with. This is a normal stage of development for children, but as the child matures they realize that no one's power is unlimited. A healthy amount of this omnipotence should remain in us all and contributes to feelings of efficacy and competence in life. For both narcissists and psychopaths, the need to feel this omnipotence, and to interpret experiences as a result of their own power, is more attractive than reality. Because treat-

ment considerations are quite different for the two groups (e.g., sympathetic mirroring comforts most narcissistic people but antagonizes antisocial ones) despite the things they have in common and the number of people who have aspects of each orientation, it may be useful to differentiate carefully between them.

McWilliams N. *Psychoanalytic Diagnosis: Understanding Personality Structure in the Clinical Process*. New York: Guilford Press; 1994:103–105, 153–155, 166, 173–174.

174. Answer: E. Risk factors most consistently associated with PSD are a past history of depression, past personal psychiatric history, dysphasia, functional impairments, living alone, and poststroke social isolation. Risk factors not associated with PSD are dementia and cognitive impairment. Controversial risk factors are age, socioeconomic status, prior social distress, dependency in regard to activities of daily living, and sex.

1. Ouimet MA, Primeau F, Cole MG. Psychosocial risk factors in poststroke depression: a systematic review. *Can J Psychiatry*. 2001;46:819–828.
2. Williams LS. Depression and stroke: cause or consequence? *Semin Neurol*. 2005;25:396–409.

175. Answer: E. Currently, hypnosis is largely used as an adjunctive technique that can be integrated with cognitive, behavioral, or psychodynamic therapies. Although such integration has been feasible, it is still unclear whether the inclusion of the hypnosis increases the efficacy of the primary treatment. However, a recent metaanalysis comparing CBT with the same treatment supplemented by hypnosis found the mean effect size for the CBT treatment supplemented by hypnosis to be significantly larger than CBT alone. Still no hypnotically augmented CBT has met the criteria for well established treatment and the mechanisms of action of hypnosis are still not well understood. Although hypnosis has been shown to be helpful in treating some of the symptoms of PTSD, it would not be appropriate to state that it has the best evidence.

Alladin A, Sabatini L, Amundson JK. What should we mean by empirical validation in hypnotherapy: evidence-based practice in clinical hypnosis. *Int J Clin Exp Hypn*. 2007;55:115–130.

176. Answer: E. Ventromedial nucleus, when stimulated, inhibits the urge to eat. Destruction of this nucleus (bilaterally) results in hyperphagia, obesity, and savage behaviors. Anterior nucleus is excitatory to the parasympathetic nervous system and is involved in temperature regulation. Destruction of this nucleus results in hyperthermia. Posterior nucleus plays a role in conservation and increased heat production.

Lesions of this nucleus result in the inability to regulate heat (i.e., poikilothermia). Mamillary nucleus is part of the Papez circuit and receives input from the hippocampal formation and projects fibers to the anterior nucleus of the thalamus via the mamillothalamic tract. Lesions of the mamillary nucleus are seen in patients with Wernicke's encephalopathy (WE) and in alcoholic patients. Suprachiasmatic nucleus receives direct input from the retina and is responsible for the regulation of the circadian rhythms.

Fix JD. *High-Yield Neuroanatomy*. Philadelphia: Lippincott Williams & Wilkins; 1995:84–87.

177. Answer: B. The syndrome with the above characteristics is known as Kluver-Bucy syndrome and is a result of bilateral damage to the amygdala, located in the temporal lobe. The arcuate fasciculus is important for language in that it connects the temporal with the frontal lobes, and a lesion here will result in conduction aphasia. Wernicke-Korsakoff's encephalopathy (confabulations and anterograde amnesia) is associated with damage to the bilateral mamillary bodies in chronic alcoholics. Lethargy or coma follows damage to the reticular activating system, which is a diffuse set of neurons that appears to set the level of consciousness. Lesions in the STN (part of basal ganglia) yield ballistic movements.

1. Kaplan HI, Sadock BJ. *Kaplan & Sadock's Synopsis of Psychiatry*. 8th ed. Philadelphia: Lippincott Williams & Wilkins; 1998:87, 90–93.
2. Patten J. *Neurological Differential Diagnosis*. 2nd ed. New York: Springer; 2003:156.
3. Rowland LP. *Merritt's Neurology*. 11th ed. Philadelphia: Lippincott Williams & Wilkins; 2005:8.

178. Answer: C. Cognitive dysfunctions are seen in about 65% of patients with MS. These patients present with problems in short-term memory, attention, concentration, and processing of information. Abnormalities of language, as well as immediate and long-term memory are also seen. Cognitive difficulties also lead to disability independent of physical disability and can cause dependence on others. These patients are also more likely to be socially withdrawn or unemployed. Patients with cognitive impairment have more disease burden, as measured by lesions on MRI and measurements of brain volume. Cognitive dysfunctions can also occur early in the course of the disease. Drugs like beta-interferons and glatiramer may be helpful in slowing down the progression of the cognitive decline. These symptoms may also be seen in depressed patients and fatigued patients. Neuropsychological testing may be needed to differentiate true cognitive dysfunction from cognitive dysfunction seen in patients with depression and fatigue symptoms. Cognitive therapy and retraining may be beneficial in some patients. Preliminary evidence suggests that cholinesterase inhibitors like donepezil, rivastigmine, or galantamine may be of benefit in patients with MS and cognitive impairment.

Schwendimann RN. Treatment of symptoms in multiple sclerosis. *Neurol Res*. 2006;28:306–315.

179. Answer: B. Although Schizophrenia exists worldwide, it is not equally distributed and, in fact, the presence of clusters of Schizophrenia has led to the hypothesis by some researchers of an infectious etiology. It is equally prevalent in men and women. And people born in the winter and early spring are more likely to develop it. Although suicide completion is 10% to 15%, half of all patients with schizophrenia will attempt suicide during their lifetimes.

Kaplan HI, Sadock BJ. *Kaplan & Sadock's Synopsis of Psychiatry*. 8th ed. Philadelphia: Lippincott Williams & Wilkins; 1998:457–459.

180. Answer: D. All four of these neurotransmitters (dopamine, glutamate, norepinephrine, and GABA) have been implicated in pathogenesis of schizophrenia.

Kaplan HI, Sadock BJ. *Kaplan & Sadock's Synopsis of Psychiatry*. 8th ed. Philadelphia: Lippincott Williams & Wilkins; 1998:460–461.

181. Answer: E. A diagnosis of Schizophrenia requires two active core symptoms (such as delusions, hallucinations, disorganized speech or behavior, catatonic behavior, or negative symptoms) for a period of a month or more, or only one symptom if delusions are bizarre or if voices consist of conversing or a running commentary. There also must be some symptoms continuously apparent for the past six months, social dysfunction, and no evidence of contributing/explanatory mood disorder, medical illness, or drug use. Although her prominent delusion lasted more than a month, delusional disorder is not appropriate in this case, because there are other prominent symptoms, and the delusions are bizarre in nature. Schizoaffective Disorder requires mood episode symptoms with active phase Schizophrenia symptoms, and a 2-week period of psychosis without prominent mood symptoms. This patient does not currently have mood symptoms, and may eventually develop a schizoaffective disorder, but does not currently meet the criteria. Schizophreniform disorder is similar to Schizophrenia, only the total duration of symptoms is between 1 and 6 months. Brief

Psychotic Disorder has psychotic symptoms that remit between 1 day and 1 month.

1. American Psychiatric Association. *Diagnostic and Statistical Manual of Mental Disorders American Psychiatric Association*. 4th ed. (Text revision). http://www.psychiatryonline.com/content.aspx?aID=8939. Accessed February 15, 2007.
2. Hales RE, Yudofsky SC. *Textbook of Clinical Psychiatry*. 4th ed. Washington: American Psychiatric Publishing; 2003:379–439.

182. Answer: C. Urine porphobilinogens and δ-amino-levulinic acid are elevated during acute attacks of acute intermittent porphyria. It is autosomal dominantly inherited, so family history is important, and may present with acute psychosis, often with abdominal pain or other symptoms. Serum ceruloplasmin or slit-lamp exam for Kaiser-Fleischer rings would be useful for evaluation if you suspected Wilson's disease, a derangement in copper metabolism. ANA is a nonspecific rheumatologic/immunologic laboratory exam. Spinal tap for CSF evaluation is not yet indicated or necessary, although it may be if other tests return negative and the clinical picture worsens or changes. MS would not likely present with this full cluster of symptoms, including abdominal pain and a positive family history.

1. Cassem NH, Stern TA, Rosenbaum JF, et al. *Massachusetts General Hospital Handbook of General Hospital Psychiatry*. 4th ed. St. Louis: Mosby; 1997:149–171.
2. Croarkin P. From King George to neuroglobin: the psychiatric aspects of acute intermittent porphyria. *J Psychiatr Pract*. 2002;8:398–405.
3. Ellencweig N, Schoenfeld N, Zemishlany Z. Acute intermittent porphyria: psychosis as the only clinical manifestation. *Isr J Psychiatry Relat Sci*. 2006;43:52–56.

183. Answer: C. Methadone substitution and maintenance therapy is becoming increasingly common. While the dosing schedules of such therapy are not universal, the consensus appears to favor a dose high enough to eliminate craving (and hence the possibility of resorting to external use) and low enough to decrease neonatal withdrawal symptoms at birth. A daily dose of 20 mg is generally recommended. If an expectant mother stable on daily methadone doses higher than 20 mg is admitted to a methadone maintenance program, the goal is to attempt to taper this by 1 to 2 mg weekly at gestation week 14 through week 32. Patients on methadone replacement and maintenance therapy require close monitoring as some of these patients have been known to ingest additional amounts of opiate derived from "non-treatment" sources, potentially leading to opiate intoxication. Although postdelivery volume shifts may affect the bioavailability of pharmacologic agents, in a patient previously tolerant of a given dose of methadone, an external source of opiate is the most likely explanation for sudden onset of intoxication. Acute opioid intoxication accompanied by respiratory suppression or coma is a medical emergency and treatment is best accomplished in the hospital setting. Therapeutic strategies include cardiopulmonary resuscitation and the administration of intravenous naloxone at a dosage of 0.4 mg to be repeated several times at intervals of 2 minutes until adequate spontaneous respiratory effort is achieved. Owing to the short half-life of naloxone, failure to administer repeated doses may result in reversal of cardiopulmonary stability.

1. Galanter M, Kleber HD. *Textbook of Substance Abuse Treatment*. 2nd ed. Washington: American Psychiatric Press; 1999:271–279.
2. Wilbourne P, Wallerstedt C, Dorato V, et al. Clinical management of methadone dependence during pregnancy. *J Perinat Neonatal Nurs*. 2001;14:26–45.

184. Answer: C. Individuals with obsessive-compulsive personality structure believe that their aggression is dangerous, and it must be controlled. Psychoanalytic clinical experience and research suggest that obsessive-compulsive people fear that their impulses, especially their aggressive urges, will get out of control. Most obsessive thoughts and compulsive actions involve efforts to undo or counteract impulses towards messiness, destructiveness, and greed. They seem to have identified with caregivers who expected them to be more grown-up than was possible at the time. They regard expressions of affect or subjectivity as "immature."

In contrast, individuals with anxious personality structure believe that they are in constant danger from forces unknown. They experience a "free-floating," global sense of anxiety, often with no idea what frightens them.

1. McWilliams N. *Psychoanalytic Diagnosis: Understanding Personality Structure in the Clinical Process*. New York: Guilford Press; 1994:279–300.
2. PDM Task Force. *Psychodynamic Diagnostic Manual*. Silver Spring: Alliance of Psychoanalytic Organizations; 2006:56, 57–59.

185. Answer: B. Phototherapy has been the most widely studied treatment for SAD. Studies of light therapy indicate that an average dosage of 2,500 lux daily for 1 week was superior to placebo, as indicated by improvements on a depression rating scale. The dosage most often found to be effective is 5,000 lux per day, given as 2,500 lux for 2 hours or 10,000 lux for 30 minutes. A recent meta-analysis of twenty-three studies of light therapy found that the odds ratio for remission was 2.9 (95% CI: 1.6 to 5.4), which is similar to ratio of pharmacotherapy for depression. Similar to drug therapy for depression, phototherapy carries some risk of precipitating mania. Light therapy generally is most effective when administered earlier in the day. Early morning light therapy regulates the circadian pattern of melatonin secretion, whereas the use of light in the evening delays the normal melatonin phase shift. To ensure adequate light exposure, patients should be treated with phototherapy units that are specifically designed to treat SAD.

1. Golden RN, Gaynes BN, Ekstrom RD, et al. The efficacy of light therapy in the treatment of mood disorders: a review and meta-analysis of the evidence. *Am J Psychiatry.* 2005;162:656–662.
2. Lurie SJ, Gawinski B, Pierce D, et al. Seasonal affective disorder. *Am Fam Physician.* 2006;74:1521–1524.

186. Answer: B. Duloxetine is a serotonin and norepinephrine reuptake inhibitor effective in the treatment of major depression and diabetic neuropathy. It is metabolized by the cytochrome P 4502D6 and 1A2 hepatic microsomal enzyme system and has a half-life of 12 hours. It can cause a discontinuation syndrome if abruptly discontinued. However, no dosage adjustments are needed in elderly patients. Average dose of Duloxetine is 30 mg twice a day orally.

Albers LJ, Hahn RK, Reist C. *Handbook of Psychiatric Drugs.* Laguna Hills: Current Clinical Strategies Publishing; 2005:17–18.

187. Answer: C. Of all the choices, the only one that is not an indication for couple's therapy is couple problems that are ego syntonic.

Hales RE, Yudofsky SC. *American Psychiatric Publishing Textbook of Clinical Psychiatry.* 4th ed. http://www.psychiatryonline.com/content.aspx?aID=94999. Accessed April 4, 2007.

188. Answer: C. The paraventricular nucleus regulates the water balance. It produces the antidiuretic hormone, the corticotrophin-releasing hormone, and oxytocin. It projects to the neurohypophysis via the supraopticohypophyseal tract. Lesion of this nucleus results in diabetes mellitus. Suprachiasmatic nucleus receives direct input from the retina and is responsible for the regulation of the circadian rhythms. Stimulation of the lateral nucleus results in the urge to eat. Bilateral destruction of this nucleus results in starvation and emaciation. The arcuate nucleus is also called the *infundibular nucleus* and contains the neurons that produce the hypothalamic releasing and inhibiting factors. It also gives rise to tuberohypophysial tract, which ends in the median eminence. This nucleus

also contains neurons that produce dopamine. Inhibition of these neurons results in hyperprolactinemia. Medial preoptic nucleus regulates the release of gonadotropic hormones from the adenohypophysis.

Fix JD. *High-Yield Neuroanatomy.* Philadelphia: Lippincott Williams & Wilkins; 1995:84–87.

189. Answer: A. Depression is very common in patients with MS. Severe depression in MS is however highly correlated with cerebral involvement.

1. Kaufman DM. *Clinical Neurology for Psychiatrists.* 5th ed. Philadelphia: WB Saunders; 2001:375–376.
2. Rowland LP. *Merritt's Neurology.* 11th ed. Philadelphia: Lippincott Williams & Wilkins; 2005:950.

190. Answer: D. This patient has developed WE due to the deficiency of thiamine. The clinical features of WE include a sub-acute onset of ocular palsies, nystagmus, gait ataxia, and confusion. Other features include hypothermia and orthostatic hypotension. More than 80% of these patients may also have an associated peripheral neuropathy. Starting intravenous glucose infusion in patients who have thiamine deficiency may consume the available thiamine and precipitate an acute WE. At-risk patients should always receive parenteral thiamine before administration of glucose or parenteral nutrition. The recommended dose of thiamine is 100 mg intravenously for 5 days followed by oral maintenance doses of thiamine (50 to 100 mg/day). At times, high-dosage thiamine (100 mg intravenously every 8 hours) may be required in the first few days of treatment. Response to treatment in WE is variable. Ocular signs improve in a few hours, although a fine horizontal nystagmus may persist in 60% of patients. Improvement in gait ataxia and memory is variable and often delayed. Apathy and lethargy improve over days or weeks. Even with thiamine treatment, the mortality rate remains at about 10% to 20%. Following appropriate treatment, some patients are left with Korsakoff's psychosis a disorder of impaired memory and learning.

1. Kumar N. Nutritional neuropathies. *Neurol Clin.* 2007;25:209–255.
2. Thomson AD, Marshall EJ. The natural history and pathophysiology of Wernicke's Encephalopathy and Korsakoff's Psychosis. *Alcohol Alcohol.* 2006;41:151–158.

191. Answer: E. Delirium tremens occurs in approximately 5% of hospitalized patients suffering from alcohol withdrawal. Close monitoring of alcohol withdrawal symptoms and prompt initiation of treatment are key in the prevention of DTs. When DTs are detected promptly and treated appropriately, the mortality rate is approximately 1% (much less than the mortality rate of 20% that has historically been reported). When it does occur, death is typically secondary to cardiovascular collapse or comorbid infection. Treatment of DTs often includes fluid repletion and correction of nutritional deficiencies and electrolyte imbalances. As with all alcohol withdrawal syndromes, benzodiazepines (typically lorazepam or chlordiazepoxide) are the mainstay of treatment. They help reduce autonomic arousal and prevent seizures. They are also beneficial in calming agitated patients. Antipsychotic medications may be required if patients are particularly agitated from hallucinations, although careful consideration must be given to use of these medications as they can lower seizure threshold.

Wright T, Myrick H, Henderson S, et al. Risk factors for delirium tremens: a retrospective chart review. *Am J Addict*. 2006;15:213–219.

192. **Answer: C.** Social skills training is a form of behavior therapy used to help patients with schizophrenia. It is not geared towards patients' developing insight. Rather, it helps them develop behavior that enhances such things as communication skills, dating skills, and job performance skills (skills that improve their social interactions).

Kaplan HI, Sadock BJ. *Kaplan & Sadock's Synopsis of Psychiatry*. 8th ed. Philadelphia: Lippincott Williams & Wilkins; 1998:488–489.

193. **Answer: B.** The belief that a neighbor is stealing from them could be potentially true. If untrue, it may be a non-bizarre paranoid or persecutory delusion, that may add to the symptom pattern for the A criteria of schizophrenia. The A criteria for the DSM-IV-TR diagnosis of schizophrenia requires two of five symptoms: (i) hallucinations, (ii) delusions, (iii) disorganized speech, (iv) grossly disorganized or catatonic behavior, or (v) negative symptoms. Only one symptom is required if the delusions are bizarre, or if the hallucinations include conversing voices or a running commentary.

1. American Psychiatric Association. *Diagnostic and Statistical Manual of Mental Disorders American Psychiatric Association*. 4th ed. (Text revision). http://www.psychiatry-online.com/content.aspx?aID=8939. Accessed February 15, 2007.
2. Hales RE, Yudofsky SC. *Textbook of Clinical Psychiatry*. 4th ed. Washington: American Psychiatric Publishing; 2003:379–439.

194. **Answer: D.** This patient has signs and symptoms most consistent with hyperthyroidism or some other medical cause (e.g., diabetes, Cushing's syndrome, hypoglycemia, etc.) of anxiety, and appropriate laboratory testing would be the next step in evaluation. Coor-

dinating care with a primary care provider will be important in continued evaluation and management of this patient. Regardless of whether her anxiety is organic in origin, she should be followed by a primary care provider. Relaxation and cognitive therapy would be a harmless adjunct, as long as medical etiologies are also pursued, and the patient is not left with the impression that they are curative without further work-up. Dexamethasone suppression test is a sometimes useful evaluation, but other medical etiologies are likely here. Prescribing benzodiazepines or SSRIs without completing your differential, especially in a case with obvious physical signs and symptoms, may lead to missing a true underlying general medical diagnosis. A full neurological examination would also be helpful in this case.

1. Cassem NH, Stern TA, Rosenbaum JF, et al. *Massachusetts General Hospital Handbook of General Hospital Psychiatry*. 4th ed. St. Louis: Mosby; 1997:173–210.
2. Simon NM, Blacker D, Korbly NB, et al. Hypothyroidism and hyperthyroidism in anxiety disorders revisited: new data and literature review. *J Affect Disord*. 2002;69:209–217.

195. **Answer: B.** This patient is presenting with an expressive aphasia from a lesion affecting the Broca's area, which in most people resides in the left hemisphere, and thus the artery supplying this part of the brain is the left middle cerebral artery. Lesions involving the right-middle cerebral artery are usually not associated with aphasia, but are associated with spatial neglect syndrome. Posterior cerebral artery strokes and basilar strokes affect the posterior circulation of the brainstem and brain and often produce unilateral or bilateral motor/sensory deficits, and may be accompanied by cranial nerve and brainstem signs, although speech is rarely affected.

Rowland LP. *Merritt's Neurology*. 11th ed. Philadelphia: Lippincott Williams & Wilkins; 2005:295, 299–300.

196. **Answer: A.** A chemical must meet four criteria in order to be classified as a neurotransmitter. The criteria are: (a) the molecule is synthesized in a neuron, (b) the molecule is present in the presynaptic neuron and is released on depolarization in physiologically significant amounts, (c) when administered exogenously, it mimics the effects of the endogenous neurotransmitter, and (d) a mechanism in the neurons or the synaptic cleft acts to remove or deactivate the molecule. There are three major types of neurotransmitters. They include biogenic amines, amino acids, and peptides. The biogenic amine neurotransmitters are dopamine, norepinephrine, epinephrine, serotonin, acetylcholine, and histamine. Amino acid neurotransmitters include GABA, glycine, and glutamic

acid. The peptide neurotransmitters comprise neurotensin, thyrotropin-releasing hormone, and cholecystokinin octapeptide.

Sadock BJ, Sadock VA. *Kaplan and Sadock's Synopsis of Psychiatry*. 9th ed. Philadelphia: Lippincott Williams & Wilkins; 2003:88–108.

197. Answer: C. If pharmacological treatments prove to be ineffective, inadequate, or inappropriate, many patients may need nonpharmacological treatment for their migraine headaches. Clinical trials support the notion that nonpharmacological therapies can be a first choice for patients in need of prevention, either in monotherapy or as an adjunct to drugs. The most common therapies include relaxation, cognitive-behavioural therapy, and BF. Available evidence indicates that these therapies are effective in the treatment of migraine. However, no single method has been found to be clearly superior. When using the headache index (a composite score of frequency, severity, and/or duration) as a guide to treatment efficacy, these therapies reduced the headache index by 50% or more in 30% to 60% of patients, which is identical to the effect of commonly used prophylactic drugs. The initial effects from these therapies appear to be maintained for several years, but change mechanisms in these treatments have not yielded any clear results. Nonpharmacological treatments are a viable option for treatment of common migraines, but in more complicated cases, conjoint therapy should be considered.

1. Goadsby PJ. Migraine: diagnosis and management. *Intern Med J*. 2003;33:436–442.
2. Linde M. Migraine: a review and future directions for treatment. *Acta Neurol Scand*. 2006;114:71–83.

198. Answer: D. Migraine is one of the most frequent disabling neurological conditions with a major impact on the patients' quality of life. The available evidence indicates that for acute treatment of migraine attacks, oral NSAIDs and triptans are first-line treatments. Before intake of NSAIDs and triptans, oral metoclopramide or domperidone is recommended. In very severe attacks, intravenous acetylsalicylic acid or subcutaneous sumatriptan are drugs of first choice. Status migrainous can probably be treated by steroids. For the prophylaxis of migraine, beta-blockers (propranolol and metoprolol), flunarizine, valproic acid, and topiramate are drugs

of first choice. Drugs of second choice for migraine prophylaxis are amitriptyline, naproxen, petasites, and bisoprolol.

Evers S, Afra J, Frese A, et al. EFNS guideline on the drug treatment of migraine—report of an EFNS task force. *Eur J Neurol*. 2006;13:560–572.

199. Answer: C. Recovery and rehabilitation following TBI require multidisciplinary efforts and are determined by several factors. The Rancho Los Amigos Cognitive Scale is a universal tool that facilitates communication among the various specialties responsible for the rehabilitative effort. It defines and tracks the level of psychological and cognitive recovery over time. It is weighted from I (most severe deficits: unresponsive) to VIII (least severe disability: purposeful and appropriate response). A patient is said to be Ranchos Los Amigos scale VI if he is alert and inconsistently oriented to time and place and follows simple directions consistently and begins to show carryover or new learning. He is also able to recognize staff and has increased awareness or self, family, and others.

1. Center for Neuro Skills. *Rancho Los Amigos (Revised)*. http://www.neuroskills.com/rancho.shtml. Accessed March 21, 2007.
2. Rancho Los Amigos. Family Guide to The Rancho Levels of Cognitive Functioning. http://www.rancho.org/patient_education/bi_cognition.pdf. Accessed March 21, 2007.
3. RehabTeamSite. Overview of TBI: Coma Nomenclature. http://calder.med.miami.edu/pointis/tbiprov/OCCUPATIONAL/over3.html. Accessed March 21, 2007.

200. Answer: E. Psychiatric disturbances after TBI involves the interaction between premorbid personality traits, psychosocial and environmental factors, and postinjury biological changes. These risk factors can be divided into highly significant risk factors which include: preinjury history of psychiatric illness, preinjury poor social functioning, older age of onset of injury, history of alcoholism, and the presence of atherosclerosis. Less significant risk factors include: lower Glasgow Coma Scale score, lower MMSE scores, marital discord, financial instability, poor interpersonal relationship, pre-injury levels of education, and compensation claims.

Rao V, Lyketsos C. Neuropsychiatric sequelae of traumatic brain injury. *Psychosomatics*. 2000;41:95–103.

Test 9

> ## Questions

1. Ms. C is an active, healthy, 75-year-old woman who has lived alone for the past 15 years. As she enters the next two decades of her life, she can expect all of the following EXCEPT:
   A. Increased feelings of loneliness
   B. Diminished access to familiar forms of social support
   C. Increased reminiscence of the past
   D. Increased risk of loss of loved ones
   E. Increased enjoyment of solitude

2. In humans, which of the following have NOT been used to help reliably determine heritability of psychiatric disorders?
   A. Family risk studies
   B. Twin studies
   C. Adoption studies
   D. Molecular studies
   E. Randomized controlled trials (RCTs)

3. A 37-year-old Puerto Rican woman with no prior psychiatric history is taken to the emergency department by her family due to out-of-control behavior. She is observed intermittently shouting, crying, and trembling. She also complains of a feeling of heat starting in her chest and traveling to her head. Her medical workup is negative. The woman's family states that her husband moved out of their home three days prior to this presentation. What diagnosis should be considered in this patient?
   A. Amok
   B. Ataque de nervios
   C. Falling out
   D. Brain fag
   E. Koro

4. To determine the presence or absence of a particular disease outcome, a study follows two groups of subjects over a specified period of time: one that was naturally exposed to a risk factor and another that was not naturally exposed to the risk factor. What is this study design called?
   A. An RCT
   B. A case-control study
   C. A cohort study
   D. A cross-sectional study
   E. A single-blind study

5. Which is NOT included in the carbamazepine baseline pretreatment and periodic follow-up tests?
   A. Electrocardiogram (EKG)
   B. Liver function tests (LFTs)
   C. Urine pregnancy test
   D. Thyroid stimulating hormone (TSH)
   E. Complete blood count (CBC) and serum electrolytes

6. You follow a 63-year-old veteran with chronic obstructive pulmonary disease (COPD) for his anxiety symptoms. He continues to smoke, and his COPD has been worsening. His pulmonologists have continued to add trials of various bronchodilators, but he has become more hypoxic. Likewise, despite various pharmacologic and psychotherapeutic treatment strategies, his anxiety has also continued to worsen. His brother recently struggled with lung cancer and passed away last month. Given this history, which of the following may contribute to his worsening anxiety?
   A. Bereavement
   B. Chronic hypoxia
   C. Bronchodilators
   D. Adjustment to limited function
   E. All of the above

7. Which of the following is the least prominent feature of vascular dementia?
   A. Executive functioning
   B. Memory impairment
   C. Depression
   D. Attention
   E. Speed of processing information

8. A 35-year-old man presents with insomnia. He states he has had trouble falling asleep for years and denies any particular current stressors. He is very focused on his problem sleeping, and it is difficult to get him to talk about anything else. He describes lying in bed, wide awake for hours, ruminating about the issues of the day before finally falling asleep. He complains that he can only fall asleep when he isn't trying. Which of the following statements about this disorder is TRUE?

A. It is typically thought of as a type of conditioned response.

B. His polysomnogram (PSG) appears to be that of a normal sleeper.

C. These patients are rarely accurate in reporting their sleep.

D. Frequent awakenings during the night are rare.

E. Benzodiazepines and related substances are the treatment of choice for this condition.

9. If a patient meets all of the diagnostic criteria for Schizophrenia, but symptoms are present for only 6 weeks, which one of the diagnoses would be the most appropriate?

A. Schizophreniform Disorder
B. Delusional Disorder
C. Brief Psychotic Disorder
D. Schizoaffective Disorder
E. Residual type Schizophrenia

10. Which one of the following is NOT a risk factor for poor outcome for behavioral couple therapy (BCT)?

A. Younger age of the couple
B. Less-educated couples
C. Being unemployed
D. Higher degree of tradition
E. Partners' higher levels of depression

11. Which of the following is not an identified risk factor for the development of Neuroleptic Malignant Syndrome (NMS)?

A. Prominent psychomotor retardation
B. Higher doses of neuroleptics
C. Greater neuroleptic dose increment
D. Parenteral administration of the neuroleptics
E. Young age

12. Alcohol is primarily absorbed from which one of the following areas in the gut?

A. Oral mucosa
B. Stomach
C. Proximal small intestine
D. Equally from the stomach and small intestine
E. Colon

13. Which of the following is TRUE of disulfiram (Antabuse)?

A. It inhibits acetaldehyde dehydrogenase
B. It inhibits the conversion of alcohol to acetaldehyde
C. It inhibits acetylcholinesterases
D. It inhibits elimination of ethanol via kidneys
E. It is very effective in preventing relapse rates

14. Which of the following is TRUE of barbiturates?

A. They are very hydrophilic.

B. More alkaline pH increases their rate of central nervous system entry.

C. They suppress neuronal transmission via enhancing γ-aminobutyric acid (GABA) inhibition.

D. They vary widely in their chemical derivation and structure.

E. They are excreted unchanged by the kidneys.

15. In each state, court decisions based on which legal case address the clinician's potential duty to warn or protect third-party potential victims of violence. Which one of the following cases first addressed the duty of the treating psychiatrist to protect potential third party victims of violence in the United States?

A. The McNaughten ruling
B. The MacArthur ruling
C. The Tarasoff ruling
D. The Miranda ruling
E. None of the above

16. Antagonism of which dopaminergic pathway by D_2-receptor antagonists results in parkinsonian side effects?

A. Nigrostriatal tract
B. Mesolimbic tract
C. Corticospinal tract
D. Mesocortical tract
E. Tuberoinfundibular tract

17. Secretion of which of the following hormones begins at night and terminates upon retinal stimulation by sunlight?

A. Cortisol
B. Melatonin
C. Prolactin (PRL)
D. TSH
E. Testosterone

18. Which one of the following is TRUE of cognitive dysfunction in Huntington's disease (HD)?

A. It often affects long-term memory.
B. It often spares executive functions.
C. There is no delay in the acquisition of new motor skills.
D. These symptoms do not worsen over time.
E. Speech deteriorates faster than comprehension.

19. Which of the following signs is typically consistent with a dominant hemisphere lesion?

A. Hemi-inattention
B. Anosognosia
C. Constructional apraxia
D. Hemi-neglect
E. Aphasia

20. A 65-year-old man develops an infarction of the brain. He subsequently develops ptosis and miosis on

the right eyelid, right-sided ataxia, diminished pain sensation on the right side of his face, and the loss of pain sensation on his left trunk and extremities. His voice is hoarse, and his uvula deviates up into the left upon examination. Given this information, where would you expect to see a lesion on an MRI scan of his brain?

A. Right basal ganglia
B. Right brainstem
C. Spinal cord
D. Right cerebral cortex
E. Left cerebral cortex

21. Normal pressure hydrocephalus (NPH) is a clinical syndrome generally consisting of which one of the following symptoms?

A. Confusion, ataxia, and ocular motility abnormalities
B. Hallucinations, tremor, and sensitivity to neuroleptics
C. Aggression, disinhibition, and hyperorality
D. Dementia, myoclonus, and distinctive periodic electroencephalogram (EEG) complexes
E. Dementia, urinary incontinence, and gait apraxia

22. A 7-year-old boy with cerebral palsy and an IQ of 60 is brought to the clinic by his parents on account of severe self-injury. Detailed investigations reveal complete absence of hypoxanthine-guanine phosphoribosyl transferase (HGPRT) enzyme with hyperuricemia. Which one of the following is TRUE of his condition?

A. This disorder is less common in males.
B. This disorder is as common in females as it is in males.
C. The age of onset of self injury is usually about 18 years.
D. The enzyme HGPRT is present only in the brain.
E. The level of HGPRT is highest in the basal ganglia.

23. All of the following are true of mucopolysaccharidoses EXCEPT:

A. They are lysosomal storage disorders.
B. They are classified according to the type of acid hydrolase deficiency.
C. The term *gargoylism* was used in the past to describe the characteristic coarse facial features.
D. Growth retardation is seen with all mucopolysaccharidoses.
E. Mental retardation is seen in all mucopolysaccharidoses.

24. All of the following genetic disorders of lipid metabolism are transmitted via an autosomal recessive type of inheritance EXCEPT:

A. Tay-Sach's disease
B. Niemann Pick disease
C. Krabbe's disease
D. Fabry's lipogranulomatosis
E. Wolman's disease

25. All of the following are TRUE of multiple system atrophy EXCEPT:

A. It is twice as common in males as it is in females.
B. The average age of onset is in the 50s.
C. It is a syndrome of four disorders.
D. Patients usually live for 9 to 10 years after the symptoms appear.
E. A characteristic finding is the cytoplasmic inclusion bodies containing alfa-synuclein within oligodendroglial cells.

26. Which one of the following is TRUE of traumatic brain injury (TBI)?

A. Severity of functional impairments after TBI is directly related to the severity of the injury.
B. Mild TBI is defined as a blow to the head followed by a loss of consciousness (LOC) of less than 10 minutes, an altered mental status with post-traumatic amnesia (PTA) of less than 12 hours, or a Glasgow Coma Scale score of 10 to 12.
C. Patients are classified as having a moderate-to-severe TBI if they have an LOC over 15 minutes or altered mental status greater than 18 hours or a Glasgow Coma Score below 8.
D. About 15% of patients with mild TBI will continue to experience long-term cognitive, physical, and behavioral difficulties that interfere with their ability to function.
E. All of the above.

27. In a series of experiments led by Harry Harlow, infant rhesus monkeys were raised in varying degrees of social deprivation. Which one of the following behaviors was NOT observed in these monkeys?

A. Self-orality
B. Self-clasping
C. Fearful of peers
D. Ability to copulate
E. Unable to nurture young

28. Which of the following is found at increased rates in first-degree and other close relatives of probands with schizophrenia?

A. Neuropsychological deficits in the Wisconsin Card-Sort Test
B. Neurological soft signs, such as smooth pursuit eye movement dysfunction
C. Impaired suppression of p50 (50 ms) auditory evoked potentials

D. Cluster A personality traits

E. All of the above

29. Which one of the following drugs has been Food and Drug Administration (FDA) approved for the treatment of painful diabetic polyneuropathy?

A. Tricyclic antidepressants

B. Pregabalin

C. Gabapentin

D. Capsaicin cream

E. Mexiletine

30. According to the Epidemiologic Catchment Area (ECA) Study, which group of disorders has the greatest lifetime prevalence?

A. Affective Disorders

B. Schizophrenia and Schizophreniform Disorders

C. Substance Use Disorders

D. Anxiety Disorders

E. Somatization Disorder

31. Which is NOT included in the antipsychotic metabolic monitoring?

A. Blood pressure

B. Lipid panel

C. Fasting blood glucose

D. Oral Glucose Tolerance Test (OGTT)

E. Body mass index (BMI) and waist circumference

32. A 28-year-old man who complained of severe abdominal pain and tenderness was admitted to the hospital where he demanded to have an appendectomy. When a series of tests continued to return with negative results, the patient grew abusive and threatening. A review of the records indicated that this patient had been hospitalized five times in the past year with the same demands and has undergone multiple procedures including exploratory laparoscopies, all of which were negative. This person suffers from a disorder that is often characterized by all of the following EXCEPT:

A. Employment in a health-related field

B. Good prognosis once the obvious environmental goal is achieved

C. History of childhood illness leading to extensive medical treatment

D. History of early parental rejection

E. History of an important relationship with a physician

33. Who coined the term *Münchhausen syndrome*?

A. Wilford Bion

B. Sandor Ferenczi

C. Richard Asher

D. Alfred Adler

E. Eric Berne

34. Which of the following is TRUE of Avoidant Personality Disorder?

A. Experts can easily distinguish it from Social Phobia.

B. There is an equal ratio between men and women.

C. Comorbidity with other personality disorders is rare.

D. Impairment is frequently mild.

E. It is rarely encountered in outpatient practices.

35. The symptom tetrad associated with Narcolepsy includes all of the following EXCEPT:

A. Excessive daytime somnolence

B. Cataplexy

C. Sleep paralysis

D. Hypnagogic hallucinations

E. Interepisode symptoms

36. Which one of the following is NOT TRUE of psychological therapies for Borderline Personality Disorder (BPD)?

A. Dialectic behavior therapy (DBT) is more effective than treatment as usual (TAU) for the treatment of chronically parasuicidal and drug-dependent borderline women.

B. DBT-orientated therapy is also more effective than client-centred therapy (CCT) for the treatment of BPD.

C. DBT is as effective as comprehensive validation therapy plus 12-step for the treatment of opioid-dependent borderline women.

D. Manual-assisted cognitive behavioral therapy (MACT) is no more effective than TAU in the treatment of BPD.

E. Studies support the cost-effectiveness of DBT for BPD.

37. Which one of the following is not part of Freud's interpretation of dreams?

A. Archetypes

B. Condensation

C. Displacement

D. Representation

E. Symbolism

38. Which of the following is TRUE of the metabolism of alcohol?

A. It is mainly metabolized in the liver.

B. Alcohol dehydrogenase (ADH) converts alcohol into acetaldehyde.

C. Aldehyde dehydrogenase catalyzes the conversion of acetaldehyde into acetic acid.

D. Rate of alcohol metabolism by ADH is relatively constant.

E. All of the above.

39. All of the following are relative contraindications for the use of disulfiram (Antabuse) EXCEPT:

A. Active hepatic disease
B. Glaucoma
C. Coronary artery disease
D. History of psychosis
E. Chronic renal failure

40. Which of the following is NOT a common side effect of amphetamine use?

A. Hypertension
B. Respiratory depression
C. Appetite suppression
D. Paranoia
E. Tachycardia

41. Which historical figure is widely believed to have originated, and was a major developer of, psychoanalysis?

A. Jean-Martin Charcot
B. Benjamin Rush
C. Sigmund Freud
D. Adolf Meyer
E. Joseph Breuer

42. Which of the following is the rate limiting step in the synthesis of serotonin?

A. Tryptamine availability
B. Tryptophan hydroxylase
C. Tryptophan availability
D. Amino acid decarboxylase
E. Tyrosine hydroxylase

43. All of the following are TRUE of the treatment of Nicotine Dependence EXCEPT:

A. Bupropion and the nicotine patch are both first-line agents to reduce smoking.
B. Hypnosis shows efficacy for the treatment of Nicotine Dependence.
C. Combining psychosocial and pharmacologic treatments produces better outcomes than either treatment alone.
D. Clonidine is a second-line agent for Nicotine Dependence.
E. Cognitive behavioral therapy shows efficacy for treatment of Nicotine Dependence.

44. Which one of the following is TRUE of the genetics of Huntington's disease (HD)?

A. The gene for HD is located on the short arm of chromosome 19.
B. The normal alleles at gene site usually contain CCG repeats.
C. The number of trinucleotide repeats accounts for approximately 60% of the variability in the age of onset.

D. When these repeats reach 20 or more, the disease is fully penetrant.
E. All of the above.

45. Which of the following signs occur in a brainstem lesion?

A. Bowel/bladder incontinence
B. Nystagmus
C. Intention tremor
D. Parkinsonism
E. Hemi-sensory loss

46. A young woman is stabbed in the back with a knife. She develops right leg weakness and left leg numbness to temperature and pain. Upon examination, she has upgoing plantar reflex on the right and hyperactive tendon reflexes. Given this information, which of the following most appropriately describes her injury?

A. She has complete transection of the spinal cord.
B. She has hemi-transection of the right side of the spinal cord.
C. She has hemi-transection of the left side of the spinal cord.
D. She has injury to the left dorsal horn.
E. She has injury to the right dorsal horn.

47. Much to her primary physician's surprise, a 32-year-old woman reports that she has been drinking increasing amounts of alcohol recently. The woman is a successful classically trained pianist and states that she started drinking after a fine tremor began to affect her concert performances. When asked, she recalls that her father also had a tremor, which was particularly noticeable during family dinners. She is otherwise healthy and on no medications. What is the most likely cause of her tremor?

A. Parkinson's disease
B. HD
C. Essential tremor
D. Sydenham's chorea
E. Wilson's disease

48. Which one of the following is NOT TRUE of phenylketonuria (PKU)?

A. It has an autosomal recessive mode of inheritance.
B. It occurs in about 1 in 10,000 to 15,000 children in the United States.
C. Guthrie test is diagnostic of the condition.
D. The enzyme that is deficient is phenylalanine hydroxylase.
E. Approximately 50% of untreated children develop grand mal seizures.

49. All of the following mucopolysaccharidoses are transmitted via an autosomal recessive mode of inheritance EXCEPT:

A. Hunter's syndrome
B. Hurler's syndrome
C. Morquio syndrome
D. Scheie syndrome
E. Maroteaux-Lamy syndrome

50. Dietary treatment of maple syrup urine disease involves the restriction of which one of the following essential amino acids?

A. Valine, leucine, and phenylalanine
B. Histidine, valine, and tryptophan
C. Methionone, lysine, and threonine
D. Leucine, isoluecine, and valine
E. Leucine, lysine, and tryptophan

51. A 28-year-old woman with no significant past medical history presents with weakness and numbness in her left leg. Further history elicits increasing fatigue, intermittent tingling sensations in her extremities, and an episode of blurry vision in her right eye for several days that resolved on its own without treatment. A lumbar puncture and magnetic resonance imaging (MRI) support the suspected diagnosis. Which of the following statements about the etiology and epidemiology of this disease are correct?

A. There is an increasing risk of developing disease in equatorial areas.
B. The highest familial concordance is between mother and daughter.
C. Immigrants from a high-risk to a low-risk zone carry part of their increased risk.
D. The majority of cases have their onset before the age of 20.
E. There is firm evidence of a relation with environmental factors and disease.

52. A 42-year-old white woman is seen in the emergency room (ER) for sudden onset of confusion, paranoia, and agitation. Her husband reports to you that she has a history of Addison's disease and you suspect that she is currently in an Addisonian crisis. Given this information, which one of the following is NOT an important step in the acute management of her condition?

A. Confirm diagnosis with adrenal autoantibody tests and imaging of the adrenal glands
B. Draw blood for serum cortisol, adrenocorticotropic hormone (ACTH), and serum chemistry
C. Start an infusion of IV saline
D. Start treatment with dexamethasone immediately
E. Do a short corticotropin stimulation test after treatment with dexamethasone

53. According to Piaget, which one of the following is TRUE of moral development?

A. Moral judgment can be divided into three stages.
B. Younger children regard rules as being relativistic.
C. Younger children base their moral judgments on intentions.
D. Moral issues to continue to develop throughout adolescence.
E. All of the above.

54. Which of the following is the most likely mode of genetic transmission for susceptibility to Schizophrenia?

A. Polygenetic multifactorial mode
B. Autosomal dominant monogenetic mode
C. Autosomal recessive monogenetic mode
D. Sex-linked monogenetic mode
E. Tri-nucleotide repeat mode

55. Which of the following is TRUE of respondent conditioning?

A. Extinction occurs when a conditioned response is transferred from one stimulus to another.
B. Stimulus generalization occurs when the conditioned stimulus is constantly repeated without the unconditioned stimulus until the response generated by the stimulus weakens and then disappears.
C. Extinction is the process of recognizing and responding to differences between same stimuli.
D. Discrimination is the process of recognizing and responding to the differences between similar stimuli.
E. The neutral stimulus is also referred to as unconditioned stimuli.

56. According to the National Comorbidity Survey (NCS), which disorder group had the highest lifetime prevalence?

A. Affective Disorders
B. Substance Use Disorders
C. Anxiety Disorders
D. Psychotic Disorders
E. Personality Disorders

57. Which one of the statements about depression rating scales is NOT TRUE?

A. Beck Depression Inventory (BDI) score below 10 reflects minimal depression.
B. BDI score of 30 or above reflects severe depression.
C. Hamilton Depression Scale (HAM-D) is a self-report scale.

D. HAM-D 17 score below 8 reflects remission of depression.

E. HAM-D 17 score above 18 reflects severe depression.

58. Which one of the following statements is TRUE of Factitious Disorders?

A. They are synonymous with malingering and include Ganser's syndrome.

B. They have a good prognosis and respond well to psychiatric therapy.

C. The illness is intentionally feigned for either primary or secondary gains.

D. The type of disorder is based on predominantly psychological versus physical signs and symptoms.

E. It usually begins in childhood after experiencing rejection from parents.

59. A 24-year-old single, white woman has brought herself to the ER, complaining of a sharp pain in her abdomen. She also reports nausea, vomiting, and fever, which have been getting progressively worse over the past few days. As she was being worked up and no significant findings were noted, the patient started getting annoyed and argumentative with the medical staff. The medical team requests a psychiatric consult. When the psychiatrist arrives to do the evaluation, the patient gets furious, refuses to participate in the evaluation stating that "I am not crazy," and demands to be discharged against medical advice. In the brief encounter with the patient, the psychiatrist recognizes the patient as someone he had met a couple of weeks ago in the ER of a community hospital where he was moonlighting. After doing a background check, it is noted that the patient has had multiple visits to ERs, sometimes being admitted for further tests and other times being discharged from the ER. What is the distinguishing feature that makes Factitious Disorder the most likely diagnosis?

A. Intentional production of symptoms with no secondary gain

B. Intentional production of symptoms for secondary gain

C. History of many physical complaints

D. Symptoms affecting voluntary motor or sensory function suggesting a neurological or other general medical condition

E. Preoccupation with imagined defect in appearance or markedly excessive concern with slight physical anomaly

60. Which of the following statements about sleep state misperception is TRUE?

A. The PSG is usually abnormal.

B. There is a high correlation between PSG and the patient's report of sleep quality.

C. Such patients are easily aroused by an auditory stimulus.

D. There is usually a limited response to placebo.

E. Gentle reassurance is usually helpful.

61. Which one of the following is NOT typically considered to be good sleep hygiene?

A. A warm bath before sleep

B. Avoidance of alcohol before sleep

C. Avoidance of daytime naps

D. Early evening exercise routine

E. Eating at regular times, no meals before sleep

62. Which one of the following is NOT TRUE of the description of interpersonal therapy (IPT)?

A. It is time-limited and structured psychotherapy.

B. It does not rely on extensive paperwork.

C. It evokes transference issues.

D. It incorporates psychoeducation.

E. It agrees with a medical model of psychiatric illness.

63. According to Freud, which one of the following describes the process in dreams by which events and scenes are linked and made orderly?

A. Condensation

B. Displacement

C. Wish fulfilment

D. Manifest content

E. Secondary revision

64. The physiological effects of alcohol are produced by its action on which of the following receptors?

A. GABA-A receptors

B. N-methyl-D-aspartic acid (NMDA) receptors

C. Dopamine-containing neurons

D. 5-Hydroxytryptamine3 (5-HT3) receptors

E. All of the above

65. A disulfiram (Antabuse)-like reaction may be produced by which of the following drugs?

A. Metronidazole

B. Oral hypoglycemics

C. Trichomonacides

D. Carbimides

E. All of the above

66. Alternative methods of chronic pain management include all of the following EXCEPT:

A. Behavioral modification

B. Hypnosis

C. Biofeedback

D. Placebo

E. Cognitive and other psychotherapies

67. Who became the first psychiatrist to win a Nobel Prize?

A. Sigmund Freud
B. Egas Moniz
C. Julius von Wagner-Jauregg
D. Eric Kandel
E. Carl Jung

68. Where is the major site of serotonin cell bodies located?

A. Raphe nucleus
B. Locus ceruleus
C. Ventral tegmental area
D. Nucleus basalis of Meynert
E. Substantia nigra

69. Which of the following opioids CANNOT be detected with a routine urine toxicity screen?

A. Buprenorphine
B. Oxycodone
C. Hydrocodone
D. Fentanyl
E. All of the above

70. Which one of the following has an autosomal dominant form of inheritance?

A. Spinocerebellar ataxia type 3 (SCA3) in those of African descent
B. Spinocerebellar ataxia type 2 (SCA2) in those of Asian descent
C. Microtubule-associated protein tau (MAPT) mutations associated with frontotemporal dementia
D. All of the above
E. None of the above

71. Where would you expect to see a lesion on an MRI scan of the brain of a patient with new onset partial seizures?

A. Brainstem
B. Cerebellum
C. Basal ganglia
D. One cerebral hemisphere
E. Both cerebral hemispheres

72. In which of the following situations is MRI of the brain preferred over computed tomography (CT)?

A. Distinguishing white from gray matter
B. Cost is an issue
C. Screening for an intracranial bleed
D. Indwelling ferrous metal is present from an old injury
E. Time is an issue

73. Which of the following is TRUE of the neuropsychiatric manifestations of Wilson's disease?

A. Neuropsychiatric symptoms may occur in young patients even before the disease affects the liver.
B. Neurologic disorders may occur in up to 35% of patients with this disorder.
C. Parkinsonian symptoms with mood changes are associated with dilatation of the third ventricle.
D. Dyskinesia, dysarthria, and personality changes are associated with focal lesions in the putamen and pallidum.
E. All of the above.

74. The gene for the enzyme phenyl alanine hydroxylase is located on which one of the following chromosomes?

A. Chromosome 15p
B. Chromosome 8q
C. Chromosome 17p
D. Chromosome 12q
E. Chromosome 21p

75. Which one of the following is the most common type of mucopolysaccharidosis?

A. Maroteaux-Lamy syndrome
B. Morquio syndrome
C. Hunter's syndrome
D. Sanfilippo syndrome
E. Sly syndrome

76. A 13-year-old boy has an IQ of 49 and attends a special school for the mentally retarded. His reading, writing, and math skills are comparable to those of a child in the first grade. His visuospatial skills are those of a 5-year-old child. His linguistic function is relatively intact with good performance on formal language tests. He has a diagnosis of William's syndrome. All of the following are TRUE of this condition EXCEPT:

A. It is an autosomal dominant mode of inheritance.
B. Supravalvular aortic stenosis is the predominant form of congenital heart disease associated with this condition.
C. The biochemical abnormality associated with this syndrome is hypocalcemia.
D. Hyperacusis is seen in 90% of the cases.
E. The dissociation between verbal skills and visuospatial abilities is characteristic of this condition.

77. In the neuropsychological evaluation of a patient with suspected mild dementia, which of the following would be best to test attention?

A. National Adult Reading Test (NART)
B. Boston Naming Test
C. Digit Span Forward and Backward
D. Wisconsin Card-Sorting Test
E. Finger Tapping Test

78. A 40-year-old white woman was recently diagnosed with myasthenia gravis (MG). She meets with you to discuss the available treatments for this condition. When discussing all treatment options with her, which one of the following will you NOT be telling her?

A. Anticholinesterase drugs improve myasthenic symptoms in nearly all patients, but they do not fully relieve the symptoms in many patients.

B. Corticosteroids are the immunosuppressive agents most commonly used in the treatment of MG and the most consistently effective.

C. Clinical response from azathioprine may be delayed for up to 15 months.

D. Plasma exchange (plasmapheresis) and intravenous immunoglobulins (IVIGs) are used for acute management of severe muscular weakness.

E. Usually, thymectomy is performed on patients late in the course of their disease and is restricted to patients older than 60 years of age.

79. Which of the following is TRUE of Kohlberg's stages of moral development?

A. This theory postulates that moral reasoning has five identifiable developmental stages.

B. These stages are further divided into two levels.

C. In stage 2, children are no longer so impressed by any single authority and they see that there are different sides to any issue.

D. At stage 5, the concern shifts toward obeying laws to maintain the society as a whole.

E. All of the above.

80. Which of the following findings has been well-replicated regarding the inheritance of affective disorders?

A. First-degree relatives of unipolar depressed probands have an increased risk of both Unipolar Depression and Bipolar Disorder.

B. First-degree relatives of bipolar probands have an increased risk of both Bipolar Disorder and Unipolar Depression.

C. Relatives of probands with Schizoaffective Disorder of the depressive type have greater rates of Bipolar Disorder.

D. First-degree relatives of probands with Schizoaffective Disorder of the depressed type have lower rates of Schizophrenia.

E. All of the above.

81. A 30-year-old woman comes to see her psychiatrist and sits through most of the session saying little or nothing. This patient may be exhibiting which one of the following psychological processes?

A. Denial

B. Transference
C. Displacement
D. Resistance
E. Identification

82. Which of the following is an example of a secondary preventive intervention that may be utilized in mental health?

A. Genetic counseling for prospective parents

B. Gene therapy to manipulate the developing brain in utero

C. Supplementation to reduce early exposure to nutritional deficiencies

D. Pharmacologic intervention after the disease becomes symptomatic

E. Depression screening in primary care settings

83. In a patient presenting with a change in mental status, autonomic instability, hyperthermia, and muscle rigidity in the setting of neuroleptic medication, all of the following laboratory data would be consistent with this presentation EXCEPT:

A. Elevated creatinine phosphokinase (CPK)
B. Elevated LFTs
C. Elevated white blood cell (WBC) count
D. Low serum iron level
E. Increased urine output

84. Which of the following is the most common comorbidity associated with Obsessive Compulsive Disorder (OCD)?

A. Schizophrenia
B. Major Depressive Disorder (MDD)
C. Post-traumatic Stress Disorder (PTSD)
D. Dysthymia
E. None of the above

85. Which of the following statements is NOT TRUE about Factitious Disorder?

A. Factitious disorders are more frequently seen in females than in males; however, in the more severe and chronic cases, it is more common in males.

B. Factitious Disorders are diagnosed in approximately 1% of patients on whom mental health professionals are consulted.

C. Presentations with predominantly psychological signs and symptoms are reported much less commonly than those with predominantly physical signs and symptoms.

D. The onset is usually in late life.

E. The course of Factitious Disorders usually consist of intermittent episodes.

86. In working with a patient with Schizophrenia, you find that the most prominent symptoms are loosening of associations, flat affect, and disheveled appearance. Which subtype of Schizophrenia does this patient most likely suffer from according to the DSM-IV-TR classification?

A. Paranoid
B. Disorganized
C. Catatonic
D. Undifferentiated
E. Residual

87. Which one of the following is TRUE of traits associated with a Personality Disorder?

A. These traits have to be present for a prolonged period of time.
B. These traits usually manifest in various aspects of ones life.
C. These traits are autoplastic.
D. These traits are ego syntonic.
E. These traits are usually inflexible.

88. Which one of the following is NOT TRUE of IPT?

A. It has three specific stages.
B. A key feature of the first part is the compiling of an interpersonal inventory that lists and examines all the patient's relationships.
C. The therapist holds the focus and relates symptom change to interpersonal events.
D. It conceptualizes painful feelings as symptoms and expects them to diminish when negative cognitions are challenged.
E. The full benefits of IPT do not appear immediately, but after a lag.

89. Which of the following corresponds to the doctrine of respondeat superior?

A. A psychiatrist managing an agitated patient must use the least restrictive means available.
B. When a defendant has a mental illness for which medications may have been reasonably indicated, psychiatrists in the eyes of the law are the only appropriate expert witnesses.
C. A person is not legally responsible for a criminal act if, secondary to a mental illness, she could not appreciate the wrongfulness of her conduct or conform it to the requirements of the law.
D. An attending who supervises a resident is responsible for the resident's actions while under her supervision.
E. A psychiatrist who fails to adequately address a patient's stated suicidal intentions can be sued for negligence should the patient attempt suicide.

90. When treating patients with Attention-Deficit/Hyperactivity Disorder (ADHD) with amphetamines, you need to consider all of the following EXCEPT:

A. Methamphetamine, a derivative of amphetamine, is the most commonly abused prescription stimulant.
B. Amphetamines are usually abused by oral or intravenous route.
C. Methamphetamine can be produced by reducing ephedrine or pseudoephedrine.
D. Amphetamines are the drugs associated most often with emergency department visit.
E. Amphetamine and methamphetamine are schedule II drugs due to a high abuse potential.

91. Which of the following is NOT TRUE of the pharmacotherapy of Alcohol Dependence?

A. Topiramate has shown efficacy in the treatment of this disorder.
B. Gabapentin and valproate have shown efficacy in the treatment of this disorder.
C. Ondansetron has been shown to improve abstinence from alcohol.
D. Selective serotonin reuptake inhibitors (SSRIs) significantly reduce the intake of alcohol in these patients, even in the absence of Major Depression.
E. None of the above.

92. Non-opioid analgesics are considered effective for which type of pain?

A. Mild acute pain
B. Severe acute pain
C. Severe chronic pain
D. Neuropathic pain
E. All of the above

93. Who first described the tenets of classical conditioning with his studies of canine saliva production?

A. B.F. Skinner
B. Ivan Pavlov
C. Harry Stack Sullivan
D. John Watson
E. None of the above

94. Approximately 90% of the body's serotonin is found in which one of the following organs?

A. Brain
B. Liver
C. Spinal cord
D. Bones
E. Intestines

95. Each of the following medications is correctly matched with its activity or biochemical properties EXCEPT:

A. Naltrexone: Opiate receptor antagonist
B. Acamprosate: GABA analog
C. Clonidine: Alpha-1 adrenergic receptor antagonist

D. Bupropion: Dopamine reuptake inhibitor
E. Disulfiram: Aldehyde dehyrdogenase inhibitor

96. Which of the following can present with parkinsonism?

A. SCA3 in those of African descent
B. SCA2 in those of Asian descent
C. MAPT mutations associated with frontotemporal dementia
D. All of the above
E. None of the above

97. A man has weakness of his right arm, right leg, and right lower face, but his forehead muscles are unaffected. His right arm is flexed at the elbow, wrist, and fingers. His right leg is externally rotated with hip and knee flexion. Given this information, where would you expect to see the lesion on an MRI scan of his brain?

A. Right cerebellum
B. Right thalamus
C. Brainstem
D. Left cerebral cortex
E. Right cerebral cortex

98. In which of the following situations is CT preferred over MRI?

A. Differential diagnosis of multiple sclerosis (MS)
B. Posterior fossa is the area of interest
C. Pregnant patient strongly requests not to have ionizing radiation exposure
D. Differential diagnosis of spinal cord pathology
E. The patient has indwelling ferrous metal and is on life-support equipment

99. Which one of the following is NOT TRUE of physiological tremors?

A. They are seen in all normal people when muscles are activated.
B. They are typically resting tremors.
C. They usually do not interfere with activities of daily living (ADLs).
D. Stress and anxiety can exacerbate these tremors.
E. In general, no drug treatment is warranted for this condition.

100. Which one of the following is NOT TRUE of galactosemia?

A. It has an autosomal recessive mode of inheritance.
B. The deficiency of galactose-1-phosphate uridyltransferase (GALT) is the most common cause of this disorder.
C. The triad of symptoms in classical galactosemia is hepatomegaly, cataracts, and mental retardation.
D. Classical galactosemia is the least common type.

E. Failure to thrive is the most common initial symptom.

101. All of the following are features of mucopolysaccharidoses EXCEPT:

A. Affected babies appear normal at birth.
B. Developmental delays are usually mild at 12 months.
C. Coarse facial features become apparent usually by the eighth year.
D. Intelligence may be normal in some mild variants.
E. In severe forms, death may occur in the school age years and early teens.

102. A 39-year-old woman presents with emotional lability and grandiose delusions. She exhibits mild tremors and abnormal LFTs at the time of assessment. Ophthalmological examination reveals bilateral golden brown rings around the cornea. All of the following are TRUE of her condition EXCEPT:

A. The genetic defect is localized to chromosome 14.
B. The onset of symptoms is usually in childhood or early adolescence.
C. It has an autosomal recessive mode of inheritance.
D. Of these patients, 20% may present with psychiatric symptoms.
E. The presence of Kayser-Fleischer ring indicates brain damage.

103. An 80-year-old man is brought into the psychiatrist's office by his wife for follow-up of dementia. An interview with the patient and his wife reveals that he is independent in all of his activities of daily living (ADLs). The psychiatrist now wishes to assess the patient's ability to perform instrumental activities of daily living (IADLs). She will need to ask about each of the following EXCEPT:

A. Ability to feed himself
B. Ability to manage medications
C. Ability to drive
D. Ability to use the telephone
E. Ability to write a check

104. Which of the following correctly describes the mechanism of action of nonsteroidal anti-inflammatory drugs (NSAIDs) in reducing pain?

A. They inhibit the synthesis of arachidonic acid by inhibiting phospholipase A_{22}.
B. They inhibit the synthesis of arachidonic acid by inhibiting cyclooxygenase.
C. They inhibit cyclooxygenase at the $m\mu$ receptor.
D. They inhibit phospholipase A_{22} at the $m\mu$ receptor.
E. They inhibit cyclooxygenase ultimately inhibiting the synthesis of prostaglandins.

105. According to Holmes and Rahe, which one of the following is the most stressful life event?
    A. Divorce
    B. Death of a close family member
    C. Death of a spouse
    D. Marital separation
    E. Imprisonment

106. Which of the following disorders currently has the weakest body of evidence supporting its genetic transmission?
    A. Bipolar Disorders
    B. Schizophrenia
    C. Panic Disorder
    D. PTSD
    E. Alcohol Dependence

107. *Super ego lacuna* is a term some have applied to which of the following psychopathology?
    A. Borderline Personality Disorder (BPD)
    B. Narcissistic Personality Disorder
    C. Antisocial Personality Disorder (ASPD)
    D. Schizophreniform Disorder
    E. Schizoaffective Disorder

108. Which of the following deals with physician reimbursement for patients with Medicare?
    A. Medicare Part A
    B. Medicare Part B
    C. Medicare Part C
    D. Medicare Part D
    E. Medicaid

109. Which of the following symptoms is more commonly seen in Neuroleptic Malignant Syndrome (NMS) as compared to Serotonin Syndrome?
    A. Hyperkinesia
    B. Hyperreflexia
    C. Clonus
    D. Lead pipe rigidity
    E. All of the above

110. Which of the following Personality Disorders is most frequently associated with positive psychotic symptoms?
    A. Dependent
    B. Schizoid
    C. Antisocial
    D. Histrionic
    E. Schizotypal

111. A 6-year-old boy is brought to the ER by his mother. She reports that the child has been having fever and diarrhea and has not been eating very well for the past 2 days. Upon examination the child appears in no acute distress, however is very quiet. A review of records reveals that the child has had several ER visits over the past year. The mother has brought the child in for various problems. The child's pediatrician is contacted and she reports that the child has had extensive workup for various medical problems and all the reports have been noncontributory to the presentation. The pediatrician also reported to the ER resident that although the child's parents are married, the father has been significantly absent during crisis situations. After the resident orders a routine workup and notes no significant findings, he informs the mother of his findings. At this time, the mother insists that additional tests need to be done because she feels a "maternal instinct" that there is something seriously wrong with her son and it needs to be investigated immediately and treated. What is the most appropriate next step in the management of this patient if you suspect a diagnosis of Factitious Disorder By Proxy?
    A. Order additional invasive tests for the child
    B. Commit the mother for psychiatric treatment
    C. Consult with the hospital legal department and child protective services
    D. Discharge the patient home to the care of the mother
    E. Arrange foster care for the child

112. Which of the following statements about the epidemiology of Schizophrenia is NOT TRUE?
    A. It has a lifetime prevalence of approximately 1%.
    B. Male to female ratio is approximately 1:2.
    C. Most cases present between the ages of 15 to 35 years.
    D. There appears to be a higher incidence in lower socioeconomic groups.
    E. Jews are affected less commonly than Catholics or Protestants.

113. Which of the following statements regarding suicide in late life is TRUE?
    A. Substance abuse is the most common diagnosis in elderly suicide victims.
    B. Overdose is more common than violent means of suicide in the elderly.
    C. Older adults with major medical illnesses are at lowest risk of suicide.
    D. Suicide victims rarely communicate their suicidal thoughts to family or friends prior to the suicide.
    E. Over a third of suicide victims see their physician within a week of their suicide.

114. Which of the following statements is TRUE of hypothyroidism and psychiatric disorders?
    A. It can be associated with depression.

B. It can cause changes in cognition.

C. It can cause apathy.

D. It can be associated with rapid cycling bipolar disorder.

E. All of the above.

115. A comprehensive psychiatric interview involves gathering information in various areas. The topics to be covered are vast and the psychiatrist usually has a restricted time frame. In order to accomplish this task, one has to master the range between disorder-centered and patient-centered interviewing styles. Which of the following is a key feature of patient-centered interviewing style?

A. This style views psychiatric disorders as similar to medical disorders, using criteria for diagnosis as identifiable clusters of occurrences from a restricted menu of symptoms, signs, and behaviors that cause morbidity and mortality.

B. In this interview style, the interviewer chooses proven, symptom-oriented, open-ended questions with a relatively narrow scope followed up by closed-ended, nonleading questions centering on the disorder.

C. This interview style works for most cooperative patients, and patients whose communication skills are not impaired by their axis I and II disorders or their defense mechanisms.

D. This interview style is driven by the patient's help-seeking behavior.

E. This interview style is based on the introspective model, which emphasizes the individuality of the patient's experience.

116. When starting a patient on an amphetamine compound for the treatment of ADHD, you need to warn him about all of the following possible side effects EXCEPT:

A. Euphoria

B. Psychosis

C. Seizures

D. Decreased penile erection

E. Myoglobinuria

117. Which of the following is NOT a known potential adverse effect of barbiturate overdose?

A. Coma

B. Nystagmus

C. Ataxia

D. Suppressed deep tendon reflexes

E. Impaired pupillary light reflex

118. Opioid pain medication is NOT appropriate for which of the following conditions?

A. Fractures

B. Tension headaches

C. Myocardial infarction

D. Surgery

E. Cancer

119. The past few nights, while on call in the ER, there have been an unusual number of overdose cases. You decide to review toxicology antidotes to feel more prepared. Which of the following toxins is incorrectly paired with its antidote?

A. Acetaminophen: Acetylcysteine

B. Benzodiazepines: Flumazenil

C. Beta-Blocker: Glucagon

D. Anticholinergics: Pralidoxime (2-PAM)

E. Ethylene Glycol: Fomepizole

120. Excessive stimulation of glutamate receptors leads to prolonged and excessive intraneuronal concentrations of which one of the following ions?

A. Chloride

B. Calcium

C. Sodium

D. Potassium

E. Magnesium

121. Which one of the following improves in substance abusers, when social skills training is used as a treatment modality?

A. Their listening skills

B. Their understanding of other people's feelings

C. Self-awareness of their nonverbal behaviors

D. Assertiveness

E. All of the above

122. Which one of the following is TRUE of Mendelian genes for Parkinson's disease/parkinsonism?

A. SNCA (PARK1/4), has an autosomal dominant form of inheritance.

B. LRRK2 (PARK8), has an autosomal recessive form of inheritance.

C. PINK1 (PARK6) has an autosomal dominant form of inheritance.

D. DJ-1 (PARK7) has an autosomal dominant form of inheritance.

E. All of the above.

123. A woman loses vision by not being able to see out of the left field of both eyes. Given this information, where in the brain do you expect to find a lesion responsible for her symptom?

A. Optic chiasm

B. Optic nerves

C. Right cerebral hemisphere

D. Left cerebral hemisphere

E. Left brainstem

124. Which one of the following procedures provides the most detailed images of the brain's metabolic activity, chemistry, and physiology?

A. CT Scan
B. Positron emission tomography (PET)
C. MRI
D. Single photon emission computed tomography (SPECT)
E. Angiography

125. All of the following are TRUE of Lesch-Nyhan syndrome EXCEPT:

A. It is a sex-linked autosomal recessive disease.
B. It is caused by the deficiency of HGPRT.
C. It is an inborn error of pyrimidine nucleotide metabolism.
D. Self-injury is the major behavioral manifestation.
E. The self injurious behavior is not caused by hyperuricemia.

126. All of the following are true of complications seen in galactosemia EXCEPT:

A. Aldose reductase may be implicated in the development of nuclear opacities seen in lenticular cataracts.
B. Sepsis is common and may lead to death in the first weeks of life.
C. Ovarian failure and premature menopause may even occur in affected women who follow strict dietary restrictions.
D. Problems in social adaptation occur as late complications.
E. Neurological symptoms develop only on nonadherence to a galactose-free diet.

127. All of the following are true of dietary treatment in Phenylketonuria (PKU) EXCEPT:

A. It should be best started before the child is 6 months old.
B. Dietary treatment can lead to anemia and even death.
C. This can improve the level of mental retardation in untreated older children.
D. A low phenylalanine diet decreases irritability.
E. It increases social responsiveness and attention span.

128. All of the following are TRUE of Wilson's disease EXCEPT:

A. Serum ceruloplasmin levels are usually reduced.
B. Urinary copper is increased.
C. Total serum copper is usually increased.
D. A CT brain scan may demonstrate hypodense areas in the basal ganglia.
E. MRI of the brain may detect early lesions of Wilson's disease.

129. Which one of the following is NOT a manifestation of acquired immunodeficiency syndrome (AIDS) dementia?

A. Rapid decline, over weeks to months, in concentration and memory
B. Impaired language function early in the disease course
C. Gait difficulties and slow limb movements
D. Blunted affect and social withdrawal
E. Hyperactive reflexes

130. Which of the following correctly describes the mechanism of action of capsaicin in reducing pain?

A. It inhibits the synthesis of arachidonic acid by inhibiting phospholipase A_{22}.
B. It depletes nociceptors of substance P.
C. It acts as an agonist at $m\mu$ receptors.
D. It acts as an agonist at delta receptors.
E. It acts as an agonist at kappa receptors.

131. Which one of the following is NOT TRUE of Kohut's concepts of the personality development?

A. He proposed the concept of *self psychology*.
B. He developed his ideas around what he called the *tripartite self*.
C. He linked the origin of the self to narcissism.
D. He proposed that that narcissism develops through object libido and object relations.
E. Kohut postulated that the course of development is based on empathic interactions with selfobjects.

132. Which of the following study types have leant support to theories that Alcohol and Drug Dependence are heritable?

A. Adoption studies
B. Twin studies
C. Family studies
D. Genetic studies
E. All of the above

133. Which is the appropriate sequence for a Medicare provider to bill a patient with Medicare as their primary insurance?

A. Bill the secondary insurance, bill Medicare, and then bill the patient the remainder of the total charges.
B. Bill Medicare, bill the secondary insurance, and then bill the patient the remainder of the allowable charges.
C. Bill your total charges to Medicare, the secondary insurance, and the patient simultaneously and separately.
D. Bill the patient for your total charges and then require them to arrange filing for reimbursement.

E. Bill Medicare only, but not the secondary insurance or the patient.

134. Clinically, what is the most prominent cognitive disturbance associated with delirium?

   A. Acalculia
   B. Inattention
   C. Amnesia
   D. Dysexecutive syndrome
   E. None of the above

135. Which of the following statements regarding ASPD and MDD is TRUE?

   A. ASPD is associated with MDD and with completed suicide.
   B. Incidence of MDD is less frequent in ASPD patients than in the general population.
   C. All patients with ASPD suffer from MDD at some point in their life span.
   D. ASPD patients never experience depressive episodes.
   E. None of the above.

136. A 48-year-old man presents to your clinic at the behest of his wife. He is initially reticent about why he came, but admits to compulsive trips to the casino. Upon further interview, he admits to being $35,000 in debt, but insists that he has just run into a "bad stretch." He also admits that he is in danger of losing his job, because he has overdrawn his expense account to cover the losses. Given this history, which one of the following is TRUE of this person's condition?

   A. Over 10% of the population worldwide meets the criteria for this disorder.
   B. Approximately one third of pathological gamblers are women.
   C. Full-blown OCD is common.
   D. Psychotic symptoms are common in pathological gambling.
   E. Most pathological gamblers meet criteria for ASPD.

137. Which one of the following models describes the concept that patients with Schizophrenia are born with a specific biological vulnerability, which is activated by factors in the environment?

   A. Double hit hypothesis
   B. Consanguinity
   C. Stress diathesis model
   D. Polygenic model
   E. Mixed inheritability

138. A 70-year-old woman presents to her physician's office complaining of severe sadness since the death of her husband 3 months ago. She reports insomnia, poor appetite, a 20-pound weight loss, anhedonia, and severe preoccupation with guilt and worthlessness. She reports that she just "knows" that she caused her husband's death, although doctors have told her that he died of natural causes. She says she hears a strange voice telling her that she is evil for killing her husband. Given this history, which one of the following is her most likely diagnosis for her symptoms?

   A. Bereavement
   B. Major Depressive Episode with Psychotic Features
   C. Acute Stress Disorder
   D. Brief Psychotic Disorder with Marked Stressor
   E. Adjustment Disorder with Depressed Mood

139. Which one of the following statements is TRUE of hyperprolactinemia caused by antipsychotics?

   A. It is caused by their effects on the D_2 receptors in the mesolimbic system.
   B. The antipsychotic potency of the phenothiazines, butyrophenones, and dibenzoxazepine was found to parallel their potency in increasing prolactin levels.
   C. The level of elevated prolactin found with the typical antipsychotic medications is usually greater than 100 μg/L.
   D. Clozapine is known to cause elevations in prolactin level even higher than those caused by the typical antipsychotics.
   E. All of the above.

140. Which of the following factors increase a person's risk of suicide?

   A. Depressed mood
   B. Substance abuse
   C. Poor social support system
   D. Prior suicide attempt
   E. All of the above

141. The FDA has approved all of the following as indications for treatment with a stimulant compound EXCEPT?

   A. ADHD in children
   B. ADHD in adults
   C. Depression
   D. Narcolepsy
   E. Weight control in obesity

142. Which of the following is NOT a side effect of benzodiazepine use?

   A. Ataxia
   B. Drowsiness
   C. Tremor
   D. Confusion
   E. Memory impairment

143. A patient has been taking a stable dose of methadone for chronic pain. He was just started on an adjuvant medication for his pain and subsequently developed opiate withdrawal symptoms. Which of the following adjuvant pain medications may have precipitated the opiate withdrawal?
    A. Sertraline
    B. Nortriptyline
    C. Phenytoin
    D. Gabapentin
    E. Clonazepam

144. Which one of the following neurohormone-hormone stimulated pairs is matched incorrectly?
    A. Corticotropin-releasing hormone (CRH) → ACTH
    B. Thyrotropin-releasing hormone (TRH) → TSH
    C. Somatostatin (SRIF) → Growth hormone (GH)
    D. Growth hormone-releasing hormone (GHRH) → Growth hormone (GH)
    E. Gonadotropin-releasing hormone (GnRH) → Estrogen

145. How does Substance Abuse/Dependence affect the outcome of Bipolar Disorder?
    A. Increase the severity of symptoms in a mood episode
    B. Increase the occurrence of Mixed Episodes
    C. Leading to earlier onset of Bipolar Disorder
    D. Increase the frequency of mood episodes
    E. All of the above

146. An elderly woman with vascular disease develops the symptoms of intermittent flinging of her right arm and leg. Her symptoms are most likely the result of a lesion in which one of the following locations?
    A. Cerebral cortex
    B. Cerebellum
    C. Brainstem
    D. Basal ganglia
    E. Spinal cord

147. Which one of the following is NOT a limitation for the routine clinical use of PET?
    A. PET is prohibitively expensive.
    B. PET requires cyclotrons to produce ligands.
    C. PET radioligands must be appropriately matched to the pathology being studied.
    D. PET has limited resolution.
    E. PET is unable to distinguish between Alzheimer's and vascular dementias.

148. Which of the following is the mechanism of action of pramipexole in the treatment of restless legs syndrome (RLS)?
    A. It is a dopamine agonist.
    B. It is a precursor of dopamine and is converted to dopamine by an enzyme which is abundant in human tissues.
    C. It increases the synthesis of dopamine through unknown mechanisms.
    D. It enhances the actions of GABA on chloride channels.
    E. It inhibits the excitatory actions of glutamate.

149. Which one of the following is NOT TRUE of personality organization according to Kernberg?
    A. The self is an intrapsychic structure consisting of multiple self representations.
    B. The self consists of a structure that has both libidinal and aggressive components.
    C. Pathological narcissism is the libidinal investment of self.
    D. Failing the developmental task of psychic clarification of self leads to an increased risk of developing psychosis.
    E. The realistic self integrates both the good and bad self-images.

150. Which of the following are the deepest stages of sleep, referred to as "slow wave sleep" (SWS)?
    I.   Non-REM stage 1 sleep
    II. Non-REM stage 2 sleep
    III. Non-REM stage 3 sleep
    IV. Non-REM stage 4 sleep
    V.   REM sleep

    A. I and II
    B. III and IV
    C. IV and V
    D. V only
    E. None of the above

151. Which one of the following questions regarding sleep physiology is NOT TRUE?
    A. SWS occurs in stages 3 and 4 of NREM sleep.
    B. Atonia during REM sleep is maintained by the dorsolateral prefrontal cortex.
    C. During REM sleep, physiologic processes rise and may reach awakening levels.
    D. Duration of SWS periods decrease while duration of REM periods increase as an individual's sleep progresses from cycle to cycle through the night.
    E. Greater heart rate and respiratory variability, relative poikilothermia, and penile erections all occur during REM sleep.

152. Which one of the following Personality Disorders is most likely to occur in a male relative of a woman with Somatization Disorder?
    A. Schizoid
    B. Borderline

C. Antisocial
D. Narcissistic
E. Obsessive-Compulsive

153. An 18-year-old patient with Anorexia Nervosa states she has not experienced menstrual bleeding in the last 6 months. A serum pregnancy test is negative. Given this information, which one of the following statements is TRUE about this patient?

A. Her follicle stimulating hormone (FSH) levels are elevated.
B. Her amenorrhea will be permanent despite weight gain.
C. She would experience withdrawal bleeding with a progesterone challenge.
D. Her luteinizing hormone (LH) levels are elevated.
E. Her menses will resume after an appropriate weight gain.

154. Which of the following neurochemical abnormalities likely contributes to the positive symptoms of Schizophrenia?

A. Increased dopamine activity in the limbic system
B. Decreased dopamine activity in the limbic system
C. Increased dopamine activity in the frontal lobes
D. Decreased dopamine activity in the frontal lobes
E. None of the above

155. What is the lifetime prevalence of Bipolar Disorder?

A. 0.1%
B. 1%
C. 5%
D. 10%
E. 25%

156. Which one of the following drugs has an active metabolite?

A. Quetiapine
B. Aripiprazole
C. Clonazepam
D. Lorazepam
E. Oxazepam

157. You are on the psychiatric consultation-liaison service at a tertiary care medical center. You are called to evaluate a woman who has just given birth to a stillborn infant. The obstetrics service is concerned that the mother may be suicidal after this traumatic event. Given this information, which of the following is TRUE of pregnancy, the postpartum state, and suicidality?

A. The rate of suicide among pregnant women is five-fold greater than the rate of suicide among women in the general population.

B. The rate of suicide among women who give birth to stillborn infants is fivefold greater than the rate of suicide among women in the general population.
C. The rate of suicide among pregnant teenage girls is fivefold greater than nonpregnant teenage girls.
D. Postpartum admission to a psychiatric hospital increases the risk of suicide by 70-fold in the first postpartum year.
E. Pregnant women are at greater risk of dying by their own hand than by the hand of someone else.

158. All of the following are TRUE of the management of alcohol withdrawal EXCEPT:

A. Maintenance of fluid, electrolyte, and nutrition is essential.
B. Clinical Institute Withdrawal Assessment-Alcohol (Revised) scale is a valid and reliable instrument for measuring the severity of withdrawal symptoms.
C. Benzodiazepines are the treatment of choice for detoxification.
D. Beta-blockers and clonidine are as effective as benzodiazepines for the treatment of withdrawal symptoms.
E. Phenytoin is effective in preventing recurrent withdrawal seizures.

159. Typical antipsychotic medications are commonly used in the treatment of which of the following syndromes?

A. NMS
B. Gilles de la Tourette's syndrome
C. Parkinson's disease
D. MS
E. Seizure disorders

160. Which one of the following is TRUE of antipsychotics and seizures?

A. Molindone has the highest risk of seizures among antipsychotics.
B. Olanzapine can be safely used in untreated epileptic patients.
C. Ziprasidone is not safe even in moderate doses in epileptic patients.
D. Clozapine has a dose-related risk of causing seizures in nonepileptic patients.
E. All of the above.

161. The mood enhancing property of estrogen is due in part to which one of the following?

A. Its influence on neural activity in the hypothalamus
B. Its stimulation of antiglucocorticoid activity
C. Its increase in sensitivity to serotonin

D. Its ability to help neurons metabolize glucose

E. Its enhancement of the activity of the limbic system

162. A 40-year-old man with Heroin Dependence last used an opioid substance 2 days ago. He enrolls in an opioid treatment program that is licensed to provide methadone and buprenorphine. All of the following are methods of treating opioid withdrawal in this patient EXCEPT:

A. Methadone

B. Buprenorphine

C. Clonidine

D. Naltrexone

E. Naltrexone with clonidine

163. You have just diagnosed an 8-year-old boy with Tourette's syndrome. You begin treatment with clonidine. Which of the following most correctly describes the mechanism of action of clonidine?

A. It is an alpha1 agonist.

B. It is an alpha1 antagonist.

C. It is an alpha2 agonist.

D. It is an alpha2 antagonist.

E. It is a nonselective alpha antagonist.

164. Which of the following is TRUE of cognitive changes associated with aging?

A. Mental speed declines

B. Verbal intelligence declines

C. Language skills declines

D. Calculation ability declines

E. All of the above

165. Which of the following brain structures is most responsible for maintaining the circadian rhythms associated with sleep?

A. Pons

B. Amygdala

C. Hypothalamus

D. Pituitary gland

E. Pineal gland

166. Which one of the following conditions is not usually associated with the atypical antipsychotic induced "metabolic syndrome"?

A. Diabetes

B. Dyslipidemia

C. Hypertension

D. Obesity

E. Gout

167. Which of the following associations is NOT TRUE?

A. Avoidant Personality: Fears rejection and criticism

B. Dependent Personality: Fears separation

C. Borderline Personality: Fears abandonment

D. Schizoid Personality: Fears social isolation

E. Social Phobic: Fears embarrassment and humiliation

168. Elevation of which of the following laboratory values is most likely to be seen in a patient with Bulimia Nervosa?

A. Potassium

B. Fasting glucose

C. Amylase

D. Calcium

E. Magnesium

169. The rule of thirds in Schizophrenia refers to which of the following phenomenon?

A. A third of the patients with schizophrenia will respond to a typical neuroleptic, one third will require an atypical agent, and the other third will require Clozaril.

B. A third of the patients will lead relatively normal lives, one third will have persistent symptoms but can function independently, and one third will require frequent hospitalizations.

C. A third of the patients will present in their teens, one third will present in their twenties, and one third will present in their thirties.

D. A third of the patients are white, one third are black, and one third are from other racial backgrounds.

E. A third of the patients experience prominent positive symptoms, one third experience prominent negative symptoms, and one third experience a mixture of both.

170. Which one of the following statements regarding the course of Bipolar Disorder is NOT TRUE?

A. Depressive episodes tend to last longer than manic episodes.

B. Manic episodes occur more in the summer with depressive episodes occurring more in the winter and spring.

C. Rapid cycling bipolar disorder refers to patients with four or more mood episodes per year.

D. The interval between mood episodes increases with time, then often plateaus.

E. Bipolar disorder is considered a chronic and recurrent condition.

171. Which one of the following psychotherapeutic modalities has the best evidence for the treatment of Anxiety Disorders in older adults?

A. Behavior therapy

B. Cognitive therapy

C. Cognitive-behavioral therapy (CBT)

D. Relaxation training
E. Supportive therapy

172. Which of the following figures in the history of psychiatry was most noteworthy for viewing the unconscious as being structured like a language?
    A. Heinz Kohut
    B. Jacques Lacan
    C. Wilfred Bion
    D. Melanie Klein
    E. Franz Alexander

173. Which of the following is TRUE of naltrexone?
    A. It is an opioid receptor antagonist.
    B. It is approved by FDA for the treatment of Alcohol Dependence.
    C. It reduces the reinforcing effects of alcohol by blocking μ-opioid receptors.
    D. It is effective for the short-term relapse prevention of alcohol dependence in conjunction with psychosocial treatments.
    E. All of the above.

174. Which one of the following is NOT a known side effect of corticosteroid therapy?
    A. Muscle weakness
    B. Hyperglycemia
    C. Weight gain
    D. Hypertension
    E. Hyperkalemia

175. Which of the following is the most common side effect of metoclopramide?
    A. Tardive dyskinesia (TD)
    B. Galactorrhea
    C. Methemoglobinemia
    D. Priapism
    E. Dystonias

176. Melatonin is a pineal hormone that is derived from which of the following hormones?
    A. Tryptophan
    B. Oxytocin
    C. Dopamine
    D. Epinine
    E. Tyramine

177. All of the following statements regarding combining antidepressants are true EXCEPT:
    A. Adding fluoxetine to desipramine can decrease desipramine blood levels.
    B. Bupropion can augment citalopram by inhibiting dopamine reuptake.
    C. Adding bupropion to venlafaxine can increase venlafaxine blood levels.

    D. Venlafaxine can augment bupropion by inhibiting serotonin reuptake.
    E. Increasing the number of antidepressants used can adversely effect compliance.

178. A 23-year-old woman was started on oxcarbazepine for the treatment of partial complex seizures. While educating the patient about the side effects of oxcarbazepine, the physician should keep in mind that the incidence of side effects is less common with this medication in comparison with carbamazepine, except for which of the following?
    A. Seizures
    B. Cardiac arrhythmias
    C. Hyponatremia
    D. Ataxia
    E. Mydriasis

179. When full criteria for MDD is met, the DSM-IV-TR includes "specifiers" to describe the current features of the depressive episode. Which of the following symptoms needs to be present in order to describe a depressive episode as Melancholic?
    A. Anhedonia
    B. Hypersomnia
    C. Hyperphagia
    D. Fatigue
    E. Leaden paralysis

180. A friend of the family is asking you for your professional opinion regarding her 6-year-old son. Following the recommendation of his teachers, he was recently evaluated by a psychiatrist for ADHD. The psychiatrist made the diagnosis of ADHD and prescribed a medication. After researching the medication's side effects, your friend asks you if you know of any other nonstimulant medications that are helpful in the treatment of this disorder. Which one of the following does NOT have empirical support for the treatment of ADHD?
    A. Clonidine
    B. Atomoxetine
    C. Imipramine
    D. Bupropion
    E. Venlafaxine

181. Which one of the following is a poor prognostic indicator for Schizophrenia?
    A. Late onset
    B. Good premorbid functioning
    C. Mood symptoms, especially depression
    D. Positive symptoms
    E. Insidious onset

182. A 4-year-old boy is brought to see his primary care physician. The boy's mother is concerned that her

son has continued to wet his bed several times per month. The boy is medically healthy and currently is not on any medications. According to the DSM-IV-TR, what is the most appropriate diagnosis for his condition?

A. Encopresis

B. Enuresis, Nocturnal Only

C. Enuresis, Diurnal Only

D. Enuresis, Nocturnal and Diurnal

E. No DSM-IV-TR diagnosis

183. Which one of the following statements is TRUE of treatments for TD?

A. Reduction in antipsychotic dosing consistently reduces the severity of TD in patients with established TD.

B. Using quetiapine in patients with established TD consistently reduces the severity of TD.

C. Routine use of adjunctive benzodiazepine in the treatment of TD is clinically indicated.

D. All of the above.

E. None of the above.

184. Which of the following is NOT TRUE of victimization, violence, and psychiatric illness?

A. Child abuse is usually associated with violent criminal offending in adolescence and adulthood.

B. Psychiatric patients have higher rates than the general population of both child abuse and victimization as adults.

C. Severe and persistent mental illness is more predictive of violence.

D. Recent criminal victimization is more predictive of violence.

E. Only those who are victims of violent crimes are significantly more likely to engage in violent behavior.

185. All of the following are TRUE of acamprosate (calcium homotaurinate) EXCEPT:

A. It blocks glutaminergic NMDA receptors.

B. It activates GABA-A receptors.

C. It reduces short- and long-term relapse rates in patients with Alcohol Dependence.

D. It is not contraindicated in renal insufficiency.

E. It does not interact with alcohol, diazepam, disulfiram, or imipramine.

186. Which of the following is NOT a known side effect of opiate use?

A. Diarrhea

B. Hypoventilation

C. Nausea

D. Dysphoria

E. Mental status changes

187. Which of the following is TRUE of monoamine oxidase (MAO)-B inhibitors in Parkinson's disease?

A. They delay disease progression.

B. They do not have beneficial effects on motor fluctuations.

C. They are not associated with a significant increase in deaths.

D. They should be recommended for routine use in the treatment of early Parkinson's disease.

E. All of the above.

188. Viral infection during fetal neural development may be involved in the pathogenesis of which one of the following illnesses?

A. Schizophrenia

B. MDD

C. Alzheimer's disease

D. Dysthymia

E. Chronic Fatigue Syndrome

189. Which of the following is TRUE of the Clinical Antipsychotic Trials of Intervention Effectiveness (CATIE) in Schizophrenia?

A. Multiple antipsychotic medications were compared for efficacy.

B. The majority of patients in the study discontinued the antipsychotic that they were assigned to take in the first place.

C. At least one typical antipsychotic medication was included in the study.

D. Patients with a Schizoaffective Disorder diagnosis were excluded from the study.

E. All of the above.

190. A 55-year-old man, recently diagnosed with Parkinson's disease (PD) comes with his wife for an appointment because he has some questions about his newly prescribed medications. The doctor wants to be as thorough as possible when explaining the benefits and risks of levodopa to improve the patient's compliance with treatment. Which of the following statements regarding the levodopa is NOT TRUE?

A. If levodopa is administered alone, more than 90% penetrates the brain.

B. Early in the disease, levodopa can have a dramatic effect in the symptoms of PD.

C. The on/off phenomena seen with levodopa may be mediated through brain adaptation.

D. Levodopa is converted to dopamine in the brain.

E. Levodopa has a short half-life.

191. When full criteria for MDD is met, the DSM-IV-TR includes "specifiers" to describe the current features of the depressive episode. Which of the following

symptoms needs to be present in order to describe a depressive episode as Atypical?

A. Mood reactivity
B. Early morning awakening
C. Anorexia or weight loss
D. Psychomotor agitation
E. Excessive guilt

192. Which of the following best distinguishes a Major Depression Episode from Bereavement?

A. A sustained depressed mood
B. Guilt of omission
C. Marked psychomotor retardation
D. Severe crying spells
E. Poor concentration

193. What is the approximate yearly rate of developing TD for patients treated with typical antipsychotics?

A. 1%
B. 5%
C. 10%
D. 20%
E. 50%

194. According to the DSM-IV-TR, which of the following is considered a Paraphilia?

A. Transvestic Fetishism
B. Gender Identity Disorder
C. Vaginismus
D. Sexual Aversion Disorder
E. Premature Ejaculation

195. Cases of all of the following illnesses have been associated with an infectious etiology EXCEPT?

A. Dementia
B. Mental retardation
C. Lyme disease
D. Delirium
E. Multiple Sclerosis (MS)

196. Which one of the following correctly matches the types of long-term memory with their associated brain areas?

A. Explicit memory: medial temporal lobe
B. Procedural memory: amygdale
C. Emotional associations: cerebellum
D. Classical conditioning: striatum
E. All of the above

197. A 28-year-old man has been treated with valproate for absence seizures with a good response to treatment. He has been seizure-free for 18 months. However, he is very worried about the side effects of valproic acid and he does not like to have to monitor

his blood levels regularly. He would like to know if he could stop his pharmacological treatment after a year without seizures. Which of the following would be the best recommendation for this patient?

A. It is recommended to stop pharmacological treatment after 1 year without seizures.
B. An abnormal EEG is a poor prognostic factor for recurrence of seizures after stopping medications.
C. He should wait for at least 5 years without seizures before thinking about stopping medications.
D. Most recurrences occur 1 year after following discontinuation of pharmacological treatment.
E. The risk of recurrence of seizures is approximately 80% after stopping medications.

198. A 30-year-old man presented with an acute onset of generalized weakness, spasticity, dysarthria, and dysphagia. Upon physical and neurological examination, the patient was noted to have muscle atrophy and fasciculations, but with intact sensory and autonomic functions. The patient scored 30/30 in the Mini Mental State Examination (MMSE). Given this information, which of the following medications has shown to have some effects on survival in patients with this illness?

A. Interferon
B. Dantrolene
C. Riluzole
D. Tizanidine
E. Clonazepam

199. Which of the following medications does NOT inhibit the cytochrome P450 system?

A. Phenobarbital
B. Phenytoin
C. Carbamazepine
D. Modafinil
E. All of the above

200. A 19-year-old woman is brought to your office because she was recently diagnosed with a seizure disorder. The patient has episodes of sudden turning movements of the head and eyes to the left side. The patient denies any loss of consciousness during these episodes. After a full workup that confirms the diagnosis of epilepsy, what would be your treatment of choice?

A. Lamotrigine
B. Oxcarbazepine
C. Ethosuximide
D. Valproic acid
E. Carbamazepine

Answers

1. Answer: A. As people age, they are at increased risk of loss of loved ones, including their spouse, friends, and family. This results in diminished access to familiar forms of social support. Often, older adults respond to this with an increase in reminiscence of the past. Reminiscence serves as a source of comfort as well as a means of coping with adversity. As adults grow older, the physical demand of their daily routine lessens and there is an increased enjoyment of solitude, which should not be mistaken for purposeful social isolation. It is important to distinguish between being alone and being lonely. Several studies of the elderly have reported no greater feelings of loneliness than in early life (exceptions may include widowed men and women who had lived with a spouse for several years contrasted to those who lived alone).

Sadavoy J, Jarvik LF, Grossberg GT, and Meyers BS. *Comprehensive Textbook of Geriatric Psychiatry*. New York: WW Norton & Company; 2004:159–201.

2. Answer: E. RCTs are usually prospective studies, often for evaluation of treatment modalities or other interventions. Especially with ethical concerns, RCTs are currently of limited use in determining heritability in humans. Observational and naturalistic studies have so far provided the strongest evidence in humans. Twin studies (comparing rates of disorders in monozygotic and dizygotic twins) and adoption studies (comparing twins separated from birth) help to separate genetic from shared environmental influences. Family risk studies definitely help determine heritability, but cannot as clearly separate how much a given disorder may be due to shared environment, and how much may be due to genetic transmission. Molecular studies use various techniques (linkage studies, genetic association studies, and other genome studies) to help determine heritability, and isolate involved genes. Some of the strongest evidence for heritability of psychiatric conditions has been found in Bipolar Disorder and Schizophrenia. Other disorders such as Major Depression, Alcoholism, Somatization/sociopathy, Personality Traits, and possibly Anxiety and Eating Disorders have shown some results suggestive of being heritable.

Hales RE, Yudofsky SC. *Textbook of Clinical Psychiatry*. 4th ed. Washington: American Psychiatric Publishing; 2003: 3–65.

3. Answer: B. *Ataque de nervios* is a Latin culture-bound syndrome characterized by behavioral dyscontrol, emotional expression, and disrupted consciousness often seen as a result of a stressful event relating to the family. Amok is a dissociative episode characterized by a period of brooding followed by a violent outburst. *Brain fag*, or *brain fatigue*, is a West African term used to describe difficulty with concentration and memory. Falling out is a culture-bound syndrome seen in the southern United States and the Caribbean characterized by a sudden collapse and an inability to see despite open eyes. Koro is a syndrome reported in South and East Asia in which there is a sudden, intense anxiety that the penis or vulva and nipples will recede into the body.

Sadock BJ, Sadock VA. *Kaplan and Sadock's Comprehensive Textbook of Psychiatry*. 8th ed. Philadelphia: Lippincott Williams & Wilkins; 2005:2287–2288.

4. Answer: C. The study described is a cohort study, which is prospective in nature. Case-control studies are similar, but retrospective. Cross-sectional studies simply gather data from a population at a particular point in time. An RCT follows at least two different populations prospectively over time, but the intervention (exposure) is manipulated in a randomized fashion. Single blind studies are a form of RCT where only the subjects are unaware of their intervention (exposure) status. In double-blind RCTs, the subjects and investigators are blinded. In triple-blind RCTs, the subjects, investigators and statisticians are blinded to the interventions.

Tohen M, Bromet E, Murphy JM, et al. Psychiatric epidemiology. *Harv Rev Psychiatry*. 2000;8:111–125.

5. Answer: D. Carbamazepine (Tegretol) may produce anemia, aplastic anemia, leukopenia, and thrombocytopenia so pretreatment evaluation typically includes a CBC. Many clinicians monitor the CBC every 2 weeks for the first 2 months of administration. Then, if the counts have been within normal limits, the CBC is monitored every quarter. Carbamazepine should be discontinued if the WBC count is less than 3,000 per mm^3, the erythrocyte count is less than 4.0×10^6 per mm^3, hemoglobin is less than 11 mg/dL, the neutrophil count is less than 1,500 per mm^3, and the platelet count is less than 100,000 per mm^3. Because carbamazepine may cause hepatitis, baseline LFTs also are indicated. Carbamazepine has a molecular structure similar to TCAs and has the same propensity as TCAs to effect cardiac conduction (QTc and QRS prolongation). Many clinicians obtain pretreatment EKGs before starting carbamazepine. Patients with a QTc of longer than 0.440 second are at an increased risk for serious cardiac arrhythmias with carbamazepine treatment. Carbamazepine may produce hyponatremia and the syndrome of inappropriate secretion of antidiuretic hormone (SIADH) and hence serum electrolytes should be monitored. Carbamazepine may produce a variety of congenital abnormalities, including spina bifida and anomalies of the fingers. A pretreatment urine pregnancy test is usually obtained in women of childbearing years. Women should be cautioned to use adequate contraception when taking carbamazepine. TSH is monitored with lithium therapy, not carbamazepine.

1. Albers LJ, Hahn RK, Reist C. *Handbook of Psychiatric Drugs*. Laguna Hills: Current Clinical Strategies Publishing; 2005:74–77.
2. Sadock BJ, Sadock VA. *Kaplan and Sadock's Comprehensive Textbook of Psychiatry*. 8th ed. Philadelphia: Lippincott Williams & Wilkins; 2005:923.

6. Answer: E. Anxiety is common in patients with respiratory illness, and is often multi-factorial in nature. Hypoxia itself causes anxiety, and many treatments to improve hypoxia (e.g., albuterol, theophylline) will worsen anxiety. Difficulty adjusting to an illness is a common exacerbating factor, and patients always must deal with difficult stressors such as bereavement, often reacting with anxiety.

Cassem NH, Stern TA, Rosenbaum JF, et al. *Massachusetts General Hospital Handbook of General Hospital Psychiatry*. 4th ed. St. Louis: Mosby-Year Book; 1997:173–210.

7. Answer: B. Memory impairment is the most prominent feature of Alzheimer's disease. Vascular dementia is characterized by poor attention, decreased speed of processing, decline in executive functioning, and "non-cognitive" changes, such as depression and anxiety.

1. Braaten AJ, Parsons TD, McCue R, et al. Neurocognitive differential diagnosis of dementing diseases: Alzheimer's dementia, vascular dementia, frontotemporal dementia, and major depressive disorder. *Int J Neurosci*. 2006;116:1271–1293.
2. Looi JC, Sachdev PS. Differentiation of vascular dementia from AD on neuropsychological tests. *Neurology*. 1999;53:670–678.

8. Answer: A. This patient likely has psychophysiological insomnia. The question highlights a typical scenario. Patients with psychophysiological insomnia have a conditioned state of heightened arousal associated with the act of going to bed or the environment in which sleep typically occurs, which often develops after some emotionally traumatic event. Long after the event has been forgotten, the patient associates going to bed with an uncomfortable condition generating anxiety and heightened arousal, which are incompatible with sleep. This heightened arousal is often specific to their bedroom. The PSG usually indicates objectively disturbed sleep with a relatively long sleep latency, shortened total sleep time, or frequent awakenings during the night. These patients are usually fairly accurate on the amount and quality of sleep they get.

Sadock BJ, Sadock VA. *Kaplan and Sadock's Comprehensive Textbook of Psychiatry*. 8th ed. Philadelphia: Lippincott Williams & Wilkins; 2005:2023–2024.

9. Answer: A. If all of the criteria are met for schizophrenia, but symptoms are present for less than 6 months, the most appropriate diagnosis is Schizophreniform disorder. Patients with Delusional Disorder report non bizarre delusions, but have relatively intact functioning. Brief Psychotic Disorder typically presents with psychotic symptoms for less than 1 month, and clearly following a stressful event. Both Schizoaffective Disorder and Residual Type Schizophrenia require the presence of psychotic symptoms for greater than 6 months.

American Psychiatric Association. *Quick Reference to the Diagnostic Criteria from DSM-IV-TR*. Washington: American Psychiatric Association; 2000:153–165.

10. Answer: A. Several studies have found that younger couples respond more favorably to BCT. In addition, less-educated couples had better response to BCT than those with higher education. Being unemployed or being employed in a position of unskilled labor also predicts poorer treatment outcome. Couples who are married longer also showed the greater treatment gains. Couples having the greatest difficulties in their relationship are less likely to benefit from treatment. Lack of commitment and behavioral steps taken toward divorce have been associated with poor treatment outcome to BCT. Poor outcome was also predicted by negative communication behavior, lower relationship quality, greater negative relationship affect and disengagement, and greater desired change in the relationship. Inequality prior to the therapy predicted positive treatment outcome at posttest and at six-month follow-up. Wife-dominant couples improved the most in response to couple therapy in terms of increased satisfaction and improved communication. Greater interpersonal sensitivity and emotional expressiveness—as determined by measures of "femininity"—have been found to predict better outcome at termination. Couples in which partners exhibit a higher degree of traditionality (i.e., higher affiliation needs in the wife and higher independence needs in the husband) have been shown to have poorer response to BCT. Partners' higher levels of depressed affect have been linked to poorer outcome.

1. Atkins DC, Berns SB, George WH, et al. Prediction of response to treatment in a randomized clinical trial of marital therapy. *J Consult Clin Psychol.* 2005;73:893–903.
2. Snyder DK, Castellani AM, Whisman MA. Current status and future directions in couple therapy. *Annu Rev Psychol.* 2006;57:317–344.

11. Answer: A. The most consistently identified risk factors for developing NMS are prominent psychomotor agitation, higher doses of neuroleptics (mean and maximum dose), greater neuroleptic dose increments over a short time period (increased dose within 5 days), the magnitude of increase from initial dose, and parenteral administration of the drugs (for example, intramuscular injections). Combination of two or more neuroleptics may also precipitate NMS. Other psychotropic drugs like lithium, when administered concomitantly with neuroleptics, are also reported to be associated with NMS. Psychiatric illness, including affective disorders, altered sensorium, psychomotor agitation, acute disorganization, and catatonia are also potential risk factors for the development of NMS. Infectious encephalitis, AIDS, organic brain disorders, and tumors also increases the susceptibility for NMS. Young age and male gender and the development of dehydration are also considered risk factors for the development of NMS. Other factors, such as trauma, infection, malnutrition, alcoholism leading to malnutrition, premenstrual phase in females, and sympathoadrenal hyperactivity (e.g., thyrotoxicosis) also have been implicated independently in cases of NMS.

Bhanushali MJ, Tuite PJ. The evaluation and management of patients with neuroleptic malignant syndrome. *Neurol Clin.* 2004;22:389–411.

12. Answer: C. The most prominent area of alcohol absorption is the proximal small intestine. It is also absorbed through the mucosal lining in the mouth, esophagus, and the stomach. The rate of absorption can be delayed by the presence of food in the small intestine.

Sadock BJ, Sadock VA. *Kaplan and Sadock's Comprehensive Textbook of Psychiatry.* 7th ed. Philadelphia: Lippincott Williams & Wilkins; 2000:955.

13. Answer: A. Disulfiram inhibits acetaldehyde dehydrogenase and, therefore, prevents metabolism of acetaldehyde to acetate. Although it has been used to treat alcohol dependence for more than 40 years, the evidence for its effectiveness is weak. It is usually used in the dosage range of 250 to 500 mg per day. Disulfiram is administered only after the patient has been abstinent from alcohol for at least 12 hours, and it is recommended to avoid alcohol for at least 2 weeks from the last usage of disulfiram. It is not generally recommended to be used in the primary care setting. It is FDA approved, and is category C in pregnancy.

1. Graham AW, Schultz TK, Mayo-Smith MF, et al. *Principles of Addiction Medicine.* 3rd ed. Chevy Chase, Maryland: American Society of Addiction Medicine; 2003:701–703.
2. Williams SH. Medications for treating alcohol dependence. *Am Fam Physician.* 2005;72:1775–1780.

14. Answer: C. Most barbiturates are derived from barbituric acid with various side chains from the parent molecule. Barbiturates presumably work by enhancing pre- and postsynaptic GABA receptors to reduce postsynaptic excitatory potentials. Barbiturates are typically very lipophilic (not hydrophilic), and the higher their lipid solubility, the greater the potency, and the quicker and briefer the action. The ionized forms of barbiturates enter the brain faster, and lower blood pH (more acidic) increases the entry of barbiturates into the brain. Barbiturates are mostly metabolized in the liver, and metabolites are then excreted by the kidneys.

Ropper AH, Brown RH. *Adams and Victor's Principles of Neurology.* 8th ed. New York: McGraw-Hill; 2005:1017–1045.

15. Answer: C. The Tarasoff issue is based on an initial 1974 ruling by the California supreme court that clinicians have a duty to warn potential victims of violence, which was subsequently reconsidered with a new 1976 ruling that clinicians have a duty to protect potential victims. Interpretation of the Tarasoff ruling varies from state to state, and you should be familiar with the laws in your state. The ruling is based on what obligation a clinician has to a third party based on knowledge gained in a "special relationship." Duty to protect may be interpreted more vaguely than duty to warn. Protection may arise from hospitalization, medication adjustments, changing frequency of meetings, involving family, increasing social support, notification of police, involving the potential victim, or various other means, but should be individualized for the patient in question. The MacArthur studies examined risk factors for violent behavior. The McNaughten ruling involves the potential for absolution of guilt by reason of insanity.

The Miranda rulings relate to being informed of your rights.

Cohen BJ. *Theory and Practice of Psychiatry*. New York: Oxford University Press; 2003:445–466.

16. **Answer: A.** Dopamine is a biogenic amine neurotransmitter. There are four major dopamine pathways in the brain: the nigrostriatal tract, the mesolimbic tract, the mesocortical tract, and the tuberoinfundibular tract. The nigrostriatal tract projects from the substantia nigra to the corpus striatum. When D_2 receptors at the end of the pathway are antagonized, Parkinsonian side effects can emerge. Moreover, in Parkinson's disease, this tract degenerates causing the motor symptoms of the disease. The mesolimbic tract links the ventral tegmentum in the midbrain to the nucleus accumbens in the limbic system. Excess dopamine in this area has been linked to psychosis and the positive symptoms of schizophrenia. The mesocortical pathway connects the ventral tegmentum to the cortex and especially to the frontal lobes. The tract is essential to normal cognitive function and may be involved in motivation and emotional responses. Through this relationship, it may be associated with the negative symptoms of Schizophrenia. The tuberoinfundibular pathway innervates the median eminence and the posterior and intermediate lobes of the pituitary. Dopamine released at this site regulates the section of PRL from the anterior pituitary gland. Drugs that block dopamine in this tract can cause an increase in PRL levels. The corticospinal tract contains motor axons and is not one of the four major dopamine pathways.

Sadock BJ, Sadock VA. *Kaplan and Sadock's Synopsis of Psychiatry*. 9th ed. Philadelphia: Lippincott Williams & Wilkins; 2003:88–108.

17. **Answer: B.** The circadian rhythm is set by both internal and external forces called *zeitgebers* or time clues. The main influences on the cycle stem from the suprachiasmatic nuclei (SCN) of the hypothalamus and the pontine reticular formation. The typical period of human circadian rhythms is 24.5 hours. The sleep-wake cycle is linked to changes in levels of several circulating hormones, particularly melatonin, and to light. Melatonin is secreted at night and terminates upon retinal stimulation by sunlight. Other hormones whose concentrations are affected by sleep include cortisol, TSH, GH, PRL, and LH. Specifically, serum cortisol levels are lowest at sleep onset and the highest in the morning. TSH secretion is suppressed by sleep onset. GH levels surge during deep sleep. PRL and LH also reach their highest levels during sleep. Other hormones such as testosterone vary throughout the day. The circadian rhythm begins in the first few months of life and starts to fragment in old age. In terms of psychiatric disorders, depression has most often been associated with disruptions of biological rhythms. Early morning awakening, decreased latency of rapid eye movement (REM) sleep, and neuroendocrine perturbations all account for this change.

Sadock BJ, Sadock VA. *Kaplan and Sadock's Synopsis of Psychiatry*. 9th ed. Philadelphia: Lippincott Williams & Wilkins; 2003:128–135.

18. **Answer: E.** Cognitive dysfunction in HD usually spares long-term memory, but impairs executive functions, such as organizing, planning, checking, or adapting alternatives. It also delays the acquisition of new motor skills. These features worsen over time with speech deteriorating faster than comprehension.

Walker FO. Huntington's disease. *Lancet*. 2007;369:218–228.

19. **Answer: E.** Aphasias (fluent, nonfluent, conduction, isolation) are generally signs of dominant hemisphere lesions, because language function is usually associated with the dominant hemisphere. The remaining answers (hemi-inattention, hemineglect, anosognosia, and constructional apraxia) are generally characteristic of nondominant hemisphere lesions.

Kaufman DM. *Clinical Neurology for Psychiatrists*. 5th ed. Philadelphia: WB Saunders; 2001:8–25.

20. **Answer: B.** This patient most likely has a right-sided medullary infarct (brainstem). Remember: cranial nerve palsies with "alternating hypalgesia" is usually a medullary lesion (lower brainstem). Wallenberg syndrome results from a posterior inferior cerebellar artery occlusion, which results in a medullary infarct with the following complex symptom cluster: paralysis of ipsilateral palate (nucleus ambiguous of CN IX and XI damage), ipsilateral face hypalgias (trigeminal nucleus/cranial nerve V damage) with contralateral body anesthesia (due to ascending spinothalamic tract damage), ipsilateral ataxia (cerebellar damage), and sympathetic fiber damage, which may also cause a Horner's syndrome (ptosis and miosis). The ipsilateral face hypalgesia combined with contralateral body anesthesia has been termed "alternating hypalgesia." Infarct to neither cortex could cause this complex symptom pattern. Basal ganglia lesions are usually associated with motor disturbances more than weakness

and sensory changes. Spinal cord lesions would not result in cranial nerve signs.

Kaufman DM. *Clinical Neurology for Psychiatrists*. 5th ed. Philadelphia: WB Saunders; 2001:8–25.

21. Answer: E. NPH is a clinical syndrome which is characterized by dementia, urinary incontinence, and gait apraxia. Gait apraxia is usually the first and most prominent symptom and is generally the first symptom to improve with treatment. Urinary incontinence and gait abnormality present at the onset of dementia generally distinguish NPH from Alzheimer's disease. Classically, the acute presentation of Wernicke's encephalopathy is characterized by confusion, ataxia, and ocular motility abnormalities which include conjugate gaze paresis, abducens nerve paresis, and nystagmus. The dementia of Lewy body disease is often accompanied by a combination of Parkinsonian-like features (including resting tremor and bradykinesia), sensitivity to neuroleptics, and visual hallucinations. The noncognitive symptoms of frontotemporal dementia include aggression or apathy, disinhibition, hyperorality, and other aspects of Klüver-Bucy syndrome. In most cases, Creutzfeldt-Jacob disease causes a triad of dementia, myoclonus, and distinctive periodic EEG complexes.

Kaufman DM. *Clinical Neurology for Psychiatrists*. 5th ed. Philadelphia: WB Saunders; 2001:141–149.

22. Answer: E. This patient has Lesch-Nyhan syndrome, which is a sex-linked autosomal recessive inborn error of purine nucleotide metabolism. The gene involved is on the X chromosome and so the disorder occurs almost entirely in males. Occurrence in females is very rare. The onset of self-injury occurs as early as 1 year or rarely as the late teens. The enzyme HGPRT is present in all cells, but is highest in the brain, especially the basal ganglia. Its absence prevents the normal metabolism of hypoxanthine, resulting in hyperuricemia and manifestations of gout without specific treatment. HGPRT levels are related to the extent of motor symptoms, presence or absence of self-injury, and possibly cognitive function. Hypoxanthine accumulates in the brain; uric acid does not accumulate in the brain, because it is not produced in the brain and does not cross the blood–brain barrier.

Harris JC. *Developmental Neuropsychiatry*. Vol II. Oxford: Oxford University Press; 1998:306–308.

23. Answer: D. Mucopolysaccharidoses are inherited disorders leading to the incomplete breakdown and storage of mucopolysaccharides or glycosaminoglycans. The storage product is heparan sulphate, keratin sulphate, dermatan sulphate, or chondroitin 4/6 sulphates. Although mental retardation is seen with all mucopolysaccharidoses, growth retardation is not seen in the Sanfilippo and Scheie syndromes where linear growth is unaffected. Carrier detection and prenatal diagnoses are available for each of the mucopolysaccharidoses.

Harris JC. *Developmental Neuropsychiatry*. Vol II. Oxford: Oxford University Press; 1998:356.

24. Answer: D. Fabry's disease is transmitted via an X-linked recessive mode of inheritance.

Kaplan HI, Sadock BJ. *Kaplan and Sadock's Synopsis of Psychiatry*. 9th ed. Philadelphia: Lippincott Williams & Wilkins; 2003:1167.

25. Answer: C. Multiple system atrophy is a progressive neurodegenerative disorder causing pyramidal, cerebellar, and autonomic dysfunction. It includes three disorders previously thought to be distinct: olivopontocerebellar atrophy, striatonigral degeneration, and Shy-Drager syndrome. Parkinsonian symptoms (predominant in striatonigral degeneration) include rigidity, bradykinesia, postural instability, and jerky postural tremor. High-pitched, quavering dysarthria is common. In contrast to Parkinson's disease, resting tremor and dyskinesia are uncommon, and symptoms respond poorly and transiently to levodopa. Symptoms of cerebellar dysfunction (predominant in olivopontocerebellar atrophy) include ataxia, dysmetria, dysdiadochokinesia, poor coordination, and abnormal eye movements. Typical symptoms of autonomic failure are orthostatic hypotension often with syncope urinary retention or incontinence, constipation, and erectile dysfunction. Sleep apnea and respiratory stridor are common. Diagnosis is suspected clinically based on the combination of autonomic failure and Parkinsonism or cerebellar symptoms. Similar symptoms may result from Parkinson's disease, Lewy body dementia, pure autonomic failure, autonomic neuropathies, progressive supranuclear palsy, multiple cerebral infarcts, or drug-induced parkinsonism. No diagnostic test is definitive, but MRI abnormalities in the striatum, pons, and cerebellum are highly suggestive. Multiple system atrophy can be diagnosed based on these findings plus symptoms of generalized autonomic failure and lack of response to levodopa.

1. Lishman WA. *Organic Psychiatry*. 3rd ed. Oxford: Blackwell Science; 1996:668–669.
2. Rodnitzky RL. *Parkinson's Disease Dementia*. http://www.uptodateonline.com/utd/content/topic.do?topicKey=nuroegen/8264. Accessed March 7, 2007.

26. Answer: D. Severity of TBI severity is defined by the LOC, altered mental status (e.g., confusion) or PTA.

However, the severity of functional impairments after TBI often is not related to the severity of the injury. Mild TBI is defined as a blow to the head followed by an LOC of less than 30 minutes, an altered mental status with PTA of less than 24 hours or Glasgow Coma Scale score of 13 to 15. Patients are classified as having a moderate-to-severe TBI if they have an LOC over 30 minutes or altered mental status greater than 24 hours or Glasgow Coma Score below 12. For majority of those with a mild TBI, they attain full recovery within 3 to 6 months; however, approximately 15% of patients will continue to experience long-term cognitive, physical, and behavioral difficulties that interfere with their ability to function. This condition is known as persistent postconcussion syndrome. Because these consequences are not well understood, many family members and professionals assume that these individuals are exaggerating or "faking" their symptoms and emotional or behavioral problems are seen as psychogenic. However, these symptoms are most likely secondary to neurological events and not due to an underlying psychiatric disorder.

Ashman TA, Gordon WA, Cantor JB, et al. Neurobehavioral consequences of traumatic brain injury. *Mt Sinai J Med.* 2006;73:999–1005.

27. **Answer: D.** Harry Harlow studied social learning and the effects of social isolation in monkeys. In a series of experiments, monkeys were raised in various degrees of isolation (e.g., total isolation, mother-only reared, peer-only reared, partial isolation, and separation from caretaker after a bond had developed). The effects seen in those monkeys raised in total isolation (not allowed to develop caretaker or peer bonds) included self-orality, self-clasping, fearfulness of peers, and inability to copulate. If impregnated, females were unable to nurture their own young. If the duration of total isolation lasted beyond 6 months, no recovery was found to be possible.

Sadock BJ, Sadock VA. *Kaplan and Sadock's Synopsis of Psychiatry.* 9th ed. Philadelphia: Lippincott Williams & Wilkins; 2003:28, 159–161.

28. **Answer: E.** Several neuropsychological deficits have been found in relatives of Schizophrenics, including (but not limited to) the Wisconsin Card-Sort Test, Minnesota Multiphasic Personality Inventory, and tests of sustained attention (e.g., Continuous Performance Test). Various psychotic spectrum personality traits (Cluster A) have also been found in relatives of schizophrenics. More objective physiological findings, such as smooth pursuit eye movement dysfunction or impaired p50 suppression on auditory evoked potentials, have even been found in nonaffected relatives of schizophrenics.

Hales RE, Yudofsky SC. *Textbook of Clinical Psychiatry.* 4th ed. Washington: American Psychiatric Publishing; 2003: 3–65.

29. **Answer: B.** While smaller clinical trials have reported on the efficacy of tricyclic antidepressants, gabapentin, capsaicin cream, mexiletine, and opiates for the treatment of painful diabetic polyneuropathy, none of them are formally approved by the FDA for the treatment of this condition. Only duloxetine and pregabalin are the drugs that are approved by the FDA for the treatment of painful diabetic polyneuropathy. Both drugs appear to have equal efficacy in treating this condition.

Feldman EL, McCulloch DK. *Treatment of Diabetic Neuropathy.* http://www.uptodateonline.com/utd/content/topic.do?topicKey=neuropat/6605&type=A&selectedTitle=9~37. Accessed December 9, 2007.

30. **Answer: C.** According to the ECA study, Substance Use Disorders had a lifetime prevalence of 16.4%, bolstered largely by Alcohol Abuse and Dependence Disorders with a prevalence of 13.3%. Substance Use Disorders were followed closely by Anxiety Disorders, which had a 14.6% lifetime prevalence (phobias alone had a 12.5% lifetime prevalence). Perhaps pointing to their chronic nature, the 1-month prevalence of anxiety disorders was highest at 7.3%. Lifetime prevalence in the ECA study for the remaining disorders were: Affective Disorders 8.3%, Schizophrenia and Schizophreniform Disorders 1.5%, and Somatization Disorder 0.1%. Conducted in the 1980s, the ECA study included subjects from the community and institutions who were 18 years of age to elderly, but were limited to five study sites.

Tohen M, Bromet E, Murphy JM, et al. Psychiatric epidemiology. *Harv Rev Psychiatry.* 2000;8:111–125.

31. **Answer: D.** Antipsychotic treatment is associated with metabolic side effects that include weight gain, dyslipidemia, and type 2 diabetes. In addition, patients with chronic psychotic disorders have increased coronary heart disease (CHD) mortality. Obesity is a major risk factor for hypertension, diabetes, cardiovascular disease, cerebrovascular disease, and lipid abnormalities. Weight gain also contributes to medication noncompliance and poor self-image. Weight and waist circumference should be monitored *weekly* in hospital care and *monthly* in ambulatory care. Intervention is recommended in the form of nutritional counseling, exercise program, or change in antipsychotic medication when BMI increases by one

unit or when waist circumference measures greater than 35 inches for a woman or 40 inches for a man. Hyperlipidemia is associated with cardiovascular and cerebrovascular disease. Total cholesterol, high-density lipoprotein cholesterol, low-density lipoprotein cholesterol, and triglycerides should be monitored every 3 MONTHS for the first year of treatment, then ANNUALLY. Although antipsychotics do not cause hypertension directly, it is a major contributing factor in the development of CHD. In clinical trials, antihypertensive therapy has been associated with up to a 25% reduction in myocardial infarction, a 50% reduction in heart failure, and a 40% reduction in stroke incidence. Hence, blood pressure should be monitored every 3 MONTHS in patients on antipsychotics. Antipsychotic agents have been associated with abnormalities in serum glucose levels, including the development of diabetes mellitus. Fasting blood glucose should be monitored depending on risk factors and drugs—monthly in patients with family history of diabetes/obesity and/or with manifested overweight or obesity, and/or with impaired fasting glucose. In patients without risk factors, fasting blood glucose (FBG) should be monitored after 6 and 12 weeks, and then quarterly. The usual diagnostic test for diabetes is the fasting plasma glucose (FPG) (> 7.0 mmol/L, or 126 mg/dL). The 2-hour plasma glucose level taken after a 75-gm glucose drink (> 11.1 mmol/L, or 200 mg/dL), that is, the postload plasma glucose in the OGTT, is also diagnostic, as is the random glucose level (> 11.1 mmol/L, or 200 mg/dL) when there are clear symptoms of diabetes. Any abnormal result should be confirmed by a repeat test on a different day. The OGTT is not used for routine monitoring of patients on antipsychotics, although it is considered the gold standard test and has greater diagnostic sensitivity than FBG. The fasting glucose level is the favored screening test for diabetes because of its diagnostic specificity and its ease of use.

1. Cohn TA, Sernyak MJ. Metabolic monitoring for patients treated with antipsychotic medications. *Can J Psychiatry*. 2006;51:492–501.
2. De Hert M, van Eyck D, De Nayer A. Metabolic abnormalities associated with second generation antipsychotics: fact or fiction? Development of guidelines for screening and monitoring. *Int Clin Psychopharmacol*. 2006;21 (Suppl 2):S11–S115.
3. Sadock BJ, Sadock VA. *Kaplan and Sadock's Comprehensive Textbook of Psychiatry*. 8th ed. Philadelphia: Lippincott Williams & Wilkins; 2005:925–926.

32. Answer: B. This patient has Factitious Disorder with predominantly physical signs and symptoms, also known as Münchhausen syndrome, hospital addiction, polysurgical addiction, and professional patient syndrome. In this disorder, patients intentionally misrepresent medical signs and symptoms with the objective of assuming the role of a patient without any external incentive, and are able to present physical symptoms so well that they can gain admission to and stay in a hospital. Such patients often insist on surgery, and continue to be demanding and difficult in the hospital. As each test is returned with a negative result, they may become generally abusive and even accuse doctors of incompetence. Anecdotal case reports indicate that many patients with Factitious Disorder suffered childhood abuse or deprivation, and that the patient perceived one or both parents as rejecting figures. Other specific predisposing factors include: true physical disorders during childhood leading to extensive medical treatment, or a family history of serious illness or disability, a grudge against the medical profession, employment as a medical paraprofessional, and an important relationship with a physician in the past. Factitious Disorders usually have a poor prognosis. Factitious Disorder is distinguished from Malingering, in which there is an obvious, recognizable environmental incentive, and patients can stop producing their signs and symptoms when they are no longer considered profitable or when the risk becomes too great.

Kaplan HI, Sadock BJ. *Kaplan & Sadock's Synopsis of Psychiatry*. 8th ed. Philadelphia: Lippincott Williams & Wilkins; 1998:654–658.

33. Answer: C. Richard Asher, in a 1951 article in the *Lancet*, coined the term *Münchhausen syndrome* to refer to a syndrome in which patients chronically embellish their personal history and fabricate symptoms to gain hospital admission and move from hospital to hospital. Wilford Bion expanded the concept of projective identification to include an interpersonal process in which the therapist feels forced by a patient to play a role in their internal world. Sandor Ferenczi developed a procedure known as active therapy, in which the patients developed an awareness of reality through active confrontation by the therapist. Alfred Adler coined the term inferiority complex. Eric Berne developed transactional analysis.

1. Kaplan HI, Sadock BJ. *Kaplan & Sadock's Synopsis of Psychiatry*. 8th ed. Philadelphia: Lippincott Williams & Wilkins; 1998:223–229.
2. Sadock BJ, Sadock VA. *Kaplan & Sadock's Concise Textbook of Clinical Psychiatry*. 2nd ed. Philadelphia: Lippincott Williams & Wilkins; 2004:261.

34. Answer: B. The characteristics of Avoidant Personality Disorder include pervasive and excessive hypersensitivity to negative evaluation, social inhibition, and feelings of inadequacy. There is an equal sex ratio between men and women. There is an increased risk for mood and anxiety disorders, but the most frequent comorbidities are Schizotypal, Schizoid, Paranoid, Dependent, and Borderline Personality Disorders (BPD). Impairment is often severe and includes occupational and social difficulties. Prevalence rates of 10% for psychiatric outpatients are reported. Avoidant Personality Disorder is hard to differentiate from Social Phobia, and many experts believe that they represent the same disorder. Disfiguring illness and shyness in childhood predispose children for this personality disorder.

Sadock BJ, Sadock VA. *Kaplan and Sadock's Comprehensive Textbook of Psychiatry.* 7th ed. Philadelphia: Lippincott Williams & Wilkins; 2000:1747.

35. Answer: E. Excessive daytime somnolence, cataplexy, sleep paralysis, and hypnogogic hallucinations are commonly referred to as the tetrad of symptoms seen in narcolepsy. Interepisodic symptoms are not seen in these patients.

American Psychiatric Association. *Quick Reference to the Diagnostic Criteria from DSM-IV-TR.* Washington: American Psychiatric Association; 2000:269.

36. Answers: E. The available evidence on the clinical and cost-effectiveness of psychological therapies for BPD indicates that there is some evidence that DBT is more effective than TAU for the treatment of chronically parasuicidal and drug-dependent borderline women. DBT-orientated therapy is also more effective than CCT for the treatment of BPD. DBT is also as effective as comprehensive validation therapy plus 12-step for the treatment of opioid-dependent borderline women. There was also some evidence that partial hospitalization is more effective than TAU in the treatment of BPD. There is also good evidence that MACT is no more effective than TAU in the treatment of BPD and some evidence that interpersonal group therapy is no more effective than individual mentalization-based partial hospitalization (MBT) for the treatment of BPD. However, these results should be interpreted with caution as not all of these studies were primarily targeted to borderline symptoms and there were considerable differences between the studies. Studies do not support the cost-effectiveness of DBT, although, they suggest it has the potential to be cost-effective. The results for MBT are promising, although again surrounded by a high degree of uncertainty and for MACT the

analysis suggests that the intervention is unlikely to be cost-effective.

Brazier J, Tumur I, Holmes M, et al. Psychological therapies including dialectical behavior therapy for borderline personality disorder: a systematic review and preliminary economic evaluation. *Health Technol Assess.* 2006;10:iii, ix–xii, 1–117.

37. Answer: A. It was Carl Gustav Jung who believed that archetypes such as the animus, the anima, the shadow and others manifested themselves in dreams, as dream symbols or figures. In his book, *The Interpretation of Dreams*, Sigmund Freud stated that the foundation of all dream content is the fulfillment of wishes, conscious or otherwise. He described the conflict between superego and id that leads to "censorship" of dreams. Freud listed four transformations applied to wishes in the dreams to avoid censorship. These are: condensation—one dream object stands for several thoughts; displacement—a dream object's psychical importance is assigned to an object that does not raise the censor's suspicions; representation—a thought is translated to visual images; and symbolism—a symbol replaces an action, person, or idea. These transformations help to disguise the latent content, transforming it into the manifest content, what is actually seen by the dreamer. The basis for all of these systems, he claimed, was "transference," in which a would-be censored wish of the unconscious is given undeserved "psychical energy" (the quantum of attention from consciousness) by attaching to "innocent" thoughts. Freud indicated that the wishes are not revealed in dream analysis for the sake of conscious fulfillment, but instead for conscious resolution of the inner conflict.

1. Crisp T. *Sigmund Freud.* http://www.dreamhawk.com/d-freud.htm. Accessed April 19, 2007.
2. Sadock BJ, Sadock VA. *Kaplan and Sadock's Comprehensive Textbook of Psychiatry.* 8th ed. Philadelphia: Lippincott Williams & Wilkins; 2005:709–712.

38. Answer: E. Alcohol is metabolized primarily in the liver by the action of ADH, which converts alcohol to acetaldehyde. Aldehyde dehydrogenase, subsequently, catalyzes the conversion of acetaldehyde into acetic acid. Alcohol metabolism follows the zero order kinetics, that is, a constant amount is oxidized per unit of time.

Graham AW, Schultz TK, Mayo-Smith MF, et al. *Principles of Addiction Medicine.* 3rd ed. Chevy Chase, Maryland: American Society of Addiction Medicine; 2003:102.

39. Answer: B. Glaucoma is not a relative contraindication for the use of disulfiram. Consumption of alcohol after taking disulfiram results in a reaction that results in palpitation, flushing, nausea, vomiting, hypotension, sweating, dizziness, blurry vision, and headaches. Most reactions are short and self-limited, lasting about thirty minutes. However, a more severe reaction may occur, presenting with congestive heart failure, myocardial infarction, respiratory depression, convulsions, and death. It is, therefore, contraindicated in patients who have taken alcohol or metronidazole, have psychosis or cardiovascular disease, severe pulmonary disease, chronic renal failure, diabetes, or those older than 60 years of age. It is also not recommended in patients with peripheral neuropathy, seizures, or cirrhosis with portal hypertension. Hepatotoxicity is a rare but potentially fatal adverse effect. It is, therefore, recommended to closely monitor liver functions in patients receiving disulfiram.

1. Graham AW, Schultz TK, Mayo-Smith MF, et al. *Principles of Addiction Medicine*. 3rd ed. Chevy Chase, Maryland: American Society of Addiction Medicine; 2003:701–703.
2. Williams SH. Medications for treating alcohol dependence. *Am Fam Physician*. 2005;72:1775–1780.

40. Answer: B. Amphetamines stimulate respiration and suppress appetite. Cardiac effects include tachycardia and hypertension. Subjective effects include anxiety and psychosis, and amphetamines are particularly known to induce paranoia. Amphetamines may produce an initial euphoric effect and can be highly addictive in some patients. Amphetamines have been widely used for a variety of indications (e.g., including obesity, depression, and fatigue), but rebound and withdrawal effects may counteract their intended use. Amphetamines' therapeutic usefulness is best known in narcolepsy (by promoting wakefulness) and ADHD (by enhancing focus and concentration).

Ropper AH, Brown RH. *Adams and Victor's Principles of Neurology*. 8th ed. New York: McGraw-Hill; 2005:1017–1045.

41. Answer: C. Sigmund Freud (1856–1939) is generally believed to have created the field of psychoanalysis. Freud studied under the famous neurologist Charcot (1825–1893), and utilized hypnosis along with Breuer (1841–1925), but is believed to have initiated psychoanalytic theory, beginning with his technique of free association. Freud coined the term *psychoanalysis* in 1896. Rush (1745–1813) is known as the "father of American psychiatry," and believed in somatic causation of mental illness, not accepting the moral treatments popular in his day. Meyer (1866–1950) was a prominent American psychiatrist of the early 20th century who espoused psychobiology, a belief that mental illness was neither purely biological nor purely psychological. Meyer's influence on modern American psychiatry is profound and deep-rooted.

Sadock BJ, Sadock VA. *Kaplan & Sadock's Comprehensive Textbook of Psychiatry*. 7th ed. Philadelphia: Lippincott Williams & Wilkins; 2000:3301–3333.

42. Answer: C. Serotonin is synthesized in the axonal terminal. Its precursor amino acid is tryptophan. The availability of tryptophan is the rate-limiting step in its synthesis. The enzyme tryptophan hydroxylase is not rate limiting. Tryptophan hydroxylase converts tryptophan to 5-hydroxytryptophan, which is then converted to serotonin by the enzyme amino acid decarboxylase. Because tryptophan concentrations are rate limiting in the synthesis of serotonin, dietary variations in tryptophan can measurably affect serotonin levels in the brain. Tryptophan depletion causes irritability and hunger, while tryptophan supplementation can relieve anxiety, induce sleep, and promote a sense of well-being. The key enzyme involved in the metabolism of serotonin is MAO, preferentially MAO_A, and the main metabolite is 5-hydroxyindoleacetic acid (5-HIAA). Norepinephrine, epinephrine, and dopamine are all catecholamines. They are synthesized from tyrosine. The rate limiting step in their production is the enzyme tyrosine hydroxylase. In neurons which release norepinephrine and dopamine, β-hydroxylase converts dopamine to norepinephrine. In neurons that release epinephrine, phenylethanolamine-N-methyltransferase (PNMT) further converts norepinephrine into epinephrine. The major routes of deactivation of dopamine, epinephrine, and norepinephrine are through uptake back into the presynaptic neuron and metabolism by MAO_A and catechol-O-methyl transferase (COMT).

Sadock BJ, Sadock VA. *Kaplan and Sadock's Synopsis of Psychiatry*. 9th ed. Philadelphia: Lippincott Williams & Wilkins; 2003:88–108.

43. Answer: B. Bupropion and nicotine replacement therapies (such as nicotine gum or patches) are first-line agents for reducing nicotine use and withdrawal symptoms. Clonidine and nortriptyline are considered second-line agents for treating Nicotine Dependence. The best outcomes combine medication and psychosocial therapies, such as CBT, motivational enhancement therapy, brief interventions, and behavioral therapy. Choice B is false because hypnosis and 12-step programs have not shown significant efficacy in treating nicotine dependence.

Kleber HD, Weiss RD, Anton RF, et al. Treatment of patients with substance use disorders, second edition.

American Psychiatric Association. www.psychiatryonline. com/content.aspx?aID=141810. Accessed December 10, 2007.

44. Answer: C. The gene for HD is located on the short arm of chromosome four. It is associated with an expanded trinucleotide repeat. The normal alleles at this site contain CAG repeats. When these repeats reach 41 or more, the disease becomes fully penetrant. Incomplete penetrance happens with 36 to 40 repeats, and 35 or less are not associated with the disorder. The number of CAG repeats accounts for about 60% of the variation in age of onset, with the remainder represented by modifying genes and environment.

Walker FO. Huntington's disease. *Lancet.* 2007;369:218–228.

45. Answer: B. Nystagmus is often a sign of brainstem lesion, eye movements are controlled by cranial nerves whose nuclei reside in the brainstem. Incontinence usually denotes a spinal cord injury. Intention tremor usually results from cerebellar dysfunction. Basal ganglia lesions result in Parkinsonism. Any sensory loss may occur with unilateral cerebral hemisphere lesions, or possibly with loss to a "level" secondary to a spinal cord injury. Cortical sensory loss usually consists of deficits in contralateral position sense, two-point discrimination, and stereognosis. Pain sensation remains intact as it is localized to the thalamus at the uppermost portion of the brainstem.

Kaufman DM. *Clinical Neurology for Psychiatrists.* 5th ed. Philadelphia: WB Saunders; 2001:8–25.

46. Answer: B. This case describes classic Brown-Séquard syndrome. Brown-Séquard syndrome is the result of the hemi-transection of the spinal cord. Transection of cortical spinal tracks causes ipsilateral weakness from that level down. Injury to the spinothalamic tract results in contralateral loss of temperature and pain below the level of the lesion. This is because the fibers of the spinothalamic tract cross over in the spinal cord. If the dorsal columns are affected, ipsilateral impairment of vibration and position sense occurs. Complete transection of the cord would result in all symptoms bilaterally. Injury of the anterior or dorsal horns may cause deficits of either motor or sensory function, but typically not a mixture of both, and are separated anatomically so that such an injury becomes more improbable than Brown-Séquard syndrome.

Kaufman DM. *Clinical Neurology for Psychiatrists.* 5th ed. Philadelphia: WB Saunders; 2001:8–25.

47. Answer: C. Patients with essential tremor generally present with fine oscillations of their wrists, hands, or fingers. (They may also display a head tremor or tremor in their voice.) Certain actions or postures characteristically elicit the tremor, which is usually in a single plane. Essential tremor is the most common involuntary movement disorder and usually develops in young and middle-aged adults. It follows a pattern of autosomal dominant inheritance with variable penetrance, and about 30% of patients will endorse a positive family history. In 50% of affected individuals, alcohol-containing beverages suppress the tremor. Anxiety generally intensifies it. Essential tremor must be differentiated from those with other etiologies, including the few listed above. In contrast with essential tremor, the pill-rolling tremor of Parkinson's disease occurs characteristically at rest and is diminished by movement. Wilson's disease characteristically produces a "wing-beating" tremor, which is course and centered at the shoulders. Patients with Huntington's disease demonstrate chorea, which consists of random, discrete, brisk movements which jerk the pelvis, trunk, and limbs. Sydenham's chorea is a major diagnostic criterion of rheumatic fever and almost exclusively affects children between the ages of 5 and 15 years. It generally begins insidiously as grimaces and limb movements and has a duration of approximately several weeks.

Kaufman DM. *Clinical Neurology for Psychiatrists.* 5th ed. Philadelphia: WB Saunders; 2001:458–475.

48. Answer: E. A quarter to a third of untreated children with PKU develop seizures. In classical untreated PKU, the clinical features include mental retardation, neurological symptoms and varying degrees of systemic symptoms. In classical untreated PKU, the most consistent feature is mental retardation which becomes evident in mid-infancy. Behavioral problems such as hyperactivity, impulsivity, and self-injury have been reported. Autism and schizophrenia-like psychoses have also been documented. The affected child usually has fair, lightly pigmented skin, blonde hair and blue eyes. Photosensitivity and eczematous rash have been reported. A mousy odor may be present. Brain damage from untreated PKU is irreversible; however, dietary treatment with low phenylalanine foods may reduce behavioral disturbance. Guthrie test or heel-prick test is done on the fourth and seventh day to screen for PKU in the newborn.

1. Harris JC. *Developmental Neuropsychiatry.* Vol II. Oxford: Oxford University Press; 1998:332–335.
2. Kaplan HI, Sadock BJ. *Kaplan and Sadock's Synopsis of Psychiatry.* 9th ed. Philadelphia: Lippincott Williams & Wilkins; 2003:1166.

49. Answer: A. Hunter's syndrome is transmitted via an X-linked recessive mode of inheritance.

1. Harris JC. *Developmental Neuropsychiatry*. Vol II. Oxford: Oxford University Press; 1998:356.
2. Kaplan HI, Sadock BJ. *Kaplan and Sadock's Synopsis of Psychiatry*. 9th ed. Philadelphia: 2003:1172.

50. Answer: D. Maple syrup urine disease is an autosomal recessive disorder of aminoacid metabolism that causes acidosis (in the first week of life in severe cases) and central nervous system symptoms. The urine of these patients smell like maple syrup due to their inability to metabolize the branched-chain amino acids leucine, isoleucine, and valine due to deficiency of branched chain ketoacid decarboxylase. Symptoms of this disorder appear in the first week of life. It can lead to decerebrate rigidity, seizures, respiratory irregularity, hypoglycemia, recurrent ketoacidosis, and death, if untreated. Death usually occurs in the first few months of life, if untreated. Survivors are usually severely mentally retarded. Dietary treatment of maple syrup urine disease follows principles similar to that for PKU. The diet in this case should be low in leucine, isoleucine, and valine.

Kaplan HI, Sadock BJ. *Kaplan and Sadock's Synopsis of Psychiatry*. 9th ed. Philadelphia: Lippincott Williams & Wilkins; 2003:1167.

51. Answer: C. This patient has the signs and symptoms of MS. It has a prevalence of less than 1 per 100,000 in equatorial areas, and 30 to 80 per 100,000 in northern latitudes with a less well-defined gradient in the Southern Hemisphere. Immigrants from a high-risk to a low-risk zone carry with them at least part of the risk of their country of origin, even though the disease may not become apparent until 20 years after migration. The critical age of immigration appears to be about 15 years. A familial concordance of MS is also seen, with 15% having an affected relative, with the greatest concordance between siblings. About two thirds of the cases of MS have their onset between 20 and 40 years of age. Although many environmental factors have been proposed as causative (e.g., surgical operations, trauma, anesthesia, exposure to household pets [small dogs], mercury in silver amalgam fillings in teeth), these are unsupported by evidence.

1. Ebers GC. Genetic factors in multiple sclerosis. *Neurol Clin*. 1983;1(3):645–654.
2. Ropper AH, Brown RH. *Adams and Victor's Principles of Neurology*. 8th ed. New York: McGraw-Hill; 2005:773–775.

52. Answer: A. When a patient presents with Addisonian crisis, treatment with glucocorticoids must not be delayed. Blood for serum cortisol, ACTH and serum chemistry should be drawn, and therapy with IV saline and dexamethasone should be initiated immediately. A short corticotropin stimulation test can then be performed as dexamethasone does not interfere with cortisol radioimmunoassay. Following testing, therapy with dexamethasone can be replaced with hydrocortisone. Low aldosterone and high renin are consistent with the diagnosis of Addison's disease. If the cause of primary adrenal insufficiency is unknown, adrenal autoantibody tests and imaging of the adrenal glands can be performed, but is not an important test in the acute management of this patient's condition.

Anglin RE, Rosebush PI, Mazurek MF. The neuropsychiatric profile of Addison's disease: revisiting a forgotten phenomenon. *J Neuropsychiatry Clin Neurosci*. 2006;18:450–459.

53. Answer: D. According to Piaget, moral judgment can be divided into two stages. Children younger than 10 years of age think about moral dilemmas in one way and older children consider them differently. Younger children regard rules as being fixed and absolute. They believe that rules are handed down by adults or by God and that one cannot change them according to the needs of the situation. The older children view these rules as being more relativistic. They understand that it is permissible to change rules, with everyone's agreement. Rules are not sacred and absolute, but are devices by which humans use to get along cooperatively. Younger children base their moral judgments more on consequences, whereas older children base their judgments on intentions. Younger children primarily consider the amount of damage and hence the consequence, while the older child is more likely to judge wrongness in terms of the motives underlying the act. Moral issues continue to develop throughout adolescence.

Crain WC. *Theories of Development*. New Jersey: Prentice-Hall; 1985:118–136.

54. Answer: A. Polygenetic multifactorial transmission is now believed to be the most likely mode of inheritance for susceptibility to development of schizophrenia. Possible contributing loci have been found at multiple chromosome sites (1q, 6p, 8p, 22q, etc.). Most monogenetic models have been rejected. Although tri-nucleotide repeat model explanations of some rarer forms of psychosis may be valid, they do not explain Schizophrenia.

Hales RE, Yudofsky SC. *Textbook of Clinical Psychiatry*. 4th ed. Washington: American Psychiatric Publishing; 2003:3–65.

55. Answer: D. The ability to learn to recognize differences between similar but different stimuli is an important characteristic of learning. If two stimuli are significantly different, an animal could respond to one and not the other. This is termed discrimination. Studies show that dogs respond differently to similar bell sounds. A related but diametrically opposite phenomenon is stimulus generalization which occurs when a conditioned response is transferred from one stimulus to the other. According to learning theory, generalization explains phobias and PTSD: in both disorders, patients are not able to discriminate between the phobic object or cues of trauma on one hand and the inducing feared object or precipitating trauma on the other hand. Extinction occurs when a conditioned stimulus is constantly repeated without the unconditioned stimulus until the response generated by the stimulus weakens and then disappears. In the "Pavlovian" experiment, ringing the bell (conditioned stimulus) without presenting the piece of meat (unconditioned stimulus) following an initial period of pairing these two stimuli did not result in salivation. The neutral stimulus (bell) is the conditioned stimulus, because it would not on its own induce the response.

1. Lovibond PF. Animal learning theory and the future of human Pavlovian conditioning. *Biol Psychol*. 1988;27:199–202.
2. Windholz G. Pavlov's conceptualization of learning. *Am J Psychol*. 1992;105:459–469.

56. Answer: B. According to the NCS, Substance Use Disorders had a lifetime prevalence of 26.6% (highest in men), closely followed by Anxiety Disorders (highest in women) at 24.9% lifetime prevalence. Lifetime prevalence for Affective Disorders was 19.3% (higher in women), and for Psychotic Disorders was 0.7% (relatively equally distributed between sexes). Personality Disorders as a class were not broadly studied, though the NCS did study Antisocial Personality Disorders (ASPD). Anxiety disorders did have the highest 12-month prevalence, likely reflecting their chronic nature. The NCS included subjects from all 48 contiguous states, but was limited to ages of 15 to 54 years and only considered non-institutionalized people and people living in the community.

Tohen M, Bromet E, Murphy JM, et al. Psychiatric epidemiology. *Harv Rev Psychiatry*. 2000;8:111–125.

57. Answer: C. The HAM-D is a clinician-rated scale with a focus on somatic symptoms of depression. The version in most common use has 17 items, but it does not include some of the symptoms for depression in DSM-IV, most notably the so-called reverse neurovegetative signs (increased sleep, increased appetite, and psychomotor retardation). HAM-D total score ranges from 0 to 50. Scores of 7 or less may be considered normal; 8 to 13, mild; 14 to 18, moderate; 19 to 22, severe; and 23 and above, very severe depression. Ratings are completed by the examiner based on patient interview and observations. The BDI is a self-report scale with a focus on behavioral and cognitive dimensions of depression. The current version, the Beck-II, has added more coverage of somatic symptoms to be compatible with DSM-IV. The BDI includes 21 self-report items, each of which has four statements describing increasing levels of severity and the total score ranges from 0 to 84. Scores of 0 to 9 are considered minimal; 10 to 16, mild; 17 to 29, moderate; and 30 to 63, severe. Internal consistency has been high but the test–retest reliability is not consistently high, but this may reflect changes in underlying symptoms. Validity is supported by correlation with other depression measures. The instrument's strength lies in measuring the depth of depression and in its comprehensive coverage of the cognitive dimension of depression.

1. Sadock BJ, Sadock VA. *Kaplan and Sadock's Comprehensive Textbook of Psychiatry*. 8th ed. Philadelphia: Lippincott Williams & Wilkins; 2005:944–945.
2. Stein DJ, Kupfer DJ, Schatzberg AF. *Textbook of Mood Disorders*. Washington: American Psychiatric Publishing; 2006:76–80.

58. Answer: D. Factitious Disorders are distinguished from Malingering because in Factitious Disorders, patients intentionally misrepresent signs and symptoms with the objective of assuming the role of a patient (primary gain) without any external incentive, whereas in Malingering, there is an obvious, recognizable environmental incentive (secondary gain), and patients can stop producing their signs and symptoms when they are no longer considered profitable or when the risk becomes too great. Ganser's syndrome may be a variant of Malingering in which patients respond to simple questions with astonishingly incorrect answers. Factitious Disorders usually begin in early adult life, although they may appear during childhood or adolescence. Anecdotal case reports indicate that many patients with Factitious Disorder suffered childhood abuse or deprivation, and that the patient perceived one or both parents as rejecting figures. Factitious Disorders usually have a poor prognosis, and no specific psychiatric therapy has been effective. The type of Factitious Disorder is based on the presence of predominantly psychological versus physical signs and symptoms.

Kaplan HI, Sadock BJ. *Kaplan & Sadock's Synopsis of Psychiatry*. 8th ed. Philadelphia: Lippincott Williams & Wilkins; 1998:654–659.

59. Answer: A. According to the DSM-IV-TR diagnostic criteria, choice A is the definition of factitious disorder. The diagnosis of Malingering (choice B) is made when there is evidence of secondary gain. Choice C represents the diagnostic criteria for Somatization Disorder, choice D is Conversion Disorder, and choice E represents Body Dysmorphic Disorder. Choices C, D, and E are classified under Somatoform Disorders. In contrast to Factitious Disorders and Malingering, Somatoform Disorder symptoms are *not* under voluntary control.

American Psychiatric Association. *Quick Reference to the Diagnostic Criteria from DSM-IV-TR.* Washington: American Psychiatric Association; 2000:229–243.

60. Answer: D. Patients with sleep state misperception (also known as subjective insomnia) have a disconnect between objective and subjective measures of sleep. Patients claim to have slept only 1 to 2 hours in a night, but have a normal PSG. This disorder is not related to being a light sleeper, as patients are not easier to awaken by an auditory stimulus than normal sleepers. The misperception does not appear to be intentional or psychological, because there is a limited placebo response. After receiving placebo, subjective insomniacs generally report that they had been awake when asked after being awakened from nonrapid eye movement (NREM) sleep by an auditory tone. After receiving a hypnotic, the same patients respond similarly to normal sleepers, having a good match between subjective and objective measures. Despite the normal PSG, patients with sleep state misperception tend to respond poorly to hearing that there is nothing objectively wrong with their sleep. This often leads to alienating the patient.

Sadock BJ, Sadock VA. *Kaplan and Sadock's Comprehensive Textbook of Psychiatry.* 8th ed. Philadelphia: Lippincott Williams & Wilkins; 2005:2024.

61. Answer: D. While establishing a regular exercise routine is thought to contribute to good sleep hygiene, it is likely best to engage in physical exercise in the morning.

Sadock B, Sadock V. *Kaplan and Sadock's Pocket Handbook of Clinical Psychiatry.* 3rd ed. Philadelphia: Lippincott Williams & Wilkins; 2001:210.

62. Answer: C. IPT designed by Klerman and Weissman is a flexible, integrative, time-limited, and structured psychotherapy. IPT is based on interpersonal theories with the main principle abstracted from these theories is that life events occurring after the early childhood years influence psychopathology. This model incorporates psychoeducation, is "medication friendly," and agrees with a medical model of psychiatric illness. Similar to CBT, it is structured and open, using a collaborative therapeutic relationship without invoking transference issues. Rating scales monitor each patient's progress. IPT does not involve formal "homework" or rely on extensive paperwork. However, patients are encouraged to develop skills and experiment actively with these between sessions. IPT is particularly accessible to patients who find dynamic approaches mystifying and/or the "homework" demands of CBT difficult. It has been manualized as a treatment for depression, bulimia nervosa, as a group treatment for binge eating disorder, and modified and extended for treatment of anxiety, dysthymia, primary care disorders, chronic fatigue, mood disorders associated with human immunodeficiency virus (HIV), somatization, adolescent disorders and depression of later life, and for use with couples and groups. However, this model has not so far been modified for the management of psychoses.

1. Hales RE, Yudofsky SC. *American Psychiatric Publishing Textbook of Clinical Psychiatry.* 4th ed. http://www.psychiatryonline.com/content.aspx?aID=91986. Accessed April 5, 2007.
2. Morris J. Interpersonal psychotherapy: a trainee's ABC. *Psychiatric Bulletin.* 2002;26:26–28.

63. Answer: E. In his book, *The Interpretation of Dreams*, Sigmund Freud stated that the foundation of all dream content is the fulfillment of wishes, conscious or otherwise. He described the conflict between superego and id leads to "censorship" of dreams. Freud listed four transformations applied to wishes in the dreams to avoid censorship. These are: condensation—one dream object stands for several thoughts; displacement—a dream object's psychical importance is assigned to an object that does not raise the censor's suspicions; representation—a thought is translated to visual images; and symbolism—a symbol replaces an action, person, or idea. These transformations help to disguise the latent content, transforming it into the manifest content, what is actually seen by the dreamer. Freud indicated that the wishes are not revealed in dream analysis for the sake of conscious fulfillment, but instead for conscious resolution of the inner conflict. Wish fulfillment is a process by which one might dream of fulfilling desires or wishes, even symbolically that are socially or personally prohibited. The manifest content of a dream is that part of the dream which we can remember and report. Secondary revision is the process by which events and scenes are linked and made orderly.

1. Crisp T. *Sigmund Freud.* http://www.dreamhawk.com/d-freud.htm. Accessed April 19, 2007.

2. Sadock BJ, Sadock VA. *Kaplan and Sadock's Comprehensive Textbook of Psychiatry.* 8th ed. Philadelphia: Lippincott Williams & Wilkins; 2005:709–712

64. Answer: E. Important targets for the action of alcohol in the brain include the GABA-A (inhibitory) and NMDA receptors (excitatory). Alcohol has been shown to increase mesolimbic dopamine, which is thought to be associated with its reinforcing effects. Animal studies suggest involvement of 5-HT3 receptors in the subjective effects of alcohol.

Graham AW, Schultz TK, Mayo-Smith MF, et al. *Principles of Addiction Medicine.* 3rd ed. Chevy Chase, Maryland: American Society of Addiction Medicine; 2003:105–111.

65. Answer: E. In addition to disulfiram, a variety of agents such as metronidazole, oral hypoglycemics, trichomonacides, and carbimides can produce Antabuse-like reaction when alcohol is consumed during treatment with these drugs due to their inhibition of aldehyde dehydrogenase (ALDH).

Kranzler HR, Jaffe JH. Pharmacologic interventions for alcoholism. In: Graham AW, Schultz TK, Mayo-Smith MF, et al., eds. *Principles of Addiction Medicine.* 3rd ed. Chevy Chase, Maryland: American Society of Addiction Medicine; 2003:701–702.

66. Answer: D. Although placebo may be effective in the treatment of pain (especially acute pain), their use is often considered unethical. Hypnosis, biofeedback, behavioral modification, cognitive therapy, and other psychotherapies are accepted alternative treatments for chronic pain, usually as augmenting strategies.

Kaufman DM. *Clinical Neurology for Psychiatrists.* 5th ed. Philadelphia: WB Saunders; 2001:357.

67. Answer: C. Practicing in the pre-antibiotic era, von Wagner-Jauregg (1857–1940) caused remissions in general paresis (tertiary syphilis), beginning in 1917, by using malaria-induced fevers. In 1927, von Wagner-Jauregg became the first psychiatrist to win a Nobel Prize for his work. Penicillin became the treatment of choice for general paresis in the 1940s. Moniz (1874–1955) was a neurologist who helped pioneer the lobotomy, and shared the Nobel Prize in 1949 with neurophysiologist Walter Hess. Incidentally, psychotropic drugs were introduced about the same time (lithium in 1949, chlorpromazine in 1952, etc.). Freud (1856–1939) developed psychoanalysis, and though arguably the most popularly famous of those list, he never won a Nobel Prize. Jung (1875–1961) began as a follower of Freud's theories, but broke off to develop his own psychological theories. Also, psychiatrist Eric Kandel (1929-present) shared the 2000 Nobel Prize "for their discover-

ies concerning signal transduction in the nervous system" with two nonpsychiatrists, Arvid Carlsson and Paul Greengard.

1. Nobel Web. *The Official Web Site of the Nobel Foundation.* http://nobelprize.org. Accessed February 15, 2007.
2. Sadock BJ, Sadock VA. *Kaplan & Sadock's Comprehensive Textbook of Psychiatry.* 7th ed. Philadelphia: Lippincott Williams & Wilkins; 2000: 3301–3333.

68. Answer: A. Each biogenic amine neurotransmitter system originates in a subcortical nucleus and sends projections to higher brain regions. The major site of serotonergic cell bodies is in the median and dorsal raphe nuclei and to a lesser extent, the locus ceruleus, the area postrema (the brainstem vomiting center), and the interpeduncular area. These neurons project to the basal ganglia, the limbic system, and the cerebral cortex. The major concentration of noradrenergic and adrenergic cell bodies is in the locus ceruleus in the pons. Axons from these neurons project through the medial forebrain bundle to the cerebral cortex, the limbic system, the thalamus, and the hypothalamus. Cell bodies of the dopamine system reside in the substantia nigra and ventral tegmental area. Acetylcholine system cell bodies reside in the nucleus basalis of Meynert.

Sadock BJ, Sadock VA. *Kaplan and Sadock's Synopsis of Psychiatry.* 9th ed. Philadelphia: Lippincott Williams & Wilkins; 2003:88–108.

69. Answer: E. Buprenorphine, oxycodone, hydrocodone, and fentanyl all require a special assay to be detected, because they will not show on a routine urine drug screen.

Kleber HD, Weiss RD, Anton RF, et al. Treatment of patients with substance use disorders, second edition. American Psychiatric Association. www.psychiatryonline.com/content.aspx?aID=141810. Accessed December 14, 2007.

70. Answer: D. Diseases that have an autosomal dominant mode of inheritance and manifest as clinical parkinsonism and can respond to L-dopa are SCA3 in those of African descent, SCA2 in those of Asian descent, and MAPT mutations associated with frontotemporal dementia and parkinsonism, FTDP17.

Hardy J, Cai H, Cookson MR, et al. Genetics of Parkinson's disease and parkinsonism. *Ann Neurol.* 2006;60:389–398.

71. Answer: D. Partial seizures are typically a sign of unilateral cerebral hemisphere lesions. Many varieties of partial seizures exist: elementary, complex, and secondarily generalized. Partial seizures are almost always due to cerebral lesions. Approximately 90% of partial complex lesions originate in the temporal lobe. Metabolic or other injuries to both hemispheres typically result in generalized (grand mal) seizures. Partial seizures are less likely to be the result of brainstem, basal ganglia, or cerebellar lesions.

Kaufman DM. *Clinical Neurology for Psychiatrists*. 5th ed. Philadelphia: WB Saunders; 2001:8–25.

72. Answer: A. For most neurologic illnesses, an MRI is the preferred method of imaging over CT scans. MRIs give greater soft tissue resolution, and are able to distinguish white from gray matter in the brain. Because it utilizes high-powered magnets, it is dangerous to perform on patients with indwelling ferrous material. Screens for such are routinely performed before MRI. CT scan is faster, and less expensive than MRI. It also identifies fluid, fat and bones better, and hence can detect abnormalities in these structures e.g., intracranial bleeds.

1. Kaufman DM. *Clinical Neurology for Psychiatrists*. 5th ed. Philadelphia: WB Saunders; 2001:532–551.
2. Ropper AH, Brown RH. *Adams and Victor's Principles of Neurology*. 8th ed. New York: McGraw-Hill; 2005:11–38.

73. Answer: E. Neuropsychiatric symptoms may occur in young patients even before it affects the liver. Neurologic disorders may occur in up to 35% of patients with Wilson's disease. These include parkinsonian symptoms including tremor, rigidity, clumsiness of gait, slurring of speech, inappropriate and uncontrollable grinning (risus sardonicus), and drooling. About 10% of all patients may present with a range of psychiatric symptoms from subtle personality changes, deteriorating performance at school, to depression, paranoia, and catatonia. Parkinsonian symptoms with mood changes are associated with dilatation of the third ventricle. Ataxia and tremor are associated with focal thalamic lesions. Dyskinesia, dysarthria, and personality changes are associated with focal lesions in the putamen and pallidum. In these patients, the cerebrospinal fluid (CSF) copper concentrations are elevated three to fourfold as compared to controls. These levels reduce with appropriate therapy.

1. Kaplan MM. *Pathogenesis and Clinical Manifestations of Wilson's Disease*. http://www.uptodateonline.com/utd/content/topic.do?topicKey=hep_dis/9927. Accessed March 6, 2007.
2. Rosenblatt A, Leroi I. Neuropsychiatry of Huntington's disease and other basal ganglia disorders. *Psychosomatics*. 2000;41:24–30.

74. Answer: D. The gene for the enzyme phenyl alanine hydroxylase, deficient in PKU, is located on the chromosome 12q.

Harris JC. *Developmental Neuropsychiatry*. Vol II. Oxford: Oxford University Press; 1998:334.

75. Answer: D. The commonest type of mucopolysaccharidosis is the Sanfilippo syndrome.

Harris JC. *Developmental Neuropsychiatry*. Vol II. Oxford: Oxford University Press; 1998:356.

76. Answer: C. William's syndrome has a prevalence of 1 in 20,000 births. It is characterized by congenital facial ("elfin") and cardiovascular abnormalities, failure to thrive, and mental retardation. In William's syndrome, linguistic abilities are relatively spared despite the mental retardation, which can range from mild to severe. It is associated with a hemizygous deletion that includes the elastin locus on chromosome 7, which accounts for the association of congenital heart disease. Life expectancy may be reduced if there is congenital heart disease. It is accompanied by hypercalcemia in over 60% of cases. This may be treated with low calcium and vitamin D restricted diet; it may also decrease with time between the 9th and 18th month, without any dietary changes. Despite the correction of hypercalcemia, the physical and psychological symptoms persist.

1. Harris JC. *Developmental Neuropsychiatry*. Vol II. Oxford: Oxford University Press; 1998:319–332.
2. Kaplan HI, Sadock BJ. *Kaplan and Sadock's Synopsis of Psychiatry*. 9th ed. Philadelphia: Lippincott Williams & Wilkins; 2003:1166.

77. Answer: C. Each of the tests may be used during the neuropsychological evaluation of a patient with suspected mild dementia. Digit Span Forward and Backward is a commonly employed measure of attention in the elderly. Another test of attention, which also measures executive function, is the Trail Making Test-Part A. The NART, a measure of reading ability, is often used to estimate premorbid intellectual function. The Boston Naming Test asks patients to name objects from line drawings in order to assess language function. The Wisconsin Card-Sorting Test is a test of executive function, which calls upon patients' problem solving skills. Other tests of executive function include the Ruff Figural Fluency Test and the Stroop Color Word Test. Finally, the Finger Tapping Test is a test of psychomotor function, in particular, psychomotor speed. Other psychomotor function tests include the Hand Dynamometer, which assesses psychomotor strength, and the Grooved Pegboard, which assesses manual dexterity.

Sadavoy J, Jarvik LF, Grossberg GT, et al. *Comprehensive Textbook of Geriatric Psychiatry*. New York: WW Norton & Company; 2004:371–380.

78. Answer: E. Although anticholinesterase drugs improve myasthenic symptoms in nearly all patients, they do not fully relieve the symptoms in many. Thus, most patients require additional immunosuppressive treatment. Corticosteroids are the immunosuppressive agents most commonly used in the treatment of MG and the most consistently effective. They are administered at high doses for several months and at low doses for years. In patients presenting with steroid-related complications, other immunosuppressants, either as "steroid-sparing" agents or as a substitute for corticosteroids, can be used. Azathioprine, a purine analog interfering with T and B cell proliferation is used as a single immunosuppressant agent, but its major disadvantage is the delayed clinical response, which may take up to 15 months. Cyclophosphamide administered orally or intravenously is an effective treatment for MG with more than half of the patients becoming asymptomatic after 1 year of treatment. Its delayed effect and undesirable side effects like hair loss, nausea, vomiting, anorexia, and skin discoloration limits its use to the management of patients who do not respond to other immunosuppressive treatments. Cyclosporine blocks the synthesis of cytokines (and especially IL-2), IL-2 receptors, and other proteins critical in the function of CD4+ T cells. It is useful as a steroid-sparing agent. Tacrolimus, a macrolide antibiotic, with biological activity to cyclosporine has been shown in treatment-resistant patients to be useful as a steroid-sparing agent. Plasma exchange (plasmapheresis) and IVIG can be used as chronic therapy although their benefit has not been documented in rigorously designed studies. Plasmapheresis and IVIG are used for acute management of severe muscular weakness. Although therapeutic ablation of the thymus in MG has been done, its clinical efficacy is questionable. Usually, thymectomy is performed on patients early in the course of their disease and is restricted to patients younger than 60 years of age.

Conti-Fine BM, Milani M, Kaminski HJ. Myasthenia gravis: past, present, and future. *J Clin Invest*. 2006;116:2843–2854.

79. **Answer: C.** Kohlberg's stages of moral development are planes of moral adequacy to explain the development of moral reasoning and postulates that moral reasoning which is the basis for ethical behavior has six identifiable developmental stages. These six stages are further divided into into three levels: preconventional, conventional, and postconventional. His theory is based on constructive developmental stages; each stage and level is more adequate at responding to moral dilemmas than the last. These stages are as follows: the level 1, preconventional morality has the stages of (i) obedience and punishment orientation and (ii) of individualism and exchange. Level II is the stage of conventional morality, which has the stage 3 of good interpersonal rela-

tionships and stage 4 of maintaining the social order. Level III is that of postconventional morality, which has the stage 5 of social contract and individual rights and the stage 6 of universal principles. In stage 1, children think of what is right as that which authority says is right. Doing the right thing is obeying authority and avoiding punishment. In stage 2, children are no longer so impressed by any single authority and they see that there are different sides to any issue. As everything is relative, one is free to pursue one's own interests, but it is often useful to make deals and exchange favors with others. At stages 3 and 4, young people consider themselves as members of the conventional society with its values, norms, and expectations. At stage 3, the emphasis is on being a good person, which basically means having helpful motives toward people close to one. At stage 4, concerns shifts toward obeying laws to maintain society as a whole. At stages 5 and 6, people are less concerned with maintaining society for it own sake, and more concerned with the principles and values that make for a good society. At stage 5, they emphasize basic rights and the democratic processes that give everyone a say. In stage 6, the principles by which agreement will be most just are defined.

Crain WC. *Theories of Development*. 2nd rev ed. Englewood, New Jersey: Prentice-Hall; 1985:118–136.

80. **Answer: B.** Several findings of earlier studies have been replicated by the National Institute of Mental Health Collaborative Study on Affective Disorders. It has been replicated that first-degree relatives of bipolar patients are at an increased risk of both Unipolar and Bipolar mood disorders. However, regarding first-degree relatives of unipolar depressed patients, they have only increased risk for depression, not Bipolar Disorder. Schizoaffective disorder of the bipolar type is associated with increased rates of Bipolar Disorder in first-degree relatives, but such is not true for Schizoaffective Disorder of the depressive type, which is actually associated with slightly increased rates of Schizophrenia in first-degree relatives.

Hales RE, Yudofsky SC. *Textbook of Clinical Psychiatry*. 4th ed. Washington: American Psychiatric Publishing; 2003: 3–65.

81. **Answer: D.** The patient is most probably exhibiting the defense mechanism of resistance. Sigmund Freud first described this phenomenon over one hundred years ago when he discovered that his patients were opposing his technique of free association. Freud believed that some patients have an unconscious desire to frustrate their progress. Resistance as used in contemporary parlance includes ambivalence to treatment, including no shows, lateness to

appointments, silence during therapy sessions, and refusal to fill prescriptions. Denial, displacement, and identification are defense mechanisms that do not apply to this clinical scenario. Transference is the patient's displacement onto the therapist or provider of early wishes and feelings toward significant others.

Sadock BJ, Sadock VA. *Kaplan and Sadock's Comprehensive Textbook of Psychiatry*. 8th ed. Philadelphia: Lippincott Williams & Wilkins; 2005:704–708.

82. Answer: C. Primary prevention prevents the disease itself. Examples of primary prevention are genetic counseling or gene therapy to artificially introduce genetic material into the developing brain. Secondary prevention helps prevent the evolution of disease, usually targeting at-risk individuals via environmental manipulation. Examples of secondary prevention are nutritional supplementation, and reduction in exposure to viruses or early losses. Tertiary prevention focuses on preventing disease complications once the disease has occurred. Examples of tertiary prevention are pharmacologic intervention or screening.

Hales RE, Yudofsky SC. *Textbook of Clinical Psychiatry*. 4th ed. Washington: American Psychiatric Publishing; 2003:3–65.

83. Answer: E. NMS is a relatively rare but potentially fatal complication of neuroleptic treatment, whose main features are hyperthermia, severe muscular rigidity, autonomic instability, and changes in mental status. Associated findings are increased CPK, increased liver transaminase activity, increased leukocytes, and myglobinuria, which can lead to renal failure and decreased urine output. A low serum iron level is also commonly seen among NMS patients and is reported to be a 92% to 100% sensitive marker for NMS.

1. Rosenbaum JF, Arana GW, Hyman SE, et al. *Handbook of Psychiatric Drug Therapy*. 5th ed. Philadelphia: Lippincott Williams & Wilkins; 2005:43.
2. Wijdicks EFM. *Neuroleptic Malignant Syndrome*. http://www.utdol.com/utd/content/topic.do?topicKey=medneuro/5946&type=A&selectedTitle=1~17. Accessed February 22, 2007.

84. Answer: B. Depression is considered the most common comorbidity occurring with OCD. Other mood disorders and Anxiety Disorders are also frequently present in patients with OCD. Although once a controversial idea, OCD does co-occur in psychotic disorders, including Schizophrenia.

1. Bhattacharyya S, Reddy YC, Khanna S. Depressive and anxiety disorder comorbidity in obsessive compulsive disorder. *Psychopathology*. 2005;38:315–319.
2. Perugi G, Akiskal HS, Pfanner C, et al. The clinical impact of bipolar and unipolar affective comorbidity on

obsessive-compulsive disorder. *J Affect Disord*. 1997;46:15–23.
3. Tibbo P, Warneke L. Obsessive-compulsive disorder in schizophrenia: epidemiologic and biologic overlap. *J Psychiatry Neurosci*. 1999;24:15–24.

85. Answer: D. The onset of Factitious Disorders is usually in early adulthood, often after a hospitalization for a general medical condition or other mental disorder. The rest of the statements are true of Factitious Disorders.

American Psychiatric Association. *Diagnostic and Statistical Manual of Mental Disorders (DSM-IV-TR)*. 4th ed. (Revision). http://www.psychiatryonline.com/content.aspx?aID=9658. Accessed February 27, 2007.

86. Answer: B. Disorganized Schizophrenia is characterized by disorganization of speech, thought or behavior, flat affect, and early onset. The Paranoid type is associated with prominent persecutory elusions as well as hallucinations. Catatonic Schizophrenia is defined by the presence of stupor/mutism, negativism, rigidity, posturing, and echolalia/echopraxia. Those not meeting criteria for one of the subtypes are diagnosed with Undifferentiated Schizophrenia. If two or more symptoms are residual despite the absence of prominent delusions, hallucinations, incoherence, or disorganized behavior, the patient likely has the Residual type of Schizophrenia.

1. American Psychiatric Association. *Quick Reference to the Diagnostic Criteria from DSM-IV-TR*. Washington: American Psychiatric Association; 2000:153–159.
2. Sadock B, Sadock V. *Kaplan and Sadock's Pocket Handbook of Clinical Psychiatry*. 3rd ed. Philadelphia: Lippincott Williams & Wilkins; 2001:102–103.

87. Answer: C. Alloplastic refers to traits that cause a patient to try to change the environment, as opposed to trying to change him or herself (autoplastic). Traits associated with Personality Disorders are necessarily rigidly held, present for a prolonged period of time, ego syntonic, and present in several spheres of a patient's life.

Sadock B, Sadock V. *Kaplan and Sadock's Pocket Handbook of Clinical Psychiatry*. 3rd ed. Philadelphia: Lippincott Williams & Wilkins; 2001:210.

88. Answer: D. IPT usually lasts 12 to 20 sessions and is contracted in advance. It has three specific stages. The first stage closely resembles a standard psychiatric assessment. A key feature of the first part is the compiling of an interpersonal inventory that lists and examines all the patient's relationships. This is charted on rating scales or as a "spider" diagram, which becomes a key resource for future therapy. By session four, one of four prescribed foci is selected: grief, role transitions, role disputes, or interpersonal deficits. The second and longest stage comprises active work on the chosen focus. The therapist becomes less active but holds the focus, relates symptom change to interpersonal events, and encourages the patient to devise and experiment with new interpersonal strategies. Although CBT conceptualizes painful feelings as symptoms and expects them to diminish when the negative cognitions are challenged, IPT helps patients identify and deliberately tolerate feelings. The final few sessions are devoted to termination, review, relapse prevention, grief over ending, and the transition to independence. The full benefits of IPT do not appear immediately, but after a lag.

1. Hales RE, Yudofsky SC. *American Psychiatric Publishing Textbook of Clinical Psychiatry*. 4th ed. http://www.psychiatryonline.com/content.aspx?aID=92013. Accessed April 5, 2007.
2. Morris J. Interpersonal psychotherapy: a trainee's ABC. *Psychiatric Bulletin*. 2002;26:26–28.

89. Answer: D. The doctrine of respondeat superior refers to the notion that those in higher positions of responsibility are liable for actions of those below them. Thus, an attending can be held legally responsible for the actions/omissions of a resident. Choice A refers to the civil right of patients to receive the least restrictive treatment possible. Choice C refers to the Model Penal Code regarding criminal responsibility. Choice E addresses the issue of negligence. Choice B is incorrect.

Kaplan HI, Sadock BJ. *Kaplan & Sadock's Synopsis of Psychiatry*. 8th ed. Philadelphia: Lippincott Williams & Wilkins; 1998:1311–1319.

90. Answer: D. Methamphetamine is the most commonly abused prescription stimulant. The 2000 National Household Survey on Drug Abuse estimated that 4.0% of Americans (8.8 million) were lifetime methamphetamine users; 0.5% (1 million) had used methamphetamine within the past year; and 0.2% (387,000) were current users. Amphetamines are usually abused by oral or intravenous route; highly pure crystallized methamphetamine (ice) may be smoked or used intranasally. Methamphetamine can be produced by reducing ephedrine or pseudoephedrine. Cocaine is the drug most often associated with emergency department visits; amphetamine was ranked tenth and methamphetamine twelfth most common drug in emergency department visits. Amphetamine and methamphetamine are schedule II drugs due to a high abuse potential.

Graham AW, Schultz TK, Mayo-Smith MF, et al. *Principles of Addiction Medicine*. 3rd ed. Chevy Chase, Maryland: American Society of Addiction Medicine; 2003:157–192.

91. Answer: D. Recent studies suggest a role for anticonvulsants in the treatment of alcohol dependence. Topiramate inhibits mesocorticolimbic dopamine release, which is believed to be associated with cravings for alcohol. In a recent controlled study, topiramate was found be effective in initiating abstinence and reducing self-reported drinking and craving. Gabapentin and valproate have shown some promise in case studies and small trials. Selective serotonin antagonist and ondansetron, have been shown to reduce self-reported drinking and increase abstinence. However, SSRIs have not shown significant effect in patients with Alcohol Dependence without Major Depression.

1. Johnson BA, Ait-Daoud N, Bowden CL, et al. Oral topiramate for treatment of alcohol dependence: a randomised controlled trial. *Lancet*. 2003;361:1677–1685.
2. Johnson BA, Roache JD, Javors MA, et al. Ondansetron for reduction of drinking among biologically predisposed alcoholic patients: A randomized controlled trial. *JAMA*. 2000;284:963–971.
3. Williams SH. Medications for treating alcohol dependence. *Am Fam Physician*. 2005;72:1775–1780.

92. Answer: A. Non-opioid analgesics are generally considered effective for mild to moderate levels of either acute or chronic pain. They are not effective for severe pain or for neuropathic pain. Opioid analgesics are usually more effective for more severe pain. Non-opioid analgesics include acetaminophen, aspirin (and other salicylates), NSAIDs (ibuprofen, naproxen, indomethacin, ketorolac, celcoxib, rofecoxib, etc.), and others. Non-opioid analgesics act peripherally, mostly by inhibiting prostaglandin synthesis. However, NSAIDs and acetaminophen may also act centrally. Opiate mechanism of action is predominantly central. Non-opioid analgesic treatment is typically not complicated by tolerance, dependence, or withdrawal.

Kaufman DM. *Clinical Neurology for Psychiatrists*. 5th ed. Philadelphia: WB Saunders; 2001:347–368.

93. Answer: B. Classical conditioning is also named after Pavlov (1849–1936) – Pavlovian conditioning – who first described pairing a conditioned stimulus (a bell) with an unconditioned stimulus (meat powder) to produce a conditioned response (salivation) to the conditioned stimulus alone. Watson (1878–1958) was a famous behaviorist American psychologist. Skinner (1904–1990) was a behaviorist who focused on operant conditioning. Sullivan (1892–1949) developed interpersonal theory.

Sadock BJ, Sadock VA. *Kaplan & Sadock's Comprehensive Textbook of Psychiatry*. 7th ed. Philadelphia: Lippincott Williams & Wilkins; 2000:3301–3333.

94. Answer: E. Approximately 90% of the body's serotonin is found in the intestines. In the gastrointestinal tract, serotonin receptors may contribute to gastrointestinal upset and diarrhea. Other side effects related to serotonergic drugs arise from receptors in the basal ganglia, which may be responsible for akathisia and agitation; receptors in the area postrema and those in the hypothalamus may cause nausea and vomiting; in the limbic system, they may cause an initial increase in anxiety; in the brainstem sleep centers, they can contribute to insomnia or somnolence; spinal cord pathway receptors may produce sexual dysfunction; and receptors in cranial blood vessels may cause headache.

Sadock BJ, Sadock VA. *Kaplan and Sadock's Synopsis of Psychiatry*. 9th ed. Philadelphia: Lippincott Williams & Wilkins; 2003:88–108.

95. Answer: C. All of the pairings are correct except for clonidine, which is an alpha-2 adrenergic agonist not an alpha-1 adrenergic antagonist.

Kleber HD, Weiss RD, Anton RF, et al. Treatment of patients with substance use disorders, second edition. American Psychiatic Association. www.psychiatryonline.com/content.aspx?aID=14810. Accessed December 14, 2007.

96. Answer: D. Diseases that have an autosomal dominant mode of inheritance, manifest as clinical parkinsonism and respond to L-dopa are SCA3 in those of African descent, SCA2 in those of Asian descent, and MAPT mutations associated with frontotemporal dementia and parkinsonism, FTDP17.

Hardy J, Cai H, Cookson MR, et al. Genetics of Parkinson's disease and parkinsonism. *Ann Neurol*. 2006;60:389–398.

97. Answer: D. The presentation is typical of a unilateral cortical stroke. Deficits are contralateral to the site of the lesion. Forehead muscle function is intact because that portion of each cranial nerve seven (facial nerve) receives innervation from both hemispheres. Flexion is a sign of cortical release. Right thalamic or brainstem lesions would typically result in ipsilateral deficits. Cerebellar lesions usually result in incoordination of some type, not paresis.

Kaufman DM. *Clinical Neurology for Psychiatrists*. 5th ed. Philadelphia: WB Saunders; 2001:8–25.

98. Answer: E. CT scan uses ionizing radiation just as in X-rays. MRI uses a magnetic field without any ionizing radiation. CT scanning can be performed in patients with indwelling ferrous material, while this is dangerous with MRIs because of the strong magnetic field. If life-support is required, hand ventilation can be performed, and non-ferromagnetic equipment does exist. Using a CT scan, bone dis-

torts images of soft tissue, especially in the pituitary, posterior fossa, spinal cord, and optic nerves. MRI is better at distinguishing certain conditions, such as MS, progressive multifocal leukoencephalopathy, mesial temporal sclerosis, arterio venous malformations (AVMs), small gliomas, and others.

1. Kaufman DM. *Clinical Neurology for Psychiatrists*. 5th ed. Philadelphia: WB Saunders; 2001:532–551.
2. Ropper AH, Brown RH. *Adams and Victor's Principles of Neurology*. 8th ed. New York: McGraw-Hill; 2005:11–38.

99. Answer: B. Physiological tremors are seen in all normal people when the muscles are activated. They are usually action (postural) tremors and are thought to arise from the resonant oscillation of a limb as a result of mechanical factors affecting it. These tremors are barely visible to the naked eye and do not interfere with activities of daily living. The frequency of physiological tremor is about 6 to 12 Hz. The frequency usually decreases when large inertia loads are applied to the limb. Physiological tremor can be exacerbated by stress, anxiety, fatigue, lack of sleep, and excessive caffeine intake. Other conditions that can exacerbate physiological tremors include thyrotoxicosis, pheochromocytoma, hypoglycaemia, withdrawal from opioids, or sedatives. In general, no drugs are usually warranted for this condition. However, if these tremors are interfering with day to day activities, relaxation and a small dose of propranolol can be useful in reducing the intensity of these tremors.

Bhidayasiri R. Differential diagnosis of common tremor syndromes. *Postgrad Med J*. 2005;81:756–762.

100. Answer: E. Galactosemia has an autosomal recessive mode of inheritance. The deficiencies of GALT, galactokinase, and epimerase are implicated in the development of this disorder. The disease associated with the deficiency of GALT is called classical galactosemia and is the commonest and most severe type of disorder.

1. Harris JC. *Developmental Neuropsychiatry*. Vol II. Oxford: Oxford University Press; 1998:344–347.
2. Kaplan HI, Sadock BJ. *Kaplan and Sadock's Synopsis of Psychiatry*. 9th ed. Philadelphia: Lippincott Williams & Wilkins; 2003:1172.

101. Answer: C. Although appearing normal in the first 12 months of life, developmental delay and physical changes appear by the end of the first year in severe form of the disease with symptoms appearing in early childhood in milder variants. Mental retardation is characteristic of severe forms but intelligence in childhood may be normal in the milder variants. Mental retardation may not be seen in some children but will appear at a later stage. In the milder variants, survival occurs into adulthood.

Harris JC. *Developmental Neuropsychiatry*. Vol II. Oxford: Oxford University Press; 1998:356.

102. Answer: A. The genetic defect in Wilson's disease is localized to chromosome 13. It has an autosomal recessive mode of inheritance. The onset is usually in childhood or early adolescence. Approximately 40% of the patients present with hepatic symptoms, 40% with neurological symptoms, and 20% with psychiatric symptoms. Most patients who present with neuropsychiatric manifestations have cirrhosis. Kayser-Fleischer rings are formed by the deposition of copper in Descemet membrane in the limbus of the cornea and may be readily visible to the naked eye or with an ophthalmoscope. Kayser-Fleischer rings are observed in up to 90% of individuals with symptomatic Wilson's disease and are almost invariably present in those with neurologic manifestations. Although Kayser-Fleischer rings are a useful diagnostic sign, they are no longer considered pathognomonic of Wilson's disease unless accompanied by neurologic manifestations as they may also be seen in chronic cholestatic disorders such as partial biliary atresia, primary biliary cirrhosis, primary sclerosing cholangitis, and cryptogenic cirrhosis. The severity of symptoms may be reduced by D-penicillamine.

1. Kaplan HI, Sadock BJ. *Kaplan and Sadock's Synopsis of Psychiatry*. 9th ed. Philadelphia: Lippincott Williams & Wilkins; 2003:847.
2. Kaplan MM. *Pathogenesis and Clinical Manifestations of Wilson's Disease*. http://www.uptodateonline.com/utd/content/topic.do?topicKey=hep_dis/9927&type=A&selectedTitle=2~28. Accessed March 7, 2007.
3. Lishman WA. *Organic Psychiatry*. 3rd ed. Oxford: Blackwell Science; 1996:661–666.

103. Answer: A. The psychiatrist has already learnt that the patient is independent in ADLs. ADLs include the ability to feed one's self; other ADLs include toileting, grooming, dressing, and bathing. IADLs generally require higher cognitive and functional abilities. IADLs include the ability to manage one's medications, to drive or arrange transportation, to use the telephone, to drive or use public transportation, and to manage one's finances (e.g., writing checks, paying bills). The elderly typically have no difficulty performing ADLs and IADLs if they have always done so, unless they have significant cognitive deterioration (such as in Alzheimer's disease), significant physical impairment (such as a stroke), or significant perceptual impairments (such as significant hearing/visual loss). Assessment of ADLs and IADLs is of vital importance, as decline in these functional abilities are significantly associated with placement in a nursing home.

Sadavoy J, Jarvik LF, Grossberg GT, et al. *Comprehensive Textbook of Geriatric Psychiatry*. New York: WW Norton & Company; 2004:138–139.

104. Answer: E. Choices A and E refer to inhibitory steps in the pathway synthesizing eicosanoids from arachidonic acid. Corticosteroids inhibit the synthesis of arachidonic acid by inhibiting phospholipase A_2 (choice A) and inhibiting the synthesis of a type of cyclooxygenase. NSAIDs produce their analgesic affect by inhibiting cyclooxygenases as well, which are essential enzymes in the production of prostaglandins, which sensitize tissues to pain. Cyclooxygenases are not involved in the synthesis of arachidonic acid (choice B). Choices C and D are nonsensical. The mu receptor is one of the receptor types for which opioids are agonists.

1. Katzung BG, Trevor AJ. *Examination and Board Review: Pharmacology*. 5th ed. Stamford: Appleton & Lange; 1998:150–151, 272.
2. Zaidat OO, Lerner AJ. *The Little Black Book of Neurology*. 4th ed. St. Louis: Mosby, 2002:285.

105. Answer: C. Among the choices, the death of a spouse is rated as the most stressful life event on the Social Readjustment Rating Scale (SRRS) or the Holmes and Rahe Stress Scale. Psychologists Thomas Holmes and Richard Rahe examined the medical records of over 5,000 medical patients to determine whether stressful life events might cause illnesses. Thay asked patients to tally a list of 41 life events based on a relative score. A positive 0.1 correlation was found between their life events and their illnesses. Based on their findings, they developed the SRRS or the Holmes and Rahe Stress Scale. According to them, the stress adds up. Using "Life Change Units" that apply to events that people have experienced over the last year, the score that they receive gave a rough estimate of how their stress affected their health. According to Holmes and Rahe, the top ten most stressful life events are:

Life Event	Life Change Units
1. Death of a Spouse	100
2. Divorce	73
3. Marital Separation	65
4. Imprisonment	63
5. Death of a Close Family Member	63
6. Personal Injury or Illness	53
7. Marriage	50
8. Dismissal from Work	47
9. Marital Reconciliation	45
10. Retirement	45

They stated that if the cumulative score is 300 or more, the risk of illness is high. If the score is between 150 and 299, the risk of illness is moderate (reduced by 30% from the high risk) and if the score is 150 or below, there is only a slight risk of illness.

Holmes TH, Rahe RH. The social readjustment rating scale. *J Psychosom Res*. 1967;11:213–218.

106. Answer: D. Susceptibility to mood disorders, especially Bipolar Disorder, Alcohol Dependence and Schizophrenia are each well-known to be heritable, and have numerous studies supporting such. Of the Anxiety Disorders, Panic Disorder has the strongest body of evidence supporting its heritability, although not as strong as Schizophrenia and the mood disorders. Susceptibility to the development of PTSD, and possibly exposure to trauma, may be at least partially heritable, but currently there are fewer studies supporting this. Familial studies have not found aggregation of PTSD, but some genetic studies have found factors that may help explain the development of PTSD. Among the other Anxiety Disorders (e.g., OCD, generalized anxiety disorder [GAD], Phobias, Social Anxiety), current evidence for genetic transmission varies.

Hales RE, Yudofsky SC. *Textbook of Clinical Psychiatry*. 4th ed. Washington: American Psychiatric Publishing; 2003:3–65.

107. Answer: C. The lack of regard for and violation of the rights of others and the inability to conform to societal norms constitute the defining characteristics of ASPD. These are so pervasive that some regard patients with ASPD as being devoid of a conscience or having super ego deficits (super ego lacuna).

1. Niolon R. *Antisocial Personality Style and Disorder*. http://www.psychpage.com/learning/library/person/asp.html. Published March 18, 2007.
2. Sadock BJ, Sadock VA. *Kaplan and Sadock's Comprehensive Textbook of Psychiatry*. 8th ed. Philadelphia: Lippincott Williams & Wilkins; 2005:2046–2047.

108. Answer: B. Medicare Part A covers hospital and skilled nursing facility fees, also called "hospital insurance." All Medicare beneficiaries are entitled to Part A. Medicare Part B is optional for Medicare beneficiaries, and requires a premium. Part B covers physician services, specialty mental health services, outpatient care, diagnostic and laboratory tests, ambulatory services, durable medical equipment, limited home health, occupational therapy, and more. Medicare Part C are private HMO (or Medicare + Choice) alternatives to traditional fee-for-service Medicare options. Medicare Part D encompasses the newer Medicare prescription plans. Medicaid services are run jointly by federal and state governments and are for those with low income and limited resources (often children, indigent mothers, elderly, and certain disabled). Although Medicaid may cover some physician reimbursement, it is separate from Medicare.

1. Centers for Medicare & Medicaid Services. *The Centers for Medicare & Medicaid Services Website*. http://www.cms.hhs.gov/. Published February 14, 2007.
2. Sadavoy J, Jarvik LF, Grossberg GT, et al. *Comprehensive Textbook of Geriatric Psychiatry*. 3rd ed. New York: WW Norton & Company; 2004:1207–1237.

109. Answer: D. Neuroleptic malignant syndrome is usually associated with bradykinesia, lead pipe rigidity and other extrapyramidal features whereas hyperkinesia, hyperreflexia and clonus are more common in serotonin syndrome

Isbister GK, Buckley NA, Whyte IM. Serotonin toxicity: a practical approach to diagnosis and treatment. *Med J Aust*. 2007 September 17; 187(6):361–365.

110. Answer: E. Schizotypal is the Personality Disorder most closely related to Schizophrenia, particularly in the positive symptom cluster. Schizoid Personality Disorder shares overlap with Schizophrenia in the negative symptom cluster, but overall is less closely linked to Schizophrenia than Schizotypal Personality Disorder.

1. Robinson DJ. *Disordered Personalities*. 3rd ed. Port Huron: Rapid Psychler Press; 2005:56–92.
2. Seeber K, Cadenhead KS. How does studying schizotypal personality disorder inform us about the prodrome of schizophrenia? *Curr Psychiatry Rep*. 2005;7:41–50.
3. Siever LJ, Davis KL. The pathophysiology of schizophrenia disorders: perspectives from the spectrum. *Am J Psychiatry*. 2004;161:398–413.

111. Answer: C. Factitious Disorder By Proxy is a diagnosis given to the perpetrator, not the victim. The victim (usually, but not limited to child) are usually subjected to abuse. Management is usually coordinated and directed through the legal system, and protection of the child is the priority. The mother can be referred for psychiatric evaluation and treatment.

Hales RE, Yudofsky SC. *American Psychiatric Publishing Textbook of Clinical Psychiatry*. 4th ed. http://www.psychiatryonline.com/content.aspx?aID=79591. Accessed February 28, 2007.

112. Answer: B. All of the statements are correct except choice B. The rates of Schizophrenia in males and females are roughly equivalent, making the ratio 1:1. Although it appears that choice D is correct, there has been debate regarding how bias in the diagnosis of patients in lower socioeconomic classes has skewed this statistic.

Sadock B, Sadock V. *Kaplan and Sadock's Pocket Handbook of Clinical Psychiatry*. 3rd ed. Philadelphia: Lippincott Williams & Wilkins; 2001:104.

113. **Answer: E.** The rate of suicide in men consistently increases with age, reaching its highest peak in the oldest age group. For women, the suicide rate declines in late life. Whites have higher suicide rates than their minority counterparts. Elderly suicide victims are more likely to be widowed and less likely to be single or divorced compared to young adults. Depression, not substance abuse, is the most common psychiatric diagnosis in elderly suicide victims. Most elderly suicide victims have communicated their suicidal ideation to family or friends prior to the suicide, and over a third have visited a physician within a week of their suicide. Violent means of suicide are more common in the elderly, resulting in greater lethality. Elderly patients with risk factors such as major medical illnesses or a recent loss should be evaluated for depressive symptoms and suicidal ideation. Identification of those individuals with depression and suicidality can lead to proper treatment, which may ultimately reduce the risk of suicide.

Sadavoy J, Jarvik LF, Grossberg GT, et al. *Comprehensive Textbook of Geriatric Psychiatry*. New York: WW Norton & Company; 2004:619–621.

114. **Answer: E.** Psychiatric symptoms associated with hypothyroidism include depression, impaired memory functions, apathy, social withdrawal, and loss of interest in daily activities with general slowing of vocational interpersonal and social functioning. It can also be associated with poor concentration, low energy, changes in appetite, and changes in sleep. Rapid cycling bipolar disorder as well as manic episodes can also occur in hypothyroidism. Hypothyroidism was found to be associated in as many as half of the patients with rapid cycling bipolar disorder.

Khouzam HR, Weiser PM, Emes R, et al. Thyroid hormones therapy: a review of their effects in the treatment of psychiatric and medical conditions. *Compr Ther*. 2004;30:148–154.

115. **Answer: E.** Patient-centered interviewing attends to the intrapsychic battle of conflicts. It is sensitive to the patient's educational, emotional, intellectual, and social background, the personality, and the individual symptom constellations tracing their arrival to individual circumstances and the individual's unique response (cognitive-behavioral model). One example of the introspective model is the psychodynamic model. Interviewing based on the psychodynamic model uses nonstructured, open-ended questions with a broad scope, encouraging free association. The disorder-centered and patient-centered interviewing styles do not exclude each other. They are end points of a continuum. The interviewer's mobility and flexibility in gliding between the two extremes determine the efficiency, reliability, validity, and quality of data collection. The degree of the patient's impairment determines to which extent the disorder-centered interview has to be augmented by patient-centered strategies. Disorder-centered interviewing is based on a theoretical model of psychiatric disorders called the medical model, which is the official model supported by the American Psychiatric Association and the World Health Organization codified in DSM-IV-TR (2000) and the International Classification of Diseases (ICD-10). Choices A through D describe key features of this interview style.

Sadock BJ, Sadock VA. *Kaplan & Sadock's Comprehensive Textbook of Psychiatry*. 8th ed. Philadelphia: Lippincott Williams & Wilkins; 2005:795.

116. **Answer: D.** All stimulants (amphetamines, cocaine, and others) produce a similar range of physiological, psychological, and behavioral effects. Acute stimulant effects at low doses include euphoria, increased energy, increased sociability, and decreased sleep and appetite. At higher doses, stimulants cause dysphoria, anxiety/panic, irritability and agitation, movement disorders, seizures, paranoia, grandiosity, delusions, and hallucinations. Other acute stimulant effects may include rhabdomyolysis, acute renal failure from myoglobinuria, ketoacidosis in diabetics, hypothalamo-pituitary-adrenal (HPA) axis activation, increased arousal and prolonged erections, chronic rhinitis, nasal septal perforation, xerostomia, and bruxism. Stimulant induced psychosis closely resembles Schizophrenia. Stimulants can cause auditory, visual, or tactile hallucinations; tactile hallucinations are especially typical of stimulant psychosis where patients have a sensation of something crawling under their skin (formication). Chronic amphetamine and methamphetamine use, oral or intravenous, can cause paranoia and hallucinations that may persist for years after the last drug use. Psychotic flashbacks have been reported in methamphetamine use abusers up to 2 years after their last use that are often precipitated by threatening experiences. A persisting psychosis after cocaine use has not been reported. Cocaine and amphetamines are classified in pregnancy as category C.

Graham AW, Schultz TK, Mayo-Smith MF, et al. *Principles of Addiction Medicine*. 3rd ed. Maryland: American Society of Addiction Medicine; 2003:157–192.

117. Answer: E. Even with severe barbiturate intoxication, unless the patient is asphyxiated, pupillary light reflexes remain intact. In severe intoxication, pupillary meiosis may mimic poor reactivity. Barbiturate intoxication is one of the few conditions (e.g., pontine hemorrhage) that results in flaccid coma, hypothermia, and hypotension with small reactive pupils. The other signs of overdose are coma, nystagmus, ataxia, and suppressed deep tendon reflexes. Also, there is a known additive effect of barbiturates with alcohol, making this a potentially lethal combination due to possible respiratory suppression.

Ropper AH, Brown RH. *Adams and Victor's Principles of Neurology*. 8th ed. New York: McGraw-Hill; 2005:1017–1045.

118. Answer: B. Opioid pain medications are appropriate for acute moderate to severe pain due to fractures, myocardial infarction, or surgery. Chronic pain of cancer is also another indication. Use of opioid analgesics in other forms of moderate to severe refractory chronic pain is debated. Opioid analgesics may help tension headaches, but less intense forms of analgesics—such as NSAIDs, and acetaminophen, or salicylates—are considered more appropriate. Opioid analgesics may be more appropriate for more severe forms of headache, such as specific types of migraine.

Kaufman DM. *Clinical Neurology for Psychiatrists*. 5th ed. Philadelphia: WB Saunders; 2001:347–368.

119. Answer: D. The antidote to a toxic dose of anticholinergic medication is physostigmine which will inhibit acetylcholinesterase thus increasing synaptic acetylcholine. Pralidoxime (2-PAM) or atropine is the antidote to carbamates, organophosphates, and cholinergic toxicity.

Kasper DL, Braunwald E, Fauci AS. *Harrison's Principles of Internal Medicine*. 16th ed. http://www.accessmedicine.com/content.aspx?aID=110113. Accessed February 27, 2007.

120. Answer: B. The major pathophysiological conditions associated with glutamate are excitotoxicity and Schizophrenia. Excitotoxicity is the hypothesis that excessive stimulation of glutamate receptors leads to prolonged and excessive intraneuronal concentrations of calcium and nitric oxide. This, then, activates proteases that are destructive to neuronal integrity. In Schizophrenia, a reduction in NMDA receptor activity is thought to cause psychotic symptoms. It seems, therefore, that too much NMDA receptor activity kills neurons and too little NMDA receptor activity induces psychosis. Many of the remaining neurotransmitters activate sodium and/or potassium ion channels. However, GABA acting on GABA$_A$ receptors has an inhibitory physiological effect through activation of chloride ion channels. No neurotransmitter activates the magnesium channel.

Sadock BJ, Sadock VA. *Kaplan and Sadock's Synopsis of Psychiatry*. 9th ed. Philadelphia: Lippincott Williams & Wilkins; 2003:88–108.

121. Answer: E. Social skills training helps patients develop their communication and relationship skills. Development of these skills may have been impeded by substance abuse or these skills may have been acquired and then lost in the course of substance abuse.

Kleber HD, Weiss RD, Anton RF, et al. Treatment of patients with substance use disorders, second edition. American Psychiatic Association. www.psychiatryonline.com/content.aspx?aID=14810. Accessed December 14, 2007.

122. Answer: A. Five genes for Mendelian PARK loci have been cloned: SNCA (PARK1/4), parkin (PARK2), DJ-1 (PARK7), PINK1 (PARK6), and LRRK2 (PARK8). Of these, SNCA (PARK1/4), and LRRK2 (PARK8) have autosomal dominant modes of inheritance. PINK1 (PARK6) and DJ-1 (PARK7) have autosomal recessive modes of inheritance. PARK2 usually has an autosomal recessive mode of inheritance, although pseudodominant cases have been reported. At the current time, the evidence is not sufficiently strong to map the "PARK" loci to a single pathway, although there are emerging hints that one or two common processes may be of importance. This uncertainty is further complicated by the variable or unknown pathology associated with each syndrome. It is still open to discussion as to whether all or any of the PARK genes are relevant in a causative or mechanistic sense to sporadic Parkinson's disease.

Hardy J, Cai H, Cookson MR, et al. Genetics of Parkinson's disease and parkinsonism. *Ann Neurol*. 2006;60:389–398.

123. Answer: C. Homonymous hemianopsia, the inability to see at the same half-field in each eye is usually a sign of a contralateral cerebral lesion. Bilateral loss of vision of the left visual field is usually due to a lesion in the right (contralateral) cerebrum. It is theoretically possible that very precise lesions of the optic chiasm or optic nerves could cause such a deficit, but it would be extremely unlikely and unusual. The brainstem is located relatively far from the visual pathway, and would not be responsible for such a deficit.

Kaufman DM. *Clinical Neurology for Psychiatrists*. 5th ed. Philadelphia: WB Saunders; 2001:8–25.

124. Answer: B. PET scanning uses radio ligands which are produced in cyclotrons and incorporates them into organic molecules to obtain a rough picture of the brain's physiology, chemistry, and metabolism. Spatial resolution is better than with the SPECT. SPECT is a cruder, simpler, less expensive form of study than the PET, utilizing available radioligands. MRI and CT scans focus on distinguishing anatomy over function. Angiography maps blood vessels and can elucidate some of their physiology. It is not routinely used to view the brain's metabolism and chemistry.

Kaufman DM. *Clinical Neurology for Psychiatrists*. 5th ed. Philadelphia: WB Saunders; 2001:532–551.

125. Answer: C. Lesch-Nyhan syndrome is a sex-linked autosomal recessive inborn error of purine nucleotide metabolism. Self injury is the major behavioral phenotype for this disease. The disease has classical and partial variants; the classical type is associated with the complete absence of HGPRT and presents with hyperuricemia, mental retardation, cerebral palsy, early choreoathetosis with later spasticity and torsion dystonia, and compulsive self injury. The partial variants are associated with a severe form of gout with variable neurological dysfunction; the severity is inversely correlated with the amount of residual HGPRT activity. The self injurious behavior is not caused by hyperuricemia or excess hypoxanthine. Untreated hyperuricemia can lead to renal failure and death.

Harris JC. *Developmental Neuropsychiatry*. Vol II. Oxford: Oxford University Press; 1998:306–308.

126. Answer: E. Aldose reductase, which is involved in an accessory pathway in the reduction of free galactose to galactitol, is implicated in the development of cataracts and cerebral edema. Symptoms usually occur in the second half of the first week of life after initiating milk feeding. Early symptoms include edema, vomiting, jaundice, hepatosplenomegaly, increased intracranial pressure and ascites. Mental retardation becomes evident after 6 to 12 months and is not usually reversible. Despite adherence to a strict galactose-free diet, neurological and ovarian complications can occur. Likewise, cognitive deficits such as visuospatial problems and language disorders may also occur. Behavioral problems, anxiety, social withdrawal, and shyness impair social adaptation in children treated with a low galactose diet.

1. Harris JC. *Developmental Neuropsychiatry*. Vol II. Oxford: Oxford University Press; 1998:344–349.
2. Kaplan HI, Sadock BJ. *Kaplan and Sadock's Synopsis of Psychiatry*. 9th ed. Philadelphia: Lippincott Williams & Wilkins; 2003:1172.

127. Answer: C. A low phenylalanine diet can significantly improve behavior and developmental progress. Dietary treatment in PKU is not without risks. As phenylalanine is an essential amino acid, its omission can lead to anemia, hypoglycemia, edema, and even death. Dietary treatment should be continued indefinitely. If commenced before 3 months of age, some children may have normal intelligence. This treatment does not influence the level of mental retardation in untreated older children. Such a diet can also reduce irritability and abnormal EEG patterns.

Kaplan HI, Sadock BJ. *Kaplan and Sadock's Synopsis of Psychiatry*. 9th ed. Philadelphia: Lippincott Williams & Wilkins; 2003:1172.

128. Answer: C. In Wilson's disease serum ceruloplasmin level is usually reduced while the level of urinary copper is increased. Total serum copper is usually low, but free serum copper is raised, which is responsible for the symptoms. Hepatic copper is increased. MRI of the brain shows symmetrical focal areas of increased signal in the lenticular nuclei (putamen and globus pallidus), thalamus, caudate, dentate nuclei, and the brainstem.

1. Kaplan HI, Sadock BJ. *Kaplan and Sadock's Synopsis of Psychiatry*. 9th ed. Philadelphia: Lippincott Williams & Wilkins; 2003:847.
2. Kaplan MM. Pathogenesis and clinical manifestations of Wilson's disease. http://www.uptodateonline.com/utd/content/topic.do?topicKey=hep_dis/9927&type=A&selectedTitle=2~28. Accessed March 7, 2007.
3. Lishman WA. *Organic Psychiatry*. 3rd ed. Oxford: Blackwell Science; 1996:661–666.

129. Answer: B. AIDS dementia, or as the DSM-IV-TR classifies it, dementia due to HIV disease, affects 20% of all AIDS patients, making it the most frequent neurologic complication of AIDS. It is caused by the direct viral infection of the brain; macrophages and microglia (*not neurons*, unlike other viral infections of the brain) are the cells most heavily infected. AIDS dementia is manifested by a rapid decline, over weeks to a few months, in concentration and memory. Language function is generally preserved initially. Associated manifestations of AIDS dementia include blunted affect and social withdrawal, giving the patient a depressed appearance. Indeed, depression is not uncommon; the suicide rate of patients with AIDS dementia is 17 to 36 times that of the healthy population. Other clinical signs of AIDS dementia include gait difficulties, slow limb movements, ocular motility abnormalities, ataxia, clonus, and hyperactive reflexes. AIDS dementia is generally considered a late manifestation of the disease, associated with weight loss, anemia, and CD4 counts less than 200/mm^3. Disproportionately represented among those with AIDS dementia are older patients and those who acquired HIV from intravenous drug abuse.

Kaufman DM. *Clinical Neurology for Psychiatrists*. 5th ed. Philadelphia: WB Saunders; 2001:151.

130. Answer: B. Capsaicin is a derivative of hot peppers and exerts its analgesic effect by depleting nociceptors of substance P.

1. Katzung BG. *Basic and Clinical Pharmacology*. 8th ed. New York: McGraw Hill; 2001:516–517.
2. Katzung BG, Trevor AJ. *Examination and Board Review: Pharmacology*. 5th ed. Stamford: Appleton & Lange; 1998:150–151.
3. Zaidat OO, Lerner AJ. *The Little Black Book of Neurology*. 4th ed. St. Louis: Mosby; 2002:285–286.

131. Answer: D. Heinz Kohut proposed the practice of analytic and dynamic treatment approach best known as self psychology. He developed his ideas around what he called the tripartite (three-part) self. According to Kohut, this three-part self can only develop when the needs of one's "self states," including one's sense of worth and well-being, are met in relationships with others. Self psychology placed a great deal of emphasis on relationships and Kohut linked the origin of the self to narcissism. He viewed the self as the result of a separate line of narcissistic development that progresses through a series of archaic narcissistic structures toward establishing a mature and cohesive self-organization. Kohut thought that narcissism went through a separate line of development that was independent from object libido and object relations. Kohut felt that the course of development is based on empathic interactions with self-objects. The original self-object is the mother or a caregiver who provides empathic response to the self-object needs. This may be in the form of love, admiration, acceptance, joyful participation, warmth, and responsiveness, communicating a sense of valued and cherished existence to the child. Human beings will continue to seek objects to fulfill these basic self-object needs throughout life. Failures to fulfill such needs can result in the formation of a pathological psychic structure and patterns of behavior leading to the development and pathological character structures during adult life.

Sadock BJ, Sadock VA. *Kaplan & Sadock's Comprehensive Textbook of Psychiatry*. 8th ed. Philadelphia: Lippincott Williams & Wilkins; 2005:737–738.

132. Answer: E. There is strong and convincing evidence from family studies that alcoholism and substance abuse aggregates in families. Also, twin and adoption studies support that this is at least in part inherited and not explained entirely by environment.

Genetic studies have confirmed this, and responsible genes for specific molecular targets are beginning to be identified, but remain controversial. Much of the focus has been on the dopamine pathway.

Hales RE, Yudofsky SC. *Textbook of Clinical Psychiatry*. 4th ed. Washington: American Psychiatric Publishing; 2003:3–65.

133. Answer: B. The law limits a Medicare provider's total charges to an allowable amount for patients enrolled in Medicare. You do not bill the secondary (supplemental) insurance first. In fact, you will likely be denied payment until you first receive reimbursement for a service deemed medically necessary by Medicare. You do not simultaneously bill Medicare and supplemental insurances. The supplemental insurance would likely deny payment until Medicare is billed first, and secondly this may qualify as double or triple billing, and possibly fraud. Medicare providers must bill Medicare themselves. Nonproviders that a patient chooses to visit may bill the patient in certain circumstances and require the burden of filing to be placed on the patient. Medicare providers are not limited solely to Medicare reimbursement, but should also subsequently bill the supplemental insurance, followed by billing the patient the remainder of the allowable charges.

1. Centers for Medicare & Medicaid Services. *The Centers for Medicare & Medicaid Services Website*. http://www.cms.hhs.gov/. Accessed February 14, 2007.
2. Sadavoy J, Jarvik LF, Grossberg GT, et al. *Comprehensive Textbook of Geriatric Psychiatry*. 3rd ed. New York: WW Norton & Company; 2004:1207–1237.

134. Answer: B. Inattention is the hallmark of delirium. Testing three-word registration is an appropriate bedside investigation, as is the digit span test.

1. MacLeod AD. Delirium: the clinical concept. *Palliat Support Care*. 2006;4:305–312.
2. Meagher DJ. Phenomenology of delirium: assessment of 100 adult cases using standardised measures. *Br J Psychiatry*. 2007;190:135–141.

135. Answer: A. According to DSM-IV-TR, ASPD is associated with Depressive Disorders, Substance-Related Disorders, Anxiety Disorders, Somatization Disorder, Pathological Gambling, and other Impulse Control Disorders. DSM also notes that these individuals are at significantly higher risk of dying prematurely by violent outcomes (suicide, homicide, and accidents). There also seems to be a consistent relationship between antisocial behavior and Alcohol Dependence.

1. American Psychiatric Association. *Diagnostic and Statistical Manual of Mental Disorders (DSM-IV-TR)*. 4th

ed. (Text revision). http://www.psychiatryonline.com/content.aspx?aID=3928#3928. Accessed February 25, 2007.
2. Mulder R. Alcoholism and personality. *Aust N Z J Psychiatry.* 2002;36:44–52.
3. Verona E, Patrick C, Joiner T. Psychopathy, antisocial personality, and suicide risk. *J Abnorm Psychol.* 2001;110:462–470.

136. Answer: B. Pathological gambling is characterized by the failure to resist the impulse to gamble despite severe consequences. The typical pathological gambler in treatment studies is a white man from a comfortable economic background, 35 to 50 years of age, but one out of three pathological gamblers is female. Studies point to a 3% to 5% rate of problem gamblers in the general population, and an approximate 1% meeting criteria for pathological gambling. Significant comorbidity occurs with mood and substance disorders. Many patients with ASPD have gambling problems, but in comparison, the majority of pathological gamblers have a better work record, a more stable family life, and a higher moral set before the disruptions caused by chronic chasing begin. Psychosis is uncommon, and the pathological gambler's overwhelming "obsession" with play is generally, completely ego-syntonic. This is unlike the ego-dystonic obsessions of Obsessive-Compulsive Disorder.

Sadock BJ, Sadock VA. *Kaplan and Sadock's Comprehensive Textbook of Psychiatry.* 7th ed. Philadelphia: Lippincott Williams & Wilkins; 2000:1703–1705.

137. Answer: C. Consanguinity and polygenic inheritance refer to specific characteristics about the heritability of Schizophrenia. The stress diathesis model refers to an underlying predisposition to a particular disease (diathesis), which is activated by stressors in the environment.

Sadock B, Sadock V. *Kaplan and Sadock's Pocket Handbook of Clinical Psychiatry.* 3rd ed. Philadelphia: Lippincott Williams & Wilkins; 2001:105.

138. Answer: B. This patient has symptoms of a Major Depressive Episode with Psychotic Features. Although she has suffered the death of a loved one, her symptoms go beyond what would be expected for Bereavement. Bereavement may include depressive symptoms, such as sad mood, poor sleep, change in appetite, and a desire to die in order to join the lost loved one. They may even have transitory experiences of seeing or hearing the voice of the deceased loved one. If symptoms persist past 2 months or are severe enough to include morbid preoccupations with guilt or worthlessness, active suicidal ideation, or more severe psychotic symptoms, a major depres-

sive episode should be a diagnostic consideration. Acute Stress Disorder would not be diagnosed, as the patient's symptoms have lasted longer than a month and do not include reexperiencing, avoidance, or dissociative symptoms. Similarly, her symptoms would not meet criteria for Brief Psychotic Disorder as she has significant mood symptoms and her symptoms have lasted greater than 1 month. Adjustment Disorder would not be diagnosed, because the symptoms meet the criteria for another axis I disorder, Major Depressive Episode; this excludes the diagnosis of Adjustment Disorder.

American Psychiatric Association. *Desk Reference to the Diagnostic Criteria from DSM-IV-TR.* Washington: American Psychiatric Association; 2000:161, 221, 285, 311.

139. Answer: B. Medications most commonly implicated in causing hyperprolactinemia are antipsychotic agents which are dopamine receptor blockers. They cause hyperprolactinemia by via D_2 receptor blockade in the hypothalamic tuberofundibular system and on the lactotrophs. The antipsychotic potency of the older phenothiazines, butyrophenones, and dibenzoxazepine was found to parallel their potency in increasing PRL levels. The level of elevated prolactin found with these drugs is generally less than 100 μg/L. Among the atypical antipsychotic medications, risperidone is known to cause elevations in prolactin level even higher than those caused by the typical antipsychotics. In contrast, clozapine, olanzapine, quetiapine, ziprasidone, and aripiprazole are much less likely to elevate prolactin levels. It is believed that the lack of effect of these atypical agents is due to them being only transiently and weakly bound to the D_2 receptor or to them having agonist activity as well as antagonist activity at the D_2 receptor. Hyperprolactinemia causes decreased libido, erectile dysfunction in men, and galactorrhea and amenorrhea in women.

Molitch ME. Medication-induced hyperprolactinemia. *Mayo Clin Proc.* 2005;80:1050–1057.

140. Answer: E. In addition to the listed factors, hopelessness is a strong predictor of suicide. Age, gender, family history of suicide, recent inpatient psychiatric care, comorbid psychiatric disorders, a suicidal plan, access to means to harm oneself, losses or stressors, and medical illnesses are other factors to keep in mind when assessing for suicide risk.

Shea SC. *Psychiatric Interviewing: The Art of Understanding.* 2nd ed. Philadelphia: WB Saunders; 1998:463.

141. Answer: C. The FDA approved indications for prescription stimulants include ADHD in children and adults, Narcolepsy, and appetite suppression to promote weight loss in obesity. Although amphetamines, methylphenidate, and pemoline are used for their antidepressant effect in the elderly, medically ill, and those with stroke or TBI, they are not approved by FDA for these indications.

Graham AW, Schultz TK, Mayo-Smith MF, et al. *Principles of Addiction Medicine*. 3rd ed. Chevy Chase, Maryland: American Society of Addiction Medicine; 2003:165.

142. Answer: C. Tremor is not a known side effect of benzodiazepine use. However, it may appear as part of the benzodiazepine withdrawal syndrome. Drowsiness is common. Confusion may result, especially with impaired concentration, which also impairs memory encoding. Long-term use of benzodiazepines, especially in the elderly, may result in memory impairment. Ataxia and falls, including syncopal episodes, can occur.

Ropper AH, Brown RH. *Adams and Victor's Principles of Neurology*. 8th ed. New York: McGraw-Hill; 2005:1017–1045.

143. Answer: C. Carbamazepine and phenytoin are two anticonvulsant medications used as adjuvants in pain management, and each may induce the metabolism of methadone, thus precipitating a withdrawal syndrome. Gabapentin and valproate are anticonvulsants that do not significantly lower methadone levels, and may be used as adjuvant treatments in pain management. SSRIs (e.g., sertraline), tricyclic antidepressants (e.g., nortriptyline), and benzodiazepines are also used as adjuvant medications for pain management, and do not appreciably lower methadone levels by interaction.

Kaufman DM. *Clinical Neurology for Psychiatrists*. 5th ed. Philadelphia: WB Saunders; 2001:347–368.

144. Answer: E. Hormones are divided into two main classes. The first one consists of proteins, polypeptides, and glycoproteins. The second class is made up of steroids and steroid-like compounds. Hormone secretion is stimulated by the action of neurohormones, which are the secretory products of neuroendocrine transducer cells of the hypothalamus. Neurohormones include: CRH (which stimulates the release of ACTH), TRH (which excites the release of TSH), both SRIF and GHRH help to release GH, GnRH stimulates the release of both Luteinizing Hormone (LH) and Follicle Stimulating Hormone (FSH), and prolactin release is stimulated by oxytocin. Neurohormones are released from the median eminence of the hypothalamus. They then act on the anterior pituitary gland to regulate the release of their target hormones. These pituitary hormones either act directly on their target cells or stimulate the release of other hormones from peripheral endocrine organs. These last hormones often have feedback loops which help to regulate their secretion.

Sadock BJ, Sadock VA. *Kaplan and Sadock's Synopsis of Psychiatry*. 9th ed. Philadelphia: Lippincott Williams & Wilkins; 2003:128–135.

145. Answer: E. All of the choices are outcomes that can result from Substance Abuse or Dependence in patients who are diagnosed with Bipolar Disorder. The lifetime prevalence of a Substance Use Disorder in patients with Bipolar Disorder is at least 50%.

Kleber HD, Weiss RD, Anton RF, et al. Treatment of patients with substance use disorders, second edition. American Psychiatric Association. www.psychiatryonline.com/content.aspx?aID=14810. Accessed December 14, 2007.

146. Answer: D. The nuclei in the basal ganglia give rise to the extrapyramidal tract, which regulate motor tone. Her symptoms appear to be a hemiballismus. Hemiballismus is classically a result of infarction of the contralateral sub thalamic nucleus of the basal ganglia. This sounds less like chorea, but it is possible. Chorea, or jerking of the limbs and trunk, is classically the result of injury to the caudate nucleus, also in the basal ganglia. Huntington's chorea results from atrophy of the caudate nuclei; such intermittent movements would be unusual with isolated lesions of the cortex, cerebellum, brainstem, or spinal cord.

Kaufman DM. *Clinical Neurology for Psychiatrists*. 5th ed. Philadelphia: WB Saunders; 2001:8–25.

147. Answer: E. Despite its abilities to distinguish cerebral physiology, metabolism, and chemistry, certain limitations prohibit routine clinical use of PET. Most important is its scarcity as PET is found in relatively few medical centers. It is also very expensive. A cyclotrons or linear accelerator must be nearby to produce the radioligands or tracers. Radioligands must be produced to match the pathology being studied. PET cannot detect abnormalities in any systems for which you are not using the appropriate radioligand (of which there are many). Resolution is better than SPECT, but still limited, and the resolution is not nearly as good as a CT scan or MRI. PET can very well distinguish between Alzheimer's and vascular dementias, and some promote its routine clinical use for such disorders.

1. Kaufman DM. *Clinical Neurology for Psychiatrists*. 5th ed. Philadelphia: WB Saunders; 2001:532–551.
2. Ropper AH, Brown RH. *Adams and Victor's Principles of Neurology*. 8th ed. New York: McGraw-Hill; 2005: 11–38.

148. Answer: A. Pramiprexol is a dopamine agonist which has been shown to be effective in the treatment of RLS.

1. Katzung BG, Trevor AJ. *Examination and Board Review: Pharmacology.* 5th ed. Stamford: Appleton & Lange; 1998:172, 214–216.
2. Zaidat OO, Lerner AJ. *The Little Black Book of Neurology.* 4th ed. St. Louis: Mosby; 2002:332.

149. Answer: C. Otto F. Kernberg's principle contributions have been in the fields of narcissism, object relations, and personality disorders. According to Kernberg, the self is an intrapsychic structure consisting of multiple self representations. It is a realistic self which integrates both good and bad self-images. The self consists of a structure that has both libidinal and aggressive components. Kernberg described normal narcissism as the libidinal investment of self. The libidinal investment of the self is not merely derived from an instinctual source of libidinal energy, but from several relationships between the self and other intrapsychic structures, such as the ego, the superego, and the id. He described three types of narcissism: normal adult narcissism, normal infantile narcissism, and pathological narcissism. Normal adult narcissism is a normal self-esteem based on normal structures of the self. The individual has introjected whole representations of objects, has stable objects relationships, and a solid moral system. The superego is fully developed and individualized. Normal infantile narcissism regulates the self esteem through gratifications related to the age, which includes or implies a normal infantile system of values, demands, or prohibitions. In pathological narcissism, the libidinal investment is a pathological structure of the self. Kernberg also described a developmental model where he described three developmental tasks for an individual, that have to be accomplished. When one fails to accomplish a certain developmental task, they become more prone to develop certain psychopathologies. Failing the first developmental task of psychic clarification of self increases the risk of developing psychosis. Not accomplishing the second task of overcoming splitting results in an increased risk of developing a borderline personality disorder (BPD). Varieties of higher-level personality development, corresponding to Freud's description of neurosis, can develop when the first and second developmental tasks are accomplished. Self-object boundaries are established and object images are integrated and neurosis can occur as a result of the conflict between libidinal and aggressive impulses.

Sadock BJ, Sadock VA. *Kaplan & Sadock's Comprehensive Textbook of Psychiatry.* 8th ed. Philadelphia: Lippincott Williams & Wilkins; 2005:2475–2476.

150. Answer: B. NREM stages 3 and 4 are dominated by high amplitude, low frequency (0.5 to 3 Hz) delta waves on EEG, with very little eye movement, and nearly atonic muscles. These are referred to as SWS and are considered the deepest stages of sleep. Stage 1 sleep is dominated by theta (4 to 7 Hz) activity, slower than the alpha (8 to 13 Hz) and beta (>13 Hz) waves of wakefulness. During stage 2 the theta activity continues, but it also contains sleep spindles and K-complexes. REM sleep, of course, has eye movements and the most vivid dreaming.

Hales RE, Yudofsky SC. *Textbook of Clinical Psychiatry.* 4th ed. Washington, DC: American Psychiatric Publishing; 2003: 975–1000.

151. Answer: B. Paralysis during non-REM sleep is maintained in the brainstem (pons), with the diaphragm and ocular muscles being exceptions which remain active. SWS is the restorative phase of sleep, occurring in stages 3 and 4 of NREM, characterized by delta and theta waves on EEG. SWS is concentrated in the early sleep cycles, and SWS duration decreases as the night progresses. Conversely, there is less REM sleep early in the night, and REM sleep increases with successive sleep cycles. REM sleep is a period of increased cerebral activity that can approach waking levels.

Soldatos C, Paparrigopoulos T. Sleep physiology and pathology: pertinence to psychiatry. *Int Rev Psychiatry.* 2005;17:213–228.

152. Answer: C. There is substantial epidemiologic evidence documenting familial links between Antisocial Personality Disorder and Somatization Disorder, with male gender more associated with ASPD and female gender more associated with Somatization. One hypothesis about this association suggests a common underlying histrionic personality tendency, with gender influencing the outcome of ASPD or Somatization Disorder.

1. American Psychiatric Association. *Diagnostic and Statistical Manual of Mental Disorders (DSM-IV-TR).* 4th ed. (Text Revision). http://www.psychiatryonline.com/content.aspx?aID=3928#3928. Accessed February 25, 2007.
2. Cadoret R. Psychopathology in adopted-away offspring of biologic parents with antisocial behavior. *Arch Gen Psychiatry.* 1978;35:176–184.
3. Gabbard G. *Psychodynamic Psychiatry in Clinical Practice.* 4th ed. Washington: American Psychiatric Publishing; 2005:516.

153. Answer: E. In patients with Anorexia Nervosa, menses usually resume within 6 months of achieving 90% ideal body weight. Amenorrhea in this case is due to low levels of FSH and LH. A progesterone challenge will not cause withdrawal bleeding in patients with amenorrhea due to anorexia nervosa.

Forman SF. *Eating Disorders: Epidemiology, Pathogenesis, and Clinical Features*. http://www.uptodateonline.com/utd/content/topic.do?topicKey=genr_med/9522&type=A&selectedTitle=1~36. Accessed March 4, 2007.

154. Answer: A. It is thought that increased dopamine activity in the limbic system contributes to the positive symptoms of Schizophrenia. Conversely, it is thought that decreased dopamine activity in the frontal lobes plays a role in the negative symptoms of Schizophrenia.

Sadock B, Sadock V. *Kaplan and Sadock's Pocket Handbook of Clinical Psychiatry*. 3rd ed. Philadelphia: Lippincott Williams & Wilkins; 2001:105–106.

155. Answer: B. The lifetime prevalence of Bipolar Disorder is approximately 1%. Epidemiologic studies which assess for milder bipolar spectrum disorders, such as Cyclothymia and Bipolar Disorder type II, report even higher prevalence rates between 2% to 5%. Only 27% of patients identified by epidemiological studies as having Bipolar Disorder have ever received treatment. Patients with Bipolar Disorder are among the most undertreated patients with psychiatric diagnoses. Unlike MDD, which is more common in women, Bipolar Disorder is distributed equally between men and women. Comorbid psychiatric conditions are common, with 60% of patients with Bipolar Disorder developing some sort of Substance Abuse during their lifetime. Anxiety Disorders are also common and they are present in approximately half of patients with Bipolar Disorder.

Stern TA, Herman JB. *Massachusetts General Hospital Psychiatry Update and Board Preparation*. 2nd ed. New York: McGraw Hill; 2002:113.

156. Answer: B. Among the previously listed drugs, aripiprazole is the only one that has an active metabolite. It is metabolized via the cytochrome P450 2D6 and 3A4 systems to dehydro-aripiprazole. Those people who lack the cytochrome P450 2D6 enzyme have a 40% increase in the level of the active metabolite dehydro-aripiprazole when the drug is administered. Quetiapine is metabolized by the cytochrome P450 3A4 system, but it does not have an active metabolite. Clonazepam, lorazepam, and oxazepam are not metabolized by the hepatic microsomal enzyme system.

Albers LJ, Hahn RK, Reist C. *Handbook of Psychiatric Drugs*. Laguna Hills: Current Clinical Strategies Publishing; 2005:43–44, 47, 56–58.

157. Answer: D. Interestingly enough, the rate of suicide among women during both pregnancy and their first postpartum year is lower than that of women in the general population. Women who give birth to still-born infants have approximately the same level of suicide risk as women in the general population. Pregnant teens are at a lower risk for suicide than their nonpregnant counterparts, although at greater risk than pregnant women generally. Despite these statistics, a postpartum admission to a psychiatric hospital does increase a woman's risk of suicide by 70-fold in her first postpartum year and increases her lifetime risk by 17-fold. Pregnant women are particularly vulnerable to domestic violence and, rather than by suicide, are more likely to be victims of homicide.

Wyszynski AA, Wyszynski B. *Manual of Psychiatric Care for the Medically Ill*. Washington: American Psychiatric Publishing; 2005:136.

158. Answer: D. The initial step in management of alcohol withdrawal is to perform a careful assessment for the presence of medical and psychiatric problems. General management involves correction of fluid, electrolyte, and nutritional deficiencies. Parenteral administration of thiamine must precede administration of glucose in order to prevent permanent memory loss. Long acting benzodiazepines, such as chlordiazepoxide and diazepam constitute standard treatment for uncomplicated alcohol withdrawals. The short-acting agents, such as lorazepam or oxazepam, are preferable in elderly persons and patients with significant liver disease. Beta-blockers, such as atenolol and propranolol, and centrally acting alpha adrenergic agonists, such as clonidine, are effective in ameliorating only mild to moderate withdrawal, primarily by decreasing autonomic nervous system activity. Carbamazepine is equal in efficacy to benzodiazepines in treating mild to moderate withdrawal. Phenytoin has failed to show efficacy in controlling withdrawal seizures in recent trials. Neuroleptics are useful in controlling agitation in the setting of alcohol withdrawal. However, they should always be used in conjunction with a benzodiazepine since they tend to lower the seizure threshold.

Graham AW, Schultz TK, Mayo-Smith MF, et al. *Principles of Addiction Medicine*. 3rd ed. Chevy Chase, Maryland: American Society of Addiction Medicine; 2003:625–629.

159. Answer: B. Typical antipsychotics, especially pimozide and haloperidol, are commonly used to treat Tourette's syndrome. Haloperidol is also used to treat Huntington chorea. NMS is often caused or exacerbated by typical antipsychotics. Typical antipsychotics also cause parkinsonism and other extrapyramidal symptoms (dystonias, akathisia, and TD), and worsen movement abnormalities in Parkinson's disease. MS does not typically result in psychosis, nor does it typically require antipsychotic medications. Most antipsychotic medications lower the seizure threshold, and could potentially worsen management of seizure disorders.

Ropper AH, Brown RH. *Adams and Victor's Principles of Neurology*. 8th ed. New York: McGraw-Hill; 2005:1017–1045.

160. **Answer: D.** Many antipsychotics lower the seizure threshold and increase the risk of seizures. Clozapine, olanzapine, and aliphatic phenothiazines like chlorpromazine are more likely to cause seizures. More potent piperazine phenothiazines and thioxanthenes (notably fluphenazine and thiothixene), risperidone, and quetiapine are much less likely to cause seizures. Butyrophenones and molindone rarely cause seizures. Clozapine has a dose-related risk of causing seizures in nonepileptic patients. Clozapine, olanzapine, and low-potency phenothiazines and thioxanthenes, should be used with extreme caution in untreated epileptic patients. They should also be used with caution in patients undergoing withdrawal from alcohol, barbiturates, or benzodiazepines. Piperazines, aripiprazole, quetiapine, risperidone, and ziprasidone can be used safely in epileptic patients, if moderate doses are attained gradually and if concomitant anticonvulsant drug therapy is maintained.

Brunton LL, Parker KL, Buxton ILO, et al. *Goodman & Gilman's The Pharmacological Basis of Therapeutics*. 11th ed. http://www.accessmedicine.com/content.aspx?aID=939126. Accessed April 25, 2007.

161. **Answer: C.** Estrogen is a steroid hormone. It enhances mood by increasing the brain's sensitivity to serotonin. It does this possibly by inhibiting MAO. In animal studies, long-term estrogen treatment has resulted in decreased serotonin 5-HT_1 receptors and increased 5-HT_2 receptors. The association of both estrogen and progesterone with serotonin has also been hypothesized to be an important factor in premenstrual and postpartum mood disturbances. Additionally, estrogen functions to enhance neural activity in the hypothalamus and the limbic system through modulation of neuronal excitability. Dihydroepiandrosterone is the most abundant circulating steroid. It has been linked to involvement in memory and improved well being and functional status in both depressed and normal individuals. Its effects could be due to either its metabolism into estrogen or testosterone or from its antiglucocorticoid activity. Insulin increasingly has been shown to be integrally involved in memory and learning. Insulin receptors occur in high density in the hippocampus. They are thought to help neurons metabolize glu-

cose. In studies, patients with Alzheimer's dementia have been found to have lower CSF insulin concentrations than controls. Both insulin and glucose improve verbal memory.

Sadock BJ, Sadock VA. *Kaplan and Sadock's Synopsis of Psychiatry*. 9th ed. Philadelphia: Lippincott Williams & Wilkins; 2003:128–135.

162. **Answer: D.** Naltrexone is an opioid antagonist that cannot be given by itself to patients who have used a short-acting opioid, such as heroin, within the past 5 days or who have used a long-acting opioid, such as methadone, within the past 7 days. Methadone can reduce opioid withdrawal symptoms. Buprenorphine, a mixed agonist-antagonist at the opioid receptor, can be given alone or combined with naloxone for opioid withdrawal symptoms. Clonidine is an alpha-2-adrenergic receptor agonist that can suppress the noradrenergic hyperactivity and thus decreases sweating and gastrointestinal symptoms of opioid withdrawal. However, it is not generally adequate to help muscle aches or insomnia, and thus adjunctive medications may be needed. Naltrexone can be given for opioid detoxification in patients who are treated first with clonidine.

Kleber HD, Weiss RD, Anton RF, et al. Treatment of patients with substance use disorders, second edition. American Psychiatric Association. www.psychiatryonline.com/content.aspx?aID=14810. Accessed December 21, 2007.

163. **Answer: C.** Clonidine is an alpha2 agonist which has been shown to be effective in the treatment of Tourette's syndrome.

1. Katzung BG, Trevor AJ. *Examination and Board Review: Pharmacology*. 5th ed. Stamford: Appleton & Lange; 1998:90, 161–162.
2. Zaidat OO, Lerner AJ. *The Little Black Book of Neurology*. 4th ed. St. Louis: Mosby; 2002:332.

164. **Answer: A.** Recent studies have shown that cognitive losses with advancing age are much more circumscribed than previously observed. Short-term memory, mental speed, and visual-perceptual and spatial skills do appear to decline gradually with advancing age. However, verbal intelligence, most language skills (e.g., vocabulary range, reading, and spelling), calculation ability, and basic attention appear to be generally well maintained across the life span of healthy individuals. Executive abilities, which initially were thought to be the cognitive skills most disrupted by aging, are generally found to be spared in healthy persons.

Sadock BJ, Sadock VA. *Kaplan & Sadock's Comprehensive Textbook of Psychiatry*. 8th ed. Philadelphia: Lippincott Williams & Wilkins; 2005:3632.

165. Answer: C. The SCN and other important structures reside in the hypothalamus. Destruction of the SCN eliminates regulated daily circadian rhythms, though sleep cycles may persist independently. Several areas of the pons do help regulate REM sleep, but are not thought to be as important as the suprachiasmatic nucleus (SCN) in the hypothalamus in regulating the whole circadian rhythmicity of sleep. The amygdala also appears to play a role in REM control, but not so much in overall circadian rhythmicity. The pineal gland is involved in melatonin metabolism (a *zeitgeber*, or "timekeeper"), but also is not as central as the SCN in circadian rhythmicity. The pituitary is a mainly hormonal structure inferior to the hypothalamus, and its homeostatic function is intimately related to that of the hypothalamus. However, the hypothalamus is more directly in control of regulating circadian rhythms. Another important structure not mentioned is the reticular activating system involved in wakefulness and alertness.

1. Hales RE, Yudofsky SC. *Textbook of Clinical Psychiatry*. 4th ed. Washington: American Psychiatric Publishing; 2003:975–1000.
2. Sadock BJ, Sadock VA. *Kaplan & Sadock's Comprehensive Textbook of Psychiatry*. 7th ed. Philadelphia: Lippincott Williams & Wilkins; 2000:133–142.

166. Answer: E. The metabolic syndrome is associated with weight gain, dyslipidemia, and diabetes mellitus. Additionally, obesity is a known risk factor for hypertension, elevated triglycerides, insulin resistance, and diabetes mellitus. There are clinical guidelines for monitoring BMI, waist circumference, blood pressure, fasting plasma glucose, and fasting lipid profile for patients being prescribed atypical antipsychotics. Clozapine and olanzapine may be the worst offenders.

Shirzadi AA, Ghaemi SN. Side effects of atypical antipsychotics: extrapyramidal symptoms and the metabolic syndrome. *Harv Rev Psychiatry*. 2006;14:152–164.

167. Answer: D. Schizoid patients prefer isolation. The other associations are described in the DSM-IV-TR diagnostic criteria for each respective diagnosis.

American Psychiatric Association. *Diagnostic and Statistical Manual of Mental Disorders*. 4th ed. (Text Revision). Washington: American Psychiatric Association; 2000:456, 697, 710, 721, 725.

168. Answer: C. Serum amylase may be elevated in patients with Bulimia Nervosa due to excessive purging. Elevated serum amylase is seen more often in Bulimia Nervosa than Anorexia Nervosa. The elevation results from increased secretion from the salivary gland rather than the pancreas, unless there is comorbid alcoholism present. Potassium, calcium, magnesium, and fasting glucose may be variably normal or decreased.

Sadock BJ, Sadock VA. *Kaplan and Sadock's Comprehensive Textbook of Psychiatry*. 8th ed. Philadelphia: Lippincott Williams & Wilkins; 2005:2014.

169. Answer: B. The rule of thirds in Schizophrenia refers to the approximate ratio of patients who will either be able to live relatively normal lives, live independently with persistent symptoms, and will require frequent hospitalizations and possible institutionalization.

Sadock B, Sadock V. *Kaplan and Sadock's Pocket Handbook of Clinical Psychiatry*. 3rd ed. Philadelphia: Lippincott Williams & Wilkins; 2001:105–106.

170. Answer: D. Bipolar Disorder is considered a chronic and recurrent condition, for which the majority of patients will need long-term pharmacologic treatment. The interval between mood episodes *decreases* with time before it plateaus. Untreated depressive episodes last between 6 to 12 months, whereas untreated manic episodes last 3 to 6 months. Even between clearly defined mood episodes, patients may experience depressive symptoms which affect their daily functioning. Manic episodes tend to occur more in the summer, with depressive episodes occurring more in the winter and spring. The term *rapid cycling* refers to patients whose illness includes four or more mood episodes (depressive or manic) per year.

Stern TA, Herman JB. *Massachusetts General Hospital Psychiatry Update and Board Preparation*. 2nd ed. New York: McGraw-Hill; 2002:115.

171. Answer: C. In a project for identifying evidence-based psychotherapy treatments for Anxiety Disorders in older adults, the authors identified 17 studies that met criteria for evidence-based treatments (EBTs). These studies reflected samples of adults with GAD or samples with Mixed Anxiety Disorders or symptoms. Evidence was found for efficacy for four types of EBTs: relaxation training, CBT, as well as, to a lesser extent, supportive therapy and cognitive therapy, which have support for treating subjective anxiety symptoms and disorders. CBT for late-life GAD has garnered the most consistent support, and relaxation training represents an efficacious, relatively low-cost intervention.

Ayers CR, Sorrell JT, Thorp SR, et al. Evidence-based psychological treatments for late-life anxiety. *Psychol Aging*. 2007;22:8–17.

172. Answer: B. Jacques Lacan was the noteworthy figure for approaching the study of the unconscious from the perspective of linguistics/semiotics, and stipulated that the unconscious is structured like a language. Kohut is the founder of self-psychology. Klein was notable for her seminal work in the development of object relations, and Bion expanded on her work on projective identification. Franz Alexander is known for his notion of the corrective emotional experience performed by the analyst to correct early trauma.

Kaplan HI, Sadock BJ. *Kaplan & Sadock's Synopsis of Psychiatry*. 8th ed. Philadelphia: Lippincott Williams & Wilkins; 1998:224–229.

173. **Answer: E.** Naltrexone is an opioid receptor antagonist approved for use in the treatment of Alcohol Dependence in conjunction with psychosocial treatments. It acts via blocking the μ-opioid receptors thus reducing the reinforcing effects of alcohol, leading to reduced feelings of intoxication and cravings. There is ample evidence supporting short-term benefits of naltrexone in Alcohol Dependence, the evidence for longer-term efficacy is less compelling. The recommended dose is 50 mg/day in a single dose. Most common adverse effects are nausea, headache, anxiety, and sedation. It can be associated with dose-related hepatotoxicity. Therefore, all patients should have liver transaminase levels checked monthly for the first three months and every three months thereafter. Naltrexone is FDA category C in regards to pregnancy. It is contraindicated in patients with hepatitis and liver failure. It is also contraindicated in patients receiving opioid therapy for chronic pain and those who are actively abusing opioids because it can precipitate severe withdrawal symptoms.

1. Srisurapanont M, Jarusuraisin N. Opioid antagonists for alcohol dependence. *Cochrane Database Syst Rev.* 2005;1:CD001867.
2. Williams SH. Medications for treating alcohol dependence. *Am Fam Physician.* 2005;72:1775–1780.

174. **Answer: E.** Chronic steroid use often induces hypokalemia and potassium supplementation is often suggested in these cases. Hyperglycemia and diabetes may also develop with chronic use. Muscle weakness (especially proximal) or steroid myopathy is possible, and often difficult to distinguish from the myasthenia gravis. Weight gain and elevated blood pressure are common with chronic corticosteroid use. Side effects may be reduced by slowly decreasing doses or trying alternate day dosing.

Ropper AH, Brown RH. *Adams and Victor's Principles of Neurology*. 8th ed. New York: McGraw-Hill; 2005:1250–1264.

175. **Answer: E.** Metoclopramide is a dopamine antagonist used in the treatment of nausea, vomiting, and gastroparesis. Some of its most common side effects include constipation, somnolence, tremor, and dystonias (1%). TD has been reported rarely and it usually occurs after months or years of treatment. Metoclopramide, like other dopamine antagonists, can produce galactorrhea. Methamoglobinemia has been reported in neonates. Priapism has not been associated with the use of metoclopramide.

Pasricha PJ. *Treatment of Disorders of Bowel Motility and Water Flux; Antiemetics; Agents Used in Biliary and Pancreatic Disease.* http://www.accessmedicine.com/content.aspx?aID=946737. Accessed March 28, 2007.

176. **Answer: A.** Melatonin is a pineal hormone. It is derived from serotonin, which is derived from tryptophan. It is involved in the circadian-rhythm and also helps to regulate diverse body functions such as the immune system, mood, and reproductive performance. It functions too as an antioxidant. It can be used as a therapeutic agent in the treatment of Circadian Phase Disorders such as Jet Lag. Oxytocin is a posterior pituitary neurohormone. It stimulates the release of prolactin and is involved in osmoregulation, the milk ejection reflex, food intake, and female maternal and sexual behaviors. Dopamine is a biogenic amine neurotransmitter. The chemical pathway involved in the formation of catecholamines includes dopamine, tyrosine, tyramine, epinine, epinephrine, and norepinephrine.

Sadock BJ, Sadock VA. *Kaplan and Sadock's Synopsis of Psychiatry*. 9th ed. Philadelphia: Lippincott Williams & Wilkins; 2003:128–135.

177. **Answer: A.** Adding fluoxetine to desipramine can increase desipramine levels, which can lead to serious side effects such as delirium, cardiotoxicity, or seizures. Therefore, monitoring of desipramine levels is important in this combination. The other choices are all true.

Lam RW, Wan DD, Cohen NL, et al. Combining antidepressants for treatment-resistant depression: a review. *J Clin Psychiatry.* 2002;63:685–693.

178. **Answer: C.** Oxcarbazepine is a pro-drug with a principal metabolite, 10-hydroxycarbazepine, and it has similar therapeutic effects to those of carbamazepine. This medication seems to lack the toxicity profile of carbamazepine, mainly because it has a limited rate of production of active metabolites. However, the incidence of dose-related hyponatremia is similar to the one for carbamazepine. In severe cases, it has been associated with seizures and coma. Seizures, cardiac arrhythmias, ataxia, and

anticholinergic signs and symptoms can be seen in cases of carbamazepine toxicity.

Katzung BG. *Basic and Clinical Pharmacology*. 10th ed. http://www.accessmedicine.com/content.aspx?aID=2503457. Accessed March 26, 2007.

179. Answer: A. Melancholic Features can be applied to any Major Depressive Episode in either Unipolar or Bipolar Depression if anhedonia is present as well as three or more of the following: (i) depression regularly worse in the morning, (ii) early morning awakening (at least 2 hours before the usual time of awakening), (iii) marked psychomotor retardation or agitation, (iv) significant anorexia or weight loss, and (v) excessive or inappropriate guilt.

American Psychiatric Association. *Desk Reference to the Diagnostic Criteria from DSM-IV-TR*. Washington: American Psychiatric Association; 2000:202–203.

180. Answer: E. ADHD is a disorder of inattention, impulsivity, and hyperactivity affecting about 8% to 12% of children worldwide. Although the rates of ADHD decrease with age, about half of all children with this disorder will have impairing symptoms in adulthood. Twin, adoption, and molecular genetic studies have shown that ADHD is highly heritable. Obstetric complications and psychosocial adversity are also known predisposing risk factors for this disorder. Research studies indicate that the dysregulation of frontal-subcortical-cerebellar catecholaminergic circuits are involved in the pathophysiology of ADHD, with molecular imaging studies suggesting that abnormalities of the dopamine transporter lead to impaired neurotransmission. Studies over the past decade have shown the safety and effectiveness of new nonstimulant drugs and long-acting formulations of methylphenidate and amphetamine. Targeted psychosocial treatments in the context of ongoing pharmacotherapy also help patients in controlling their symptoms. Among all the listed medications, venlafaxine is the only one that has not yet been shown to be effective in treating ADHD.

Biederman J, Faraone SV. Attention-deficit hyperactivity disorder. *Lancet*. 2005;366:237–248.

181. Answer: E. While late-onset, good premorbid functioning, mood symptoms, and positive symptoms are good prognostic factors, an insidious onset is usually a poor prognostic factor for Schizophrenia. Other factors that are associated with poor outcomes include early onset, no precipitating factors, negative symptoms, and findings of neurologic deficits.

Sadock B, Sadock V. *Kaplan and Sadock's Pocket Handbook of Clinical Psychiatry*. 3rd ed. Philadelphia: Lippincott Williams & Wilkins; 2001:105–106.

182. Answer: E. Enuresis is the repeated voiding of urine into the bed or clothes; the voiding may be involuntary or intentional. For a DSM-IV-TR diagnosis to be made, the child must have a chronological age of at least 5 years (or equivalent developmental level). The behavior must occur twice weekly for a period of at least 3 months, or must cause clinically significant distress or impairment in functioning. Enuresis is diagnosed only if the behavior is not due to a medical condition. The DSM-IV-TR defines three types: Nocturnal only (passage of urine only during nighttime sleep), Diurnal only (passage of urine during waking hours), and Nocturnal and Diurnal (a combination of the other two subtypes). The child in this scenario is too young to receive a DSM-IV-TR diagnosis of Enuresis and may indeed cease to exhibit this behavior as he develops over the coming year.

1. American Psychiatric Association. *Quick Reference to the Diagnostic Criteria from DSM-IV-TR*. Washington: American Psychiatric Association; 2000:76.
2. Sadock BJ, Sadock VA. *Kaplan and Sadock's Synopsis of Psychiatry*. 9th ed. Philadelphia: Lippincott Williams & Wilkins; 2003:238–242,1256–1258.

183. Answer: E. Since the 1950s antipsychotic medications have been extensively used to treat people with chronic mental illnesses like Schizophrenia. These drugs have been also associated with a wide range of adverse effects, including movement disorders such as TD. A recent Cochrane review determined whether a reduction or cessation of antipsychotic medications is associated with a reduction in TD for people with Schizophrenia (or other chronic mental illnesses) who have existing TD. The secondary aim of the study was to determine whether the use of specific neuroleptics for similar groups of people could be a treatment for TD that was already established. One small 2-week study (n=18), reported on the "masking" effects of molindone and haloperidol on TD, which favored haloperidol (relative risk [RR]: 3.44; confidence interval (CI): 1.1 to 5.8). Two (total n=17) studies found no reduction in TD associated with antipsychotic reduction (RR: 0.38; CI: 0.1 to 1.0). One study (n=20) found no significant differences in oral dyskinesia (RR: 2.45; CI: 0.3 to 19.7) when neuroleptics were compared as a specific treatment for TD. TD was found to be not significantly different (n=32, RR: 0.62; CI: 0.3 to 1.26) between quetiapine and haloperidol when these neuroleptics were used as specific treatments for TD, although the need for additional neuroleptics was significantly lower in the quetiapine group (n=47, RR: 0.49; CI: 0.2 to 1.0) than in those given haloperidol. The authors concluded that limited data from small studies using antipsychotic reduction or specific antipsychotic drugs as treatments for TD did not provide any convincing evidence of the value of these approaches. A more recent Cochrane review concluded that inconclusive results from their study meant that routine clinical use of adjunctive benzodiazepine in the treatment of TD is not indicated.

1. Bhoopathi PS, Soares-Weiser K. Benzodiazepines for neuroleptic-induced tardive dyskinesia. *Cochrane Database Syst Rev*. 2006;3:CD000205.
2. Soares-Weiser K, Rathbone J. Antipsychotic reduction and/or cessation and neuroleptics as specific treatments for tardive dyskinesia. *Cochrane Database Syst Rev*. 2006;1:CD000459.

184. Answer: E. Child abuse leads to negative mental health outcomes including depression, anxiety, substance abuse, and PTSD. However, little attention has been given to victimization as a reason for violence among people with major mental illness. Child abuse is usually associated with angry reactive violence and with expressive violence in childhood, adolescence, and adulthood, and with violent criminal offending in adolescence and adulthood. Psychiatric patients have higher rates than the general population of both child abuse and victimization as adults. Childhood physical abuse is highly significant in predicting adult violence. Severe and persistent mental illness and recent criminal victimization is more predictive of violence in multivariate analysis than any other variable other than substance abuse. Those who are victims of violent or nonviolent crimes are significantly more likely to engage in violent behavior of both the more serious and less serious forms.

1. Hiday VA. Putting community risk in perspective: a look at correlations, causes, and controls. *Int J Law Psychiatry*. 2006;29:316–331.
2. Hiday VA, Swanson JW, Swartz MS, et al. Victimization: a link between mental illness and violence? *Int J Law Psychiatry*. 2001;24:559–572.

185. Answer: D. Acamprosate blocks glutaminergic NMDA receptors and activates the GABA-A receptors. It has been shown to reduce both short and long-term (more than 6 months) relapse rates in patients with alcohol dependence. It was recently approved by the FDA for the treatment of Alcohol Dependence. It is generally well tolerated, with the most common side effect being transient diarrhea. There are no interactions with the concomitant use of alcohol, diazepam, disulfiram, or imipramine so patients can continue to use it during a relapse. It should not be administered to patients with renal insufficiency or advanced cirrhosis.

1. Mason BJ. Acamprosate in the treatment of alcohol dependence. *Expert Opin Pharmacother*. 2005;6:2103–2115.

2. Williams SH. Medications for treating alcohol dependence. *Am Fam Physician*. 2005;72:1775–1780.

186. Answer: A. Constipation is a typical side effect to opiate use, although diarrhea may occur during opiate withdrawal. Laxatives and stool softeners may be used to treat the constipation. Opiates can cause respiratory suppression. A tolerance to this effect does not develop in the same way as tolerance to other effects of opiates. Hypoventilation is a potentially lethal effect of opioid use. Nausea and dysphoria are common side effects of opiate use. Opiates may affect mood, but also at greater doses may produce more profound mental status changes.

Kaufman DM. *Clinical Neurology for Psychiatrists*. 5th ed. Philadelphia: WB Saunders; 2001:347–368.

187. Answer: C. MAO-B inhibitors are thought to alter disease progression in Parkinson's disease, but clinical trials have produced conflicting results. A recent Cochrane review on the use of MAO-B inhibitors included ten trials (a total of 2,422 patients), with nine using selegiline and one using lazabemide. The mean follow-up was for 5.8 years. MAO-B inhibitors were not associated with a significant increase in deaths (odds ratio [OR]: 1.15; 95% CI: 0.92 to 1.44). They provided small benefits over control in impairment (weighted mean difference for change in motor Unified Parkinson's Disease Rating Scale Activities of Daily Living [UPDRS ADL] score was 3.81 points less with MAO-B inhibitors; 95% CI: 2.27 to 5.36) and disability (weighted mean difference for change in UPDRS ADL score was 1.50 less; 95% CI: 0.48 to 2.53) at one year which, although statistically significant, were not clinically significant. There was a marked levodopa-sparing effect with MAO-B inhibitors which was associated with a significant reduction in motor fluctuations (OR: 0.75; 95% CI: 0.59 to 0.94) but not dyskinesia (OR: 0.97; 95% CI: 0.76 to 1.25). The reduction in motor fluctuations was, however, not robust in sensitivity analyses. Although adverse events were generally mild and infrequent, withdrawals due to side effects were higher (OR: 2.36; 95% CI: 1.32 to 4.20) with MAO-B inhibitors. The authors concluded that MAO-B inhibitors do not appear to delay disease progression but may have a beneficial effect on motor fluctuations. There was no statistically significant effect on deaths although the confidence interval does not exclude a small increase with MAO-B inhibitors. It was indicated that these drugs should not be recommended for routine use in the treatment of early Parkinson's disease.

Macleod AD, Counsell CE, Ives N, et al. Monoamine oxidase B inhibitors for early Parkinson's disease. *Cochrane Database Syst Rev*. 2005;3:CD004898.

188. Answer: A. Schizophrenia in some cases may be the result of viral infection during fetal neural development. Data supporting this assertion include: (i) more patient births in late winter and early spring suggesting potential in utero exposure to viral illness, (ii) association between exposure to viral epidemics in utero and later development of Schizophrenia, (iii) there is an increased probability for Schizophrenic patients to have been raised with older siblings who may have served as a potential source of infection, and (iv) geographic variation in prevalence, since Schizophrenia becomes more common with greater distance from the equator. There has also been evidence for alterations in various immune markers and increased CSF immunoglobulins in patients with Schizophrenia. MDD has been associated with immune activation of an unknown source. Inflammatory processes may play a role in Alzheimer's disease. This claim has been bolstered by studies showing that long-term NSAID use is negatively correlated with the development of Alzheimer's disease. Lastly, Chronic Fatigue Syndrome is characterized by persistent fatigue, depression, and sleep disturbance. Its etiology is controversial, but some evidence suggests both immune activation and immunosuppression. Although acute viral infection often precedes development of chronic fatigue syndrome, no infectious agent, or in utero viral exposure, has been associated with the disease.

Sadock BJ, Sadock VA. *Kaplan and Sadock's Synopsis of Psychiatry.* 9th ed. Philadelphia: Lippincott Williams & Wilkins; 2003:128–135.

189. Answer: E. The CATIE study included almost 1,500 patients who had Schizophrenia and compared perphenazine (a typical antipsychotic medication) with multiple atypical antipsychotic medications. Seventy-four percent of patients discontinued their initially assigned study medication, with olanzapine having the lowest discontinuation rate. Patients with Schizoaffective Disorder or who had only one Schizophrenic episode were excluded from the study.

Lieberman JA, Stroup TS, McEvoy JP, et al. Effectiveness of antipsychotic drugs in patients with chronic schizophrenia. *N Engl J Med.* 2005;353:1209–1223.

190. Answer: A. Levodopa is one of the first-line agents for the treatment of Parkinson's disease. It is converted to dopamine in the brain and it has to be administered in combination with carbidopa, which doesn't penetrate well into the CNS. If levodopa is administered alone, most of the medication is decarboxylated in the intestinal mucosa, and only about 1% to 3% penetrates the CNS. Early in the disease

levodopa can have a dramatic effect in all the signs of symptoms of Parkinson's disease. However, with time patients tend to develop an on/off phenomenon, where levodopa improves symptoms for a very short period of time after a dose, but symptoms such as rigidity return soon before the patient receives the next dose. The plasma half-life of levodopa is between 1 to 3 hours.

Katzung BG. *Basic and Clinical Pharmacology.* 10th ed. http://www.accessmedicine.com/content.aspx?aID=2504332. Accessed December 18, 2007.

191. Answer: A. Atypical features can be applied to any Major Depressive Episode in either Unipolar or Bipolar Depression if mood reactivity is present as well as two or more of the following: weight gain or increase in appetite, hypersomnia, leaden paralysis, and rejection sensitivity.

American Psychiatric Association. *Desk Reference to the Diagnostic Criteria from DSM-IV-TR.* Washington: American Psychiatric Association; 2000:203–204.

192. Answer: C. Everyone experiences some form of normal bereavement after a loss, and some depressive symptoms can linger for 1 or 2 years. Several factors help distinguish grief from depression. Marked psychomotor retardation is not seen in normal grief. Grief is generally viewed as a normal reaction, but depressed people often view themselves as sick. The grieving person is reactive and shows a range of positive affects. Guilt about not having done more to have saved the life of their loved one (guilt of omission) is seen in normal bereavement, but guilt of commission is unusual. Psychotic experiences and active suicidal ideation are rare in grief.

Sadock BJ, Sadock VA. *Kaplan and Sadock's Comprehensive Textbook of Psychiatry.* 8th ed. Philadelphia: Lippincott Williams & Wilkins; 2005:1368.

193. Answer: B. It is thought that the risk of developing TD is 5% per year, if the patient is taking a typical antipsychotic.

Sadock B, Sadock V. *Kaplan and Sadock's Pocket Handbook of Clinical Psychiatry.* 3rd ed. Philadelphia: Lippincott Williams & Wilkins; 2001:112.

194. Answer: A. Paraphilias are abnormal expressions of sexuality. They can range from nearly normal behavior to behavior that is destructive or hurtful. The DSM-IV-TR addresses these differences by designating impulses toward Pedophilia, Frotteurism, Voyeurism, Exhibitionism, and Sexual Sadism. They become clinically significant if the person has acted on these fantasies or if these fantasies cause marked distress or interpersonal difficulty. The remaining

Paraphilias, such as Transvestic Fetishism and Sexual Masochism, meet DSM-IV-TR criteria only if they cause clinically significant distress or functional impairment, even if the urges have been expressed behaviorally. Gender Identity Disorders are not considered Paraphilias and involve the persistent desire to be, or the insistence that one is, of the other sex, as well as extreme discomfort with one's assigned sex and gender role. Vaginismus is a sexual pain disorder, together with dyspareunia. There are two Sexual Desire Disorders described in the DSM-IV-TR: Hypoactive Sexual Desire Disorder and Sexual Aversion Disorder. Orgasmic disorders include Female and Male Orgasmic Disorders and Premature Ejaculation.

1. American Psychiatric Association. *Quick Reference to the Diagnostic Criteria from DSM-IV-TR*. Washington: American Psychiatric Association; 2000:245–262.
2. Sadock BJ, Sadock VA. *Kaplan and Sadock's Synopsis of Psychiatry*. 9th ed. Philadelphia: Lippincott Williams & Wilkins; 2003:701–738.

195. Answer: E. Infectious agents can lead to neuropsychiatric illness. Some examples include: congenital infection with *rubella* or *cytomegalovirus* leading to mental retardation, delirium accompanying acute meningitis after infection with herpes simplex virus type I, dementia resulting from slow virus such as kuro or Creutzfeldt-Jakob disease, neuropsychiatric manifestations of neurosyphilis, and the tick-born spirochete *Borrelia burgdorferi* causing Lyme disease, which commonly results in the neuropsychiatric symptoms of sleep disturbance, depression, anxiety, irritability, obsessions, compulsions, hallucinations, and cognitive deficits. On the other hand, MS is a demyelinating disease characterized by disseminated white matter inflammatory lesions, which destroy myelin in the brain. Although disruption of the blood brain barrier and infiltration of T-cells, B-cells, plasma cells, and macrophages is associated with lesion formation, a specific infectious source contributing to the pathogenesis of MS has not been elucidated.

Sadock BJ, Sadock VA. *Kaplan and Sadock's Synopsis of Psychiatry*. 9th ed. Philadelphia: Lippincott Williams & Wilkins; 2003:128–135.

196. Answer: A. Long-term memory can be divided into two types: explicit (or declarative) and implicit (or non-declarative) memory. Explicit memory, such as those required for remembering facts or events, are stored in the medial temporal lobe. Both procedural memory, which involves the striatum, and emotional responses to memories, which involves the amygdala, are branches of implicit memory. Classical conditioning can be classified under implicit memory and engages the amygdala and cerebellum.

Milner B, Squire LR, Kandel ER. Cognitive neuroscience and the study of memory. *Neuron*. 1998;20:445–468.

197. Answer: B. Literature suggests that patients should wait for at least 2 years without seizures before thinking about tapering off their medications. The following factors have been associated with a high risk for recurrence after stopping pharmacological treatment: EEG abnormalities, known structural lesions, abnormal neurological exam, and a history of refractory seizures. The risk of recurrence of seizures is approximately 25% in low-risk individuals and 50% in high-risk patients. Most recurrences (80%) occur within 4 months of stopping medications.

McNamara JO. *Pharmacotherapy of the Epilepsies*. http://www.accessmedicine.com/content.aspx?aID=939993. Accessed March 26, 2007.

198. Answer: C. Amyotrophic lateral sclerosis (ALS) is a neurological disorder that affects motor neurons of the ventral horn of the spinal cord. Clinical signs and symptoms include acute onset of progressive weakness, muscle atrophy and fasciculations, spasticity, dysarthria, and dysphagia. The illness is progressive and fatal, and many patients develop respiratory compromise. Riluzole inhibits glutamate release, which has been implicated in the pathophysiology of amyotrophic lateral sclerosis. It is the only medication that has shown to have modest effects on survival of patients with this illness. Dantrolene, tizanidine, and clonazepam are symptomatic medications used to control muscle spasticity in this illness. Interferon does not play a role in the treatment of amyotrophic lateral sclerosis.

Standaert DG, Young AB. *Treatment of Central Nervous System Degenerative Disorders*. http://www.accessmedicine.com/content.aspx?aID=940556. Published March 26, 2007.

199. Answer: E. Many medications depend on the cytochrome P450 system to be metabolized. The rate in which a drug is metabolized, and thus their blood level, can change significantly when two medications that are metabolized by the same enzyme are co-administered. Other drugs can inhibit the CYP system apart from being substrates. When the CYP450 is inhibited, blood levels of medications that are metabolized by these enzymes can increase sometimes to toxic levels. Therefore, it is important to be aware of which medications inhibit or induce the different CYPs to prevent dangerous drug-drug interactions. Phenobarbital, phenytoin, carbamazepine and modafinil are all inducers of cytochrome P450 system. Common inhibitors of cytochrome P450 system include fluoxetine, parasetine fluvoxamine and HIV antivirus.

Gonzalez FJ, Tukey RH. *Drug Metabolism*. http://www.accessmedicine.com/content.aspx?aID=943988. Published March 26, 2007.

200. Answer: E. The treatment of choice for partial simple seizures is considered to be carbamazepine or phenytoin. Lamotrigine is used as a second-line agent for tonic-clonic seizures, myoclonus partial, and absence seizures. Oxcarbazepine has been successfully used for the treatment of tonic-clonic seizures and partial seizures, but there is insufficient data to consider it a first-line agent yet. Ethosuximide is frequently used for the treatment of absence seizures. Valproic acid is used as a first-line agent for many seizure disorders, but it is not a first-line agent for partial simple seizures.

Ropper AH, Brown RH. *Adams and Victor's Principles of Neurology*. 8th ed. http://www.accessmedicine.com/content.aspx?aID=969583. Published March 26, 2007.

Questions

1. Which one of the following is generally TRUE of cognitive differences between men and women?

   A. Women appear to have a slight advantage in mathematical calculations.

   B. Men appear to have a slight advantage in fund of general information.

   C. Women appear to have a slight advantage in select visual-perceptual and spatial tasks.

   D. Men may show a minor advantage on select executive skills.

   E. Men may show a minor advantage in speeded eye-hand coordination.

2. Which of the following statements regarding the development of the sleep-wake cycle throughout the lifespan is TRUE?

   A. Latency age children have relatively greater amounts of rapid eye movement (REM) sleep and high amplitude, slow-wave sleep.

   B. Humans are born with an intact circadian sleep-wake rhythm.

   C. Slow-wave sleep increases throughout adolescence.

   D. Sleep efficiency during adulthood improves with age.

   E. Diurnal sleep-wake patterns become more ingrained and consolidated with advancing age.

3. What defense mechanism is commonly utilized by patients with Obsessive-Compulsive Disorder (OCD)?

   A. Denial

   B. Regression

   C. Isolation of affect

   D. Projection

   E. All the above

4. Which of the following is the most appropriate statement about giving confidential information about a patient's psychiatric care to a third-party payer and their agents?

   A. The psychiatrist does not need to talk to the third-party payer or their agents, as it is not their job.

   B. The psychiatrist must obtain the patient's specific consent to talk to the third-party payer or their agents.

   C. The psychiatrist does not need the patient's consent to talk to the third-party payer or their agents.

   D. The psychiatrist must give all information regarding the patient's care, as the patient has signed on to the specific insurance plan.

   E. None of the above.

5. At a major, tertiary-care facility you are requested to provide psychiatric consultation for a 40-year-old gentleman who was admitted 2 days prior to the medical intensive care unit. He was found unconscious on the street and was brought to an emergency department (ED). He was thought to be intoxicated on alcohol. Psychiatry service was consulted because a few hours ago the patient started becoming agitated, was belligerent with the staff, and demanding to leave the hospital immediately. You were told by the medical team that there is limited history about the patient as he has not been able to provide a cohesive history and it has not been possible to contact anyone for collateral information. You meet with the patient and note that he is extremely agitated and during the course of the interview tells you to make the "little people in the corner of the room stop talking." He further goes on to tell you that "if they must talk, not to call out his name and disturb him." A few minutes later he appears slightly calmer and looks at you and asks you "who are you, what are you doing here?" After you make the appropriate pharmacologic recommendations, you proceed to write the note. While writing the mental status examination, particular attention must be paid to which of the following categories?

   A. Appearance and mood

   B. Behavior and thought process

   C. Perception and behavior

   D. Speech and mood

   E. Appearance and thought content

6. A 27-year-old single woman presents to her primary care physician for an annual check-up. In the course of their conversation, she reveals that she has been struggling to complete her Master's thesis over the past several years and is worried that she will soon be asked to leave the program. Each day when she attempts to make progress on the thesis, she is frequently overcome by the irresistible urge to sleep. She is afraid that she might be "going crazy," as she sometimes sees figures in her apartment when she is awakening from sleep. During times of significant

561

stress (e.g., when presenting to her Master's supervisory committee), she has felt suddenly weak and has narrowly averted falling to the ground. What is the term used in DSM-IV-TR to describe this patient's experience of feeling "suddenly weak?"

A. Catatonia
B. Cataplexy
C. Catalepsy
D. Narcolepsy
E. Sleep paralysis

7. All of the following will enhance optimum treatment outcomes for a patient with Unipolar Depression EXCEPT:

A. Treatment adherence
B. Good therapeutic alliance
C. Lack of significant adverse effects of somatic treatment
D. Partial remission of symptoms
E. None of the above

8. Which one of the following is TRUE of the physiology of glutamate and the N-methyl-D-aspartate (NMDA) receptor?

A. Glutamate is the main inhibitory neurotransmitter in the central nervous system (CNS).
B. Glutamate excitotoxicity, mediated via excessive activation of NMDA receptors, is believed to play a role in neuronal death observed in several degenerative diseases, including Parkinson's disease.
C. In Alzheimer's disease (AD), excessive activation of NMDA receptors has been reported to cause increase in extracellular calcium ions, leading to a cascade of events that ultimately cause neurodegeneration.
D. Memantine acts as a high affinity competitive inhibitor of the NMDA receptor.
E. None of the above.

9. Which one of the following is NOT TRUE of Nicotine Dependence in the United States?

A. An estimated 22.5% of adults (46 million Americans) are cigarette smokers.
B. The highest prevalence of smoking is among African-Americans.
C. Nicotine replacement therapies (e.g., gum, lozenges, nasal spray, inhaler, and transdermal) are United States Food and Drug Administration (FDA) approved for the treatment of Nicotine Dependence.
D. Bupropion is FDA approved for the treatment of Nicotine Dependence.
E. Anxiolytic drug mecamylamine is FDA approved for the treatment of Nicotine Dependence.

10. Which one of the following statements is TRUE of the pharmacological treatments for OCD?

A. Clomipramine has superior efficacy over selective serotonin reuptake inhibitors (SSRIs) in the treatment of OCD.
B. SSRIs have more cardiotoxicity than clomipramine.
C. SSRIs are responsible for more asthenia, insomnia, and nausea than clomipramine.
D. SSRIs are more effective at relieving obsessional thoughts than compulsive rituals.
E. Clomipramine is considered the treatment of choice for OCD.

11. Which of the following is TRUE of interventions for insomnia in middle-aged adults and older adults?

A. Cognitive behavior therapy (CBT) is superior to behavior therapy.
B. CBT is as good as behavior therapy.
C. CBT is superior to relaxation.
D. CBT is inferior to relaxation.
E. Relaxation is superior to behavior therapy.

12. Which of the following is NOT an effective treatment for Nicotine Dependence?

A. Haloperidol
B. Bupropion
C. Nicotine replacement
D. Nortriptyline
E. Clonidine

13. Which of the following drugs has the lowest risk of discontinuation syndrome, when abruptly discontinued?

A. Fluoxetine
B. Fluvoxamine
C. Paroxetine
D. Sertraline
E. Citalopram

14. Adverse effects of valproate include all of the following EXCEPT:

A. Constipation
B. Weight gain
C. Hair loss
D. Agranulocytosis
E. Hepatotoxicity

15. Who is best known for the theory of *degeneration*, which holds that a variety of psychiatric conditions get worse as they are passed from generation to generation?

A. Eugen Bleuler
B. Antoine Boyle
C. Benedict-Augustin Morel

D. Jean Etienne Dominique Esquirol
E. Ugo Cerletti

16. A 70-year-old white man with a history of malabsorption syndrome due to ileal resection now presents to a neurology clinic with a 1-year history of weakness in both legs. On examination, he is found to have impaired perception of position and vibration sense and extensor plantar response in both lower limbs. Given this history, which one of the following is NOT TRUE of his condition?
    A. He has a myelopathy that involves the posterior and the lateral columns of the spinal cord in the cervical and upper thoracic region.
    B. In this condition, involvement of the anterior column of spinal cord is very common.
    C. Pathological changes in this condition include spongiform changes and foci of myelin and axon destruction in the spinal cord white matter.
    D. He will subsequently develop loss of myelin sheath followed by axonal degeneration and gliosis.
    E. All of the above.

17. Which of the following is a possible application of polymerase chain reaction (PRC) in clinical and experimental settings?
    A. Genetic fingerprinting
    B. Paternity testing
    C. Detection of hereditary disease
    D. Gene cloning
    E. All of the above

18. Which one of the following statements is TRUE of movement disorders caused by dopamine-receptor blocker (DRB) drugs?
    A. Acute dystonic reactions usually occur after a week of treatment with these drugs.
    B. Young women are at a particularly high risk of developing dystonias from these drugs.
    C. Neuroleptic malignant syndrome may occur at any time during treatment with DRB.
    D. Akathisia usually occurs within the first 24 hours of treatment with these drugs.
    E. All of the above.

19. Which one of the following has NOT shown to be a predictor of successful aging?
    A. High education
    B. Social class
    C. Maintenance of appropriate weight
    D. Regular exercise
    E. Absence of depression

20. Which of the following regarding the *zeitgeber* ("timekeeper") melatonin is NOT TRUE?

A. Melatonin is secreted in the pineal gland and the retina.
B. Circulating melatonin levels are greatest during the night.
C. Melatonin is required for sleep in humans.
D. Melatonin levels generally decline with age.
E. Melatonin release by the pineal gland is regulated by the suprachiasmatic nucleus.

21. The parents of a 3-year-old girl were walking in a park, pushing the child in her stroller, when she began to cry inconsolably. After ascertaining that she was not in any physical danger, her father noticed that her stuffed rabbit was missing. The child was very attached to the stuffed animal, taking it with her everywhere, and would have a temper tantrum when it was taken away to be washed. From the perspective of psychoanalytic theory, the stuffed rabbit is a *transitional object*. Which of the following authors first described the concept of the transitional object?
    A. Anna Freud
    B. Wilfred Bion
    C. Otto Kernberg
    D. D.W. Winnicott
    E. Melanie Klein

22. Which one of the following need NOT be demonstrated in order to prove psychiatric malpractice?
    A. A doctor-patient relationship existed, creating a duty of care
    B. The doctor has a history of prior malpractice claims
    C. A deviation from the standard of care occurred
    D. The patient was damaged
    E. Deviation from the standard of care caused damage

23. When documenting a mental status examination of a patient all of the following features may be used to describe the thought process EXCEPT:
    A. Flight of ideas
    B. Loosening of association
    C. Circumstantiality
    D. Delusions
    E. Tangentiality

24. Which of the following is a characteristic of Type A Alcohol Dependence?
    A. Late onset
    B. Numerous childhood risk factors
    C. Severe alcohol dependence
    D. Strong family history of alcohol abuse
    E. Significant comorbid psychopathology

25. Which one of the following is the peak age for the incidence of traumatic brain injury (TBI)?
    A. 4- to 5-year-olds

B. 15- to 25-year olds
C. 25- to 35-year olds
D. 35- to 45-year olds
E. All of the above

26. A 32-year-old white woman is referred to you for a psychiatric evaluation. During the initial visit the patient reports that she has noticed that she is "worried a lot lately." She goes on to describe that she has always been a "worrier," but over the past year, it has been getting worse. She is the vice president of a banking company and is well liked by her colleagues. However, she is very fearful that she would potentially lose her job and would never be able to find another job. Recently, these worries have been preoccupying her and she has been having difficulty concentrating at work. She has also been feeling very tired, restless, and has had difficulty sleeping. She has tried taking vitamin supplements, drinking tea, and taking deep breaths to combat some of these symptoms. When this was not alleviating the symptoms, she made an appointment to see her primary care physician. A complete medical workup was noncontributory. Given this history, what is the most likely diagnosis for this patient's symptoms?

   A. Malingering
   B. Acute Mania
   C. Schizophrenia
   D. Generalized Anxiety Disorder (GAD)
   E. Major Depressive Disorder (MDD)

27. A 45-year-old woman comes to your office for an initial evaluation. She is wearing a bright, pink dress with matching shoes, as well as big, white sunglasses and a yellow scarf. She reports a long standing history of having constant problems in her work because she thinks that her boss pays more attention to her coworkers than to herself. She talks about many very intense and close friendships, although she only met most of these friends a few months ago. During the interview she keeps eye contact and seductively smiles. Which of the following criteria is NOT included in the diagnosis of this patient's disorder as per the DSM-IV-TR criteria?

   A. Patients display rapidly shifting and shallow expressions of emotion.
   B. Patients are uncomfortable in situations in which they are not the center of attention.
   C. Patients often interact with inappropriate sexually seductive or provocative behavior.
   D. Patients are easily influenced by others.
   E. Patients require excessive admiration.

28. Which one of the following statements is TRUE of the treatment of OCD?

   A. CBT is recommended as the first-line treatment for children and adolescents.
   B. CBT can be offered as first-line treatment for adults with OCD.
   C. Pharmacotherapy can be offered as first-line treatment for adults with OCD.
   D. The superiority of pharmacotherapy combined with CBT being superior to either treatment modality is controversial.
   E. All of the above.

29. Management of Opioid Intoxication involves which of the following?

   A. Intravenous (IV) access and fluids
   B. Ventilatory support
   C. Support of cardiac function
   D. Parenteral naloxone
   E. All of the above

30. Which one of the following tricyclic antidepressants (TCAs) shows the most biochemical selectivity?

   A. Imipramine
   B. Desipramine
   C. Amitriptyline
   D. Clomipramine
   E. Doxepin

31. Which of the following is a selective norepinephrine-reuptake inhibitor (SNRI)?

   A. Bupropion
   B. Imipramine
   C. Reboxetine
   D. Sertraline
   E. None of the above

32. Which one of the following statements is TRUE of anticonvulsant mood stabilizers?

   A. Controlled studies have shown efficacy of gabapentin in Bipolar Disorder.
   B. Lamotrigine acts at voltage-sensitive calcium channels.
   C. Valproate increases the metabolism of lamotrigine.
   D. Topiramate has been confirmed to be an effective mood stabilizer.
   E. All of the above.

33. Which of the following is NOT included in the DSM-IV-TR diagnostic criteria for Premenstrual Dysphoric Disorder (PMDD)?

   A. Increased energy
   B. Markedly depressed mood
   C. Increased anxiety
   D. Persistent anger or irritability
   E. Difficulty concentrating

34. A 50-year-old white woman with a diagnosis of human immunodeficiency virus (HIV) infection now presents to a neurology clinic with a 6-month history of weakness in both legs. On examination, she is found to have impaired perception of position and vibration sense, and extensor plantar response in both lower limbs. A magnetic resonance imaging (MRI) of the brain and spinal cord shows a signal change in the subcortical white matter and posterior and lateral columns. There is also contrast enhancement involving the dorsal or lateral columns in the spinal cord. Given this history, which one of the following is NOT TRUE of the diagnostic tests for the cause of her symptoms?

    A. Serum vitamin B_{12} level determination is the mainstay for evaluating vitamin B_{12} status.

    B. Serum vitamin B_{12} measurement has technical and interpretive problems and lacks sensitivity and specificity for the diagnosis of vitamin B_{12} deficiency.

    C. Falsely elevated vitamin B_{12} levels may be seen with pregnancy, or with oral contraceptive and anticonvulsant use.

    D. Levels of serum methylmalonic acid (MMA) and plasma total homocysteine are elevated in vitamin B_{12} deficiency.

    E. The specificity of elevated MMA level is greater than the specificity of elevated plasma homocysteine level in vitamin B_{12} deficiency.

35. A 55-year-old Vietnam War veteran has been recently diagnosed with hepatitis C. He is referred to your consultation liaison service because of "anxiety" symptoms. You are told that he is being considered for interferon alpha therapy. On examination he says he is worried about "all possible psychiatric side effects of interferon treatment." Patients with hepatitis C virus infection are at the greatest risk for which of the following psychiatric disorder?

    A. Antisocial Personality Disorder

    B. Depressive Disorders

    C. Borderline Personality Disorder (BPD)

    D. Anxiety Disorders

    E. Somatoform Disorders

36. Which one of the following statements is NOT TRUE of drug induced akathisia?

    A. Acute akathisia develops in 20% to 40% of patients receiving DRB.

    B. In 75% of patients, acute akathisia develops within three days after therapy initiation with DRB.

    C. It is usually more common in older patients.

    D. It may be caused by serotonin reuptake inhibitors.

    E. It may be caused by cocaine.

37. Which one of the following is considered an absolute contraindication for receiving an MRI?

    A. The patient is pregnant.

    B. The patient requires ventilation.

    C. The patient has an implanted cardiac pacemaker or defibrillator.

    D. The patient has a newer, weakly ferromagnetic prosthetic heart valve.

    E. The patient has a nonferrous, metal joint prosthesis.

38. All of the following are TRUE of Marchiafava-Bignami disease EXCEPT:

    A. It is caused by demyelinating lesions in the corpus callosum.

    B. It is rapidly progressive and fatal.

    C. It is associated with alcohol abuse.

    D. It can cause depression, mania, paranoia, and dementia may be present.

    E. Seizures are uncommon in this disorder.

39. Which of the following is TRUE of the neuropsychiatric manifestations of vitamin B_{12} deficiency?

    A. Neurologic manifestations may be the earliest and only manifestation of vitamin B_{12} deficiency.

    B. These patients may present with a myelopathy with or without an associated neuropathy.

    C. The severity of the hematologic and neurologic manifestations may be inversely related in a particular patient.

    D. Relapses in the illness are often associated with the same neurologic phenotype.

    E. All of the above.

40. A 45-year-old unemployed Gulf War veteran is referred by his primary care physician for evaluation of this patient's complaints of "difficult to manage pain." His pain involves the right lower leg and foot. He describes persistent burning pain superimposed on irritating numbness. You are told of a healed minor fracture occurring several months before. On examination, his right leg is atrophic, smooth, and shiny, and the left leg appears normal. He goes to great length to protect the affected area and does not allow physical examination on account of "unbearable pain." You make a diagnosis of complex regional pain syndrome (reflex sympathetic dystrophy) and tell the referring physician all the following EXCEPT:

    A. Treatment consists of adjuvant medications, blockade of regional sympathetic ganglion, and physical therapy.

    B. Symptoms may include tremors and other involuntary movements.

C. This patient may develop similar symptoms on the left leg.

D. Nerve damage is often described.

E. The pain is disproportionately greater than the injury would suggest.

41. A 31-year old woman has been suffering from multiple sclerosis (MS) for 8 years. She has not developed any severe symptoms in the past 3 years. She recently got married and is contemplating pregnancy. She asked about what to expect and is concerned about a future child's risk of developing MS. Which of the following would you tell her about the relationship between pregnancy and MS?

A. Pregnancy has a protective effect from developing an MS exacerbation, and not to worry as MS is not heritable.

B. Pregnancy will not worsen her MS, but her child will likely also develop MS, as it is highly heritable.

C. Childbirth may provoke postpartum episodes by exacerbating her MS, and her child would have an increased risk of developing MS.

D. Pregnancy increases her risk of developing an MS episode, though her child will only be at risk for future MS if she develops an exacerbation during the first trimester.

E. Pregnancy may provoke an MS exacerbation in her, but her child will not be at an increased risk for developing MS.

42. A 19-year old man with a history of heart disease presents to the emergency room (ER) after developing trouble walking. On examination, his feet are noted to be very high arching. Some of his younger siblings also have similar feet, along with difficulty walking. He raises his knees high when taking steps. Given this information, what do you think is the mode of inheritance for his condition?

A. Poly-genetic

B. Autosomal recessive with trinucleotide repeat

C. Autosomal dominant

D. Sex-linked

E. Spontaneous mutation

43. A 55-year-old man, a nonsmoker, develops ataxia of the legs that spreads to the upper extremities and face. After years, he develops some symptoms of parkinsonism. An MRI of the brain shows marked atrophy of medullary olivary nuclei. There is no family history of similar problems. He is healthy, without any evidence of anemia, cardiovascular, or spinal problems. Given this history, which one of the following is the most likely diagnosis for his condition?

A. Malignancy

B. Friedreich's ataxias

C. Olivopontocerebellar atrophy

D. Stroke

E. Parkinson's disease

44. Which of the following is a side effect of topiramate?

A. Priapism

B. Renal stones

C. Hepatic adenoma

D. Respiratory acidosis

E. Coma

45. Which one of the following is NOT TRUE of social supports in the elderly?

A. Those individuals with strong social supports appear to have better outcomes than those who are isolated.

B. The elderly have reduced social networks and frequency of social contacts, as compared to younger adults.

C. Although overall social contacts decrease in late life, it is only contact with family and close friends that decreases significantly.

D. Older adults with nuclear family members tended to have social networks that are both larger and more emotionally close.

E. Social structure of the oldest-old indicates that most individuals over the age of 85 have at least one surviving relative.

46. Which of the following circadian changes in hormone metabolism is NOT TRUE?

A. Growth hormone increases with sleep onset.

B. Sleep onset reduces the secretion of adrenocorticotropic hormone (ACTH) and cortisol.

C. Cortisol levels increase toward the morning.

D. Prolactin hormone levels decrease during sleep.

E. Thyroid stimulating hormone (TSH) levels decrease after sleep onset.

47. A 26-year old automobile mechanic sought treatment for "obsessive thoughts" that were interfering with his ability to function at work. Over the past year, he had developed an extensive ritual that he had to perform before he could move to a new task, including checking to make sure all of the lug nuts were securely tightened nine times on each wheel of the car he was working on, no matter which part of the car was being serviced. On discussing the obsessive thoughts that led to his compulsive checking and counting, he stated that he had to check everything or the occupants of the car would have a fatal auto accident the day after the car was repaired. Given this information, which of the following defense mechanisms do you think that the patient is using to reduce his anxiety?

A. Splitting
B. Undoing
C. Reaction formation
D. Sublimation
E. Projective identification

48. A 31-year old man shoots and kills his neighbor. The man pleads insanity due to a psychotic disorder. Which of the following is NOT one of the four basic elements of his insanity defense?

A. Presence of a mental disorder
B. Presence of a defect of reason
C. A mental disorder demonstrated only by repeated criminal behavior
D. A lack of knowledge of the nature or wrongfulness of the act
E. An incapacity to refrain from the act

49. A 24-year old white man is brought to the psychiatric ER by his roommate. His roommate reports that the patient has been acting strangely and when he talks he does not seem to make sense. During the course of the evaluation, you notice that the patient has difficulty answering questions directly, provides a lot of details even to answer simple closed-ended questions, and is unable to come to the point. What disorder of thought process do you document on the mental status examination?

A. Circumstantiality
B. Tangentiality
C. Blocking
D. Loose Associations
E. Perseveration

50. All of the following have been documented as warning signs that should trigger the suspicion for Factitious Disorder by Proxy EXCEPT:

A. Family history of similar sibling illness or death
B. History of drug abuse in the perpetrator
C. Laboratory findings that are unusual or discrepant
D. Symptoms that do not make sense
E. Victim who remains passive to perpetrator's deeds

51. A 24-year old man is seen status post-motor-vehicle-related head trauma. He has now been referred for post-TBI rehabilitation. His wife wants to know when he will become "his old self again." In discussing his prognosis with her, you should consider which of the following issues?

A. Recovery is a slow process that may take up to 10 years.
B. She may be manifesting "caregiver burden anxiety."
C. A significant proportion of individuals with moderate to severe TBI may never recover to premor-

bid levels, and may in fact continue to manifest cognitive and behavioral difficulties.
D. Most TBI patients follow a well defined trajectory of recovery of cognitive functions following moderate to severe injury.
E. All of the above.

52. A 27-year old black man was recently referred to the psychiatric outpatient service at a community mental health center from the ED of the local community hospital. The patient was brought to the ER a week ago because his family had noted that in the past few days, the patient had "appeared to be in a daze." They report that 2 weeks prior to this, he was at a party with his friends and, while they were returning back, were stopped by some gangsters and robbed at gunpoint. According to the family, the patient came home and reported the incident to his family; however, he did not want to talk about it much more. During the evaluation at the ER, he had a complete medical workup which was noncontributory. Since the patient was not at imminent danger to himself or others, he was referred for outpatient treatment. He arrived promptly for his first session with you. He reports that he has been having difficulty sleeping and concentrating since the incident and every once in a while would have a flashback of the incident. Initially he was not able to go to work for a couple of days, but has now started going to work and has noticed that he is able to complete his work with difficulty. He reports being extremely anxious and finds himself watching over his shoulder and checking if anyone is following him. He agrees to twice a week appointments. While reevaluating the patient in 6 weeks, he reports marked improvements in his symptoms (he no longer has flashbacks and is able to talk more openly about his trauma). Given this information, what is his most likely diagnosis?

A. GAD
B. Posttraumatic Stress Disorder (PTSD)
C. Acute Stress Disorder
D. Panic Disorder
E. OCD

53. A 44-year old woman comes to your office seeking to start psychotherapy. She reports that she is currently in an abusive relationship and she is finding it very hard to leave her husband. She states that she is used to letting him make most of the decisions around the house. She works as an assistant in her husband's business, and she even chose her career because her husband thought it would be a good choice for her. Since the age of 18 years, she cannot recall a time when she didn't have a boyfriend, and she found it very hard to tolerate being alone. She fears her

husband's explosive behavior, but she is very afraid of leaving him and having to take care of herself. Which of the following criteria is NOT included in the diagnosis of this patient's disorder, as per the DSM-IV-TR criteria?

A. Subjects are unrealistically preoccupied with fears of being left to take care of self.

B. Subjects urgently seek another relationship as a source of care and support when a close relationship ends.

C. Subjects have a hard time making decisions without an excessive amount of advice from others.

D. Subjects show restraint within intimate relationships because of the fear of being shamed or ridiculed.

E. Subjects go to excessive lengths to obtain support from others.

54. Which one of the following statements is NOT TRUE of psychological therapies for GAD?

A. The CBT approach is more effective than treatment as usual/waiting list (TAU/WL) in achieving clinical response at post-treatment.

B. The CBT approach is more effective than TAU/WL in reducing anxiety at post-treatment.

C. The CBT approach is more effective than TAU/WL in reducing depressive symptoms at post-treatment.

D. CBT is superior to supportive therapy at achieving clinical response post-treatment.

E. Psychological therapy based on CBT principles is effective in reducing anxiety symptoms for short-term treatment of GAD.

55. Which of the following medications can be used for the management of Opioid Withdrawal symptoms?

A. Methadone

B. Clonidine

C. Buprenorphine

D. Naltrexone

E. All of the above

56. Which of the following statements regarding TCAs is NOT TRUE?

A. They are mainly absorbed in the stomach.

B. They are mainly metabolized in the liver.

C. Their elimination half-lives is about 24 hours.

D. They are very lipophilic.

E. None of the above.

57. Which of the following is a SNRI?

A. Bupropion

B. Venlafaxine

C. Paroxetine

D. Fluvoxamine

E. All of the above

58. What percent of women meet the criteria for PMDD, as defined by DSM-IV-TR?

A. 3% to 5%

B. 11% to 20%

C. 21% to 30%

D. 31% to 40%

E. 70% to 80%

59. Which one of the following areas of is NOT involved in Wernicke's encephalopathy (WE)?

A. Temporal lobes

B. Thalamus

C. Hypothalamus

D. Mamillary bodies

E. Cerebellar vermis

60. A 55-year old Vietnam War veteran has been recently diagnosed with hepatitis C. He is referred to your consultation liaison service because of "anxiety" symptoms. You are told that he is being considered for interferon alpha therapy. On examination he says he is worried about "all possible psychiatric side effects of interferon treatment." In educating him about the neuropsychiatric complication of this drug, you should consider all of the following EXCEPT:

A. Anxiety is the commonest psychiatric disorder in patients undergoing interferon therapy.

B. Psychosis is a common psychiatric disorder in these patients.

C. Treatment emergent depressive symptoms are frequently encountered and may be reason for premature termination of interferon therapy.

D. Prophylactic antidepressant therapy has been approved by the FDA and has become part of routine care in these patients.

E. Treatment emergent suicidal behaviors have been directly linked to INF therapy.

61. Which of the following is TRUE of electroencephalogram (EEG) recordings between seizures?

A. A single EEG recording will show a normal pattern in 30% of patients with absence seizures.

B. A single EEG recording will show a normal pattern in 50% of those with grand mal epilepsy.

C. A single EEG recording will show abnormal although nonspecific activity in 30% to 40% of epileptics.

D. All of the above.

E. None of the above.

62. Diagnosis of which type of disorder may be more readily performed via cerebral angiography?

A. Infection

B. Tumor

C. Vascular disorder

D. Fracture

E. None of the above

63. Typical findings of acute alcoholic myopathy include all of the following EXCEPT:

   A. Elevated level of serum creatine kinase

   B. Fever

   C. Rhabdomyolysis

   D. Polymyositis

   E. Muscle weakness

64. A 50-year old black man with a 30-year history of Alcohol Dependence is being seen at the ER of a tertiary care hospital for a 1-week history of worsening confusion. On examination, he is very confused and scores a 10/30 on the Folstein Mini-Mental State Examination. Staff at the ER, who have known him for the last 10 years, indicate that he is much more confused than before and is also confabulating. He is very unsteady on his feet and is exhibiting horizontal nystagmus on lateral gaze. The blood alcohol level is zero and the urine drug screen is negative for any illicit drugs. A computed tomography (CT) scan of the head does not show any acute changes and all other blood tests are normal including the liver function test. You discuss this information with the attending physician who indicates that the patient should be treated with thiamine. Which one of the following is NOT TRUE of thiamine and its importance in the pathophysiology of this patient's condition?

   A. Thiamine deficiency results in reduced synthesis of high-energy phosphates and accumulation of lactate.

   B. The highest concentrations of thiamine are found in yeast and in the pericarp of grain.

   C. The area most vulnerable to thiamine deficiency in the brain is the cerebral cortex.

   D. A continuous dietary supply of thiamine is necessary to keep up with the body's requirement.

   E. Prolonged cooking of food, baking of bread, and pasteurization of milk all are potential causes for loss of thiamine from foods.

65. A 42-year old white woman is seen in the ER for sudden onset of confusion and agitation. The laboratory work-up done at the ER indicates that the patient is in Addisonian crisis. Given this information, which of the following is NOT TRUE of her condition?

   A. Mild disturbances in mood, motivation, and behavior are core clinical features of Addison's disease.

   B. Psychosis and extensive cognitive changes (including delirium) are associated with severe disease and may be the presenting feature of Addisonian crisis.

   C. Rare presentations of Addison's disease have included catatonia and self-mutilation.

   D. In the majority of cases, symptoms usually occur after diagnosis and treatment, indicating that the mental status changes are mainly caused by treatment with cortisone.

   E. A diagnosis of Addison's disease is based on the measurement of low plasma cortisol, elevated ACTH, and the results of a corticotropin stimulation test.

66. Which one of the following is best correlated with cognitive impairment in MS?

   A. Early age at onset of MS

   B. Longer time since the onset of the disorder

   C. Severity of neurologic symptoms

   D. Total area of lesions on neuroimaging

   E. Spinal form of the disease

67. A woman presents after developing progressively unsteady gait and incoordination of her limbs. On examination, she has scanning speech and some spasticity in her trunk and limbs. Further history reveals that her father and other paternal family members developed similar illnesses. Given this history, you would most likely suspect which one of the following conditions?

   A. MS

   B. Friedrich's ataxia

   C. Spinocerebellar degeneration

   D. Infratentorial tumor

   E. Alcohol-related disorder

68. An otherwise-healthy 42-year old woman developed an arteriovenous malformation (AVM) bleed. At that time, an MRI scan of the brain was unremarkable except for signs consistent with a subarachnoid hemorrhage. After stabilization of her condition over the course of a few hours, the patient begins to complain of a headache, visual changes, and develops vomiting and bilateral upgoing plantar reflex (Babinski's signs). She also starts becoming confused. Given this information, which one of the following conditions do you suspect for this patient's condition?

   A. Ruptured aneurysm

   B. Stroke

   C. Obstructive hydrocephalus

   D. Cerebral tumor

   E. Seizure

69. Which of the following is the most frequently reported fetal malformation seen in newborn children of epileptic mothers?

   A. Urinary tract malformations

   B. Joint defects

C. Mental retardation
D. Limb contractures
E. Orofacial clefts

70. In Freud's psychoanalytic theory of development, the anal stage corresponds to which age range?

A. 0 to 12 months
B. 12 to 36 months
C. 3 to 5 years
D. 5 to 12 years
E. 12 to 18 years

71. Which of the following comparisons of physiologic parameters during REM sleep and non-REM sleep is TRUE?

A. Muscles are more relaxed during non-REM sleep than REM sleep.
B. Heart rate and blood pressure are more variable during non-REM sleep than during REM sleep.
C. Respiratory rate is decreased and steadier during non-REM sleep than during REM sleep.
D. Brain temperature is higher during non-REM sleep than during REM sleep.
E. Cerebral glucose metabolism is greater in non-REM sleep than in REM sleep.

72. The superego, ego, and id are components of which of Freud's psychoanalytic models?

A. Topographic model
B. Affect-trauma model
C. Structural model
D. Interpersonal model
E. Object relations theory

73. What is the most common claim in alleged psychiatric malpractice?

A. Incorrect treatment
B. Unnecessary hospitalization
C. Incorrect diagnosis
D. Attempted or completed suicide
E. Undue familiarity

74. Which one of the following statements about the Global Assesment of Functioning (GAF) scale is TRUE?

A. It was designed to rate the axis V on the DSM-IV.
B. Ratings should generally be made for the past month.
C. It is a pure measure of function.
D. Most non-patients should rate at or near 100.
E. Patients with acute psychotic symptoms usually score above 40 on the GAF.

75. The most common perpetrator of Münchhausen syndrome by proxy has been documented as which of the following?

A. Adopted or foster parent
B. Biological father
C. Biological mother
D. Grandparent
E. Spouse

76. A 24-year old man is seen status post-motor-vehicle-related head trauma. He has now been referred for post-TBI rehabilitation. The patient undergoes psychological testing in preparation for discharge and long-term rehabilitation. You are told that he performed very well on structured, familiar tasks, but evidenced loss of spontaneity and has "difficulty shifting set." Given this information, which area of his brain do you think has been affected by the trauma?

A. Frontal
B. Medial temporal
C. Inferior temporal
D. Right parietal
E. Limbic system

77. A 20-year old man presents to a community mental health center requesting treatment. During the intake, he reports that in the past year he has been flashing himself to unsuspecting women on the street. He reports that thoughts of flashing strange women in public places make him sexually aroused and excited. He feels guilty about his behavior and hence wants help. Given this information, what is the most likely diagnosis for his condition?

A. Fetishism
B. Pedophilia
C. Frotteurism
D. Voyeurism
E. Exhibitionism

78. Which of the following statements is NOT true regarding BPD?

A. 75% of patients with BPD are women.
B. Patients with BPD may develop psychotic-like symptoms during episodes of stress.
C. The risk of completed-suicides in patients with BPD is the same as in the general population.
D. Patients with BPD often have unstable relationships.
E. Patients with BPD have chronic feelings of emptiness.

79. Which one of the following is NOT TRUE of the treatment of Panic Disorder with or without Agoraphobia?

A. In the acute treatment phase, combined treatment of pharmacotherapy with psychotherapy is more effective than pharmacotherapy alone.
B. In the acute treatment phase, combined treatment of pharmacotherapy with psychotherapy is more

effective than psychotherapy alone in the acute treatment phase.

C. In the continuation treatment phase, combined treatment of pharmacotherapy with psychotherapy is more effective than psychotherapy alone.

D. In the maintenance treatment phase, combined treatment of pharmacotherapy with psychotherapy is more effective than psychotherapy alone.

E. In the maintenance treatment phase, combined treatment of pharmacotherapy with psychotherapy is more effective than pharmacotherapy alone.

80. Methadone maintenance treatment for Opioid Dependence is associated with all of the following EXCEPT:

A. Reduced IV drug use

B. Reduced crime rates

C. Reduced HIV seroconversion rates

D. Cognitive impairment in children born to methadone maintained women

E. All of the above

81. The use of TCAs is indicated in which of the following conditions?

A. Panic Disorder

B. OCD

C. Migraine

D. Attention Deficit Hyperactivity Disorder (ADHD)

E. All of the above

82. All of the following statements regarding bupropion are true EXCEPT:

A. It is a noradrenergic-dopaminergic agent.

B. It is associated with a higher risk of seizures.

C. It causes sexual side effects.

D. It is effective in smoking cessation.

E. It is indicated in the treatment of ADHD.

83. A 26-year old woman with a history of bipolar disorder who has been stable on valproic acid presents to her psychiatrist saying that she would like to become pregnant. While educating this patient on the treatment of bipolar disorder in pregnancy, what would you state is the FDA pregnancy safety category for valproic acid?

A. Category A

B. Category B

C. Category C

D. Category D

E. Category X

84. Which of the following psychosocial treatments have evidence of efficacy in patients with Schizophrenia?

A. Family interventions

B. Employment

C. Assertive community treatment

D. Cognitive behavioral therapy

E. All of the above

85. Depressive symptoms emerging in hepatitis C patients undergoing INF-alpha therapy is best described by all of the following EXCEPT:

A. The risk of depression increases with increasing dosage and duration of INF-alpha therapy.

B. Depressive symptoms are apparent at week 4 of treatment.

C. Depressive symptoms peak at week 24 of therapy.

D. Age, gender, and history of substance abuse are well documented predictors of treatment emergent depression.

E. Patients with mild pretreatment depressive symptoms are extremely likely to develop treatment emergent moderate to severe depression.

86. Which of the following is NOT TRUE of traumatic tap in a lumbar puncture (LP)?

A. In a traumatic tap, there is usually a decreasing number of red blood cells (RBC) in the second and third tubes done during an LP.

B. In traumatic tap, the cerebrospinal fluid (CSF) pressure is usually elevated.

C. Prompt centrifugation of bloody fluid from a traumatic tap will yield a colorless supernatant.

D. The fluid from a traumatic tap usually should contain one or two white blood cells (WBCs) per 1,000 RBC.

E. All of the above.

87. Which one of the following is the safest, most widely available and least invasive, but reliable test to evaluate the patency of the carotid arteries?

A. Magnetic resonance angiography (MRA)

B. Computed tomography angiography (CTA)

C. Conventional x-ray angiography

D. Ultrasonography

E. Physical examination

88. Which of the following is NOT clearly associated with uncomplicated aging of the CNS?

A. Memory loss

B. Hearing loss

C. Reduced motor speed

D. Depressed deep tendon reflexes (DTRs)

E. Loss of vibratory sense

89. Which one of the following is NOT TRUE of porphyrias?

A. There are two forms of porphyria, the acquired and the heritable forms.

B. The genetic categories are further divided into hepatic and erythropoietic types, depending on the site of the enzymatic disorder.

C. Neurologic manifestations are encountered only in acute intermittent porphyria (AIP).

D. Rash does not occur in AIP.

E. In AIP, women are more often affected than men.

90. Which one of the following is NOT TRUE of transient global amnesia (TGA)?

A. It is characterized by an acute inability to retain new information (anterograde amnesia).

B. During the acute stage of this disorder, patients can present with retrograde amnesia.

C. Patients with TGA repeatedly ask the same questions and seem to be confused and disoriented in time and place.

D. Patients with TGA have loss of self-awareness and consciousness.

E. The amnesic syndrome of TGA usually resolves spontaneously within 24 hours.

91. Two months postpartum, a 33-year old Canadian woman develops visual loss in her left eye that is painful, especially with movement. This resolves spontaneously, but over the next several years she develops intermittent bouts of trigeminal nerve pain, urinary incontinence, ataxia, and fatigue. Which one of the following would be the most likely finding on an MRI of this patient's brain?

A. Pituitary tumor

B. Numerous widely distributed demyelinated areas

C. Normal brain

D. Evidence of scattered old cerebrovascular infarcts

E. Right brainstem lesion

92. A 5-year old girl presents with gait disturbance. She has a history of chronic sinus infections and has become slower in achieving her developmental milestones. On her cheeks, nose, and conjunctiva are aggregations of small dilated blood vessels. Given this information, which one of the following disorders do you suspect for her presentation?

A. Ataxia-telangiectasia

B. Sturge-Weber syndrome

C. Tuberous sclerosis

D. HIV infection

E. Phenylketonuria (PKU)

93. A 4-month-old infant, who is 6-weeks premature, begins to develop an enlarged skull (greater than the 97th percentile)—making his face looked pinched and small—with tight skin and prominent distended veins. Both anterior and posterior fontanelles are tense. The infant has become more disinterested and feeds poorly. He has begun to rest with somewhat flexed arms and extended legs, but there is no papilledema. Given this information, which of the following is the most likely cause of this infant's condition?

A. Supratentorial tumor

B. Hydrocephalus

C. Fetal alcohol syndrome

D. Cerebral palsy

E. Pseudotumor cerebri

94. A 30-year old woman with long-standing generalized tonic-clonic seizures comes to your office because she is thinking about getting pregnant and wants your advice. Since she used to have several seizures per week before taking phenytoin and she has failed other medications in the past, she would like to stay on her medication during her pregnancy. You decide to warn and educate the patient in regard to the risk of the different teratogenic effects of phenytoin, including the fetal hydantoin syndrome. Which of the following clinical characteristics is NOT part of the fetal hydantoin syndrome?

A. Midfacial hypoplasia

B. Digital hypoplasia

C. Cardiac abnormalities

D. Urinary tract abnormalities

E. Facial clefts

95. In Erik Erikson's theory of development, the *initiative versus guilt stage* corresponds with which age?

A. Infancy

B. Toddlerhood

C. Preschool age

D. School age

E. Adolescence

96. Which of the following statement is NOT TRUE in describing the effects of tryptophan depletion?

A. Depressive symptoms increase in subjects with a MDD who were SSRI responders.

B. Depressive symptoms increased in subjects with MDD who were noradrenergic TCA responders.

C. Depressive symptoms increased in subjects with MDD who were mirtazapine responders.

D. Depressive symptoms increased in healthy subjects with positive family history of depression.

E. Depressive symptoms increased in subjects with seasonal affective disorder who were light therapy responders.

97. In psychoanalytic theory, the term condensation refers to which one of the following?

A. A patient's tendency to minimize troubling symptoms when beginning therapy.

B. The fusion of several different dream thoughts into one image in a dream.

C. The true meaning of a dream image.

D. Pushing back an unacceptable wish to the unconsciousness.

E. The removal of emotional content from a painful memory.

98. According to the American Psychiatric Association, which of the following is NOT an indication for seclusion and restraint?

A. Prevent clear, imminent harm to patient

B. Assist in treatment as a part of ongoing behavior therapy

C. Prevent significant disruption to treatment program or physical surroundings

D. A patient's request to maintain safety

E. Convenience of staff

99. Which one of the following statements about endocrine evaluations in psychiatry is NOT TRUE?

A. The dexamethasone-suppression test is used in routine clinical care.

B. Diabetes insipidus may develop in response to chronic lithium use.

C. Low serum prolactin could distinguish a seizure from a pseudoseizure.

D. High thyrotropin (TSH) levels in newly admitted psychiatric patients generally require treatment.

E. Measurement of insulin level is useful in antipsychotic related glucose intolerance.

100. Which of the following are important concepts to adhere to while treating patients with BPD?

A. A clear discussion of what is involved in psychotherapeutic treatment

B. Encouraging the patient to reflect or mentalize about their internal state

C. Setting limits when needed

D. Being aware of your own countertransference about the patient

E. All of the above

101. Which one of the following is TRUE of Dementia with Lewy bodies (DLB)?

A. It is characterized by the presence of Lewy bodies restricted to the subcortical areas of the brain only.

B. It is characterized by the presence of Lewy bodies restricted to the cortical areas of the brain only.

C. Neurofibrillary tangles are as common as in Alzheimer's dementia.

D. It is characterized by the presence of Lewy bodies in the subcortical and cortical areas of the brain as well as amyloid plaques.

E. Specific risk factors for DLB have been described.

102. A 35-year old man is brought for psychiatric evaluation by his fiancé. A week ago his fiancé caught him masturbating while watching his neighbors having sex. The patient reports that over the past 2 years he feels sexually aroused when he watches other people having sex. He has often felt guilty about his behavior, as he has a stable relationship with his girlfriend. Given this information, what is the most likely diagnosis for his condition?

A. Fetishism

B. Pedophilia

C. Frotteurism

D. Voyeurism

E. Exhibitionism

103. A 35-year old man was referred to a therapist by his primary physician because he wanted to work on his "shyness." The patient reports that he has been having problems with relationships for as long as he can remember. He only gets involved with people when he is certain that they like him, and he avoids going to parties or social activities because he is afraid to be rejected. He has always felt that he is inferior to others and he only rarely engages in new activities because he is afraid to be embarrassed. Which one of the following disorders is most often associated with this condition?

A. MDD

B. GAD

C. Social Phobia

D. Substance Abuse

E. Panic Disorder

104. Which of the following statements is TRUE of the treatment for established tardive dyskinesia (TD)?

A. There is good evidence that reducing the dose of the antipsychotic drug is an effective treatment for established TD.

B. There is good evidence that using specific antipsychotic drugs like quetiapine is an effective treatment for established TD.

C. There is no evidence that using specific antipsychotic drugs like quetiapine is an effective treatment for established TD.

D. There is good evidence that reducing the dose of antipsychotic worsens established TD.

E. There is good evidence that using specific antipsychotic drugs like quetiapine worsens established TD.

105. Which of the following agents is least effective in maintenance pharmacotherapy of Opioid Dependence?

A. Methadone

B. Naltrexone
C. Buprenorphine
D. Levo-α-acetylmethadol (LAAM)
E. Buprenorphine-naloxone combination

106. Which of the following is NOT a side effect of TCAs?

A. Tachycardia
B. Orthostatic hypotension
C. Slowed cardiac conduction
D. Hypersalivation
E. Urinary retention

107. All of the following are appropriate pharmacologic augmentation strategies for the treatment of refractory depression EXCEPT:

A. Antidepressants and stimulants
B. Antidepressants and lithium
C. Antidepressants and pramipexole
D. Antidepressants and inositol
E. Antidepressants and thyroid hormone

108. Who is credited with developing the concept of adult identity?

A. Leo Kanner
B. B.F. Skinner
C. Donald Winnicott
D. Sigmund Freud
E. Erik Erikson

109. Which of the following is an indication for inpatient treatment of anorexia nervosa in adults?

A. A pulse rate of 50 beats per minute
B. A potassium level of 2.5 mEq/L
C. A blood glucose level of 65 mg/dL
D. A body weight of 80% of expected weight
E. A serum creatinine of 1.3 mg/dL

110. Which one of the following regarding the NMDA receptor is TRUE?

A. Excitotoxicity due to understimulation of this receptor may underlie neuronal damage in several neurodegenerative disorders.
B. Cellular proliferation due to overstimulation of this receptor may underlie neuronal damage in several neurodegenerative disorders.
C. Excitotoxicity due to excessive glutamatergic stimulation may account for the neuronal damage in several neurodegenerative disorders.
D. Excitotoxicity secondary to serotonergic overstimulation may account for the neuronal damage in several neurodegenerative disorders.
E. None of the above.

111. Which one of the following is the greatest risk factor for a cerebrovascular accident (CVA)?

A. Age

B. Hypertension
C. Smoking
D. Diabetes mellitus
E. Migraines

112. Which of the following is true of postsynaptic potentials?

A. Excitatory postsynaptic potentials are frequently generated by the opening of chloride channels, a process often mediated by glutamate.
B. Excitatory postsynaptic potentials are frequently generated by the opening of sodium channels, a process often mediated by γ-aminobutyric acid (GABA).
C. Excitatory postsynaptic potentials are frequently generated by the opening of chloride channels, a process often mediated by glycine.
D. Inhibitory postsynaptic potentials are frequently generated by the opening of chloride channels, a process often mediated by GABA.
E. Inhibitory postsynaptic potentials are frequently generated by the opening of sodium channels, a process often mediated by glutamate.

113. Which one of the following gait abnormalities is correctly paired?

A. Normal pressure hydrocephalus (NPH): Festinating gait
B. Parkinson's disease: Steppage gait
C. Cerebellar damage: Ataxic gait
D. CVA: Apraxic gait
E. All of the above

114. Which one of the following is TRUE of AIP?

A. Psychiatric symptoms are the most common presentation.
B. Patients rarely present with abdominal pain.
C. A higher incidence of psychosis has been found in asymptomatic carrier family members.
D. Symptoms of the neuropathy are mainly sensory and occur without abdominal pain.
E. None of the above.

115. Which of the following is NOT TRUE of myasthenia gravis (MG)?

A. The demonstration of serum anti-AChR antibodies proves the diagnosis of MG.
B. The absence of serum anti-AChR antibodies excludes the diagnosis of MG.
C. In patients with MG symptoms who do not have detectable anti-AChR antibodies, serologic diagnosis of MG can be made by determining the presence of anti-MuSK antibodies.
D. In about 5% of patients with MG, they neither have anti-AChR nor anti-MuSK antibodies.

E. The most sensitive electrodiagnostic test for MG is single-fiber electromyography.

116. Which one of the following tests is diagnostic of MS?

A. CSF oligoclonal bands
B. CSF myelin basic protein
C. Increased latency on evoked responses
D. Characteristic lesions on brain MRI with gadolinium enhancement
E. None of the above

117. An 8-year-old girl develops gait problems abruptly after a febrile illness. This gradually progresses over the next few years to clumsiness of hands and dysarthric speech. Past history is remarkable only for a history of unspecified cardiac arrhythmia. Examination is remarkable for hammertoes and kyphoscoliosis. Given this information, what is the most likely diagnosis for her condition?

A. Guillain-Barré syndrome
B. Friedrich's ataxia
C. MG
D. Acute cerebellitis
E. Amyotrophic lateral sclerosis (ALS)

118. Which one of the following is NOT a typical clinical sign in the presentation of NPH?

A. Ataxia
B. Dementia
C. Papilledema
D. Urinary incontinence
E. None of the above, as they are all typical clinical signs of NPH

119. A 33-year old woman presents to your office complaining of intermittent weakness and tingling of the right leg. She also reports that for the past few weeks she has been getting tired easily and has lost some weight. On neurological examination, you notice bilateral Babinski sign. An MRI of the brain shows T2-intense periventricular abnormalities and discrete white matter lesions. Which of the following statements is NOT TRUE in regard to the treatment of this patient's condition?

A. Corticosteroids are beneficial in the treatment of acute attacks.
B. Interferon beta can decrease the severity and frequency of relapses.
C. Natalizumab is considered a first-line agent in the treatment of this condition.
D. Amantadine has been shown to help with fatigue in this condition.
E. Bethanecol helps to treat urinary retention in this condition.

120. Normally, at what age should a child be able to ride a tricycle using pedals, and turn pages singly in a book?

A. 15 months
B. 18 months
C. 30 months
D. 48 months
E. 60 months

121. Which clinician-rated dimensional scales for mood disorder have the highest reliability and validity?

A. Hamilton Rating Scale for Depression and Montgomery-Asberg Depression Rating Scale
B. Mania Diagnostic and Severity Scale and Clinician-Administered Rating Scale for Mania
C. Young Mania Rating Scale and Manic-State Rating Scale
D. A and C
E. A and B

122. To prove medical malpractice, the plaintiff must establish all but which one of the following?

A. Duty of care within a doctor-patient relationship
B. Deviation from the standard of care
C. Deliberate intention to harm
D. Damage to the patient
E. Causation (damage directly caused by deviation)

123. Within a mental status examination, circumstantiality, flight of ideas, perseveration, and thought blocking are all considered abnormalities of which of the following?

A. Thought content
B. Thought form
C. Speech
D. Concentration
E. Insight

124. A 35-year old male patient has a long history of inflexible, maladaptive personality traits that have caused significant difficulties in his relationships and occupation. He is exhibiting paranoia that is suggestive of a micropsychotic episode in your office today. Which of the following personality disorders is/are consistent with a transient psychotic episode?

A. BPD
B. Schizotypal Personality Disorder
C. Paranoid Personality Disorder
D. All of the above
E. None of the above

125. Which one of the following is NOT associated with dementia with Lewy bodies (DLB)?

A. Fluctuating cognition
B. Visual hallucinations

C. Parkinsonism
D. REM sleep behavior disorder
E. Restless leg syndrome

126. Which of the following is NOT TRUE of paraphilias?
    A. Features of a paraphilia are recurrent, intense, sexually-arousing fantasies, urges, or behaviors generally involving nonhuman objects, the suffering or humiliation of oneself or one's partner, or children or other nonconsenting persons that occur over a period of at least 6 months.
    B. These disorders tend to be acute and self-limited.
    C. Paraphilic imagery may be acted out with a nonconsenting partner in a way that may be injurious to the partner (sexual sadism or pedophilia) or self (sexual masochism).
    D. The individual may be subject to arrest and incarceration.
    E. Approximately one half of the individuals evaluated for paraphilias are married.

127. Which of the following statements is NOT true regarding Antisocial Personality Disorder?
    A. Its overall prevalence is approximately 8% in males.
    B. It is more common in urban settings.
    C. Individuals with this disorder lack empathy.
    D. Individuals with this disorder have increased irritability or aggressiveness.
    E. Individuals must be at least 18 years old to meet diagnostic criteria for this disorder.

128. Which of the following is an established treatment for serotonin syndrome?
    A. Using IV electrolyte infusion
    B. Using β-blockers
    C. Using cyproheptadine
    D. Using chlorpromazine
    E. Using ziprasidone

129. Which one of the following is NOT TRUE of methadone?
    A. It acts as a mu-opioid receptor agonist.
    B. It is a long-acting agent.
    C. It is highly lipophilic.
    D. It has poor bioavailability with oral use.
    E. It is metabolized by demethylation and cyclization in the liver.

130. Which of the following statements regarding monoamine oxidase inhibitors (MAOIs) is NOT TRUE?
    A. They produce a reduction of β-adrenoreceptors.
    B. They are indicated for the treatment of depression.
    C. The MAOIs are classified according to their structure.

D. Selegiline is a monoamine oxidase (MAO)-A inhibitor.
    E. Moclobemide is a reversible MAO-A inhibitor.

131. A 65-year old woman with a history of Bipolar Disorder, in remission of manic symptoms on lithium therapy, was recently started on an antihypertensive agent. A few days later, she was brought to the ED due to dysarthria, confusion, ataxia, and tremors. Laboratory study revealed a lithium level of 2.5 mEq/L. Which one of the following agents is least likely to contribute to lithium toxicity?
    A. Propranolol
    B. Calcium channel blockers
    C. Thiazide diuretic
    D. Angiotensin-Converting Enzyme (ACE) inhibitors
    E. Furosemide

132. You make a diagnosis of spasmodic torticollis in a 46-year-old man and decide to administer botulinum toxin injection. Which of the following is the mechanism of action of "Botox"?
    A. It blocks acetylcholine reuptake.
    B. It enhances acetylcholine activity.
    C. It depletes epinephrine.
    D. It inhibits acetylcholine presynaptic release at the neuromuscular junction.
    E. It stimulates postsynaptic receptors.

133. All the following describe the NMDA receptor in health and disease EXCEPT:
    A. It has binding sites for glutamate, glycine, phencyclidine (PCP), and ketamine.
    B. Disease states linked to NMDA receptor include epilepsy, stroke, and Parkinson's disease.
    C. Memantin an NMDA receptor antagonist is approved for the treatment of moderate to severe AD.
    D. Lamotrigine and riluzole may act by decreasing glutamate activity.
    E. PCP stimulates the NMDA receptors.

134. Which one of the following is TRUE of DTRs elicited during a neuropsychiatric examination?
    A. They are graded from 0 to 5.
    B. Briskness of reflexes indicates upper motor neuron lesion.
    C. Withdrawal from alcohol suppresses these reflexes.
    D. An up-going toe with or without fanning of the other toes is referred to as a Babinski sign.
    E. All of the following.

135. On the physical examination of a patient with a lesion of the extrapyramidal tract, which of the following would you NOT expect to see?
    A. Paresis

B. Abnormal DTRs
C. Babinski's sign
D. All of the above
E. None of the above

136. A 45-year old unemployed Gulf War veteran is referred by his primary care physician for evaluation of this patient's complaints of "difficult to manage pain." His pain involves the right lower leg and foot. He describes persistent burning pain superimposed on irritating numbness. You are told of a healed minor fracture occurring several months before. On examination, his right leg is atrophic, smooth, and shiny, and the left leg appears normal. He goes to great length to protect the affected area and does not allow physical examination on account of "unbearable pain." This patient has which one of the following conditions?

A. Complex regional pain syndrome
B. Somatization Disorder
C. Irritation of the posterior tibia nerve
D. Post herpetic neuralgia
E. Psychotic Disorder, Not Otherwise Specified

137. Which of the following is the strongest risk factor for the exacerbation of an episode of multiple selerosis (MS)?

A. Childbirth
B. Cold-weather
C. Hypoxia
D. Psychological stress
E. Vaccinations

138. A 39-year old woman with a confirmed history of MS is on your inpatient service after becoming psychotic on over-the-counter diet pills she was using to self-treat her fatigue. After gaining education, she asks for safer and recognized alternative treatments. Which of the following is NOT a widely accepted treatment for fatigue in MS?

A. Modafinil
B. Amantadine
C. Pemoline
D. Levothyroxine
E. All of the above

139. An otherwise healthy 17-year old honor student presents with an acute onset ataxia. Testing for Friedreich's ataxias and its variants are negative. He also reports some difficulty reading, and on examination has some eye movement abnormalities. He remains cognitively intact. Given this history, which one of the following is the most likely cause of his ataxia?

A. Alcohol related nutritional deficiency
B. Stroke
C. Autosomal dominant gene mutation
D. Paraneoplastic syndrome
E. Prion disease

140. An overweight 19-year old woman presents with unremitting fluctuating headaches, blurred vision, and dizziness. The headache is dull and generalized. On physical examination, the only significant finding is unilateral papilledema. An MRI of the head is unremarkable. CSF studies are within normal limits, but with an opening pressure of 350 mm H_2O (elevated). Given this information, which of the following do you suspect is the cause of this patient's presentation?

A. Pseudotumor cerebri
B. Cluster headaches
C. Migraine
D. Brain tumor
E. Temporal arteritis

141. Which one of the following is the mechanism of action of phenytoin?

A. It slows the rate of recovery of voltage-activated sodium channels.
B. It reduces low threshold calcium currents in thalamic neurons.
C. Its mechanism of action involves potentiation of synaptic inhibition through an action on the GABA-A receptor.
D. Its mechanism of action involves a nonvesicular release of GABA.
E. It slows the rate of recovery of chloride channels.

142. Which of Piaget's cognitive developmental stages typically occurs between 7 and 10 years of age?

A. Sensorimotor
B. Preoperational
C. Concrete operational
D. Formal operational
E. None of the above

143. Which one of the following statements about circadian rhythms is TRUE?

A. Most species have three distinct periods of activity during a 24-hour period.
B. The circadian rhythm of humans needs to be adjusted on a daily basis.
C. Body temperature typically rises during sleep.
D. High light exposure in the middle of the day typically delays onset of sleep.
E. The circadian rhythm of humans is typically around 23 hours.

144. Which one of the following models describes the concept that patients with Schizophrenia are born with a specific biological vulnerability, which is activated by factors in the environment?
   A. Double hit hypothesis
   B. Consanguinity
   C. Stress diathesis model
   D. Polygenic model
   E. Mixed inheritability

145. A 50-year old man who has been in psychotherapy for 1 year appears to have little empathy for others. He has fired employees for relatively minor issues, harshly disparages strangers who cause him any amount of delay or discomfort, and expects that his family will rearrange their schedules around his plans every weekend. Which of the following personality disorders is/are characterized by a low or absent level of empathy for others?
   A. Antisocial Personality Disorder
   B. Narcissistic Personality Disorder
   C. Schizoid Personality Disorder
   D. Histrionic Personality Disorder
   E. All of the above

146. Which of the following is characteristic of the pseudo-delirium of DLB?
   A. It occurs in 50% to 75% of patients with DLB
   B. Daytime sleep of 2–3 hours
   C. Staring into space for long periods of time episodes of disorganized speech
   D. Episodes of disorganized speech
   E. All of the above

147. Which of the following opioids may require multiple and higher dose treatments with naloxone in case of an overdose?
   A. Heroin
   B. Methadone
   C. Oxycodone
   D. Hydromorphone
   E. Morphine

148. Which one of the following is NOT TRUE of the treatment of Paraphilias and Hypersexual Disorders?
   A. Psychoanalytic therapy is the most effective non-pharmacological treatment.
   B. Twelve-step programs are also helpful in these disorders.
   C. Couples therapy has a role in the treatment of these disorders.
   D. SSRIs have some efficacy in the treatment of these disorders.
   E. Gonadotropin-releasing hormones have the advantage over the earlier treatments of being available in long-acting depot formulations and having fewer side effects.

149. Which one of the following is NOT TRUE of oxcarbazepine?
   A. It is a structural analog of carbamazepine.
   B. It is rapidly converted to its monohydroxy derivative (MHD).
   C. It has the property of autoinduction.
   D. It has a more selective induction of P450 enzyme system compared to carbamazepine.
   E. It does not interact with propoxyphene.

150. All of the following benzodiazepines are suitable for use in patients with abnormal hepatic function EXCEPT:
   A. Lorazepam
   B. Diazepam
   C. Lormetazepam
   D. Temazepam
   E. None of the above

151. Which of the following is TRUE of MG and the Lambert-Eaton syndrome?
   A. They are both paraneoplastic syndromes.
   B. Repetitive stimulation alleviates muscle weakness in Lambert-Eaton syndrome while exacerbating the weakness in MG.
   C. They result from rapid acetylcholine receptor inactivation.
   D. They are autoimmune disorders due largely to thymomas.
   E. Extraocular muscle palsy and dysarthria are frequent symptoms of both disorders.

152. Which one of the following is NOT a monoamine neurotransmitter?
   A. Serotonin
   B. Histamine
   C. Norepinephrine
   D. Dopamine
   E. Acetylcholine

153. Which of the following choices is incorrectly matched?

Presentation	Depression	Dementia
A. History	Subacute onset	Chronic
B. History of Depression	Most likely	Less likely
C. Awareness of memory loss	Usually absent	Usually present
D. Mood	Depressed	Variable
E. Cognitive testing	Patchy and variable	Global impairment

154. A 23-year old man was recently evaluated for suspected meningitis. His workup included an MRI scan, LP, and complete blood count and electrolytes were within normal limits. Most of his symptoms subsided with symptomatic treatment. However, he subsequently develops a headache that lasts for days, somewhat relieved when he lies down, with some neck pain, nausea, and fatigue. Another LP is performed, and the results are remarkable only for an opening pressure of 25 mm H_2O (low). Given this information, which of the following best explains his persisting symptoms?

A. Aseptic meningitis
B. Post-LP meningitis
C. LP headache
D. Migraine
E. None of the above

155. When administered together, valproic acid has the potential to inhibit the metabolism of which one of the following drugs?

A. Carbamazepine
B. Ethosuximide
C. Phenytoin
D. Oxcarbazepine
E. Gabapentin

156. According to Bowlby's theory of attachment, with appropriate caretaking, during which time does an infant or child begin the first formative "attachment making" process?

A. Birth to 6 weeks of age
B. 6 weeks old to 8 months of age
C. 8 months old to 2 years of age
D. 2 years old to 5 years of age
E. 5 years old and older

157. Which of the following statements about neuroimmunology is TRUE?

A. There is a high level of B-lymphocytes in the brain during an infection.
B. There is no evidence to support a viral cause of Schizophrenia.
C. There is no evidence to support a role for inflammation in AD.
D. Elevated immune markers have been found in Major Depression.
E. There is no intrinsic immune response in the human brain.

158. All of the following are associated with tobacco withdrawal EXCEPT:

A. Irritability
B. Weight gain
C. Tachycardia

D. Impaired concentration
E. None of the above

159. In addition to the time-course of illness, what else differentiates Acute Stress Disorder from PTSD?

A. Dissociation
B. Avoidance
C. Hyperarousal
D. Reexperiencing
E. All of the above

160. Which of the following is TRUE of frontotemporal lobar degeneration (FTLD)?

A. It is the second most common cause of cortical dementia.
B. Pick's bodies are the defining histopathologic feature of FTLD.
C. FTLD encompasses two pathologic substrates and three prototypic neurobehavioral syndromes.
D. Patients are often clinically amnestic.
E. None of the above.

161. Which stage in the addiction process is incorrectly paired with its predominant neurotransmitters, brain structures, and neural circuits?

A. Initiation: Corticotrophin-releasing hormone in orbitofrontal cortex, endorphins in ventral tegmental area, and dopamine in nucleus accumbens.
B. Continuation: Dopamine in nucleus accumbens, corticotrophin-releasing hormone in amygdala, and glutamate in frontal-cingulate circuit.
C. Withdrawal: Glutamate and norepinephrine in locus coeruleus.
D. Stress-induced relapse: Norepinephrine and corticotrophin-releasing hormone in orbitofrontal cortex, anterior cingulate gyrus, and amygdala.
E. Cue-induced relapse: GABA acid and glutamate in orbitofrontal cortex, anterior cingulate gyrus, and amygdala.

162. Which one of the following is found in most patients with Intermittent Explosive Disorder?

A. Slowing of the EEG
B. Executive dysfunction on neuropsychological testing
C. Low mean 5-hydroxyindoleacetic acid (5-HIAA) concentrations in the CSF
D. Neurological soft signs
E. None of the above

163. Which one of the following is TRUE of the treatments for Body Dysmorphic Disorder (BDD)?

A. Cognitive-behavioral therapy (CBT) is a promising approach for BDD.

B. CBT has demonstrated effectiveness only in the individual and not group format.

C. Studies indicate that pharmacotherapy with SSRI is more effective than CBT alone.

D. Studies indicate that CBT alone is more efficacious than pharmacotherapy with SSRI.

E. All of the above

164. Which of the following is NOT TRUE of LAAM?

A. It is a derivative of methadone.

B. It has a duration of action up to 3 days.

C. Its metabolites are potent and longer acting than the parent drug.

D. It is safe in cardiac patients.

E. It has a slow onset of action.

165. All of the following are contraindicated with MAOIs EXCEPT?

A. Tyramine containing food items

B. SSRIs

C. TCAs

D. Meperidine

E. Lithium

166. Which one of the following does NOT increase lithium clearance?

A. Mannitol

B. Urea

C. Aminophylline

D. Acetazolamide

E. Valproate

167. A 9-year old boy has had generalized muscle weakness for the last 5 years. On examination, his calf muscles appear very well developed, but he has great difficulty standing up from the sitting position and has to hold on to the arms of chairs to do so. Given this information, which one of the following do you NOT expect in his condition?

A. Waddling gait

B. Inability to raise his hands above the head

C. Positive Gower's sign

D. Absence of dystrophin staining on muscle biopsy

E. Chromosomal analysis demonstrating deletion on the Y chromosome

168. Which one of the following is the characteristic neuropathological change in the brain of a patient with Huntington's disease?

A. A decline in the number of medium spiny neurons in the striatum

B. Atrophy of caudate nucleus

C. Atrophy of frontal lobes

D. Atrophy of putamen

E. Atrophy of globus pallidus

169. A 70-year old man with history of gradual and progressive memory decline, as well as hypertension and diabetes mellitus type 2, is brought to your office for an evaluation of his memory decline. After a routine workup for dementia, you diagnose Alzheimer's dementia of moderate severity and decide to start him on donepezil. The patient's family members would like to know how that drug works. Which one of the following would be the most accurate answer for their question?

A. It produces a blockade of the NMDA receptors.

B. It is a reversible inhibitor of acetylcholinesterase (AChE) in the CNS.

C. It directly destroys the β-amyloid in the brain.

D. Its mechanism of action is unknown.

E. It increases levels of dopamine in the brain.

170. Which one of the following statements regarding adolescent substance abuse is NOT TRUE?

A. Urban adolescents are at greater risk compared to suburban youth.

B. Conduct Disorder diagnosis predicts substance use.

C. Peer group substance use is a risk factor.

D. Adolescents with ADHD who are prescribed stimulants have no greater risk of substance abuse.

E. None of the above.

171. Which of the following differentiates FTLD from AD?

A. A predominantly "senile" onset

B. Absence of severe amnesia, visuospatial impairment and myoclonus

C. The preponderance of neurofibrillary tangles (NFTs) over amyloid plaques

D. The presence of "bradyphrenia"

E. All of the above

172. Of the patients entering treatment for heroin dependence, what percentage are white, Hispanic, and black?

A. 50% black, 25% Hispanic, 22% white

B. 50% Hispanic, 25% white, 22% black

C. 50% white, 25% black, 22% Hispanic

D. 50% black, 25% white, 22% Hispanic

E. 50% white, 25% Hispanic, 22% black

173. Which one of the following is TRUE of dependant personality disorder?

A. It is diagnosed more often in men.

B. These patients are at higher risk of developing Alcohol Dependence.

C. It often co-occurs with Narcissistic Personality Disorder.
D. Chronic physical illness or Separation Anxiety Disorder in childhood or adolescence may predispose individuals to develop this disorder.
E. All of the above.

174. Which one of the following has the best evidence for the treatment of Chronic Fatigue Syndrome?
    A. CBT
    B. Antidepressants
    C. Steroids
    D. Analgesics
    E. Opioids

175. Which one of the following is NOT TRUE of buprenorphine?
    A. It is a morphine derivative.
    B. It is a partial agonist at mu-receptors.
    C. It has high affinity for mu-receptors.
    D. It has slow dissociation from mu-receptors.
    E. It has good bioavailability with sublingual use.

176. MAOI-induced hypertensive crisis can be treated with which of the following drugs?
    A. Phentolamine
    B. Furosemide
    C. Propranolol
    D. Nifedipine
    E. All of the above

177. Adverse effects from lithium include all of the following EXCEPT:
    A. Memory problems
    B. Hypoparathyroidism
    C. Hypothyroidism
    D. Diabetes insipidus
    E. Acne

178. Tardive Dyskinesia (TD) is least likely to be associated with which one of the following antipsychotic agents?
    A. Thioridazine
    B. Haloperidol
    C. Clozapine
    D. Trifluoperazine
    E. Fluphenazine

179. Fragile X syndrome is characterized by which one of the following?
    A. Dinucleotide repeats
    B. Higher incidence in Italian Americans
    C. Occasional expression in girls
    D. Microorchidism
    E. Normal developmental milestones

180. While evaluating a patient in the neurology clinic, you notice that the patient has a dilated pupil, ptosis, and is unable to abduct her right eye. Her left eye is normal. A lesion of which of the following cranial nerves is most likely to be responsible for these findings?
    A. Left oculomotor nerve
    B. Right oculomotor nerve
    C. Right trochlear nerve
    D. Left trochlear nerve
    E. Right abducens nerve

181. Which one of the following statements is TRUE of Pramipexole?
    A. It is a dopamine antagonist used in the treatment of Schizophrenia.
    B. It is a catechol-o-methyl transferase (COMT) inhibitor used in the treatment of Parkinson's disease.
    C. It is an AChE inhibitor used in the treatment of AD.
    D. It is a dopamine receptor agonist used in the treatment of Parkinson's disease.
    E. It is an MAO-B inhibitor used in the treatment of affective disorders.

182. All of the following help distinguish Body Dysmorphic Disorder (BDD) from OCD EXCEPT:
    A. The two conditions have different phenomenology.
    B. The beliefs in BDD are egosyntonic compared to those in OCD.
    C. Higher rates of delusional conviction is seen in BDD.
    D. Patients with BDD do not respond to serotoninergic antidepressants.
    E. None of the above.

183. Which one of the following is TRUE of the pathogenesis of AD?
    A. Neuritic plaques and NFTs are pathognomonic of AD.
    B. Neuritic plaques are intracellular lesions composed of a central core of aggregated amyloid-β peptide surrounded by neurites, activated microglia, and reactive astrocytes.
    C. Neurofibrillary tangles are extracellular bundles of paired helical filaments and straight filaments.
    D. Neuritic plaques and neurofibrillary tangles are at the root of the pathogenesis of AD and targeting the genesis of these proteinaceous lesions is believed to hold out hope for disease modifying therapeutic options.

E. Neuritic plaques and neurofibrillary tangles are peripheral to the pathogenesis of AD.

184. Which of the following is NOT TRUE of cocaine and its effect on the heart?

A. Cocaine use is associated with both acute and chronic cardiovascular disease.
B. The risk of acute myocardial infarction (MI) is highest within the 1st hour of cocaine use.
C. There is no clear relationship between dose or pattern of use and the occurrence of MI.
D. Beta-blockers should be administered with caution in patients using cocaine.
E. More than 25% of cocaine-induced chest pain is due to acute MI.

185. Which of the following is TRUE of Antisocial Personality Disorder?

A. It is more common in people of lower socioeconomic status.
B. It is more common in rural settings.
C. It is more common in women.
D. It does not become less evident or remit as the individual grows older.
E. All of the above.

186. Which of the following is TRUE of the treatments for irritable bowel syndrome?

A. Bulking agents have the best evidence of efficacy.
B. Loperamide has the best evidence of efficacy.
C. Antidepressants have no evidence of efficacy.
D. There is not enough evidence to differentiate between different forms of psychotherapy.
E. None of the above.

187. Which of the following is TRUE of the treatments for Hallucinogen Intoxication?

A. Haloperidol is the treatment of choice.
B. Benzodiazepines are the treatment of choice.
C. It should always be treated in a hospital setting.
D. Supportive therapy is never sufficient.
E. None of the above.

188. SSRIs are indicated in the treatment of which of the following conditions?

A. Dysthymia
B. OCD
C. Premature ejaculation
D. Fibromyalgia
E. All of the above

189. Common adverse effects of carbamazepine include all of the following EXCEPT:

A. Diplopia
B. Agranulocytosis
C. Hepatic failure

D. Pancreatitis
E. Weight gain

190. A patient presents to ED with feelings of restlessness, inability to sit still, pacing, and jitteriness after receiving a medication for the treatment of auditory hallucinations. Which one of the following agents is most effective in treating his symptoms?

A. Bromocriptine
B. Amantadine
C. Benztropine
D. L-dopa
E. Propranolol

191. A patient presents to the ED with fever, muscular rigidity, tachycardia, and impaired consciousness after being treated with a high dose of haloperidol. All of the following agents are effective in treating this condition EXCEPT:

A. Dantrolene
B. Amantadine
C. Bromocriptine
D. Thioridazine
E. None of the above

192. Which one of the following best describes polymerase chain reaction (PCR)?

A. It is a molecular biology procedure for enzymatically replicating DNA without using living organism.
B. It is a biochemistry technique for enzymatically replicating DNA using living organism.
C. It is identical to amplification.
D. It is an *in vivo* technique.
E. None of the above.

193. Many months after treatment for a subarachnoid hemorrhage, an 83-year old man develops a progressive shuffling and short-stepped gait, patchy memory problems, and urinary incontinence. On examination, he has a mild tremor in his hands, but no cogwheeling or stiffness. Which of the following is the diagnostic test of choice for this patient's condition?

A. An MRI or CT scan of the brain
B. A trial of AChE inhibitors
C. A trial of L-dopa/carbidopa
D. An LP with pressure measurements
E. An EEG

194. Which one of the following statements is TRUE of Selegiline?

A. Selegiline is a nonspecific MAOI.
B. Metabolites of selegiline include amphetamines.
C. Selegiline inhibits peripheral metabolism of catecholamines.

D. Selegiline is a first-line agent for treatment of Parkinson's disease.

E. At low doses, selegiline produces inhibition of MAO-A.

195. A 35-year old man with severe ALS is complaining of disabling muscle spasticity. His physician decides to start the patient on baclofen. Which of the following statements is TRUE regarding this medication?

A. Baclofen works at the GABA-A receptor.

B. Baclofen can only be used through the oral route.

C. Baclofen is a first-line agent for the treatment of spasticity in ALS.

D. The time of onset of action of baclofen is approximately 4 hours.

E. Baclofen works by inhibiting calcium channels.

196. All of the following adverse effects are associated with clozapine EXCEPT:

A. Agranulocytosis

B. Sialorrhea

C. Seizures

D. Anticholinergic effects

E. Weight loss

197. Psychostimulants are indicated for which of the following conditions?

A. ADHD

B. Narcolepsy

C. Obesity

D. Depression

E. All of the above

198. A 19-year old woman comes to her physician because she does not want to continue taking valproic acid for her generalized tonic-clonic seizures. The patient states that she has gained a significant amount of weight, and she is also concerned about developing ovarian problems. You decide to discuss the option of switching her to lamotrigine. Which of the following statements is TRUE in regard to lamotrigine?

A. Lamotrigine resembles phenytoin in its anticonvulsant activity and toxicity.

B. Lamotrigine works by blocking delayed calcium channels.

C. Lamotrigine causes a rash in approximately 20% of patients.

D. The addition of valproic acid greatly reduces plasma levels of lamotrigine.

E. Lamotrigine is a first-line agent for absence seizures.

199. A 24-year old woman who was recently diagnosed with MS was started on interferon-β. The patient wishes to know how this medication works. Which of the following would be the best answer for this patient's question?

A. Interferon-β suppresses the proliferation and the migration to the CNS of T lymphocytes.

B. Interferon-β alters signals through the T-cell receptor complex and thus decreases the immune response.

C. Interferon-β forms DNA-DNA crosslinks and thus inactivates parts of DNA.

D. Interferon-β works as a monoclonal antibody.

E. Interferon-β specifically blocks the migration of monocytes.

200. A 22-year old man is referred to your clinic for an evaluation of headache that has not responded to nonsteroidal anti-inflammatory drugs (NSAIDs). The patient reports several episodes a week of sudden onset of hemicranial headache, nausea, and vomiting that last for hours. During those attacks he has to stay in a closed room without light, because any noise or light make the pain worse. The pain is usually throbbing in nature and it is very disabling. Since the patient has not responded to conventional NSAIDs, you decide to start him on sumatriptan for acute attacks. Which one of the following is the mechanism of action of sumatriptan?

A. Sumatriptan is a 5-HT1D receptor antagonist.

B. Sumatriptan is a 5-HT1D receptor agonist.

C. Sumatriptan is a 5-HT1A receptor agonist.

D. Sumatriptan is a 5HT3 receptor agonist.

E. Sumatriptan is a 5HT3 receptor antagonist.

Answers

1. Answer: B. Men and women display differences in cognitive skills. Men appear to have a slight advantage in mathematical calculations, fund of general information, and select visual-perceptual and spatial tasks, whereas women may show a minor advantage on rote verbal memory tasks, select executive skills, and speeded eye-hand coordination. These may become more pronounced with advancing age.

Sadock BJ, Sadock VA. *Kaplan and Sadock's Comprehensive Textbook of Psychiatry*. 8th ed. Philadelphia: Lippincott Williams & Wilkins; 2005:3633.

2. Answer: A. Humans are born with an ultradian sleep-wake pattern, which develops into a circadian rhythm during the first few years of life. Slow-wave sleep declines precipitously during adolescence, likely related to pruning phenomena. Sleep efficiency gradually declines through adulthood. In addition to lighter sleep, it becomes more fragmented with age, with a greater percentage of daytime naps. The incidence of insomnia and many sleep-wake disorders increases with age.

1. Hales RE, Yudofsky SC. *Textbook of Clinical Psychiatry*. 4th ed. Washington: American Psychiatric Publishing; 2003:975–1000.
2. Sadock BJ, Sadock VA. *Kaplan and Sadock's Comprehensive Textbook of Psychiatry*. 7th ed. Philadelphia: Lippincott Williams & Wilkins; 2000:199–209.

3. Answer: E. Isolation of affect, reaction formation, and undoing are common defense mechanisms utilized by patient with diagnosis of OCD. Isolation of affect is the unconscious process in which there is dissociation of affect from an impulse. If isolation of affect fails to control anxiety associated with a given impulse, patients with OCD resort to compulsive acts, which are unconscious attempts to neutralize anxiety. In reaction formation, patients exhibit attitudes that are diametrically opposite to underlying impulse. Denial is a narcissistic defense in which some painful aspects of reality are avoided, while regression is an attempt to return to an earlier libidinal stage of functioning to avoid conflict, it is an immature defense. These latter defenses are not commonly utilized in OCD. Denial is common in patients with substance-related disorders, and regression is frequently utilized by the severely mentally ill.

Projection is an immature defense mechanism used by patients with Borderline Personality Disorder or psychotic illness.

Sadock BJ, Sadock VA. *Kaplan and Sadock's Comprehensive Textbook of Psychiatry*. 8th ed. Philadelphia: Lippincott Williams & Wilkins; 2005:721–722.

4. Answer: B. Third-party payers and their agents may request data from psychiatric evaluations to make determinations about whether a hospital admission or a specific treatment will be covered by a particular insurance plan. When such information is requested the psychiatrist must obtain the patient's consent for such communications. It is necessary to inform the patient about the specific information that has been requested and obtain specific consent for the release of that information. The psychiatrist may also withhold information about the patient not directly relevant to the utilization review or preauthorization decisions.

American Psychiatric Association. *American Psychiatric Association Practice Guidelines for the Treatment of Psychiatric Disorders*. http://www.psychiatryonline.com/content. aspx?aID=138119. Accessed February 15, 2007.

5. Answer: C. The mental status examination is the part of the clinical assessment that describes the sum total of the examiner's observations and impressions of the psychiatric patient at the time of the interview. Hallucinations (visual, auditory, olfactory, or tactile) are described as perceptual abnormalities, as are feelings of depersonalization and derealization (extreme feeling of detachment from the self or the environment). Agitation is characterized as behavior in the general description of the patient. Other aspects that are included in this category include mannerisms, tics, gestures, stereotyped behavior, and psychomotor retardation.

Sadock BJ, Sadock VA. *Kaplan & Sadock's Concise Textbook of Clinical Psychiatry*. 2nd ed. Philadelphia: Lippincott Williams & Wilkins; 2004:6–7.

6. Answer: B. Cataplexy is described in the DSM-IV-TR as brief episodes of sudden bilateral loss of muscle tone, most often in association with intense emotion. Cataplexy is present in approximately 50% of cases of Narcolepsy, a primary sleep disorder that consists of irresistible sleep attacks and one or both of cataplexy and abnormal manifestations of REM sleep. Sleep paralysis is an uncommon symptom that occurs most often upon awakening in the morning. During sleep paralysis, patients are apparently awake and conscious, but unable to move a muscle. In contrast, Catatonia can be seen in various psychiatric (and medical) disorders and is usually manifested by a combination of motoric immobility, excessive motor activity (which is apparently purposeless and not influenced by external stimuli), extreme negativism or mutism, peculiarities of voluntary movement, and echolalia/echopraxia. Catalepsy is a general term for an immobile position that is constantly maintained.

1. American Psychiatric Association. *Quick Reference to the Diagnostic Criteria from DSM-IV-TR*. Washington: American Psychiatric Association; 2000:267–279.
2. Sadock BJ, Sadock VA. *Kaplan and Sadock's Synopsis of Psychiatry*. 9th ed. Philadelphia: Lippincott Williams & Wilkins; 2003:281, 768–769.

7. Answer: D. The goal of treatment for Unipolar Depression is the complete remission of symptoms. Partially remitted symptoms are powerful predictors of relapse. These findings have led to the hypothesis that residual symptoms upon recovery may progress to become prodromal symptoms of relapse.

1. Fava GA, Fabbri S, Sonino N. Residual symptoms in depression: an emerging therapeutic target. *Prog Neuropsychopharmacol Biol Psychiatry*. 2002;26:1019–1027.
2. Fava GA, Ruini C, Belaise C. The concept of recovery in major depression. *Psychol Med*. 2007;37:307–317.

8. Answer: B. Glutamate is the main excitatory neurotransmitter in the CNS. Its physiologic and excitotoxic activities are mediated through stimulation of the NMDA receptor and result from the influx of calcium ions. Excitotoxicity is believed to play a role in the pathogenesis of several diseases, including Parkinson's disease and AD. Several NMDA receptor antagonists have been described. PCP and MK-801 cause psychotomimetic side effects, due to their activities on the NMDA receptors. Memantine, approved by the FDA for the treatment of moderate to severe AD, is a noncompetitive NMDA receptor antagonist with moderate affinity that protects against excessive stimulation of the receptor while allowing normal physiologic activities unhindered.

1. Hynd MR, Scott HL, Dodd PR. Glutamate-mediated excitotoxicity and neurodegeneration in Alzheimer's disease. *Neurochem Int*. 2004;45:583–595.
2. Kornhuber J, Weller M. Psychotogenicity and N-methyl-D-aspartate receptor antagonism: implications for neuroprotective pharmacotherapy. *Biol Psychiatry*. 1997;41:135–144.

3. Sonkusare SK, Kaul CL, Ramarao P. Dementia of Alzheimer's disease and other neurodegenerative disorders—memantine, a new hope. *Pharmacol Res*. 2005;51:1–17.

9. Answer: B. Cigarette use is the single most preventable cause of death in our society, causing 1 of every 5 deaths. By the 2004 estimate, about 22.5% of adults (46 million Americans) were cigarette smokers, with the highest prevalence among Native Americans and Alaska natives (40.8%); followed by whites (23.6%). Available data indicates that the use of pharmacotherapy by smokers in conjunction with behavioral modification can produce long-term abstinence at up to double the rate achieved by smokers without pharmacotherapy. Pharmacotherapies that have approved by the FDA for treatment of Nicotine Dependence include nicotine replacement therapies (e.g., gum, lozenges, nasal spray, inhaler, and transdermal), antidepressants (e.g., bupropion), and anxiolytic drugs (e.g., clonidine, nortriptyline, and mecamylamine), although anxiolytics have been used as second-line agents. Varenicline was approved by the FDA on May 11, 2006 for the treatment of Nicotine Dependence.

Zierler-Brown SL, Kyle JA. Oral varenicline for smoking cessation. *Ann Pharmacother*. 2007;41:95–99

10. Answer: C. The evidence is not strong enough to support superior efficacy of clomipramine over SSRIs. SSRIs have a better side effect profile compared to clomipramine resulting in improved acceptability and tolerability. In a comparator study, the drop-out rate from adverse effects on clomipramine (approx. 17%) was consistently higher than for paroxetine (9%). Clomipramine is associated with significantly more early withdrawals associated with side-effects than fluvoxamine. The risk of dangerous side effects such as convulsions (occurring in up to 2% on clomipramine, compared to 0.1% to 0.5% on high-dose SSRIs), cardiotoxicity, and cognitive impairment is substantially lower with SSRIs. Clomipramine is associated with dry mouth, constipation, and blurred vision, and is lethal in overdose. All SSRIs are associated with impaired sexual performance, but clomipramine (80% cases) appears more problematic than SSRIs (up to 30% cases). SSRIs are responsible for more asthenia, insomnia, and nausea. Weight gain is more with clomipramine as compared to SSRIs. SSRIs are equally effective at relieving obsessional thoughts and compulsive rituals. Their improved safety and tolerability offer considerable benefits for the long-term treatment of OCD. SSRIs should usually be considered the treatments of choice, with clomipramine reserved for those who cannot tolerate or who have failed to respond to them.

1. Fineberg NA, Gale TM. Evidence-based pharmacotherapy of obsessive-compulsive disorder. *Int J Neuropsychopharmacol.* 2005;8:107–129.
2. Zohar J, Judge R. Paroxetine versus clomipramine in the treatment of obsessive-compulsive disorder. OCD Paroxetine Study Investigators. *Br J Psychiatry.* 1996;169:468–474.

11. Answer: B. A recent meta-analysis supports the effectiveness of behavioral interventions for the treatment of insomnia in older patients. This meta-analysis of randomized controlled trials (n=23), found cognitive-behavioral treatment, relaxation, and behavioral therapy to have similar effects. Both middle-aged and persons older than 55 years of age showed similar robust improvements in sleep quality, sleep latency, and wakening after sleep onset.

Irwin MR, Cole JC, Nicassio PM. Comparative meta-analysis of behavioral interventions for insomnia and their efficacy in middle-aged adults and in older adults 55+ years of age. *Health Psychol.* 2006;25:3–14.

12. Answer: A. Bupropion, a dopamine and norepinephrine reuptake inhibitor, has been found to significantly improve abstinence from smoking. Nicotine gum, inhaler, nasal spray, and transdermal patch appear to be equally effective and approximately double the abstinence rates as compared to placebo. Both bupropion and nicotine replacement therapy has been approved by the FDA for Nicotine Dependence. Nortriptyline and clonidine are second-line medications for treatment of Nicotine Dependence and are not approved by the FDA. Several behavioral therapies including practical counseling (problem solving training, coping skills, and relapse prevention), intratreatment support (encourage patients to quit, and communicate care and concern), extra-treatment support (encourage patient to solicit social support, and arrange outside support), and aversive smoking procedures (rapid smoking, rapid puffing) have been found to be effective in increasing abstinence from smoking compared to no-contact controls.

Lowinson JH, Ruiz P, Millman RB, et al. *Substance Abuse: A Comprehensive Textbook.* 4th ed. Philadelphia: Lippincott Williams & Wilkins; 2005:387–403.

13. Answer: A. Fluoxetine has a half-life of about 4 to 6 days, therefore, has the lowest risk of discontinuation symptoms with abrupt discontinuation. The half-lives of other SSRIs (fluvoxamine: 15 hours, paroxetine: 21 hours, sertraline: 26 hours, and citalopram: 35 hours) are shorter. Therefore, sudden discontinuation of shorter-acting agents can result in anxiety, irritability, crying spells, dizziness, nausea and vomiting, lethargy, sleep disturbances, and flu-like symptoms.

1. Sadock BJ, Sadock VA. *Kaplan and Sadock's Comprehensive Textbook of Psychiatry.* 7th ed. Philadelphia: Lippincott Williams & Wilkins; 2000:2433–2438.
2. Schatzberg AF, Nemeroff CB. *Textbook of Psychopharmacology.* 2nd ed. Washington: American Psychiatric Press; 1998:219–237.

14. Answer: A. Most frequent adverse effects associated with valproate are gastrointestinal effects (nausea, vomiting, and diarrhea) and neurological effects (tremors, sedation, and ataxia). It is also commonly associated with weight gain. Hair loss is usually transient, but total alopecia has been rarely associated with valproate therapy. Reversible thrombocytopenia may occur in the initial phase of valproate treatment. It often produces modest elevations of hepatic enzymes. On rare occasions, valproate may be associated with agranulocytosis, severe hepatotoxicity, and hemorrhagic pancreatitis. Unlike carbamazepine, it does not potentiate hepatic metabolism of concomitant drugs. It can cause neural tube defect with use in pregnancy. Hematologic and hepatic parameters should be regularly monitored in patients receiving valproate.

Sadock BJ, Sadock VA. *Kaplan and Sadock's Comprehensive Textbook of Psychiatry.* 7th ed. Philadelphia: Lippincott Williams & Wilkins; 2000:2289–2299.

15. Answer: C. Benedict-Augustin Morel (1809–1873) was a French psychiatrist who proposed an early version of biological psychiatry which held that mental illness is congenitally inherited and can be activated by the environment. Bleuler coined the term *Schizophrenia*, and introduced *autism* and *ambivalence* to the psychosis literature. Boyle suggested in 1826 that the general paresis (of syphilis) was an organic disease, which was not conclusively demonstrated until 1912. Esquirol expanded the theory of moral therapy, wrote an influential textbook, coined the concept of *hallucination*, and wrote a law detailing provisions for patient care. Cerletti and Lucio Bini developed electroshock therapy in 1938.

Sadock BJ, Sadock VA. *Kaplan and Sadock's Comprehensive Textbook of Psychiatry.* 7th ed. Philadelphia: Lippincott Williams & Wilkins; 2000:3304–3305.

16. Answer: B. This patient has sub-acute combined degeneration of spinal cord. It is a neurologic manifestation of vitamin B_{12} deficiency and is characterized by a myelopathy that involves the posterior and lateral columns of the spinal cord in the cervical and upper thoracic regions. The involvement of anterior columns of the spinal cord is rare. Pathological changes include spongiform changes and foci of myelin and axon destruction in the spinal cord white matter. There is also loss of myelin followed by axonal degeneration and gliosis. Clinical features include spastic paraparesis, extensor plantar response, and impaired perception of position and vibration. Symptoms usually start in the feet and are symmetric. Other neuropsychiatric manifestations include decreased memory, personality change, psychosis, and delirium. Majority of patients who develop vitamin B_{12} deficiency have pernicious anemia. It is also more common in the elderly and can be seen after gastric surgery, as well as with acid reduction therapy with H_2-blockers. It may also be caused by malabsorption syndromes due to ileal disease or resection, bacterial overgrowth, and tropical sprue. Vitamin B_{12} deficiency is also seen in HIV-infected patients. Vitamin B_{12} deficiency can also occur in strict vegetarians. This phenomenon is usually rare and the consequences of this deficiency are often mild and subclinical. Clinical manifest disease occurs only when poor intake begins in childhood.

Kumar N. Nutritional neuropathies. *Neurol Clin*. 2007;25: 209–255.

17. **Answer: E.** The technique of PRC has a wide range of applications in diagnostic, experimental, and forensic settings. In genetic fingerprinting, for example, an accused may either be virtually placed on a crime scene or excluded as a suspect by comparing DNA from a crime scene with his or her sample. Given that the crime scene sample may contain a tiny amount of DNA, the task is accomplished by first fragmenting the sample from the crime scene and then amplifying these fragments by several magnitudes. By utilizing several genetic fingerprints, the relationship between parent and child may be established in a paternity case. Using the methods of gene amplification and sequencing, disease causing mutations can be detected in a given genome. Gene cloning is another potential use of PCR. This utilizes gene engineering and amplification.

Cheng S, Fockler C, Barnes WM, et al. Effective amplification of long targets from cloned inserts and human genomic DNA. *Proc Natl Acad Sci USA*. 1994;91:5695–5699.

18. **Answer: C.** Drug-induced movement disorders are mainly caused by DRB that are used as antipsychotics (neuroleptics) and antiemetics. Acute dystonic reactions usually occur within the first 4 days of treatment with these drugs. Usually, cranial, pharyn-

geal, and cervical muscles are affected. Young men are at a particularly high risk of developing this disorder. The use of anticholinergics produces a prompt relief in symptoms. Neuroleptic malignant syndrome is a rare, but life-threatening, adverse reaction to DRB, which may occur at any time during treatment with DRB. It is characterized by hyperthermia, rigidity, reduced consciousness, and autonomic failure. Therapeutically immediate DRB withdrawal is crucial. Additional dantrolene or bromocriptine application together with symptomatic treatment may be necessary. Akathisia is also a common side effect of DRB, and is characterized by exceedingly bothersome feeling of restlessness and the inability to remain still. It usually occurs within a few days after the initiation of treatment with DRB and subsides when the DRB is discontinued.

Dressler D, Benecke R. Diagnosis and management of acute movement disorders. *J Neurol*. 2005;252:1299–1306.

19. **Answer: B.** The new paradigm in gerontology views aging not as an inevitable deterioration, but one that includes the potential for development and growth. Recent studies examining both objective and subjective indicators of successful aging found that only 10% of the sample could be classified as "successfully aged" when based on objective criteria that included quantitative assessments of physical, cognitive, and social functioning and measures of well being. However, when successful aging was defined as a subjective sense of having adapted well to the demands of life, many more individuals could be classified as having aged successfully. Recent research studies determining predictors of successful aging indicate that high education, absence of alcohol abuse and cigarette smoking, absence of depression, maintenance of appropriate weight, regular exercise, and social support are all predictors of successful aging. Social class, however, does not appear to be an important predictor for successful aging.

Sadock BJ, Sadock VA. *Kaplan and Sadock's Comprehensive Textbook of Psychiatry*. 8th ed. Philadelphia: Lippincott Williams & Wilkins; 2005:3629.

20. **Answer: C.** Melatonin is a hormone chemical produced and secreted by the pineal gland, and in smaller amounts by the retina. Melatonin levels in the CSF may be up to twenty times greater than serum levels. Its levels increase in the evenings, and decrease during the day. Melatonin is not required for sleep in humans, and without it (e.g., removal of the pineal gland) there may be little change in the sleep-wake cycle. Regardless, it is an important hormone in synchronizing the onset of sleep

and environmental light signals. Although melatonin production generally declines with age, how such a decline occurs is debated. Some say it occurs gradually, and others say there is a large decline in adolescence, and again with the CNS degeneration of advancing age. Release of melatonin is via a complex multisynaptic system regulated by the suprachiasmatic nucleus, and culminates in noradrenergic projections from the superior cervical ganglion to pinealocytes.

Turek FW, Gillette MU. Melatonin, sleep, and circadian rhythms: rationale for development of specific melatonin agonists. *Sleep Med.* 2004;5:523–532.

21. **Answer: D.** The transitional object is a blanket, pacifier, song, or other object that a child uses to comfort herself when separated from her parents, such as a "security blanket." The concept was put forth by Winnicott, a pediatrician and psychoanalyst of the British object relations school, who theorized that the transitional object was a representation of the object of the original relationship (mother or breast), and provides a transition from the physical relationship with the original object, to a physical relationship with the transitional object, to a symbolic representation of the original object. The transitional object is used as a defense against anxiety, frequently when the child is going to sleep.

1. Dell'Orto S, Caruso E. [W. D. Winnicott and the transitional object in infancy.] *Pediatr Med Chir.* 2003;25:106–112.
2. Sadock BJ, Sadock VA. *Kaplan and Sadock's Comprehensive Textbook of Psychiatry.* 8th ed. Philadelphia: Lippincott Williams & Wilkins; 2005:4026–4046.

22. **Answer: B.** A history of prior malpractice claims is not needed to prove malpractice. The elements of a malpractice claim are called the four Ds: duty, deviation, damage, and direct causation.

Sadock BJ, Sadock VA. *Kaplan and Sadock's Comprehensive Textbook of Psychiatry.* 8th ed. Philadelphia: Lippincott Williams & Wilkins; 2005:3969.

23. **Answer: D.** Delusions are described as thought content and not as process of thought. Flight of ideas, loosening of association, circumstantiality, along with thought blocking, word salad, clang associations, punning, and neologism are all used to describe abnormalities in thought process.

Sadock BJ, Sadock VA. *Kaplan & Sadock's Concise Textbook of Clinical Psychiatry.* 2nd ed. Philadelphia: Lippincott Williams & Wilkins; 2004:7–8.

24. **Answer: A.** Various researchers have attempted to divide Alcohol Dependence into subtypes based pri-

marily on phenomenological characteristics. One relatively recent classification denotes *Type A Alcohol Dependence* as characterized by a late onset, few childhood risk factors, relatively mild dependence, few alcohol-related problems, and little psychopathology. In contrast, *Type B Alcohol Dependence* is characterized by many childhood risk factors, severe dependence, an early onset of alcohol-related problems, much psychopathology, a strong family history of alcohol abuse, frequent polysubstance abuse, a long history of alcohol treatment, and a high number of severe life stresses. Some research has suggested that patients with Type A Alcohol Dependence may respond better to interactional psychotherapies, whereas patients with Type B Alcohol Dependence may respond better to coping skills training.

Sadock BJ, Sadock VA. *Kaplan and Sadock's Synopsis of Psychiatry.* 9th ed. Philadelphia: Lippincott Williams & Wilkins; 2003:402–403.

25. **Answer: B.** Over a million Americans sustain TBIs every year, making it a leading cause of morbidity and mortality. TBI exhibits a bimodal age frequency. It is more prevalent in people between the ages of 15 to 25 years and those 75 years and older. While motor vehicle accidents account for a large proportion of TBI in younger people, a majority of elderly patients sustain TBI by way of falls.

1. Day H, Roesler J, Gaichas A, et al. Epidemiology of ED-treated traumatic brain injury in Minnesota. *Minn Med.* 2006;89:40–44.
2. Rutland-Brown W, Langlois JA, Thomas KE, et al. Incidence of traumatic brain injury in the United States, 2003. *J Head Trauma Rehabil.* 2006;21:544–548.

26. **Answer: D.** DSM-IV-TR criteria for GAD include excessive anxiety and worry about a number of events or activities occurring more days than not for at least 6 months. The person finds it difficult to control the worry. The anxiety and worry are associated with three (or more) of the following six symptoms (with at least some symptoms present for more days than not for the past 6 months): restlessness, being easily fatigued, difficulty concentrating, irritability, muscle tension, and sleep disturbance. The focus of the anxiety and worry is not confined to features of an axis I disorder. The anxiety, worry, or physical symptoms cause clinically significant distress or impairment in social, occupational, or other important areas of functioning. The disturbance is not due to the direct physiological effects of a substance (e.g., a drug of abuse, a medication) or a general medical condition (e.g., hypothyroidism) and does not occur exclusively

during a mood disorder, a psychotic disorder, or a pervasive developmental disorder.

American Psychiatric Association. *Diagnostic and Statistical Manual of Mental Disorders (DSM-IV-TR).* 4th ed. (Text Revision). http://www.psychiatryonline.com/content.aspx?aID=3476#3476. Accessed March 14, 2007.

27. **Answer: E.** Patients with Histrionic Personality Disorder have pervasive and excessive emotionality and attention-seeking behavior. The following are the DSM-IV-TR criteria for the diagnosis of this personality disorder: (a) these individuals are uncomfortable in situations in which they are not the center of attention, (b) they often exhibit inappropriate sexually seductive or provocative behaviors, (c) they display rapidly shifting and shallow expressions of emotions and consistently use physical appearance to draw attention to self, (d) they have a style of speech that is excessively impressionistic and lacking in detail, (e) they show self-dramatization and exaggerated expression of emotion, and (f) others easily influence them, and they consider relationships to be more intimate than they actually are. Furthermore, patients with Narcissistic Personality Disorder require excessive admiration from others.

American Psychiatric Association. *Diagnostic and Statistical Manual of Mental Disorders (DSM-IV-TR).* 4th ed. (Text Revision). http://www.psychiatryonline.com/content.aspx?aID=4017. Accessed March 28, 2007.

28. **Answer: E.** The available evidence indicates that psychological and drug treatments appear to be equally effective for children, adolescents, and adults. CBT is recommended as the first-line treatment for children and adolescents, because of the assumption that it has fewer risks than SSRIs. For adults, CBT or pharmacotherapy can be offered as first-line treatments. There is still uncertainty as to whether pharmacotherapy combined with CBT is superior to either treatment modality provided alone.

Heyman I, Mataix-Cols D, Fineberg NA. Obsessive-compulsive disorder. *BMJ.* 2006;333:424–429.

29. **Answer: E.** Management of Opioid Intoxication involves general supportive measures, as well as institution of the specific antidote, naloxone. An adequate airway is established, and respiratory and cardiac functions are assessed and maintained. IV access is essential for fluids and nutrition. Naloxone hydrochloride, a pure opioid antagonist, is used to reverse the CNS effects of opioid intoxication. An initial IV dose of 0.4 to 0.8 mg is administered to counteract neurologic and cardiorespiratory depression. The onset of action of intravenously administered naloxone is approximately 2 minutes. The subcutaneous route has been found to be equally effective since the slower rate of absorption via this route is offset by the delay in establishing IV access. Overdose with opioids that are more potent, such a fentanyl or longer acting agents like methadone, require higher doses of naloxone administered over prolonged periods.

Graham AW, Schultz TK, Mayo-Smith MF, et al. *Principles of Addiction Medicine.* 3rd ed. Chevy Chase, Maryland: American Society of Addiction Medicine; 2003:651–669.

30. **Answer: B.** TCAs derive their name from their three-ring structure. The tertiary amine tricyclic compounds, such as amitriptyline and imipramine, have two methyl groups at the end of the side chain. These compounds are demethylated to secondary amines, such as desipramine and nortriptyline. The tertiary amines are more potent as inhibitors of serotonin reuptake, and the secondary amines are more potent than norepinephrine inhibitors. The TCAs also possess cholinergic and histaminergic receptor blocking property. Desipramine is the most biochemically selective compound that blocks norepinephrine reuptake, and is unlikely to affect serotonin reuptake. Additionally, desipramine has little affinity for muscarinic-cholinergic, histaminergic, and α1-adrenergic receptors. The tetracyclic compounds, maprotiline and amoxapine, have a four-ring structure.

1. Sadock BJ, Sadock VA. *Kaplan and Sadock's Comprehensive Textbook of Psychiatry.* 7th ed. Philadelphia: Lippincott Williams & Wilkins; 2000:2491–2502.
2. Schatzberg AF, Nemeroff CB. *Textbook of Psychopharmacology.* 2nd ed. Washington: American Psychiatric Press; 1998:199–218.

31. **Answer: C.** Reboxetine is an SNRI that has been shown to be effective for the treatment of major depression. It is rapidly absorbed after oral administration, and is metabolized by P450 isoenzyme 3A4. It is generally well tolerated, and has fewer side effects (dry mouth, constipation, and other anticholinergic side effects) as compared to the TCAs. Reboxetine does not adversely affect the cardiac conduction, and is safer in overdose. Atomoxetine is another SNRI that has shown efficacy in the treatment of ADHD. Among TCAs, desipramine is the most biochemically selective compound that blocks norepinephrine reuptake. Bupropion is a norepinephrine-dopamine reuptake inhibitor, imipramine is a tricyclic agent, and sertraline is an SSRI.

Sadock BJ, Sadock VA. *Kaplan and Sadock's Comprehensive Textbook of Psychiatry.* 7th ed. Philadelphia: Lippincott Williams & Wilkins; 2000:2521–2531.

32. **Answer: B.** Controlled studies have not confirmed the efficacy of gabapentin or topiramate as

effective mood stabilizers. Lamotrigine has been found to be effective in treating both mania and depression. It acts at voltage-sensitive sodium channels, and inhibits the presynaptic release of glutamate and aspartate. Most common side effects of lamotrigine include ataxia, dizziness, headache, diplopia, blurred vision, nausea, vomiting, and rash. Lamotrigine does not cause weight gain. It is rarely associated with Stevens-Johnson syndrome and toxic epidermal necrolysis. Valproate inhibits the metabolism of lamotrigine, and carbamazepine and phenobarbitone enhance its metabolism.

Sadock BJ, Sadock VA. *Kaplan and Sadock's Comprehensive Textbook of Psychiatry.* 7th ed. Philadelphia: Lippincott Williams & Wilkins; 2000:2299–2304.

33. Answer: A. PMDD is characterized by lethargy and easy fatigability. Other symptoms of PMDD include depressed mood, increased anxiety, difficulty concentrating, and persistent anger or irritability.

American Psychiatric Association. *Quick Reference to the Diagnostic Criteria from DSM-IV-TR.* Washington: American Psychiatric Association; 2000:178–179.

34. Answer: C. This patient has sub-acute, combined degeneration of spinal cord, a neurologic manifestation of vitamin B_{12} deficiency, which is characterized by a myelopathy that involves the posterior and lateral columns of the spinal cord in the cervical and upper thoracic regions. The involvement of anterior columns of the spinal cord is rare. Pathological changes include spongiform changes and foci of myelin and axon destruction in the spinal cord white matter. There is also loss of myelin followed by axonal degeneration and gliosis. Majority of patients who develop vitamin B_{12} deficiency have pernicious anemia. It is also more common in the elderly, after gastric surgery, with H_2-blockers therapy, malabsorption syndromes, bacterial overgrowth, and tropical sprue. Clinical features include spastic paraparesis, extensor plantar response, and impaired perception of position and vibration. Symptoms usually start in the feet and are symmetric. Serum vitamin B_{12} level determination is the mainstay for evaluating vitamin B_{12} status. Serum vitamin B_{12} measurement has technical and interpretive problems, and it lacks sensitivity and specificity for the diagnosis of vitamin B_{12} deficiency. Low levels may often be seen in pregnancy, with oral contraceptive or anticonvulsant use, with transcobalamine deficiency, with folate deficiency, in association with HIV infection, and in multiple myeloma. Falsely elevated vitamin B_{12} levels may be seen with renal failure, liver disease, and myeloproliferative disorders. Levels of serum MMA and plasma total homocysteine are useful an-

cillary diagnostic tests for vitamin B_{12} deficiency. MMA is a byproduct of methylmalonyl-CoA and it accumulates in vitamin B_{12} deficiency. Its specificity is superior to that of plasma homocysteine in vitamin B_{12} deficiency.

Kumar N. Nutritional neuropathies. *Neurol Clin.* 2007;25:209–255.

35. Answer: B. Hepatitis C virus infection has been associated with depression independent of therapeutic complications. Personality Disorders, Anxiety and Somatization Disorders are no more prevalent in hepatitis patients than in the general population. Interferon-α is a cytokine host defense protein and immune modulator. Produced by lymphocytes, it is indicated for the treatment of hepatitis C, melanoma, and renal cell carcinoma. Interferon-α therapy is associated with a variety of psychiatric symptoms. For example, some studies indicate depression rates as high as 40%. Other less well documented neuropsychiatric symptoms include poor concentration, memory deficits, anxiety, and rarely psychosis. Treatment emergent depression is a frequent reason for premature termination of INF therapy. There is evidence suggesting well defined risk factors for the development of depression in these patients. Dose and duration of INF therapy and pretreatment depressive symptoms, particularly mild depression, have been shown to be risk factors for INF-induced depression. Age, gender, and history of substance use have not been shown to impact this risk. Depression occurring in INF-treated patients typically becomes evident and peaks at week 4 and week 24, respectively. Although there are studies suggesting that prophylactic antidepressant therapy may lead to significant reduction in depression rates among patients undergoing INF therapy, this mode of intervention is currently not approved by the FDA nor is it routine standard of care.

1. Dieperink E, Willenbring M, Ho SB. Neuropsychiatric symptoms associated with hepatitis C and interferon alpha: a review. *Am J Psychiatry.* 2000;157:867–876.
2. Hauser P, Khosla J, Aurora H, et al. A prospective study of the incidence and open-label treatment of interferon-induced major depressive disorder in patients with hepatitis C. *Mol Psychiatry.* 2002;7:942–947.
3. Raison CL, Borisov AS, Broadwell SD, et al. Depression during pegylated interferon-alpha plus ribavirin therapy: prevalence and prediction. *J Clin Psychiatry.* 2005;66: 41–48.

36. Answer: C. *Akathisia* is the Greek word for the inability to sit down. It is one of the most common movement disorders induced by DRB. Patients often suffer from a feeling of restlessness and the inability to remain still. Objectively, they present with increased motor activity, consisting of complex, semi-purposeful, stereotypic, and repetitive movements. They have the urge to move. Acute akathisia develops in 20% to 40% of patients receiving DRB. In 75% of patients acute akathisia develops within three days after therapy initiation. There are direct correlation between the potency of the neuroleptics, the neuroleptic dose and the rate of dosage increase, and the risk and severity of akathisia. There is no age or gender predisposition to developing akathisia. Acute akathisia usually tends to continue for as long as the neuroleptic medication is maintained and subsides shortly after cessation of treatment. It is very bothersome to the patients and often limits the patient's compliance. Anticholinergics, amantadines, and benztropines may be helpful as may be clonazepam and clonidine. Acute akathisia may also be caused by serotonergic agents, SSRIs, or cocaine.

Dressler D, Benecke R. Diagnosis and management of acute movement disorders. *J Neurol*. 2005;252:1299–1306.

37. Answer: C. Currently, implantation of cardiac pacemakers, defibrillators, and brain and spinal cord stimulators are all considered absolute contraindications to undergoing an MRI, because the strong magnets may induce unwanted currents in these devices. Ventilation may be performed by hand or by non-ferromagnetic machines. Newer, weakly ferromagnetic heart valves, access ports, and aneurysm clips are typically not a problem with MRI. Joint prostheses, even metal ones (as long as they are not significantly ferromagnetic), are typically okay for MRI. Some animal studies have reported the development of cataracts in fetuses exposed to MRI in utero. Human studies have not borne this out, and when the situation warrants, MRI may be performed on a pregnant patient.

Ropper AH, Brown RH. *Adams and Victor's Principles of Neurology*. 8th ed. New York: McGraw-Hill; 2005:11–38.

38. Answer: E. Marchiafava-Bignami disease is a demyelinating condition of the corpus callosum. It presents with rapidly progressive neurologic symptoms and ends fatally within a few months. It is specifically associated with alcoholism. Psychiatric manifestations include depression, mania, paranoia, and dementia predominate. Seizures are common, and hemiparesis, aphasia, dyskinesia, and ataxia are variably present.

Graham AW, Schultz TK, Mayo-Smith MF, et al. *Principles of Addiction Medicine*. 3rd ed. Chevy Chase, Maryland: American Society of Addiction Medicine; 2003:1152.

39. Answer: E. Neurologic manifestations may be the earliest and often the only manifestation of vitamin B$_{12}$

deficiency. The neurologic manifestations of this deficiency include a myelopathy with or without an associated neuropathy, cognitive dysfunction, optic neuropathy, and paresthesias without abnormal signs. Studies have also demonstrated that the severity of the hematologic and neurologic manifestations may be inversely related in a particular patient. Relapses in the illness are usually associated with the same neurologic phenotype.

Kumar N. Nutritional neuropathies. *Neurol Clin*. 2007;25:209–255.

40. Answer: D. Complex regional pain syndrome is an emerging diagnostic entity comprising reflex sympathetically mediated pain, regional sympathetic dystrophy (RSD) and causalgia. Autonomic dysfunction, disproportionate pain and soft tissue alteration are the common factors underlying these entities. Precipitating injuries are largely minor but may include fractures, peripheral vascular disease, and gun shot wounds. Of these entities, RSD is the commonest. It is not associated with direct nerve damage and treatment consists of blockade of regional sympathetic nerve ganglion, physical therapy, and adjunctive medications. An interesting phenomenon in RSD is pain extending far beyond the precipitating injury, as in this case. The most commonly used agents to treat this condition include anticonvulsants, antidepressants, steroids, biphosphates, and opiates, but they have not been adequately studied in the treatment of complex regional pain syndrome. All these agents should be used in conjunction with a comprehensive interdisciplinary approach aimed at functional restoration and improved quality of life of the patient.

1. Harden RN, Bruehl SP. Diagnosis of complex regional pain syndrome: signs, symptoms, and new empirically derived diagnostic criteria. *Clin J Pain*. 2006;22:415–419.
2. Mackey S, Feinberg S. Pharmacologic therapies for complex regional pain syndrome. *Curr Pain Headache Rep*. 2007;11:38–43.
3. Schwartzman RJ. New treatments for reflex sympathetic dystrophy. *N Engl J Med*. 2000;343:654–656.

41. Answer: C. Her child is at increased risk of developing MS as there is a genetic susceptibility for developing MS. Monozygotic twins have a greater than 30% concordance rate for developing MS while dizygotic twins have 4% to 5% concordance rates. Environmental factors also play a significant role in development of MS. Spending your childhood in cool temperate latitudes of the Northern Hemisphere increases the risk of developing MS. Pregnancy can precipitate an MS episode especially in the first 3 postpartum months. MS is not known to increase the risk of obstetric complications, fetal malformations, or spontaneous abortions. Exacerbations of MS in pregnancy are not believed to affect outcome of the fetus. Pregnancy also does not affect the long-term outcome or prognosis of MS.

1. Ropper AH, Brown RH. *Adams and Victor's Principles of Neurology*. 8th ed. New York: McGraw-Hill; 2005:771–796.
2. Kaufman DM. *Clinical Neurology for Psychiatrists*. 5th ed. Philadelphia: WB Saunders; 2001:369–391.

42. Answer: B. Friedreich's ataxia is an autosomal, recessive disorder of trinucleotide repeats that presents in late childhood. This condition should be distinguished from the spinocerebellar degenerations or types of spinocerebellar ataxias (SCAs), which are transmitted in an autosomal dominant fashion with trinucleotide repeat expansion on various chromosomes. Some consider the pes cavus foot deformity pathognomonic (high arch, elevated first dorsum, and retracted first metatarsal) of Friedreich's ataxia. Another feature of Friedreich's ataxia is that it is often associated with cardiomyopathy and posterior column sensory deficits. A "steppage gait" of raising the feet high is common in Friedreich's and other ataxias associated with damage to posterior column of the spinal cord. His younger siblings are at risk to develop his symptoms later on in their lives.

Kaufman DM. *Clinical Neurology for Psychiatrists*. 5th ed. Philadelphia: WB Saunders; 2001:8–25.

43. Answer: C. Olivopontocerebellar atrophy may be familial (sometimes autosomal dominant or recessive) or sporadic. They often present in the 40s. The sporadic form is more common, and presents at a younger age. Progressive ataxias, often beginning in the lower limbs, may develop into parkinsonism in half the cases. It may be related to multiple system atrophy in some cases. Pathologically there is extensive degeneration in middle cerebellar peduncles, cerebellar white matter, and specific nuclei (pontine, olivary, and arcuate). This may be secondary to myelin degeneration. Other associated features may include retinal degeneration, spastic paraplegia, areflexia, dementia, ophthalmoplegia, neuropathies, and dystonias. Lesions to olivary nuclei are characteristic of olivopontocerebellar atrophy. Friedreich's ataxia is a more common hereditary form of ataxia, and it presents earlier and with different associated findings. Lack of cardiac and spinal problems makes the diagnosis of Friedreich's ataxia less likely. Stroke could present similarly, but the patient is healthy and without evidence of vascular disease. It would also be unusual to have a lesion specific to the olivary nuclei presenting with progressive ataxia. Parkinson's disease does not typically present with prominent ataxia. No tumors are seen on MRI, and paraneoplastic ataxias are more common in women with ovarian and breast cancers.

Ropper AH, Brown RH. *Adams and Victor's Principles of Neurology*. 8th ed. New York: McGraw-Hill; 2005:931–938.

44. Answer: B. Topiramate is a new anticonvulsant drug that has been used for both partial and generalized seizures. It can precipitate renal stones in patients taking the medication. It has also been associated with hyperchloremic metabolic acidosis and angle-closure glaucoma. It can produce rashes, especially when used with valproic acid. This medication has not been commonly associated with priapism, hepatic adenomas, or coma.

Ropper AH, Brown RH. *Adams and Victor's Principles of Neurology*. 8th ed. http://www.accessmedicine.com/content.aspx?aID=969583. Published March 26, 2007.

45. Answer: C. Given equivalent stressors, those individuals with strong social supports appear to have better outcomes than those who are isolated or those who perceive that support is unavailable or unhelpful from those in their social network. The elderly have reduced social networks and the frequency of their social contacts as compared to younger adults. This is true for the oldest-old, whose social networks have been shown to be one half the size of the young-old. For many older adults, this reduction in social contact is not voluntary and may be more related to disability and reduced mobility than preference. Although overall social contacts decrease in late life, it is only contact with acquaintances and other peripheral individuals that decreases significantly. Social contacts with very close friends and family remain stable, and older adults' satisfaction with these close relationships remains high. Older adults with nuclear family members tended to have social networks that were both larger, as well as more emotionally close, than older adults without nuclear family. However, those without nuclear family report greater feelings of closeness to friends than those with nuclear family, suggesting that older adults can adapt to the absence of family by creating satisfying relationships with others. Recent studies of the social structure of the oldest-old indicate that most individuals over the age of 85 have at least one surviving relative, but approximately one fourth had little or no contact with that relative. For the oldest-old the family, especially adult children, appears to play a crucial role in providing social support.

Sadock BJ, Sadock VA. *Kaplan and Sadock's Comprehensive Textbook of Psychiatry*. 8th ed. Philadelphia: Lippincott Williams & Wilkins; 2005:3627.

46. Answer: D. Many hormones have a diurnal pattern. Prolactin levels usually increase during the sleep period, as do luteinizing hormones (especially in adolescents). Growth hormone has a similar pattern. TSH has a different pattern, with increased levels in the evening hours, which decrease after sleep onset. Cortisol production usually decreases at night, and increases toward morning. This pattern may be disrupted by depression.

Sadock BJ, Sadock VA. *Kaplan and Sadock's Comprehensive Textbook of Psychiatry*. 7th ed. Philadelphia: Lippincott Williams & Wilkins; 2000:199–209.

47. Answer: B. Also called "doing and undoing," *undoing* is a defense mechanism employed to essentially attempt to reverse unconscious hostile wishes by recreating and "re-writing" a situation, to remove the aggressive thoughts before they are enacted. In this case, obsessive thoughts about the driver of the car being killed in an accident lead the man to perform an elaborate ritual to maintain the driver's safety. From a psychoanalytic perspective, the auto mechanic's behavior could be interpreted as a defense against unconscious impulses to cause harm to the driver by performing an action (loosening the lug nuts) that must then be "undone." Splitting is a primitive defense mechanism that results in division of good and bad aspects of an object into two separate objects, allowing the patient to avoid the ambivalent conflict of maintaining contradictory aspects of an object together. Reaction formation refers to a defense mechanism in which the person acts in a way diametrically opposed to their inner wishes, such as being excessively friendly to a person he dislikes. In sublimation, unconscious urges are partially expressed in a socially acceptable way, such as the channeling of aggressive impulses to competitive sports. Projective identification is a complicated form of primitive defense, in which the patient projects intolerable feelings to the therapist, which can then be identified by the therapist and processed, reducing anxiety. Sudden feelings experienced by the therapist during a session that seem foreign can be reflections of the inner world of the patient, projected onto the therapist.

Bateman A and Holmes J. *Introduction to Psychoanalysis: Contemporary Theory and Practice*. London: Routledge; 1995:76–94.

48. Answer: C. The core of the insanity defense is the presence of a mental disorder. Mental disorders that meet criteria for the insanity defense do not include symptoms manifested solely as criminal behavior or antisocial acts. Presence of a defect of reason, lack of knowledge of wrongfulness, and incapacity to refrain from the criminal act are basic components of the insanity defense. However, the importance of these elements may vary depending on jurisdiction.

Sadock BJ, Sadock VA. *Kaplan and Sadock's Comprehensive Textbook of Psychiatry*. 8th ed. Philadelphia: Lippincott Williams & Wilkins; 2005:3984.

49. Answer: A. All of the choices are disorders of thought process. Circumstantiality is a disorder in which the patient is unable to be goal directed and incorporates exhausting details that are unnecessary, and has difficulty in arriving at an end point. Tangentiality describes a thought process in which the patient digresses from the subject and introduces thoughts that seem unrelated, skewed, and irrelevant. Blocking is a sudden cessation in the middle of a sentence, at which point a patient cannot recover what was said and is unable to complete their thoughts. Loose associations refer to switching from one topic to another with no apparent connection between the topics. Perseveration refers to repeating the same response to any questions with an inability to change the response or topic.

Hales RE, Yudofsky SC. *American Psychiatric Publishing Textbook of Clinical Psychiatry*. 4th ed. 2003. http://www.psychiatryonline.com/content.aspx?aID=68501. Accessed February 22, 2007.

50. Answer: B. A history of drug abuse has no connection with Factitious Disorder by Proxy. This disorder is also known as *Münchhausen syndrome by proxy*, and involves the intentional feigning or production of physical or psychological symptoms in another person who is under a perpetrator's care, where the perpetrator's motive is to assume the sick role by proxy. The perpetrator may give a false medical history and provide symptoms that do not make sense, as well as alter records or contaminate laboratory samples while the victim remains passive to the perpetrator's deeds, and there is often a family history of similar sibling illness.

1. Sadock BJ, Sadock VA. *Kaplan and Sadock's Comprehensive Textbook of Psychiatry*. 8th ed. Philadelphia: Lippincott Williams & Wilkins; 2005:1834.
2. Thomas K. Münchhausen syndrome by proxy: identification and diagnosis. *J Pediatr Nurs*. 2003;18:174–180.

51. Answer: C. Although post-TBI recovery is a gradual process, most patients show significant recovery within 3 years, while most of the recovery occurring within 6 months as the brain regenerates. Recovery following the more severe TBI is individualized and depends on nature, location, and severity of the injury. Most spouses of patients with moderate to severe TBI are appropriately concerned and perhaps apprehensive, thus this behavior falls within the norm.

1. Rao V, Lyketsos C. Neuropsychiatric sequelae of traumatic brain injury. *Psychosomatics*. 2000;41:95–103.
2. Rao V, Lyketsos CG. Psychiatric aspects of traumatic brain injury. *Psychiatr Clin North Am*. 2002;25:43–69.

52. **Answer: C.** The feature of acute stress disorder is the development of characteristic anxiety, dissociative, and other symptoms that occurs within 1 month after exposure to a traumatic stressor. Either while experiencing the traumatic event or after the event, the individual has at least three of the following dissociative symptoms: (i) a subjective sense of numbing, detachment, or absence of emotional responsiveness, (ii) a reduction in awareness of his or her surroundings, (iii) derealization, (iv) depersonalization, or (v) dissociative amnesia. Following the trauma, the traumatic event is persistently reexperienced, and the individual displays marked avoidance of stimuli that may arouse recollections of the trauma and has marked symptoms of anxiety or increased arousal. The symptoms must cause clinically significant distress, significantly interfere with normal functioning, or impair the individual's ability to pursue necessary tasks. The disturbance lasts for a minimum of 2 days and a maximum of 4 weeks after the traumatic event. If symptoms persist beyond 4 weeks, the diagnosis of PTSD may be applied. The symptoms are not due to the direct physiological effects of a substance or a general medical condition, are not better accounted for by brief psychotic disorder, and are not merely an exacerbation of a preexisting mental disorder.

American Psychiatric Association. *Diagnostic and Statistical Manual of Mental Disorders (DSM-IV-TR)*. 4th ed. (Text Revision). http://www.psychiatryonline.com/content.aspx?aID=3432#3432. Accessed March 15, 2007.

53. **Answer: D.** Subjects with Dependent Personality Disorder have an excessive need to be taken care of, and show submissive behavior and fear of separation. They think that they would be unable to function without the help of others and actively seek this help. They have unrealistic fears of being left to take care of themselves and they urgently seek other relationships as a source of support. They also have a hard time making decisions and need constant advice and support. Patients with avoidant personality disorder show restraint within intimate relationships because of the fear of being shamed or ridiculed.

American Psychiatric Association. *Diagnostic and Statistical Manual of Mental Disorders (DSM-IV-TR)*. 4th ed. (Text Revision). http://www.psychiatryonline.com/content.aspx?aID=4125. Accessed March 28, 2007.

54. **Answer: D.** A recent Cochrane review included twenty-two studies with 1,060 participants with GAD. Based on thirteen studies, psychological therapies, all using a CBT approach, were more effective than TAU/WL in achieving clinical response at posttreatment (relative risk [RR]: 0.63; 95% confidence interval [CI]: 0.55 to 0.73), and also in reducing anxiety, worry, and depression symptoms. No studies conducted longer-term assessments of CBT against TAU/WL. Six studies compared CBT against supportive therapy (nondirective therapy and attention-placebo conditions). No significant difference in clinical response was indicated between CBT and supportive therapy at posttreatment (RR: 0.86; 95% CI: 0.70 to 1.06). Based on their findings, the authors concluded that psychological therapy based on CBT principles is effective in reducing anxiety symptoms for short-term treatment of GAD. The body of evidence comparing CBT with other psychological therapies is small and heterogeneous, which precludes drawing conclusions about which psychological therapy is more effective.

Hunot V, Churchill R, Silva de Lima M, et al. Psychological therapies for generalised anxiety disorder. *Cochrane Database Syst Rev*. 2007;1:CD001848.

55. **Answer: E.** Pharmacologic agents used for assisting patients through a safer and more comfortable opioid withdrawal include use of an opioid agonist (methadone), α2-adrenergic agonist (clonidine), and a mixed opioid agonist/antagonist (buprenorphine). In addition, opioid antagonists, such as naltrexone and naloxone, are use in combination with clonidine or general anesthesia for rapid withdrawal from opiates.

Graham AW, Schultz TK, Mayo-Smith MF, et al. *Principles of Addiction Medicine*. 3rd ed. Chery Chase, Maryland: American Society of Addiction Medicine; 2003:651–669.

56. **Answer: A.** TCAs are absorbed rapidly and completely in the small intestine. They are extensively bound to plasma proteins. They are mainly metabolized in the liver by demethylation of the side chain and hydroxylation of the ring structure. Elimination half-lives for most tricyclics is about 24 hours, therefore, they can be administered in once a day dosing schedule. The tricyclic and tetracyclic compound are lipophilic amines, therefore, have a high volume of distribution. They are concentrated in a variety of tissues in the body, and their concentration in cardiac tissues exceeds those in plasma.

Sadock BJ, Sadock VA. *Kaplan and Sadock's Comprehensive Textbook of Psychiatry*. 7th ed. Philadelphia: Lippincott Williams & Wilkins; 2000:2491–2502.

57. Answer: B. Venlafaxine is an SNRI, which is well absorbed in the gastrointestinal tract, and metabolized by P450 isoenzymes 2D6 and 3A4. Other SNRIs include milnacipran and duloxetine. Venlafaxine and milnacipran have been shown to be safe and effective antidepressants. In addition, research studies have suggested a role of venlafaxine in GAD, OCD, Panic Disorder, Social Phobia, Agoraphobia, and ADHD. Most common adverse effects observed with venlafaxine include asthenia, sweating, nausea, constipation, anorexia, vomiting, somnolence, dizziness, anxiety, tremor, blurred vision, impaired orgasm or ejaculation, and impotence in men. Venlafaxine is associated with sustained hypertension in patients treated with more than 300 mg/day. Duloxetine has been shown to be effective in treating depression and pain syndromes.

Sadock BJ, Sadock VA. *Kaplan and Sadock's Comprehensive Textbook of Psychiatry*. 7th ed. Philadelphia: Lippincott Williams & Wilkins; 2000:2521–2531.

58. Answer: A. Although statistics vary, approximately 3% to 5% of women meet criteria for PMDD. Most women of childbearing age experience some symptoms of MDD during the course of some of their menstrual cycles. PMDD is best determined by prospective daily symptom rating scales completed over a 2-month interval.

1. American Psychiatric Association. *DSM-IV-TR, Diagnostic and Statistical Manual of Mental Disorders*. 4th ed. (Text Revision). http://www.psychiatryonline.com/content.aspx?aID=5272#5272. Accessed March 4, 2007.
2. Hales RE, Yudofsky SC. *The American Psychiatric Publishing Textbook of Clinical Psychiatry*. 4th ed. http://www.psychiatryonline.com/content.aspx?aID=5285&searchStr=premenstrual+dysphoric+disorder#5285. Accessed March 4, 2007.

59. Answer: A. Temporal lobes are unaffected in Wernicke's encephalopathy. Symmetric lesions are usually seen in the periventricular regions of the thalamus and hypothalamus, the nuclei at the level of the third and fourth ventricle, superior cerebellar vermis, and the mammillary bodies. The changes seen include necrosis, neuronal loss, edema, prominent capillaries with endothelial proliferation, and hemorrhage. In the late stages of the illness, cell loss with astrocytic and microglial proliferation may also be seen.

Kumar N. Nutritional neuropathies. *Neurol Clin*. 2007;25:209–255.

60. Answer: D. Hepatitis C virus infection has been associated with depression independent of therapeutic complications. Personality Disorders, anxiety, and Somatization Disorders are no more prevalent in hepatitis patients than in the general population. Interferon-α is a cytokine host defense protein and immune modulator. Produced by lymphocytes, it is indicated for the treatment of hepatitis C, melanoma, and renal cell carcinoma. Interferon-α therapy is associated with a variety of psychiatric symptoms. For example, some studies indicate depression rates as high as 40%. Other less well documented neuropsychiatric symptoms include poor concentration, memory deficits, anxiety, and rarely psychosis. Treatment emergent depression is a frequent reason for premature termination of INF therapy. Well defined risk factors for depression in these patients have been documented. Dose and duration of INF therapy, pretreatment depressive symptoms particularly mild depression have been shown to be risk factors for INF-induced depression. Age, gender, and substance use history have not been shown to impact this risk. Depression occurring in INF-treated patients typically becomes evident and peaks at week 4 and week 24, respectively. Although there are studies suggesting that prophylactic antidepressant therapy may lead to significant reduction in depression rates among patients undergoing INF therapy, this mode of intervention is currently not approved by the FDA, nor is it routine standard of care.

1. Dieperink E, Willenbring M, Ho SB. Neuropsychiatric symptoms associated with hepatitis C and interferon alpha: a review. *Am J Psychiatry*. 2000;157:867–876.
2. Hauser P, Khosla J, Aurora H, et al. A prospective study of the incidence and open-label treatment of interferon-induced major depressive disorder in patients with hepatitis C. *Mol Psychiatry*. 2002;7:942–947.
3. Raison CL, Borisov AS, Broadwell SD, et al. Depression during pegylated interferon-alpha plus ribavirin therapy: prevalence and prediction. *J Clin Psychiatry*. 2005;66:41–48.

61. Answer: D. In between seizures, a single EEG recording will show a normal pattern in 30% of patients with absence seizures and 50% of those with grand mal epilepsy. Another 30% to 40% of epileptics, though abnormal between seizures, are nonspecific. Therefore, the diagnosis of epilepsy can be made only by the correct interpretation of clinical data in relation to the EEG abnormality.

Ropper AH, Brown RH. *Adams and Victor's Principles of Neurology*. 8th ed. http://www.accessmedicine.com/content.aspx?aID=970327. Accessed May 9, 2007.

62. Answer: C. Cerebral angiography (using dye and x-rays) is most useful in diagnosing cerebrovascular disorders. This does not necessarily include stroke or certain types of hemorrhages, for which CT and MRI are extremely useful. Conventional angiography is particularly useful in diagnosing aneurysms, vascular malformations, arterial and venous occlusion, angiitis, and dissection. CTA and a CTA (CTangiography) and MRA (MRangiography) may eventually replace traditional angiography, but for now it is still used, particularly in interventional procedures. It is a potentially dangerous and invasive technique. Tumors are best visualized on MRI (sometimes CT, e.g., men and genome is), fractures on CT. Certain infections can be seen on CT or MRI (e.g., cysticercosis, toxoplasmosis, and the effects of meningitis), but LP remains vital.

Ropper AH, Brown RH. *Adams and Victor's Principles of Neurology*. 8th ed. New York: McGraw-Hill; 2005:11–38.

63. Answer: B. Alcoholic myopathy ranges in severity from asymptomatic elevation of serum creatine kinase, to a progressive polymyolysis-like presentation, to acute rhabdomyolysis. Muscle weakness is common, but fever is not typically present.

Graham AW, Schultz TK, Mayo-Smith MF, et al. *Principles of Addiction Medicine*. 3rd ed. Chevy Chase, Maryland: American Society of Addiction Medicine; 2003:1153.

64. Answer: C. This patient has developed Wernicke's encephalopathy due to the deficiency of thiamine. The clinical features of Wernicke's encephalopathy include a subacute onset of ocular palsies, nystagmus, gait ataxia, and confusion. Thiamine functions as a coenzyme in the metabolism of carbohydrates and branched-chain amino acids. Thiamine deficiency results in reduced synthesis of high-energy phosphates and causes an accumulation of lactate. The recommended daily requirement for adults is 1.2 mg/day for men and 1.1 mg/day for women, and its highest concentrations are found in yeast and in the pericarp of grain. Most cereals and breads available in the United States are fortified with thiamine. Organ meats are good sources of thiamine, while dairy products, seafood, and fruits are poor sources. Prolonged cooking of food, baking of bread, and pasteurization of milk remain potential causes of thiamine loss. The areas most vulnerable to thiamine deficiency in the brain are those with the highest turnover rates like the caudal part of the brain and the cerebellum. As its turnover rate is rapid (half-life of 10 to 14 days) and there is lack of storage, a continuous dietary supply of thiamine is necessary to balance the body's requirement. In some cases thiamine deficiency may manifest in just 2 to 3 weeks on a deficient diet. Thiamine deficiency in alcoholism occurs because of inadequate dietary intake, reduced gastrointestinal absorption, and reduced liver thiamine stores. Additionally, alcohol also inhibits the transport of thiamine in the gastrointestinal system and blocks phosphorylation of thiamine to thiamine diphosphate, the active form of thiamine.

1. Kumar N. Nutritional neuropathies. *Neurol Clin*. 2007;25:209–255.
2. Thomson AD, Marshall EJ. The natural history and pathophysiology of Wernicke's encephalopathy and Korsakoff's psychosis. *Alcohol Alcohol*. 2006;41:151–158.

65. Answer: D. Four case series have documented mental status changes associated with cases of Addison's disease. Mood symptoms and decreased motivation are common in less severe cases, and an "acute organic brain syndrome" is associated with severe cases. These series indicates that mild disturbances in mood, motivation, and behavior are core clinical features of Addison's disease. Psychosis and extensive cognitive changes (including delirium) do occur, but are associated with severe disease and may be the presenting feature of Addisonian crisis. Rare presentations of Addison's disease have included catatonia and self-mutilation. In 80% of the case reports, symptoms occurred before diagnosis and treatment, indicating that the mental status changes are a feature of Addison's disease and not caused by treatment with cortisone. In the majority of cases, both physical and mental symptoms were resolved with cortisone treatment in 1 week. A diagnosis of Addison's disease is based on the measurement of low plasma cortisol, elevated ACTH, and the results of a corticotropin stimulation test. In a short corticotropin stimulation test, 250g of cosyntropin (a synthetic form of ACTH) is given before 10 AM, and plasma cortisol is measured before the test and 60 minutes after the injection. In patients with Addison's disease, the adrenal cortex is unable to increase cortisol secretion in response to cosyntropin. When patients present with an Addisonian crisis, glucocorticoid treatment must not be delayed. Blood for serum cortisol, ACTH, and serum chemistry should be drawn, and therapy with IV saline and dexamethasone should be initiated immediately. A short corticotropin stimulation test can then be performed as dexamethasone does not interfere with cortisol radioimmunoassay. Following testing, therapy with dexamethasone can be replaced with hydrocortisone. Low aldosterone and high renin are consistent with the diagnosis of Addison's disease. If the cause of primary adrenal insufficiency is unknown, adrenal autoantibody tests and imaging of the adrenal glands can be performed.

Anglin RE, Rosebush PI, Mazurek MF. The neuropsychiatric profile of Addison's disease: revisiting a forgotten phenomenon. *J Neuropsychiatry Clin Neurosci*. 2006;18: 450–459.

66. Answer: D. In MS, total "lesion load" assessed via imaging is the most predictive of cognitive deficits. Total physical disability also correlates with cognitive deficits. Location of lesions often corresponds well with specific deficits (commonly enlarged ventricles, corpus callosum atrophy, and periventricular white matter demyelination). However, many lesions are clinically asymptomatic. Initially the patient usually appears cognitively normal, despite MS symptoms that interfere with full assessment. Subtle deficits may be found early on more sophisticated testing. Impairments are often first noted in memory and concentration, but may eventually deteriorate to dementia. Age of onset and length of time since onset are less well correlated with cognitive impairment. The spinal form of MS is less likely to be associated with "subcortical" cognitive deficits or dementia, which may occur in advanced MS.

1. Kaufman DM. *Clinical Neurology for Psychiatrists*. 5th ed. Philadelphia: WB Saunders; 2001:369–391.
2. Ropper AH, Brown RH. *Adams and Victor's Principles of Neurology*. 8th ed. New York: McGraw-Hill; 2005: 771–796.

67. Answer: C. Spinocerebellar degenerations are autosomal dominant progressive neurodegenerative diseases of trinucleotide repeat expansions. They are now classified as Spinocerebellar ataxias (SCAs), and have been located to various genes. SCAs present with degenerative cerebellar dysfunction, such as progressive ataxias and incoordination of limbs, possibly scanning speech. Depending on the type of SCA, other systems are often involved (e.g., sensory deficits, movement problems, and spasticity). Alcohol-related neurologic dysfunction, possibly related to vitamin B_{12} deficiency, might fit a similar pattern, but usually without spasticity.

Kaufman DM. *Clinical Neurology for Psychiatrists*. 5th ed. Philadelphia: WB Saunders; 2001:8–25.

68. Answer: C. Obstructive hydrocephalus, also known as *tension* or *noncommunicating hydrocephalus*, commonly presents following subarachnoid hemorrhage, AVM bleeds, aneurysm ruptures, deep hemisphere bleeds, and with meningeal neoplasms. Imaging usually shows ventricular enlargement. Ventricular expansion is greatest in the frontal horns, thus resulting in frontal dysfunction. The patient is relatively young, and otherwise healthy, so a stroke would be of less concern. A tumor is less likely if imaging was negative, though some neoplasms may invade the meninges. A ruptured aneurysm is possible, but the patient was just treated, and there is no mention of other possible aneurysms. Treatment of acute obstructive hydrocephalus or CSF drainage by LP, or often via a ventricular catheter.

Ropper AH, Brown RH. *Adams and Victor's Principles of Neurology*. 8th ed. New York: McGraw-Hill; 2005:529–545.

69. Answer: E. Along with cardiac malformations, orofacial clefts are the most frequently reported defects in newborn children of epileptic mothers. Clefts develop approximately ten times more frequently in children of epileptic mothers than in the general population. Other common teratogenic effects of anticonvulsants include the fetal hydantoin syndrome with the use of phenytoin or carbamazepine, microcephaly with the use of trimethadione, and neural tube defects with the use of valproic acid.

Cunningham FG, Leveno KL, Bloom SL. *Williams Obstetrics*. 22nd ed. http://www.accessmedicine.com/content.aspx?aID=722696. Accessed March 26, 2007.

70. Answer: B. The anal stage corresponds to toddlerhood, and typically occurs from 12 to 36 months of age. During Freud's anal stage, the child is able to control their bowels, begins to understand gender labels in relation to themselves, and understands activities related to gender. The oral stage occurs in infancy (0 to 12 months), the anal stage and toddlerhood (12 to 36 months), the phallic and Oedipal stages and preschool (3 to 5 years), and the latency stage during school age (5 to 12 years). Adolescence and the genital stage are thought to occur from 12 to 18 years.

1. Hales RE, Yudofsky SC. *Textbook of Clinical Psychiatry*. 4th ed. Washington: American Psychiatric Publishing; 2003:67–105.
2. Sadock BJ, Sadock VA. *Kaplan and Sadock's Comprehensive Textbook of Psychiatry*. 7th ed. Philadelphia: Lippincott Williams & Wilkins; 2000:2534–2550.

71. Answer: C. Respirations are more variable during REM sleep. Also, while muscles are usually partially relaxed during non-REM sleep, muscles are most relaxed during REM sleep, and may in fact actually be atonic. Heart rate and blood pressure are both typically decreased and steady during non-REM sleep, but are more variable during REM sleep. Brain temperature is decreased during non-REM sleep. Cerebral glucose is unchanged to mildly increased during REM sleep, and decreased during non-REM sleep. For most of the physiological parameters listed, with the exception of the protective muscle atonia, the REM state more closely resembles the awakened state than does the non-REM state.

Sadock BJ, Sadock VA. *Kaplan and Sadock's Comprehensive Textbook of Psychiatry*. 7th ed. Philadelphia: Lippincott Williams & Wilkins; 2000:199–209.

72. Answer: C. In formulating his theories, Freud developed three different models for the structure of the mind and built on each of these models. In his first model, the affect-trauma model, Freud viewed symptoms such as hysteria as a release of "built-up" affect that resulted from a prior trauma, causing an imbalance in psychological functioning. He next devised the topographical model, defining a division of the mind into the unconscious, the preconscious, and the conscious, in which the preconscious served as a reservoir for unconscious thoughts and drives to be modified so that they are acceptable to the conscious. The structural model was the next of Freud's models to be developed, outlining the id, ego, and superego. The id refers to basic innate drives and instincts, such as aggression and libido, which are then regulated by the ego to make them consistent with external reality and acceptable. The superego provides conscience and ideals to the personality.

Bateman A and Holmes J. *Introduction to Psychoanalysis: Contemporary Theory and Practice*. London: Routledge; 1995:27–47.

73. Answer: A. Approximately one third of allegations of psychiatric malpractice are claims of incorrect treatment. Twenty percent of claims are due to attempted or completed suicide. Eleven percent of claims are allegations of incorrect diagnosis. Allegations of undue familiarity and unnecessary hospitalization each comprise less than 5% of claims.

Sadock BJ, Sadock VA. *Kaplan and Sadock's Comprehensive Textbook of Psychiatry*. 8th ed. Philadelphia: Lippincott Williams & Wilkins; 2005:3970.

74. Answer: A. The GAF score was designed to rate axis V on the DSM-IV. It is a 100-point scale based on all available information, with clear descriptions of each ten-point interval. Ratings are normally made for the past week, but longer intervals (e.g., highest during the past year) can be used. The GAF shows fair to good reliability and good validity. The main problem with the GAF is a tendency to confound symptoms and functioning, leading to low scores even with a relative sparing of social and occupational functioning (e.g., positive symptoms in schizophrenia necessitate a score below 40).

1. Sadock BJ, Sadock VA. *Kaplan and Sadock's Comprehensive Textbook of Psychiatry*. 7th ed. Philadelphia: Lippincott Williams & Wilkins; 2000:758–760.
2. American Psychiatric Association. *Diagnostic and Statistical Manual of Mental Disorders (DSM-IV-TR)*. 4th ed. (Text revision). http://www.psychiatryonline.com/content.aspx?aID=16921. Published March 1, 2007.

75. Answer: C. Münchhausen syndrome by proxy, also known as *factitious disorder by proxy*, is the intentional feigning or production of physical or psychological symptoms in another person who is under a perpetrator's care, where the perpetrator's motive is to assume the sick role by proxy. Biological mothers have been reported to be the most common culprits, and these mothers are mostly white, most are married, and between 20 to 30 years old. Many have also had some form of health care training background. Fathers, adopted/foster parents, grandparents, babysitters, and spouses (in the cases of older victims) have also been implicated as perpetrators, but are less common than biological mothers.

1. Sadock BJ, Sadock VA. *Kaplan and Sadock's Comprehensive Textbook of Psychiatry*. 8th ed. Philadelphia: Lippincott Williams & Wilkins; 2005:1838.
2. Thomas K. Munchausen syndrome by proxy: identification and diagnosis. *J Pediatr Nurs*. 2003;18:174–180.

76. Answer: A. Patients with frontal lobe injury manifest loss of spontaneity, difficulty "shifting set," perseveration, poor generative thinking, lack of initiative and drive, poor anticipation and planning. They perform well on highly structured and familiar tasks however. The temporal lobe mediates memory and receptive speech while the parietal lobe functions to integrate various associative modalities.

1. Rao V, Lyketsos C. Neuropsychiatric sequelae of traumatic brain injury. *Psychosomatics*. 2000;41:95–103.
2. Rao V, Lyketsos CG. Psychiatric aspects of traumatic brain injury. *Psychiatr Clin North Am*. 2002;25:43–69.

77. Answer: E. All of the above choices are types of paraphilias. Exhibitionism is a type of paraphilia in which an individual experiences recurrent, intense sexually arousing fantasies, urges, or behaviors involving the exposure of one's genitals to an unsuspecting stranger over a period of at least 6 months. Fetishism involves recurrent, intense sexually arousing fantasies, sexual urges, or behaviors involving the use of nonliving objects (e.g., female undergarments). Pedophilia involves recurrent, intense sexually arousing fantasies, sexual urges, or behaviors involving sexual activity with a prepubescent child or children. The person is at least 16 years of age and at least 5 years older than the child or children involved in the act. Voyeurism involves getting intense sexually arousing fantasies, sexual urges, or behaviors involving the act of observing an unsuspecting person who is naked, in the process of disrobing or engaging in sexual activity. In order to make a diagnosis of a paraphilia, the time frame must be at least

6 months, and the individual must have experienced marked distress and interpersonal difficulties due to acting on these urges or fantasies.

American Psychiatric Association. *Quick Reference to the Diagnostic Criteria from DSM-IV-TR*. Washington: American Psychiatric Association; 2000:255–258.

78. Answer: C. Patients with Borderline Personality Disorder have a pervasive pattern of instability of interpersonal relationships, affect, and self-image. Seventy-five percent of patients with BPD are women. Patients often engage in self-mutilating and suicidal behaviors, and completed suicide occurs in 8% to 10% of these individuals. Some individuals present with psychotic-like symptoms, such as hallucinations or ideas of reference, during moments of stress. They have a hard time dealing with real or imagined abandonment, and suffer from chronic feelings of emptiness.

American Psychiatric Association. *Diagnostic and Statistical Manual of Mental Disorders (DSM-IV-TR)*. 4th ed. (Text revision). http://www.psychiatryonline.com/content.aspx?aID=3974. Accessed March 28, 2007.

79. Answer: D. In a recent Cochrane review, twenty-three randomized comparisons (representing 21 trials, 1,709 patients), twenty-one of which involved behavior or cognitive-behavior therapies for the treatment of panic disorder with or without agoraphobia were identified. In the acute phase treatment, combined therapy was superior to antidepressant pharmacotherapy (RR: 1.24; 95% CI: 1.02 to 1.52) or psychotherapy (RR: 1.17; 95% CI: 1.05 to 1.31). The combined therapy produced more dropouts due to side effects than psychotherapy (number needed to harm around 26). After the acute phase treatment, as long as the drug was continued, the superiority of the combination over either monotherapy appeared to persist. After termination of the acute phase and continuation of treatment, the combined therapy was more effective than pharmacotherapy alone (RR: 1.61; 95% CI: 1.23 to 2.11) and was as effective as psychotherapy (RR: 0.96; 95% CI: 0.79 to 1.16). The authors concluded that either combined therapy or psychotherapy alone may be chosen as first-line treatment for panic disorder with or without agoraphobia, depending on patient preference.

Furukawa TA, Watanabe N, Churchill R. Combined psychotherapy plus antidepressants for panic disorder with or without agoraphobia. *Cochrane Database Syst Rev*. 2007;1:CD004364.

80. Answer: D. Methadone maintenance treatment for Opioid Dependence is associated with reduced IV drug use, reduced relapse to IV drug use, reduction in crime days, reduced death rates, and a reduced HIV seroconversion rates. Long-term follow up of children who were exposed to methadone *in utero* found no cognitive impairment in preschool years. There are no serious adverse effects associated with methadone maintenance treatment. Minor side effects include constipation, excessive sweating, drowsiness, and decreased sexual interest and performance. A maintenance dose of 60 mg/day or more of methadone has been shown to have better outcome than lower doses. The initial dose of methadone should not exceed 30 mg for the first dose and 40 mg for the first day. After the initial dose, methadone dose is carefully adjusted over 4 to 5 days (the induction phase) to achieve a plasma steady state. The risk of overdose and intoxication is highest during this phase, and any sign of overmedication warrants a dose reduction.

Graham AW, Schultz TK, Mayo-Smith MF, et al. *Principles of Addiction Medicine*. 3rd ed. Chevy Chase, Maryland: American Society of Addiction Medicine; 2003:735–758.

81. Answer: E. All tricyclic and tetracyclic antidepressants are approved by the FDA for the treatment of depression. Due to its potent serotonin reuptake blockade, clomipramine has been found to be effective in OCD, and is approved by the FDA for use in this condition. Tricyclics are used for a variety of other conditions without FDA approval including Panic Disorder, Bulimia, Narcolepsy, Enuresis, migraine prophylaxis, neuralgia, peptic ulcer, urticaria, and ADHD. The reports of sudden death in children under 12 years of age (most likely of the cardiac origin) have substantially reduced the use of these agents in younger patients.

1. Sadock BJ, Sadock VA. *Kaplan and Sadock's Comprehensive Textbook of Psychiatry*. 7th ed. Philadelphia: Lippincott Williams & Wilkins; 2000:2491–2502.
2. Schatzberg AF, Nemeroff CB. *Textbook of Psychopharmacology*. 2nd ed. Washington: American Psychiatric Press; 1998:199–218.

82. Answer: C. The exact mechanism of action of bupropion is unclear. However, it is thought to exert its effect by enhancing noradrenergic and dopaminergic activity. It is rapidly absorbed after oral administration, and undergoes extensive hepatic metabolism. Therapeutic indications of bupropion include major depression, ADHD, and smoking cessation. It is rarely associated with the side effect of seizure induction. The use of bupropion should be avoided in patients with bulimia nervosa due to reports of grand mal seizures. Unlike SSRIs and SNRIs, bupropion does not cause sexual side effects.

Schatzberg AF, Nemeroff CB. *Textbook of Psychopharmacology*. 2nd ed. Washington: American Psychiatric Press; 1998:257–261.

83. Answer: E. Valproic acid falls under category X. It has proved fetal risk in humans and is contraindicated in pregnancy, even in life-threatening situations. One to two percent of fetuses exposed to valproic acid develop neural tube-like defects, a 10- to 20-fold increase over the general population.

1. Sadock BJ, Sadock VA. *Kaplan and Sadock's Comprehensive Textbook of Psychiatry*. 8th ed. Philadelphia: Lippincott Williams & Wilkins; 2005:2309.
2. Schachter SC. *Risks Associated With Epilepsy and Pregnancy*. http://www.uptodateonline.com/utd/content/topic.do?topicKey=epil_eeg/3066&type=A&selectedTitle=8~268. Accessed March 4, 2007.

84. Answer: E. All of the answers listed and social skills training are helpful for the chronic management of patients with Schizophrenia.

Lehman AF, Lieberman JA, Dixon LB, et al. *Quick Reference to the American Psychiatric Association Practice Guidelines for the Treatment of Psychiatric Disorders*. Arlington: American Psychiatric Association; 2004:77.

85. Answer: D. Interferon-α is a cytokine host defense protein and immune modulator produced by the lymphocytes and is indicated for the treatment of hepatitis C, melanoma, and renal cell carcinoma. Interferon-α therapy is associated with a variety of psychiatric symptoms. Treatment emergent depression is a frequent reason for premature termination of INF therapy. Dose and duration of INF therapy, pretreatment depressive symptoms, particularly mild depression, have been shown to be risk factors for INF-induced depression. Age, gender, and history of substance use have not been shown to impact this risk for depression. Depression occurring in INF-treated patients typically becomes evident and peaks at week 4 and week 24 respectively. Although there are studies suggesting that prophylactic antidepressant therapy may lead to significant reduction in depression rates among patients undergoing INF therapy, this mode of intervention is currently not approved by the FDA nor is it routine standard of care.

1. Dieperink E, Willenbring M, Ho SB. Neuropsychiatric symptoms associated with hepatitis C and interferon alpha: a review. *Am J Psychiatry*. 2000;157:867–876.
2. Hauser P, Khosla J, Aurora H, et al. A prospective study of the incidence and open-label treatment of interferon-

induced major depressive disorder in patients with hepatitis C. *Mol Psychiatry*. 2002;7:942–947.
3. Raison CL, Borisov AS, Broadwell SD, et al. Depression during pegylated interferon-alpha plus ribavirin therapy: prevalence and prediction. *J Clin Psychiatry*. 2005;66: 41–48.

86. Answer: B. Normally the CSF is clear and colorless. A traumatic tap (in which blood from the epidural venous plexus has been introduced into the spinal fluid) may seriously confuse the diagnosis, if it is incorrectly interpreted. To distinguish between two types of "bloody tap," two or three serial samples of fluid should be taken at the time of the LP. With a traumatic tap, there is usually a decreasing number of RBC in the second and third tubes. In a traumatic tap, the CSF pressure is usually normal. If a large amount of blood is mixed with the fluid, it will clot or form fibrinous webs. Prompt centrifugation of bloody fluid from a traumatic tap will yield a colorless supernatant. Only large amounts of blood will result in the supernatant being xanthochromic, due to contamination with serum bilirubin and lipochromes. The fluid from a traumatic tap usually should contain one or two WBCs per 1,000 RBC. These changes are not seen with preexistent hemorrhage because the blood has been greatly diluted with CSF and defibrinated. In subarachnoid hemorrhage, the RBC begins to hemolyze within a few hours, imparting a pink-red discoloration (erythrochromia) to the supernatant fluid. If allowed to stand for a day or more, the fluid becomes yellow-brown (xanthochromia).

Ropper AH, Brown RH. *Adams and Victor's Principles of Neurology*. 8th ed. http://www.accessmedicine.com/content.aspx?aID=970233. Accessed May 9, 2007.

87. Answer: D. Carotid ultrasound (carotid duplex) is a test that is widely available, inexpensive, noninvasive, and reliable in determining carotid artery patency. It uses sound waves to map the carotid arteries, and the flow of blood through them. MRA and CTA are not yet as widely available, though are quickly becoming more popular. MRA and CTA are more expensive and require more equipment, thus are less portable. Although generally safe, they may require dye for certain procedures. Conventional x-ray angiography is capable of testing carotid artery patency, possibly providing the most precise and reliable images, but is the most invasive and least safe of the alternatives. Because of this, its use is limited to special situations. It is widely available, but not as frequently utilized as ultrasound for evaluating the carotids. Physical examination, including palpation and auscultation for bruits is safe, available, inexpensive, and noninvasive. However, it is possibly the least reliable and most inconsistent of the listed techniques in measuring carotid patency.

Ropper AH, Brown RH. *Adams and Victor's Principles of Neurology*. 8th ed. New York: McGraw-Hill; 2005:11–38.

88. Answer: A. Memory loss has not clearly been associated with uncomplicated aging, and may be more appropriately considered as a complication of aging. Early studies on cognition and aging may not have separated out those with pathology related to memory loss, when studying the elderly, thus biasing results. There is still some debate, but it is not clear how much memory loss is truly due to aging alone of the nervous system. Study results are variable. Even ideas such as the "be nine" cognitive loss of *age-associated memory impairment* or *mild cognitive impairment* may actually represent incipient pathology, such as a very early AD. It is likely that some other cognitive changes do occur with normal aging, possibly decreased cognitive flexibility, slowed processing speed, or decline in verbal abilities. These may affect or mimic memory problems. Other more clear signs of uncomplicated neurologic aging include loss of vibratory sense (especially in the lower extremities), depression of DTRs, reduced motor speed and activity, impairment of fine coordination, reduced muscle power, losses in anterior horn cells, loss of the sense of smell (and also possibly taste), progressive hearing loss (especially higher pitches) and speech discrimination, as well as multiple visual changes.

Ropper AH, Brown RH. *Adams and Victor's Principles of Neurology*. 8th Ed. New York: McGraw-Hill; 2005:519–525.

89. Answer: C. There are two forms of porphyria, the acquired and the heritable forms. The genetic categories are further divided into hepatic and erythropoietic types, depending on the site of the enzymatic disorder. Neurologic manifestations are encountered in the AIP and variegate porphyria. These two forms differ primarily in that a rash occurs in the variegate form, but not in AIP. Both are inherited as autosomal dominant traits, with low penetrance. AIP is a disorder of heme biosynthesis that causes intermittent elevations in porphobilinogen and other related porphyrins. The prevalence of AIP is about 1:100,000. All races seem to be affected with women being more often affected than men. Symptoms are rare in childhood and most likely occur in adolescents or young adults.

Rowland LP. *Merritt's Neurology*. 11th ed. Philadelphia: Lippincott Williams & Wilkins; 2005:668–669.

90. Answer: D. *Transient global amnesia* (TGA) is a term that was coined by Fisher and Adams over 40 years ago. It is characterized by an acute inability to retain new information (anterograde amnesia). During the acute stage of this disorder, retrograde amnesia can extend as far back as weeks or months. Many of the patients with TGA repeatedly ask the same questions and seem to be confused and disoriented in time and place. However, loss of self-awareness and consciousness is not seen in typical TGA and patients are able to do complex activities like cooking and driving during these episodes. During an attack, some patients report nausea, vertigo, and headaches. The amnesic syndrome usually resolves spontaneously within 24 hours. The incidence of TGA is five to eleven per 100,000 people per year. The mean age of symptom onset is about 60 years. Although TGA is a benign syndrome, there may be persistent impairment of cognitive functions. Recent evaluation using single-photon-emission CT found persistent hypoperfusion in patients with TGA with recurrent attacks.

Sander K, Sander D. New insights into transient global amnesia: recent imaging and clinical findings. *Lancet Neurol*. 2005;4:437–444.

91. Answer: B. This is a classic presentation of MS. Incidents of MS is two to three times higher in females, and the mean age at onset is 33 years old. Two thirds of the cases have onset between 20 and 40 years old. Pregnancy is one of the best-known precipitating/exacerbating factors. Spending the first 15 years of your life in cool temperate climates increases the risk. Though multiple neurologic symptoms are possible, initial presentation of optic neuritis may occur in up to 25% of patients, and up to 80% may develop it during the course of their illness. Other common symptoms include trigeminal neuralgia, ataxia, incontinence, as well as internuclear ophthalmoplegia (MLF syndrome), the cerebellar disturbance, fatigue, impotence, muscle spasms. A relapsing-remitting course is the most common clinical presentation of MS. MRI shows lesions in 90% of patients with clinically definite MS. Widespread demyelination is the most common MRI finding, ranging from cerebrum, to cerebellum, to spinal cord. Gadolinium enhancement shows active lesions, and T2 weighting reveals lesions of various ages. At least three white matter lesions, especially periventricular, are indicative of MS.

1. Kaufman DM. *Clinical Neurology for Psychiatrists*. 5th ed. Philadelphia: WB Saunders; 2001:369–391.
2. Ropper AH, Brown RH. *Adams and Victor's Principles of Neurology*. 8th ed. New York: McGraw-Hill; 2005: 771–796.

92. Answer: A. Ataxia-telangiectasia is a neurocutaneous disorder with a defect on chromosome 11. They present with immunodeficiency or recurrent/chronic infections due to defects in both cellular and humoral immunity. They may eventually develop lymphomas (as in HIV-related immunodeficiency). Neurologic deficits, often ataxias related to cerebellar vermis degeneration, develops from age 3 to 5; cognitive impairment follows. Telangiectasias (small dilated vessels) aggregate on the conjunctiva, nose, and cheeks. Sturge-Weber syndrome has port-wine stains in trigeminal nerve distribution, and unilateral cerebral atrophy and calcification, often focal deficits, and mental retardation, and seizures. Children with tuberous sclerosis (TS) may have hypopigmented ash-leaf areas on the skin, scaly shagreen patches on the trunk and periungual fibromas, and develop malar angiofibromas in adolescence. Early on, with speech and language delay, some develop mental retardation and seizures, possibly dementia. TS is often due to defects on chromosome 9 or 16. They develop 1 to 3 cm potato-like tubers in the cerebrum, or even retinas, kidneys, or heart. Most children in the United States are screened for PKU shortly after birth. PKU is an autosomal recessive defect on chromosome 12, which results in any buildup of phenylalanine, a deficiency in tyrosine. Undetected and untreated, MR may develop at 8 months old, some develop profound mental retardation. Treatment is via phenylalanine-free diet.

Kaufman DM. *Clinical Neurology for Psychiatrists*. 5th ed. Philadelphia: WB Saunders; 2001:320–346.

93. Answer: B. This is a classic presentation of the overt hydrocephalus. Congenital or infantile hydrocephalus may become a chronic condition. It usually presents in the first months of life. Common etiologies are intraventricular matrix hemorrhages in preemies, infections (especially fetal and neonatal), Arnold-Chiari II malformations, Dandy-Walker syndrome, and aqueductal atresia/stenosis. Eventually, such patients may develop vomiting, poor feeding, downward gaze (setting sun sign), feeble movements, tremulous, and clumsiness. Acute exacerbations may occur. Because the sutures are not fused in infants, the skull may expand, and papilledema may be absent early in the course. This does not mean the findings are normal. Cerebral palsy would not likely present with an enlarged skull. Infratentorial tumors would be more likely to lead to hydrocephalus. Fetal alcohol syndrome fits a separate pattern. Although, pseudotumor cerebri is not common in infants, it can occur in some children, more so in adolescent females. It often presents with papilledema and headaches.

Ropper AH, Brown RH. *Adams and Victor's Principles of Neurology*. 8th ed. New York: McGraw-Hill; 2005:529–545.

94. Answer: D. Fetal hydantoin syndrome is a teratogenic effect caused by the use of phenytoin and carbamazepine during pregnancy. This syndrome consists of craniofacial abnormalities including midfacial hypoplasia, fingernail and lower distal digital hypoplasia, cardiac abnormalities, growth deficiency, developmental delay, and facial clefts. The use of phenobarbital during pregnancy has been associated with urinary tract malformations.

Cunningham FG, Leveno KL, Bloom SL. *Williams Obstetrics*. 22nd ed. http://www.accessmedicine.com/content.aspx?aID=722696. Accessed March 26, 2007.

95. Answer: C. Erikson's stage of "initiative versus guilt" occurs during the preschool age, ranging from approximately 3 to 5 years of age. "Trust versus mistrust" occurs during infancy, "autonomy versus shame and doubt" occurs during toddlerhood, "initiative versus guilt" in preschool years, "industry versus inferiority" during school-age years, and "identity versus role confusion" during adolescence.

Hales RE, Yudofsky SC. *Textbook of Clinical Psychiatry*. 4th ed. Washington: American Psychiatric Publishing; 2003:67–105.

96. Answer: B. Amino acid tryptophan depletion studies have explored the role of serotonin in development of mood disorders and have contributed to some of the best evidence for the "serotonin hypothesis" of depression. This hypothesis posits that serotonin system deficiency contributes to the development of depression. According to this hypothesis, one would expect tryptophan depletion to result in worsening of depression, since agents that increase brain serotonin (like SSRIs and MAOIs) improve depression. However, research shows that not all patients develop depression with serotonin depletion and not all depressed patients recover with SSRIs or MAOIs. Thus, the etiology of depression may include other factors than serotonin. Among depressed patients with MDD who responded to SSRIs (such as fluoxetine), tryptophan depletion transiently reverses antidepressant response and causes a brief return of core depressive symptoms during the maximal depletion relative to the patients who received placebo. Similar increase in depression occurred among patients with MDD who responded to mirtazapine, among seasonal affective disorder patients who responded to light therapy, and among healthy subjects with positive family history for depression. In contrast, patients with MDD who responded to TCAs (noradrenergic antidepressants, such as desipramine) were less likely to have depressive symptoms on tryptophan depletion. This data speaks to the importance of both serotonergic and noradrenergic systems in mediating development of depression.

1. Delgado PL, Miller HL, Salomon RM, et al. Tryptophan-depletion challenge in depressed patients treated with desipramine or fluoxetine: implications for the role of serotonin in the mechanism of antidepressant action. *Biol Psychiatry*. 1999;46:212–220.
2. Stein DJ, Kupfer DJ, Schatzberg AF. *Textbook of Mood Disorders*. Washington: American Psychiatric Publishing; 2006:104–106.

97. Answer: B. In dream interpretation, the term condensation refers to the melding or fusing of several dream thoughts or symbols into one image. The true meaning of a dream image is called the *latent content*, while the manifest content is the surface representation. Repression is a defense mechanism used to keep unacceptable wishes and desires from conscious thought. Preservation of a painful memory, with no connected emotional reaction to it, is achieved through the use of the defense mechanism, isolation of affect.

Bateman A, Holmes J. *Introduction to Psychoanalysis: Contemporary Theory and Practice*. London: Routledge; 1995:76–94, 118–135.

98. Answer: E. Seclusion and restraint use is contraindicated for the purposes of staff convenience or as a means of punishment. Indications for seclusion and restraint include imminent harm, minimization of significant disruption, patient request to maintain safety, and assistance in ongoing behavior therapy.

Sadock BJ, Sadock VA. *Kaplan and Sadock's Comprehensive Textbook of Psychiatry*. 8th ed. Philadelphia: Lippincott Williams & Wilkins; 2005:3980.

99. Answer: B. Management of psychiatric illness can be complicated by comorbid endocrine disease, and knowledge of various endocrine abnormalities can be useful. The dexamethasone-suppression test, while not recommended for routine clinical use, is sometimes useful in severe or psychotic depression. Lithium has been shown to decrease the sensitivity of renal tubules to antidiuretic hormone, which may lead to an acquired form of nephrogenic diabetes insipidus (excessive clearance of water by the kidneys). Prolactin levels often become elevated by antipsychotic agents, particularly risperidone and typical antipsychotics. Additionally, prolactin levels may

briefly rise after a seizure, which can help distinguish a seizure from a pseudoseizure. Disease of the thyroid is associated with many psychiatric manifestations, particularly depression and anxiety. Interpretation of thyroid function tests is made difficult by transient abnormalities of thyroid function in many newly admitted psychiatric patients. These abnormalities normalize over time without treatment and may be related to stress. Measurement of insulin level is helpful in detecting antipsychotic related glucose intolerance.

Sadock BJ, Sadock VA. *Kaplan and Sadock's Comprehensive Textbook of Psychiatry*. 8th ed. Philadelphia: Lippincott Williams & Wilkins; 2005:924–926.

100. Answer: E. Patients with Borderline Personality Disorder require stability, which may involve an explicit discussion of the nature and limits of a psychotherapy relationship, as well as attention to rapport and countertransference feelings. While some flexibility is needed, setting limits or boundaries is often also an important component of treating these patients. Patients with Borderline Personality Disorder can be impulsive and therefore an increase in self-reflection, especially before impulsive actions, should be encouraged.

Gabbard GO. *Psychodynamic Psychiatry in Clinical Practice*. 3rd ed. Washington: American Psychiatric Press; 2000:438–446.

101. Answer: D. Emerging consensus suggests that DLB represents a distinct pathologic entity that lies somewhere between AD and Parkinson's disease pathologically. Whereas AD is associated with amyloid plaques and NFTs in the parietal, parieto-occipital and temporal cortex, Parkinson's disease is characterized by the presence of Lewy bodies in the subcortical regions of locus ceruleus and substantia nigra. On the other hand, DLB is associated with the presence of Lewy bodies in the subcortical and cortical areas, predominantly frontotemporal regions of the brain and amyloid plaques. Neurofibrillary tangles are not common findings in DLB. No specific risk factors have been identified in DLB.

1. McKeith I, Mintzer J, Aarsland D, et al. Dementia with Lewy bodies. *Lancet Neurol*. 2004;3:19–28.
2. Nussbaum RL, Ellis CE. Alzheimer's disease and Parkinson's disease. *N Engl J Med*. 2003;348:1356–1364.

102. Answer: D. All of the choices are types of paraphilias. Voyeurism involves intense sexually arousing fantasies, sexual urges, or behaviors involving the act of observing an unsuspecting person who is naked, in the process of disrobing, or engaging in sexual activity. Fetishism involves recurrent, intense sexually arousing fantasies, sexual urges, or behaviors involving the use of nonliving objects (e.g., female undergarments). Pedophilia involves recurrent, intense sexually arousing fantasies, sexual urges, or behaviors involving sexual activity with a prepubescent child or children. The person is at least age 16 years and at least 5 years older than the child or children. Frotteurism involves recurrent, intense sexually arousing fantasies, sexual urges, or behaviors involving touching and rubbing against a nonconsenting person. Exhibitionism is a type of paraphilia in which an individual experiences recurrent, intense sexually arousing fantasies, urges, or behaviors involving the exposure of one's genitals to an unsuspecting stranger. In order to make a diagnosis of a paraphilia, the timeframe must be at least 6 months, and the individual must have experienced marked distress and interpersonal difficulties due to acting on these urges or fantasies.

American Psychiatric Association. *Quick Reference to the Diagnostic Criteria from DSM-IV-TR*. Washington: American Psychiatric Association; 2000:255–258.

103. **Answer: C.** Mood and anxiety disorders are commonly associated with Avoidant Personality Disorder. Of these, the most frequently associated disorder is Social Phobia of the Generalized Type. Avoidant Personality Disorder has also been associated with Dependent Personality Disorder, because these individuals become very attached and dependent on the few people that they can trust and consider friends.

American Psychiatric Association. *Diagnostic and Statistical Manual of Mental Disorders (DSM-IV-TR)*. 4th ed. (Text revision). http://www.psychiatryonline.com/content.aspx?aID=4125. Accessed March 28, 2007.

104. **Answer: C.** A Cochrane review determining whether the use of specific antipsychotics for similar groups of people could be a treatment for established TD, included five trials. One small 2-week study (n=18), reported on the 'masking' effects of molindone and haloperidol on TD, which favored haloperidol (RR: 3.44; 95% CI: 1.1 to 5.8). Two (total n=17) studies found no reduction in TD associated with neuroleptic reduction (RR: 0.38; 95% CI: 0.1 to 1.0). One study (n=20) found no significant differences in oral dyskinesia (RR: 2.45; 95% CI: 0.3 to 19.7) when antipsychotics were compared as a specific treatment for TD. There was no significant difference in dyskinesia (n=32; RR: 0.62; 95% CI: 0.3 to 1.26) between quetiapine and haloperidol, when these antipsychotics were used as specific treatments for TD. However, the need for additional antipsychotics was significantly lower in the quetiapine group (n=47; RR: 0.49; 95%

CI: 0.2 to 1.0) than in those given haloperidol. The authors concluded that the limited data available from small studies using antipsychotic reduction or specific antipsychotic drugs as treatments for TD did not provide any convincing evidence of the value of these approaches. There is a need for larger trials of a longer duration in order to fully investigate this area.

Soares-Weiser K, Rathbone J. Neuroleptic reduction and/or cessation and neuroleptics as specific treatments for tardive dyskinesia. *Cochrane Database Syst Rev*. 2006;1:CD000459.

105. **Answer: B.** Naltrexone is a long-acting opioid antagonist that provides a complete blockade of the reinforcing properties of opioids, and therefore, is an ideal maintenance agent. However, the treatment retention rate for this agent is only 20% to 30% at 6 months and 10% to 20% at 1 year. The one-year retention rates for methadone (50% to 60%), buprenorphine-naloxone (40% to 50%), and LAAM (50% to 80%) are significantly higher as compared to naltrexone treatment. Buprenorphine is used for short-term detoxification from opioids, and is combined with naloxone for maintenance treatment to obviate IV abuse. However, it is used for maintenance treatment in pregnancy.

1. Graham AW, Schultz TK, Mayo-Smith MF, et al. *Principles of Addiction Medicine*. 3rd ed. Chevy Chase, Maryland: American Society of Addiction Medicine; 2003:735–748.
2. Kirchmayer U, Davoli M, Verster AD, et al. A systematic review on the efficacy of naltrexone maintenance treatment in opioid dependence. *Addiction*. 2002;97:1241–1249.

106. **Answer: D.** TCAs can cause postural hypotension and reflex tachycardia by blocking $\alpha 1$- adrenergic receptors. Tachycardia is also believed to occur because of norepinephrine reuptake blockade. Most dangerous side effect of the TCAs is a quinidine-like, membrane-stabilizing effect resulting in slowed impulse conduction. Patients with a QTc interval of 450 milliseconds or more are at increased risk for conduction delay and heart-block, and therefore, should not be treated with TCAs. They are lethal in overdose most commonly due to cardiac toxicity. Blockade of muscarinic receptors produce blurred vision, dry mouth due to decreased salivation, constipation, urinary retention, and cognitive dysfunction. At blood concentrations above 300 ng/ml, they can cause delirium (therapeutic level: 50 to 150 ng/ml). TCAs cause extrapyramidal movement disorders by blocking D2 receptors, and sedation and weight gain by blockade of histamine (H1) receptors.

1. Sadock BJ, Sadock VA. *Kaplan and Sadock's Comprehensive Textbook of Psychiatry*. 7th ed. Philadelphia: Lippincott Williams & Wilkins; 2000:2491–2502.

606 TEST X · Answers

2. Schatzberg AF, Nemeroff CB. *Textbook of Psychopharmacology*. 2nd ed. Washington: American Psychiatric Press; 1998:199–218.

107. Answer: D. Stimulants in combination with TCAs or SSRIs have been shown to be effective for the treatment of refractory depression. Several studies support the use of lithium in combination with antidepressants in resistant depression. Lithium can be safely combined with MAOIs as well for treating refractory depression. Other augmentation strategies include combining antidepressants with atypical antipsychotic agents, triiodothyronine, buspirone, pindolol, and dopaminergic agonists (pergolide, amantadine, pramipexole, and ropinirole). One small, double-blind study reported positive results from the use of testosterone gel (1% gel, 10 g/d) in men, and estrogen has limited support from mostly anecdotal evidence. Inositol was found to be no better than placebo in a double-blind study.

Nierenberg AA, Katz J, Fava M. A critical overview of the pharmacologic management of treatment-resistant depression. *Psychiatr Clin North Am*. 2007;30:13–29.

108. Answer: E. Erik Erikson developed the concepts of adult identity and identity crisis. Leo Kanner wrote the first English-language textbook of child psychiatry. Donald Winnicott first described the concept of transitional objects. Burrhus Skinner described operant conditioning. Sigmund Freud first described the unconscious and infantile sexuality, laying the foundation of psychoanalysis.

Sadock BJ, Sadock VA. *Kaplan and Sadock's Comprehensive Textbook of Psychiatry*. 8th ed. Philadelphia: Lippincott Williams & Wilkins; 2005:4026.

109. Answer: B. Indications for inpatient treatment of anorexia nervosa in adults, according to the American Psychiatric Association Practice Guidelines, include weight less than 75% of the expected or standard weight, a pulse of less than 40 beats per minute, blood pressure less than 90/60 mm of Hg, blood glucose less than 60 mg/dL, potassium less than 3 mEq/L, electrolyte imbalance, dehydration, temperature less than 97.0°F, or significant hepatic, renal, or cardiovascular compromise. Suicidality, comorbid psychiatric disorders, and noncompliance with care in less structured settings are also important factors to consider when determining if inpatient hospitalization is indicated.

Yager J, Devlin MJ, Halmi KA, et al. *Quick Reference to the American Psychiatric Association Practice Guidelines for the Treatment of Psychiatric Disorders*. Arlington: American Psychiatric Association; 2004:149.

110. Answer: C. A major glutamate receptor, NMDA is a multimolecular protein with binding sites for several neurotransmitters and drugs including glycine, PCP, ketamine, lamotrigine and riluzole. Several of these either stimulate or inhibit the NMDA receptor resulting in far reaching physiologic and pathologic consequences. In healthy humans, this receptor under the modulation of the inhibitory neurotransmitter, glycine, regulates calcium channels. A number of neurotransmitters and drugs mediate various pathologic and therapeutic activities. For example, glutamate (the brain's major excitatory neurotransmitter) may lead to overstimulation, excitotoxicity, and neuron death. This is believed to be the pathologic basis of several neurodegenerative diseases including AD, Parkinson's disease, stroke, and ALS. This has therapeutic implications. For example, memantine (a medication approved for treating Alzheimer's disease) is an NMDA receptor antagonist, while riluzole (which slows progress of ALS) acts by decreasing glutamate activity, as does lamotrigine (the antiepileptic drug). PCP acts by binding to the NMDA receptor and prevents the stimulating activity of glutamate.

1. Greenamyre JT, Porter RH, Greenamyre JT, et al. Anatomy and physiology of glutamate in the CNS. *Neurology*. 1994;44(suppl 8):S7–S13.
2. Lipton SA, Rosenberg PA. Excitatory amino acids as a final common pathway for neurologic disorders. *N Engl J Med*. 1994;330:613–622.

111. Answer: A. The greatest risk factor for a CVA is age. About 75% of the strokes occur after the age of 65 years. Hypertension leads to CVA in middle aged and older people. Both systolic and diastolic hypertension is associated with CVA. Smokers are four times more likely to have a CVA compared to non-smokers. Smokers who are also hypertensive have a twenty-fold increased risk of having a CVA. Migraines are a risk factor in younger adults, accounting for about 25% of the CVAs in this population.

Kaufman DM. *Clinical Neurology for Psychiatrists*. 5th ed. Philadelphia: WB Saunders; 2001:274.

112. Answer: D. Excitatory postsynaptic potentials and inhibitory postsynaptic potentials are depolarizing or polarizing potentials respectively that either induce or inhibit the firing of an action potential in a summative fashion. For example, an excitatory action potential itself does not typically generate an action potential, but several excitatory postsynaptic potentials combined will provide enough depolarization to generate an action potential. Excitatory postsynaptic potentials are usually produced by the opening of sodium and calcium channels, whereas inhibitory postsynaptic potentials are generated by the opening of chloride and potassium channels. The neurotransmitter glutamate mediates excitatory action potentials and GABA and glycine mediate inhibitory postsynaptic potentials.

1. Kandel ER, Schwartz JH, Jessel TM. *Principles of Neural Science*. 4th ed. New York: McGraw Hill; 2000:209–218.
2. Katzung BG, Trevor AJ. *Examination and Board Review: Pharmacology*. 5th ed. Stamford: Appleton & Lange; 1998:165–166.

113. Answer: C. Of those listed, only cerebellar damage is correctly paired with ataxic gait. In NPH, gait apraxia is noted. Parkinson's disease is associated with festinating gait. Hemiparetic gait is seen CVA. Steppage gait is seen in tabes dorsalis and peripheral neuropathies.

Kaufman DM. *Clinical Neurology for Psychiatrists*. 5th ed. Philadelphia: WB Saunders; 2001:15.

114. Answer: E. None of these facts are true of AIP. The symptoms of an attack of AIP are most commonly gastrointestinal (attributed to autonomic neuropathy) in nature. Abdominal pain is most common and may occur alone or with a neurologic or psychiatric disorder. There is usually no abdominal rigidity, but fever, leukocytosis, and diarrhea or constipation are often present. Common psychiatric presentations may include conversion reaction, acute delirium, mood change, or an acute or chronic psychosis. During such attacks, MRI studies reveal transient cerebral lesions. AIP may be mistaken for Schizophrenia, as neurological signs may be absent and the psychiatric symptoms may be the most prominent presentation. A higher incidence of Anxiety Disorders was found in asymptomatic carrier family members (indicating that even mild elevations in porpholbilinogen concentration may cause significant psychological symptoms. The diagnosis of AIP is important as many psychotropic medications may induce or exacerbate an acute attack. Symptoms of the neuropathy may be purely motor and are almost always associated with abdominal pain. Only 25% recover completely with others being left with some neurologic disability. Survivors may have recurrent attacks. Cerebral manifestations are unusual, except for the syndrome of inappropriate secretion of antidiuretic hormone.

1. Rowland LP. *Merritt's Neurology*. 11th ed. Philadelphia: Lippincott Williams & Wilkins; 2005:668–669.
2. Estrov Y, Scaglia F, Bodamer OA. Psychiatric symptoms of inherited metabolic disease. *J Inherit Metab Dis*. 2000;23:2–6.

115. Answer: B. The diagnosis of MG is confirmed by serological tests that detect anti-AChR or anti-MuSK antibodies and sometimes antibodies against other muscle proteins (actin, striational protein) and electrodiagnostic tests that detect characteristic defects in neuromuscular transmission. The demonstration of serum anti-AChR antibodies proves the diagnosis of MG. However, their absence does not exclude MG because anti-AChR antibodies are detectable only in 80% to 90% of MG patients generalized symptoms and 30% to 50% of MG patients with ocular symptoms. In patients with MG symptoms who do not have detectable anti-AChR antibodies, serologic diagnosis of MG can be made by determining the presence of anti-MuSK antibodies. In about 5% of MG patients, they neither have anti-AChR nor anti-MuSK antibodies. Standard electrodiagnostic tests that utilize repetitive stimulation of peripheral nerves are commonly used to detect neuromuscular transmission defect in MG. They are relatively sensitive and reliable. The most sensitive electrodiagnostic test for MG is single-fiber electromyography, which reveals deficits of neuromuscular transmission in 95% to 99% of MG patients and excludes the diagnosis of MG when it yields normal results.

Conti-Fine BM, Milani M, Kaminski HJ. Myasthenia gravis: past, present, and future. *J Clin Invest*. 2006;116:2843–2854.

116. Answer: E. No single laboratory or imaging test alone is diagnostic of MS. Characteristic clinical picture combined with objective testing (especially MRI) has a 90% diagnostic accuracy. CSF findings of elevated IgG oligoclonal bands or IgG index, or myelin basic protein from the breakdown of myelin, are nonspecific findings for CNS illness. Increased latencies on various evoked response tests may be found in MS and they may help localize these deficits or lesions that are detectable on the neurological examination. However, none of these findings are diagnostic of MS. Common tests, also called *evoked potential tests*, are visual evoked responses, brainstem auditory evoked responses, and somatosensory evoked responses. CT imaging is insensitive and often not useful in MS. MRI is much more sensitive and the most important diagnostic test. It may reveal asymptomatic as well as symptomatic lesions. T1 gadolinium enhancement (open rings) shows active lesions and T2 imaging shows new and old lesions. Three lesions in the heavily demyelinated areas are suggestive of MS. MRI may allow monitoring for the development of new lesions. Common MRI findings include enlarged ventricles, corpus callosum atrophy, and periventricular white matter demyelination.

1. Kaufman DM. *Clinical Neurology for Psychiatrists*. 5th ed. Philadelphia: WB Saunders; 2001:369–391.
2. Ropper AH, Brown RH. *Adams and Victor's Principles of Neurology*. 8th ed. New York: McGraw-Hill; 2005:771–796.

117. **Answer: B.** This is a classic presentation of Friedreich's ataxia, of the early onset type. Friedreich's ataxia comprises about half the cases of hereditary ataxias. It has been traced to a GAA trinucleotide repeat on and autosomal recessive intron of a gene coding for the protein "frataxin" on chromosome 9. Pes cavus (with hammertoes) and kyphoscoliosis (which can restrict respirations) are found in some patients. Over half the patients with Friedreich's ataxia will have a cardiomyopathy, and may develop (and/or die from) congestive heart failure or arrhythmias. Mentation is usually preserved, but emotional lability may be noticeable. Little affective therapy is known. Guillain-Barré syndrome is an acute ascending inflammatory polyneuropathy, which occurs after an illness, without the findings characteristic for Friedreich's ataxia, and without prominent ataxia. MG produces weakness and fatigue ability more than ataxia. Acute cerebellitis can occur with febrile illness, but would not be progressive, though may have residual symptoms. ALS presents later and with more weakness than ataxia.

Kaufman DM. *Clinical Neurology for Psychiatrists*. 5th ed. Philadelphia: WB Saunders; 2001:641, 931–938.

118. **Answer: C.** NPH occurs when hydrocephalus reaches equilibrium, CSF formation decreases (due to downstream pressure), CSF reabsorption increases (due to upstream pressure), and intracranial pressure gradually falls to a high normal level. The classic triad of findings in NPH is an early progressive gait apraxia, followed by impaired cognition, and then urinary incontinence. Pedal grasp reflexes and falling attacks may occur. Complaints of weakness and tiredness of the legs are common. Headaches are infrequent. Papilledema and Babinski signs are not present. Gait may appear Parkinsonian (shuffling, stooped, and short steps), but the entire clinical picture for Parkinson's disease is not met. The gait has been described as a "magnetic gait" (with trouble at steps and curbs), and in more advanced states as *astasia-abasia*. Cognitive difficulties are often consistent with frontal dysfunction, but may also include memory deficits. Urinary urgency, frequency, and incontinence typically appear later in the syndrome.

1. Kaufman DM. *Clinical Neurology for Psychiatrists*. 5th ed. Philadelphia: WB Saunders; 2001:145–147.
2. Ropper AH, Brown RH. *Adams and Victor's Principles of Neurology*. 8th ed. New York: McGraw-Hill; 2005:529–545.

119. **Answer: C.** MS is a chronic illness characterized by episodes of focal neurological disorders of the optic nerves, the spinal cord, and the brain. Multiple therapies have been used to treat acute attacks and to try to slow the progression of this illness. These treatments include corticosteroids, ACTH, cyclophosphamide, interferon-β, mitoxantrone, and natalizumab, among others. Corticosteroids are the treatment of choice for acute attacks. However, their prolonged use after an acute attack has not shown any beneficial effect. Interferon-β has shown to have a modest effect on decreasing the severity and frequency of relapses in MS. Natalizumab is a novel treatment that has shown to have a slight effect in reducing the number of relapses and decreasing the MRI lesions. However, it is not considered a first-line agent in the treatment of MS. Amantadine has shown to help with fatigue in patients with MS. Bethanecol is a very helpful agent to treat urinary retention in MS.

Ropper AH, Brown RH. *Adams and Victor's Principles of Neurology*. 8th ed. http://www.accessmedicine.com/content.aspx?aID=974933. Accessed March 26, 2007.

120. **Answer: C.** According to Gesell's developmental schedules, with typical gross and fine motor skills, a 30-month-old can ride a tricycle using pedals, turn pages singly, alternate feet going up stairs, and build a tower of nine blocks. Other developmental landmarks at 30 months (2 1/2 years) include:

Adaptive function: Naming his/her own drawings, imitating horizontal strokes and circles, and repeating two digits.
Language: Speaking in eight to nine word sentences, using "he/she" correctly, relating events of 2 to 3 days ago, and carrying a tune.
Personal/Social: Pour from glass to glass, keep time to music, pull up pants, put shoes on, and name self in the mirror.

Hales RE, Yudofsky SC. *Textbook of Clinical Psychiatry*. 4th ed. Washington: American Psychiatric Publishing; 2003:67–105.

121. **Answer: D.** Reliability is the extent to which a measurement instrument yields consistent results over repeated observations or measurements under the same conditions each time. There are three ways that reliability is usually estimated: interrater, test/retest, and internal consistency. Validity is the degree to which a measurement instrument yields the best available approximation to the truth of a given conclusion. Validity estimates include convergent, discriminant, and responsive to change validity. The Hamilton Rating Scale for Depression and the Montgomery-Asberg Depression Rating Scale have the highest reliability and validity of all of the clinician-rated dimensional scales for depression.

The Hamilton Rating Scale for Depression's reliability is good to excellent, including internal consistency and interrater assessments. The Hamilton Rating Scale for Depression's validity appears good based on correlation with other depression symptom measures. It is more problematic in the elderly and the medically ill, in whom the presence of somatic symptoms may not be indicative of major depression. The Montgomery-Asberg Depression Rating Scale has adequate reliability and excellent validity. Overall, mania rating scales have less reliability and validity than depression rating scales. Of all of the clinician-rated dimensional scales for mania, the Young Mania Rating Scale and the Manic-State Rating Scale have the highest reliability and validity. The Young Mania Rating Scale reliability is good based on interrater reliability and internal consistency studies. Validity also appears good based on correlation with other mania measures.

1. Stein DJ, Kupfer DJ, Schatzberg AF. *Textbook of Mood Disorders*. Washington: American Psychiatric Publishing; 2006:76–80.
2. Sadock BJ, Sadock VA. *Kaplan and Sadock's Comprehensive Textbook of Psychiatry*. 8th ed. Philadelphia: Lippincott Williams & Wilkins; 2005:944.

122. Answer: C. Medical malpractice is a civil wrong resulting from a physician's negligence (doing something that the physician should not have done or failing to do something that should have been done). To prove malpractice, the plaintiff (e.g., patient, family, or estate) must establish by a preponderance of the evidence that (a) a doctor-patient relationship existed which created a *duty* of care, (b) there was a *deviation* from the standard of care, (c) the patient was *damaged*, and (d) the deviation *directly* caused the damage. These elements of a malpractice claim are sometimes referred to as the four D's (duty, deviation, damage, and direct causation). In addition to malpractice negligence suits, physicians can also be sued for the intentional torts of assault, battery, false imprisonment, defamation, fraud or misrepresentation, invasion of privacy, and intentional infliction of emotional distress. In an intentional tort, wrongdoers are motivated by the intent to harm another person or realize/should have realized that such harm was likely to result from their actions.

Sadock BJ, Sadock VA. *Kaplan and Sadock's Synopsis of Psychiatry*. 9th ed. Philadelphia: Lippincott Williams & Wilkins; 2003:1351–1352.

123. Answer: B. Within the structure of a mental status examination, thought is usually divided into process (or form) and content. Process or form refers to the way in which a person puts together ideas and associations. Thought process/form may range from logical and coherent to completely illogical and even incomprehensible. Formal thought disorders include circumstantiality, clang associations, derailment, flight of ideas, perseveration, tangentiality, and thought blocking. Content refers to what a person is actually thinking about (e.g., ideas, beliefs, preoccupations, and obsessions). Within a mental status examination, "speech" describes the physical characteristics of verbal output. Speech can be described in terms of its quantity, rate of production, and quality. Concentration is generally considered when describing the sensorium and cognition of the patient. Insight may be defined as a patient's degree of awareness and understanding about being ill.

Sadock BJ, Sadock VA. *Kaplan and Sadock's Synopsis of Psychiatry*. 9th ed. Philadelphia Lippincott Williams & Wilkins; 2003:238–242.

124. Answer: D. In general, the following personality disorders are associated with micropsychotic episodes: schizotypal, paranoid, and borderline personality disorders, and less commonly with narcissistic and histrionic personality disorders.

Shea SC. *Psychiatric Interviewing: The Art of Understanding*. 2nd ed. Philadelphia: WB Saunders; 1998:333.

125. Answer: E. Although the core symptoms of DLB are dementia, delirium, and visual hallucinations with Parkinsonism, a significant proportion of patients manifest extreme sensitivity to antipsychotic medications and REM sleep behavior disorder. An association between restless leg syndrome and LBD has not been described.

1. Knopman DS, Boeve BF, Petersen RC. Essentials of the proper diagnoses of mild cognitive impairment, dementia, and major subtypes of dementia. *Mayo Clin Proc*. 2003;78:1290–1308.
2. Stewart JT. Defining diffuse Lewy body disease. Tetrad of symptoms distinguishes illness from other dementias. *Postgrad Med*. 2003;113:71–75.

126. Answer: B. All of the choices about paraphilias are true except choice B. These disorders tend to be chronic and lifelong. However, both the fantasies and the behaviors often diminish with advancing age in adults.

American Psychiatric Association. *Diagnostic and Statistical Manual of Mental Disorders (DSM-IV-TR)*. 4th ed. (Text revision). http://www.psychiatryonline.com/content.aspx?aID=10252#10252. Accessed March 18, 2007.

127. Answer: A. Individuals with Antisocial Personality Disorder show a pervasive pattern of lack of empathy, disregard, and violation of the rights of others. They don't conform to social norms and show an increased level of irritability and aggressiveness. This personality disorder has been associated with low socioeconomic status and urban settings. Individuals must be at least 18-years-old to be diagnosed with this personality disorder. The overall prevalence of antisocial personality disorder is approximately 3% in males and 1% in females.

American Psychiatric Association. *Diagnostic and Statistical Manual of Mental Disorders (DSM-IV-TR)*. 4th ed. (Text revision). http://www.psychiatryonline.com/content.aspx?aID=3928. Accessed March 28, 2007.

128. Answer: A. In cases of serotonin syndrome, the serotonergic agents must be discontinued. Monitored IV electrolyte solution should also be administered in a hospital environment to maintain diuresis between 50 to 100 mL/h and to avoid the risk of myoglobinuria. β-blockers, which block 5-HT1A receptors, may be helpful in treatment, but their efficacy is not established. Resuscitation (cooling off, mechanical ventilation, anticonvulsant agents, and antihypertensive agents) may be required for serious cases. The effectiveness of cyproheptadine and chlorpromazine has not yet been established in the treatment for serotonin syndrome. Cyproheptadine is a H1-receptor antagonist with anticholinergic and antiserotonergic characteristics. It can cause drowsiness. Chlorpromazine is a 5-HT1A and 5-HT2 receptor antagonist that can have anticholinergic effects and cause hypotension, dystonias, or neuroleptic malignant syndrome. The data for using ziprasidone, for its power for blocking of 5-HT1A receptors, is also not yet established.

Birmes P, Coppin D, Schmitt L, et al. Serotonin syndrome: a brief review. *CMAJ*. 2003;168:1439–1442.

129. Answer: D. Methadone is mu-receptor agonist with a half-life of 24 to 36 hours. The pharmacologic properties of methadone are similar to morphine. It is absorbed well from the gastrointestinal tract, and has a bioavailability of 80% to 90% with oral use. Peak plasma levels occur at 2 to 4 hours. It is highly lipophilic, about 90% of methadone is protein bound after therapeutic doses. It is extensively metabolized in the liver via N-demethylation and cyclization into pyrrolidines and pyrroline. The metabolites are essentially inactive, and are excreted in bile and urine. Repeated administration leads to accumulation of methadone in liver and other tissues, and low concentrations are released into circulation upon discontinuation of methadone administration (reservoir effect), which probably accounts for the mild, protracted withdrawal.

1. Brunton LL, Lazo JS, Parker KL. *Goodman & Gilman's*

The Pharmacological Basis of Therapeutics. 11th ed. New York: McGraw-Hill; 2006:572–573.
2. Graham AW, Schultz TK, Mayo-Smith MF, et al. *Principles of Addiction Medicine*. 3rd ed. Chevy Chase, Maryland: American Society of Addiction Medicine; 2003:751–748.

130. Answer: D. Classic MAOIs (tranylcypromine, phenelzine, and isocarboxazid) exert their effects by inhibiting the breakdown of amines (epinephrine, norepinephrine, serotonin, tyramine, etc.), leading to a reduction in the number of β-adrenoreceptors, α1- and α2-adrenergic receptors, and serotonin-1 and serotonin-2 receptors. They are indicated in the treatment of Major Depressive Disorder, atypical and anergic depression, Dysthymia, Panic Disorder, Social Phobia, OCD, PTSD, dysphoria, Bulimia, and atypical facial pain. The MAOIs are classified according to their structure (hydrazine versus nonhydrazine), by affinity for their substrates (reversible versus nonreversible), or by their selectivity for the A or B MAO isoenzymes. Selegiline is an irreversible MAO-B inhibitor used in the treatment of Parkinson's disease. Moclobemide is a reversible inhibitor of MAO-A, and has been found to be effective in treating various depressive disorders.

1. Sadock BJ, Sadock VA. *Kaplan and Sadock's Comprehensive Textbook of Psychiatry*. 7th ed. Philadelphia: Lippincott Williams & Wilkins; 2000:2397–2407.
2. Schatzberg AF, Nemeroff CB. *Textbook of Psychopharmacology*. 2nd ed. Washington: American Psychiatric Press; 1998:239–249.

131. Answer: A. The serum concentration of lithium can be increased by thiazide diuretics, loop-diuretic (furosemide), and potassium-sparing diuretics. Angiotensin-converting enzyme inhibitors reduce lithium clearance and can contribute to lithium toxicity. There are case reports of neurotoxicity from calcium channel blockers and methyldopa. Propranolol is used for lithium-induced tremors, and is unlikely to cause lithium toxicity. Most of the NSAIDs, with the exception of aspirin and sulindac, reduce renal clearance of lithium, and can cause lithium toxicity. Lithium toxicity usually presents with coarse tremors, dysarthria, ataxia, and may progress to neuromuscular irritability (fasciculations, myoclonus), seizures, coma, and death. It can occur within the therapeutic range (0.6 to 1.2 mEq/L). However, the severity of lithium toxicity generally correlates with the serum concentration of lithium and the length of exposure. The risk factors for lithium toxicity include excessive intake, reduced excretion, drug-interactions, dehydration, and old age. Treatment consists of gastric lavage, correction of dehydration, polystyrene sulfonate (Kayexalate), and polyethylene glycol solution (GoLYTELY).

Hemodialysis is the treatment of choice for severe intoxication.

Sadock BJ, Sadock VA. *Kaplan and Sadock's Comprehensive Textbook of Psychiatry*. 7th ed. Philadelphia: Lippincott Williams & Wilkins; 2000:2377–2390.

132. Answer: D. Focal dystonias including torticollis are localized sustained muscle contraction. They occur spasmodically and are found in middle aged and older patients. The pathogenesis includes hyperactive neuromuscular system. An effective remedy, butulinum toxin acts by binding irreversibly to the presynaptic membrane, where it inhibits the release of acetylcholine and thereby weakens the muscle. Although injected muscles weaken, they remain functional. Botox injection has to be repeated every 3 months if continuing relief of torticollis is to be achieved as Botox is degraded slowly over several weeks.

1. Kaufman DM. Use of botulinum toxin injections for spasmodic torticollis of tardive dystonia. *J Neuropsychiatry Clin Neurosci*. 1994;6:50–53.
2. Tarsy D, Kaufman D, Sethi KD, et al. An open-label study of botulinum toxin A for treatment of tardive dystonia. *Clin Neuropharmacol*. 1997;20:90–93.

133. Answer: D. A major glutamate receptor, NMDA is a multimolecular protein with binding sites for several neurotransmitters and drugs including glycine, PCP, ketamine, lamotrigine, and riluzole. Several of these either stimulate or inhibit the NMDA receptor resulting in far reaching physiologic and pathologic consequences. In healthy humans, this receptor under the modulation of the inhibitory neurotransmitter, glycine, regulates calcium channels. A number of neurotransmitters and drugs mediate various pathologic and therapeutic activities. For example, glutamate (the brain's major excitatory neurotransmitter) may lead to overstimulation, excitotoxicity, and neuron death. This is believed to be the pathologic basis of several neurodegenerative diseases including AD, Parkinson's disease, stroke, and ALS. This has therapeutic implications. For example, memantine (a medication approved for treating Alzheimer's) is an NMDA receptor antagonist, while riluzole (which slows progress of ALS) acts by decreasing glutamate activity, as does lamotrigine (the antiepileptic drug). PCP acts by binding to the NMDA receptor and prevents the stimulating activity of glutamate.

1. Greenamyre JT, Porter RH, Greenamyre JT, et al. Anatomy and physiology of glutamate in the CNS. *Neurology*. 1994;44(suppl 8):S7–S13.
2. Lipton SA, Rosenberg PA. Excitatory amino acids as a final common pathway for neurologic disorders. *N Engl J Med*. 1994;330:613–622.

134. Answer: D. Tendon reflexes are graded from 0 to 4, with 2 being the average. Briskness of reflexes varies in any healthy normal individual. Absence of reflexes (areflexia) that is not asymmetric and not associated with any other neurological problems is not necessarily pathologic. In individuals who are anxious, treated with benzodiazepines, or withdrawing from alcohol, these reflexes may be diffusely increased. In a healthy adult, stimulation of the plantar surface of the foot can result in either no response or plantar flexion (a down-going toe). In individuals with upper motor neuron lesion (e.g., a pyramidal tract lesion), the great toe may dorsiflex (i.e., extend) and the toes fan out. An up-going toe with or without fanning of the other toes is referred to as a *Babinski sign*. The Babinski sign in an adult usually implies structural disease of the CNS or a toxic metabolic encephalopathy.

Schiffer RB, Rao SM, Fogel BS. *Neuropsychiatry*. 2nd ed. Philadelphia: Lippincott Williams & Wilkins; 2003:17.

135. Answer: E. Lesions of the extrapyramidal tract produce Parkinsonism, athetosis, chorea, and hemiballismus. Paresis, abnormal DTRs and Babinski's sign are seen due to damage to the corticospinal (pyramidal) tract.

Kaufman DM. *Clinical Neurology for Psychiatrists*. 5th ed. Philadelphia: WB Saunders; 2001:15.

136. Answer: A. Complex regional pain syndrome (CRPS) is a diagnostic entity comprising reflex sympathetically mediated pain, RSD, and causalgia. Autonomic dysfunction, disproportionate pain, and soft tissue alteration are the common factors underlying these entities. Precipitating injuries are largely minor but may include fractures, peripheral vascular disease, and gun shot wounds. Of these entities, RSD is the commonest. It is not associated with direct nerve damage and treatment consists of blockade of regional sympathetic nerve ganglion, physical therapy, and adjunctive medications. An interesting phenomenon in RSD is pain extending far beyond the precipitating injury as in this case. The most commonly used agents include anticonvulsants, antidepressants, systemic steroids, biphosphates, and opiates, but they have not been adequately studied in the treatment of CRPS. All these agents should be used in conjunction with a comprehensive interdisciplinary approach aimed at functional restoration and improved quality of life of the patient.

1. Harden RN, Bruehl SP. Diagnosis of complex regional pain syndrome: signs, symptoms, and new empirically derived diagnostic criteria. *Clin J Pain*. 2006;22:415–419.

2. Mackey S, Feinberg S. Pharmacologic therapies for complex regional pain syndrome. *Curr Pain Headache Rep.* 2007;11:38–43.
3. Schwartzman RJ. New treatments for reflex sympathetic dystrophy. *N Engl J Med.* 2000;343:654–656.

137. Answer: A. Childbirth is the best-known and most accepted exacerbating factor for developing and triggering MS symptoms. This occurs most commonly during the first 3 months postpartum. In fact, exacerbation rates decreased some during the third trimester. However, keep in mind that no precipitating factor is definitely proven. Other factors that may trigger MS include: infection, head/spine trauma, intervertebral disc surgery, and electrical injury. Smoking, fatigue, and hyperventilation, may also temporally induce neurologic symptoms. Strong data or studies supporting any of these factors are limited. No vaccination has been definitely linked to MS outbreaks.

1. Kaufman DM. *Clinical Neurology for Psychiatrists.* 5th ed. Philadelphia: WB Saunders; 2001:369–391.
2. Ropper AH, Brown RH. *Adams and Victor's Principles of Neurology.* 8th ed. New York: McGraw-Hill; 2005: 771–796.

138. Answer: D. Multiple treatments are used for fatigue in MS. Recognized treatments include amantadine, modafinil, and pemoline. Whether levothyroxine is helpful for MS fatigue is unclear. Potassium channel blockers may be helpful, but are not FDA approved and may provoke seizures. Although depression is common in MS and may present with fatigue, antidepressants usually do not alleviate that fatigue.

1. Kaufman DM. *Clinical Neurology for Psychiatrists.* 5th ed. Philadelphia: WB Saunders; 2001:369–391.
2. Ropper AH, Brown RH. *Adams and Victor's Principles of Neurology.* 8th ed. New York: McGraw-Hill; 2005:771–796.

139. Answer: C. Spinocerebellar ataxias (SCAs) are a group of late onset (often in teens), autosomal dominant cerebellar ataxias, with mutant genes identified in at least fourteen different loci. An expanded polyglutamine molecule leads to cell death. Since each molecule has a different locus, they affect different subpopulations of neurons, and they often have various clinical presentations. Each disorder may have its own associated features: neuropathies, spasticity, and eye movement abnormalities are common. Treatment options are limited, and focus mostly on fall prevention. Friedreich's ataxia is an autosomal recessive mode of inheritance, and often has an earlier onset in childhood. Paraneoplastic ataxias are usually associated with breast and ovarian cancer (anti-Yo antibodies) and is unlikely in this male. This patient is young and unlikely to have developed nu-tritional ataxias, even if drinking alcohol regularly. A stroke is also unlikely due to his age. Prion diseases, such as Creutzfeldt-Jakob disease, can present with ataxia and myoclonus, and often progress rapidly over days to weeks or months, with eventual dementia, and generally affects adults. Some SCAs do have cognitive decline as an associated component.

Ropper AH, Brown RH. *Adams and Victor's Principles of Neurology.* 8th ed. New York: McGraw-Hill; 2005:931–938.

140. Answer: A. Pseudotumor cerebri is a syndrome of headache, papilledema (unilateral or bilateral), with few focal neurologic signs, possibly due to elevated CSF pressure but normal of composition, with normal imaging findings. It is more common in overweight adolescent females, and is often associated with menstrual irregularities. Various etiologies have been described, but the most common is idiopathic ("benign") intracranial hypertension. Other etiologies include cerebral venous hypertension (e.g., venous sinus occlusion), meningeal disease, toxicity (hypervitaminosis A, lead, and tetracycline), corticosteroid use, myxedema, hypoparathyroidism, adrenal dysfunction, Guillain-Barré Syndrome (GBS), and Systemic lupus erythematosus (SLE). Sustained papilledema may result in blindness. Treatments include diuretics, carbonic anhydrase inhibitors, dieting, CSF drainage (LP or shunt), and steroids. Cluster headaches and migraines would not typically present with papilledema and elevated CSF pressure. It is unlikely to be a brain tumor with a normal MRI of the brain. Temporal arteritis usually occurs in patients greater than 50 years of age, with a persistent throbbing headache, and a thickened/tender temporal artery.

1. Kaufman DM. *Clinical Neurology for Psychiatrists.* 5th ed. Philadelphia: WB Saunders; 2001: 216–217.
2. Ropper AH, Brown RH. *Adams and Victor's Principles of Neurology.* 8th ed. New York: McGraw-Hill; 2005: 529–545.

141. Answer: A. The anticonvulsant mechanism of action of phenytoin involves slowing the rate of recovery of voltage-activated sodium channels. Ethosuximide reduces low threshold calcium currents in thalamic neurons. Phenobarbital's mechanism of action involves potentiation of synaptic inhibition through an action on the GABA-A receptor. Although the exact mechanism of action of gabapentin is largely unknown, it may promote nonvesicular release of GABA. Phenytoin does not slow the recovery of chloride channels.

McNamara JO. *Goodman & Gilman's Pharmacological Basis of Therapeutics.* http://www.accessmedicine.com/content.aspx?aID=939716. Accessed March 28, 2007.

142. Answer: C. Piaget developed a theory of cognitive growth that occurs in stages. Piaget's sensorimotor stage occurs from birth to 2 years (using body senses and activity to explore the environment), the pre-operational stage occurs from 2 to 7 years (thinking symbolically but illogically), the concrete operational stage occurs from ages 7 to 10 years (thinking logically and in an organized way), and formal operational development occurs during adolescence from 11 to 19 years (abstract thought develops).

Sadock BJ, Sadock VA. *Kaplan and Sadock's Comprehensive Textbook of Psychiatry*. 7th ed. Philadelphia: Lippincott Williams & Wilkins; 2000:2534–2550.

143. Answer: B. Circadian rhythms exist in most species to help adjust between two periods of distinct activity, diurnal and nocturnal. Human rhythm is slightly longer than 24 hours, and needs to be adjusted by daylight on a daily basis. Light in the evening typically delays sleep onset, but midday light usually has no effect.

Sadock BJ, Sadock VA. *Kaplan and Sadock's Comprehensive Textbook of Psychiatry*. 7th ed. Philadelphia: Lippincott Williams & Wilkins; 2000:133–134.

144. Answer: C. Consanguinity and polygenic inheritance refer to specific characteristics about the heritability of Schizophrenia. The stress diathesis model refers to an underlying predisposition to a particular disease (diathesis), which is activated by stressors in the environment.

Sadock B, Sadock V. *Kaplan and Sadock's Pocket Handbook of Clinical Psychiatry*. 3rd ed. Philadelphia: Lippincott Williams & Wilkins; 2001:105.

145. Answer: E. Antisocial, Narcissistic, and Schizoid Personality Disorders can all be characterized by a low level of empathy for others. Patients with Histrionic Personality Disorder can also exhibit poor empathy for others.

Shea SC. *Psychiatric Interviewing: The Art of Understanding*. 2nd ed. Philadelphia: WB Saunders; 1998:419.

146. Answer: E. Fluctuating mental status occurs frequently in DLB. Some studies suggesting a prevalence of 50% to 70% in these patients. Fluctuations are often dramatic and can mimic delirium, and are often referred to as *pseudodelirium*. The delirium associated with DLB is characterized by daytime drowsiness and lethargy, daytime sleep of 2 or more hours, persistent motionless stare, and episodic disorganized verbalization.

1. Ferman TJ, Smith GE, Boeve BF, et al. DLB fluctuations: specific features that reliably differentiate DLB from AD and normal aging. *Neurology*. 2004;62:181–187.
2. McKeith I, Mintzer J, Aarsland D, et al. Dementia with Lewy bodies. *Lancet Neurol*. 2004;3:19–28.

147. Answer: B. Heroin overdose is one of the leading causes of death among heroin addicts. It is well established that nonfatal overdoses are highly prevalent among those with opioid addiction. One study showed that 23% to 33% of injecting heroin users had taken a nonfatal overdose in the last year and that 43% witnessed a heroin overdose in another user within the last year.

The short-acting opioid antagonist naloxone is an effective substance for treating respiratory depression and coma in patients with an overdose. Treatment of overdose patients should always take into account the specific opioid that caused the overdose, with special emphasis on the half-life of the different opioids. Heroin and prescription opioids such as hydromorphone, morphine, oxycodone, and codeine have a relatively short half-life (2 to 6 hours), and a single dose of naloxone (half-life: 1 to 2 hours) is generally sufficient to solve the problem. However, methadone has a much longer half-life (16 to 48 hours), and multiple treatments with naloxone may be necessary to guarantee a stable solution of a potentially life-threatening situation.

Finally, the partial opioid agonist buprenorphine has a relatively short half-life (3 to 4 hours), but it has a very strong and long-lasting affinity to the mu-opioid receptors and requires higher dosages of naloxone in the case of an overdose. Taken together, it is crucial to ascertain the type of opioid or the combination of opioids responsible for the overdose and to provide adequate dosages of the antidote along with clinical observation of the patient for at least 24 hours.

1. Clarke S, Dargan P. Towards evidence based emergency medicine: best BETs from the Manchester Royal Infirmary. Intravenous bolus or infusion of naloxone in opioid overdose. *Emerg Med J*. 2002;19:249–250.
2. Sporer KA. Acute heroin overdose. *Ann Intern Med*. 1999;130:584–590.
3. Van den Brink W, Haasen C. Evidenced-based treatment of opioid-dependent patients. *Can J Psychiatry*. 2006;51:635–646.
4. Warner-Smith M, Darke S, Lynskey M, et al. Heroin overdose: causes and consequences. *Addiction*. 2001;96:1113–1125.

148. Answer: A. CBT appears to be the most effective nonpharmacological strategy for treatment of Paraphilias and Hyperactive Sexual Disorders. CBT techniques for decreasing and/or controlling sexual urges include satiation, covert sensitization, fading, cognitive restructuring, and victim empathy therapy, as well as methods for enhancing appropriate sexual interest and arousal (e.g., social skills training, assertiveness skills training, sex education, and couples therapy). Twelve-step programs and surveillance networks are also effective modes of treatment of these patients. SSRIs have been studied for the treatment of these disorders in uncontrolled trials and appear promising. Antiandrogens (e.g., estrogen, progesterone, and cyproterone acetate) have demonstrated efficacy in the treatment of paraphilias. The newer gonadotropin-releasing hormone agonists have the advantage over the earlier treatments of being available in long-acting depot formulations and having fewer side effects. Preliminary studies and case reports with these agents appear promising. The treatment algorithm should begin with less restrictive treatments (e.g., behavioral or verbal therapies), if possible, and moving to more restrictive alternatives (e.g., biological therapies and institutionalization) as needed.

Krueger RB, Kaplan MS. Behavioral and psychopharmacological treatment of the paraphilic and hypersexual disorders. *J Psychiatr Pract*. 2002;8:21–32.

149. **Answer: C.** Oxcarbazepine is a structural analog of carbamazepine. In the body, it is rapidly converted to its MHD, which is its main active metabolite. MHD has several pharmacokinetic advantages over carbamazepine, including the absence of autoinduction, less pronounced and more selective induction of P450 enzyme system, and the absence of interaction with agents such as erythromycin or propoxyphene. These drugs usually result in excessive accumulation of carbamazepine.

Abou-Khalil BW, ed. Oxcarbazepine and carbamazepine: expected and unexpected differences and similarities. *Epilepsy Curr*. 2007;7:74–76.

150. **Answer: B.** Most benzodiazepines (diazepam, chlordiazepoxide, and clorazepate) are metabolized in the liver by oxidation (phase I metabolism), each forming multiple active metabolites. Some benzodiazepines such as lorazepam, temazepam, and lormetazepam are biotransformed by glucuronidation (phase 2 metabolism) to inactive glucuronides or other sulfated or acetylated compounds. Patients with impaired liver function, elderly patients, and smokers better tolerate those metabolized by phase 2, which involves simpler biotransformation to inactive metabolites.

Sadock BJ, Sadock VA. *Kaplan and Sadock's Comprehensive Textbook of Psychiatry*. 7th ed. Philadelphia: Lippincott Williams & Wilkins; 2000: 2317–2324.

151. **Answer: B.** Although Lambert-Eaton syndrome and MG are both neuromuscular diseases, they differ in several aspects. Lambert-Eaton syndrome is a paraneoplastic disease characterized by weakness (primarily in the limbs), autonomic dysfunction, and increasing strength with repetitive stimulation or exertion. On a cellular level, it results from the presynaptic inhibition of acetylcholine release. On the other hand, MG is an autoimmune disease with fluctuating asymmetric weakness of extraocular, facial, and bulbar muscles, worsened or induced by repeated stimulation. It results from autoimmune-induced inactivation or destruction of postsynaptic, acetylcholine receptors.

1. Dalmau JO, Posner JB. Paraneoplastic syndromes affecting the nervous system. *Semin Oncol*. 1997;24: 318–328.
2. Posner JB, Dalmau JO. Paraneoplastic syndromes affecting the central nervous system. *Annu Rev Med*. 1997;48:157–166.

152. **Answer: E.** Among the listed neurotransmitters, acetylcholine is the only nonmonamine neurotransmitter. These monoamine neurotransmitters and acetylcholine play an important role in the etiology and treatment of various neuropsychiatric disorders. They are widely distributed throughout the CNS and each neurotransmitter system modulates multiple neuronal pathways.

Sadock BJ, Sadock VA. *Kaplan and Sadock's Comprehensive Textbook of Psychiatry*. 8th ed. Philadelphia: Lippincott Williams & Wilkins; 2005:49.

153. **Answer: C.** Clinical features that are thought to differentiate patients with depressive "pseudodementia" and progressive dementia include a subacute onset, a history of depression, a personal awareness of memory loss, a consistently depressed mood, and patchy and variable cognitive impairment. However, depression is now a recognized risk factor for dementia and is much more likely to occur in patients with a pseudodementia. Hence, these features probably represent more differences in degree rather than absolutes, and it is very important to keep in mind that overlap in features may occur in many cases.

O'Brien J. Dementia associated with psychiatric disorders. *Int Psychogeriatr*. 2005;17 (suppl 1):S207–S221.

154. **Answer: C.** LP headaches are a common phenomenon attributable to intracranial hypotension (low CSF pressure), presumably due to a leak of CSF through the needle insertion site or into adjacent tissue. The headaches often worsen while standing upright, and may be quickly relieved upon lying down. Other possible symptoms include pain at the base of the skull, cervical and thoracic spine, neck stiffness, nausea, or vomiting. Upon repeat LP, there may be signs of

meningeal irritation, even some WBCs in the CSF. Shaking of the head worsens the pain. MRI with gadolinium may show dural enhancement, or fusions in severe cases. Prevention is by using the smallest gauge needles as possible. Treatment is usually via "blood patch." The patient is now afebrile, and aseptic meningitis would be less likely, as would LP-introduced meningitis (post-LP meningitis). Migraines are possible after LP, but would not have the characteristic postural changes.

Ropper AH, Brown RH. *Adams and Victor's Principles of Neurology.* 8th ed. New York: McGraw-Hill; 2005: 529–545.

155. **Answer: C.** Valproic acid inhibits the metabolism of medications that are substrates for CYP2C9, such as phenytoin and phenobarbital. It also inhibits the metabolism of drugs, such as lamotrigine. Valproic acid may increase the metabolism of carbamazepine by inducing CYP3A4 system. Oxcarbazepine can produce increased blood levels of valproic acid through reduced induction of hepatic enzymes. Gabapentin does not interact with other anticonvulsants.

McNamara JO. *Goodman & Gilman's Pharmacological Basis of Therapeutics.* http://www.accessmedicine.com/content.aspx?aID=939876. Accessed March 28, 2007.

156. **Answer: B.** According to Bowlby's theory of attachment, the *pre-attachment* stage occurs from birth to 6 weeks. From that time until 8 months, *attachment-making* begins. With appropriate caretaking, the infant develops a preference for a particular individual. This is the first formative attachment making process. From 8 months to 2 years, Bowlby described a phase of *clear-cut attachment*. After these things have been successfully achieved, children 2-years-old and older understand trust, reciprocity, and acceptance. They may then expand their attachments to form additional *reciprocal relationships*.

Sadock BJ, Sadock VA. *Kaplan and Sadock's Comprehensive Textbook of Psychiatry.* 7th ed. Philadelphia: Lippincott Williams & Wilkins; 2000:2534–2550.

157. **Answer: D.** Neuroimmunology studies the relation between cytokines/inflammatory modulators and the CNS. Elevated immune markers have been found in Major Depression, including cytokines IL-1, IL-6, and C-reactive protein. While brain lacks conventional lymphatics and has low levels of traditional lymphocytes, during infection or injury of the CNS, glia are induced to express MHC I and II. While circumstantial, several lines of evidence support a potential infectious role in Schizophrenia, including higher rates in cold climates and higher prevalence after epidemics. AD is partially an inflammatory disease, with increased levels of proinflammatory cytokines found in an around plaques.

Sadock BJ, Sadock VA. *Kaplan and Sadock's Comprehensive Textbook of Psychiatry.* 7th ed. Philadelphia: Lippincott Williams & Wilkins; 2000:130–131.

158. **Answer: C.** Bradycardia is associated with nicotine withdrawal, as are the other answer choices. Increased appetite is thought to persist longer than other symptoms.

Karnath B. Smoking cessation. *Am J Med.* 2002;112:399–405.

159. **Answer: A.** Dissociative symptoms are part of the DSM-IV-TR diagnostic criteria for Acute Stress disorder, but not for PTSD. The other three symptom clusters are shared between both diagnoses (choices B, C, and D).

American Psychiatric Association. *American Psychiatric Association: Diagnostic and Statistical Manual of Mental Disorders.* 4th ed. (Text revision). Washington: American Psychiatric Association; 2000:463–472.

160. **Answer: C.** FTLD is the third most common cause of cortical dementia (after AD and DLB type). It encompasses two major pathologic substrates affecting the frontal or temporal cortex, sometimes asymmetrically. Three clinical syndromes are produced by FTLD (frontotemporal dementia, progressive nonfluent aphasia, and semantic dementia). Although for a long time Pick's disease was used synonymously with FTLD, two histologic types have been described with the same underlying histopathologic features: prominent microvascular change devoid of specific histologic features and severe astrocytic gliosis with or without ballooned cells and inclusion bodies (Pick's disease).

1. The Lund and Manchester Groups. Clinical and neuropathological criteria for frontotemporal dementia. *J Neurol Neurosurg Psychiatry.* 1994;57:416–418.
2. Thompson JC, Stopford CL, Snowden JS, et al. Qualitative neuropsychological performance characteristics in frontotemporal dementia and Alzheimer's disease. *J Neurol Neurosurg Psychiatry.* 2005;76:920–927.

161. **Answer: A.** Different stages in the addiction process have been identified and are often indicated with terms like initiation, continuation, withdrawal, and relapse. These phases are characterized by predominant actions of specific neurotransmitters, involvement of specific brain structures, and activities in specific neural circuits. In the first phase, *initiation*, mu-opioid receptors (endorphins) and dopamine play an important role in the acute reinforcing effects of drug abuse, with the ventral tegmental area and the nucleus accumbens as the

primary structures of interest. In the second phase of continued drug use, *conditioned responses and drug craving*, several neurotransmitters are involved, including dopamine in the nucleus accumbens, corticotrophin-releasing hormone in the amygdala, and glutamate in the frontal-cingulate circuit. In the third phase, *detoxification and withdrawal*, glutamate and norepinephrine in the locus coeruleus seem to be crucial. In the fourth phase, relapse after sustained abstinence, the orbitofrontal cortex, the anterior cingulate gyrus, and the amygdala are important brain regions, with norepinephrine and corticotrophin-releasing hormone representing the brain stress system (stress-induced relapse) and GABA and glutamate representing the compulsive and habit system (cue-induced relapse). The roles of these different processes, the related neurotransmitters, and their interactions are crucial for understanding the therapeutic strategies for the treatment of drug addiction.

1. Bossert JM, Ghitza UE, Lu L, et al. Neurobiology of relapse to heroin and cocaine seeking: an update and clinical implications. *Eur J Pharmacol.* 2005;526: 36–50.
2. Kreek MJ, LaForge KS, Butelman E. Pharmacotherapy of addictions. *Nat Rev Drug Discov.* 2002;1:710–726.
3. Van den Brink W, Haasen C. Evidenced-based treatment of opioid-dependent patients. *Can J Psychiatry.* 2006;51:635–646.

162. Answer: E. Nonspecific EEG findings (e.g., slowing) or evidence of abnormalities on neuropsychological testing, e.g., difficulty with letter reversal, may be seen in some patients with Intermittent Explosive Disorder. Signs of altered serotonin metabolism (e.g., low mean 5-HIAA concentrations) have been found in the CSF of some impulsive and temper-prone individuals, but the specific relationship of these findings to Intermittent Explosive Disorder remains unclear. There may also be nonspecific or "soft" findings on neurological examinations (e.g., reflex asymmetries or mirror movements). Some patients may present with developmental difficulties indicative of cerebral dysfunction (i.e., delayed speech or poor coordination). A history of neurological conditions (e.g., migraine headaches, head injury, and episodes of unconsciousness) or febrile seizures in childhood may also be present is some patients. If the clinician judges that the aggressive behavior is a consequence of the direct physiological effects of a diagnosable general medical condition, then a mental disorder due to a General Medical Condition should be diagnosed instead of Intermittent Explosive Disorder.

Although these findings may be seen in some patients with intermittent explosive disorder, it would be incorrect to say that they are seen in most patients with this disorder.

American Psychiatric Association. *Diagnostic and Statistical Manual of Mental Disorders (DSM-IV-TR)* American Psychiatric Association. 4th ed. (Text revision). http://www.psychiatryonline.com/content.aspx?aID=11056#11056. Accessed April 16, 2007.

163. Answer: A. CBT is a promising approach to treat BDD. Studies have found that BDD often improves when cognitive restructuring (e.g., developing more accurate and helpful beliefs about appearance), exposure (e.g., exposing the perceived defect in social situations and preventing avoidance behaviors), response prevention (e.g., stopping compulsive behaviors, such as mirror checking), and behavioral experiments (empirically testing hypotheses; i.e., dysfunctional thoughts and beliefs) are used. Additional components, such as mirror retraining and mindfulness, may also be used in the treatment of BDD. CBT has demonstrated effectiveness in treating BDD in both the individual and group format. No studies have examined the relative efficacy of medication versus CBT, or their combination, for BDD.

Grant JE, Phillips KA. Recognizing and treating body dysmorphic disorder. *Ann Clin Psychiatry.* 2005;17:205–210.

164. Answer: D. LAAM is a derivative of methadone, approve by the FDA for use in the treatment of opioid addiction. Compared to methadone, it has a long duration of action (three days) and a slower onset of action. The long half-life (2.6 days) obviates the need for daily dosing, and permits a 3 days/week dosing schedule. The extended action of LAAM is due to its metabolites, nor-LAAM and dinor-LAAM, both of which are more potent and longer acting than the parent drug. The main disadvantage of such a long duration of action is the time necessary to reach a steady-state plasma concentration (4 to 5 half-lives), and stabilize the patient at an appropriate comfort level. Due to the slow onset of action, the patient may find it hard to wait for the agonist effects and be tempted to use illicit opiates during the induction phase posing a serious risk of overdose. LAAM has been shown to increase the risk of sudden cardiac death due to prolongation of QT interval, and is contraindicated in males with a QTc > 430 milliseconds, and females with a QTc > 450 milliseconds. It has not been studied in pregnancy, and is not recommended for nursing mothers or patients younger than 18 years. Therefore, LAAM is not the treatment of choice for most patients with opioid addiction.

Graham AW, Schultz TK, Mayo-Smith MF, et al. *Principles of Addiction Medicine*. 3rd ed. Chevy Chase, Maryland: American Society of Addiction Medicine; 2003:735–758.

165. Answer: E. The most dangerous adverse effect of irreversible MAOIs is hypertensive crisis, characterized by hypertension, palpitations, occipital headache, nausea, vomiting, neck rigidity, dilated pupils, and motor agitation. This can be caused by consumption of tyramine containing food items such a red wine, tap beer, cheese, yeast extracts, pickled fish, aged meat, overripe aged fruits, fava beans, etc. Tyramine is sympathomimetic amine, which is normally broken down by the MAO-A in the gut. In patients taking MAOIs, unbroken tyramine results in displacement of intracellular norepinephrine resulting in hypertensive crisis. Hypertensive crisis can result with simultaneous use of MAOIs and stimulants (dextroamphetamines, methylphenidate), TCAs and bupropion, other MAOIs (furazolidone, pargyline), carbamazepines, buspirone, direct sympathomimetic (L-dopa), and indirect sympathomimetic agents. Serotonin syndrome (confusion, agitation, hypomania, sweating, myoclonus, fever, and coma) can occur when SSRIs, clomipramine, imipramine, meperidine, dextromethorphan, propoxyphene, venlafaxine, and sumatriptan are use in conjunction with MAOIs. Lithium can be safely combined with MAOIs for the treatment of resistant depression. When switching from an irreversible MAOI to a tricyclic agent or SSRIs, a minimum washout period of 2 weeks should be allowed for return to normal MAO activity. When switching from TCAs or SSRIs to an MAOI, a washout period of 10 to 14 days is sufficient, except in the case of fluoxetine, which requires a washout period of 5 weeks.

1. Sadock BJ, Sadock VA. *Kaplan and Sadock's Comprehensive Textbook of Psychiatry*. 7th ed. Philadelphia: Lippincott Williams & Wilkins; 2000:2397–2407.
2. Schatzberg AF, Nemeroff CB. *Textbook of Psychopharmacology*. 2nd ed. Washington: American Psychiatric Press; 1998:239–249.

166. Answer: E. Osmotic-diuretics (mannitol and urea), xanthines (aminophylline, caffeine, and theophylline), carbonic anhydrase inhibitor (acetazolamide), and sodium bicarbonate increase renal lithium clearance and decrease serum lithium concentration. Anticonvulsants (valproate and carbamazepine) do not have significant pharmacokinetic interaction with lithium.

Sadock BJ, Sadock VA. *Kaplan and Sadock's Comprehensive Textbook of Psychiatry*. 7th ed. Philadelphia: Lippincott Williams & Wilkins; 2000:2377–2390.

167. Answer: E. This patient has Duchenne muscular dystrophy, the most frequently occurring myopathy becoming evident in early childhood. It is a sex-linked disorder (transmitted from mothers to boys on the X chromosome). It is slowly progressive but incapacitating and ultimately fatal disease. It begins as a proximal myopathy, accounting for waddling gaits (thigh weakness) and inability to raise hands above the head (shoulder weakness). Proximal myopathy also explains difficulty standing up from a sitting position and the basis for the Gower's sign: patients pulling themselves up or climbing up on themselves when attempting to stand up. The cellular basis for Duchenne's muscular dystrophy is the absence of a membrane protein, dystrophin.

McDonald CM, Abresch RT, Carter GT, et al. Profiles of neuromuscular diseases. Duchenne muscular dystrophy. *Am J Phys Med Rehabil*. 1995;74(5 suppl):S70–S92.

168. Answer: A. The characteristic neuropathological change in Huntington's disease is the decline in the number of medium spiny neurons in the striatum, but changes in the caudate nucleus are most impressive. Cell death also occurs in the globus pallidus. As the disease advances, cell death occurs in the caudate nucleus, frontal lobes, putamen, and other regions of the brain.

Anderson KE. Huntington's disease and related disorders. *Psychiatr Clin North Am*. 2005;28:275–290.

169. Answer: B. Inhibitors of AChE are used frequently in the treatment of Alzheimer's dementia and they have shown mild and transitory improvement of memory in such patients. There are four major AChE inhibitors, which include donepezil, rivastigmine, tacrine, and galantamine. Donepezil is a selective inhibitor of AChE in the CNS with little effect on AChE in peripheral tissues. Memantine produces a dose-dependent blockade of NMDA receptors. There are no medications that directly destroy β-amyloid in the brain. Donepezil does not increase levels of dopamine in the brain.

Standaert DG, Young AB. *Goodman & Gilman's Pharmacological Basis of Therapeutics*. http://www.accessmedicine.com/content.aspx?aID=940520. Accessed March 28, 2007.

170. Answer: A. Studies have shown no greater risk for substance use in urban versus suburban youth. Conduct

Disorder diagnosis and peer group substance use are both risk factors for adolescent substance use. There are multiple sources indicating that adolescents with ADHD who are treated with stimulants are not at higher risk of substance use.

1. Deas D, Brown ES. Adolescent substance abuse and psychiatric comorbidities. *J Clin Psychiatry*. 2006;67:E02.
2. Levine SB, Coupey SM. Adolescent substance use, sexual behavior, and metropolitan status: is "urban" a risk factor? *J Adolesc Health*. 2003;32:350–355.
3. Schubiner H. Substance abuse in patients with attention-deficit hyperactivity disorder: therapeutic implications. *CNS Drugs*. 2005;19:643–655.

171. Answer: B. Patients with FTLD are occasionally misdiagnosed as Alzheimer's dementia. Careful history taking and attention to certain aspects of presentation are likely to clarify diagnosis. FTLD has a predominantly "presenile" onset whereas AD is more common in the elderly. Severe amnesia, visuospatial deficits and myoclonus are characteristic of AD and often not described in the early stages of FTLD. Patients with FTLD are typically oriented and do not evidence significant deficits in negotiating their local environment. Profound alteration in personality in the early stages of a dementing illness suggests FTLD rather than AD. Bradyphrenia is typical of subcortical vascular dementia.

1. Knibb JA, Kipps CM, Hodges JR. Frontotemporal dementia. *Curr Opin Neurol*. 2006;19:565–571.
2. Neary D, Snowden J, Mann D. Frontotemporal dementia. *Lancet Neurol*. 2005;4:771–780.

172. Answer: E. There are an estimated 800,000 Opioid-Dependent persons in the United States. Of patients entering treatment for Heroin Dependence in 1998, 50% were non-Hispanic white, 25% were Hispanic, and 22% were non-Hispanic black. Sixty-two percent had at least a 12th-grade education, and 36% had health insurance. Almost half the patients beginning methadone maintenance therapy had coexisting psychiatric conditions.

Fiellin DA, O'Connor PG. Clinical practice. Office-based treatment of opioid-dependent patients. *N Engl J Med*. 2002;347:817–823.

173. Answer: D. Patients with Dependent Personality Disorder are at increased risk of developing Mood Disorders, Anxiety Disorders, and Adjustment Disorder. They often co-occur with other personality disorders, especially Borderline, Avoidant, and Histrionic Personality Disorders. Chronic physical illness or separation anxiety disorder in childhood or adolescence may predispose individuals to the development of this disorder. The degree to which dependent behaviors is appropriate varies across different age groups and sociocultural groups. Dependent behavior should be considered characteristic of the disorder, only when it is clearly in excess of the individual's cultural norms or reflects unrealistic concerns. Emphasis on passivity, politeness, and deferential treatment is characteristic of some societies and may be misinterpreted as traits of Dependent Personality Disorder. Some societies may differentially foster and discourage dependent behavior. This disorder has been diagnosed more frequently in women, although some studies report similar prevalence rates among men and women.

American Psychiatric Association. *Diagnostic and Statistical Manual of Mental Disorders (DSM-IV-TR)*. 4th ed. (Text revision). http://www.psychiatryonline.com/content.aspx?aID=4125#4125. Accessed April 16, 2007.

174. Answer: A. Two treatments with best evidence for efficacy for the treatment of Chronic Fatigue Syndrome are graded exercise and cognitive behavioral therapy. There is little evidence to support the use of antidepressants, opioids, and immunological agents including steroids for the treatment of this condition.

Henningsen P, Zipfel S, Herzog W. Management of functional somatic syndromes. *Lancet*. 2007;369:946–955.

175. Answer: A. Buprenorphine is a thebaine derivative, which is highly lipophilic, and twenty-five to fifty times more potent than morphine. It is a partial mu-receptor agonist. It has a high affinity for mu-opioid receptors, therefore, competes with other opioids and blocks their effects. It dissociates very slowly from opioid receptors. Buprenorphine is metabolized in the liver via N-dealkylation (by cytochrome P450 3A4 enzyme system) into an active metabolite, norbuprenorphine. It has good bioavailability when administered sublingually, whereas naloxone has poor bioavailability by sublingual route. It is approved by the FDA for the treatment of Opioid Dependence. Treatment is initiated with buprenorphine alone, followed by maintenance therapy with buprenorphine and naloxone combination to minimize abuse potential. The target dose is 8 to 16 mg/day. An 8 mg/day dose of buprenorphine is equivalent to 35 to 60 mg of methadone in maintenance treatment. Since buprenorphine is a partial agonist, it is associated with a ceiling effect, and there is no added benefit above 32 mg/day dose. It is a highly safe medication for both acute and chronic use.

1. Brunton LL, Lazo JS, Parker KL. *Goodman & Gilman's The Pharmacological Basis of Therapeutics*. 11th ed. New York: McGraw-Hill; 2006:572–573.

2. Graham AW, Schultz TK, Mayo-Smith MF, et al. *Principles of Addiction Medicine*. 3rd ed. Chevy Chase, Maryland: American Society of Addiction Medicine; 2003:751–758.

176. Answer: E. Phentolamine, an α-adrenergic antagonist, is the mainstay treatment of MAOI-induced hypertensive crisis. It has a rapid onset of action, usually less than five minutes, and a single dose of 5 mg of phentolamine administered intravenously or intramuscularly is generally sufficient. If needed, additional doses of phentolamine can be administered over several hours. More recently, nifedipine, a calcium channel blocker, has been shown to be effective in the treatment of hypertensive crisis. It has a rapid onset of action with sublingual use (about 5 minutes), and the effect lasts for about 3 to 5 hours. Usually, 10 mg of sublingual nifedipine is administered, with a repeat dose after 20 minutes if required. A diuretic such as furosemide can be given to avoid fluid retention, and a β-adrenergic receptor antagonist such as propranolol can be given to control tachycardia.

Sadock BJ, Sadock VA. *Kaplan and Sadock's Comprehensive Textbook of Psychiatry*. 7th ed. Philadelphia: Lippincott Williams & Wilkins; 2000:2397–2407.

177. Answer: B. Neurologic adverse effects of lithium are memory difficulty, slowed reaction time, tremors, occasional extrapyramidal symptoms, and peripheral neuropathy. Lithium toxicity can present with more severe neurologic symptoms, as described previously. Lithium can cause hypothyroidism, goiter, exophthalmos, and rarely hyperthyroidism. It is associated with parathyroid adenoma and hyperparathyroidism. Cardiovascular adverse effects are benign T-wave changes and sinus node dysfunction. Lithium use can result in polyuria (nephrogenic diabetes insipidus), concentrating defects, reduced GFR, nephritic syndrome, and renal tubular acidosis. It can cause acne, rash, hair loss, and psoriasis. Gastrointestinal side effects include nausea, vomiting, diarrhea, and appetite loss. Lithium can also cause altered carbohydrate metabolism, weight gain, and fluid retention.

Sadock BJ, Sadock VA. *Kaplan and Sadock's Comprehensive Textbook of Psychiatry*. 7th ed. Philadelphia: Lippincott Williams & Wilkins; 2000:2377–2390.

178. Answer: C. TD is a movement disorder characterized by abnormal mouth and tongue movements (lip smacking, sucking, puckering, and facial grimacing), choreoathetoid-like movements of the fingers and toes, and slow writhing movements of the trunk. Approximately 5% of patients undergoing treatment with antipsychotic drugs develop TD each year. The

risk factors for TD include old age, female gender, and dosage of antipsychotic medications and duration of treatment with these drugs. It has been hypothesized to be related to increased sensitivity of dopamine type 2 (D2) receptors in the basal ganglia associated with use of typical antipsychotics, such as thioridazine, haloperidol, trifluoperazine, and fluphenazine. Clozapine is less likely to cause TD, possibly due to a relatively low affinity for D2 receptors.

Sadock BJ, Sadock VA. *Kaplan and Sadock's Comprehensive Textbook of Psychiatry*. 7th ed. Philadelphia: Lippincott Williams & Wilkins; 2000:2356–2377.

179. Answer: C. Fragile X syndrome is probably the most common genetically based cause of mental retardation. It is transmitted on the X chromosome and therefore occurs most often in boys although it has been described in girls who inherit two abnormal X chromosomes. Genetically, fragile X syndrome consists of excessive trinucleotide repeats (more than 60). It has not been associated with a specific ethnic group. Clinical features include moderate to severe mental retardation (70% of affected boys), long thin face, prominent jaw, large everted, low set ears, and macroorchidism and autistic behaviors.

Freund LS, Reiss AL, Abrams MT. Psychiatric disorders associated with fragile X in the young female. *Pediatrics*. 1993;91:321–329.

180. Answer: B. The oculomotor nerve (third cranial nerve) supplies the pupil constrictor, eye lid, and adductor and elevator muscles of each eye. Lesion of this nerve causes ipsilateral-dilated pupil, ptosis, and outward deviation of the eye. The trochlear nerve (fourth cranial nerve) supplies the superior oblique muscle and is responsible for the adduction of the eye. It is usually difficult to diagnose a trochlear nerve injury in isolation. The abducens nerve (sixth cranial nerve) innervates the lateral rectus muscle and is responsible for the abduction of the ipsilateral eye. Lesion of this nerve causes ipsilateral adduction of the eye, but no ptosis or pupillary changes.

Kaufman DM. *Clinical Neurology for Psychiatrists*. 5th ed. Philadelphia: WB Saunders; 2001:37–39.

181. Answer: D. Pramipexole is a dopamine receptor agonist used in the treatment of Parkinson's disease. It has selective activity on D2- and D3-receptor proteins and little or no activity at D1 receptors. Dopamine agonists can actually worsen or mimic some positive symptoms of Schizophrenia, such as hallucinations. Tolcapone and entacapone are COMT inhibitors used in the treatment of Parkinson's disease. Selegiline is a selective MAO-B inhibitor, which is also used in the treatment of Parkinson's disease.

Standaert DG, Young AB. *Goodman & Gilman's Pharmacological Basis of Therapeutics*. http://www.accessmedicine.com/content.aspx?aID=940486. Accessed March 28, 2007.

182. **Answer: D.** Both BDD and OCD respond to serotonergic antidepressants. Answer choices A, B, and C are distinguishing characteristics when comparing BDD to OCD. BDD is thought to be related to, but distinct from, OCD. BDD is also linked to mood disorders, social anxiety disorder, and the eating disorders. Some have postulated that Anorexia Nervosa may be a subtype of BDD, as the two conditions are disorders of body image with substantial overlap. However, Anorexia Nervosa and BDD differ in gender ratio, treatment response, psychiatric comorbidity, and familial aggregation. In family members of OCD probands, BDD (but not anorexia nervosa) is overrepresented. When BDD patients' beliefs reach delusional intensity, DSM-IV-TR provides for a second diagnosis: Delusional Disorder, Somatic Subtype. These delusions are usually not bizarre, but a more intense degree of the same beliefs. Some suggest there is no substantial difference between delusional and non-delusional BDD patients, with the distinction that the delusional BDD patients have less insight and more severe illness. Considering BDD from a dimensional rather than categorical perspective may help clarify the condition as well. There is talk of moving BDD from its current *Somatoform* classification and, for example, placing it with *Obsessive spectrum* disorders in DSM-V.

1. Castle DJ, Rossell SL. An update on body dysmorphic disorder. *Curr Opin Psychiatry*. 2006;19:74–78.
2. Castle DJ, Rossell S, Kyrios M. Body dysmorphic disorder. *Psychiatr Clin North Am*. 2006;29:521–538.
3. Mataix-Cols D, van den Heuvel O. Common and distinct neural correlates of obsessive-compulsive and related disorders. *Psychiatr Clin North Am*. 2006;29:391–410.

183. **Answer: D.** Neuritic plaques and NFTs are characteristic hallmarks of AD and are considered central to its pathogenesis, making them targets of prospect and novel therapeutic interventions. However, they are by no means pathognomic of the disease, as they are found in varying degrees in normal aging, mild cognitive impairment, and several other dementias. Neuritic plaques are extracellular lesions composed of a central core of aggregated amyloid-β peptide, while NFTs are intracellular bundles of paired and straight filaments.

Mott RT, Hulette CM. Neuropathology of Alzheimer's disease. *Neuroimaging Clin N Am*. 2005;15:755–765.

184. **Answer: E.** Cocaine users have a lifetime risk of non-fatal MI that is seven times the risk of nonusers. The use of cocaine accounts for about 25% of acute MIs in patients 18 to 45 years of age. Cocaine use is associated with both acute and chronic cardiovascular diseases. Cocaine blocks epinephrine and norepinephrine reuptake. Acute effects of cocaine are due to α-adrenergic effects of cocaine which lead to coronary spasm and decreased oxygen delivery to myocardium. α-adrenergic effects of cocaine also lead to peripheral vasoconstriction and increased blood pressure. β-adrenergic effects lead to increased heart rate. Increased blood pressure and heart rate both lead to increased oxygen demand. The combination of increased demand with decreased supply results in cardiac ischemia, arrhythmia, and infarction. Chronic effects of cocaine use include accelerated atherosclerosis, hypertension, arrhythmias, contraction-band necrosis, cardiomyopathy, and myocarditis. The risk of acute MI is highest within the first hour of cocaine use. During the hour after cocaine is used, the risk of MI is twenty-four times the base-line risk. However, some reports suggest that MI can occur as early as minutes after cocaine administration and as late as several days afterward. β-blockers should be administered with caution since their use may worsen unopposed stimulation of alpha receptors. In a prospective multicenter study of patients presenting with chest pain following cocaine use, about 6% had MI. ECG abnormalities occur in 90% of patients with cocaine induced MI and include ST-segment elevation, T-wave inversion, and Q waves. An ECG revealing ischemia or infarction had a sensitivity of about 36% for predicting an MI. The specificity, positive predictive value, and negative predictive value of the ECGs were 90%, 18%, and 96%, respectively.

1. Hollander JE, Hoffman RS, Gennis P, et al. Prospective multicenter evaluation of cocaine-associated chest pain. Cocaine Associated Chest Pain (COCHPA) Study Group. *Acad Emerg Med*. 1994;1:330–339.
2. Kloner RA, Rezkalla SH. Cocaine and the heart. *N Engl J Med*. 2003;348:487–488.
3. Mittleman MA, Mintzer D, Maclure M, et al. Triggering of myocardial infarction by cocaine. *Circulation*. 1999;99:2737–2741.
4. Qureshi AI, Suri MF, Guterman LR, et al. Cocaine use and the likelihood of nonfatal MI and stroke: data from the Third National Health and Nutrition Examination Survey. *Circulation*. 2001;103:502–506.

185. **Answer: A.** Antisocial Personality Disorder appears to be associated with low socioeconomic status and urban settings. It is much more common in males than in females. The prevalence of Antisocial Personality

Disorder in the community is about 3% in males and about 1% in females. They are more prevalent in psychiatric clinics with a prevalence varying from 3% to 30%, depending on the predominant characteristics of the populations being sampled. Higher prevalence rates are seen in substance abuse treatment settings, prisons, and forensic settings. Although Antisocial Personality Disorder has a chronic course, it may become less evident or remit as the individual grows older (i.e., by the fourth decade of life). This remission tends to be particularly evident for engaging in criminal behavior, but there may also be a decrease in the full spectrum of antisocial behaviors and substance abuse.

American Psychiatric Association. *Diagnostic and Statistical Manual of Mental Disorders (DSM-IV-TR).* 4th ed. (Text revision). http://www.psychiatryonline.com/content.aspx?aID=3928. Accessed April 16, 2007.

186. Answer: D. Current evidence is unequivocal on the value or not for some peripheral pharmacological agents: bulking agents and loperamide seem ineffective, the 5-HT$_4$-agonist tegaserod and the 5-HT$_3$-antagonist alosetron seem effective in selected subgroups (female patients with irritable bowel syndrome dominated by constipation or diarrhoea, respectively). There is moderate evidence for the efficacy of antidepressants and psychotherapy. For the latter, there is not enough evidence to differentiate between different forms of psychotherapy.

Henningsen P, Zipfel S, Herzog W. Management of functional somatic syndromes. *Lancet.* 2007;369:946–955.

187. Answer: E. Most patients with Hallucinogen Intoxication can be treated effectively with "talk-down" therapy, which involves minimizing stimulation and providing non-judgmental support. They usually respond positively to a reminder that they are under the influence of a drug, and the effects are transient. The treatment can usually be accomplished outside a hospital and without medications. However, if talk-down therapy does not provide sufficient relief, intramuscular haloperidol or lorazepam along with continued support is indicated.

Graham AW, Schultz TK, Mayo-Smith MF, et al. *Principles of Addiction Medicine.* 3rd ed. Chevy Chase, Maryland: American Society of Addiction Medicine; 2003:286.

188. Answer: E. SSRIs (fluoxetine, citalopram, escitalopram, fluvoxamine, paroxetine, and sertraline) are indicated in the treatment of MDD, Dysthymia, Seasonal Affective Disorder, Trichotillomania, OCD, Bulimia Nervosa, Anorexia Nervosa, Panic Disorder, PTSD, Social Phobia, Alcoholism, and pain syndromes including fibromyalgia and diabetic neu-

ropathy. Sexual dysfunction is a common adverse effect of SSRIs, which can be used for treating premature ejaculation. Fluvoxamine is approved for treating OCD, but is also indicated in MDD, Panic Disorder, Social Phobia, and Binge-Eating Disorders.

Sadock BJ, Sadock VA. *Kaplan and Sadock's Comprehensive Textbook of Psychiatry.* 7th ed. Philadelphia: Lippincott Williams & Wilkins; 2000:2433–2438.

189. Answer: E. Common neurologic adverse effects of carbamazepine include sedation, ataxia, dizziness, and dipolopia. The hematologic adverse effects range from mild leucopenia to agranulocytosis and aplastic anemia. Carbamazepine can cause hepatic enzyme elevation, and is rarely associated with severe hepatitis and hepatic failure. It induces hepatic microsomal enzymes, which leads to an accelerated elimination of drugs including barbiturates and oral contraceptives. By stimulating vasopressin receptor function, carbamazepine can cause hyponatremia and water intoxication. It is occasionally associated with cardiac conduction disturbances including bradycardia and Stoke-Adams syndrome. Dermatologic reactions range from benign rashes to exfoliative dermatitis and Stevens-Johnson syndrome. Rare idiosyncratic adverse effects include mania/psychosis, pancreatitis, and renal problems. Unlike some other mood stabilizers, such as lithium and valproate, carbamazepine does not appear to cause significant weight gain. It can cause neural tube defect with use in pregnancy. Hematologic and hepatic parameters should be regularly monitored in patients receiving carbamazepine.

Sadock BJ, Sadock VA. *Kaplan and Sadock's Comprehensive Textbook of Psychiatry.* 7th ed. Philadelphia: Lippincott Williams & Wilkins; 2000:2282–2288.

190. Answer: E. Antipsychotic drugs, due to their dopamine receptor blockade, are associated with acute extrapyramidal adverse effects including akathisia, acute dystonia, and parkinsonism. Akathisia is the most common and often the most distressing acute extrapyramidal adverse effect, and manifests with an inability to keep the legs still, feelings of inner restlessness, frequent shifting of posture, walking in place, and shifting of weight from one foot to another. Akathisia is a disturbance in the normal balance between dopamine and norepinephrine. β-adrenergic receptor antagonist, such as propranolol and benzodiazepines have been found to be effective in treating this condition. Acute dystonias respond well by intravenous or intramuscular administration of anticholinergic drugs such as diphenhydramine or benztropine. Oral anticholinergic drugs are usually effective for treating Parkinsonism. Amantadine alleviates extrapyramidal adverse effects by releasing dopamine. Direct dopamine agonists (bromocriptine) and indirect dopamine agonists (L-dopa) may exacerbate psychosis, and therefore, are not preferred for the treatment of extrapyramidal adverse effects of antipsychotics.

Sadock BJ, Sadock VA. *Kaplan and Sadock's Comprehensive Textbook of Psychiatry*. 7th ed. Philadelphia: Lippincott Williams & Wilkins; 2000:2356–2377.

191. **Answer: D.** This patient appears to have developed neuroleptic malignant syndrome (NMS). NMS is a rare, but potentially fatal condition associated with high dosage and rapid titration of high-potency dopamine blocking agent such as haloperidol. The clinical manifestations of NMS include hyperthermia, severe muscular rigidity, autonomic instability (tachycardia, high blood pressure, tachypnea, and diaphoresis), and changing level of consciousness. It is associated with increased creatine phosphokinase and aldolase activity, increased liver transaminase activity, leukocytosis, myoglobinemia and myoglobinuria, acute renal failure, and is fatal in 20% to 30% patients. Management of NMS includes discontinuation of antipsychotic medications, such as thioridazine, treating extrapyramidal adverse effects with antiparkinsonian medications, and supportive treatment for fever, cardiovascular symptoms, and the correction of fluid and electrolyte imbalance. Dantrolene is effective in treating severe NMS. Bromocriptine and amantadine are also helpful in the treatment of this condition.

Sadock BJ, Sadock VA. *Kaplan and Sadock's Comprehensive Textbook of Psychiatry*. 7th ed. Philadelphia: Lippincott Williams & Wilkins; 2000:2356–2377.

192. **Answer: A.** PCR is a biochemical and molecular biology technique used to ezymatically replicate DNA without using a living organism. While both amplification and PCR allow a small amount of DNA to be amplified exponentially, the former uses living organisms and the latter occurs *in vitro*.

Cheng S, Fockler C, Barnes WM, et al. Effective amplification of long targets from cloned inserts and human genomic DNA. *Proc Natl Acad Sci USA*. 1994;91:5695–5699.

193. **Answer: D.** This patient has the classic triad of NPH-ataxia, dementia, and urinary incontinence. Most cases of NPH are believed to be due to asymptomatic fibrosising meningitis. However, NPH often follows a subarachnoid hemorrhage, head trauma, meningitis, Paget's disease, and achondroplasia. When NPH is suspected, the first true diagnostic step is LP to evaluate CSF pressure, and possible removal of CSF

to assess response. If you selected imaging, you are not entirely incorrect, but it is not the diagnostic test of choice. Often imaging (CT or MRI) is performed first to help determine any risks for herniation on performing LP. This is the typical next choice and tests, although imaging is often nonspecific for the diagnosis of NPH. Typical findings will be ventricles enlarged disproportionate to the cortical atrophy, especially in the frontal and temporal areas. Referral to a neurosurgeon for evaluation for ventriculoperitoneal shunt placement may follow. Diagnostic electroencephalogram is generally not helpful in the diagnosis of NPH. NPH may appear like Parkinson's disease, but complete examination and clinical picture would differentiate the two. Tremors are common in elderly patients, and not specific to Parkinson's disease. An L-dopa/carbidopa trial is not yet appropriate. Neither would be a trial of an AChE inhibitor for dementia, especially at the expense of missing a diagnosis of NPH.

1. Kaufman DM. *Clinical Neurology for Psychiatrists*. 5th ed. Philadelphia: WB Saunders; 2001:145–147.
2. Ropper AH, Brown RH. *Adams and Victor's Principles of Neurology*. 8th ed. New York: McGraw-Hill; 2005:529–545.

194. **Answer: B.** Selegiline is a selective inhibitor of MAO-B. It is used in the treatment of Parkinson's disease, and it is thought to retard the breakdown of dopamine in the striatum. Although it is beneficial in the treatment if Parkinson's disease, its effect is only modest and it is not considered the drug of choice for the treatment of this condition. At low doses it acts as a selective MAO-B inhibitor. However at higher doses, it can produce inhibition of MAO-A. Metabolites of Seleqiline include amphetamine and methamphetamine, which can produce anxiety or insomnia. Selegiline does not inhibit the peripheral metabolism of catecholamines and it can be safely used with L-dopa.

Standaert BG, Young AB. *Goodman & Gilman's Pharmacological Basis of Therapeutics*. http://www.accessmedicine.com/content.aspx?aID=940486. Accessed March 28, 2007.

195. **Answer: C.** Baclofen is considered the best treatment for spasticity in ALS. It is a GABA-B receptor agonist and it can be administered by the oral or intrathecal route. The time of onset of action of baclofen is approximately 0.5 to 1 hour and its peak effect occurs at 4 hours. This medication does not work through calcium channels.

Standaert BG, Young AB. *Goodman & Gilman's Pharmacological Basis of Therapeutics*. http://www.accessmedicine.com/content.aspx?aID=940556. Accessed March 28, 2007.

196. Answer: E. Clozapine has a lower risk for extrapyramidal adverse effects compared to other antipsychotics. However, it is associated with agranulocytosis in 1% to 2% patients. Clozapine therapy should be discontinued whenever the total WBC count falls below 3000 cell per cubic mm or the granulocyte count falls below 1500 cells per cubic mm. Carbamazepine should not be administered concurrently with clozapine due to a higher risk of agranulocytosis. Hypersalivation is a bothersome side effect, which is treated with clonidine or amitriptyline. Clozapine treatment is associated with grand mal seizures that are dose dependent. Anticholinergic effects include dry mouth, blurred vision, constipation, and urinary retention. Metabolic disturbances including weight gain, diabetes, and hyperlipidemia have been reported with clozapine. The incidence of weight gain is higher with clozapine and other atypical antipsychotic agents likely due to a higher affinity for 5-HT1 and histamine type-1 receptors. The most frequent cardiovascular adverse effects are tachycardia and postural hypotension. Urogenital effects include enuresis, frequency and urgency, hesitancy, urinary retention, and impotence. Sedation is the most common adverse effect believed to be due to the α1- and Ha-blocking effects of clozapine.

Sadock BJ, Sadock VA. *Kaplan and Sadock's Comprehensive Textbook of Psychiatry.* 7th ed. Philadelphia: Lippincott Williams & Wilkins; 2000:2455–2474.

197. Answer: E. Psychostimulant drugs, such as amphetamine and methylphenidate, are similar in structure to the catecholamines (dopamine and norepinephrine). All stimulants act as indirect-sympathomimetics by increasing the release and blocking reuptake of catecholamines. Amphetamine is approved for the treatment of ADHD, Narcolepsy, and exogenous obesity. Methylphenidate is approved by the FDA for ADHD and Narcolepsy. Pemoline is also approved for treating ADHD. In addition, research studies support the use of amphetamine and methylphenidate for depression secondary to medical conditions, apathy, and depression secondary to CNS disease or trauma, augmentation of analgesic effects of opioids in cancer patients, and augmentation of antidepressants in treatment-resistant depression.

Sadock BJ, Sadock VA. *Kaplan and Sadock's Comprehensive Textbook of Psychiatry.* 7th ed. Philadelphia: Lippincott Williams & Wilkins; 2000:2474–2478.

198. Answer: A. Lamotrigine is an anticonvulsant that resembles phenytoin in its anticonvulsant activity and its toxicity. It selectively blocks the slow sodium channels and prevents the release of glutamate and aspartate. It can cause serious rashes in approximately 1% of patients and minor rashes in 12% of patients. The addition of valproic acid increases the serum level of lamotrigine. Lamotrigine is considered a first-line or adjunctive agent for generalized and focal seizures. Valproic acid and ethosuximide are considered first-line agents for the treatment of absence seizures.

Ropper AH, Brown RH. *Adams and Victor's Principles of Neurology.* 8th ed. http://www.accessmedicine.com/ content.aspx?aID=969583. Accessed March 28, 2007.

199. Answer: A. Several types of immunotherapies have been used for the treatment of MS, with varying degrees of success. Interferon-β suppresses the proliferation and the migration to the CNS of T lymphocytes. Glatiramer diminishes the autoimmune response by altering signals through the T-cell receptor complex. Cyclophosphamide forms intra-strand and inter-strand DNA-DNA cross-links, which then inactivate the DNA. Natalizumab is a monoclonal antibody directed against an adhesion molecule integrin, which is expressed in lymphocytes and monocytes.

Kasper DL, Braunwald E, Fauci AS. *Harrison's Principles of Internal Medicine.* 16th ed. http://www.accessmedicine.com/ content.aspx?aID=106923. Accessed March 28, 2007.

200. Answer: B. The triptans, which include sumatriptan, zolmitriptan, naratriptan, and rizatriptan, are important medications in the treatment of migraine headaches. This class of medications is a 5HT-1D receptor agonists that produce a selective vasoconstriction of the cranial circulation. Buspirone is a 5-HT1A partial agonist that is used in the treatment of anxiety and depression. Ondansetron is a 5-HT3 antagonist, which is used in the treatment of chemotherapy-induced emesis.

1. Ropper AH, Brown RH. *Adams and Victor's Principles of Neurology.* 8th ed. http://www.accessmedicine.com/ content.aspx?aID=968133. Accessed March 28, 2007.
2. Sanders-Bush E, Mayer SE. *Goodman & Gilman's Pharmacological Basis of Therapeutics.* http://www.accessmedicine.com/content.aspx?aID=937147. Accessed March 28, 2007.

INDEX